MEDICAL MICROBIOLOGY

A GUIDE TO MICROBIAL INFECTIONS:

PATHOGENESIS, IMMUNITY, LABORATORY INVESTIGATION AND CONTROL

Commissioning Editor: Jeremy Bowes
Development Editors: Sam Crowe/Joshua Mearns
Project Managers: Atiyaah Muskaan/V. Apoorva
Designer: Renee Duenow
Illustration Manager: Amy Heyden-Faith
Illustrator: Toppan Best-set Premedia Limited

NINETEENTH EDITION

MEDICAL MICROBIOLOGY

A GUIDE TO MICROBIAL INFECTIONS:
PATHOGENESIS, IMMUNITY, LABORATORY
INVESTIGATION AND CONTROL

EDITED BY

MICHAEL R. BARER

Professor of Clinical Microbiology, Department of Infection, Immunity and Inflammation, University of Leicester Medical School, Leicester, UK

WILL IRVING

Professor and Honorary Consultant in Virology, University of Nottingham and Nottingham University Hospitals NHS Trust, Department of Microbiology, Queen's Medical Centre, Nottingham, UK

ANDREW SWANN

Consultant Microbiologist, Clinical Microbiology, University Hospitals of Leicester NHS Trust, Leicester, UK

NELUN PERERA

Consultant Microbiologist and Honorary Associate Professor, University Hospitals of Leicester and University of Leicester, Department of Clinical Microbiology, Leicester Royal Infirmary, Leicester, UK

ELSEVIER

ELSEVIER

First edition 1925
Second edition 1928
Third edition 1931
Fourth edition 1934
Fifth edition 1938
Sixth edition 1942
Seventh edition 1945
Eighth edition 1948
Ninth edition 1953
Tenth edition 1960
Eleventh edition 1965

Twelfth edition (Vol. 1) 1973
Twelfth edition (Vol. 2) 1975
Thirteenth edition (Vol. 1) 1978
Thirteenth edition (Vol. 2) 1980
Fourteenth edition 1992
Fifteenth edition 1997
Sixteenth edition 2002
Seventeenth edition 2007
Eighteenth edition 2012
Nineteenth edition 2018

Notices

Practitioners and researchers must always rely on their own experience and knowledge in evaluating and using any information, methods, compounds or experiments described herein. Because of rapid advances in the medical sciences, in particular, independent verification of diagnoses and drug dosages should be made. To the fullest extent of the law, no responsibility is assumed by Elsevier, authors, editors or contributors for any injury and/or damage to persons or property as a matter of products liability, negligence or otherwise, or from any use or operation of any methods, products, instructions, or ideas contained in the material herein.

ISBN: 978-0-7020-7200-0

your source for books,
journals and multimedia
in the health sciences

www.elsevierhealth.com

 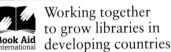

Working together
to grow libraries in
developing countries

www.elsevier.com • www.bookaid.org

The
publisher's
policy is to use
paper manufactured
from sustainable forests

Printed in China

Last digit is the print number: 9   8   7   6   5   4   3   2   1

Preface

In revising this classic introductory text, now evolved over 90 years, the imprint of the past keeps our focus on the nature and significance of microbes that concern us in medicine but looks to the future in contemplating the constantly changing threat of infection.

Though consistently raised in previous editions, the spectre of antimicrobial resistance (AMR) has been given public prominence, notably by the O'Neill review[1] and the responses of the UK Chief Medical Officer. That, without concerted action, we face a projected global annual death toll of 10 million attributable to drug-resistant infections by 2050 stands out as the stark headline. This timeline could encourage procrastination in our actions, but the current mortality and morbidity statistics show AMR as a pressing but remediable problem requiring insight into all areas of microbial life.

In the face of AMR and other emergent threats such as Ebola and Zika virus, human ingenuity has brought new tools such as whole genome sequencing within the grasp of well-resourced laboratories and public health systems. This information is transforming our insights into chains of transmission and AMR profiling.

In preparing this edition we have brought both the emerging problems and the potential technological solutions into focus at a level suitable for both students and specialist trainees concerned with infection. Sections dealing with molecular methods and developments in antimicrobial stewardship illustrate how we have combined the foundations of our subject with the leading edges of technology and clinical practice.

As with the 18th edition we cannot improve on the historical perspective set out in an earlier preface, which is reproduced below. This reference to aspects of the past needing no improvement brings us to note with great sadness the death of David Greenwood in 2015[2]. David, a scientific pioneer in antimicrobial chemotherapy, led the production of four editions of this book with clarity and charm. He is sorely missed, but we are sure he would welcome two new editors, Nelun Perera and Andrew Swann, to the team.

We commend this book to all those who aspire to reduce the scourge of infection through knowledge and reason based in persistent critical enquiry.

MRB
WI
NP
AWS
Leicester, Nottingham
December 2017

From the Preface to the 17th edition (2006): It is now more than 80 years since the first appearance of this textbook's illustrious forerunner – Mackie and McCartney's *Introduction to Practical Bacteriology as Applied to Medicine and Public Health*. When that classic text first appeared in 1925, the requirements of medical students, then thought to include a need to be fully conversant with laboratory methods, could be encompassed in a small-format handbook of less than 300 pages. At that time, virology scarcely existed, immunology was in its infancy, parasitology was regarded as a subject of study necessary only for prospective colonial doctors, effective treatment of microbial disease was almost non-existent and molecular biology was unknown. Medical students are, thankfully, no longer expected to be familiar with what goes on in microbiology laboratories, except insofar as they need to be able to use laboratory services and interpret the results emanating from them in an intelligent fashion, but this has been replaced by an unmanageable corpus of clinical knowledge that encompasses not only the burgeoning subjects of bacteriology, virology, mycology and parasitology, but also the related disciplines of immunology, antimicrobial chemotherapy and epidemiology. Such has been the explosion in knowledge that one can only sympathize with today's student doctors in their struggle to master the basic facets of medical microbiology that will impinge daily on their professional lives.

Of course, all the information one could ever need is now available at the click of a mouse via the internet – that vast, unregulated agglomeration of the good, the bad and the ugly – yet textbooks remain stubbornly popular with students, at least for core subjects. This should not be surprising, as a good textbook offers a uniquely user-friendly source of knowledge, assembled by experts familiar with the needs of students and presented in an accessible format, clearly written and logically arranged. Such, at any rate, have been the defining features of

[1] https://amr-review.org/ Last accessed 18 December 2017.
[2] Richard Slack (2016). Professor David Greenwood, 25 August 1935-9 July 2015. Journal of Antimicrobial Chemotherapy **71**:1433-1434.

previous manifestations of this textbook, a tradition that we believe this new edition fully upholds.

As before, the 17th edition of *Medical Microbiology* strives to bridge the gap between texts that deal with microbiology in a traditional organism-based way and the more modern approaches that take microbial diseases as the starting point or attempt to view the subject from an immunological or epidemiological perspective. Thus, a thorough overview of microbial biology is followed by a consideration of the principles of the body's immunological response to various types of microorganisms, before moving on to consider bacteria, viruses, fungi and parasites individually. The content of these 'systematic' chapters is heavily biased towards understanding the associated diseases, their pathogenesis, clinical features, epidemiology and control. A final section integrates what has gone before in terms of the day-to-day practicalities of the diagnosis of infection, its treatment and avoidance.

In our experience, students of medicine and allied health-care sciences are among the most motivated of all students: it is rare to find one who does not harbour a genuine desire to become a safe and knowledgeable doctor or health-care professional. For our part we sincerely hope that we have provided a text that will help them to fulfil these ambitions in the context of the intrinsically fascinating subject of medical microbiology. For the first time, we have included 'key point' boxes in each chapter to highlight issues that are of particular relevance to the topic. These are intended to provide students with signposts to a wider understanding of key issues and are certainly not meant to represent 'all the student needs to remember' on a particular theme. To use them in such a way would impoverish the student's understanding of the subject and negate the whole purpose of the text. Make no mistake: a thorough knowledge of infection in all its guises is as necessary to the practice of medicine today as it ever was.

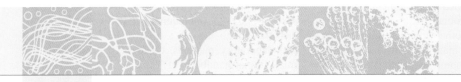

Acknowledgements

In addition to expressing our heartfelt thanks to the editorial team at Elsevier for their patience and persistence, we wish to thank past contributors who have enabled the evolution of the text into its current form. In particular we recognise those whose previous contributions have been taken on by new authors and thank them for their diligence in the past. We are particularly grateful to Sharon Koo, Felicia Lim and Fiona Price of University Hospitals of Leicester NHS Trust for developing many of the clinical scenarios. As frontline clinical microbiologists their insights have been invaluable in bringing infective agent sections authored by non-clinical colleagues into greater clinical perspective.

Contributors

Robert P. Allaker
Professor of Mucocutaneous Microbiology
Institute of Dentistry
Queen Mary University of London
London, UK

David J. Allen
Assistant Professor
Department of Pathogen Molecular Biology
London School of Hygiene and Tropical Medicine
London, UK

Gayatri Amirthalingam
Consultant Medical Epidemiologist
Immunisation, Hepatitis and Blood Safety department
Public Health England
London, UK

Ashley C. Banyard
Rhabdovirus Research Team Leader
Wildlife Zoonoses and Vector Borne Disease Research
Group
Animal and Plant Health Agency (APHA)
Surrey, UK

Michael R. Barer
Professor of Clinical Microbiology
Department of Infection, Immunity and Inflammation
University of Leicester Medical School
Leicester, UK

Eleanor Barnes
Professor of Hepatology and Experimental Medicine
Experimental Medicine Division
Peter Medawar Building
Oxford, UK

Alan D. T. Barrett
Director
World Health Organization Collaborating Center for
Vaccine Research, Evaluation, and Training in
Emerging Infectious Diseases;
Director
Sealy Center for Vaccine Development;
Professor
Pathology and Microbiology and Immunology
University of Texas Medical Branch
Galveston, TX, USA

Christopher D. Bayliss
Reader
Department of Genetics
University of Leicester
Leicester, UK

David W. Brown
Virus Reference Department
Public Health England
London, UK;
Laboratory for Measles and respiratory viruses
Instituto oswaldo cruz
Rio de Janeiro, Brazil

Kevin E. Brown
Virus Reference Department
Public Health England
London, UK

Rebecca Brown
Global Health Research Institute
Southampton University
Southampton, UK

Vicki J. Chalker
Respiratory and Vaccine Preventable Bacteria
Reference Unit
Bacterial Reference Department
Public Health England
London, UK

Ian A. Cooper
CBR Division
Defence Science and Technology Laboratories
Wiltshire, UK

David J. Cousins
Professor of Immunology
Department of Infection, Immunity and Inflammation
University of Leicester
Leicester, UK

Nigel Cunliffe
Professor
Clinical Infection, Microbiology and Immunology
University of Liverpool
Liverpool, UK

Kate Cuschieri
Professor
Scottish HPV Reference Laboratory
Laboratory Medicine
Royal Infirmary of Edinburgh
Edinburgh, UK

Nilanthi R. de Silva
Professor
Department of Parasitology
Faculty of Medicine
University of Kelaniya
Ragama, Sri Lanka

Mathew A. Diggle
Consultant Clinical Scientist
Clinical Microbiology
Nottingham University Hospitals NHS Trust
Nottingham, UK

Matthew Dryden
Consultant in Microbiology and Infection
Rare and Imported Pathogens Department
Public Health England
Salisbury, UK;
Consultant
Hampshire Hospitals Foundation Trust
Winchester, UK

Darryl Falzarano
Research Scientist II
Vaccine and Infectious Disease Organization -
International Vaccine Centre
University of Saskatchewan
Saskatchewan, Canada

Heinz Feldmann
Chief
Laboratory of Virology
National Institute of Health
Hamilton, MT, USA

Anthony R. Fooks
Lead Scientist for International Development
Animal and Plant Health Agency (APHA)
Surrey, UK

Norman K. Fry
Respiratory and Vaccine Preventable Bacteria
Reference Unit
Public Health England National Infection Service
London, UK

Sheila Graham
Professor of Molecular Virology
Centre for Virus Research
University of Glasgow
Glasgow, UK

Luke R. Green
Department of Genetics
University of Leicester
Leicester, UK

Tanzina Haque
Clinical lead consultant virologist and honorary senior
lecturer
Royal Free Hospital
London, UK

Heli Harvala
Consultant Medical Virologist
Laboratory Medicine
University College of London Hospital Trust
London, UK

Mark W. Head
The National CJD Research and Surveillance Unit
Centre for Clinical Brain Sciences
The University of Edinburgh
Edinburgh, UK

Albert Heim
Institute for Virology
Hannover Medical School
Hannover, Germany

Hilary Humphreys
Professor of Clinical Microbiology
Royal College of Surgeons in Ireland;
Professor of Microbiology
Beaumont Hospital
Dublin, Ireland

Joseph P. Icenogle
Rubella Virus Laboratory Team Leader
Division of Viral Diseases
Centers for Disease Control and Prevention
Atlanta, GA, USA

Samreen Ijaz
Virus Reference Department
Public Health England
London, UK

James W. Ironside
Professor of Clinical Neuropathology
Centre for Clinical Brain Sciences
University of Edinburgh
Edinburgh, UK

William L. Irving
Professor and Honorary Consultant in Virology
University of Nottingham and Nottingham University
Hospitals NHS Trust
Department of Microbiology
Queen's Medical Centre
Nottingham, UK

Miren Iturriza-Gómara
Professor
Institute of Infection and Global Health
University of Liverpool
Liverpool, UK

Claire Jenkins
Gastrointestinal Bacteria Reference Unit
Public Health England
London, UK

David R. Jenkins
Consultant Medical Microbiologist
Clinical Microbiology
University Hospitals of Leicester NHS Trust
Leicester, UK

Ingólfur Johannessen
Director
Laboratory Medicine
NHS Lothian
Royal Infirmary of Edinburgh;
Honorary Clinical Senior Lecturer
Edinburgh Medical School
University of Edinburgh
Edinburgh, UK

Nadira D. Karunaweera
Professor
Department of Parasitology
Faculty of Medicine
University of Colombo
Colombo, Sri Lanka;

Julian M. Ketley
Professor of Genetics
University of Leicester
Leicester, UK

Mogens Kilian
Professor of Medical Microbiology
Department of Biomedicine
Aarhus University
Aarhus, Denmark

David Mabey
Professor of Communicable Diseases
Infectious and Tropical Diseases
London School of Hygiene and Tropical Medicine
London, UK

Jim McLauchlin
Professor
Food Water and Environmental Microbiology Services
Public Health England
London, UK

Osamu Nakagomi
Professor
Molecular Epidemiology
Nagasaki University Medical School
Nagasaki, Japan

Marco Rinaldo Oggioni
Professor
Department of Genetics
University of Leicester
Leicester, UK

Petra Oyston
Defence Science and Technology Laboratory
Salisbury, UK

Manish Pareek
NIHR Post-doctoral Fellow/Senior Clinical Lecturer
Department of Infection, Immunity and Inflammation
University of Leicester
Leicester, UK

Rosanna W. Peeling
Diagnostic Research
London School of Hygiene and Tropical Medicine
London, UK

J. S. Malik Peiris
Professor
School of Public Health
The University of Hong Kong
Pokfulam, Hong Kong

T. Hugh Pennington
Emeritus Professor of Bacteriology
University of Aberdeen
Aberdeen, UK

Ludmila Perelygina
Senior Researcher
Division of Viral Diseases
Centers for Disease Control and Prevention
Atlanta, GA, USA

Nelun Perera
Consultant Microbiologist and Honorary Associate
Professor
University Hospitals of Leicester and University of
Leicester
Department of Clinical Microbiology
Leicester Royal Infirmary
Leicester, UK

Mathieu Picardeau
Head of the Biology of Spirochetes unit
Institut Pasteur
Paris, France

Ann M. Powers
Division of Vector-Borne Infectious Disease
Centers for Disease Control and Prevention
Fort Collins, CO, USA

Philippe Riegel
Laboratory of Bacteriology
University hospitals of Strasbourg
Strasbourg, France

Thomas V. Riley
Senior Clinical Scientist
PathWest Laboratory Medicine
Queen Elizabeth II Medical Centre
Nedlands, Western Australia

Andrew Rosser
Consultant
Infectious Diseases and Medical Microbiology
University Hospitals of Southampton
Southampton, UK

Richard C. Russell
Professor of Medical Entomology
Public Health
University of Sydney
Sydney, Australia

Paul Russell
Principal Medical Officer (Research), DSTL Porton
Down
Consultant Medical Microbiology and Virology
Salisbury District Hospital
Salisbury, UK

David Safronetz
Chief of Special Pathogens
National Microbiology Laboratory
Public Health Agency of Canada
Winnipeg, Canada

Marilda M. Sequeira
Titular Researcher
Oswaldo Cruz Foundation
Rio de Janeiro, Brazil

Peter Simmonds
Professor of Virology, Group Head / PI and Fellow
Experimental Medicine Division
Peter Medawar Building
Oxford, UK

Mary P.E. Slack
Professor
School of Medicine
Queensland, Australia

Iain Stephenson
Consultant
Infectious Diseases Unit
Leicester Royal infirmary
Leicester, UK

Andrew Swann
Consultant Microbiologist
Clinical Microbiology
University Hospitals of Leicester NHS Trust
Leicester, UK

Yusri Taha
Departments of Microbiology and Infectious Diseases
Newcastle upon Tyne Hospitals NHS Trust (Freeman
Hospital)
Newcastle upon Tyne, UK

Richard S. Tedder
Virologist
Public Health England
London, UK

Joanne E. Thwaite
Chemical, Biological and Radiological Division
Defence Science and Technology Laboratory
Salisbury, UK

C. Y. William Tong
Infection
Barts Health NHS Trust
London, UK

Arnoud H. M. van Vliet
University of Surrey
School of Veterinary Medicine
Faculty of Health and Medical Sciences
Surrey, UK

David H. Walker
Professor of Pathology
Executive Director
Center for Biodefense and Emerging Infectious
Diseases
University of Texas Medical Branch
Galveston, TX, USA

David W. Warnock
Former Director
U.S. CDC, Division of Foodborne, Bacterial and
Mycotic Diseases;
Adjunct Professor of Pathology and Laboratory
Medicine
Emory University School of Medicine
Atlanta, GA, USA;
Visiting Professor
The University of Manchester
Manchester, UK

Adrian M. Whatmore
Department of Bacteriology
Animal and Plant Health Agency
Surrey, UK

Craig Winstanley
Professor
Institute of Infection and Global Health
University of Liverpool
Liverpool, UK

Karl G. Wooldridge
Associate Professor
School of Life Sciences
University of Nottingham
Nottingham, UK

Guanghui Wu
Wildlife Zoonoses and Vector-Borne Diseases
Research Group
Department of Virology
Animal and Plant Health Agency (APHA)
Surrey, UK

Xue-Jie Yu
Professor
Departments of Pathology and Microbiology and
Immunology
The University of Texas Medical Branch
Galveston, TX, USA

Maria Zambon
Deputy Director National Infection Service
Public Health England
London, UK

Contents

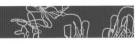

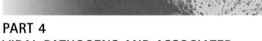

PART 4
VIRAL PATHOGENS AND ASSOCIATED DISEASES

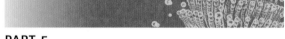

PART 5
FUNGAL PATHOGENS, PARASITIC INFECTIONS AND MEDICAL ENTOMOLOGY

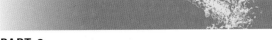

PART 6
DIAGNOSIS, TREATMENT AND CONTROL OF INFECTION

PART 1
MICROBIAL BIOLOGY

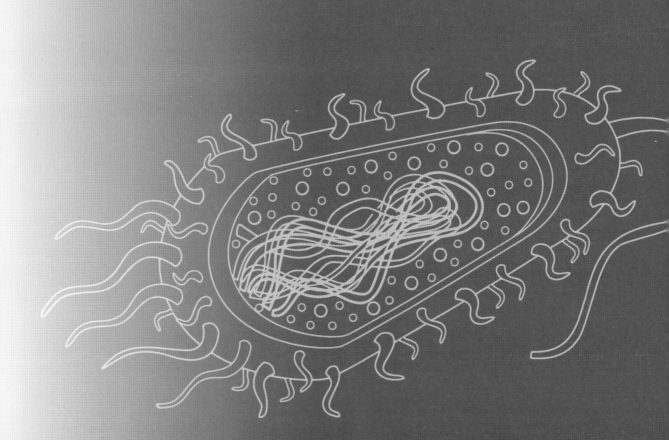

1 Microbiology and medicine

MICHAEL R. BARER

KEY POINTS

- Microbes are too small to be seen directly, and special methods are needed to investigate them. In daily life and in clinical practice we are forced to use our imagination to understand how human behaviour influences and is influenced by them.
- Infections and microbes were considered as separate phenomena until the late 19th century when Pasteur reconciled previous observations on the physical requirements for the transmission of infection with the nature of microbes and established the necessity of a chain of transmission in infection.
- Some infections can be prevented by interrupting transmission and/or by immunisation.
- The role of specific microbes in specific infective conditions may be established by propagating the microbe in pure laboratory culture and subsequently reproducing the disease in a suitable model.
- Nucleic acid-based analytical methods have opened up new ways of identifying microbes and establishing causality in infection.
- Transmission of infection is related to the *reservoir, immediate source* and mode of transmission of the causal agent.
- Close to 10^{14} bacterial, fungal and protozoan cells live on and in healthy human bodies. Most are harmless or even beneficial. Those that cause disease in otherwise healthy individuals are termed *pathogens*. The normal microbiota constitutes the reservoir and immediate source for *endogenous* infection. Infections in which the source of the causal organism is external are termed *exogenous* infections.
- Many infections can now be treated with antimicrobial agents that possess *selective toxicity*. Nonetheless, infection remains the most common cause of morbidity and premature death in the world.

Read this paragraph and, then close your eyes and think through the following: on and in you there reside more than one thousand billion (10^{12}) microbial cells—at least 10-fold more than the number of cells that make up your body. We are not conscious of these companions any more than we are conscious of passing them round every time we shake hands, speak or touch a surface. Inoculation with just one microbe of the wrong type in the wrong way may kill you, yet we tolerate and indeed thrive on constant appropriate exposure to this unseen world.

Because microbes are generally hidden from our senses, an appreciation of microbiology and infection demands imagination. Our forebears who established the discipline lavished imagination on the problems they studied. Sadly it is lack of imagination that now underpins serious problems such as hospital-acquired infection and antibiotic resistance.

Hard-won advances in microbiology have transformed the diagnosis, prevention and cure of infection and have made key contributions to improved human health and a doubling in life expectancy. The conquest of epidemic and fatal infections has sometimes seemed so conclusive that infections may be dismissed as of minor concern to modern doctors in wealthy countries. However, infection is far from defeated. In resource-poor settings, an estimated 10 million young children die each year from the effects of pneumonia, diarrhoea, measles, malaria, tetanus, diphtheria and whooping cough alone. Many other classical scourges, such as tuberculosis, cholera, typhoid and leprosy, continue to take their toll. Although we have the potential to prevent nearly all of these deaths, political and social issues constantly hinder progress, and more effective and economic means of delivery provide a constant challenge.

Even in wealthy nations, infection is still extremely common: at least a quarter of all illnesses for which patients consult their doctors in the United Kingdom are infective and around 1 in 10 patients acquire infection while in hospital, sometimes with multiresistant organisms. Global communications and changes in production systems, particularly those affecting food, can have a profound effect on the spread of infectious disease. Current levels of bacterial pathogens resistant to multiple antimicrobial agents are estimated to be responsible for 25,000 deaths annually across Europe (and very likely to increase), and the emergence of severe acute respiratory syndrome (SARS), avian influenza, Middle East respiratory syndrome (MERS), Ebola and Zika all illustrate the need for continued vigilance.

The relative freedom of wealthy societies from fatal infections has been won through great struggles, which are all too easily forgotten. As generations grow up without the experience of losing friends and relatives through infection, so the balance of perceived risk and benefit looks different. So now, in addition to the old threats that are ever present, we constantly face pressure to drop or modify measures such as public immunisation. A historical understanding of infection is as important in maintaining and improving the present status as is knowledge of contemporary progress.

AN OUTLINE HISTORY OF MICROBIOLOGY AND INFECTION

MICROORGANISMS AND INFECTION

Infection and microbiology followed different strands of development for centuries (Fig. 1.1). We tend to map this story against the recorded efforts of prominent individuals, though many others doubtless contributed.

Ideas of infection and epidemics were recorded by Hippocrates, but it was nearly 2000 years before Girolamo Fracastoro (1478–1553) proposed in his classic tome 'De Contagione' that 'seeds of contagion' (as opposed to spirits in the ether) might be responsible. Quite separately, the early microscopists began to make observations on objects too small to be seen by the naked eye. Foremost among these was the Dutchman Antonie van Leeuwenhoek (1632–1723). With his remarkable homemade and handheld microscope, he found many microorganisms in materials such as water, mud, saliva and the intestinal contents of healthy subjects and recognised them as living creatures ('animalcules') because they swam about actively. That he saw bacteria as well as the larger microbes is known from his measurements of their size ('one-sixth the diameter of a red blood corpuscle').

Before the discipline of microbiology was formally established in the second half of the 19th century, three key aspects of infection were brought into stark relief by publicly acknowledged demonstrations:

1. John Hunter (1728–1793) inoculated secretions from sores around a prostitute's genitals into a penis (his own according to some sources) and

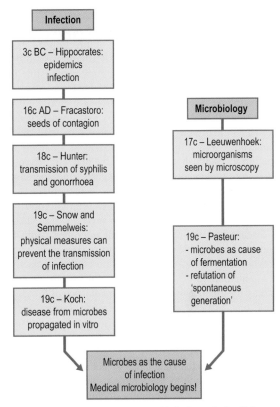

Fig. 1.1 Timelines for the history of infection and microbiology.

demonstrated a physical reality to the transmission of infection, in this case syphilis and gonorrhoea (the prostitute had both, leading to a mistaken belief that the distinctive symptoms were manifestations of the same disease).

2. Edward Jenner (1749–1823) adapted the long-established oriental practice of variolation (inoculation with material from a mild case of smallpox) for the prevention of smallpox, by showing that cowpox was as effective and safer. The procedure, termed *vaccination* (Latin *vacca* = cow) established the concept of *immunisation* in Europe.

3. John Snow (1813–1858) showed that, by preventing access to a water source epidemiologically linked to a cholera outbreak, further infections could be terminated. This established that physical measures could prevent the transmission of infection, a point further illustrated by Ignaz Semmelweis (1818–1865) in Vienna and others who showed that fatal streptococcal infections (puerperal fever) affecting mothers following childbirth could be substantially reduced if those attending the birth applied simple hygienic measures (breaking the chain of transmission).

Later, two towering figures, Louis Pasteur (1822–1895) and Robert Koch (1843–1910), played central roles in establishing the microbial causation of infectious disease. The brilliant French chemist Louis Pasteur crushed two prevailing dogmas: that the fermentation responsible for alcohol formation was a purely chemical process (by demonstrating that the presence of living microorganisms was essential), and that life could be spontaneously generated (by showing that nutrient solutions remained sterile if microbes were excluded). Refutation of spontaneous generation established unequivocally that all life must come from progenitors of the same species and, therefore, the need for a *chain of transmission* where infection is concerned. Pasteur made many other seminal contributions, including the identification of several causal agents of disease and the recognition that microbes could be rendered less capable of causing disease (less *virulent*) or *attenuated* by artificial subculture. He used the principle of attenuation to develop a successful vaccine against anthrax for use in animals. It was the influence of Pasteur's work that inspired the British surgeon Joseph Lister (1827–1912) to establish *antisepsis,* aimed at destroying the microorganisms responsible for infection during surgery.

The other great founding father of medical microbiology, Robert Koch, came to microbiology through medicine. Working originally as a country doctor in East Prussia, Koch established the techniques required to isolate and propagate pure cultures of specific bacteria. His numerous contributions include establishment of the bacterial causes of anthrax, tuberculosis and cholera. He also formulated more precisely, proposals first put forward by one of his mentors, Jacob Henle (1809–1885), describing how specific microbes might be recognised as the cause of specific diseases. These principles, often referred to as *Koch's postulates,* are used to substantiate claims that a particular organism causes a specific ailment. They require that:

- The organism is demonstrable in every case of the disease.
- It can be isolated and propagated in pure culture in vitro.
- Inoculation of the pure culture by a suitable route into a suitable host should reproduce the disease.
- The organism can be reisolated from the new host.

For various reasons, universal application of the postulates is impossible, and greater subtleties in establishing causal relationships in infection are now recognised. Austin Bradford Hill (1897–1991) developed a sophisticated algorithm to recognise a biological gradient of association; most recently, an approach to determining the role of specific molecules in pathogenesis has been enshrined in Koch's molecular postulates.

Organisms for which Koch's postulates and later modifications have been fulfiled are clearly capable of inducing disease and are designated as *pathogens* to distinguish them from the vast majority of *nonpathogenic* microorganisms. It should be emphasised that fulfilment of the postulates and the diagnostic process in which a given patient's illness is attributed to a known pathogen, are profoundly different processes. In the former, many experiments are done to provide robust scientific evidence, whereas, in the latter, circumstantial evidence is obtained, which, in the light of experience, identifies a particular microorganism as the most likely cause of the illness.

In the century following Pasteur and Koch's work, the list of specific human pathogens has extended to include several hundred organisms. Early on, fungal and protozoan pathogens were recognised, as were macroscopic agents including parasitic worms and insects. Technological breakthroughs, including tissue culture and electron microscopy, were required to enable recognition of viruses. In the early days, viral pathogens were termed *filterable agents* because they passed through filters designed to retain bacteria. In many cases, pathogens of insects, animals or even plants were described before their medical equivalents were recognised.

Many further advances in technology through the 20th and into the 21st century provided more precise understanding of the nature and function of microbes. The revolution in molecular biology that followed the elucidation of the structure of DNA by Rosalind Franklin, James Watson, Francis Crick and Maurice Wilkins in 1953 ultimately enabled a leap forward in analytical capability. For three decades this did not radically change the understanding of microbes and infection. However, almost exactly a century after Pasteur and Koch initiated what has been called the 'golden era of bacteriology', four interconnected breakthroughs once again altered our perspective:

1. The recognition, principally by the American molecular biologist Carl Woese, that ribosomal ribonucleic acid (rRNA), which has essentially the same core structure in all cells, carries unique signatures indicating its evolutionary relationships. It transpires that all cellular forms of life can be classified according to the DNA sequence encoding their rRNA (rDNA). Determination of this sequence provides a means of identifying all cellular microbes and has led to the discovery of a previously unsuspected third 'domain' of life, the *Archaea* (see Ch. 2).
2. Technological advances made possible by molecular genetics. The molecular basis for the pathogenesis of infection now enables recognition of the specific roles of individual genes and their products in both

the pathogen and the host. This offers the promise of new approaches to treatment and prevention of infection. The discovery of mobile genetic elements that convey genes from one organism to another (see Ch. 6) confronted our biological sense of what makes up an individual. Bacterial genes located on mobile genetic elements and encoding antibiotic resistance present an emerging crisis threatening the practice of medicine.

3. The development of ultrasensitive means of detecting specific DNA or RNA sequences and the development, by Kary Mullis, of the polymerase chain reaction (PCR) in 1986. The analytical capacity of nucleic acid amplification techniques, robust kit formulations and high-throughput analytical platforms offers the increasing prospect that the aetiology of all infections will be routinely determined by these methods. While there are many challenges to be met before we abandon laboratory cultures, the possibility that this will become a specialist, research or minority activity is a real prospect.

4. Stimulated first by Fred Sanger's breakthrough in DNA sequencing and latterly with the emergence of massively parallel nucleotide sequencing technologies (so-called next-generation sequencing [NGS] or high-throughput sequencing [HTS]), it seems very likely that genomic and polymorphism analyses will become routinely established in well-resourced laboratories.

HYGIENE, TREATMENT AND PREVENTION OF INFECTION

The work of Snow, Semmelweis, Lister and others led to an appreciation of the benefits of hygiene in the prevention of infection. Nursing practices rooted in necessarily obsessive cleanliness became the norm and *aseptic* practice (avoidance of contact between sterile body tissues and materials contaminated with live microorganisms) was introduced to supplement the use of antisepsis. Before the advent of antibiotics, hygiene was a matter of life and death; institutes of hygiene were established around the world. When treatment of infection later became reliable and routine, hygiene standards were often allowed to drop, leading to present problems, notably with hospital-acquired infection.

The discovery of phagocytic cells and humoral immunity (antibodies) as natural defence mechanisms at the end of the 19th century led to a reassessment of the response to infection. One outcome was the use of antibodies produced in one host for the protection of another *(serum therapy)*. This produced some spectacular successes, notably in the lifesaving use of antitoxin in diphtheria and tetanus.

Unfortunately these foreign proteins often caused hypersensitivity reactions *(serum sickness)*, and few diseases responded reliably to serum therapy. Nevertheless, the capacity of the immune system to achieve *selective toxicity*, and observations by the brilliant German doctor Paul Ehrlich (1854–1915) that dyes used to stain infected tissues selectively labelled parasites in preference to host tissues, contributed to the notion that systemic chemotherapy might be achievable.

In 1909, Ehrlich and his colleagues introduced the arsenical drug Salvarsan for the treatment of syphilis, but it fell short of his ideal of a *magic bullet* that would destroy the parasite without harming the host. A more important breakthrough than Ehrlich's came in 1935 with the publication of a paper by Gerhard Domagk (1895–1964) of the German dyestuffs consortium, IG Farbenindustrie. Domagk described the remarkable activity against streptococci of a dye derivative, prontosil, which turned out to owe its activity to a sulphonamide substituent previously unsuspected of antibacterial activity. Earlier, in 1928, Alexander Fleming had accidentally discovered the antibacterial properties of a fungal mould *Penicillium notatum*, but he was unable to purify the active component or exploit the therapeutic potential of his discovery. This was left to a team of scientists at Oxford (Florey, Chain and Heatley), heralding the start of the antibiotic era—the most important therapeutic development of the 20th century.

Meanwhile, in America, the Ukrainian-born soil microbiologist Selman Waksman (1888–1973) undertook a systematic search for antibiotic substances produced by soil microorganisms that achieved its greatest success in 1943 with the discovery of streptomycin by one of his PhD students, Albert Schatz (1920–2005). The hunt for antibiotics intensified after the Second World War, yielding chloramphenicol, tetracyclines and many other natural, synthetic and semi-synthetic antibacterial compounds. These developments were brought to fruition in the 1970s, and the following 40 years brought no new classes of antimicrobials until the introduction of the cyclic lipopeptides and the oxazolidinones in the first decade of this century. This dearth of new agents has been met by a build-up in antimicrobial resistance that many regard as the greatest public health threat of the present century.

Similar histories may be told of the agents used to treat infections due to protozoa, fungi, helminths and viruses. The threat of resistance is there too. The emergence of HIV in the 1980s, the extraordinary effort in developing antivirals and the outstanding success of highly active antiretroviral therapy in the 1990s was and is a great triumph, tarnished only by the gap between its first availability and its delivery to the poorest populations.

SOURCES AND SPREAD OF INFECTION

To adequately grasp the ways in which the microbial world intersects with human lives it is necessary to understand different microbial lifestyles and the degree to which they depend on human beings. Thus there are some pathogens for which an association with humans is essential in order for them to propagate, whereas for others human association is of little significance compared with their propagation in other species or environments. Microbes that depend on human beings are *obligate parasites*. A few actually need to cause disease to propagate themselves; these are termed *obligate pathogens*. In most cases, disease is accidental, or even detrimental, to the microbe's long-term survival. Viruses that cause disease in humans are obligate parasites, although they often cause inapparent, subclinical or *asymptomatic* infection. Many viruses rely on infecting a particular host species. Smallpox was eradicated, not only because of the availability of an effective vaccine, but also because humans were the only host. Some bacteria, fungi, protozoa and helminths are also species-specific. Among bacteria, the agent of tuberculosis, which is harboured by one-third of humanity, has an absolute requirement to cause disease for its natural transmission to continue.

Since Pasteur established the need for a chain of transmission in infection, it has been possible to fit the sources and spread of infection into a relatively simple framework. All infection recently transmitted has an *immediate source* and reaches the newly infected individual via one or more specific *mode(s) of transmission*. Behind these events, the organism, which of course does not care how we choose to classify it or its activities, lives and propagates in its natural habitat(s). These may or may not be the same as the immediate source but, in considering the control of infection, the natural habitat of the causal organism constitutes the *reservoir of infection*. These points are illustrated in Fig. 1.2. Elimination of the organism from the reservoir will lead to eradication of the infection, whereas elimination from the immediate source, if this is distinct from the reservoir, provides one means by which control of infection can be achieved.

The mode of transmission can involve other infected individuals in the case of contagious infections; food in the case of foodborne infections; water in water-borne infection; aerosol generation by an infected individual or from a water source in airborne infection; or contamination of an inanimate object *(fomites)* such as medical equipment or bed linen. The possible sources and modes of transmission of infection are enormous, and new variants are continually being recognised, often as a consequence of ways of processing material connected with the immediate source or reservoir for the organism concerned.

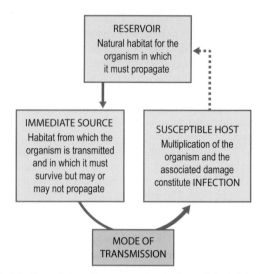

Fig. 1.2   Reservoir, immediate source and mode of transmission in infection.

Engagement of all health-care workers in recognising and controlling these hazards is a vital part of medical practice. Fortunately, most infections are transmitted by well-recognised pathways (Table 1.1), and these must be clearly understood and learnt.

In the public mind, most infection is seen as contagious, but a large proportion of infections result from *endogenous infection* with a bacterium or fungus that is normally resident in the patient concerned. These resident organisms constitute the *normal microbiota* of the host (the term *normal flora* cannot be considered appropriate any longer as it denotes plant life and does not reflect the relationships between microbes and other organisms). These abundant fellow travellers generally cause infection when they get into the wrong place, often as a result of traumatic wounds (including surgery) or impairment of natural clearance mechanisms (e.g., in the lungs or urinary tract). Disturbance of the normal microbiota by antibiotics may also allow unaffected *opportunist* pathogens from the endogenous microbiota or the environment to cause infection.

In the case of endogenous infection, the reservoir and source of infection are the same and transmission is unnecessary. When infection comes from an external source it is termed *exogenous infection*, and the reservoir reflects the natural habitat of the organism. Where other animals constitute that habitat, the infection is termed a *zoonosis*. In many countries, bacteria, protozoa, helminths and viruses are commonly transmitted by insects or other arthropods, and the conditions they cause are classified as *vector-borne* diseases.

Study of the ecology and transmission of disease, including infectious disease, is the province of the important public health discipline of *epidemiology*. Important tools

Table 1.1 Examples of reservoirs, sources and modes of transmission

Infective disease	Agent of infection	Reservoir	Immediate source	Mode of transmission
Sore throat	*Streptococcus pyogenes*[a] (bacterium)	Human upper respiratory tract	Human upper respiratory tract	Exogenous: airborne droplets
Oral thrush	*Candida albicans* (fungus)	Most human mucosal surfaces	Normal microbiota of oral mucosa	Endogenous: overgrowth in antibiotic-treated or immunocompromised patient
Tetanus	*Clostridium tetani* (bacterium)	Soil or animal intestine	Any environment contaminated with soil or animal faeces	Exogenous: penetrating injury
Syphilis	*Treponema pallidum* (bacterium)	Infected humans	Patients with genital ulcers or secondary syphilis	Exogenous: sexual contact
Yellow fever[b]	Yellow fever virus (virus)	Monkeys	Usually infected humans, occasionally monkeys	Exogenous: mosquito-borne
AIDS	Human immunodeficiency virus (virus)	Infected humans	Usually human blood	Exogenous: mainly blood-borne and by sexual contact
Toxoplasmosis[b]	*Toxoplasma gondii* (protozoon)	Cats	Undercooked meat or contact with areas contaminated by cat faeces	Exogenous: ingestion

AIDS, Acquired immune deficiency syndrome.
[a]One of many causes of sore throat.
[b]Example of a zoonosis.

include surveillance of the *prevalence* (total cases in a defined population at a particular time) and *incidence* (number of new cases occurring during a defined period) of disease. Knowledge of the ways in which microorganisms spread and cause disease in communities has produced vital insights that can be used to inform effective control programmes in hospitals and the wider community. Monitoring of the prevalence and incidence of infection on an institutional, local, national or global basis can similarly help in the formulation of policies that reduce the impact of specific infections (monitoring of influenza virus variants to forestall global pandemics is a good example) or of drug-resistant microorganisms such as those causing malaria, tuberculosis or staphylococcal infections. The World Health Organization and other national or international surveillance agencies carry out much of this important work and deserve full support. For, make no mistake, despite antibiotics, immunisation and—for the fortunate—improved living conditions and effective health services, infection will remain a common cause of sickness and premature death for the foreseeable future.

RECOMMENDED READING

Brachman, P. S., & Abrutyn, E. (Eds.). (1999). *Bacterial infections of humans: Epidemiology*. New York: Springer.

Brock, T. D. (Ed.). (1999). *Milestones in microbiology*. Washington, DC: American Society for Microbiology.

Bulloch, W. (1938). *The history of bacteriology*. Oxford: Oxford University Press.

Collard, P. (1976). *The development of microbiology*. Cambridge: Cambridge University Press.

Cox, F. E. G. (Ed.). (1996). *Illustrated history of tropical diseases*. London: Wellcome Trust.

Foster, W. D. (1970). *A history of medical bacteriology and immunology*. London: Cox and Wyman.

Greenwood, D. (2008). *Antimicrobial drugs: Chronicle of a twentieth century medical triumph*. Oxford: Oxford University Press.

Grove, D. I. (1990). *A history of human helminthology*. Oxford: CAB International, Wallingford.

Mann, J. (1999). *The elusive magic bullet: The search for the perfect drug*. Oxford: Oxford University Press.

Waterson, A. P., & Wilkinson, L. (1978). *An introduction to the history of virology*. Cambridge: Cambridge University Press.

Zinsser, H. (1935). *Rats, lice and history*. London: Routledge.

Websites

Train Online. EBI. Next generation sequencing practical course. Available at https://www.ebi.ac.uk/training/online/course/ebi -next-generation-sequencing-practical-course/how-take -course. (Accessed Aug 2017).

United Nations Children's Fund. The State of the World's Children 2009. Available at http://www.unicef.org/sowc09/. (Accessed Aug 2017).

World Health Organization. Infectious diseases. Available at http://www .who.int/topics/infectious_diseases/en/. (Accessed Aug 2017).

2 Morphology and nature of microorganisms

MICHAEL R. BARER

KEY POINTS

- Agents of infection include cellular organisms belonging to two of the three *domains* of life, the *Bacteria* and the *Eukarya*. The latter include fungi and protozoa. The subcellular entities *viruses, viroids* and *prions* also cause infection but depend on host cells and tissues for propagation.
- Bacterial and eukaryotic microorganisms can be detected by light microscopy, whereas electron microscopy is required for viruses. Adult stages of multicellular eukaryotic agents of infection or infestation, such as *helminths* (worms) and insects, are generally visible to the naked eye.
- Most pathogenic bacteria can be recognised as either *Gram-positive* or *Gram-negative* after staining. These properties reflect, respectively, the relatively thick *peptidoglycan* layer and the thin peptidoglycan plus outer membrane cell wall structures possessed by cells belonging to these two groups.
- The mycobacteria, which include the global pathogens causing tuberculosis and leprosy, have a different staining property, described as *acid fast*.
- In addition to the cell wall, key bacterial structures with biological and medical significance include the *nucleoid, inclusion granules* and *spores* within the cell, and *flagella, fimbriae* or *pili* and *capsules* on the cell surface.
- Bacterial *endospores* are highly resistant cells that result from a differentiation process in some Gram-positive bacteria.
- Viruses are obligate intracellular parasites that use the host cell's machinery to replicate. They contain a nucleic acid core comprising DNA or RNA (not both) in single- or double-stranded form.
- The core is surrounded by a protein *capsid* comprising multiple *capsomeres*; an envelope derived from the host cell membrane surrounds the capsid of some viruses.

Microorganisms are beyond doubt the most successful forms of life; they have been here the longest, they are the most numerous and their distribution defines the limits of the biosphere, encompassing environments previously thought incapable of sustaining life. Here, we are concerned with the tiny fraction of microorganisms that form associations with human beings and these encompass the cellular entities, *bacteria, archaea, fungi* and *protozoa,* and the subcellular entities, *viruses, viroids and prions*. Whether the last three can be considered organisms or even living entities is a matter for debate. Nonetheless, their transmissible nature, the immune responses they provoke and our inability to detect them with the naked eye place them firmly within the province of medical microbiology. The first two of these criteria also require us to consider some multicellular macroscopically visible organisms (members of the helminths) as agents of infection (see Ch. 60). Most of this chapter is concerned with bacteria. The subcellular entities are introduced briefly and the remaining medically significant groups are considered in more specialised chapters.

Medical microbiology has been founded on recognising microorganisms that are associated with human disease. This recognition has relied predominantly on two techniques:

- microscopy
- propagation in laboratory cultures

Over the last quarter of the 20th century, it became possible to detect, describe and differentiate microorganisms by biochemical and genetic methods, and this had two profound effects on microbiology. First, due largely to the work of Carl Woese (see Ch. 1), it is now possible to make a reasonable assessment of the evolutionary relationships between microorganisms, a task that previously could be achieved for macroorganisms only by examining fossil records (microorganisms have not left interpretable fossils). Woese's approach led to the recognition of an entire 'new' *domain* (a group ranking above kingdom level) of cellular organisms, the *Archaea* and a fundamental review of how we classify all of life. While the nature of the LUCA, the

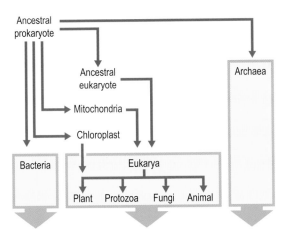

Bacteria

Eukarya

Plant Protozoa Fungi Animal

Ancestral
prokaryote

Ancestral
eukaryote

Mitochondria

Chloroplast

Archaea

Fig. 2.1 Diagram illustrating proposed evolutionary pathways from a putative last universal common ancestor (LUCA) to the present. The points at which lineages diverged are not intended to be precise. Definition of the lineages is made difficult by the influence of horizontal gene transfer (Ch. 6) and variations in the rates of evolutionary change. The Archaea were not recognised as a separate lineage until Woese's work.

last universal common ancestor of all living organisms, and the origin of eukaryotic (nucleated) cells remain subjects of active current research the key branches of life and the origin of mitochondria and chloroplasts are now generally accepted (Fig. 2.1). Second, we have now amassed an enormous body of nucleotide sequence and other molecular data describing microbes. In the previous edition of this text, we reported the availability of complete genome sequences for all the major bacterial and viral pathogens and most of the pathogenic protozoa and fungi. Obtaining sufficiently accurate sequence data from an isolated pathogen to recognise single nucleotide differences between isolates is now relatively straightforward so that strain and evolutionary relationships can be inferred within a short timescale. Such facilities are available now in major centres, thus large numbers of full genome sequences are now available documenting the population structures of many major pathogens.

Although genomic information has impacted substantially on classification and identification of microbes (see Ch. 3), morphology and cultural characteristics remain important in the routine practice of clinical laboratories. However, as we learn more about them, some of the "certainties established" in the pre DNA sequencing era are undermined. Thus, we will see examples of how classification and nomenclature has needed to change in the next chapter, while some bacterial structures that have not been revealed by conventional laboratory studies have been recognised first through genomic sequence data. The capsule (see later in the chapter) of *Campylobacter jejuni* provides one prominent example of this.

We are currently in a transitional, information-gathering phase. Molecular descriptions and detection methods are coming to dominate our view of the microbial world. However, at present it must be emphasised that Gram stain–based morphological classification provides a basic structure to bacteriology that is understood by clinicians and will remain as a basis for communication, at least in the medium term. Moreover, although this is changing, in many instances light and fluorescence microscopy remain competitively cheap and rapid compared with molecular methods as means of providing information relevant to the clinical management of infection. Finally, the discipline of medical microbiology requires the understanding of the basic structural properties and physiology of microorganisms to underpin our approach to infections.

PROKARYOTIC AND EUKARYOTIC CELLS

Microorganisms are microscopic in size and are usually unicellular. The diameter of the smallest body that can be resolved and seen clearly with the naked eye is about 100 μm. All medically relevant bacteria are smaller than this and a microscope is therefore necessary to see individual cells. When propagated on solid media, bacteria (and fungi) form macroscopically visible structures comprising at least 10^8 cells, which are known as *colonies*.

Woese's insights provided for the first time a coherent view of the evolutionary pathways behind the diversity of all living organisms. In particular, a satisfactory explanation was offered for the existence and diversity of *prokaryotic* and *eukaryotic* cells, and all living forms are seen to fall within three *domains* of life: the *Bacteria*, the *Archaea* and the *Eukarya*. This division is of practical significance, as the earlier the point of divergence, the greater the difference in metabolic properties between the present-day representatives of the two lineages. These differences can be exploited by directing treatments at processes unique to the target organism. Some key differences between the three domains of life are summarised in Table 2.1. Although human beings are colonised with members of the Archaea and there is little doubt that they contribute to health and disease, these roles have yet to be defined. Thus beyond noting that there are key chemical distinctions between the composition and physiology of *Bacteria* and *Archaea,* the latter group will not be discussed in detail.

It is worth noting that while the term *prokaryote* has value in orienting our grasp of cell biology, its value in classification is questionable, as it reflects a crude assessment of phenotype that does not reflect evolutionary pathways (see Ch. 3).

Table 2.1   General characteristics of cellular microorganisms in the three domains of life

| Domains | Prokaryotes | | Eukaryotes |
	Bacteria	Archaea	Eukarya
Major groups (examples only)	Gram positives, Proteobacteria	*Methanococcus, Thermococcus*	Fungi, entamoebae, ciliates, flagellates
Cell diameter	≈1 μm	≈1 μm	≈10 μm
Membrane-bound organelles	–	–	+ (e.g., mitochondria, nucleus, Golgi, etc.)
Chromosomes	Single, closed circular	Single, closed circular	Multiple, linear
Introns	Very rare	Rare	Common
Transcription/translation	Coupled	Coupled	Compartmentalised
mRNA	Very labile	Very labile	Stable and labile
Ribosomes	70S	70S	80S
Protein synthesis inhibited by:			
Chloramphenicol	+	–	–
Diphtheria toxin	–	+	+
Peptidoglycan cell wall	+	–	–

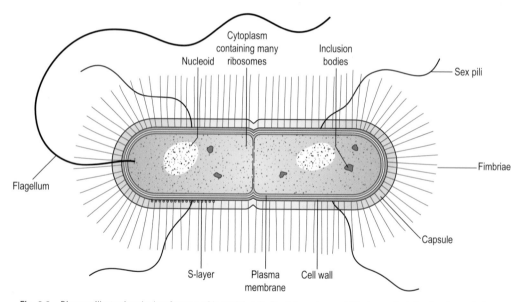

Fig. 2.2   Diagram illustrating the key features of bacterial cells. The S-layer is a variably demonstrated ordered protein layer.

ANATOMY OF THE BACTERIAL CELL

The principal structures of a typical bacterial cell revealed by long established methods are shown in Fig. 2.2. Over the last two decades, developments in genetic manipulation combined with advances in fluorescence and electron microscopy have opened up our understanding of microbial cytology to the point where many key macromolecular assemblies can be described in great and dynamic detail. Some of these will be mentioned below, but, for the most part, this account is rooted in well-established descriptions.

The cytoplasm is bounded peripherally by a very thin, elastic and semipermeable cytoplasmic (or plasma) membrane (a conventional phospholipid bilayer). Outside, and closely covering this, lies the rigid, supporting *cell wall,* which is porous and relatively permeable. Cell division occurs by the development of constrictions mediated by the assembly of an actin-like protein, FtsZ. The constrictions proceed from the periphery inwards and, in some cases, produce a transverse cell wall known as a *septum* or *cross-wall.*

The exact pattern of cell division and the structures associated with the cell wall and cytoplasmic membrane (collectively the cell envelope) combine to produce the

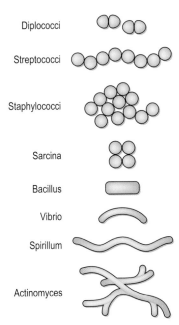

Diplococci

Streptococci

Staphylococci

Sarcina

Bacillus

Vibrio

Spirillum

Actinomyces

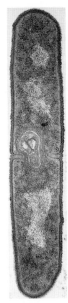

Fig. 2.4 Thin section of a dividing bacillus showing cell wall, cytoplasmic membrane, ribosomes, a developing cross-wall and a mesosome, a membranous structure now generally considered to be an artifact or reflecting some form of cell damage. Magnification ×50,000. (Courtesy Dr P. J. Highton and the editors of *Journal of Ultrastructure Research*.)

Fig. 2.3 The shapes and characteristic groupings of various bacterial cells.

cell morphology and characteristic patterns of cell arrangement. The recognition of these features by oil-immersion light microscopy remains of great practical value in making presumptive identifications of bacteria associated with human infections. Bacterial cells may have two basic shapes, spherical *(coccus)* or rod shaped *(bacillus)*; the rod-shaped bacteria show variants that are comma shaped *(vibrio)*, spiral *(spirillum* and *spirochaete)* or filamentous (Fig. 2.3).

The *cytoplasm* is a predominantly aqueous environment packed with ribosomes and numerous other protein and nucleotide–protein complexes. The cytoplasmic contents are not normally visible by light microscopy. Although bacterial cytoplasm has traditionally been viewed as devoid of structure, it is now clear that, like eukaryotes, bacteria have an extensive cytoskeletal network, which, in different genera, includes structures corresponding to eukaryotic actin, tubulin and intermediate filaments (e.g., MreB, FtsZ and crescentin, respectively). The importance of these is emerging in determining cell shape, division and spore formation (see later in the chapter) and, as we obtain more detailed information concerning their function, so we may consider them as potential new targets for chemotherapy.

Some larger structures such as spores or *inclusion bodies* of storage products such as volutin (polyphosphate), lipid (e.g., poly-β-hydroxyalkanoate or triacylglycerol), glycogen or starch occur in some species under specific growth conditions. Specialised labelling techniques (generally requiring fluorescence imaging) enable visualisation of the nuclear material or *nucleoid* and other structures (e.g., the forming cell division annulus). Fig. 2.4 is an electron micrograph of a thin section of a dividing bacterial cell. Outside the cell wall there may be a protective gelatinous covering layer called a *capsule* or, when it is too thin to be resolved with the light microscope, a *microcapsule*. Soluble large-molecular material may be dispersed by the bacterium into the environment as *loose slime*. Many bacteria bear, protruding outwards from the cell wall, one or more kinds of protein-based filamentous appendages called *flagella*, which are organs of locomotion, and hairlike structures termed *fimbriae* or *pili*, which, via specific receptor–ligand interactions at their tip, mediate adhesion.

Bacterial nucleoid

The genetic information of a bacterial cell is mostly contained (with a few exceptions) in a single, long molecule of double-stranded DNA, which can be extracted in the form of a closed circular thread about 1 mm long. The cell solves the problem of packaging this enormous macromolecule by condensing and looping it into a *supercoiled* state. As well as the chromosome, the bacterium may contain one or more additional fragments of *episomal* (extrachromosomal) DNA, known as *plasmids*. Bacteria are essentially haploid organisms with only one allele of each gene per cell, although gene dosage (copies of a single gene) is affected by multiple copies of plasmids and the presence during rapid growth of several rounds of chromosome replication in progress (see Ch. 4). Unlike the mitotic or meiotic divisions of eukaryotic cells, chromosomal segregation in bacteria at the time of cell division (or fission) does not involve structures that can be resolved by light microscopy. Nonetheless, the speed at which replication can occur (cell divisions more frequently than 1 every 15 minutes in some cases) and the simultaneous requirement for multiple rounds of chromosome replication in one cell provide a mind-boggling challenge for the segregation machinery. (Imagine unravelling two 1-m threads inside a 1-mm sphere!)

The bacterial nucleoid lies within the cytoplasm and is associated with several nucleoid-associated proteins (NAPs). Although these were originally referred to as histone-like, they are not structurally related and they function in the cytoplasm rather than within a membrane-bound nucleus. The NAPs such as H-NS and IHF exert important influences on prokaryotic gene expression (see Chs 4 and 6). The cytoplasmic location of the nucleoid means that as DNA-dependent RNA polymerase makes RNA, ribosomes may attach and initiate protein synthesis on the still attached (nascent) messenger RNA. Synthesis of mRNA and protein (transcription and translation) are therefore seen to be directly coupled in bacteria. In contrast, complete transcripts in eukaryotic cells have to be spliced (to remove the noncoding introns) and capped with poly-adenine (this rarely occurs with bacterial mRNA) before the posttranscriptionally modified message is translocated to the cytoplasm.

Ribosomes

Bacterial ribosomes are slightly smaller (10–20 nm) than those of eukaryotic cells, and they have a sedimentation coefficient of 70S, being composed of a 30S and a 50S subunit (cf. 40S and 60S in the 80S eukaryotic counterparts). They may be seen by electron microscopy and number many thousands in most growing cells. Multiple ribosomes attach to single mRNA molecules to form *polysomes*. It was the nucleotide sequencing of DNA encoding small-subunit ribosomal RNA (rDNA) that led Woese to postulate the evolutionary pathways shown in Fig. 2.1. Essentially all cellular organisms can now be classified, at least down to genus level, by their small-subunit rRNA (SSrRNA) nucleotide sequences. Subsequently, it was recognised that, as growing cells contain so many ribosomes, it should be possible to detect unique identifying (or determinative) SSrRNA sequences by complementary in situ hybridisation with fluorescently labelled oligonucleotide probes. Indeed, it is now possible to apply this approach to natural samples, and this has enabled recognition of bacteria that have never been grown in laboratory culture. Finally, it should be noted that, reflecting their bacterial origin, two key organelles in eukaryotes, mitochondria and chloroplasts, both contain 70S ribosomes. When the SSrRNA-encoding genes on the circular chromosomes of these organelles were sequenced, their original free-living bacterial origin was clearly indicated and the proposed endosymbiotic route by which they became organelles confirmed.

Cytoplasmic membrane

The bacterial cytoplasmic membrane is 5–10 nm thick and consists mainly of phospholipids and proteins. Its structure can be resolved in some ultra-thin sections examined by electron microscopy. *Membranes* generally appear in suitably stained electron microscope preparations as two dark lines about 2.5 nm wide, separated by a lighter area of similar width. Integral, transmembrane and peripheral or anchored proteins occur in abundance and perform similar functions to those described in eukaryotes (e.g., transport and signal transduction). A key feature differentiating prokaryotic cytoplasmic membranes from those of eukaryotes is their multifunctional nature. Thus while in eukaryotic cells the endoplasmic reticulum and Golgi apparatus are involved in protein secretion, packaging and processing, and the mitochondrial inner membrane is the site of electron transport and oxidative phosphorylation, all of these functions must be performed by one membrane in prokaryotes. It is hardly surprising that prokaryotic cell membranes are relatively protein rich, allowing relatively little space for phospholipids.

An important emerging field in bacteriology is the recognition that bacteria produce *membrane vesicles* (MVs) composed of the cytoplasmic membrane and enclosing specific proteins. Although the mechanisms of MV production are not well established, the result could be considered analogous to the exocytosis that occurs in eukaryotes. MVs are involved in pathogenesis, elicit immune responses and interact with other microbes.

Cell wall

The cell wall (Figs. 2.5 and 2.6) lies immediately external to the cytoplasmic membrane. It is 10–25 nm thick, strong and relatively rigid, though with some elasticity, and openly porous, being freely permeable to solute molecules smaller than 10 kDa in mass and 1 nm in diameter. It is strong but elastic and supports the weak cytoplasmic membrane against the high internal osmotic pressure (25 and 5 atm in Gram-positive and Gram-negative cells, respectively) and maintains the characteristic shape of the bacterium in its coccal, bacillary, filamentous or spiral form.

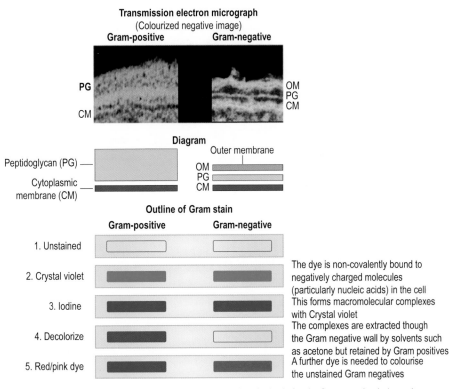

Fig. 2.5   Electron micrograph and diagrams illustrating the basis for the Gram reaction in bacteria.

Except under defined osmotic conditions, cell survival is dependent on the integrity of the cell wall. If the wall is weakened or ruptured, the cytoplasm may swell from osmotic inflow of water and burst the weak cytoplasmic membrane. This process of lethal disintegration and dissolution is termed *lysis*.

The chemical composition of the cell wall differs considerably between different bacterial species, but in all species, the main strengthening component is *peptidoglycan* (syn. *mucopeptide* or *murein*). Peptidoglycan is composed of *N*-acetylglucosamine and *N*-acetylmuramic acid molecules linked alternately in a chain (Fig. 2.7). This heteropolymer forms a single molecular continuous sac external to the cytoplasmic membrane (described as the murein sacculus). The thickness of the peptidoglycan layer turns out to be of great practical importance in differentiating medically significant bacteria. In the late 19th century a Danish physician, Christian Gram, immortalised himself by devising a staining procedure that we now know distinguishes bacteria with a thick (Gram-positive) and a thin (Gram-negative) murein sacculus (see Fig. 2.5). The traditional classification of bacteria is fundamentally rooted in this dichotomy, which has, fortunately, largely been supported by rRNA-based classification.

The rapid (<5 minutes) Gram-stain procedure remains a cornerstone of day-to-day practice in detecting and identifying bacteria in clinical laboratories. *Gram's stain* distinguishes bacteria as Gram-positive or Gram-negative, according to whether or not they resist decolouration with acetone, alcohol or aniline oil after staining with a triphenyl methane dye, such as crystal violet, and subsequent treatment with iodine. The Gram-positive bacteria resist decolouration and remain stained a dark purple colour. The Gram-negative bacteria are decolourised and are then counterstained light pink by the subsequent application of safranin, neutral red or dilute carbol fuchsin. In routine diagnostic work a Gram-stained smear is often the only preparation examined microscopically, as it shows clearly the general morphology of the bacteria as well as revealing their Gram reaction. It should be noted that characteristically Gram-positive species may sometimes appear Gram-negative under certain conditions of growth, especially in ageing cultures on nutrient agar or after exposure to antibiotics.

The *N*-acetylmuramic acid units of peptidoglycan each carry a short peptide, usually consisting of L-alanine, D-glutamic acid, either *meso*-diaminopimelic acid (in Gram-negative bacteria) or L-lysine (in Gram-positive bacteria) and D-alanyl-D-alanine. The wall is given its strength by cross-links that form between adjacent strands.

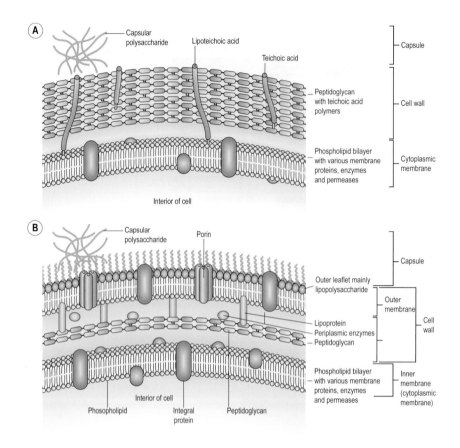

Fig. 2.6 The envelope of (A) the Gram-positive cell wall and (B) the Gram-negative cell wall.

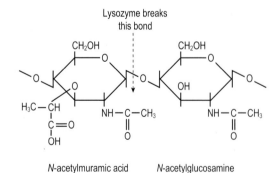

Fig. 2.7 The basic building block of bacterial cell wall peptidoglycan. *N*-acetylmuramic acid is derived from *N*-acetylglucosamine by the addition of a lactic acid unit. Each *N*-acetylmuramic acid molecule is substituted with a pentapeptide; an *N*-acetylglucosamine molecule is joined to the muramylpentapeptide within the cell membrane, and the unit is transferred to growth points in the existing peptidoglycan, where adjacent strands are cross-linked (see also Fig. 2.8).

These may be formed directly between the *meso*-diaminopimelic acid or L-lysine of one strand and the penultimate D-alanine of the next, or (the usual form in Gram-positive organisms) through an interpeptide bridge composed of up to five amino acids; in either case, the terminal D-alanine is lost in the cross-linking reaction (Fig. 2.8). Several antibiotics interfere with the construction of the cell wall peptidoglycan (see Ch. 5).

The bacterial cell wall also contains other components whose nature and amount vary with the species. Many Gram-positive bacteria contain relatively large amounts of *teichoic acid* (a polymer of ribitol or glycerol phosphate complexed with sugar residues) interspersed with the peptidoglycan; some of this material *(lipoteichoic acid)* is linked to lipids buried in the cell membrane.

Electron microscopy reveals that Gram-negative bacteria possess a second *outer membrane* external to the peptidoglycan layer. This is essentially another unit membrane in which the outer leaflet is largely composed of a molecule referred to as lipopolysaccharide (LPS).

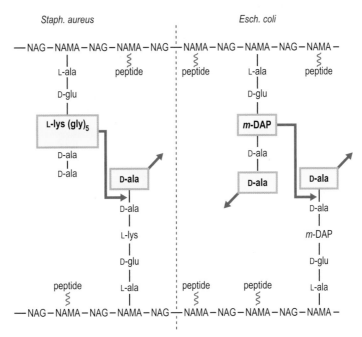

Fig. 2.8 Schematic representation of the peptidoglycan of a representative Gram-positive organism *(Staphylococcus aureus)* and a representative Gram-negative organism *(Escherichia coli)*. Note that in the Gram-positive bacterium cross-linking occurs through a peptide bridge (pentaglycine in *Staph. aureus*), whereas direct cross-linking occurs in *E. coli*. In both cases, the terminal D-alanine is lost. Not all peptides are engaged in cross-linking in *E. coli*, and carboxypeptidases remove redundant D-alanine residues. *NAG*, N-acetylglucosamine; *NAMA*, N-acetylmuramic acid; m-*DAP*, meso-diaminopimelic acid.

Like the cytoplasmic membrane, this membrane contains many associated proteins whose functions include selective permeability (porins) and attachment (adhesins). The outer membrane confers several important properties on Gram-negative bacteria:

- It protects the peptidoglycan from the effects of lysozyme (a natural body defence substance that cleaves the link between *N*-acetylglucosamine and *N*-acetylmuramic acid (see Fig. 2.7).
- It impedes the ingress of many antibiotics.

Components of the LPS, in particular the core structure, lipid A, form endotoxin, which, when released into the bloodstream, may give rise to endotoxic shock (see Ch. 10).

In addition to the basic Gram stain–related properties outlined above, a third type of cell envelope is characteristic of mycobacteria, a group that includes the causal agents of tuberculosis and leprosy. Mycobacteria are related to Gram-positive bacteria, though they can rarely be demonstrated as such. The peptidoglycan layer is covalently linked on its outer aspect to arabinogalactan, which is itself substituted with unique lipids known as *mycolic acids*. These β-hydroxy fatty acids consist of 60–90 carbon residues and, together with noncovalently linked free lipids, form an extremely hydrophobic external layer. This layer

has some properties in common with the Gram-negative outer membrane (indeed, porins have recently been detected therein). The whole envelope structure confers the property of *acid-fast staining* by methods such as the Ziehl–Neelsen (ZN) and phenol–auramine procedures.

The ZN method is of great value in the detection of the tubercle bacillus and other mycobacteria. The mycolic acids referred to above provide a barrier to simple aqueous stains, but when permeability is altered by heating or phenol (or both), concentrated solutions of basic fuchsin, and the fluorescent dyes auramine and rhodamine, can produce well-stained cells that subsequently resist decolourisation by strong acid in alcohol. Any decoloured non–acid-fast organisms are counterstained in a contrasting colour with methylene blue or malachite green. Modifications of the ZN method are also useful for the demonstration of bacterial endospores and organisms such as *Nocardia* spp. and cysts of some protozoa, notably *Cryptosporidium* spp.

The recognition that some bacterial genera have two boundary lipid layers while others have one has led to the recommendation that the descriptive term *diderm* (two skin) be applied to Gram-negative bacteria and to a number of other groups, such as the mycobacteria. In this nomenclature, bacteria with a single lipid boundary, such as conventional Gram-positive bacteria, are referred to as monoderms.

The cell envelope is a highly dynamic structure in growing bacterial cultures. Its components are subject to rapid turnover (synthesis, assembly, disassembly and degradation), and there is busy molecular traffic in and out of the cytoplasm. Although the diagrammatic and photographic representations here give it a somewhat monolithic and immutable character, the envelope and other surface structures can change very rapidly (within minutes) in response to environmental signals. The cell surface receives and transmits many signals from the surrounding environment, including those involving other bacteria, particularly those belonging to the same strain. This latter phenomenon is known as *quorum sensing* and appears to be important in regulating gene expression in groups of bacteria.

The structures involved in the molecular traffic through the cell envelope are the subject of intense investigation. In particular, the outward secretion of proteins attracts much current interest. At least seven distinct processes have been identified; all involve impressive macromolecular complexes anchored in the cytoplasmic membrane. Of particular interest here are the *type III secretion systems* in Gram-negative bacteria. The fully assembled multiprotein complex spans the cytoplasmic membrane, the periplasmic space, the murein sacculus and the outer membrane and in some cases projects from the cell surface into an adjacent host (human) cell. These impressive delivery systems are capable of injecting *effector molecules* into the host cell and thereby subvert the function of the latter to the advantage of the microbe.

Extracellular polysaccharides: capsules, microcapsules and loose slime

Many bacteria have been demonstrated to possess a more or less continuous but relatively amorphous layer external to the Gram-negative and Gram-positive envelopes described earlier. Although these are detected quite readily in some bacteria grown under laboratory conditions, they are somewhat ephemeral in others. These structures appear to be important in mediating contact with potentially hostile environments and may be subject to strict environmental control.

When this layer is fully hydrated and resolvable by light microscopy, it is called a *capsule* (Fig. 2.9). When it is narrower, and detectable only by indirect, serological means or by electron microscopy, it may be termed a *microcapsule*. The capsular gel consists largely of water and has only a small content (e.g., 2%) of solids. In most species, the solid material is a complex polysaccharide, although in some species its main constituent is polypeptide.

Loose slime, or free slime, is an amorphous, viscid, colloidal material that is secreted extracellularly by some bacteria. In bacteria that also possess a demonstrable

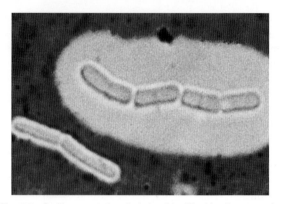

Fig. 2.9 *Bacillus megaterium.* A chain of bacilli with a large capsule, and a pair with a very small capsule. Wet film with India ink, ×3500.

capsule, the slime is generally similar in chemical composition and antigenic character to the capsular substance. When slime-forming bacteria are grown on a solid culture medium, the slime remains around the bacteria as a matrix in which they are embedded, and its presence confers on the growths a watery and sticky 'mucoid' character. The slime is freely soluble in water and, when the bacteria are grown or suspended in a liquid medium, it passes away from them and disperses through the medium.

All of these features appear to have some role in interactions with the external environment. In some cases, capsules have been shown to protect against phagocytosis, the lytic action of complement and bacteriophage invasion. In at least three instances, antibodies directed against capsular antigens have been shown to protect against infection and, indeed, capsular preparations are used in several vaccines. Capsules also appear to have a role in protecting cells against desiccation. The production of extracellular polysaccharides in general provides a matrix within which *biofilm* formation can take place.

S-layers

A rather more structured (paracrystalline) protein layer has been demonstrated in some bacteria. This S-layer can be shown by electron microscopy and appears to share at least some functional properties with capsules.

Flagella and motility

Motile bacteria possess filamentous appendages known as *flagella* (singular, *flagellum*), which act as organs of locomotion. The flagellum is a long, thin filament, twisted spirally in an open, regular waveform. It is about 0.02 μm thick and is usually several times the length of the bacterial cell. It originates in the bacterial cytooplasm and the structure projects through the cell envelope. According to the species, there may be one, or up to 20, flagella per cell. In elongated bacteria the arrangement of the flagella may be *peritrichous,* or *lateral,* when they originate from the sides of the cell, or *polar,* when they originate from one or both ends. Where several occur on a cell, they may function coiled together as a single 'tail'. The external portion of a flagellum is essentially a polymer of a single protein, *flagellin,* whereas the basal region inserted into the cytoplasmic membrane comprises multiple subunits that anchor and power the organ. In a remarkably elegant manner, the flagellar motor is powered directly (as opposed to indirectly via adenosine triphosphate) by the proton gradient created across the cytoplasmic membrane by electron transport. In *E. coli,* alternation between the anticlockwise and clockwise motion of the flagella effects, respectively, linear or tumbling motility. The intervals between these two patterns are modulated by chemical signals in the environment and the end result is that the bacterium shows *chemotactic behaviour* (movement towards or away from certain stimuli).

Flagella are invisible in ordinary light microscope preparations, but may be shown by the use of special staining methods, and in special circumstances by dark-ground illumination. Because of the difficulties of these methods, the presence of flagella is commonly inferred from the observation of motility. They can be demonstrated easily and clearly with the electron microscope, usually appearing as simple fibrils without internal differentiation (Fig. 2.10). In some preparations the flagellum appears as a hollow tube formed of helically twisted fibrils, and the flagella of some bacteria (e.g., vibrios) have an outer sheath. In the spirochaetes the flagellum is located in the periplasm, and hence is referred to as an endoflagellum, and this presumably underpins their characteristic spiral motion.

Motility is clearly important to many bacteria and probably serves mainly to place the cell in environments favourable to growth and free from noxious influences. In some cases, possession of flagella is thought to contribute to the pathogenesis of disease.

Fimbriae and pili

Many bacteria possess filamentous appendages called *fimbriae* or *pili*. These terms are often used interchangeably, although the latter was originally reserved for structures involved in genetic exchange between bacteria (*sex pili*; see later in the chapter). Fimbriae are far more numerous than flagella (e.g., 100–500, being borne peritrichously by each cell) and are much shorter and only about half as thick (e.g., varying from 0.1–1.5 μm in length and having a uniform width between 4 and 8 nm). They do not have the smoothly curved spiral form of flagella and are mostly more or less straight. They cannot be seen

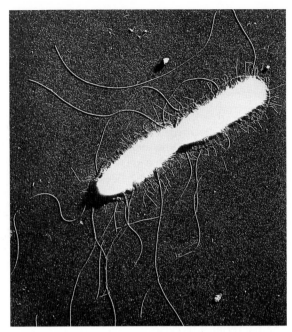

Fig. 2.10 *Salmonella enterica* serotype Typhi. Dividing bacillus from log-phase culture bears about 15 long wavy flagella and >100 short fimbriae. Note the dense *(white)* protoplast shrunken away from the cell wall. Whole bacillus dried and shadow-cast. Electron micrograph, ×16,000. (From Duguid, J. P., & Wilkinson, J. F. (1961). Environmentally induced changes in bacterial morphology. *Symposia of the Society for General Microbiology* 11, 69–99.)

with the light microscope but are clearly seen with the electron microscope in preparations (see Fig. 2.10). The molecular structure of pili has been studied extensively and reveals many features required to span the bacterial cell envelope that are common to different bacterial groups and different cell structures.

Multiple types (e.g., types 1 and 2, P type, etc.) of fimbriae have been recognised according to their dimensions, antigenic and phenotypic properties. Until recently it was thought that they were confined to Gram-negative bacteria, but now they have been demonstrated in many Gram-positive bacteria. In medical and veterinary contexts, fimbriae are recognised to be important in mediating adhesion between the bacterium and host cells (classically this was recognised in the phenomenon of haemagglutination, a property of type 1, mannose-sensitive pili). In contrast, sex pili are structurally similar to other fimbriae but are longer and confer the ability to attach specifically to other bacteria that lack these appendages. Sex pili initiate the process of conjugation (see Ch. 6); they also act as receptor sites for certain bacteriophages described as being 'donor specific'.

It should be noted that fimbriae are not the only means by which bacteria can be involved in specific adhesion events. *Nonfimbrial adhesins* (generally proteins or glycoproteins) are also important in this regard. Receptor-specific interactions are very important in infective disease, as they are thought to determine much of the tissue tropism of the pathological process.

Importance of microbial surface structures in infection

The structures described have significance for the function of bacteria and their identification by clinical microbiologists, but the surface structures of all microorganisms (not just bacteria) are of critical importance in the process of infection. They are vital in initiating the contact that occurs during the encounter and establishment of infection (see Ch. 13). Moreover, in addition to substances secreted by microorganisms, surface structures are exposed to the actions of the innate and adaptive immune systems (see Ch. 8) and, among pathogens, their composition, variability and function reflect these selection pressures and provide opportunities for immunisation.

The bacterial 'life cycle'

Multicellular organisms have long been recognised to pass through many different stages. These may include many immature forms (cf. the larval stages of helminth parasitic worms) or dormant forms (e.g., plant seeds). Even protozoa and fungi may show multiple developmental stages. In contrast, bacteria have been viewed as growing *(vegetative)*, stationary or dead. With the exception of spore-forming genera (see later in the chapter), because they do not undergo morphological differentiation, bacterial cells have been considered essentially uniform in their properties. As indicated previously, it is now recognised that all bacteria adapt extensively and rapidly to their environment. This adaptation takes place at both phenotypic (gene expression) and genotypic (genetic complement and arrangement) levels. It seems clear that there are many more physiological states in which bacteria can exist than previously acknowledged and that these states may influence the capacity of the immune system and antimicrobial agents to eliminate them. In particular, the possibility that nonsporulating bacteria are capable of dormancy (a reversible state of metabolic shutdown) has attracted much interest. Spore formation, however, is the key paradigm of differentiation and dormancy in bacteria.

The different forms taken on by organisms at different stages in the life cycle are of course important in their recognition. The range of basic cellular forms of bacteria was mentioned previously. It is difficult to generalise, but important to mention that bacterial cell morphology does alter with the physiological state. Characteristically, the cells of bacteria that are growing rapidly are larger than their non- or slowly growing counterparts. Although this does not alter basic coccal morphology, it may make bacilli appear more intermediate (cocco-bacillary) or spherical (coccoid) in shape. Bacilli exposed to certain noxious influences (notably some antibiotics) may produce extended forms that are sometimes described as filamentous. Bacteria that are characterised as essentially filamentous produce a mat of intertwining filaments known as a mycelium (one characteristic form of fungal growth). This form of growth is also associated with fragmentation in which coccal forms may be released, and this results in highly *pleomorphic* cultures. All of these alternative growth forms are undoubtedly under the influence of environmental signals, although their identities have yet to be determined in most cases.

Bacterial spores

Some bacteria, notably those of the genera *Bacillus* and *Clostridium,* develop a highly resistant resting phase or *endospore,* whereby the organism can survive in a dormant state through a long period of starvation or other adverse environmental conditions (resuscitation of spores several thousand years old has been claimed). The process does not involve multiplication: in *sporulation,* each vegetative cell forms only one spore, and in subsequent *germination,* each spore gives rise to a single vegetative cell. Geneticists have viewed sporulation as a paradigm of a simple differentiation process, and the key molecular processes required in *Bacillus subtilis* are now understood in detail. In the face of sporulation stimuli, classically starvation or transition from growth to stationary phase, a programme of sequential expression of specific genes is triggered. The end result is a morphologically distinct structure, the endospore, within the *mother cell.*

In unstained preparations the spore is recognised within the parent cell by its greater refractility. It is larger than lipid inclusion granules and is often ovoid, in contrast to the spherical shape of the lipid granules. Mature ungerminated spores are 'phase bright' when viewed by phase-contrast microscopy; immature or germinated spores are 'phase dark'. When mature, the spore resists colouration by simple stains, appearing as a clear space within the stained cell. Spores are slightly acid-fast and may be stained differentially by a modification of the ZN method. The appearance of the mature spores varies according to the species, being spherical, ovoid or elongated, occupying a terminal, subterminal or central position, and being narrower than the cell or broader and bulging it. Spores of some species have an additional, apparently loose, covering known as the *exosporium* (Fig. 2.11).

Spores are much more resistant than the vegetative forms to exposure to disinfectants, drying and heating. Thus application of moist heat at 100–120°C or more for a period

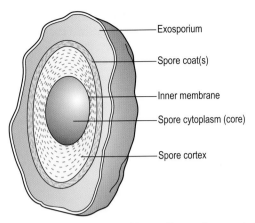

— Exosporium

— Spore coat(s)

— Inner membrane

— Spore cytoplasm (core)

— Spore cortex

Fig. 2.11 Cross-section of a bacterial spore. The core is surrounded by the inner spore membrane. The cortex, a laminated structure, is protected by a more resistant layer or multiple layers forming the spore coat. In some cases, a loose outer covering (exosporium) can be defined.

of 10–20 minutes may be needed to kill spores, whereas heating at 60°C suffices to kill most vegetative cells. In the dry state, or in moist conditions unfavourable to growth, spores may remain viable for many years. The marked resistance of spores has been attributed to several factors in which they differ from vegetative cells: the impermeability of their cortex and outer coat, their high content of calcium and dipicolinic acid, their low content of water and their very low metabolic and enzymic activity.

Reactivation of the spore is termed *germination* and it should be noted that this is not just a reversal of the process by which the spore was formed. Germination of the spore occurs in response to specific stimuli that are generally related to external conditions favourable to growth. It is irreversible and involves rapid degradative changes. The spore successively loses its heat resistance and its dipicolinic acid; it loses calcium, it becomes permeable to dyes and its refractivity changes. Spores that have survived exposure to severe adverse influences such as heat are much more exacting than normal spores in their requirements for germination. For this reason, specially enriched culture media are used when testing the sterility of materials, such as surgical catgut, that have been exposed to disinfecting procedures. In the process of germination, the spore swells, its cortex disintegrates, its coat is broken open and a single vegetative cell emerges.

The initiation of germination *(activation)* is incompletely understood. It is clear that the state of dormancy of spores may be altered by various treatments, such as transient exposure to heat at 80°C, so that germination can then proceed more rapidly in the individual cells or more completely in a spore population. Activation is distinct from germination and is reversible if germination does not proceed.

After germination, cell growth leading up to the formation of the first vegetative cell and before the first cell division is referred to as *outgrowth*. The conditions required for successful outgrowth may differ markedly from those that allow germination.

Conidia (exospores)

Some of the mycelial bacteria *(Actinomycetales)* and many filamentous fungi form *conidia*, resting spores of a kind different from endospores. The conidia are borne *externally* by abstriction from the ends of the parent cells (conidiophores) and are disseminated by the air or other means to fresh habitats. They are not especially resistant to heat and disinfectants.

Pleomorphism and involution

During growth, bacteria of a single strain may show considerable variation in size and shape or form a proportion of cells that are swollen, spherical, elongated or pear shaped. This pleomorphism occurs most readily in certain species (e.g., *Streptobacillus moniliformis* and *Yersinia pestis*) in ageing cultures, on artificial medium and especially in the presence of antagonistic substances such as penicillin, glycine, lithium chloride, sodium chloride in high concentrations and organic acids at low pH. The abnormal cells are generally regarded as degenerate or *involution* forms; some are nonviable, whereas others may grow and revert to the normal form when transferred to a suitable environment. In many cases the abnormal shape seems to be the result of defective cell wall synthesis and produces a grotesquely swollen cell, comparable to a spheroplast (see later in the chapter), that later usually bursts and lyses.

Spheroplasts, protoplasts and L-forms

If bacteria have their cell walls removed or weakened while they are held in a solution of sufficient osmolarity to prevent them taking up water by osmosis, they may escape being lysed and, instead, may become converted into viable spherical bodies. If all the cell wall material has been removed from them, the spheres are *free protoplasts*. If they remain enclosed by an intact, but weakened, residual cell wall, they are called *spheroplasts*. Protoplasts and spheroplasts are osmotically sensitive; they vary in size with the osmotic pressure of the suspending medium and, if the medium is much diluted, they swell up and perish by lysis. In contrast to these laboratory-generated forms (which may be made deliberately for research or biotechnological applications), *L-forms* of bacteria may arise spontaneously and are also cell wall deficient. There is much controversy about the contribution of L-forms to infection. They are difficult to demonstrate as they do not stain with Gram or acid-fast methods and may not propagate in vitro. In common with another controversial area in bacteriology, the 'nanobacteria', L-forms may pass through standard bacteria-stopping filters.

with icosahedral symmetry are enclosed by an outer envelope. The poxviruses are large and complex and do not show either type of symmetry; they are referred to as complex. The size of virions varies considerably, from 25–300 nm, in different families (Fig. 2.14).

THE NATURE AND COMPOSITION OF VIRUSES

Structure

The basic infectious particle of a virus is known as the *virion*. In the simplest viruses, this consists of nucleic acid and a surrounding coat of protein called the *capsid*. Some viruses are enclosed within an *envelope* derived from host cell membranes but modified by the inclusion of viral glycoproteins. The capsid is composed of distinct morphological units or *capsomeres,* which are assembled from viral proteins. Depending on the arrangement of these proteins, the capsomeres may be spherical, cylindrical or ring-like in appearance. The *nucleocapsid* is the combination of nucleic acid and capsid. The arrangement of the capsomeres around the nucleic acid determines the *symmetry* of the virion. When the capsomeres are applied directly to the helical nucleic acid, a coil-like structure with the appearance of a hollow tube is formed. Viruses with this arrangement are said to have *helical symmetry*. Most helical viruses enclose the nucleocapsid within an envelope, and thus do not have a rigid appearance. The other major type is shown by the viruses with *icosahedral symmetry* (Fig. 2.12), in which the capsomeres are arranged as if lying on the faces of an icosahedron with 20 equilateral triangular faces and 12 corners or apices (Fig. 2.13). Capsomeres on the faces and edges of this figure are called hexons, as they always link with six adjacent capsomeres; those positioned at the apices are the pentons, as they always join to five capsomeres. Viruses with icosahedral symmetry have a rigid structure and, under the electron microscope, have a characteristic hexagonal outline with triangular faces. However, if the diameter of the virion is less than about 50 nm the particle will appear spherical. Many viruses

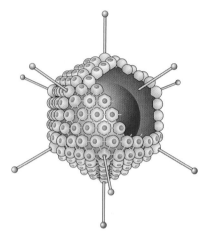

Fig. 2.13   Icosahedron of an adenovirus. The core of DNA is represented by a circular mass. Some of the pentamers at the 12 vertices have been indicated with protruding fibres and terminal knobs. The remaining 240 hexamer capsids are, for the most part, shown as compressed into hollow spheres linked to one another by divalent bonds. The hexagonal shape of a few of the capsomeres is seen in the centre of the diagram.

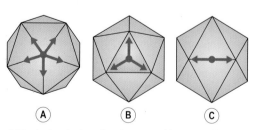

Fig. 2.12   An icosahedron viewed along its (A) five-fold, (B) three-fold and (C) two-fold axes of symmetry.

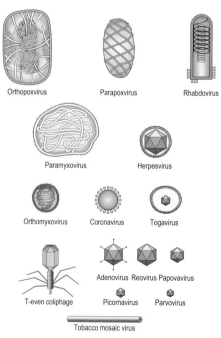

Fig. 2.14   Morphology of viruses.

Viral nucleic acid

The most common types of nucleic acid in viruses of human beings are single-stranded RNA and double-stranded DNA. However, both double-stranded RNA and single-stranded DNA occur in the reoviruses and parvoviruses, respectively. The genomes of RNA viruses may be present as a single strand as in paramyxoviruses, or as two copies as in the retroviruses, or exist as a specific number of fragments as in the orthomyxoviruses and reoviruses. Circular molecules of DNA are present in the virions of papovaviruses and hepadnaviruses. The amount of nucleic acid in virions is constant for a particular virus but shows considerable variation; thus, the genome can vary from 5 kilobase pairs in parvoviruses to 375 kilobase pairs in the largest poxviruses.

Virion enzymes

Several viruses carry essential enzymes in the virion. As discussed in Ch. 7, an RNA-dependent RNA polymerase or transcriptase is an essential component of the virion in several virus families, including the negative-strand RNA viruses. Among DNA viruses, only the poxviruses carry a DNA-dependent RNA polymerase. The hepadnaviruses have a virion polymerase complex that has some similarity to the reverse transcriptase complex found in the retroviruses.

Viral proteins

Analysis of the proteins produced in a cell during viral infection shows that some are essential components of the virion; these are the structural proteins and include capsid proteins and enzymes as well as basic core proteins that may be necessary to package the nucleic acid within the capsid. Other proteins such as enzymes are needed for the production of viral components but are not part of the virion; these are the nonstructural proteins. The essential steps of virus attachment and penetration of the host cell are known to depend on regions of the outer capsid, such as the apical fibres and knobs of adenoviruses, or on parts of the envelope glycoproteins of viruses, such as influenza A and B and the human immunodeficiency virus.

Viroids, defective viruses and prions

Our concept of the organismal nature of infectious agents is stretched to the limit by these infective entities. Viroids are essentially circular RNA molecules that have been associated with several plant diseases; they do not encode proteins or possess a capsid. The hepatitis delta agent has some features in common with viroids and defective viruses (viruses that need the help of another virus for the formation of infectious particles). In the case of the delta agent, these features result in an infective agent that can be transmitted in parallel with hepatitis B.

Prions are proteinaceous infective agents that are responsible for the transmissible spongiform encephalopathies (see Ch. 57). An increase in the number of prion proteins in a new host seems to result from the capacity of the introduced protein to induce abnormal conformational changes in a closely related host protein, rather than by replication. Accumulation of the protein in the induced conformation produces the characteristic pathology of the disease.

RECOMMENDED READING

Fagan, R. P., & Fairweather, N. F. (2014). Biogenesis and functions of bacterial S-layers. *Nature Reviews. Microbiology, 12*(3), 211–222. doi:10.1038/nrmicro3213.

O'Donoghue, E. J., & Krachler, A. M. (2016). Mechanisms of outer membrane vesicle entry into host cells. *Cellular Microbiology, 18*(11), 1508–1517. doi:10.1111/cmi.12655.

Swanson, M., Reguera, G., & Schaechter, M. (2016). *Microbe* (p. 833). Washington, DC: ASM Press.

Websites

CELLS alive! Available at Tree of Life Web Project. Available at http://tolweb.org/tree/.

3 Classification, identification, typing and diversity of bacteria

MICHAEL R. BARER AND ANDREW SWANN

KEY POINTS

- Microbial taxonomy is a branch of science embracing the classification, nomenclature and identification of microbes. The Linnean naming of organisms by genus and species is governed by an international code.
- The Gram stain remains an important phenotypic method by which bacteria can be separated into two major divisions that exhibit a range of shapes and sizes including spherical (cocci), rod shaped (bacilli), filaments and spirals.
- The modern classification of bacteria based on DNA sequence relatedness and inferred evolutionary lineage places most medically important bacteria into phyla with names currently unfamiliar in clinical practice. These include the major phyla *Proteobacteria* (Gram-negative), *Firmicutes* (mainly Gram-positive) and *Bacteroidetes* (Gram-negative anaerobes).
- In clinical practice, bacteria are recognised by colony and microscopic morphology, their requirement for oxygen and specific growth media and by their activity in phenotypic tests.
- Where required, a full identification of most clinically relevant bacteria can now be achieved by a form of high throughput mass spectrometry (MALDI-TOF MS), which is increasingly available in well-resourced laboratories.
- Bacterial species may be highly diverse (panmictic) or relatively uniform (clonal) depending mainly on the frequency of horizontal gene transfer (see Ch. 6).
- Recognition of the relationships between bacteria associated with different patients, potential sources and reservoirs (typing) is now predominantly achieved by DNA sequence-based analyses. Phenotypic typing of bacterial isolates may still be valuable but provides less discrimination than most sequence-based methods.

The central paradigm of medical microbiology has been that the identities of infecting microbes define their pathogenic potential and the selection of appropriate therapies. Soon after the initiation of the antibiotic era in the 1950s it was realised that identity did not satisfactorily predict antibiotic susceptibility, particularly in Gram-negative organisms. This first breakdown between identity and medical significance has continued with the recognition that the genetic complement of organisms meeting a single species definition could be highly variable, as could the disease states with which different isolates could be linked. The capacity of *E. coli* to be associated with harmless commensalism, endogenous infections and both modest and life-threatening exogenous enteric infections stands testimony to this phenomenon.

What then is the value of identifying microbes isolated from clinical specimens? The case remains strong:

1. We need a structure to our description of microbes that is meaningful to clinicians and that informs our management strategies. We also need to be certain that workers in different places are referring to the same organism!
2. While accepting that new analytical methods may link the presence of specific genes or polymorphisms in a clinical sample to specific diagnoses, clinical discussions about microbial aetiology are conducted with reference to the biology of particular organisms.
3. Microbial identity is still sufficient to guide initial therapy; moreover, the threat of antimicrobial resistance and the desirability of not disrupting the normal microbiota makes use of narrow spectrum, ideally specific pathogen-directed, therapy highly desirable.
4. A recognisable identity is the essential first step in detecting and controlling outbreaks and wider epidemics.

The focus of this book is on microbes that cause human disease. These are members of the domains *Bacteria* and

Eukarya as well as the viruses (see Ch. 2). To date, although many members of the domain Archaea have been detected in human samples, they have not been clearly associated with disease. Pathogens (including opportunists) within the Eukarya include Fungi (yeasts and moulds; Ch. 58), Protozoa (Ch. 59) and the multicellular (non-microbial) agents (roundworms and flatworms; Ch. 60) as well as arthropods affecting humans (Ch. 61).

Viruses are noncellular infective agents incapable of independent replication. Their detection and classification are now almost entirely achievable by nucleotide sequence-based methods. They represent the most complex version of molecular infective agents that include viroids, protein-free fragments of single-stranded circular RNA that cause disease in plants and prions, the causative agents of fatal neurodegenerative disorders in animals and humans (see Ch. 57).

The remainder of this chapter is concerned only with bacteria.

TAXONOMY

Taxonomy comprises classification, nomenclature and identification. Classification allows the orderly grouping of microorganisms, whereas nomenclature concerns the naming of these organisms and requires agreement so that names are used unambiguously. Changes in nomenclature may give rise to confusion and are subject to internationally agreed rules. In clinical practice, microbiologists are generally concerned with identification—the correct naming of isolates according to agreed systems of classification. These components, together with taxonomy, make up the overarching discipline of systematics, which is concerned with evolution, genetics and speciation of organisms together with their environmental adaptations, and is commonly referred to as *phylogenetics*.

Like all cellular organisms, bacteria are classified and named according to the standard rules of classification and nomenclature that have been developed following the pioneering work of the 18th century Swedish botanist Linnaeus (Carl von Linné). Large subdivisions (class, order, family, etc.) are finally classified into individual species designated by a Latin binomial, the first term of which is the genus, e.g., *Staphylococcus* (genus) *aureus* (species). In some species, it is useful to recognise subspecies levels as these may be associated with very different biological effects. Thus *Salmonella* (genus) *enterica* (species) *enterica* (subspecies), conventionally written *Salmonella enterica* subsp. *enterica* includes enteric pathogens regularly seen in human samples. The subspecies *enterica* is further subdivided into variants that show distinct antigenic, pathogenic and epidemiological features and these are recognised by their surface antigens and

include the serovars Typhi and Typhimurium that are, respectively, causal agents of typhoid and food poisoning (see Ch. 17).

These points emphasise that even differences within species can be associated with substantial differences in medical significance. It is worth noting that organisms that engage extensively in horizontal gene transfer (see Ch. 6) reproduce asexually and show a high frequency of spontaneous mutation provide a significant challenge to the species concept. Nonetheless, species-level classification and identification remain the reference point for medical and biological assessment of bacteria and the background to this is outlined in the next section.

There remains no 'official' classification of bacteria that is universally accepted and applied. However, most clinical laboratories adhere to defined national standards for identifying medically significant bacteria. Bacterial nomenclature is governed by an international code prepared by the International Committee on Systematic Bacteriology and published as *Approved Lists of Bacterial Names* in the *International Journal of Systematic and Evolutionary Microbiology*. Most new species are also first described in this journal, and a species is considered to be validly published only if it appears on a validation list in this journal.

Multiple taxonomic ranks are recognised. The term *kingdom* is still widely used in biology but the traditional recognition of plants and animals at this level does not fit comfortably with currently recognised DNA relatedness and evolutionary lineages (see later in the chapter). The ranks currently used in the classification of bacteria are shown in Table 3.1.

METHODS OF CLASSIFICATION

There remains an unresolved tension in biological classification that is particularly prominent in microbiology. Should classification reflect the evolutionary pathway and distances between organisms or should it reflect their current properties and practical significance in the real

Table 3.1 Ranks used to classify bacteria and the threshold of similarity in 16S rDNA sequence accepted for allocation to that rank

Category	Example	
Domain	Bacteria	16S % similarity
Phylum	Firmicutes	75.0
Class	Bacilli	78.5
Order	Bacillales	82.0
Family	Staphylococcaceae	86.5
Genus	*Staphylococcus*	94.5
Species	*Staphylococcus aureus*	98.7

world? This tension is encompassed by the terms *cladistic* (evolutionary) and *phenetic* (phenotypic), referring to the way in which a particular classification has been achieved. Both approaches have their shortcomings.

Cladistic approaches are based on DNA sequencing and this works well for establishing the relatedness between individual molecules. However, different molecules within the same organism can sometimes clearly be shown to have different phylogenies (evolutionary pathways); how is this possible? The observation suggests that genes in one organism have come from more than one progenitor, an apparent transgression of the laws of inheritance. This multiple inheritance is in fact the case and reflects the phenomenon of *horizontal gene transfer* (HGT) across bacterial cells, species and indeed higher order classes (see Ch. 6). This complicates cladistic classifications, particularly where attempts are made to infer deep evolutionary relationships. The strength of the approach is recovered by the observation that certain genes (particularly 16S) appear to be infrequently involved in HGT and that, while all bacterial genomes reflect this phenomenon, the core genome has been inherited through a recognisable lineage.

The phenetic approach is subject to different problems. We tend to think in biology that related organisms have related roles in and impacts on their environments. While there are some themes in medical bacteriology where this view is helpful, small genetic differences can be associated with very different phenotypes, particularly in pathogenic potential. Moreover, the tests we apply to establish the phenotype and identity of a bacterial isolate are not directly related to the medical significance of that organism so there can be large discrepancies between what we measure in the laboratory and medical importance.

In the end, we need a classification that is practically workable, that reflects our best understanding of biological relationships and that serves clinical needs.

Polyphasic approaches

Until the 1980s, bacterial classification was developed using a combination of phenotypic characteristics, including cell morphology and tests such as motility and biochemical reactions, while genetic relationships were determined by G+C ratios and DNA homology (see later in the chapter). In 1794, Michel Adanson proposed that biological classifications should be based on many characteristics and this was the guiding 'Adansonian' approach adopted by most bacteriologists. However, there was much argument between authorities regarding appropriate classifications because different criteria were used in different labs and characteristics were given different weight by different schools of thought. The situation was greatly improved by the introduction of *Numerical Taxonomy* methods in the 1960s by Peter Sneath and colleagues. In this approach

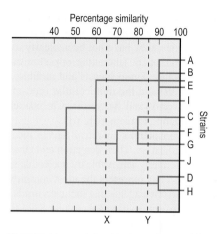

Fig. 3.1 Hierarchical taxonomic tree (dendrogram) prepared from similarity matrix data. The dashed lines *X* and *Y* indicate levels of similarity at which separation into genera and species might be possible.

all measured characteristics were given equal weight but many (usually >50) were assessed. Phenotypic relatedness could then be calculated on the basis of a similarity coefficient representing the proportion of characteristics held in common by any two isolates. When these pairwise comparisons are entered into a similarity matrix, charts or dendrograms can be drawn showing the hierarchy of relationships across a set of tested organisms (Fig. 3.1).

DNA composition

The hydrogen bonding between guanine and cytosine (G–C) base pairs in DNA is stronger than that between adenine and thymine (A–T). Thus the melting or denaturation temperature of DNA (at which the two strands separate) is determined primarily by the G + C content. At the melting temperature the separation of the strands brings about a marked change in the light absorption characteristics at a wavelength of 260 nm, and this is readily detected by spectrophotometry. There is a very wide range in the G + C component of bacterial DNA, varying from about 25%–80% in different genera. However, for any one species, the G + C content is relatively fixed or falls within a very narrow range, and this provides a basis for classification. Note also that regions in sequenced genomes often show substantial variation in G + C% against the overall ratio and this is generally taken to indicate that these *genomic islands* have been acquired from other (unrelated) bacteria by HGT (see Ch. 6).

DNA homology (DNA:DNA hybridisation)

Another approach to classification is to arrange individual organisms into groups on the basis of the *homology* of their DNA base sequences. This exploits the fact that double strands re-form (anneal) from separated strands during controlled cooling of a heated preparation of DNA. This process can be readily demonstrated with purified and suitably heated homologous DNA extracted from a single species, but it can also occur with DNA from two related species, so that hybrid pairs of DNA strands are produced. These hybrid pairings occur with high frequency between complementary regions of DNA, and the degree of hybridisation can be assessed if labelled DNA preparations are used. Binding studies with messenger RNA (mRNA) can also give information to complement these observations, which provide genetic evidence of relatedness among bacteria. Organisms with different G + C ratios are unlikely to show significant DNA homology. However, organisms with the same, or close, G + C ratios do not necessarily show homology. Species-level identity is generally accepted at homologies above 70% by this method.

Sequencing of genes encoding 16S ribosomal RNA and other housekeeping genes

As noted in the previous chapter, ribosomes in all cells function by near identical mechanisms. The nucleotide sequence of small subunit rRNA includes regions that are conserved across all bacteria and indeed some that are conserved across eukaryotes and bacteria. While sequencing of the entire 16S encoding gene provides good resolution in the classification of most bacteria, there are some groups where this is not the case. In these cases, sequencing of other highly conserved housekeeping genes such as *rpoB, recA, groEL,* or *gyrB* may provide better resolution. Alternatively, the 23S rDNA and the 16S–23S internal transcribed sequences may be analysed. In practice, the DNA of the test organism is extracted and amplified by PCR using universal primers. The DNA sequence of the product is determined and the sequence compared against databases to find the closest fit. It is generally accepted that sequence similarity between 0.5% and 1.0% (with the type species) is required for the identification of an unknown organism.

The major advantage of the 16S target is the availability of extensive and well-curated databases against which a new sequence can be compared.

Whole genome sequencing (WGS)

The establishment of reliable massively parallel DNA sequencing platforms in the second decade of this century has transformed the high-resolution classification of bacteria. If sufficient growth of the organism can be obtained, a first pass genome sequence can be obtained within a few hours and at a modest price such that WGS is rapidly

making other approaches to typing strains redundant (see later in the chapter). The challenge in classification is to have sufficient relevant comparative data from related and distantly related organisms to achieve a robust classification. It seems inevitable that WGS data will be required to classify newly identified bacterial groups in future, and this process will be greatly assisted by the development of computational tools that are more accessible to workers with limited bioinformatic expertise. At present there is no standard way of including WGS data in classification, rather individual gene sequences, such as those identified above, are used. At the whole genome level, virtually every isolate is unique and inclusion of the complete sequence is complicated by HGT (see Ch. 6).

CLASSIFICATION IN CLINICAL PRACTICE

For many years, approaches to classification could be somewhat different in academic and clinical/diagnostic circles; the aim of the former was to achieve a robust and defensible structure, while the latter needed to work with the clinical community using names that enable effective clinical and public health decisions. To some extent, this situation was perpetuated by the need for clinical laboratories to use highly abbreviated phenotypic schemes to achieve presumptive rather than definitive identifications and the recognition that, in many circumstances, identification to family or genus level was sufficient to meet clinical needs.

Two technologies have now changed this situation in well-resourced laboratories, the advent of DNA sequence-based classification and the use of mass spectrometry profiling of isolates to achieve phenotypic identification. This means that, where required, more or less definitive identities can be obtained on the same day that colonies are seen on an agar plate. These identifications are supported by reference to regularly updated databases using formally approved names.

Nonetheless, many practical problems remain. The underlying debate between phenetic and cladistic classifications is now played out between these near ultimate technologies. In the medical context, contemporary resolution must reflect practical application. We need to place medically significant organisms into a classification scheme that informs medical understanding and practice. Classically, a scheme based on Gram stain morphology has been the mainstay of our approach. However, both the more sophisticated identification methods now deployed and the emerging clinical significance of microbiomics bring unfamiliar names into medical discourse where Gram morphology is a secondary consideration. Thus our current need is to serve both sources of information set within a classification system that may be considered sound. This we attempt later in the chapter and in Table 3.2.

Table 3.2 Cladistic classification of medically important bacteria

Gram-	Phylum and shape	Genus names
POSITIVE	**Actinobacteria** (High G+C, mainly bacilli)	*Actinomyces, Streptomyces, Corynebacterium, Nocardia, Mycobacterium[2], Micrococcus*
	Firmicutes (Low G+C) (Includes some Gram-negative groups[1])	
	Bacilli	*Listeria, Bacillus, Clostridium*, Lactobacillus*, Eubacterium**
	Cocci	*Staphylococcus, Streptococcus, Enterococcus*
NEGATIVE	Cocci	*Veillonella*[1], Mycoplasma[2]*
	Proteobacteria (5 subdivisions assigned α, β, γ, δ, and ε)	
	Cocci: Betaproteobacteria Gammaproteobacteria	*Neisseria* *Moraxella*
	Bacilli: Alphaproteobacteria Betaproteobacteria Gammaproteobacteria " " Epsilonproteobacteria	*Brucella, Rickettsia,* *Burkholderia, Bordetella, Spirillum* *Escherichia, Klebsiella, Proteus, Salmonella, Shigella, Yersinia, Pseudomonas, Stenotrophomonas, Haemophilus, Legionella, Coxiella, Francisella, Vibrio* *Campylobacter, Helicobacter*
	Bacteroidetetes	*Bacteroides*, Prevotella**
	Spirochaetes	*Borrelia, Treponema[2], Brachyspira[2], Leptospira[2]*
	Chlamydia	*Chlamydia[2]*

*Anaerobes. 1 – Some members of the Firmicutes have a Gram-negative diderm cell envelope including LPS. Recent evidence supports the view that Firmicutes evolved from diderms and that most lost their outer membranes. 2 – Do not stain with the Gram method.
Note that many traditional phenotypic relationships based on Gram morphology growth atmosphere are disrupted by the evolutionary relationships reflected here.

One important consequence of bringing microbial classification into better order in light of evolutionary insights is that established names of certain organisms cannot be justified by nomenclatural rules and are therefore changed. Thus a medically significant streptococcus formerly named *S. bovis* (because it was isolated from cattle) was increasingly recognised on phenotypic grounds to be part of a group of related but distinct strains. The former *S. bovis* was known, when isolated from patients' bloodstreams, to be associated with an increased risk of colon cancer. When isolates were reexamined in light of the distinctions recognised above, only one of the phenotypes (designated biotypes), which had the property of degrading gallic acid, was found to have the association with cancer; the risk ratio for these isolates was found to be ~seven-fold above the population average, much higher than the bovis group as a whole. Thus it makes sense to differentiate these gallic acid degrading strains with the formally justified name of *S. gallolyticus*. These transitions need to be actively managed by clinical microbiologists so that clinicians appreciate their significance.

A second consequence is that organisms formerly considered closely or distantly related on phenotypic grounds show very different relationships on cladistics grounds. Some examples of this are apparent in Table 3.2.

The major phyla and some example genera and species of medically significant bacteria are listed below.

Actinobacteria

These are generally considered Gram-positive (although many do not take up the stain), and their basic cell wall structure includes external features additional to peptidoglycan. They have a high G + C content and many are capable of filamentous growth with true branching that may produce a type of mycelium. They include antibiotic-producing bacteria and a small number of highly significant pathogens.

- *Actinomyces.* Gram-positive, non–acid-fast, tend to fragment into short coccal and bacillary forms and not to form conidia; anaerobic (e.g., *Actinomyces israelii*).
- *Streptomyces.* Vegetative mycelium does not fragment into short forms; conidia form in chains from aerial hyphae (e.g., *Streptomyces griseus*).

- *Mycobacterium.* Acid-fast; most do not take up the Gram stain; usually bacillary, rarely branching; make mycolic acids (e.g., *Mycobacterium tuberculosis*).
- *Nocardia.* Similar to *Actinomyces* but aerobic and mostly acid-fast; make mycolic acids (e.g., *Nocardia asteroides*).
- *Corynebacterium.* Pleiomorphic (variably shaped) Gram-positive bacilli; make mycolic acids (e.g., *Corynebacterium diphtheriae*).

Firmicutes

- *Streptococcus.* Gram-positive cocci; generally occur in chains due to successive cell divisions occurring in the same axis (e.g., *Streptococcus pyogenes*); diplococci also occur (e.g., *Streptococcus pneumoniae*).
- *Staphylococcus.* Gram-positive cocci; generally occur in irregular clusters due to successive divisions occurring in different planes (e.g., *Staph. aureus*).
- *Mycoplasma and Ureaplasma.* Pleiomorphic cocci that do not make peptidoglycan.
- *Veillonella.* Gram-negative; generally very small cocci arranged mainly in clusters and pairs; anaerobic (e.g., *Veillonella parvula*).
- *Gram-positive spore-forming bacilli.* The key medically relevant genera here are the genera *Bacillus* and *Clostridium* (anaerobic). They are Gram-positive but liable to become Gram-negative in ageing cultures. The size, shape and position of the spore may assist recognition of the species, for example the bulging, spherical, terminal spore ('drumstick' form) of *Clostridium tetani*.
- *Gram-positive nonsporing bacilli.* These include several genera. *Erysipelothrix* and *Lactobacillus* are distinguished by a tendency to grow in chains and filaments, and *Listeria* by flagella that confer motility.

Proteobacteria

A very large of group of Gram-negative bacteria (bacilli and cocci) with generally reactogenic LPS or LOS (Chs 2 and 10) in their outer membranes and five subdivisions (alpha, beta, gamma, delta and epsilon).

- *Alphaproteobacteria.* Include the cell-dependent *Rickettsia* group, the facultatively intracellular *Brucella* group and the *Bartonella* group.
- *Betaproteobacteria. Neisseria* – cocci, mainly adherent in pairs and slightly elongated at right angles to axis of pairs (e.g., *Neisseria meningitidis*). *Burkholderia* – bacilli (*Burkholderia pseudomallei*).
- *Gammaproteobacteria.* Bacilli including the enterobacteria (*Escherichia coli*), and the genera *Pseudomonas, Legionella* and the curved vibrios (e.g., *Vibrio cholerae*).
- *Deltaproteobacteria.* No medically significant bacteria.
- *Epsilonproteobacteria.* Curved and loosely spiral bacilli including the genera *Helicobacter* and *Campylobacter*.

Bacteroidetes

Gram-negative nonsporing anaerobic bacilli.

- *Bacteroides, Prevotella* and *Porphyromonas* are major genera.

Spirochaetes

These organisms differ from the other groups in being slender flexuous spiral filaments that, unlike the spirilla, are motile without possession of flagella. They have a Gram-negative cell wall. The different varieties are recognised by their size, shape, waveform and refractility, observed in the natural state in unstained wet films by dark-ground microscopy. Genera of medical importance include *Borrelia, Treponema* and *Leptospira*.

Chlamydiae

Chlamydiae are obligate intracellular parasites with a distinctive cell envelope structure including an extensively cross-linked outer membrane complex and probable trace amounts of peptidoglycan. (e.g., *Chlamydia trachomatis*).

IDENTIFICATION OF BACTERIA

The principal driver for a microbiology lab serving an acute medical facility must be the provision of microbiological results on a timescale that enables appropriate clinical and public health management decisions. In the present era, when antibiotic resistance threatens their therapeutic value, the microbiology lab must strive to provide microbial aetiologies at the earliest possible time so that narrow- rather than broad-spectrum antimicrobials can be used.

For most clinical purposes, clear, rapid guidance on the likely cause of an infection is required and, consequently, microbiologists usually rely on a few simple procedures, notably microscopy and culture, backed up, when necessary, by a few supplementary tests to achieve a presumptive identification. As noted earlier in the chapter, the technologies of DNA analysis and mass spectrometry have brought definitive identifications within reach of some well-resourced clinical laboratories. Nonetheless, use of these technologies is usually confined to particularly significant isolates, such as those found in deep-seated infections or those isolated from blood.

Microscopy is rapid (minutes), but culture generally takes at least 18 hours, sometimes longer. More rapid tests are constantly being sought and near-patient microbial antigen detection methods (bedside or office diagnostics) are gaining popularity.

Most specimens for bacteriological examination, whether from human beings, animals or the environment, contain mixtures of bacteria, and it is essential to obtain pure cultures of individual isolates before embarking on identification. Noncultural methods, such as antigen or nucleic acid–based detection, do not have this disadvantage; however, in most cases, they do not distinguish between live and dead microbes.

Microscopy

Morphology and staining reactions of individual organisms generally provide sufficient results to place an unknown species in its appropriate biological group. Accumulation of analyses over many years has led to a situation in which we recognise a limited range of likely organisms in particular specimen types such that a presumptive identification may be achieved even at this early stage.

A Gram-stain smear suffices to show the Gram reaction, size, shape and grouping of the bacteria and the arrangement of any endospores. An unstained wet film may be examined with dark-ground illumination in the microscope to observe the morphology of delicate spirochaetes; an unstained wet film, or 'hanging-drop', preparation is examined with ordinary bright-field illumination for observation of motility. Capsules surrounding bacterial cells are demonstrated by 'negative staining' with India ink; the capsules remain unstained against the background of ink particles. To identify mycobacteria, or other acid-fast organisms, a preparation is stained by the Ziehl–Neelsen or Auramine fluorescence method or one of its modifications. The microscopic characters of certain organisms in pathological specimens may be sufficient for presumptive identification, for example tubercle bacilli in sputum, or *T. pallidum* in exudate from a chancre. However, many bacteria share similar morphological features, and further tests must be applied to differentiate them.

Cultural characteristics

The appearance of colonial growth on the surface of a solid medium, such as nutrient agar, is often very characteristic. Attention is paid to the diameter of the colonies, their outline, their elevation, their translucency (clear, translucent or opaque) and colour. Changes brought about in the medium (e.g., haemolysis in a blood agar medium) may also be significant. The range of conditions that support growth is characteristic of particular organisms. These include optimum growth temperature, ability or inability of the organism to grow in the presence (aerobe) or absence (anaerobe) of oxygen, in a reduced oxygen atmosphere (microaerophile) or requirement for carbon dioxide (capnophile). Growth on media containing selective inhibitory factors (e.g., bile salt, specific antimicrobial agents, or low or high pH) may also be of diagnostic significance (see Table 4.1).

Biochemical reactions

Species that cannot be distinguished by morphology and cultural characters may exhibit metabolic differences that can be exploited. It is usual to test the ability of the organism to produce acidic and gaseous end-products when presented with individual carbohydrates (glucose, lactose, sucrose, mannitol, etc.) as the sole carbon source. Other tests determine whether the bacterium produces particular end-products (e.g., indole or hydrogen sulphide) when grown in suitable culture media, and whether it possesses certain enzyme activities, such as oxidase, catalase, urease, gelatinase or lecithinase. Traditionally, such tests have been performed selectively and individually according to the recommendations of standard guides. For most of the 20th century such guides, including the two classics produced by Cowan and Steel and by MacFaddin, have served as the mainstay for service labs when more than simple presumptive identifications were required. Towards the end of this era this approach was progressively replaced by microgalleries of identification tests that combine simplicity and accuracy with, in some cases, automated reading. These testing systems are still widely used but take second place in labs that support matrix-assisted laser desorption ionisation-time of flight (MALDI-TOF) mass spectrometry analyses.

Matrix–assisted laser desorption ionisation-time of flight mass spectrometry (MALDI-TOF MS)

This approach, developed for bacterial identification over the last 30 years, has revolutionised phenotypic identification of bacteria into a one-step procedure yielding, in most cases, a more or less definitive species-level output and a probability that the assignment is correct. A small amount of solid medium growth (e.g., a colony) is applied to a target plate (an array of spots allowing multiple isolates to be processed in a single run). The bacterial biomass is then overlaid with a matrix reagent with or without prior formic acid treatment. When dry the preparation is placed in the vaporising chamber, exposed to a vacuum then scanned with a laser beam that vaporises (desorbs) it. The matrix has the remarkable capacity to reliably and consistently transfer positive charges to most of the vaporised macromolecules while maintaining their integrity. The vapour phase and charged molecules are accelerated within an electrostatic field and move towards a detector at a rate determined by their charge to mass ratio.

The end result is a succession of impacts on the detector at different times (time of flight) and with different intensities. The pattern is effectively a fingerprint that can be very closely related to the identity of the organism, probably mainly related to its protein content. Very large databases have been built by the manufacturers of these instruments such that the vast majority of medically important (and many other) bacteria can be identified with a few minutes of laboratory scientist benchwork. As the databases build up their discriminatory capacity increases and new organisms can be included. In addition to bacteria, this already applies to yeasts and filamentous fungi and is being considered with protozoa; the approach also has discriminatory power to identify viruses in cell culture. Methods are also available to prepare isolates in broth cultures (particularly blood cultures) for direct identification without solid medium growth.

We use the abbreviation MALDI in the rest of this book to denote the MALDI-TOF approach.

Nucleotide sequence–based identification

The application of these methods both for identification of isolates and for direct application to clinical samples has become so important that a separate chapter has been devoted to this area (Ch. 64). At this point we note that bacterial identification is generally achieved by full-length 16S rDNA analysis. As noted earlier in the chapter, in some fields this may be insufficient to provide necessary differentiation (e.g., in *Salmonella* spp.). In these cases, WGS may be the most readily deliverable next step or further phenotypic analyses, such as antigenic characterisation, may be required.

Antigenic characterisation

Species and types of microorganism can often be identified by specific serological (antigen–antibody) reactions. These depend on the fact that the serum from an animal immunised against a microorganism contains antibodies specific for the homologous species or type that react in a characteristic manner with the particular microorganism. Such simple in vitro tests have been used for many years in microbiology, notably in the formal identification of presumptive isolates of pathogens (e.g., salmonellae) from clinical material. The specificity and range of antibody tests have been greatly improved by the availability of highly specific monoclonal antibodies. Antibody–antigen complexes denoting a positive reaction can be detected in a variety of ways including slide agglutination, immunofluorescence and enzyme-linked immunosorbent assay (ELISA). Similar technologies are also used to detect patients' antibody responses using antigens specific to individual organisms.

TYPING OF BACTERIA

Different bacterial species exhibit different population structures. Some species are characterised by highly diverse populations at one extreme and closely similar members at the other. The frequency of recombination of chromosomal genes (see Ch. 6) is the major determinant of a population structure of a given species, and this frequency ranges from negligible to very high. Highly recombining populations are termed *panmictic*, in contrast to *clonal* populations where recombination is infrequent (Table 3.3). Species such as *Neisseria gonorrhoeae* and *Haemophilus influenzae* are naturally transformable, that is, they are able to take up DNA (foreign and native) from their environment, and their populations are characterised by a high frequency of recombination. In clonal populations such as *Salmonella enterica*, recombination is rare and there is nonrandom association of alleles in a background of limited genetic exchange. Mutations occur as a result of natural and selective pressures, but these are not sufficient to disrupt the clonal lineage and daughter cells continue to resemble the ancestral parent. Bacterial clones are therefore not identical to their parents but display a number of characteristics in common with their ancestors. Many species are characterised by considerable genetic diversity but with clonal expansion of a subpopulation. Some of these clones may be transient, although others may persist and spread nationally and globally.

Table 3.3 Panmictic versus clonal populations					
	Reproduction	Recombination	Allele arrangement	Mutation	Selective pressures
Panmictic	Sexual*	Frequent	Segregated	Normal	Natural selection
Clonal	Asexual	Rare	Nonrandom association	Normal	Environmental
*Refers to recombination between genetic elements from different organisms in bacteria.					

By typing we identify a recognisable subdivision of a species that serves as a reference marker against which other isolates of the same species can be compared. A population of bacteria presumed to descend from a single bacterium, as found in a natural habitat, in primary cultures from the habitat, and in subcultures from the primary cultures, is called a *strain*. Each primary culture from a natural source is called an *isolate*. The distinction between strains and isolates may be important; for example, cultures of typhoid bacilli isolated from 10 different patients should be regarded simply as 10 different *isolates* unless epidemiological or other evidence indicates that the patients have been infected from a common source with the same *strain*. The ability to discriminate between similar strains may be of great epidemiological value in tracing sources or modes of spread of infection in a community or hospital ward, and various typing methods have been devised.

Typing may inform different levels of epidemiological investigation, ranging from micro-epidemiology (local investigation), macroepidemiology (regional, national, international) to population structure analysis (evolution of strains and global patterns of spread). The data derived may assist in the control of infection by excluding sources, identifying carriers and establishing the prevalence of individual strains and in developing national and global vaccination strategies. Common reasons for microbial typing are to identify common or point sources, discriminate between mixed strain infections, distinguish reinfection from relapse and occasionally to identify a type and disease association (e.g., *Escherichia coli* O157 and haemolytic uraemic syndrome, skin and throat types of group A *Str. pyogenes*, etc.).

Typing methods should be reproducible both in the laboratory and clinically. The former is easily established by repeated tests on a sample of experimental strains, but should also be established in vivo by examining multiple pairs of isolates from single sources to determine the stability of the strain characteristics probed by the typing method used. A typing method should also discriminate adequately and clearly between different populations and be comprehensive, that is, assign most populations to a type. The typing data should be in a format that is easily assimilated into databases and should be able to be incorporated into the national picture to inform other workers in the field. In the past, very few phenotypic typing methods met these criteria and there was a need to utilise multiple methods, preferably directed at unlinked targets and always in the context of an epidemiological investigation.

Phenotypic typing methods used extensively in the 20th century are now largely redundant because of the availability of genotypic methods. There remains the need, in some cases, to reconcile the results of older methods with genotyping methods in order to track changing epidemiological patterns. In clinical practice a first guess at the relatedness of isolates can be gained from their antibiotic susceptibility profiles (antibiogram- or resistotyping) and serotyping remains an important front-line method for enteric pathogens, particularly salmonellas.

The classical methods include biotyping, phage typing, bacteriocin typing and protein typing and can all still be applied, but they require considerable expertise and maintenance of critical reagents. They will not be discussed further here, and the reader is referred to earlier editions of this text for explanations of these methods. DNA sequence-based typing is now generally cheaper and provides results that are globally comparable and deliverable on a rapid timescale.

Restriction endonuclease typing

Restriction endonucleases are a family of enzymes that each cut DNA at a specific sequence recognition site, which may be rare or frequent in the DNA of the species being examined. The frequency with which an enzyme cuts in a particular species is dependent on the oligonucleotide sequence, the frequency of the restriction site, and the percentage G + C content of the species. For example, the recognition site of enzyme *Sma*I is 5′-CCC↓GGG-3′ (↓ site of cleavage) and this cuts infrequently in the AT-rich genome of *Staph. aureus,* whereas enzyme *Xba*I (5′-T↓CTAGA-3′) is a rare cutter in most Gram-negative species with a high GC content. Both plasmid and chromosomal DNA can be analysed by this means. Frequent-cutting endonucleases generate numerous small fragments that can be resolved by conventional electrophoresis in agarose gel and detected by staining with a dye. The resolution of conventional agarose gel electrophoresis does not exceed 20 kb and optimal separation in standard length gels is achieved between 1 and 15 kb.

The large DNA fragments produced by infrequent-cutting enzymes need to be separated in special electrical fields with a pulsed current (pulsed-field gel electrophoresis; PFGE). In this technique, bacteria are encased in an agarose plug (to minimise shearing of DNA) and the cells are digested with proteinase K enzyme before the DNA is digested with the enzyme. By introducing a pulse or change in the direction of the electric field, fragments as large as 10 Mb can be separated. The time taken by fragments to reorient to the alternate electric field is proportional to their molecular size and where they migrate in the electric field. The most widely used apparatus is the contour-clamped homogeneous electric field (CHEF), which has 24 electrodes arranged in a hexagonal array. Run times are often of the order of 30–40 hours, but shorter, more rapid, protocols have been described. A number of factors influence the quality of results, including DNA quality and concentration, agarose concentration, voltage and pulse times and buffer strength and temperature.

Interpretation of PFGE profiles can be problematic. For some species the criteria of Tenover (see recommended reading list) can be applied to establish the significance of differences in banding profiles of strains. As a rule of thumb, isolates from an incident under investigation that show no difference in profiles can be considered indistinguishable, those with one to three band differences as closely related, four to six bands as possibly related and seven or more band differences as indicating distinct strains. However, this rule should be applied with a degree of caution, as some species (e.g., *Enterococcus faecium*) can exhibit significant variation (6–10 band differences) apparently within members of the same clone. A number of computer-assisted analysis packages are available that calculate coefficients of similarity between strains and represent these as dendrograms (Fig. 3.1). Two commonly employed coefficients, the Jaccard and Dice, use the number of concordant bands in profiles and the total number of possible band positions to calculate the percentage similarity between the isolates. The Pearson coefficient gives the advantage that specific band positions do not have to be defined. A cut-off point of 85% similarity is often used, but, as for the band difference rule, this should be set by experiment with related and unrelated strain sets.

Gene probe typing

DNA probes (see earlier in the chapter) for strain typing consist of cloned specific, random or universal sequences that can detect restriction site heterogeneity in the target DNA. The detection of variation in rDNA gene loci is the basis of ribotyping, and this method has been universally applied to the typing of various species. Other commonly used probes target insertion sequences (lengths of DNA involved in transposition; see Ch. 6) that may define clonal structures of populations.

Polymerase chain reaction–based methods

These methods have generally passed through a number of generations. Polymerase chain reaction (PCR) is a technique that allows specific sequences of DNA to be amplified. Multiple copies of regions of the genome defined by specific oligonucleotide primers are made by repeated cycles of amplification under controlled conditions. Such methods can be used to study DNA from any source.

PCR-mediated DNA fingerprinting makes use of the variable regions in DNA molecules. These may be variable numbers of tandem repeat regions or areas with restriction endonuclease recognition sequences. To perform PCR

typing, it is necessary to know the sequences of the bordering regions so that specific oligonucleotide primers can be synthesised.

Multilocus sequence typing

This technique indexes allelic variation in several housekeeping genes by nucleotide sequencing, rather than indirectly from the electrophoretic mobilities of their gene products, as was the case with its parent technique, multilocus enzyme electrophoresis. Housekeeping genes are not subject to selective forces as are variable genes and they diversify slowly. Multiple genes (usually seven) are employed to overcome the effects of recombination in a single locus, which might distort the interpretation of the relationship of the strains being compared. Multilocus sequence typing (MLST) can rightly be referred to as definitive genotyping, as sequence data are unambiguous and databases of allelic profiles of isolates of individual species are accessible via the Internet. The level of discrimination of MLST depends on the degree of diversity within the population to generate alleles at each locus, but some highly uniform species such as *M. tuberculosis* are not amenable to analysis by the technique. Recently, increased discrimination has been sought in virulence-associated genes necessary for survival and spread of the organism on the basis that these genes are exposed to frequent environmental changes and thus provide a higher degree of sequence variation. Intergenic regions of selected genes are amplified by PCR and a 500-bp internal fragment sequenced to identify allelic polymorphisms.

A variant of MLST termed *multilocus restriction typing* introduces restriction digestion of amplified housekeeping genes and removes the need for sequencing. The restriction fragment length polymorphisms (RFLPs) can be sorted into type patterns and reveal population structures similar to those with MLST.

Variable number tandem repeat analysis

Variable number tandem repeats (VNTRs) are short nucleotide sequences (20–100 bp) that vary in copy number in bacterial genomes. They are thought to arise through DNA strand slippage during replication and are of unknown function. Separate VNTR loci are identified from published sequences and are often located in intergenic regions and annotated open reading frames. Primers are designed to amplify five to eight loci and the products sequenced to generate a digital profile. VNTR typing is rapid and reproducible and relatively simple to perform. Improved discrimination may be achieved by identification of more loci, but there is debate about their stability over time.

Whole genome–based typing

The advent of new high throughput DNA sequencing methods is ushering in a new era in which it is becoming feasible to compare and type bacteria based on entire genome sequence data. These massively parallel sequencing technologies produce relatively short nucleotide sequence reads but on such a scale that these can be assembled into a sequence matched against those obtained from previous isolates of that organism. This enables a genome-wide comparison to be made and a more or less definitive evolutionary relationship to be established to other contemporaneous and historical isolates. The costs of such analyses are rapidly becoming competitive with traditional typing methods. Such analyses have the potential to transform medical bacteriology by producing unambiguous epidemiological information and by identifying genetic elements such as those encoding antibiotic resistance and significant antigens under selection pressures.

RECOMMENDED READING

Baltrus, D. A. (2016). Divorcing strain classification from species names. *Trends in Microbiology, 24*(6), 431–439. doi:10.1016/j.tim.2016.02.004.

Barrow, G. I., & Feltham, R. K. A. (Eds.). (1993). *Cowan and Steel's Manual for the Identification of Medical Bacteria* (3rd ed.). Cambridge: Cambridge University Press.

Beiko, R. G. (2015). Microbial malaise: How can we classify the microbiome? *Trends in Microbiology, 23*(11), 671–679. doi:10.1016/j.tim.2015.08.009.

Bentley, S. D., & Parkhill, J. (2015). Genomic perspectives on the evolution and spread of bacterial pathogens. *Proceedings of the Royal Society of Biological Sciences, 282*(1821), doi:10.1098/rspb.2015.0488.

Carrico, J. A., Sabat, A. J., & Friedrich, A. W. (2013). Bioinformatics in bacterial molecular epidemiology and public health: databases, tools and the next-generation sequencing revolution. *Euro Surveillance, 18*(4), 32–40.

Jorgensen, J. H., Pfaller, M. A., & Carroll, K. C. (Eds.). (2015). *Manual of Clinical Microbiology* (11th ed.). Washington, DC: ASM Press.

Goodfellow, M., Sutcliffe, I., & Chun, J. (Eds.). (2014). *New Approaches to Prokaryotic Systematics.* San Diego: Elsevier Academic Press Inc.

Gupta, R. S. (2016). Impact of genomics on the understanding of microbial evolution and classification: the importance of Darwin's views on classification. *FEMS Microbiology Reviews, 40*(4), 520–553. doi:10.1093/femsre/fuw011.

Logan, N. A. (2009). *Bacterial systematics.* London: Wiley.

Patel, R. (2015). MALDI-TOF MS for the Diagnosis of Infectious Diseases. *Clinical Chemistry, 61*(1), 100–111. doi:10.1373/clinchem.2014.221770.

Polz, M. F., Alm, E. J., & Hanage, W. P. (2013). Horizontal gene transfer and the evolution of bacterial and archaeal population structure. *Trends in Genetics, 29*(3), 170–175. doi:10.1016/j.tig.2012.12.006.

Sentausa, E., & Fournier, P. E. (2013). Advantages and limitations of genomics in prokaryotic taxonomy. *Clinical Microbiology and Infection, 19*(9), 790–795. doi:10.1111/1469-0691.12181.

Spratt, B. G., Feil, E. J., & Smith, N. H. (2002). Population genetics of bacterial pathogens. In M. Sussman (Ed.), *Molecular medical microbiology* (pp. 445–484). San Diego: Academic Press.

Tenover, F. C., Arbeit, R. D., Goering, R. V., Mickelsen, P. A., Murray, B. E., Persing, D. H., & Swaminathan, B. (1995). Interpreting chromosomal DNA restriction patterns produced by pulsed-field gel electrophoresis: criteria for strain typing. *Journal of Clinical Microbiology, 33*(9), 2233–2239.

Van Regenmortel, M. H., V, Fauquet, C. M., & Bishop, D. H. L. (Eds.). (2000). *Virus taxonomy. Classification and nomenclature of viruses.* San Diego: Academic Press.

Woese, C. R. (2000). Interpreting the universal phylogenetic tree. *Proceedings of the National Academy of Sciences of the USA, 97*(15), 8392–8396.

Websites

Genotyping database at Oxford University. Available at http://www.mlst.net/

National Center for Biotechnology information for rRNA sequence analysis. Available at http://www.ncbi.nlm.nih.gov/Genbank/

Universal virus database of the International Committee on Taxonomy of Viruses. Available at http://www.ictvdb.org/

4 Bacterial growth, physiology and death

MICHAEL R. BARER

KEY POINTS

- Bacterial growth and multiplication are of practical value in the detection and identification of pathogens, and are generally necessary components of infection.
- Bacteria divide asexually through a process of *binary fission*, passing through *lag*, *exponential* and *stationary* phases of *planktonic* growth in broth cultures. Bacterial growth can also be recognised in *sessile* form as *colonies* or *biofilms*. A given bacterial strain may have profoundly different physiological properties in each of these growth states.
- Recovery of pure bacterial cultures was greatly enhanced by the development of solidified agar media. Different medium designs enable *selection, enrichment, identification or defined* growth conditions.
- Different bacteria have evolved to grow and survive in widely differing habitats and these define their potential reservoirs and sources of infection. The growth atmospheres required by different bacteria are an important defining characteristic, and *obligate*

aerobes, obligate anaerobes, microaerophilic and *facultative* organisms are recognised.
- Bacterial viability is generally recognised and quantified by detecting growth of single cells into colonies in colony-forming unit (cfu) counts. Discrepancies between cfu counts and the number of cells seen by microscopy have led to recognition that many cells in natural samples do not form colonies.
- Bacteria may die through senescence in stationary cultures, through genetically programmed or prophage-induced cell death, or as result of external noxious influences such as antibiotics or the deliberate processes of *sterilisation* and *disinfection*.
- Sterilisation involves the destruction of all propagating biological entities, whereas disinfection involves a reduction in microbial load to an acceptable level. Both processes can be achieved by application of *moist and dry heat, ionising radiation, filtration, gaseous chemical agents* and *liquid chemical agents*.

Most of what we know about bacteria derives from their growth. Their ability to propagate may be seen as a supreme achievement that enables them to attain enormous populations at rates that are breathtaking from a human perspective. These properties underpin their capacity for change by mutation and the rapidity with which some infections develop.

Bacterial growth involves both an increase in the size of organisms and an increase in their number. Whatever the balance between these two processes, the net effect is an increase in the total mass (biomass) of the culture. Medical microbiologists have traditionally concentrated on the number of individuals in growth studies. Whether this emphasis on cell number is appropriate remains uncertain; nonetheless, it will be adopted here, as the number of individual bacteria involved is important in the course and outcome of infections and in the measurement of the effects of antibiotics.

Students of medicine may be surprised and even dismayed to hear that organisms as small as bacteria have a physiology. However, the complement of enzymes and the biochemical and biophysical processes occurring in a bacterial cell at any one time represent the product of genetic and biochemical control mechanisms that are every bit as sophisticated and tightly regulated as those in eukaryotic cells. Moreover, the recognition and definition of the mechanisms by which bacteria sense and adapt to nutritional and noxious stimuli in their environments have provided insights that are likely to translate into medically significant advances in the foreseeable future.

In some sense, asexual organisms such as bacteria appear to be immortal, but bacterial death or loss of viability occurs in many natural settings. This has practical consequences, as only viable bacteria can initiate infections and most microscopic, molecular and immunological detection methods do not differentiate between live and dead organisms. Of course, we often need to assess the lethal effects of antibiotics and processes aimed at sterilisation, disinfection and antisepsis. The practical approach to assessing the effects of antibiotics is introduced in Ch. 5, but the principles of sterilisation and disinfection are introduced here.

Although this chapter discusses growth and physiology only from a bacteriological perspective, some of the principles are also applicable to fungi, particularly yeasts. The central difference between their growths is that cell division is generally achieved in bacteria by binary fission to produce identical offspring that cannot be distinguished as parents and progeny, whereas fungi divide by budding in the case of yeast growth and hyphal septation in the mould form. In contrast, the principles of sterilisation and disinfection refer to all infective agents. Their application is considered further in Ch. 67.

BACTERIAL GROWTH

When placed in a suitable nutritious environment and maintained under appropriate physical and chemical conditions, a bacterial cell begins to grow; when it has manufactured approximately twice the amount of component materials that it started with, it divides. The range of specific components that define 'suitable' and 'appropriate' for all known bacteria (and *Archaea*) is so broad that it actually defines the global biosphere (those environments that can sustain life), and includes temperatures and pressures present at the opening of hydrothermal vents on the ocean floor to the outer reaches of the atmosphere. Although these conditions do not regularly occur in humans, they serve to illustrate that no part of the body or medical device with which it may come in contact is too difficult for bacteria to colonise and that bacteria may lurk in surprising environmental niches. Conversely, the conditions required for some organisms to grow are so precise that, so far, we have not been able to reproduce them in artificial laboratory media. This applies to some well-known organisms such as the agents of leprosy and syphilis, but also to many other potential pathogens about which we are beginning to learn through molecular methods that do not depend on growth. In fact, it is estimated that we have not yet isolated >1% of all the bacterial species that exist, and it is almost certain that there are many medically important organisms among the 'as yet uncultivated' microorganisms.

As the central technique in bacteriology, growth in the laboratory has been used to serve many different purposes. From the clinical perspective, growth is used for detection and identification, and for the assessment of antibiotic effects, whereas scientific and industrial objectives are often served by growth in bulk to obtain sufficient biomass for detailed biochemical analysis and to produce the desirable products of the brewing and biotechnology industries.

Types of growth

In the laboratory, bacterial growth can be seen in three main forms:

1. By the development of colonies, the macroscopic product of 20–30 cell divisions of a single cell.
2. By the transformation of a clear broth medium to a turbid suspension of 10^7–10^9 cells per mL.
3. In biofilm formation, in which growth is spread thinly (300–400 μm thick) over an inert surface and nutrition obtained from a bathing fluid.

In natural systems, only biofilms, such as those that develop on the surfaces of intravascular cannulae, appear to function in a manner comparable to biofilms produced in the laboratory, whereas colonies, the other form of sessile growth, rarely reach macroscopic dimensions. Turbid liquid systems caused by planktonic growth of a single organism are also a rarity in nature. Single organism infections affecting normally sterile sites in the body are one exception to this, whereas most natural microbial communities are complex assemblies of microorganisms competing, and in many cases cooperating, to exploit the local resources. However, in spite of these unrepresentative features, pure growth of single organisms in monocultures to produce macroscopic colonies or high cell densities in broth offer great practical advantages and remain central techniques.

While much has been learned about the nature of bacteria by studying them in lab cultures, it is clear that they change their properties in different patterns of growth and nongrowth and in response to their environment. Thus when we try to treat or immunise by targeting properties revealed in standard lab cultures, we often fail because the organism is not expressing those properties. This is particularly the case for bacteria in biofilms and in nonreplicating states.

Growth phases in broth culture

Bacterial growth in broth has been studied in detail and has provided a framework within which the growth state or growth phase of any given pure culture of a single organism can be placed; these phases are summarised in the idealised growth curve shown in Fig. 4.1. When growth is initiated by inoculation into appropriate broth conditions, the number of cells present appears to remain constant for the lag phase, during which cells are thought to be

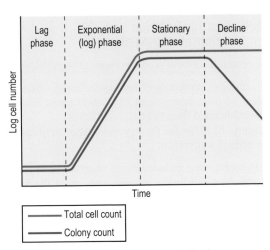

Fig. 4.1 Phases of growth in a broth culture.

preparing for growth. Increase in cell number then becomes detectable, and its rate accelerates rapidly until it is established at the maximum achievable rate for the available conditions. This is known as the *exponential phase* because the number of cells is increasing exponentially with time. To accommodate the astronomic changes in number, the growth curve is normally displayed on a logarithmic scale, which shows a linear increase in log cell number with time (hence the older term, *log phase*). This log–linear relationship is sufficiently constant for a given bacterial strain under one set of conditions that it can be defined mathematically and is often quoted as the *doubling time* for that organism. Doubling times have been measured at anything between 13 minutes for *Vibrio cholerae* and 24 hours for *Mycobacterium tuberculosis*. On this basis, it is not surprising that cholera is a disease that can kill within 12 hours, whereas tuberculosis takes months to develop. A further consequence is that, when specimens are submitted to diagnostic laboratories for the detection of these organisms by culture, a result is usually available for *V. cholerae* the next day, whereas several weeks are required for conventional culture of *M. tuberculosis*.

It is often difficult to grasp fully the scale of exponential microbial growth; the message may be strengthened by considering that the progeny of a lecture theatre containing 150 students would exceed the global population of humanity (7×10^9) in under 9 hours if they were able to breed like *Escherichia coli*!

Exponential growth cannot be sustained indefinitely in a closed (batch) system with limited available nutrients. Eventually growth slows down, and the total bacterial cell number reaches a maximum and stabilises. This is known as the *stationary* or *postexponential phase*. At

this stage it becomes important to know what method has been used to determine the growth curve. If a direct method that assesses the total number of cells present is used then the count remains constant. Such methods include counting cells in a volumetric chamber observed by microscopy, electronic particle counters and measurement of turbidity. If, however, the growth potential of the individual cells present in the culture is assessed by taking regular samples, making 10-fold dilutions of these and inoculating them on to agar, the number of colony-forming units (cfus) per unit volume can be determined at each sample time. Although such cfu counts closely parallel the results obtained by direct counting methods in the exponential and early stationary phases, a divergence begins to emerge towards the end of the latter; the total cell number remains constant, whereas the colony count declines. This marks the beginning of the final, decline phase in the sequence of growth states that can be observed in broth. The discrepancy between the total and cfu counts is conventionally held to represent the death of cells because of nutrient exhaustion and accumulation of detrimental metabolic end-products. However, there is some doubt concerning this interpretation (see later in the chapter).

As noted earlier, there has been increased interest in the properties of bacteria in non-growing states. While there are many different systems for studying nonreplicating bacteria and their separate relevance to infection is argued, one phenomenon is of particular interest as it illustrates their capacity for adaptation based on mutation. The growth advantage in stationary phase (GASP) phenomenon is now well established and illustrates that while total cell numbers in a population may remain constant or decline, multiple genetic variants arise, some of which come to dominate the population. The genes and polymorphisms that lead to the growth advantage have been informative in improving our understanding of survival and competition under nutrient-limited conditions.

The study of bacterial growth in broth provides a valuable point of reference to which practical, experimental and routine diagnostic procedures are often related. For example, the length of the lag phase and rates of exponential growth in different circumstances are used to make predictions and contribute to safety standards for storage in the food industry. An important feature to emerge is that cultures inoculated with cells prepared at different stages in the growth curve yield different results. The exponential phase is the most reproducible and readily identified and is therefore used most frequently. It can be extended in an open system known as *continuous culture* using a chemostat in which cells of a growing culture are harvested continuously and nutrients replenished continuously. Chemostat studies have provided very detailed information on the chemistry of microbial growth and the way in which different organisms convert specific substrates into biomass. The extraordinary efficiency of this process has made natural and genetically manipulated microbes a powerful resource for the biotechnology industry.

In contrast to growth in broth, far less is known about the state of the bacteria in a mature macroscopic colony on an agar plate. Such a colony presents a wide range of environments, from an abundance of oxygen and nutrients at the edge to almost no oxygen or nutrients available to cells in the centre. It is likely that all phases of growth are represented in colonies, depending on the location of a particular cell and the age of the culture. Although in practice, colonies can be used reliably to inoculate routine tests of antimicrobial susceptibility in clinical laboratories, they cannot be considered a defined starting point for experimental work because they comprise such a heterogeneous population of cells. In fact, colonies are complex and dynamic communities in which cells at different locations can show startlingly different phenotypes. In spite of its complexity, the capacity for and quality of colonial growth of specific organisms on specialised media is central to the laboratory description of medically important bacteria.

MEDIA FOR BACTERIAL GROWTH

The media used in a medical diagnostic bacteriology laboratory have their origins, for the most part, back in the 'golden age of bacteriology' in the late 19th and early 20th centuries. A vast amount of experience and knowledge has accrued from their use and, apart from better standardisation and quality control in their production, little has changed in their basic design. The objectives of early media design were to grow pathogenic bacteria, separate them from other organisms present in samples and, ultimately, differentiate their phenotypic properties so that they could be identified. A critical development was the introduction of solidifying agents, most particularly the largely indigestible polysaccharide extract of seaweed known as agar. Alternative solidifying agents include gelatine and egg albumen. Before the development of solid media, pure cultures could be achieved only by dilution of inocula so that only one growing cell or clump of cells was present at the initiation of growth, a very laborious and unreliable procedure. In contrast, solid media in Petri dishes provided a growth substrate on to which mixed cultures could be inoculated and, provided the population density could be made low enough to allow development of well-separated colonies, the different organisms present could be differentiated and subsequently separated into pure cultures.

Media used for isolation and identification of pathogens

The central features of media in medical bacteriology are:

1. a source of protein or protein hydrolysate, often derived from casein or an infusion of brain, heart or liver obtained from the nearest butcher
2. control of pH in the final product (after sterilisation)
3. a defined salt content

Early media often included blood or serum in an attempt to reproduce nutritional features present in the human body. Growth of some pathogens was found to be dependent on such supplements, and it was recognised that these relatively fastidious or nutritionally exacting organisms were dependent on growth factors. The identity of many of the growth factors is now known (e.g., haemin and several coenzymes), but blood often remains their most convenient source.

Selective and indicator media

Tremendous ingenuity has gone into designing growth media that provide information relevant to patient management as early as possible. There are two main approaches, both of which depend on adding supplements to the basal medium. Selective media contain substances such as bile salts or antibiotics that inhibit the growth of some organisms but have little or no effect on the organisms for whose isolation they were designed. They are essential for samples containing a normal microbiota such as faeces. The inclusion of components or specific reagents that show whether the bacteria possess a particular biochemical property characterises an indicator medium. Such media are critical to the rapid presumptive identification of isolates. Combinations of selective and indicator supplements in agar media have led to formulations with some remarkably elegant differential properties that effectively colour code the colonies according to their biochemical properties and restrict growth to a desired range of organisms. Broth indicator media tend to be much simpler, as they generally require a pure inoculum of a single organism and reveal only one property per formulation. Broth media with selective properties are usually referred to as *enrichment media* as they change the balance of organisms inoculated in favour of the desired range of organisms, thereby enriching them.

MEDIA FOR LABORATORY STUDIES

Most of the objectives of a clinical diagnostic laboratory can be fulfilled with the range of media outlined earlier in the chapter. However, the composition of these media is not defined, and this poses problems for some investigations, including the detailed analysis of antibiotic action. Wherever possible, such investigations are based on a defined or synthetic medium where every chemical component is carefully regulated. In genetic experiments, use is often made of a minimal medium in which every component is required for the growth of the organism under investigation, so that if one component is removed growth cannot occur. Minimal media also prevent the growth of mutants that have additional nutritional requirements to those of the parent strain. For some organisms, particularly those that can grow outside the human body, minimal media may comprise as little as an ammonium salt to provide nitrogen, a carbon source, which in some cases can be as simple as methane or carbon monoxide, trace amounts of iron and other essential elements, and pH adjustment to within an appropriate range. Defined and minimal media generally have to be developed for small groups of closely related organisms and should not be used for other organisms.

Relatively well-defined media are preferred, even for routine antibiotic tests, because quantitative aspects of bacterial biochemistry, growth and susceptibility to noxious stimuli can be influenced substantially by minor changes in medium composition. The use of fully defined media has underpinned almost all of what we know about bacterial physiology. Rather curiously, however, it is well recognised that defined media are often suboptimal for the recovery of bacteria from environments in which they have been stressed. This may reflect the support provided to injured bacteria by complex media. Defined media can really be optimised only for bacteria in a single physiological state, whereas complex media have greater potential to cope with the diversity of states present in natural samples.

BACTERIAL PHYSIOLOGY

The complement of processes that enable an organism to occupy and thrive in a particular environment places certain requirements on its physiology. Traditional descriptions of bacterial groups emphasise features that place a microbe in particular ecological niches. Thus we have acidophiles for organisms such as *Lactobacillus* spp. that grow at lower pH levels than most other organisms, and halophiles for organisms that grow at high salt concentrations. The environments that can be colonised by a pathogen are, of course, critical in determining its reservoirs and potential modes of transmission. More recently it has been recognised that individual bacteria are not restricted to a single physiological state. Rather, they respond to environmental stimuli and undergo adaptive responses that confer improved capacity for survival in adverse conditions. All of these properties sustain the viability of the organism.

However, it has become apparent that our ability to measure viability by conventional means may be inadequate.

The specific means by which a particular organism obtains energy and raw materials to sustain its growth (its nutritional type) and the physical conditions it requires reflect its fundamental physiological characteristics. Placing an organism into the groups defined by these characteristics is an important step in its conventional classification.

Nutritional types

Traditionally, all living organisms have been divided into two nutritional groups: heterotrophs and autotrophs. The former depend on the latter to produce organic molecules by fixing carbon dioxide, predominantly by photosynthesis. Bacterial metabolism is now recognised to be so diverse that it cannot be encompassed by these two terms. Three basic features are used in the present terminology: the *energy source,* the *hydrogen donors* and the *carbon source.*

Energy for adenosine triphosphate (ATP) synthesis may be obtained from light in a *phototrophic* organism and from chemical oxidations in the case of a *chemotrophic* organism. The hydrogen donor type characterises an organism as an *organotroph* if it requires organic sources of hydrogen and as a *lithotroph* if it can use inorganic sources (e.g., ammonia or hydrogen sulphide). Finally, the terms *autotroph* and *heterotroph* are reserved for the carbon source; the former can fix carbon dioxide directly, whereas the latter require an organic source. In general, only the energy and hydrogen donor designations are referred to routinely by combining the two terms. Hence we refer to *chemoorganotrophs* (the vast majority of currently recognised medically important organisms) and *chemolithotrophs* (e.g., some *Pseudomonas* spp.). Surprisingly, there are even some *photolithotrophs* with medical significance; the cyanobacteria are now known to produce many toxins that can affect humans.

Physical conditions required for growth

All living organisms use oxidation to transfer energy to compounds that participate in their internal biochemical and biophysical processes. Oxidation of a molecule is equivalent to the removal of hydrogen and requires another molecule to receive electrons in the process. In aerobic respiration the final electron recipient in the oxidation process is molecular oxygen (i.e., O_2), whereas under anaerobic conditions (in the absence of oxygen) most medically important organisms use an organic molecule as the final electron recipient, and the oxidative process is referred to as *fermentation*. There are also some forms of anaerobic respiration that use inorganic electron acceptors such as nitrates. Respiration in this context is generally used to denote involvement of a membrane-associated electron transport chain in the oxidation. In the early period of development of life on Earth, there was no oxygen in the atmosphere; thus, at this time, all bacteria were *anaerobes*. Subsequently, following the development of photoautotrophic organisms, atmospheric oxygen became abundant, and organisms capable of using oxygen evolved.

Although aerobic metabolism is a more efficient means of obtaining energy than anaerobiosis, it is not without its cost. Some oxidation–reduction (redox) reactions occurring in the presence of oxygen commonly result in the formation of the reactive superoxide (O_2^-) and hydroxyl (OH^-) radicals as well as hydrogen peroxide (H_2O_2), all of which are highly toxic. To cope with this, aerobic organisms or *aerobes* have developed two enzymes that detoxify these molecules. *Superoxide dismutase* converts superoxide radicals to hydrogen peroxide ($2\ O_2^- + 2H^+ \rightarrow H_2O_2 + O_2$), whereas *catalase* converts hydrogen peroxide to water and oxygen in the reaction $2\ H_2O_2 \rightarrow H_2O + O_2$. Possession or lack of these enzymes has the important consequence of defining the atmosphere necessary for growth and survival of different organisms. Moreover, when produced in large amounts, the enzymes also provide protection for pathogenic organisms against the reactive oxygen intermediates deliberately produced as a defence mechanism by phagocytic cells.

Growth atmosphere

These oxygen-related features underpin the major practical grouping of bacteria according to their atmospheric requirements (Table 4.1). Thus strict or obligate aerobes require oxygen, usually at ambient levels (≈20%), and strict or obligate anaerobes require the complete absence of oxygen. Many organisms exhibit intermediate properties: facultative anaerobes generally grow better in oxygen but are still able to grow well in its absence; microaerophilic organisms require a reduced oxygen level (≈5%); aerotolerant anaerobes have a fermentative pattern of metabolism but can tolerate the presence of oxygen because they possess superoxide dismutase. Many medically important organisms are facultative anaerobes. There is a mixture of aerobic and anaerobic microenvironments in the human body, and the capacity to replicate in both is clearly advantageous. For obvious reasons, strict anaerobes are particularly associated with infection of tissues where the blood supply has been interrupted.

Among the various physical requirements for the growth of different bacterial groups, atmosphere assumes particular importance because, in practice, agar cultures from most clinical specimens are set up aerobically and anaerobically. Thus when growth is first inspected after overnight incubation, the isolates can readily be differentiated into strict aerobes, anaerobes and facultative anaerobes according to the conditions under which they have grown. Various atmospheric conditions can also be obtained in broth media. If the medium is unstirred, strict aerobes tend to grow on the surface, microaerophiles just under the surface and anaerobes in the body of the medium away from the surface. Growth of anaerobes is often improved by the addition of a reducing agent such as cysteine or thioglycollate to mop up any free oxygen.

Growth temperature

The other significant physical condition for bacterial growth from the medical perspective is temperature (see Table 4.1). Pathogens that actually replicate on or in the human body must be able to grow within the temperature range of 20–40°C and are generally referred to as *mesophiles*. Organisms that can grow outside this range are either *psychrophiles* (cold loving) or *thermophiles* (heat loving). The former may be capable of growth in food or

---

Table 4.1   Key descriptive terms used to categorise bacteria according to their growth requirements

Descriptive term	Property	Example
Growth atmosphere		
Strict (obligate) aerobe	Requires atmospheric oxygen for growth	*Pseudomonas aeruginosa*
Strict (obligate) anaerobe	Will not tolerate oxygen	*Bacteroides fragilis*
Facultative anaerobe	Grows best aerobically, but can grow anaerobically	*Staphylococcus* spp., *E. coli*, etc.
Aerotolerant anaerobe	Anaerobic, but tolerates exposure to oxygen	*Clostridium perfringens*
Microaerophilic organism	Requires or prefers reduced oxygen levels	*Campylobacter* spp., *Helicobacter* spp.
Capnophilic organism	Requires or prefers increased carbon dioxide levels	*Neisseria* spp.
Growth temperature		
Psychrophile	Grows best at low temperature (e.g., <10°C)	*Flavobacterium* spp.
Thermophile	Grows best at high temperature (e.g., >60°C)	*Bacillus stearothermophilus*[a]
Mesophile	Grows best between 20–40°C	Most bacterial pathogens

[a]Not a pathogen; its spores are very heat resistant and are used for testing the efficiency of heat sterilisation.

pharmaceuticals stored at normal refrigeration temperatures (0–8°C), whereas the latter can be a source of proteins with remarkable thermotolerant properties, such as Taq polymerase, the key enzyme used in the polymerase chain reaction. Organisms such as the leprosy bacillus that prefer lower growth temperatures are often associated with skin and superficial infections, whereas organisms that grow in the colon (often a few degrees warmer than normal body temperature) can grow well up to 44°C.

Extremophiles

Some bacteria require ostensibly bizarre physical conditions for growth. For example, *barophiles* isolated from the ocean floor may require enormous pressures before they can replicate. Such organisms are often referred to as *extremophiles*. The properties of these organisms serve to remind us that microbes have the potential to occupy any environmental niche where energy and nutrition are available. It should be noted that most extremophiles actually turn out to belong to the *Archaea* (see Ch. 2).

Bacterial metabolism

Although some bacteria are able to obtain their resources for growth in ways that seem alien to us, the core of their metabolism is essentially very similar to that of mammalian cells. The basic details of glycolysis, the tricarboxylic acid cycle, oxidative phosphorylation, ATP biosynthesis and amino acid metabolism are constant, although some notable minor differences occur. Variations in the pathways that feed into and flow from these core processes are readily detected by what are loosely termed *biochemical tests* in medical laboratories. These detect traits such as the ability to use individual carbohydrate sources to produce acid and the possession of specific enzymes.

The common nature of central catabolic and anabolic pathways in bacteria and multicellular organisms reflects the economy of biology and evolution. Processes that work well cannot be outcompeted and tend to be preserved in the genetic stock. Thus many of the specific enzymes involved in bacterial metabolism show remarkable levels of conservation in their amino acid sequences across very substantial distances in evolutionary terms. DNA sequencing has enabled the identification of molecular families of proteins with a common evolutionary origin. In addition to the metabolic enzymes, it has been recognised that many transport proteins responsible for importing and exporting specific substrates into and out of the bacterial cytoplasm are closely related in their structure and mode of function to those present in mammalian cells. Of course, because bacteria generally have only one cell compartment in which to operate, the location of these proteins is often

different; for example, as they have no mitochondria, the cytoplasmic membrane contains the components of the electron transport chain, and the proton gradient across the inner mitochondrial membrane is generated across the cytoplasmic membrane instead. This feature actually means that bacteria can perform some energy-requiring processes at the cell surface, notably flagellar rotation (motility), by directly exploiting the proton gradient rather than consuming ATP.

Aside from its role in identification and intrinsic biological interest, bacterial metabolism has real consequences for humans. In direct terms, the resident microbiota have impact on human health and disease. For example, the bacteria in dental plaque produce acid when presented with certain carbohydrate sources, and this acid is responsible for tooth decay; on the positive side, bacteria in the intestines deconjugate bile salts and thereby contribute to the enterohepatic circulation. It seems likely that the importance of such bioconversions will be recognised increasingly in the future. In particular, the role of bacteria in recovering nitrogen excreted into the colon in marginal human nutritional states and metabolic activity leading to the formation of carcinogens or other biologically active molecules are both areas where there is much room for further work. The totality of microbes (and their genomes) within the human body is referred to as the *microbiome* and the role of this assemblage in human health and disease will be discussed further in Ch. 11.

Human beings are also indirectly affected by microbial metabolism. At one level, the chemistry of our environment has been shaped extensively by microbes; the original development of oxygen in our atmosphere, the availability of elemental sulphur and the flow of nitrogen are all critically dependent on microbial metabolism. Exploitation of microbial metabolism in industry has, of course, given us ethanol, and many of the other alcohols and acids that result from fermentation have commercial value. Finally, bacteria have been used to combat the deleterious effects of environmental pollution in the process referred to as *bioremediation*.

Adaptive responses in bacteria

The extent to which bacteria respond to environmental stimuli was originally recognised by monitoring gross phenotypic, biochemical and behavioural changes. Much of the genetic basis for how bacteria change their phenotypes was established in the 1960s and 1970s following on from the paradigm established for β-galactosidase regulation in *E. coli* by Jacob and Monod. This work began to open up our understanding of how gene expression is regulated. It clearly makes no sense that all genes should be expressed continuously. Some appear to be, and their expression is termed *constitutive,* while others are only expressed in response to certain stimuli and this is termed *inducible* (see Ch. 6).

The scale and rapidity (major changes can be seen in seconds) of bacterial responses became apparent through the 1980s and 1990s as the use of global analytical approaches that attempt to characterise the instantaneous expression of every gene the organism carries became established. At the translational level, the use of two-dimensional gel electrophoresis has now been replaced by sophisticated forms of mass spectrometry and this now underpins the so-called *proteomic* approach. This technique reveals and separates most of the several hundred proteins that are being synthesised by a pure culture at a particular time. The catalogue of different proteins detected represents those proteins that the organism requires to function in the circumstances from which the sample was drawn. Assays of this type have shown that different sets of proteins are made in the exponential and stationary phases of the growth cycle and, indeed, in response to almost any environmental change. This finding underpins the recognition of just how different the phenotype of a single organism can be in different physiological states and reinforces the need to define the inoculum used in laboratory experiments. The development of DNA arrays and high throughput nucleotide sequencing (RNAseq) have enabled global analysis of responses at the transcriptional level by detecting messenger RNA (mRNA) molecules relating to every gene in the organism in a single analysis. The complement of RNA species present in an organism at a given time is referred to as the *transcriptome*.

The comprehensive analyses achieved by transcriptome and proteome analyses followed on from the recognition that global genome analyses and comparisons or genomics (see Ch. 6) have the potential to explain many—some would say most—biological and medical phenomena. The complexities linking genotype to phenotype remain overwhelming in most instances; nonetheless, we have now entered an era where global analyses of mRNA, proteome and metabolic function (the metabolome) are being addressed enthusiastically in an integrative computational approach pooling data from different analyses in what has been termed the *systems biology* approach.

The effects of specific sublethal but noxious stimuli on gene expression are the subject of intense current study. Each different stimulus leads to an adaptive stress response, which is to some extent specific to the stimulus applied. Heat shock (the effects of raising temperature to 45°C and above for a few minutes) has been studied most extensively. The newly synthesised proteins elicited in this response are referred to as *heat shock proteins*. When the amino acid sequences of the principal heat shock proteins were determined, they were found to belong to a molecular family now recognised in all prokaryotic and eukaryotic cells. Apart from their role in improving the ability of bacteria to survive heat shock, these proteins, by virtue of their similarity to analogous host cell antigens, seem to be involved in initiating autoimmune damage and immune dysfunction. A very important feature of the stress response in bacteria is that many of the stimuli used are prominent aspects of the stresses applied by the human immune system to an invading pathogen. Thus acid stress is provided by the stomach and the hostile environment of phagolysosomes includes both oxidative and pH stress.

The information built up from studying stress responses has made it possible to identify sets of proteins that are made in response to several different stresses and those that appear exclusive to one stress. Together with other approaches, this has allowed recognition of global regulatory systems or networks within bacteria that are responsible for differential gene expression under different circumstances. The hierarchy of specific control mechanisms involved has spawned two important new terms, *stimulon* and *regulon*. A stimulon denotes all the genes whose expression is increased or decreased by a specific external stimulus, whereas a regulon refers to all the genes under the influence of a specific regulatory protein. A regulon may affect several operons (see Ch. 6), and there may be many regulons in one stimulon.

Regulatory networks have been identified in almost every area of bacterial physiology. Thus, in addition to the stimuli cited above, osmotic stress, cold shock, nutrient limitation (separate responses for carbon, nitrogen and phosphate), anaerobic and many other stimulons are recognised. These control systems are responsible for making sure the organism synthesises only those proteins appropriate to its current circumstances. Particularly important medical examples of this are the regulation of proteins concerned with an organism's progress in an infection (virulence factors) and those made in response to sublethal levels of antibiotics. Equally important from the scientific perspective is the recognition that chemicals secreted by an organism can themselves act as regulatory stimuli to individuals of the same species in a way analogous to the pheromones released by insects.

Although it is still important to recognise that different organisms are particularly adapted to special environmental niches with descriptive terms such as *mesophile, acidophile* and *halophile*, the discovery of adaptive responses in bacteria has pushed us into an uncertain period where much of what has been established about the tolerance of microorganisms to noxious stresses will have to be reexamined. Furthermore, as the extent to which bacteria modulate their phenotype according to their circumstances is now clear, the need for caution in concluding that any property detected in the laboratory is significant in a natural infection is unavoidably obvious.

Bacterial defence against antibiotics and other noxious chemicals

The features outlined above all contribute to the well-being of bacteria. In the natural world, microorganisms encounter many chemicals that could cause their destruction, and in their 3.5 billion years on Earth, they have evolved numerous protective mechanisms. In clinical practice, these are recognised as biochemical mechanisms of antibiotic resistance, and four basic categories are recognised:

1. *Preventing access:* achieved by low cell envelope permeability or efflux pumps affecting the chemical concerned.
2. *Destruction:* achieved by enzymes that modify or degrade the chemical.
3. *Lack of target:* many chemicals that damage bacteria work through specific targets. The target may be absent or be altered by mutation (see Ch. 6).
4. *Bypass of target:* in some cases, an alternate or modified pathway can be used.

These mechanisms may be intrinsic to the organism concerned or they may be acquired through mutation or gene transfer (see Ch. 6). It should also be noted that expression of some resistance mechanisms outlined above may be inducible and may not be apparent with assays that do not take this into account.

Not all resistance to noxious molecules is mediated by the mechanisms listed above. In certain nonreplicating states and in biofilms, bacteria classified as sensitive to certain agents by standard tests become resistant, particularly to the lethal action of the agent concerned. This phenotypic resistance or tolerance appears to be a significant factor in the recalcitrance of certain chronic infections to antibiotic treatment, and the survivors against antibiotic exposures that might reasonably be expected to be effective from conventional susceptibility tests are termed *persisters*. It is important to appreciate that these survivors are no more antibiotic-resistant than their forebears.

Bacterial viability

A central feature of the general and adaptive physiology of bacteria is the capacity to preserve the viability of a particular organism. There is, however, a persistent problem—how do we define viability in practical terms? Traditionally, the operational definition of the capacity of a cell to form a colony on an appropriate agar medium (the colony or cfu count) has been almost universally accepted. It is also often expressed as the proportion of cells within a population that are capable of forming colonies. This has been used extensively in recognising the cidal (lethal) and static (growth inhibitory) activities of antibiotics. In the former case, cfu counts decline, and

in the latter they remain constant. However, it must be emphasised that viability is not a clearly measurable property. At the individual level it expresses the expectation that, in a suitable environment, a particular cell has the capacity to grow and undergo binary fission and that its progeny will have the same potential. The key assumption is that colony counts provide an accurate measure of viability.

The central problem can be stated as follows: it is self-evident that if a bacterial cell produces a colony it must have been viable, but to what extent is it true that a cell that fails to do this is nonviable or dead? Immediately, contradictions to this proposal can be identified. The bacterial pathogens, such as *Mycobacterium leprae* and *Treponema pallidum,* which cannot be induced to form colonies on available agar media, are clearly viable. Similarly, all the 'as yet uncultivated organisms' (possibly as many as 99% of all bacterial species) are clearly able to propagate themselves. They simply have not been sporting enough to do it on our laboratory media. A further exception is the phenomenon of bacterial recovery from injury (e.g., cold or osmotic shock) in which colony counts can be shown to rise in the absence of cell division.

It is possible that some organisms that are readily cultivable may be able to switch to a physiological state in which they cannot be induced to form colonies. A popular terminology for cells in this putative state is *viable but nonculturable* (VBNC).

Epidemiological and laboratory evidence provide some support for the existence of a VBNC state. In particular, the occurrence of several infectious diseases acquired from environmental sources, notably cholera, is at variance with our ability to recover the causal organisms from the implicated source. Environmental studies have demonstrated cells with immunological properties compatible with those of the cholera vibrio, while failing to recover the organism in culture, and laboratory studies have indicated that the organism can persist in a nonculturable form. There is also evidence that nonculturable forms may revert to their 'normal' culturable state.

A major attraction of the VBNC hypothesis is that it may resolve a number of important mysteries in medical microbiology. In general, these are situations in which we know the organism must be present but are unable to culture it. This is particularly so with diseases, such as tuberculosis, that have latent phases.

The most significant problem for the VBNC hypothesis is that it has not been defined in physiological, biochemical or genetic terms. On the face of it, one might expect transition to the VBNC state to result from an adaptive response such as those described in the previous section. Alternatively, transition might be the result of a programme of gene expression such as that observed in spore formation or starvation. From this standpoint the stationary and decline phases in the growth cycle outlined above (when spore formation is induced in sporulating bacteria) may represent the initiation of and transition to a nonculturable phase rather than loss of viability (the traditional view). In spite of their popularity, these ideas must presently be viewed as interesting speculations for which there is circumstantial but no conclusive evidence.

Measurement of viability has been of great practical value in medical microbiology. Colony counts performed to investigate the action of antibiotics and other disruptive influences such as heat, and those performed at different stages during experimental infections in animal models of human infections, have provided a wealth of valuable information. Moreover, there is no reason to doubt that this approach will continue to be extremely useful.

Nonetheless, it is necessary to maintain a clear view of the limitations of bacterial culture as a measure of the organisms present in a sample and of their viability. Studies often use the term *viability* when in fact growth on agar or in broth was measured, and confusion would be prevented if the terms *culturability* and *colony counts* were used instead.

We are now entering an era in which many diagnostic and investigational techniques may be replaced by molecular detection procedures. The fact that signals based on such techniques may come from culturable, dead and potentially VBNC cells should be recognised. Unravelling these three possibilities presents ample challenge for medical and nonmedical microbiologists alike.

Bacterial death

Notwithstanding the problems outlined in the previous section, the ability to recognise and quantify bacterial death is of great practical significance in the practice of medicine. At present, except in highly defined circumstances, the cfu count remains the cornerstone for such measurements. In natural systems where no actively noxious environmental conditions pertain, if bacterial growth ceases, as in the stationary phase described earlier, after a variable period of time depending on the conditions and the organism concerned, then cfu counts begin to decline. In some cases this may lead to complete loss of viability, whereas in others a stable but lower cfu count is established. For example, *E. coli* appears to survive indefinitely in buffered salt solutions, the constant lysis of dying cells apparently providing for a balancing level of cell replication. Even after adaptation to starvation or other conditions leading to stasis, the rate at which viability is lost seems to follow a well-defined pattern. Cells in stasis are clearly getting older and this provides a bacterial correlate of senescence. Although the study of bacterial cell senescence is relatively new, it is emerging that cumulative oxidative damage to cell proteins and other

key macromolecules is one critical determinant of survival. This observation fits very well with the observation that one can often recover higher cfu counts of stressed facultative organisms on media containing catalase or other reagents that provide protection against reactive oxygen intermediates or following incubation under microaerophilic conditions.

It is not widely appreciated that many (probably all) bacteria carry genes encoding for programmed cell death. While several mechanisms are involved, these are distinct from the process of apoptosis that occurs in eukaryotic cells. These systems were first identified as toxin–antitoxin pairs functioning to maintain particular genes in the bacterial cell. However, it now seems likely that their occurrence cannot be explained solely on this basis and that, over time, they become integrated into the regulatory networks of the cell, particularly in controlling growth rate under certain conditions. It should be noted that the activation of latent prophages (see Ch. 6) constitutes another endogenous mechanism by which bacteria can initiate their own demise.

In addition to killing bacteria with antibiotics, medical practice is frequently concerned with decontaminating locations and materials that have been in contact with infectious patients. Moreover, the safe practice of surgery, parenteral administration of therapy and the preparation of media and sampling materials for bacteriological studies all require the reduction or complete elimination of bacteria from key locations and devices. Although the methods applied to remove live bacteria may be checked with tests of biological efficacy, the relatively predictable rate of decline achieved with specific methods and target organisms enables safe practice. Because the cfu count is relatively convenient, it has been used in the establishment of most methodologies. However, removal or destruction of all infective agents is necessary to achieve sterility, and tests directed to all of these are required to some extent in establishing safe practice.

STERILISATION AND DISINFECTION

Key definitions

Sterilisation

- The inactivation of all self-propagating biological entities (e.g., bacteria, viruses, prions) associated with the materials or areas under consideration.

Disinfection

- The reduction of pathogenic organisms to a level at which they no longer constitute a risk.

Antisepsis

- Term used to describe disinfection applied to living tissue such as a wound.

Methods used in sterilisation and disinfection

In practice, all processes of sterilisation have a finite probability of failure. By convention, an article may be regarded as sterile if it can be demonstrated that there is a probability of less than one in a million of there being viable microorganisms on it. As will be seen later in the chapter, the level of microbial killing achieved by applying a particular method is dependent on the intensity with which the method is applied and its duration. Five main approaches are used.

Heat

The only method of sterilisation that is both reliable and widely applicable is heating under carefully controlled conditions at temperatures above 100°C to ensure that bacterial spores are killed. There is some concern that even this temperature is insufficient to destroy prions. Shorter applications of lower temperatures, such as in pasteurisation, can effectively remove specific infection hazards.

Ionising radiation

Both β (electrons) and γ-irradiation (photons) are employed industrially for the sterilisation of single-use disposable items such as needles and syringes, latex catheters and surgical gloves, and in the food industry to reduce spoilage and remove pathogens. Ultraviolet irradiation can be used to cut down the level of contamination but is generally too mild to achieve sterility.

Filtration

Filters are used to remove bacteria and all larger microorganisms from liquids that are liable to be spoiled by heating, for instance blood serum and antibiotic solutions in which contamination with filter-passing viruses is improbable or unimportant. Industrial-scale filtration is used widely to reduce bacterial load and remove cysts of protozoa that are not killed by chlorination in the production of drinking water.

Gaseous chemical agents

Ethylene oxide is used mainly by industry for the sterilisation of plastics and other thermolabile materials that cannot withstand heating. Formaldehyde in combination with subatmospheric steam is used more commonly in hospitals for reprocessing thermolabile equipment. Both processes carry toxic and other hazards for the user and the patient. More recently, hydrogen peroxide, ozone and nitrogen dioxide have been used.

Liquid chemical agents

Use of liquids such as glutaraldehyde is generally the least effective and most unreliable method. Such methods should be regarded as high-grade disinfection only, to be applied when no other sterilisation method is available, for example for heat-labile fibreoptic instruments such as flexible endoscopes. Various chemicals with antimicrobial properties are used as disinfectants. They are all liable to be inactivated by excessive dilution and contact with organic materials such as dirt or blood, or a variety of other materials. Nevertheless, they may provide a convenient method for environmental disinfection and other specific applications.

Incorporation of agents into solids for surface antisepsis

Both silver and copper have been used in this regard. Silver has been used on surfaces and in indwelling medical devices, copper in the former but not as yet in the latter.

Choice of method

The choice of method of sterilisation or disinfection depends on:

- the nature of the item to be treated
- the likely microbial contamination
- the risk of transmitting infection to patients or staff in contact with the item

Choice is based on an assessment of risk according to different categories of patient (e.g., immunocompromised), the equipment involved and its application. The selection of sterilisation, disinfection or simple cleaning processes for individual items of equipment and the environment should be agreed as part of the infection control policy of a hospital (see Ch. 67). The preferred option wherever possible, for both sterilisation and disinfection, is heat rather than chemicals. This relates not only to the antimicrobial efficacy but also to safety considerations, which are more difficult to control in some chemical processes. Wherever chemicals are to be used for disinfection and sterilisation, the safety of persons involved directly or indirectly in the procedure must be considered. It should be remembered that all sterilising and disinfecting agents have some action on human cells. No method should be assumed to be safe unless appropriate precautions are taken.

Measurement of microbial inactivation

Every method used must be validated to demonstrate the required degree of microbial kill. With heat sterilisation and irradiation, a biological test may not be required if the physical conditions are sufficiently well defined and controlled.

When microorganisms are subjected to a lethal process, the number of viable cells decreases exponentially in relationship to the extent of exposure. If the logarithm of the number of survivors is plotted against the lethal dose received (e.g., time of heating at a particular temperature), the resulting curve is described as the *survivor curve*. This is independent of the size of the original population and is approximately linear. The linear survivor curve is an idealised concept and, in practice, minor variations, such as an initial shoulder or final tail, occur (Fig. 4.2).

D *value*

The *D* value or decimal reduction value is the dose required to inactivate 90% of the initial population. From Fig. 4.2, it can be seen that the time (dose) required to reduce the population from 10^6 to 10^5 is the same as the time (dose) required to reduce the population from 10^5 to 10^4; that is, the *D* value remains constant over the full range of the survivor curve. Extending the treatment beyond the point at which there is one surviving cell does not give rise to fractions of a surviving cell but rather to a statement of the probability of finding one survivor. Thus, by extrapolation from the experimental data, it is possible to determine the lethal dose required to give a probability of $<10^{-6}$, which is required to meet the pharmacopoeial definition of 'sterile'. Note that in preparations intended for mass use, if the probability of a single live organism in a batch from which 10 million doses are to be administered is 10^{-6}, then it is likely that around 10 people will receive doses containing live organisms! Another consequence recognisable from Fig. 4.2 is that the greater the number of microbes in the material to be sterilised, the longer the required exposure time. Thus, where efficient decontamination is the target, thorough cleansing can reduce the microbial load by several orders of magnitude and dramatically reduce both the time required and the level of certainty that sterility or adequate disinfection has been achieved.

Resistance to sterilisation and disinfection

Many common factors affect the ability of microorganisms to withstand the lethal effects of sterilisation or disinfection processes. Factors specific to individual processes are considered in the description of those processes. In general, vegetative bacteria and viruses are more susceptible and bacterial spores the most resistant to sterilising and disinfecting agents. However, within different species and strains of species there may be wide variation in intrinsic resistance. For example, within the Enterobacteriaceae, *D* values at 60°C range from a few minutes *(E. coli)* to 1 hour (*Salmonella enterica* serotype Senftenberg). The typical *D* value for *Staphylococcus aureus* at 70°C is <1 minute, compared with 3 minutes for *Staph. epidermidis*. However, an unusual strain of *Staph. aureus* has been isolated with a *D* value of 14 minutes at 70°C. Such variations may be attributed to morphological or physiological changes such as alterations in cell proteins or specific targets in the cell envelope affecting permeability.

Inactivation data obtained for one microorganism should not be extrapolated to another; thus it should not be assumed that bactericidal disinfectants are also potent against viruses. The inactivation data for scrapie, bovine spongiform encephalopathy and Creutzfeldt–Jakob disease (CJD) suggest that prions are highly resistant agents, requiring six times the normal heat sterilisation cycle (134°C for 18 minutes). This has led to requirements for the mandatory use of disposable instruments that are in direct contact with brain or other nervous tissue (including the retina) or tonsils where the risk of exposure to the prion causing CJD is high.

Owing to the adaptive processes described above, the conditions under which the microorganisms were grown or maintained before exposure to the lethal process have a marked effect on their resistance. Organisms grown under nutrient-limiting conditions are typically more resistant than those grown under nutrient-rich conditions. Resistance usually increases through the late logarithmic

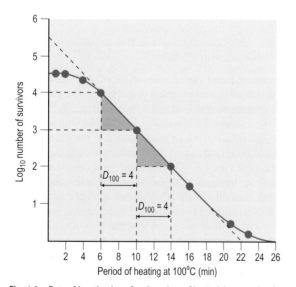

Fig. 4.2 Rate of inactivation of an inoculum of bacterial spores showing the decimal reduction time (*D* value) at 100°C and the nonlinear 'shoulder and tail' effects.

phase of growth of vegetative cells and declines erratically during the stationary phase. Finally, bacterial endospores, formed principally by *Bacillus* and *Clostridium* species, are relatively resistant to most processes. Similarly, fungal spores are more resistant than the vegetative mycelium, although they are not usually as resistant as bacterial spores. Bacterial spores were used to define the sterilisation processes in current use, and preparations of bacterial spores (biological indicators) are used to monitor the efficacy of ethylene oxide sterilisation, in which physical monitoring is inadequate. In general, disinfection processes have little or no activity against bacterial spores.

The microenvironment of the organism during exposure to the lethal process has a profound effect on its resistance. Thus microorganisms occluded in salt have greatly enhanced resistance to ethylene oxide; the presence of blood or other organic material will reduce the effectiveness of hypochlorite solution.

Sterilisation by moist heat

Moist heat is much more effective than dry heat because hydrated proteins can be denatured with less energy than dehydrated semicrystalline proteins. Further, where steam is used, its condensation delivers the latent heat of vaporisation to the surface concerned. It is therefore necessary that all parts of the load to be sterilised are in direct contact with the water molecules in steam. Sterilisation requires, in most cases, exposure to moist heat at 121°C for 15 minutes.

Moist heat sterilisation requires temperatures above that of boiling water. Such conditions are attained under controlled conditions by raising the pressure of steam in a pressure vessel (autoclave). At sea level, boiling water at atmospheric pressure (1 bar) produces steam at 98–100°C, whereas raising the pressure to 2.4 bar increases the temperature to 125°C, and at 3.0 bar to 134°C. Conversely, at subatmospheric pressures, including those at higher altitude, water boils at lower temperatures.

Steam is nontoxic and noncorrosive, but for effective sterilisation it must be saturated, which means that it holds all the water it can in the form of a transparent vapour. It must also be dry, which means that it does not contain water droplets. When dry saturated steam meets a cooler surface it condenses into a small volume of water and liberates the latent heat of vaporisation. The energy available from this latent heat is considerable; for example, 6 L of steam at a temperature of 134°C (and a corresponding pressure of 3 bar absolute) will condense into 10 mL of water and liberate 2162 J of heat energy. By comparison, <100 J of heat energy is released to an article by the sensible heat from air at 134°C.

Steam at a higher temperature than the corresponding pressure would allow is referred to as *super-heated steam*, and behaves in a similar manner to hot air. Conversely, steam that contains suspended droplets of water at the same temperature is referred to as *wet steam* and is less efficient. The presence of air in steam affects the sterilising efficiency by changing the pressure–temperature relationship.

As can be seen from the foregoing, sterilisation by moist heat requires delivery of steam at exactly the right temperature and pressure, and for the right time. This places considerable demands on the engineering and maintenance of autoclaves, and in critical situations, such as provision of sterile materials for clinical practice, their performance must be monitored continually and precisely. Physical measurements of temperature, pressure and time with thermometers and pressure gauges are recorded for every load, and periodic detailed tests are undertaken with temperature-sensitive probes (thermocouples) inserted into standard test packs. Biological indicators comprising dried spore suspensions of a reference heat-resistant bacterium, *Bacillus stearothermophilus,* are no longer considered appropriate for routine testing, although spore indicators are essential for low-temperature gaseous processes in which the physical measurements are not reliable.

Sterilisation by dry heat

Dry heat is believed to kill microorganisms by causing a destructive oxidation of essential cell constituents. Killing of the most resistant spores by dry heat requires a temperature of 160°C for 2 hours. This high temperature causes slight charring of paper, cotton and other organic materials.

Incineration is an efficient method for the sterilisation and disposal of contaminated materials at a high temperature. It has a particular application for pathological waste materials, surgical dressings, sharp needles and other clinical waste. Red heat is achieved by holding inoculating wires, loops and points of forceps in the flame of a Bunsen burner until they are red hot.

Hot air sterilisers are used to process materials that can withstand high temperatures for the length of time needed for sterilisation by dry heat, but that are likely to be affected by contact with steam. Examples include oils, powders, carbon steel microsurgical instruments and empty laboratory glassware. The overall cycle of heating up and cooling may take several hours.

Disinfection by chemicals

Chemicals used in the environment or on the skin (disinfectants or antiseptics) cannot be relied on to kill or inhibit all pathogenic microorganisms. The distinction between disinfectants and antiseptics is not clear-cut; an antiseptic can be regarded as a special kind of disinfectant that is sufficiently free from injurious effects to be applied to the surface of the body, though not suitable for systemic administration. Some would restrict the term *antiseptic* to preparations applied to open wounds or abraded tissue, and prefer the term *skin disinfection* for the removal of organisms from the hands and intact skin surfaces.

The efficacy of a particular method of chemical disinfection is heavily dependent on the concentration and stability of the agent; the number, type and accessibility of microorganisms; the temperature and pH; and the presence of organic (especially protein) or other interfering substances.

In general, the rate of inactivation of a susceptible microbial population in the presence of an antimicrobial chemical is dependent on the relative concentration of the two reactants, the microorganism and the chemical. The optimum concentration required to produce a standardised microbial effect in practice is described as the *in-use* concentration. Care must always be taken in preparing an accurate in-use dilution of concentrated product. Accidental or arbitrary overdilution may result in failure of disinfection.

The velocity of the reaction depends on the number and type of organisms present. In general, Gram-positive bacteria are more sensitive to disinfectants than Gram-negative bacteria; mycobacteria and fungal spores are relatively resistant, and bacterial spores are highly resistant.

Enveloped or lipophilic viruses are relatively sensitive, whereas hydrophilic viruses such as poliovirus and other enteroviruses are less susceptible. Although difficult to test in vitro, there is evidence that hepatitis B virus is more resistant than other viruses (including human immunodeficiency virus) and most vegetative bacteria to the action of chemical disinfectants and heat.

Glutaraldehyde is highly active against bacteria, viruses and spores. Other disinfectants, such as hexachlorophane, have a relatively narrow range of activity, predominantly against Gram-positive cocci. Some disinfectants are more active or stable at a particular pH value; although glutaraldehyde is more stable under acidic conditions, use at a higher pH (8.0) improves the antimicrobial effect.

Disinfectants may be inactivated by hard tap water, cork, plastics, blood, urine, soaps and detergents or another disinfectant. Information should be sought from the manufacturer or from reference authorities to confirm that the disinfectant will remain active in the circumstances of use.

Maintenance of effective disinfection in large health-care facilities is a major challenge requiring management skills and technical understanding in equal measure. The selection of appropriate disinfectants and maintaining standards in practice is supported by the development of local disinfection policies. These points are considered further in Ch. 67.

RECOMMENDED READING

Barer, M. R., & Harwood, C. R. (1999). Bacterial viability and culturability. *Advances in Microbial Physiology, 41*, 94–138.

Bergkessel, M., Basta, D. W., & Newman, D. K. (2016). The physiology of growth arrest: uniting molecular and environmental microbiology. *Nature Reviews. Microbiology, 14*(9), 549–562. doi:10.1038/nrmicro.2016.107.

Dix, A., Vlaic, S., Guthke, R., & Linde, J. (2016). Use of systems biology to decipher host-pathogen interaction networks and predict biomarkers. *Clinical Microbiology and Infection, 21*(7), 600–606. doi:10.1016/j.cmi.2016.04.014.

Flemming, H. C., Wingender, J., Szewzyk, U., Steinberg, P., Rice, S. A., & Kjelleberg, S. (2016). Biofilms: an emergent form of bacterial life. *Nature Reviews. Microbiology, 14*(9), 563–575. doi:10.1038/nrmicro.2016.94.

Fraise, A. P., Maillard, J. Y., & Satta, S. (2013). *Russell, Hugo & Ayliffe's principles and practice of disinfection, preservation and sterilization* (p. 618). Wiley-Blackwell.

Nadell, C. D., Drescher, K., & Foster, K. R. (2016). Spatial structure, cooperation and competition in biofilms. *Nature Reviews. Microbiology, 14*(9), 589–600. doi:10.1038/nrmicro.2016.84.

Papenfort, K., & Bassler, B. L. (2016). Quorum sensing signal-response systems in Gram-negative bacteria. *Nature Reviews. Microbiology, 14*(9), 576–588. doi:10.1038/nrmicro.2016.89.

Schneider, P. M. (2013). Special edition on sterilization and disinfection. *American Journal of Infection Control, 41*(5), S1–S118.

Swanson, M., Reguera, G., Schaechter, M., & Neidhardt, F. C. (2016). *Microbe* (p. 833). Washington, DC: ASM Press.

Wallace, C. A. (2016). New developments in disinfection and sterilization. *American Journal of Infection Control, 44*(5), E23–E27. doi:10.1016/j.ajic.2016.02.022.

Websites

CDC Guideline for Disinfection and Sterilization in Healthcare Facilities, 2008. Available at https://www.cdc.gov/infectioncontrol/guidelines/disinfection/index.html.

LabWork Bacterial growth curve. Available at http://www.microbiologybytes.com/LabWork/bact/bact1.htm.

5 Antimicrobial agents

ANDREW SWANN AND WILL IRVING

KEY POINTS

- Most antimicrobial agents are active only against bacteria; smaller numbers of antifungal, antiviral, antiprotozoal and anthelminthic agents are available.
- Antimicrobial agents used in clinical medicine do not affect spores of bacteria or fungi, or latent viruses.
- The largest group of antibacterial agents are β-lactam compounds (penicillins, cephalosporins, etc.), most of which are semisynthetic derivatives of naturally occurring antibiotics. Members of this group have widely different properties.
- Other widely used antibacterial agents include aminoglycosides, tetracyclines, macrolides, glycopeptides and quinolones.
- Some antifungal agents are suitable only for topical application. Agents used for systemic therapy of fungal infection include amphotericin, azoles, flucytosine and echinocandins.
- The largest groups of antiviral compounds are the antiretroviral (anti-HIV) and the anti-herpes agents, such as aciclovir, that act on nucleic acid synthesis.
- Combinations of three or more antiretroviral drugs can effectively keep HIV levels in the circulation down below the limit of detection.

Antimicrobial agents are used not only to treat bacterial diseases but also infections with viruses, fungi, protozoa and helminths. These drugs have transformed the management of infectious disease, but none is free from unwanted side effects, and microbial resistance is a constant threat. Consequently, they must be used with discretion and understanding of their individual properties. The treatment of individual infections is dealt with in the appropriate chapters. Only antibacterial, antiviral and antifungal agents will be considered here. The general strategy of antimicrobial chemotherapy, which is crucial to the control of antimicrobial drug resistance, is covered in Ch. 65.

Antibiotics are naturally occurring microbial products; synthetic compounds such as sulphonamides, quinolones, nitrofurans and imidazoles should strictly be referred to as *chemotherapeutic* (or *antimicrobial*) *agents*. However, as some antibiotics can be manufactured synthetically, whereas others are the products of chemical manipulation of naturally occurring compounds *(semi-synthetic antibiotics)*, the distinction is ill defined. Nowadays, the term *antibiotic* is used loosely to describe agents (mainly, but not exclusively, antibacterial agents) employed to treat infection. Antimicrobial substances that are too toxic to be used other than in topical therapy or for environmental decontamination are referred to as *antiseptics* or *disinfectants* (see Ch. 4).

ANTIBACTERIAL AGENTS

The principal types of antibacterial agents are listed in Table 5.1. Because there are so many, it is convenient to group them into classes that relate to their structure and site of action.

Sites of action and mechanisms of resistance

There are four sites of action:

1. Cell wall
2. Protein synthesis
3. Nucleic acid synthesis
4. Cell membrane

Some microorganisms can evade antimicrobial activity because they have intrinsic or acquired resistance (see Ch. 6 on Bacterial Genetics). The three principal mechanisms of resistance are:

1. Drug-inactivating enzymes
2. Altered target with lower affinity for the antimicrobial
3. Altered uptake (decreased permeability for the drug or increased efflux out of the bacterium)

Table 5.1 Principal types of antibacterial agent (other than agents used exclusively in mycobacterial infection)

Agent	Site of action	Useful clinical activity[a] against:					
		Staphylococci	Streptococci	Enterobacteria	Pseudomonas aeruginosa	Mycobacterium tuberculosis	Anaerobes
Penicillins	Cell wall	+R	+	V	V	−	+[b]
Cephalosporins	Cell wall	+	+	+	V	−	+[b]
Other β-lactam agents	Cell wall	V	V	+	V	−	V
Glycopeptides	Cell wall	+	+	−	−	−	+[c]
Tetracyclines	Ribosome	+R	+R	+R	−	−	+R
Chloramphenicol	Ribosome	+	+	+	−	−	−
Aminoglycosides	Ribosome	+	−	+	V	V	−
Macrolides	Ribosome	+	+	−	−	−	-
Lincosamides	Ribosome	+	+	−	−	−	+
Fusidic acid	Ribosome	+	+	−	−	+	-
Oxazolidinones	Ribosome	+	+	−	−	−	−
Streptogramins	Ribosome	+	+[d]	−	−	−	
Rifamycins	RNA synthesis	+	+	+	−	+	+
Sulphonamides	Folate metabolism	+R	+R	+R	−	−	−
Diaminopyrimidines	Folate metabolism	+	+	+R	−	−	−
Quinolones	DNA synthesis	V	V	+	V	V	−
Nitrofurans	DNA synthesis	−	−	+	−	−	-
Nitroimidazoles	DNA synthesis	−	−	−	−	−	+

+, Active; −, inactive; V, variable activity among different agents of the group. +R indicates that acquired resistance is very common.
[a]Usual spectrum of intrinsic activity.
[b]Poor activity against anaerobes of the *Bacteroides fragilis* group.
[c]Poor activity against most Gram-negative anaerobes.
[d]Poor activity against *Enterococcus faecalis*.

Inhibitors of bacterial cell wall synthesis

As most bacteria possess a rigid cell wall that is lacking in mammalian cells (see Ch. 2), this structure is a prime target for agents that exhibit selective toxicity, the ability to inhibit or destroy the microbe without harming the host. However, the bacterial cell wall can also prevent access of agents that would otherwise be effective. Thus the complex outer envelope of Gram-negative bacteria is impermeable to large hydrophilic molecules, which may be prevented from reaching an otherwise susceptible target.

Inhibitors of bacterial cell wall synthesis act on the formation of the peptidoglycan layer (Fig. 5.1). Bacteria that lack peptidoglycan, such as mycoplasmas, are resistant to these agents.

β-lactam agents

Penicillins, cephalosporins and other compounds that feature a β-lactam ring in their structure fall into this group (Fig. 5.2). All of these compounds bind to proteins situated at the cell wall–cell membrane interface. These penicillin-binding proteins are involved in cell wall construction, including the cross-linking of the peptidoglycan strands that gives the wall its strength. Opening of the β-lactam ring by hydrolytic enzymes, collectively called *β-lactamases,* abolishes antibacterial activity. Many such enzymes are found in bacteria. Those elaborated by Gram-negative enteric bacilli are particularly diverse in their activity and properties. Most prevalent are the so-called *TEM β-lactamases* (TEM-1, TEM-2, etc.), numerous forms of which have evolved under selective pressure of β-lactam antibiotic use. Gram-negative bacteria able to produce enzymes that inactivate many different β-lactam antibiotics—so-called *extended-spectrum β-lactamases* (ESBLs)—sometimes become endemic in hospitals and have now spread into the community around the world.

Penicillins The original penicillin, benzylpenicillin (penicillin G; often called simply *penicillin*), exhibits activity against staphylococci, streptococci, neisseriae, spirochaetes and certain other organisms. However, resistance, normally due to the production of β-lactamase, has undermined its activity against staphylococci and gonococci. Bacteria, including staphylococci and pneumococci, that exhibit reduced susceptibility to penicillin by a nonenzymic mechanism are also encountered. Benzylpenicillin revolutionised the treatment of infection caused by

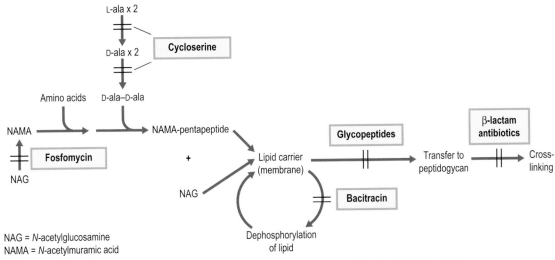

Fig. 5.1 Formation of bacterial cell wall peptidoglycan, showing the sites of action of inhibitors of the process.

some of the most virulent bacterial pathogens, but it also suffers from several shortcomings:

- breakdown by gastric acidity when given orally
- very rapid excretion by the kidney
- susceptibility to penicillinase (β-lactamase)
- restricted spectrum of activity

Further development of the penicillin family has been directed towards improving these properties. Crucial to this was the discovery that removal of the phenylacetic acid side-chain left intact the core structure, 6-aminopenicillanic acid, the starting point for the numerous semi-synthetic penicillins that have been produced. Among the most important penicillins that followed the introduction of benzylpenicillin are:

- phenoxymethylpenicillin (penicillin V), which can be given orally
- procaine penicillin, a long-acting salt of benzylpenicillin (no longer licenced in the United Kingdom)
- flucloxacillin, dicloxacillin and oxacillin, compounds resistant to staphylococcal β-lactamase
- ampicillin and amoxicillin, which are active against some enterobacteria
- ticarcillin and piperacillin (now only available in combination with β-lactamase inhibitors), which are active against *Pseudomonas aeruginosa*

Penicillins other than flucloxacillin and its relatives are inactivated by staphylococcal β-lactamase. Meticillin-resistant *Staphylococcus aureus* (MRSA; a term that has persisted, although meticillin is now obsolete) is resistant

because of alterations in the target penicillin-binding proteins; they are resistant to all penicillins and to all other β-lactam antibiotics with the exception of certain new cephalosporins (see later in the chapter) and those agents combined with β-lactamase inhibitors.

Some penicillins such as ampicillin and mecillinam are also available as esterified prodrugs (pivampicillin and pivmecillinam), a formulation providing improved absorption in the gut, where the active ingredient is released into the circulation.

Cephalosporins   Cephalosporins are close cousins of the penicillins, but the β-lactam ring is fused to a six-membered dihydrothiazine ring rather than the five-membered thiazolidine ring of penicillins. The additional carbon carries substitutions that may alter the pharmacological behaviour of the molecule, and sometimes its antibacterial activity. Some cephalosporins (e.g., cefalotin [formerly called cephalothin] and cefotaxime) carry an acetoxymethyl group on the extra carbon. This can be removed by hepatic enzymes to yield a less active derivative, but it is doubtful whether this has any therapeutic significance. Other cephalosporins (e.g., cefamandole, cefoperazone and the oxacephem, latamoxef) possess a methyltetrazole substituent. Use of compounds with this feature has been associated with hypoprothrombinaemia and bleeding in some patients, and none of these agents is used in the United Kingdom now.

Cephalosporins are generally stable to staphylococcal penicillinase (though they are differentially susceptible to hydrolysis by the various types of enterobacterial β-lactamase), but they lack activity against enterococci. They exhibit a broader spectrum than most penicillins

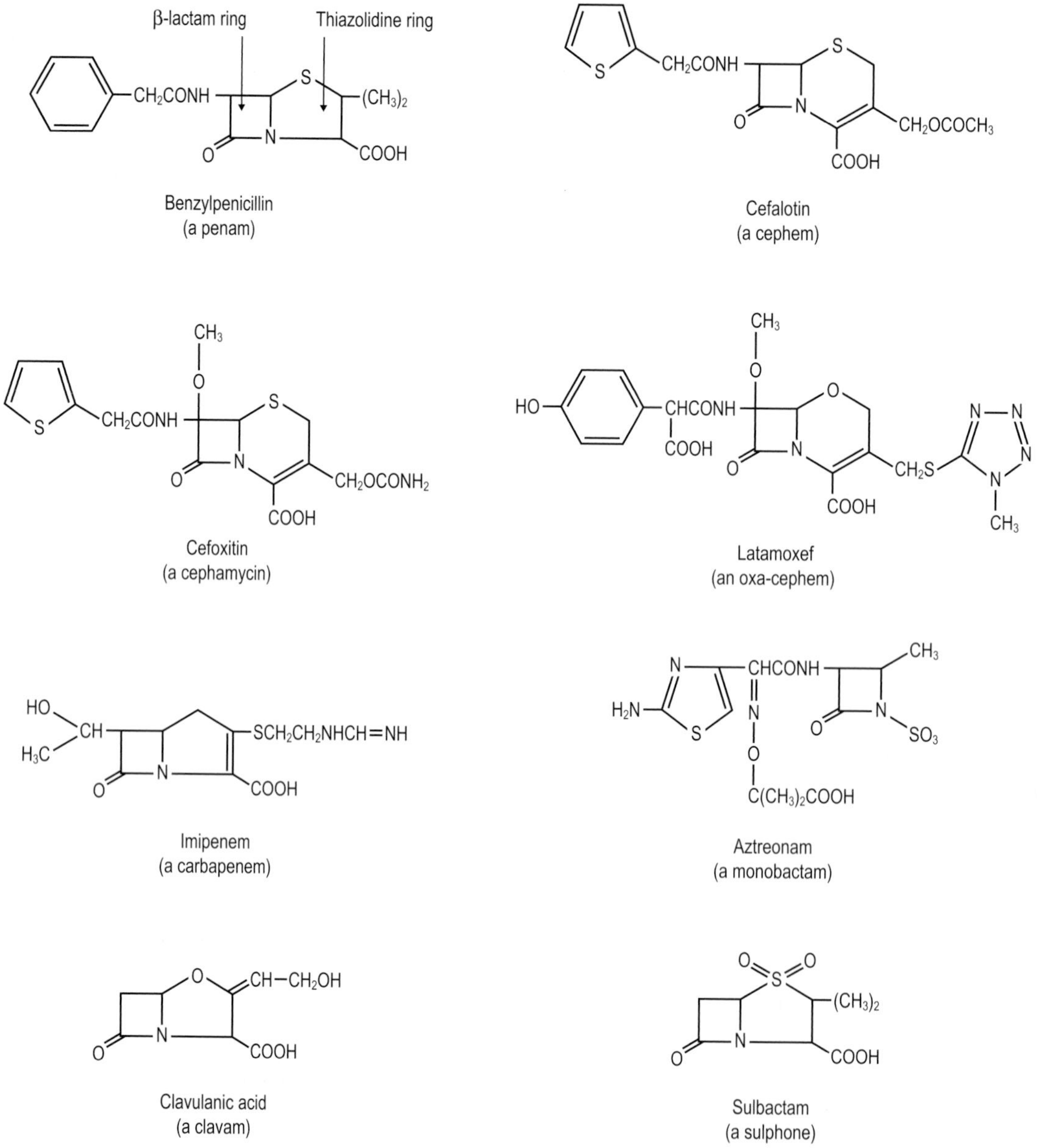

Fig. 5.2 Examples of different types of molecular structures among β-lactam antibiotics.

and are less prone to cause hypersensitivity reactions. Among the most important cephalosporins in therapeutic use are:

- cefalexin, cefradine and cefaclor, which can be given orally
- cefuroxime and cefoxitin, which are stable to many β-lactamases
- cefotaxime and ceftriaxone, which combine β-lactamase stability with high intrinsic activity

- cefpodoxime (as the proxetil prodrug) and cefixime, which combine stability to enterobacterial β-lactamases with oral absorption
- ceftazidime and cefpirome, which additionally exhibit good activity against *Ps. aeruginosa*
- ceftobiprole and ceftaroline, which are active against MRSA

Two newly introduced agents include ceftolozane (combined with the β-lactamase inhibitor tazobactam) and the combination of ceftazidime with avibactam (another β-lactamase inhibitor). Both combinations have extensive activity against Enterobacteriaceae and *Pseudomonas aeruginosa.*

Other β-lactam agents Various agents with diverse properties share the structural feature of a β-lactam ring with penicillins and cephalosporins (see Fig. 5.2):

- *Carbapenems* (e.g., imipenem, meropenem and ertapenem) have a broad spectrum of activity, embracing most Gram-positive and Gram-negative aerobic and anaerobic bacteria. Imipenem is inactivated by a dehydropeptidase in the human kidney, and is co-administered with a dehydropeptidase inhibitor, cilastatin.
- The *oxacephem* latamoxef is a broad-spectrum β-lactamase-stable compound.
- The *monobactam,* aztreonam, is a monocyclic compound with a spectrum that is restricted to aerobic Gram-negative bacteria.
- The *clavam,* clavulanic acid, exhibits poor antibacterial activity but has proved useful as a β-lactamase inhibitor when used in combination with β-lactamase-susceptible compounds such as amoxicillin (co-amoxiclav) and ticarcillin.
- The *sulphones,* sulbactam and tazobactam, also act as β-lactamase inhibitors and are marketed in combination with ampicillin (or cefoperazone) and piperacillin (or ceftolozane), respectively.

Glycopeptides

Vancomycin and teicoplanin are large molecules that are unable to penetrate the outer membrane of Gram-negative bacteria, and the spectrum is consequently restricted to Gram-positive organisms. Their chief importance resides in their action against Gram-positive cocci, with multiple resistances to other drugs. Enterococci and staphylococci, including MRSA, that exhibit resistance or reduced sensitivity to glycopeptides are being reported more frequently. Other glycopeptides (e.g., telavancin and ramoplanin) have been developed. The structurally related lipoglycopeptide dalbavancin has recently been approved for treatment of acute bacterial skin and skin structure infections. Dalbavancin has a very long half-life and is given as a single dose or a two-dose regimen separated by a week.

Other inhibitors of bacterial cell wall synthesis

- Fosfomycin is a simple phosphonic acid antibiotic used mainly for the oral treatment of urinary tract infection. However, the spread of multiply-resistant bacteria has led to some use of the intravenous formulation.
- Bacitracin is active against Gram-positive bacteria but is too toxic for systemic use. It is found in many topical preparations and is used in the laboratory in the presumptive identification of haemolytic streptococci of Lancefield group A (see Ch. 13).
- Isoniazid and some other compounds used to treat tuberculosis interfere with the formation of the mycolic acids of the mycobacterial cell wall.
- Cycloserine is an analogue of D-alanine used occasionally against multiresistant strains of *Mycobacterium tuberculosis.*

Inhibitors of bacterial protein synthesis

Bacterial ribosomes are sufficiently different from those of mammalian cells to allow selective inhibition of protein synthesis. Most agents that act at this level are true antibiotics (or derivatives thereof) produced by *Streptomyces* species or other soil organisms. Some have an effect in eukaryotic cells, which have mitochondrial ribosomes similar to those of bacteria (see Ch. 2).

Tetracyclines

These are broad-spectrum agents with important activity against chlamydiae, rickettsiae, mycoplasmas and, surprisingly, malaria parasites, as well as some conventional Gram-positive and Gram-negative bacteria. They prevent binding of amino-acyl transfer RNA (tRNA) to the ribosome and inhibit, but do not kill, susceptible bacteria. The various members of the tetracycline group are closely related and differ more in their pharmacological behaviour than in antibacterial activity. Doxycycline and minocycline are in most common use. Resistance has limited the value of tetracyclines against many Gram-positive and Gram-negative bacteria, but rickettsiae, chlamydiae and mycoplasmas are usually susceptible. Tigecycline (a glycylcycline) retains activity against many bacteria resistant to other tetracyclines.

Chloramphenicol

Chloramphenicol also possesses a very broad antibacterial spectrum. It acts by blocking the growth of the peptide chain. Use of chloramphenicol has been limited because of the occurrence of a rare but fatal side effect, aplastic anaemia. Its wide availability in some countries has been associated with increasing resistance.

Aminoglycosides

Streptomycin, the first antibiotic to be discovered by random screening of soil organisms, is predominantly active against enterobacteria and *M. tuberculosis.* Like

Table 5.2 Summary of the important differential properties of aminoglycoside antibiotics

Aminoglycoside	Activity against:		Relative susceptibility to inactivation by bacterial enzymes	Relative degree of:	
	Pseudomonas aeruginosa	*Mycobacterium tuberculosis*		Ototoxicity	Nephrotoxicity
Amikacin	+	+	±	++	+
Gentamicin	+	−	++	++	++
Kanamycin	−	+	++	++	++
Neomycin	−	±	++	+++	++
Netilmicin	+	−	+	+	+
Streptomycin	−	+	++	+++	±
Tobramycin	+	−	++	++	++

other members of the aminoglycoside family, it has no useful activity against streptococci, anaerobes or intracellular bacteria. The group also has in common a tendency to damage the eighth cranial nerve (ototoxicity) and the kidney (nephrotoxicity).

The chief properties of aminoglycosides are shown in Table 5.2. They inhibit formation of the ribosomal initiation complex and also cause misreading of messenger RNA (mRNA). They are bactericidal compounds, and some, notably gentamicin and tobramycin, exhibit good activity against *Ps. aeruginosa*. Resistance may arise from ribosomal changes (streptomycin) or alterations in drug uptake; however, it is more often caused by bacterial enzymes that phosphorylate, acetylate or adenylate exposed amino or hydroxyl groups. Enzymic resistance consequently affects the various aminoglycosides differentially, depending on the possession of exposed groups that can be attacked by the enzyme involved. Amikacin is resistant to most of the common enzymes.

Macrolides

Macrolide antibiotics have a large macrocyclic lactone ring substituted with some unusual sugars. They act by interfering with the translocation of mRNA on the bacterial ribosome. They are used mainly as antistaphylococcal and antistreptococcal agents, though some have wider applications. They have no useful activity against enteric Gram-negative bacilli. The original macrolide, erythromycin, is unstable in gastric acid and is usually administered orally as the stearate salt or as an esterified prodrug (pharmacological preparations that improve absorption and deliver the active drug into the circulation). Salts suitable for intravenous administration are also available. Certain other macrolides, for example clarithromycin and the azalide azithromycin, offer improved pharmacological properties.

Telithromycin is a ketolide that retains activity against macrolide-resistant Gram-positive cocci but has limited applications because of toxicity.

Lincosamides

The original lincosamide antibiotic, lincomycin, has been superseded by a derivative, clindamycin, that is better absorbed after oral administration and is more active against the organisms within its spectrum. These include staphylococci, streptococci and most anaerobic bacteria, against which clindamycin exhibits outstanding activity. Enthusiasm for the use of clindamycin has been tempered by an association with the occasional development of severe diarrhoea, which sometimes progresses to a life-threatening pseudomembranous colitis (see *Clostridium difficile*, Ch. 29).

Lincosamides bind to the 50S ribosomal subunit at a site closely related to that at which macrolides act. Inducible resistance to macrolides caused by enzymic modification of the ribosomal binding site also renders the cells resistant to lincosamides (and streptogramins; see later in the chapter), but only in the presence of macrolides, which alone are able to act as inducers. There is some evidence that clindamycin and other protein synthesis inhibitors such as linezolid have a role in suppressing toxin release in serious Gram-positive infections.

Fusidic acid

The structure of fusidic acid is related to that of steroids, but the antibiotic is devoid of steroid-like activity. It blocks factor G, which is involved in peptide elongation. Fusidic acid has an unusual spectrum of activity that includes corynebacteria, nocardia and *M. tuberculosis*, but the antibiotic is usually regarded simply as an antistaphylococcal agent. It penetrates well into bone and has been used (generally in combination with a β-lactam antibiotic to prevent the selection of resistant variants) in the treatment of staphylococcal osteomyelitis.

Linezolid

Linezolid is an oxazolidinone. It is a narrow-spectrum anti–Gram-positive agent that acts by preventing the formation of the ribosomal initiation complex. It is used against MRSA and other Gram-positive cocci resistant to older agents. There is some evidence that it may be of use in drug-resistant tuberculosis, but the duration of treatment is usually limited by the risk of adverse effects.

Streptogramins

This is the collective name for a family of antibiotics that occur naturally as two synergistic components. They were formerly used mainly in animal husbandry, although one member of the group, pristinamycin, is available in some countries as an antistaphylococcal agent. Use was limited by poor solubility, but derivatives suitable for parenteral administration, quinupristin and dalfopristin, have been developed. The combination exhibits bactericidal activity against most Gram-positive cocci, but has poor activity against *Enterococcus faecalis*. It is no longer available in the United Kingdom.

Mupirocin

This is an antibiotic, produced by *Pseudomonas fluorescens*, that blocks incorporation of isoleucine into proteins. Its useful activity is restricted to staphylococci and streptococci; as it is inactivated when given systemically, it is used only in topical preparations.

Inhibitors of nucleic acid synthesis

A number of important antibacterial agents act directly or indirectly on DNA or RNA synthesis.

Sulphonamides and diaminopyrimidines

These agents affect DNA synthesis because of their role in folic acid metabolism. Folic acid is used in many one-carbon transfers in living cells, including the conversion of deoxyuridine to thymidine. During this process the active form of the vitamin, tetrahydrofolate, is oxidised to dihydrofolate, and this must be reduced before it can function in further reactions.

Sulphonamides are analogues of *para*-aminobenzoic acid, and prevent the condensation of this compound with dihydropteridine during the formation of folic acid. Diaminopyrimidines, which include the broad-spectrum antibacterial agent trimethoprim and the antimalarial compounds pyrimethamine and cycloguanil (the metabolic product of proguanil), prevent the reduction of dihydrofolate to tetrahydrofolate. Sulphonamides and diaminopyrimidines thus act at sequential stages of the same metabolic pathway and interact synergistically, although in bacterial infections trimethoprim is generally sufficiently effective, and less toxic, when used alone.

Sulphonamides are broad-spectrum antibacterial agents, but resistance is common and the group also suffers from problems of toxicity. The numerous sulphonamides exhibit similar antibacterial activity but differ widely in their pharmacokinetic behaviour. They have largely been replaced by safer and more active agents, although the combination of sulfamethoxazole with trimethoprim (co-trimoxazole) is still used. Sulfadoxine or sulfadiazine combined with pyrimethamine is used in malaria and toxoplasmosis, respectively.

Quinolones

These drugs act on the α subunit of DNA gyrase. Their properties allow them to be categorised roughly into three groups (Table 5.3), although many of these are unavailable in the United Kingdom. Nalidixic acid and its early congeners are narrow-spectrum agents active only against Gram-negative bacteria. Their use is virtually restricted to urinary tract infection, although they have also been used in enteric infections. Later quinolones, such as ciprofloxacin and ofloxacin, which are 6-fluoro derivatives and are described as *fluoroquinolones,* display much enhanced activity and a broader spectrum, although activity against some Gram-positive cocci, notably *Streptococcus pneumoniae,* is unreliable. Continued development has produced compounds that lack the latter defect and, in some cases, exhibit further broadening of the spectrum and improved pharmacokinetic properties.

Quinolones are quite well absorbed when given orally and are widely distributed throughout the body. Extensive metabolisation may occur, particularly with nalidixic acid and the older derivatives. Ciprofloxacin and other fluoroquinolones are used widely despite certain problems of toxicity (which has led to limited use or product withdrawal), and resistance is becoming more prevalent.

Table 5.3 Principal types of quinolone antibacterial agents

Narrow-spectrum compounds[a]	Broad-spectrum compounds[b]	Compounds with further enhanced spectrum[c]
Cinoxacin[d]	Ciprofloxacin	Clinafloxacin[d]
Nalidixic acid	Enoxacin[d]	Gemifloxacin[d]
Oxolinic acid[d]	Levofloxacin	Moxifloxacin
Pipemidic acid[d]	Lomefloxacin[d]	Sparfloxacin[d]
	Norfloxacin	
	Ofloxacin	

[a]Spectrum restricted to enteric Gram-negative bacilli.
[b]Improved activity against *Pseudomonas aeruginosa* and Gram-positive cocci.
[c]Further improved activity against Gram-positive cocci and some anaerobes.
[d]Not available in the United Kingdom.

Nitroimidazoles

Azole derivatives feature prominently among antifungal, antiprotozoal and anthelminthic agents. Those that exhibit antibacterial activity are 5-nitroimidazoles. At low redox (E_h) values, they are reduced to a short-lived intermediate that causes DNA strand breakage. Because of the requirement for low E_h values, 5-nitroimidazoles are active only against anaerobic (and certain microaerophilic) bacteria and anaerobic protozoa. The representative of the group most commonly used clinically is metronidazole; similar derivatives include tinidazole and nimorazole.

Nitrofurans

The most familiar nitrofuran is nitrofurantoin, an agent used exclusively in urinary tract infection. Other derivatives, including furazolidone, which is used in enteric infections, are marketed for a variety of purposes in some parts of the world. These compounds probably act on DNA through a reduced metabolite, in a manner analogous to that of the nitroimidazoles.

Rifamycins

This group of antibiotics is characterised by excellent activity against mycobacteria, although other bacteria are also susceptible; staphylococci in particular are exquisitely sensitive. These compounds act by inhibiting transcription of RNA from DNA. Rifampicin, the best-known member of the group, is used in tuberculosis and leprosy and also in combination with other antibiotics in the treatment of complex staphylococcal infections. Rifapentine has similar properties, but exhibits a longer plasma half-life. Rifabutin (ansamycin) is used in infections caused by atypical mycobacteria of the avium-intracellulare group (see Ch. 28).

Disruption of cell membranes
Polymyxins

Polymyxin B and colistin (polymyxin E) act like cationic detergents to disrupt cell membranes. They exhibit potent antipseudomonal activity, but toxicity has limited their usefulness, except in topical preparations and bowel decontamination regimens. If systemic use is contemplated (for example in the treatment of multiply-resistant bacterial infections), a sulphomethylated derivative, colistin sulfomethate, is preferred.

Daptomycin

Daptomycin is a semisynthetic lipopeptide antibiotic with activity against Gram-positive cocci. It acts by disrupting multiple aspects of cell membrane function. It has a role in the treatment of infections caused by multiresistant organisms.

Antimycobacterial agents

As well as streptomycin and rifampicin (see earlier in the chapter), various agents are used exclusively for the treatment of mycobacterial infection. These include isoniazid, ethambutol and pyrazinamide, which are commonly found in antituberculosis regimens, and diaminodiphenylsulfone (dapsone) and clofazimine, which are used in leprosy. Cycloserine and *p*-aminosalicylic acid (PAS), which were formerly used in tuberculosis, have now been largely abandoned except for drug-resistant tuberculosis. Some fluoroquinolones and macrolides exhibit activity against certain mycobacteria and may have a role in treatment.

ANTIFUNGAL AGENTS

Superficial fungal infections of the skin and mucous membranes can often be treated with topical agents, including polyenes, such as nystatin, or azole derivatives, of which many (clotrimazole, miconazole, econazole, etc.) are marketed as vaginal pessaries and creams. For dermatophyte infections of the nails, oral therapy with griseofulvin or the allylamine derivative terbinafine is particularly suitable, as these agents are deposited in newly formed keratin.

Azole derivatives exhibit the broadest spectrum of activity, embracing yeasts, filamentous fungi and dimorphic fungi. They include the 2-nitroimidazole ketoconazole, and the triazoles fluconazole, itraconazole, posaconazole, voriconazole and isavuconazole. The latter four exhibit useful activity against *Aspergillus fumigatus*. Fluconazole is well distributed after oral administration and has been used successfully in systemic yeast infections, including cryptococcal meningitis.

Other agents for systemic treatment of yeasts and other fungi include the polyene, amphotericin B, which is extremely toxic. Newer formulations of the drug, in which it is complexed with liposomes or lipids, are better tolerated. The pyrimidine analogue 5-fluorocytosine is active against many types of yeast and is used in combination with amphotericin B in severe systemic yeast infections. Anidulafungin, caspofungin and micafungin are members of the echinocandin class of agents. They are active against various fungi, including *Candida*, *Aspergillus* and *Pneumocystis jirovecii* (formerly *P. carinii*), a fungus long thought to be a protozoan.

The spectrum of activity of the common antifungal compounds is shown in Table 5.4. Most act by interfering with the integrity of the fungal cell membrane, either by

Table 5.4 Summary of the clinically useful spectrum of activity of antifungal agents

Agent	Candida albicans	Cryptococcus neoformans	Dermatophytes	Aspergillus fumigatus	Dimorphic fungi
Amphotericin B	+	+	−	+	+
Echinocandins	+	−	−	+	-
Flucytosine	+	+	−	−	−
Griseofulvin	−	−	+	−	−
Imidazoles	+	+	+	−	+
Nystatin[a]	+	−	-	-	−
Terbinafine	−	−	+	-	+[b]
Triazoles	+	+	+	(+)[c]	+

[a]For topical use only.
[b]Clinical efficacy not yet established.
[c]Itraconazole, posaconazole, voriconazole and isavuconazole are active against *A. fumigatus*, but fluconazole is not.

Table 5.5 Antiviral agents in clinical use for infections other than human immunodeficiency virus or hepatitis C virus

Compound	Mode of action	Indication
Antiherpesvirus agents		
Aciclovir	Nucleoside analogue	Herpes simplex; varicella-zoster
Cidofovir	Nucleotide analogue	Cytomegalovirus retinitis
Famciclovir	Prodrug of penciclovir	Herpes simplex; varicella-zoster
Foscarnet	Inhibition of DNA polymerase	Cytomegalovirus; aciclovir-resistant herpes simplex or varicella-zoster
Ganciclovir	Nucleoside analogue	Cytomegalovirus
Penciclovir	Nucleoside analogue	Herpes simplex; varicella-zoster
Valaciclovir	Prodrug of aciclovir	Herpes simplex; varicella-zoster
Valganciclovir	Prodrug of ganciclovir	Cytomegalovirus
Antiinfluenza agents		
Amantadine (and rimantadine)	Viral uncoating	Influenza A
Oseltamivir	Neuraminidase inhibitor	Influenza A and B
Zanamivir	Neuraminidase inhibitor	Influenza A and B
Antihepatitis B agents		
Adefovir	Nucleotide analogue	Chronic hepatitis B
Entecavir	Nucleoside analogue	Chronic hepatitis B
Interferon-α	Immunomodulator	Chronic hepatitis B and C
Lamivudine	Nucleoside analogue	Chronic hepatitis B
Telbivudine	Nucleoside analogue	Chronic hepatitis B
Tenofovir	Nucleotide analogue	Chronic hepatitis B
Other antiviral agents		
Ribavirin	Nucleoside analogue	Respiratory syncytial virus; hepatitis C

binding to membrane sterols (polyenes) or by preventing the synthesis of ergosterol (azoles and allylamines). Echinocandins interfere with β-glucan synthesis in the fungal cell wall. Use in individual fungal diseases is considered in Ch. 58.

ANTIVIRAL AGENTS

Antiviral agents in clinical use are presented in Tables 5.5, 5.6 and 5.7. Some important antiviral compounds, representing a range of molecular structures, are illustrated in Fig. 5.3.

Table 5.6 Directly acting antiviral agents for chronic hepatitis C infection

HCV target gene	Protein function	Drugs
NS3	Protease	Grazoprevir, Glecaprevir, Paritaprevir, Simeprevir, Voxilaprevir
NS5a	Multifunctional (nonenzymatic)	Daclatasvir, Elbasvir, Ledipasvir, Ombitasvir, Pibrentasvir, Velpatasvir
NS5b	RNA polymerase	Nucleotide analogue: Sofosbuvir Nonnucleoside: Dasabuvir

NS, non-structural

Table 5.7 Antiretroviral agents in clinical use

Type of agent	Drug names
Nucleoside analogue reverse transcriptase inhibitor	Abacavir, Didanosine, Emtricitabine, Lamivudine, Stavudine, Zidovudine
Nucleotide analogue reverse transcriptase inhibitor	Tenofovir
Nonnucleoside reverse transcriptase inhibitor[a]	Efavirenz, Etravirine, Nevirapine, Rilpivirine
Protease inhibitor	Atazanavir, Darunavir, Fosamprenavir, Indinavir, Lopinavir (formulated with Ritonavir), Ritonavir, Saquinavir, Tipranavir
Fusion inhibitor	Enfuvirtide[a]
Entry inhibitor	Maraviroc[b]
Integrase inhibitor	Raltegravir, Dolutegravir

[a]Active against only HIV-1.
[b]Active against only those HIV strains that use CCR5 coreceptors.

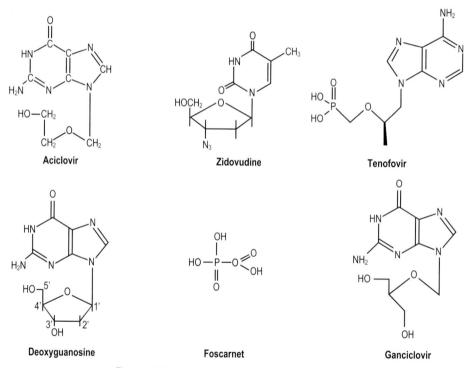

Fig. 5.3 Molecular structures of some antiviral compounds.

Treatment of herpesvirus infections

Nucleoside analogues

The most widely used antiviral agent is the nucleoside analogue acycloguanosine, otherwise known as aciclovir. This is first monophosphorylated by a virus-encoded thymidine kinase produced in cells infected by herpes simplex virus (HSV) or varicella-zoster virus (VZV). Subsequent phosphorylation steps are completed by cellular kinases to form aciclovir triphosphate. This competes with guanosine triphosphate for the viral DNA polymerase,

becomes incorporated into the viral DNA chain and inhibits further viral DNA polymerase activity (Fig. 5.4). Aciclovir lacks a 3′-hydroxyl group on its acyclic side-chain, and therefore it cannot form a phosphodiester bond with the next nucleotide due to be added to the growing herpesvirus DNA chain, which is terminated prematurely. The lack of cellular toxicity of aciclovir is a consequence of three selective features:

1. Initial phosphorylation takes place only in virus-infected cells.

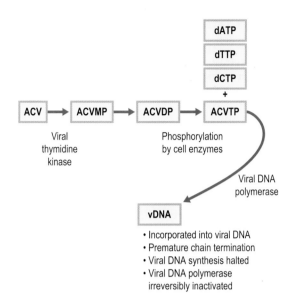

Fig. 5.4 Mode of activation and action of aciclovir *(ACV)*. *ACVMP*, Aciclovir monophosphate; *ACVDP*, aciclovir diphosphate; *ACVTP*, aciclovir triphosphate; *dATP*, deoxyadenosine triphosphate; *dTTP*, deoxythymidine triphosphate; *dCTP*, deoxycytidine triphosphate; *vDNA*, viral deoxyribonucleic acid.

2. As phosphorylation within virally infected cells reduces the intracellular concentration of free aciclovir, more drug will diffuse into the cell from the extracellular space, thereby resulting in concentration of drug specifically within virally infected cells.
3. Aciclovir triphosphate inhibits viral (but not cellular) DNA polymerase.

Aciclovir has an established record in the treatment of HSV and VZV disease, as prophylaxis against HSV reactivation after transplantation, and in the long-term suppression of recurrent genital herpes. Penciclovir is a related molecule that works through the same mechanism. Valaciclovir and famciclovir are oral prodrug formulations of aciclovir and penciclovir, respectively. They provide improved systemic drug levels and require less frequent administration.

Aciclovir has very little clinically useful activity against another herpesvirus, cytomegalovirus (CMV). However, a related compound, ganciclovir, is activated by a CMV protein kinase encoded by the viral gene *UL97* in CMV-infected cells, but there is also considerable phosphorylation in uninfected cells, and ganciclovir is much more toxic than aciclovir, particularly to the bone marrow. Ganciclovir also exhibits antiviral effects against human herpesviruses HHV-6 and HHV-7, which do not respond to aciclovir. Valganciclovir is an oral prodrug formulation providing a much improved systemic concentration of ganciclovir after oral administration.

Cidofovir is a nucleoside phosphonate and therefore does not require virus-mediated mono-phosphorylation. It is converted in cells into the diphosphate, which inhibits CMV DNA polymerase. It shows activity against a range of DNA viruses, but its main clinical use is for CMV retinitis. It is not absorbed orally, has a very long half-life (2 weeks) and is nephrotoxic. Brincidofovir, a derivative bound to a lipid moiety currently undergoing clinical trials, is orally bioavailable, has higher potency and is considerably less toxic.

These antiviral agents inhibit only replicating herpesvirus and do not eliminate latent virus. Reduced susceptibility is occasionally found in isolates of HSV, VZV or CMV, usually derived from severely immunocompromised hosts who have been receiving prolonged antiviral therapy. Clinically significant antiviral resistance arises from mutations in the viral DNA polymerases that no longer bind the antiviral triphosphate derivatives, or in the virally encoded enzymes thymidine kinase (HSV, VZV) and UL97 phosphorylase (CMV) such that the virus cannot phosphorylate the drugs.

Nonnucleoside antiherpes agents

Foscarnet, a pyrophosphate analogue, inhibits nucleic acid synthesis without requiring any activation and is an important agent for treatment of cytomegalovirus or of other herpesvirus infections that have become resistant to aciclovir or ganciclovir. It is poorly absorbed orally, and exhibits nephrotoxicity. There are a number of promising new anti-herpes drugs undergoing clinical trials including pritelivir, an inhibitor of HSV helicase-primase, maribavir, an inhibitor of the CMV UL97 kinase, and letermovir, an inhibitor of the CMV terminase enzyme complex.

Treatment of influenza
Neuraminidase inhibitors

Zanamivir and oseltamivir are agents specifically designed to block the action of the influenza virus enzyme, neuraminidase by occupying the catalytic site. They act on all influenza viruses. Neuraminidase is found on the surface of influenza virus, where it enables release of newly formed mature virus particles from the cell surface, which would otherwise remain attached through the interaction of viral haemagglutinin to cell surface sialic acid residues. Thus neuraminidase inhibitors act to prevent release of newly formed viral particles from the cell surface, reducing the spread of influenza viruses locally. Zanamivir is taken by inhalation into the oropharynx; oseltamivir is the oral prodrug form of a similar agent.

Agents that block viral uncoating

Amantadine, a symmetrical amine compound, has long been known to inhibit influenza A virus replication. Amantadine (and its derivative, rimantadine) blocks an ion channel formed by the integral membrane protein (M2) of influenza A (but not influenza B) virus, preventing uncoating of the virus within cells. Resistance arises rapidly through mutations in the *M2* gene.

Treatment of chronic hepatitis B virus infection
Interferons

Interferons, naturally occurring antiviral compounds produced by mammalian cells in response to viral infection, are now manufactured by genetic recombination. Interferon-α (given by either subcutaneous or intramuscular injection thrice weekly) is used to treat chronic infection with hepatitis B and C viruses. Modification of interferon by addition of polyethylene glycol—peginterferon—results in sustained plasma levels after just one dose per week. The mode of action of interferon-α is complex, producing an antiviral state in cells to which it binds, and interfering with the production of virus in those cells (see Ch. 9). However, interferons also act through immune modulation, upregulating the expression of major histocompatibility complex (MHC) molecules on cell surfaces. This is a significant part of the action in clearing chronic hepatitis B.

HBV DNA polymerase inhibitors

The nucleoside analogues lamivudine, entecavir and telbivudine, and the nucleotide analogues adefovir and tenofovir (used as prodrugs, adefovir dipivoxil and tenofovir disoproxil, respectively) all inhibit the reverse transcriptase activity of hepatitis B virus (HBV), thereby reducing virus replication. These drugs differ in their potency and also in the genetic barrier to development of resistance within the viral enzyme, with entecavir and tenofovir being classified as highly potent drugs with the least likelihood of emergence of resistance.

Treatment of chronic hepatitis C virus infection

Up until 2012, standard therapy for chronic HCV infection consisted of a combination of pegylated interferon and ribavirin (see later in the chapter) given for 6–12 months, with a sustained virological response rate (SVR, equates to cure) of around 50%. The precise mechanism of action of either drug in this condition was not clear. However, the past 2 years have seen a complete revolution with the development of drugs targeted against virally encoded proteins—known as directly acting antiviral

agents, or DAAs. The three main HCV targets (see Table 5.6) are:

- NS3 protease enzyme—HCV protease inhibitor drugs have the suffix: previr
- NS5a multifunctional protein—NS5a inhibitors have the suffix: asvir
- NS5b polymerase enzyme—NS5b inhibitors have the suffix: buvir.

DAAs are usually given in combination to reduce the risk of viral resistance, and ribavirin is added for particular patient groups. DAA-based therapy has several advantages over interferon-based regimens, including oral administration, very few adverse effects, shorter duration of therapy (e.g., 8–12 weeks) and, most importantly, almost unbelievable success rates, with SVR rates well in excess of 95%.

Other antiviral drugs—ribavirin

Ribavirin is a nucleoside analogue that is used in a nebulised form in the treatment of respiratory syncytial virus infection and intravenously for Lassa fever. It is also used orally in combination therapy for the treatment of chronic hepatitis C. Its mechanism of action is unclear, but the wide antiviral spectrum it exhibits, particularly in vitro, suggests that it may interfere with the processing of virally derived mRNA.

ANTIRETROVIRAL AGENTS

Seven classes of drugs are now available for the treatment of HIV infection, acting variously to inhibit viral nucleic acid synthesis, viral protein synthesis, viral entry and integration of the DNA provirus into the host genome (see Table 5.7). All inhibit only replicating HIV and do not eliminate integrated proviral DNA.

The use of multiple drugs in combination antiretroviral therapy (cART; see Ch. 52) may result in such suppression of HIV replication that virus is undetectable in the circulation. The use of cART prevents the development of immune deficiency in infected patients and may also result in immune reconstitution in patients who have already developed the acquired immunodeficiency syndrome (AIDS).

Emergence of resistant mutants has been a problem with all classes of anti-HIV agent, and has stimulated developments in the field of antiviral susceptibility testing.

Nucleoside and nucleotide reverse transcriptase inhibitors

The earliest anti-HIV agent, zidovudine (azidothymidine), and several other compounds, including didanosine (dideoxyinosine), zalcitabine (dideoxycytidine; now rarely used), lamivudine and stavudine, are nucleoside analogues. New additions include abacavir and emtricitabine and a nucleotide analogue, tenofovir. They are activated (phosphorylated) by cellular enzymes and inhibit the reverse transcriptase function of the viral polymerase of HIV-1 or HIV-2, with many terminating the chain of proviral DNA. Phosphorylation rates vary in different cell types and between resting and replicating cells.

Unlike aciclovir, these nucleoside analogues are associated with some toxicity as there is less selectivity in their activation and action.

- Initial phosphorylation is by cellular kinases.
- Some inhibition of cellular (mitochondrial) DNA polymerase occurs

Nonnucleoside reverse transcriptase inhibitors

These compounds, which include nevirapine, efavirenz, etravirine and rilpivirine, inhibit only HIV-1. They bind directly, without activation, away from the catalytic site of reverse transcriptase but exert a structural change that inhibits its action. They are not incorporated into the DNA chain.

HIV protease inhibitors

These compounds act at a late stage in the viral cycle by interfering with the cleavage of essential polyprotein precursors. The numerous derivatives now available are listed in Table 5.7. One problem with the protease inhibitors (PIs) is their tendency to interact with the liver cytochrome P450 enzyme complex and therefore give rise to drug–drug interactions. However, one advantage of this is the use of ritonavir at low dose to inhibit P450 and thereby boost the plasma levels of PIs, which would otherwise be metabolised in the liver.

HIV fusion inhibitors

Enfuvirtide is a homologue of the short peptide sequence active in fusion of the HIV-1 envelope to the cell membrane after attachment, and it inhibits that final stage of the entry process. The drug has to be given by subcutaneous injection, and its use is reserved for patients who have limited options for treatment. It is not active against HIV-2.

HIV entry inhibitors

Initial binding of HIV to CD4 molecules present on the target cell surface is followed by binding to one of a number of secondary receptors, the most commonly used of which is CCR5, a chemokine receptor. Maraviroc is a drug that binds specifically to CCR5, thereby preventing access of viral particles to this molecule.

HIV integrase inhibitors

Once viral RNA has been reverse transcribed into a DNA form (known as the provirus), integration of the provirus into the host cell genome is mediated by a viral integrase enzyme. The latest antiretroviral drugs to have been developed are integrase inhibitors (e.g., raltegravir), acting to prevent this step in the viral life cycle.

With regard to antiviral drug assays, concerns over toxic levels of aciclovir or ganciclovir arise on occasion, and these can be measured. Therapeutic drug monitoring is also practised in relation to HIV therapy, mainly to test for compliance with the onerous regimens necessary in the management of this chronic condition.

RECOMMENDED READING

De Clercq, E. (2009). In search of a selective therapy of viral infections. *Antiviral Research, 85*(1), 19–24. doi:10.1016/j.antiviral.2009.10.005.

De Clercq, E., & Li, G. (2016). Approved antiviral drugs over the past 50 years. *Clinical Microbiology Reviews, 29*(3), 695–747. doi:10.1128/CMR.00102-15.

Finch, R. G., Davey, P. G., Wilcox, M. H., & Irving, W. L. (2012). *Antimicrobial chemotherapy* (6th ed.). Oxford: Oxford University Press.

Finch, R. G., Greenwood, D., Norrby, S. R., & Whitley, R. J. (2012). *Antibiotic and chemotherapy: anti-infective agents and their use in therapy* (9th ed.). London: Saunders, Elsevier.

Franklin, T. J., & Snow, G. A. (2005). *Biochemistry and molecular biology of antimicrobial drug action* (6th ed.). New York: Springer.

Grayson, M. L., Crowe, S. M., McCarthy, J., Mills, J., Mouton, J. W., Norrby, S. R., ... Pfalle, M. A. (2010). *Kucers' the use of antibiotics: a clinical review of antibacterial, antifungal and antiviral drugs* (6th ed.). London: Hodder Arnold.

Lorian, V. (Ed.). (2005). *Antibiotics in laboratory medicine* (5th ed.). Baltimore: Lippincott Williams & Wilkins.

Volberding, P., & Deeks, S. G. (2010). Antiretroviral therapy and management of HIV infection. *Lancet, 376*(9734), 49–62. doi:10.1016/S0140-6736(10)60676-9.

Websites

National electronic library of infection. Bugs & drugs on the Web. Available at http://www.antibioticresistance.org.uk/.

United States National Library of Medicine and National Institutes of Health. Antibiotics. Available at http://www.nlm.nih.gov/medlineplus/antibiotics.html.

World Health Organization. Essential Medicines and Pharmaceutical Policies. Available at http://www.who.int/medicines/en/.

6 Bacterial genetics

MARCO RINALDO OGGIONI

KEY POINTS

- The properties of a bacterial cell are defined by the information encoded in its double-stranded DNA. The genome of a bacterial cell is composed of a single generally circular chromosome with additional information residing within extrachromosomal elements known as plasmids.
- Plasmids and several other mobile genetic elements, including bacteriophages, transposons and other integron-based entities, render the bacterial genetic complement highly susceptible to variation by the addition of new genes. Such elements are often organised into recognisable genetic clusters known as pathogenicity islands or resistance islands and which may affect the medical significance of bacterial strains when the genes they encode affect antibiotic susceptibility or virulence.
- Mobile genetic elements are transferred horizontally between related bacteria through the processes of transformation, conjugation and transduction.
- Bacterial genomes are also susceptible to change through mutation, in which the primary nucleotide sequence of one or more genes or regulatory elements is altered. Because bacterial populations grow rapidly to very large cell numbers, the possibilities for generation and selection of advantageous mutations, such as

those conferring resistance to antibiotics, are of significant impact.
- These forms of genotypic variation should be distinguished from phenotypic variation because the former are heritable, whereas the latter are not, and reflect changes in gene expression and, in the case of phase variation, genetic rearrangements leading to altered expression patterns without changing the cell's genetic complement.
- Advent of high-throughput genomic sequencing has transformed our knowledge of the genetic information and organisation of all cells, including bacteria. Sequencing of one strain of a given species reveals the complete set of genes of a given species (operational taxonomic unit, OTU) and allows us to infer the metabolic pathways and related phenotypes. The sequencing of multiple isolates sheds light on the large genetic variability within an OTU revealing the genes present in all isolates (core-genome) and the full complement of genes present in any single isolate of a given OTU (pan-genome). High-throughput sequencing has revolutionised research into gene expression (RNAsreq), revealing roles for regulatory RNAs, together with approaches to detecting drug resistance determinants and epidemiological relationships.

GENETIC ORGANISATION AND REGULATION OF THE BACTERIAL CELL

All properties of a bacterial cell, including those of medical importance, such as virulence, pathogenicity and antibiotic resistance, are determined ultimately by the genetic information contained within the cell genome. This information is normally encoded by the specific sequence of nucleotide bases comprising the DNA of the cell. There are four common nucleotide bases in DNA: adenine,

guanine, cytosine and thymine; it is the linear order in which these bases are arranged linked by a covalent sugar phosphate backbone that determines the properties of the cell. With only a few exceptions, most of the genetic information required by the bacterial cell is arranged in the form of a single generally circular double-stranded chromosome. It is worth noting that the main bacterial chromosome is not a completely stable structure but can exhibit quite dynamic reorganisation following the insertion or deletion of transposons, integrons and genomic islands (see later in the chapter) under fluctuating environmental and selective conditions. In the model organism, *Escherichia coli*, the chromosome is about 1.3 mm long (4 million base pairs) and occurs in an irregular coiled bundle in the cytoplasm of a bacillary cell sized only 2×0.5 µm. The chromosome is tightly associated with histone-like proteins as it is in eukaryotic cells, although there are many DNA binding proteins involved in regulation of gene expression, including several proteins referred to as histone-like.

In addition to the single main chromosome, bacterial cells may also carry one or more circular extrachromosomal elements termed *plasmids*. These plasmids can vary in size from a few hundred to over a million base pairs. Plasmids replicate independently of the main chromosome in the cell. Although dispensable, they often carry supplementary genetic information coding for beneficial properties (e.g., resistance to antibiotics) that enable the host cell to survive under a particular set of environmental conditions.

A third source of genetic information in a bacterial cell can be provided by the presence of certain types of bacterial viruses, bacteriophages. Bacteriophages consist essentially of just a protein coat enclosing the virus genome, and, because they are unable to multiply in the absence of their bacterial host, generally they are lethal to their host cell. In some instances, they can enter a potentially long-term state of infection, lysogeny, after integration into the bacterial chromosome. In such a state, the bacteriophage genome is referred to as a prophage and effectively becomes a temporary part of the total genetic information available to the cell and may consequently bestow additional properties on the cell (e.g., toxins).

Processes leading to protein synthesis

The character of a bacterial cell is determined essentially by the specific polypeptides that comprise its enzymes and other proteins. The DNA acts as a template for the transcription of RNA by RNA polymerase for subsequent protein production within the cell. In the transcription process the specific sequence of nucleotides in the DNA determines the corresponding sequence of nucleotides in the messenger RNA (mRNA). This, in turn, is then translated into the appropriate sequence of amino acids by ribosomes. Finally, the sequence of amino acids in the resulting polypeptide chain determines the configuration into which the polypeptide chain folds itself, which in many cases determines the enzymatic properties of the completed protein. A segment of DNA that specifies the production of a particular polypeptide chain is called a gene (a segment of DNA without stop codons; an open reading frame, ORF), and the processes of transcription and translation leading to protein synthesis are collectively termed the central dogma of molecular biology. These processes are illustrated schematically in Fig. 6.1.

Gene regulation

Bacterial genomes range in size from a few hundred thousand base pairs to many millions, but most bacteria contain enough DNA to code for the production of between 1000 and 6000 different polypeptide chains—1000–6000 different genes. However, during normal bacterial life, some polypeptides will be required in particular growth states (see Ch. 4), whereas others are only made when the cell is in particular environments providing specific conditions such as growth substrates, temperature, pH or salinity, or when it is confronted by a new challenge, such as an antibiotic. Protein production is an energy-intensive process, and therefore the expression of many genes is controlled actively to prevent waste and to optimise housekeeping of precious energy.

In bacteria the process of gene expression is best studied for controls acting at the transcriptional level, thereby conserving the energy supply and the transcription–translation apparatus. This is achieved by means of regulatory elements that either inhibit or enhance the rate of RNA chain initiation and termination for a particular gene. Numerous complex regulatory mechanisms are involved in coordinating the many biochemical reactions that proceed inside a cell, but related genes involved in a common regulatory system are often clustered on the bacterial chromosome. Such functional clusters are known as operons, of which the most well-known example is the lactose operon of *E. coli* (Fig. 6.2).

For transcription to occur as the first stage in protein synthesis, RNA polymerase has to attach to DNA at a specific promoter region and transcribe the DNA in a fixed direction. This process can be switched off by the attachment of a repressor molecule to a specific region of the DNA, known as the operator. This lies between the promoter and the structural gene(s) being transcribed; the repressor then blocks the movement of the RNA polymerase molecule so that the genes downstream are not transcribed.

The repressor is often an allosteric molecule with two active sites. One recognises the operator region so that the repressor can bind to it to prevent transcription. The other recognises an inducer molecule. When the inducer is present, it binds to the repressor and simultaneously alters the binding specificity at the other site, so that the repressor no longer binds to the operator and transcription can resume.

There are many different variations on this basic regulatory system. For example, a repressor may be normally inactive but activated by the end product of a biosynthetic pathway; thus, for example, when the end product of an operon-encoded pathway is present at a sufficient concentration, the repressor combines with the operator and switches off transcription of the operon. Alternatively,

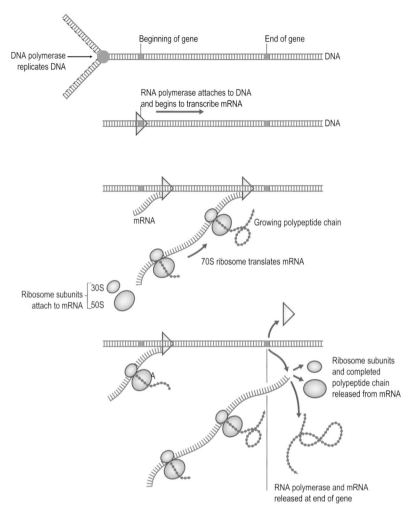

DNA polymerase → replicates DNA

Beginning of gene

End of gene

DNA

RNA polymerase attaches to DNA and begins to transcribe mRNA

DNA

mRNA

Growing polypeptide chain

70S ribosome translates mRNA

Ribosome subunits attach to mRNA ⎰30S ⎱50S

Ribosome subunits and completed polypeptide chain released from mRNA

RNA polymerase and mRNA released at end of gene

Fig. 6.1 The central dogma of molecular biology.

regulation of certain operons involves proteins that bind to the DNA and assist RNA polymerase to initiate transcription. These are just a few examples, and other regulatory systems display both minor and major differences. Finally, it should be stressed that prokaryotic gene regulation frequently involves interwoven regulatory circuits that respond to a variety of different stimuli. As noted in Ch. 4, these networks of genes are organised into functional units known as stimulons when they respond to a particular stimulus and regulons when they are regulated by a single protein or, as recently shown, a single regulatory RNA.

MUTATION

As bacteria reproduce by asexual binary fission, the genome is normally identical in all of the progeny. However, one

of the fundamental requirements for evolution is that, although gene replication must normally be completely accurate to ensure stability, there must also be occasional variation to produce new or altered characters that might be of selective value to the organism. Inaccuracies in DNA replication are a natural event during replication and are mostly corrected by specific proofreading and repair mechanisms. Nonetheless, some errors escape control and generate a slightly altered nucleotide sequence in one of the progeny cells. Such a mutation is heritable and will be passed on stably to subsequent generations. Mutations may not produce any observable effect on the structure or function of the corresponding protein, but in a small proportion of cases an enzyme with altered specificity for substrates, inhibitors or regulatory molecules may be produced. This is the kind of mutation that is most likely to be of evolutionary value to an organism; indeed, many

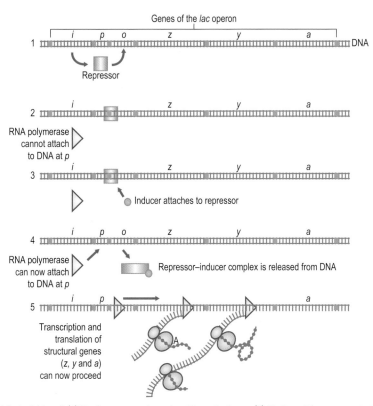

Fig. 6.2 The *lac* operon of *Escherichia coli*. (1) The *lac* repressor is produced from the *i* gene. (2) Binding of the repressor to the operator site *(o)* prevents transcription of the genes *z* (β-galactosidase), *y* (galactoside permease) and *a* (transacetylase). (3) The inducer (lactose, or a closely related derivative) can bind specifically to the repressor. (4) The repressor molecule is thereby altered at its operator-binding site, and the repressor–inducer complex is released from the DNA. (5) RNA polymerase can now attach to the promoter site *(p)* and transcribe the structural genes of the *lac* operon. Note that, in bacteria, several genes may be transcribed into a single polycistronic mRNA molecule.

examples of acquired antibiotic resistance have been shown to be of this type. Other mutations may alter a gene so that a nonfunctional protein is formed; if this protein is essential to the cell then the mutation will be lethal. As a mutation may occur in any one of the several thousand genes in the cell, and different mutations in the same gene may produce different effects, the number of possible mutations is very large. Particular mutations occur at fairly constant rates, normally between 1 per 10^4 and 1 per 10^{10} cell divisions. As a large bacterial colony contains at least 10^9 cells, even a pure bacterial culture will contain many thousands of cells with different mutations affecting many different genes. Some of these mutations will be viable and potentially selected for by particular environmental conditions during subculture. For the same reason, in an infected patient, a variety of mutants will appear spontaneously in the population that grows from the few bacteria originally entering the body. Such mutations may enhance the ability of an organism to cause infection—for example, by conferring antibiotic resistance, enhanced virulence or altered surface antigens. In such a situation, cells with

the mutation will rapidly outgrow cells without the mutation, so that selection of the mutant cells occurs and they soon become the predominant type.

Phenotypic variation

The properties of a bacterial cell at a particular time are referred to as its phenotype. These properties are determined not only by its genome (genotype) but also by its environment. Phenotypic variation occurs when the expression of genes is changed in response to the environment—for instance, by the induction or repression of synthesis of particular enzymes. Such changes in gene expression underpin the differentiation process involved in sporulation (see Ch. 4), the differing phenotypes observed during different growth phases and under different growth conditions (see Ch. 4) and the physiological adaptive responses of bacteria (see Ch. 4). The distinction between genotypic mutation and phenotypic variation is critical; the former is heritable and maintained through changes in environmental conditions, whereas the latter is reversible, being dependent

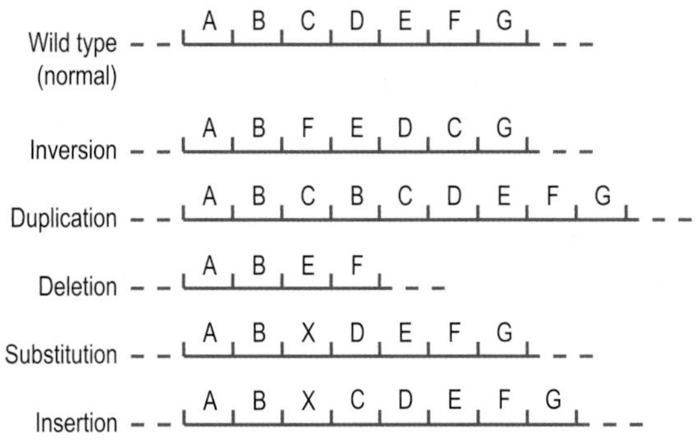

Fig. 6.3 Examples of types of mutations. The top sequence represents a portion of the wild-type chromosome from which the different mutational rearrangements shown below are derived.

on environmental conditions and altering when these change. Phenotypic variation is therefore not a form of mutation.

Types of mutations

Mutations can be divided conveniently into multisite mutations, involving extensive chromosomal rearrangements such as inversions, duplications and deletions and point mutations, which are defined as only affecting one, or very few, nucleotides. The structure of DNA is such that point mutations can be divided into one of three basic types (Fig. 6.3):

1. substitution of one nucleotide for another
2. deletion of one or more nucleotides
3. insertion of one or more nucleotides

Mutations occur spontaneously during replication of DNA, but most are corrected immediately by the cell's editing apparatus. Occasional mutations, particularly those conferring a selective advantage to the cell, will be inherited stably by the progeny, but secondary mutations can occasionally restore the original nucleotide sequence. It is important to distinguish this relatively rare event of back-mutation from the separate process of phase variation, which is readily reversible and occurs with relatively high frequency in either direction (e.g., at a cell division frequency of 10^{-3}). The variation of certain Gram-negative bacteria between a fimbriate and a non-fimbriate phase, the variation of flagellar antigens in *Salmonella enterica* serotypes and variation in the methylation target-specificity of certain restriction-modification systems are examples of phase variation. These may involve segments of DNA that are inverted or recombination to yield alternative gene products and hence different phenotypes. In some cases, promoters can initiate DNA transcription in different directions to give a flip-flop type of action. The number of such switching systems is limited, but they have high

value to the organism in providing a mechanism to produce reversible alternatives as opposed to irreversible changes.

Mutations may occur in any gene, but many individual mutations are lethal. Other mutations affect gene products that are essential only under particular cultural conditions. The detailed function and regulation of processes in the bacterial cell can often only be analysed by searching systematically for mutations that affect each separate step in a process. Thus, mutations can be found that produce increased resistance to almost any antimicrobial agent, and the study of such mutants is an essential step in understanding the modes of action of antibiotic agents and mechanisms of resistance to them.

HORIZONTAL GENE TRANSFER

A change in the genome of a bacterial cell may be caused either by a mutation in the DNA of the cell or result from the acquisition of additional DNA from an external source. DNA may be transferred between bacteria by three mechanisms:

1. transformation
2. conjugation
3. transduction

Each of these mechanisms occurs at a low frequency in nature and is central to the evolution of bacterial populations. It is important to note that acquisition by bacteria of new properties following gene transfer or mutation becomes significant and emerges in the population if the new genetic end product is subject to favourable selection by the conditions under which the bacteria are growing.

Transformation

Most species of bacteria are unable to take up exogenous DNA from the environment; indeed, most bacteria produce nucleases that recognise and break down foreign DNA. However, bacteria in some genera, notably *Streptococcus pneumoniae*, *Haemophilus influenzae* and certain *Bacillus* species, have been shown to be capable of taking up DNA either extracted artificially or released by lysis from cells of another strain. It was in particular by transforming *Streptococcus pneumoniae* that Oswald Avery discovered in 1944 that the hereditary material of cells was composed of DNA. Bacterial cells are competent for genetic transformation only under certain conditions of growth, usually in late log phase or, in *Bacillus* species, during sporulation. However, bacterial geneticists have also developed treatments by means of which organisms can be made artificially competent.

Once a piece of DNA has entered the cell by transformation, it has to become incorporated into the existing chromosome of the cell by a process of recombination in order to be inherited to the progeny. This is a complex molecular process for which the transformed DNA, entering the cell as a single strand, must have been derived from a closely related bacterium, as segments of DNA can recombine with the chromosome only when there is a high degree of nucleic acid similarity (homology).

Any gene may be transferred by transformation, as any fragment of a donor chromosome may be taken up by the recipient cells. However, a piece of DNA introduced into a cell by transformation will generally be relatively short and will contain only a small number of genes.

Conjugation

Conjugation is a process by which one cell, the donor, makes contact with another, the recipient, and DNA is transferred directly from the donor into the recipient. Certain types of plasmids carry the genetic information necessary for conjugation to occur. Only cells that contain such a plasmid can act as donors; those lacking a corresponding plasmid act as recipients.

Transfer of DNA between cells by conjugation requires direct contact between donor and recipient cells. Plasmids capable of mediating conjugation carry genes coding for the production of a 1- to 2-μm-long protein appendage, termed a *pilus*, on the surface of the donor cell. The tip of the pilus attaches to the surface of a recipient cell and holds the two cells together so that DNA can pass into the recipient cell. It is probable, at least for the type IV pili of Gram negatives, that DNA transfer actually occurs through the pilus, but other types of pili appear to act simply as a mechanism by which the donor and recipient cells are drawn together. Different types of pili are specified by different types of plasmids and can therefore be used as an aid to plasmid classification.

In the vast majority of cases, the only DNA transferred during the conjugation process is the plasmid that mediates the process. It is thought that one strand of the circular DNA of the plasmid is nicked open at a specific site and the free end is passed into the recipient cell. The DNA is replicated during transfer so that each cell receives a copy. As donor ability is dependent upon having a copy of the plasmid, the recipient strain becomes converted into a donor, able to conjugate with further recipients and convert them in turn. In this way, a plasmid may spread rapidly through an entire population of recipient cells; this process is sometimes described as infectious spread of a plasmid. During conjugation, the recipient cell thus receives a complete genetic element that can carry many genes or operons, which can confer in one single event numerous phenotypes to the recipient, as, for example, multiple antimicrobial drug resistances.

Mobilisation of chromosomal genes by conjugation

Many different types of plasmids have the ability to transfer themselves. Some (but not all) plasmids also have the ability to mobilise the chromosomal genes of bacteria. The first reported plasmid of this type was the F factor (fertility factor) of *E. coli*. Cells that contain the F plasmid free in the cytoplasm (cells) have no unusual characteristics apart from the ability to produce F pili and to transfer the F plasmid to F− cells by conjugation. In a very small proportion of F+ cells, the F plasmid becomes inserted into the bacterial chromosome. Once inserted, the entire chromosome behaves like an enormous F plasmid, and hence chromosomal genes can be transferred in the normal manner to a recipient cell at a relatively high frequency. Such cultures are termed *high-frequency recombination* (Hfr) strains.

It is important to emphasise that the F plasmid system is confined to *E. coli* and other closely related enteric bacteria. However, many bacterial species and in particular in the Gram-positive *Enterococcus* spp. and *Streptococcus* spp. have large chromosomal conjugative elements unable to replicate in the cytoplasm and that excise with an integrase-related mechanism similar to bacteriophages, replicate with a circular intermediate and then transpose to a recipient cell. As for most other mobile elements, these conjugative transposons are most known for their contribution to the spread of drug-resistance genes.

Transduction and bacteriophages

The third known mechanism of horizontal gene transfer in bacteria involves the transfer of DNA between cells by bacteriophages. Bacteriophages (phages) are viruses that infect bacteria. The number of phages in any environment outnumber the bacteria, which already are the most abundant form of cellular life. Phages may alternatively go through a lytic cycle or integrate into the host chromosome. This is the case of temperate phages, which can alternatively have a lytic cycle or a lysogenic state when integrated into the chromosome. Because of their high plasticity and continuous selective force acting on bacterial population, phages significantly contribute to microbial evolution.

Most bacteriophages carry their genetic information (the phage genome) as a double-stranded DNA coiled up inside a protein coat. Other phages are known in which the phage genome consists of single-stranded DNA or RNA, but, as far as is known, transducing phages all contain double-stranded DNA. Two major types of transductions are known to occur in bacteria: generalised and specialised transduction. In both types, bacterial genes are occasionally and accidentally incorporated into new phage particles. During generalised transduction, any bacterial gene of the chromosome being broken down during phage replication can be incorporated by error into a phage particle and transduced. In specialised transduction, any lysogenic phage integrated into the chromosome excises imprecisely including also a nearby gene, which then is packaged with the phage genome and transduced. When such a phage particle subsequently infects a second bacterial cell, the DNA that enters the cell includes a short segment of chromosome from the original host. Bacterial genes have been transduced by the phage into the second cell. Genes can be transduced only between fairly closely related strains, as particular phages usually attack only a limited range of bacteria. As well as chromosomal genes, transducing bacteriophages may also pick up and transfer plasmid DNA. As an example, the penicillinase gene in staphylococci is usually located on a plasmid, and it may be transferred into other staphylococcal strains by transduction.

Lysogenic conversion

The presence of integrated prophage DNA constitutes a genetic alteration to the host cell. Usually only the phage repressor gene is expressed, but in certain cases it can be demonstrated that other genes are also expressed by the host cell. For example, *Corynebacterium diphtheriae* produces diphtheria toxin only when it is lysogenised by β phage; the toxin is specified by one of the phage genes. This process is termed *lysogenic conversion*. It is probable that the production of many toxins by staphylococci, streptococci and clostridia is also dependent upon lysogenic conversion by specific bacteriophages. In such cases, lysogenic conversion not only gives the cell superinfection immunity but also actively influences the virulence of the bacterium for humans.

PLASMIDS

Properties encoded by plasmids

As described above, plasmids are circular extrachromosomal genetic elements that may encode a variety of supplementary genetic information, including the information for self-transfer to other cells by conjugation. Not all plasmids can transfer themselves, but nonconjugative plasmids can be mobilised by other conjugative plasmids present in the same donor cell. Apart from this optional transfer ability, all bacterial plasmids contain the basic genetic information necessary for self-replication and segregation into daughter cells at cell division. Plasmids seem to be ubiquitous in bacteria; many encode genetic information for such properties as resistance to antibiotics,

bacteriocin production, resistance to toxic metal ions, production of toxins and other virulence factors, reduced sensitivity to mutagens, or the ability to degrade complex organic molecules.

Plasmid classification

As plasmids are mobile elements and often composed of a mosaic structure, their classification has long been difficult. The classical methodology grouped the plasmids first by their host range and then by incompatibility testing. The identification of the host range—that is, the range of bacterial species in which the plasmid could replicate—can be identified experimentally by testing replication of a given plasmid in different species or simply by epidemiological association of a given plasmid to the species in which it is found.

The method of incompatibility testing relies on the fact that closely related plasmids are unable to coexist stably in the same bacterial cell. Plasmids that are sufficiently closely related to interfere with one another's replication in this manner are said to be incompatible and to belong to the same incompatibility group. In contrast, unrelated plasmids can coexist stably and are therefore said to belong to different incompatibility groups.

In the era of massive routine DNA sequencing, the nucleotide sequences of plasmids are available and allow typing of plasmids by genetic features. In general, the gene sequences of their replicase genes are used in place of the original more time-consuming process of testing the stability of pairs of plasmids in a bacterial cell.

Plasmid epidemiology and distribution

Some plasmid groups have been identified in many different countries of the world, whereas others have so far been found only in a single bacterial species isolated from a solitary ecological niche. There seem to be two major ways in which plasmids spread:

1. by direct transfer from one bacterium to another in a particular microenvironment
2. by being carried in a particular host from one environment, such as a hospital, to another

The epidemiological tracing of these pathways requires identification not just of the plasmids involved but also typing of their host bacterial strains (see Ch. 3).

TRANSPOSONS, INTEGRONS AND GENOMIC ISLANDS

As mentioned earlier in the chapter, the main bacterial chromosome can exhibit quite dynamic reorganisation following the insertion or deletion of insertion sequences, transposons, integrons and genomic islands under fluctuating environmental and selective conditions. Transposons are linear pieces of DNA, often including genes for antibiotic resistance (see later in the chapter), that can migrate between unrelated plasmids and/or the bacterial chromosome independently of the normal bacterial recombination processes. This horizontal gene transfer allows for exchange of large multiple gene-containing segments. These integrons include highly efficient gene-trap systems, which form an essential building block of many transposons and allow the rapid formation and expression of new combinations of genes in response to selection pressures. A detailed description of the properties of these elements lies outside the scope of this text, but suffice it to say that these elements seem to provide the primary mechanism for foreign gene capture and dissemination, certainly among Gram-negative bacteria. In addition to these defined mobile elements, the sequencing of bacterial genomes has revealed the presence of segments present in some strains of a given bacterial species and absent in others and which have been termed *genomic islands*. Depending on the genes contained in these islands, they may be referred to as pathogenicity islands or resistance islands. In some cases, the collection of genes included can form a highly mobile genetic element based on the island encoding transposase genes providing the capacity to excise and transpose the whole element to a new replicon or new cell. For example, highly mobile superantigen-encoding pathogenicity islands can be found in *Staphylococcus aureus*; these are characterised by a specific set of phage-related functions that enable them to use the phage reproduction cycle for their own transduction across quite large phylogenetic distances.

GENETIC BASIS OF ANTIBIOTIC RESISTANCE

All of the properties of a microorganism are determined ultimately by genes located or inserted either on the main chromosome or on plasmids or on lysogenic bacteriophages. With regard to antibiotic resistance, it is important to distinguish between intrinsic and acquired resistance. Intrinsic resistance is dependent upon the natural insusceptibility of an organism. In contrast, acquired resistance involves changes in the DNA content of a cell, such that the cell acquires a phenotype (i.e., antibiotic resistance) that is not inherent in that particular species.

Intrinsic resistance

Organisms that are naturally insensitive to a particular drug will always exist. The most obvious determinant of bacterial response to an antibiotic is the presence or absence of the target for the action of the drug. Thus, polyene antibiotics such as amphotericin B kill fungi by binding tightly to the sterols in the fungal cell membrane and altering the permeability of the fungal cell. As bacterial membranes do not contain sterols they are intrinsically resistant to this class of antibiotics. Similarly, the presence of a permeability barrier provided by the cell envelopes of Gram-negative bacteria is important in determining sensitivity patterns to many antibiotics. A very clear example is also the lack of peptidoglycan cell wall in the small obligate intracellular *Mycoplasma*, which renders these cells naturally resistant to penicillins. Intrinsic resistance is usually predictable in a clinical situation as it tightly relates to the bacterial species causing a given infection facilitating an informed and judicious choice of appropriate empirical antimicrobial therapy.

Acquired resistance

An ongoing problem of antimicrobial chemotherapy has been the appearance of resistance to particular drugs in a normally sensitive microbial population. An organism may lose its sensitivity to an antibiotic during a course of treatment. In some cases, the loss of sensitivity may be slight, but often organisms become resistant to clinically achievable concentrations of a drug. Once resistance has appeared, the continuing presence of an antibiotic exerts a selective pressure in favour of the resistant organisms. Three main factors affect the frequency of acquired resistance:

1. The amount of antibiotic that is being used
2. The frequency with which bacteria can undergo spontaneous mutations to resistance
3. The prevalence of plasmids able to transfer resistance from one bacterium to another

Chromosomal mutations

Random spontaneous mutations occur continuously at a low frequency in all bacterial populations, and some mutations may confer resistance to a particular antibiotic. The rate at which these mutations occur is not normally influenced by presence of the antibiotic, but in the presence of the drug the resistant mutant can survive, grow and eventually become the predominant, or only, member of the population. The degree of resistance conferred by chromosomal mutation depends on the biological consequences of the mutation. With single large-step mutations, the drug target is altered by mutation so that it is totally unable to bind a drug, although it can still carry out its normal biological functions sufficiently well to permit the continued survival of the cell. This type of mutation occurs with quinolones, streptomycin and rifampicin. More commonly, the target is altered so that it can no longer bind a drug as efficiently, although it still has some residual affinity. In such a case a higher concentration of antibiotic would be required to produce the same antimicrobial effect: the minimum inhibitory concentration (MIC) of the antibiotic for the organism would be increased. Once a slightly resistant organism has been produced, additional mutational events—each conferring an additional small degree of resistance—can eventually lead to the production of organisms that are highly resistant. This is called the multistep pattern of resistance. Spontaneous chromosomal mutation is of clinical importance in tuberculosis, in which mutants resistant to any single drug (e.g., streptomycin, rifampicin or isoniazid) are likely to be present in the patient before the start of treatment. If only one drug is given to the patient, the few resistant mutant bacteria will multiply and eventually cause a relapse of the disease. Combined therapy with several drugs to which the organism is sensitive is used in the treatment of tuberculosis so that each drug kills the few mutants that are resistant to the other. The frequency with which double or triple mutations occur spontaneously in the same cell is so low as to be clinically insignificant.

There are many other examples of chromosomal muta-tions to antibiotic resistance that have assumed clinical importance. Bacterial enzymes called β-lactamases are commonly responsible for resistance to penicillins, cephalosporins and related antibiotics that contain a β-lactam ring (see Ch. 5). Mutations in the genes control-ling the production of chromosomally encoded β-lactamases in Gram-negative bacteria can result in overproduction of these enzymes and consequent resistance to the cephalosporin antibiotics normally regarded as stable to β-lactamase.

Chromosomal mutations leading to antibiotic resistance are in many cases just as important clinically as the types of transferable resistance described in the next section.

Transferable antibiotic resistance

Of the three modes of gene transfer in bacteria, plasmid-mediated or transposon-mediated conjugation is of greatest significance in terms of drug resistance. Plasmids conferring resistance to one or more unrelated groups of antibiotics can be transferred rapidly by conjugation throughout the population. Resistance plasmids were first demonstrated in Japan in 1959, when it was shown that resistance to several antibiotics could be transferred by conjugation between strains of *Shigella* and *E. coli*. Many surveys since then, in all parts of the world, have shown that plasmids carrying resistance genes are extremely common and widespread.

The way in which plasmids are built up in vivo probably varies from case to case, but it is clear that simple transfer

factors can pick up resistance genes and combine them with nontransmissible resistance plasmids to produce complex transmissible plasmids that encode resistance to as many as eight or more different antimicrobial drugs. This process of plasmid evolution is accelerated considerably by the involvement of transposons and integrons (see earlier in the chapter). Depending on their host range, plasmids can transfer themselves into a wide range of commensal and pathogenic bacteria, but recombination among plasmids is frequent, thereby significantly increasing the host range for the genes transported. Once resistance to an antibiotic appears in any one of these species, the process of transposition assists the dissemination of the responsible gene among different plasmids and subsequent distribution to other bacterial species. As described earlier in the chapter, integrons form an essential building block of many transposons and allow the rapid formation and expression of new combinations of antibiotic resistance genes in response to selection pressures. These, in turn, can be assembled into resistance islands that can be found inserted into the bacterial chromosome. For example, antibiotic resistance in several *Salmonella enterica* serovars that cause gastrointestinal disease in humans is caused by the presence in the chromosome of a set of related genomic islands carrying a class 1 integron, which carries the resistance genes. *Salmonella* genomic island 1 (SGI1), the first island of this type, was found in *S. enterica* serovar *Typhimurium* DT104 isolates, which are resistant to ampicillin, chloramphenicol, flor-fenicol, streptomycin, spectinomycin, sulphonamides and tetracycline.

As the prevalence of multiple-resistance plasmids carrying transposons and integrons continues to increase, infections caused by a wide range of pathogens become more difficult to treat. In addition, resistance plasmids can also carry genes—for example, for toxin produc-tion—that confer increased virulence on a bacterial cell. Thus, use of antibiotics may select for bacteria carrying plasmids that confer not only multiple drug resistance but also increased pathogenicity.

Control of antibiotic resistance

The major cause of the spread of genes conferring antibiotic resistance is the selection pressure brought about by the increased, and often indiscriminate, use of antibiotics in humans and animals. Plasmid-encoded drug resistance is increased by the widespread use of antibiotics in animal husbandry, where antibiotics are used as animal feed supplements and whole animal populations may be treated, rather than an individual subject as occurs in medical practice. When resistance plasmids are present, the mass use of antibiotics fails to prevent the spread of resistance and selects plasmids in the gut microbiota of the whole population of animals. Resistance might thus be directly selected in humans or animals, but the environmental dispersal of the antibiotics in manure or effluents is also a risk as antibiotics do reach both surface- and ground-water, where they exert selection pressure on environmental bacteria. This newly selected resistance gene pool can then find its way back to human commensals and pathogens and provide a significant clinical risk.

The WHO and many national governments have recognised that it is important to minimise antimicrobial drug resistance. Rational use of antibiotics and sensible restriction of their availability in humans and animals could prevent further spread of resistance genes and perhaps reduce their incidence. Some plasmids are unstable and tend to lose resistance genes when the selection pressure is removed. Cells that lose a plasmid, transposon or genomic island may have a slight metabolic advantage and may slowly outgrow drug-resistant organisms. Moreover, genetic elements that evolve in one species may be unstable in another or may transfer themselves to other organisms much less efficiently. Similarly, organisms that are adapted to the gut of a calf, pig or chicken may not establish readily in human beings. Such factors may help to contain the spread of resistance genes.

THE BACTERIAL SPECIES AND MOLECULAR TYPING OF MICROORGANISMS

The concept of species, central to eukaryotic evolution, and deriving from botany and zoology is not applicable to bacteria as it defines as organisms belonging to one species those able to generate a fertile F1 generation. This works well for higher eukaryotes as there is sexual reproduction, but bacteria do divide by binary fission after mitosis. This generates populations with less defined borders and the term more appropriately used to define such homogeneous evolutionary groups of bacteria is *OTU*, which stands for operational taxonomic unit. The assignment to an OTU occurs by tracing genes conserved in all bacteria, as, for example, the gene for the 16S rRNA (16 Svedberg ribosomal RNA). A modern definition of a bacterial OTU (or species) is still under discussion, so that the classical parameter of a DNA identity of >97% of the 16S rRNA gene is still valid. The alignment of the 16S rRNA genes, termed a *molecular clock*, allows the calculations of parameters for phylogenic trees. In these trees, the number of variations in the nucleotide sequence (of the 16S rRNA gene) correlates to the diversity between the bacteria sequenced. These analyses of the 16S rRNA genes do not only allow to assign any bacterium to a given OTU (or species), but allow also to study noncultivable bacteria and bacterial communities (see Ch. 11 on the microbiome).

Typing of microorganisms is increasingly important for studying cross-infection and epidemiological relationships, particularly during outbreaks of nosocomial infection. Molecular fingerprinting methods are now the most commonly used techniques for assessing the relatedness of individual bacterial isolates in epidemiological studies. These techniques can be used to study any organism from which DNA can be prepared and offer the possibility of a unified approach to microbial typing that can be applied immediately to a new epidemiological problem with no prior knowledge of the organisms being investigated (see Ch. 3).

A complete DNA sequence forms the ultimate reference standard for identifying microorganisms and their subtypes. Increasing numbers of microorganisms are now being sequenced, and the knowledge gained is of immense value for research purposes. However, the recent substantial reduction in sequencing costs and improvement of bio-informatic tools have enabled rapid automated sequence analyses to enter routine diagnostic laboratories where they provide resources for antimicrobial susceptibility testing, epidemiology and identification of unconventional agents. Whole genome sequencing offers the prospect of using all variations (all single-nucleotide polymorphisms [SNPs]) to draw detailed phylogenetic trees of any given group of related organisms. So far, this approach is still limited to epidemiological research and did not enter the routine lab.

One of the main problems in microbial epidemiology is that for many bacteria the extent of horizontal gene transfer accounts for much of the variability and hinders construction of phylogenetic trees. Critically, the number of genetic differences does not correlate with the number of genetic events that generated them (one DNA fragment transferred by horizontal gene transfer with 100 SNPs is one genetic event; not 100 genetic events). The methodology generally used is termed *multilocus sequence typing* (MLST). The technique relies on the analysis of sequence variation in a relatively small set of housekeeping genes (usually about seven) that are present in all isolates of a particular bacterial species. The genes selected for analysis should be widely separated on the chromosome and should not be adjacent to genes that may be under selective pressure. Specific primers are designed that amplify circa 500-bp fragments of these genes, which are then sequenced to determine naturally occurring variation. The sequences can be compared with those already contained in worldwide databases in order to analyse both global and local epidemiology. MLST schemes and databases are already available for all medically relevant bacteria with frequent horizontal gene transfer. Species in which horizontal gene transfer is generally absent—for example, *Mycobacteria*—do not use this typing methodology but rely on alternative approaches that make use of repetitive DNA and thus highly variable DNA segments in their genomes (for example, variable number of tandem repeat analysis [VNTR]). MLST and VNTR are powerful approaches for the characterisation of microbial populations as they provide unambiguous data that are electronically portable among laboratories and can be used for global epidemiological studies.

MICROBIAL GENOMES AND GENOMICS

The combination of a continuing increase in the capacity of DNA sequencing and the matching reduction of costs has dramatically transformed biology and medicine. In the 1970s, Fred Sanger at the UK Medical Research Council developed the methodology of dideoxy chain termination for DNA sequencing; this is still used sequencing isolated DNA fragments. Newer methods, known collectively as next-generation sequencing (NGS) technologies include multiple approaches, which allow for massively parallel generation of nucleotide sequences on a scale that would have taken years to achieve using Sanger technology. Examples include illumina sequencing (Illumina Inc.), presently the methodology of choice for high-throughput sequencing (HTS), which allows, depending on the specific machine used, production of one flow cell of 1000 gigabases (10^{12} nucleotides) of DNA (a bacterial genome is 1–6 Mb; the human genome is 30 Gb). Multiplexing of samples on this or similar instruments allows for massively parallel sequencing bringing, at the time of writing, the cost of a human and a bacterial genome down to around 1000 and 50 dollars, respectively. Other technologies, such as single-molecule real-time sequencing (Pacbio Biosciences Inc., Menlo Park, California) allows for sequencing of single DNA fragments, of long DNA fragments up to 20 kb and the concomitant detection of base modifications such as methylation; an important tool in the study of epigenetic phenomena. An alternative methodology proposed by Oxford Nanopore makes use of a sequencing device that is only slightly larger than a USB stick; this runs directly attached to a laptop computer and potentially revolutionises the setup of sequencing laboratories and delivers leading edge technology to resource poor areas of the world and to field applications. The molecular details of these methodologies are outside the scope of this chapter and can be found online and in many reviews.

In 1995, the Institute for Genome Research (TIGR, Rockville, MD, United States) sequenced and published the first complete microbial genome of the bacterium *Haemophilus influenzae*. Twenty years after publication of that first genome sequence the open access database Genbank contains over 35,000 microbial genomes (http://www.ncbi.nlm.nih.gov/genbank/), and numbers of deposited genomes are increasing exponentially. Genomes, including microbial and eukaryotic genomes, can be queried using text queries or sequence alignment software (e.g., basic local alignment search tool [BLAST]) and can be downloaded to run standalone analyses on local computers or networks. Again, many tutorials on the basics of bioinformatics and genome analysis are available online.

When describing microbial genomes, the large evolutionary distances between organisms must be taken into account. In this regard it should be noted that Gram-negative bacteria (proteobacteria), such as the common urinary tract pathogen *E. coli*, are more closely related to our mitochondria than to any Gram-positive bacterium (firmicutes) and that the distance between proteobacteria and firmicutes equals or exceeds that between humans and any plant of fungus. This extreme diversity provides insight into the profound differences found in the organisation of prokaryotic genomes. As stated in the first paragraph of this chapter, the bacterial genome includes all elements of a cell that carry genetic information, and the bacterial chromosome and potential accessory molecules such as plasmids and bacteriophages must also be included. As in all cellular organisms, the chromosomes are composed of a single double-stranded DNA copy able to replicate autonomously. The bacterial chromosome is generally single, haploid, and circular (Box 6.1; Fig. 6.4), while accessory elements like plasmids are often present in multiple copies and have autonomous replication and partitioning systems. To this general rule, there are multiple exceptions. Examples include the linear chromosomes the genus *Streptomyces* (frequent producers of antibiotics), the spirochetes of the genus *Borrelia* (cause of Lyme borreliosis) or the alpha-proteobacterium *Agrobacterium tumefaciens* (plant root symbionts). Multiple chromosomes have been found, for example, in the spirochete *Leptospira interrogans* (4,300,000 and 360,000 base pairs, respectively), or in the proteobacterium *Burkholderia pseudomallei* (4,070,000 and 3,100,000 base pairs, respectively). The decision to classify both independent structures as chromosomes (rather than identifying one as a very large plasmid) reflects the presence of essential genes on both replicons.

Box 6.1   Common properties of most bacterial genomes

- A single circular chromosome
- A haploid chromosomal complement
- A chromosomal size between 150,000 and 9,000,000 base pairs
- An average gene length of 1000 base pairs
- Presence of continuous open reading frames (no introns)
- Each gene encoding a single protein (no polyproteins)
- Genes are separated by noncoding regions (no overlapping genes)
- Related genes are often cotranscribed in operons
- A limited presence of noncoding RNAs

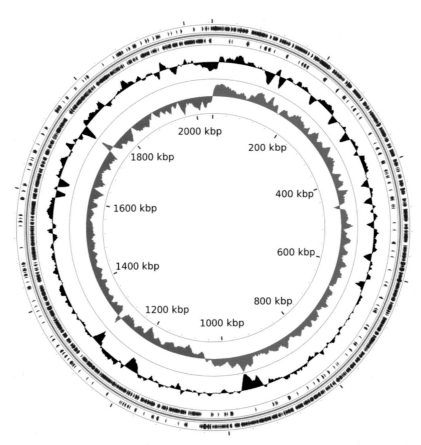

Fig. 6.4 Map of the chromosome of the Gram-positive bacterium *Streptococcus pneumoniae*. The map shows the circular chromosome of *Strep. pneumoniae* strain D39. This genome is deposited in the public database Genbank with the accession number NC_008533. The genome is 2,046,115 base pairs in size and has 2069 open reading frames (ORFs) predicted to encode 2069 proteins. On both the forward (clockwise) and reverse (anticlockwise) strands the protein encoding genes are shown in blue, and the ribosomal RNA genes are shown in pink (in-between the blue on the two outer rings). The black shading indicates the content in the bases guanine and cytosine (GC content). Large local variation in GC content often indicates the presence of recently transferred DNA or bacteriophages. The GC skew (positive in green, negative in purple) indicates the asymmetry between guanine and cytosine on the two filaments and allows recognition of the leading and lagging strand of the genome during replication. The map was visualised using the free software package CGView (http://wishart.biology.ualberta.ca/cgview/). (Stothard, P., & Wishart, D. S. (2005). Circular genome visualization and exploration using CGView. *Bioinformatics*, 21(4), 537-539.)

A further distinctive characteristic of bacterial genomes is that genes are generally intron free, do not overlap and do not encode polyproteins (Box 6.1; Fig. 6.4). In eubacteria, there are no spliceosome introns and rare group I introns, while self-splicing mobile group II introns are a bit more frequent. The latter behave as mobile genetic elements. Amongst the few genes that encode more than one protein is the gene for cytochrome B and C1 of *Bradyrhizobium japonicum*. This should not be mixed up with polycistronic transcripts of operons, where a single messenger RNA (mRNA) encodes for many sequential genes, each of which is transcribed separately. Finally, the obligate endosymbiont *Carsonella ruddii*, with the smallest known genome, shows many overlapping genes, probably due to a selective pressure to optimise the limited space available.

The size of bacterial genomes can vary widely, but as a general consideration it can be stated that bacteria that are able to encounter many environmental situations tend to have much larger genomes than species with restricted ecological niches. Extreme examples are the reduced genomes of mitochondria and chloroplasts (both are technically and evolutionarily prokaryotes), which for millions of years have been intracellular symbionts of nucleated cells, or the insect endosymbiont *Carsonella ruddii* with the smallest micoabial genome of 160,000 bp, or finally that of the human intracellular pathogen *Mycoplasma genitalium* (480,000 bp). Bacteria that live in the

Table 6.1 Examples of bacterial genomes

Species	Notes	GenBank	Form	Length (Mbp)	GC content[a]	Proteins
Carsonella ruddii	Insect endosymbiont	AP009180	Circular	0.16	16.6%	182
Mycoplasma genitalium	Urogenital infections	L43967	Circular	0.6	31.7%	477
Borrelia burgdorferi	Lyme disease	AE000783	Linear	0.9	28.6%	851
Haemophilus influenzae	Epiglottitis and otitis media	L42023	Circular	1.8	38.1%	1657
Streptococcus pneumoniae	Pneumonia and meningitis	AE005672	Circular	2.2	39.7%	2105
Mycobacterium tuberculosis	Tuberculosis	AL123456	Circular	4.4	65.6%	3989
Escherichia coli	Urinary and intestinal infections	U00096	Circular	4.6	50.8%	4243
Pseudomonas aeruginosa	Environmental organism and wound infections	AE004091	Circular	6.3	66.6%	5568
Streptomyces coelicolor	Antibiotic producer	AL645882	Linear	8.6	72.1%	7769
Bradyrhizobium japonicum	Nitrogen fixation, legume-root modulating	BA000040	Circular	9.1	64.1%	8317

[a]Percentage of guanine or cytosine bases in the genome.

environment—for example, *Pseudomonas*, *Bradyrhizobium* or *Streptomyces*—have genomes ranging in size from 6 to 9 million base pairs (Mb) and that render them metabolically versatile, allow responses to multiple external stimuli and adaptation to highly divergent situations (Table 6.1). Independent of genome size, the fundamental characteristics of cellular life, replication, transcription, translation and core energy metabolism remain essentially constant. As genome size increases, so too does the complement of genes encoding for sensor proteins, transcriptional and translational regulators and accessory metabolic pathways. All these characteristics confer a seemingly endless array of adaptive abilities to bacteria with large genomes (Table 6.1).

The sequencing of the first genome of any given species will deliver the complete gene content of the isolate and allows elucidation of a large part of its metabolic processes and its general physiology. Revealed features include the identification of many metabolic pathways, the characterisation of many of its surface proteins including transporters, adhesins and signal transduction proteins, all of which interact with the environment (the human host), and the anabolic pathways for biosynthesis of compounds (cell wall, lipopolysaccharide, capsule or secondary metabolites like antibiotics). Medical applications derived from this knowledge can include the identification of novel drug targets utilising information on metabolism or novel candidate vaccine antigens from analysis of surface exposed proteins. From an industrial point of view the genomic information on metabolic pathways may lead to optimisation of industrial fermentation processes, as in the example of biofuel production, or to biotechnological optimisation

of catabolic properties as in processes of bioremediation, where bacteria are exploited for the removal of pollutants from the environment.

As described earlier in the chapter, horizontal gene transfer (transformation, conjugation and transduction) are processes that significantly shape the structure of bacterial genomes by allowing for the addition and loss of a significant number of genes. Because bacteria divide by binary fission, all material transferred horizontally is immediately passed to the progeny. The sequencing of multiple independent isolates of the same bacterial species allows us to recognise the variability of single genes and operons by comparative analysis of the genome sequences obtained. This allows identification of the set of genes conserved in all isolates of a given species, and this is defined as the core-genome. On the contrary, the complement of all genes cumulatively present in all isolates of a given species is termed the pan-genome. The within-species genomic variability due to horizontal gene transfer is so large that two independent isolates of the same species can differ for presence or absence of >25% of their genes. This means that the core-genome of a given isolate often represents <60% of its genes, while the other genes may include essential genes (and which are present in other allelic forms in other isolates) or nonessential additions—for example, antimicrobial resistance genes. Presently, thousands of genome sequences of the most important bacterial pathogens have been generated and are being evaluated in order to assign subtle genomic differences to variations in the pathogenic potential of the bacteria linked, for example, to the severity or the type of infection caused.

RECOMMENDED READING

Avery, O. T., Macleod, C. M., & McCarty, M. (1944). Studies on the chemical nature of the substance inducing transformation of pneumococcal types. Induction of transformation by a desoxyribonucleic acid fraction isolated from *Pneumococcus* type III. *The Journal of Experimental Medicine, 79*(2), 137–158.

Fleischmann, R. D., Adams, M. D., White, O., Clayton, R. A., Kirkness, E. F., Kerlavage, A. R., & Merrick, J. M. (1995). Whole-genome random sequencing and assembly of *Haemophilus influenzae* Rd. *Science, 269*(5223), 496–512.

Sanger, F., Nicklen, S., & Coulson, A. R. (1977). DNA sequencing with chain-terminating inhibitors. *Proceedings of the National Academy of Sciences of the United States of America, 74*(12), 5463–5467.

Virus–cell interactions

WILL IRVING

KEY POINTS

- Viruses are completely dependent on the host cell for their replication.
- A part of the capsid (in the case of nonenveloped viruses) or envelope (in the case of enveloped viruses) binds to a specific receptor or receptors on the host cell to initiate entry of the virus into the cell.
- The interaction of viruses with cells can result in:
  - Acute cytolytic infection with production of new virus particles resulting in killing of the host cells
  - Chronic or persistent infection
  - Latency
  - Transformation
- In the productive replication cycle, the sequential stages are attachment (adsorption), entry (penetration) into the cytosol, uncoating, synthesis of viral macromolecules (mRNA, proteins and genomes), assembly of new viral particles, morphogenesis and release.
- In latency, the virus persists as its genome, with limited expression of selected viral genes, sometimes as RNA only.
- In viral transformation, the virus persists as its genome, with expression of selected viral proteins that induce the host cell to behave like a tumour cell.

Viruses are totally dependent on the cells they infect to provide the energy, metabolic intermediates and most (in some cases all) of the enzymes required for their replication. With advances in the techniques of molecular virology, crystallography and modelling, together with the classical methods of electron microscopy, titration and biochemical assay, it has become possible to study virus–cell interactions at a sophisticated level. The picture that has emerged, and is still emerging, is a fascinating one as viruses are found to associate with, and affect, cells in a wide variety of ways. The outcomes of virus–cell interaction that have clinical relevance are:

1. Acute cell death. Viruses infect and replicate within cells causing the cells to lyse when the progeny virions are released. This is called a *cytolytic cycle*; the infection is productive and the cell culture demonstrates cytopathic effects, which are often characteristic of the infecting virus. The host cells are termed *permissive*.
2. Chronic or persistent infection. In this instance viruses are produced from the infected cells, but the cells are not killed by the process: that is, the infection is productive but non-cytolytic and may become persistent.
3. Latency. Virus is present within cells, but there is no virus replication and progeny viruses are not produced by the infected cell. The virus is maintained within the cell in the form of DNA, which replicates in association with the host cell DNA. The host cell is termed *nonpermissive* and retains its normal properties, and the infection is nonproductive.
4. Transformation. Again, cells are infected with virus, but there is no virus replication. However, viral proteins interfere with the normal cellular controls over cell division, and the cell exhibits many of the properties of a tumour cell.

THE CYTOLYTIC OR CYTOCIDAL GROWTH CYCLE

Although there are large differences in the details of the lytic growth cycle depending on the virus studied, and to some extent on the host cell, certain features are common. In the early part of the cycle, virus particles come into contact with the cells and may then attach or adsorb to them. The virion then enters or penetrates into the host cell and is partially uncoated to reveal the viral genome. Macromolecular synthesis of viral components follows.

This can often be divided into early and late phases separated by the replication of the viral nucleic acid. Early messenger RNA (mRNA) is first transcribed and translated into proteins. These are frequently non-structural proteins and enzymes required to undertake nucleic acid synthesis and the later stages of replication. Viral nucleic acid is then produced, followed by late mRNA transcription and translation. Most proteins synthesised at this stage are structural ones and will make up part of the final virion. This phase ends with the assembly and release of newly formed virus particles. The cycle can vary from as little as 8 hours for some picornaviruses to >40 hours for human cytomegalovirus, a herpesvirus.

ATTACHMENT (ADSORPTION)

The initial interaction is by random collision and depends on the relative concentrations of virus particles and cells. Adsorption then takes place through specific binding sites on the virus (the viral ligands) and viral receptors on the plasma membrane of the cell. It is important to note that viruses have evolved to take advantage of molecules that exist on the cell surface and that have functions other than to act as a viral receptor. Viruses vary widely in the range of cells to which they can adsorb, depending on the nature of the sites to which they attach and how widespread they are among cells of different types, tissues and species. The presence of the receptor determines whether the cell will be susceptible to the virus, but the cells must also be permissive; that is, for successful production of new virions, they need to contain the range of intracellular components required by the virus for its replication. The ability of a virus to enter and replicate in a particular cell type is called tissue or cell tropism.

Many cellular receptors are protein in nature, but they can also be composed of carbohydrate or lipid. There is considerable interest in identifying receptors for particular viruses, as the attachment step is a potential target for antiviral therapy and could aid in the understanding of viral pathogenesis. Specific receptors for selected viruses have been described but have frequently been disputed. Newer techniques involving monoclonal antibodies, molecular cloning and gene transfer have helped to resolve these issues. It has become apparent that more than one type of receptor molecule may be required by the majority of viruses to complete the entry stage of the replication cycle. Indeed it is likely that there is a complex interaction between different functional domains of the virus and several receptor arrays. First there is the true attachment step whereby the virus binds to the cell receptor, and then entry itself may involve a further set of receptors called coreceptors or postbinding receptors, acting either in succession or in parallel. These interactions frequently

induce conformation changes in the surface proteins of the virus, exposing hidden domains that are required for the entry step (see next section). This more complicated view of the initial contact between the virus and the cell suggests that the primary binding receptor may not be the only determinant of tropism. In Table 7.1, examples of viruses whose cellular receptors have been identified are shown.

ENTRY (PENETRATION)

Entry occurs immediately after attachment and, unlike adsorption, requires energy and does not occur at 0°C. The speed of this stage of the replication cycle varies among different viruses, some penetrating into cells in less than a second and others taking several minutes. In

Table 7.1 Examples of viral receptors and coreceptors

Virus	Receptor
Coxsackievirus A21	CD55 (decay-accelerating protein), ICAM-1
Epstein–Barr virus	CD21 (complement receptor), HLA Class II, various integrins
Foot and mouth disease virus	Sialic acid, various integrins
Hepatitis B virus	Sodium taurocholate cotransporting polypeptide (NTCP)
Hepatitis C virus	CD81, SR-B1, Claudin 1, Occludin
Herpes simplex virus type 1	Heparan sulfate, herpesvirus entry-mediator A, nectin 1 and 2, various integrins
Human immunodeficiency virus type 1	CD4, chemokine receptors (CCR5, CXCR4)
Influenza virus A	Sialic acid
Lassa virus	β-dystroglycan
New World haemorrhagic fever arenaviruses	Transferrin receptor 1
Parvovirus B19	Erythrocyte P antigen
Rabies virus	Nicotinic acetylcholine receptor, CD56 (neuronal cell adhesion molecule), low-affinity nerve growth factor receptor
Respiratory syncytial virus	Heparan sulfate, ICAM-I
Rhinovirus	ICAM-I (majority of strains), low-density lipoprotein receptor (minority of strains)
Rotavirus	Sialic acid, various integrins, heat shock protein 70
Severe acute respiratory syndrome coronavirus	Angiotensin-converting enzyme 2

CD, cluster of differentiation; *HLA*, human leukocyte antigen; *ICAM*, intercellular adhesion molecule.

addition, the efficiency of the process varies from 50% of attached viruses entering successfully to <0.1%. Entry is complex, and, despite much study, it is still not clear exactly what the steps are for the majority of viruses.

For viruses with envelopes, penetration is accomplished by membrane fusion catalysed by fusion proteins in the viral envelope. Receptors with adsorbed virus move together (patch) to pits coated with clathrin before moving into the cytosol to form small uncoated vesicles, which then fuse together as endosomes. Viral entry via endocytosis can be independent of clathrin and dependent instead on caveolae or lipid rafts. These are areas of the membrane that are rich in cholesterol and sphingolipids. Penetration into the cytosol occurs through the endoplasmic reticulum.

For many nonenveloped viruses, the mechanism by which they deliver their genomes across the host cell membrane in the absence of fusion is poorly understood. Recent findings indicate that such viruses may undergo programmed conformational changes following attachment, resulting in capsid disassembly and the release of small membrane-interacting peptides. These breach the membrane, thus allowing the viral genome to enter the cell.

UNCOATING

Uncoating refers to the process whereby the viral genome is released into the cell. This can take place at several stages and sites in the cell and, generally, is not a well-understood process. Some viruses undergo conformational changes on attachment that result in the opening of the capsid and release of selected viral proteins and viral nucleic acid into the cell. Endosomes formed from enveloped viruses that enter by receptor-mediated endocytosis may fuse to lysosomes within the cell cytoplasm, and the resultant low pH in the endolysosome results in dissolution of the viral capsid. Uncoating can also take place in the cytosol or at the nuclear membrane.

The final step in the complex uncoating process involves transport of the capsid (or the viral genome with, in some instances, viral enzymes and proteins) to the correct site in the cell to commence synthesis of the macromolecules that will comprise the new virions. Although details are not available for many viruses, it is clear that microtubules and microtubule-dependent motors are frequently involved in the transport. Some viruses stay in the cytosol for the remainder of their replication (e.g., poliovirus), but others proceed towards the nucleus where they are uncoated at the nuclear membrane before entry into the nucleus (e.g., herpesviruses) or enter the nucleus intact (e.g., papillomaviruses). Targeting to the nucleus depends on nuclear localisation sequences found on the surface of the capsids. To gain access to the nucleus, the virus or its genome can either enter when the cell is undergoing mitosis (when the nuclear membrane is temporarily absent) or, more commonly, be delivered directly into the nucleoplasm though nuclear pore complexes.

SYNTHESIS OF VIRAL COMPONENTS

The nucleic acid in viruses is either single or double stranded, circular or linear, in one piece or segmented. In addition, viruses vary enormously in their complexity, ranging from those with nucleic acid sufficient to code for only a few proteins, such as the papillomaviruses, up to those coding for several hundred proteins, such as the poxviruses. Although every virus has a unique method of replicating and has a strict temporal control on the synthesis of components, each must present functional mRNA to the cell, so that new virally encoded polypeptides and nucleic acid can be synthesised using the normal cellular processes. Thus, only viruses that contain DNA and replicate in the nucleus can use solely cellular enzymes for transcription and translation. All other viruses must synthesise their mRNA by processes other than those found in uninfected cells. In 1970, Baltimore described a classification system for viruses, based on the nature of their genome and the ways in which each virus group replicates its genome and generates mRNA for translation into viral proteins. The Baltimore classification now has seven different classes, six of which were in the original scheme (Fig. 7.1). Conventionally, in the scheme, nucleic acid of the same polarity or sense as mRNA is called positive (+), and that of the opposite polarity or antisense is called negative (−). Rather than be exhaustive, one or two illustrative examples from each class will now be described.

Class 1: Double-stranded DNA viruses

This comprises a very large group of viruses that contain double-stranded DNA in a linear form (e.g., herpesviruses, adenoviruses and poxviruses) or a circular form (e.g., papillomaviruses). The poxviruses can be separated from the others, as their replication takes place entirely in the cytoplasm, and they can code for all the factors required for their own transcription and genomic replication. In the remaining double-stranded DNA viruses, replication occurs in the nucleus and is dependent to some extent on host cell factors. Herpes simplex virus is used as an example.

After uncoating at the nuclear pore, the viral nucleic acid enters the nucleus, and, using the normal host cell mechanisms of transcription and translation, three groups of viral polypeptides are synthesised in a strict temporal fashion. They are called immediate early (α), early (β) and late (γ). A component in the virus particle

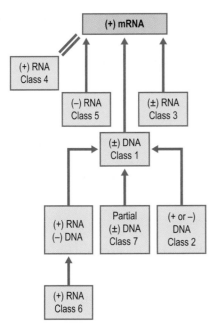

Fig. 7.1 Division of animal viruses into seven classes, based on mechanisms of transcription.

(α-transcription initiation factor [α-TIF], a γ protein), acting as a transactivator, induces the transcription of the first set of mRNAs. A second component of the viral tegument called virion host shut-off protein (VHS) inhibits host cell macromolecular synthesis, and all the metabolic energy of the cell is turned towards the production of new virus particles. Among the early gene products are thymidine kinase and a virus-specific DNA polymerase. Most of the late proteins are structural proteins that inhibit the synthesis of the α and β proteins. Between β and γ protein synthesis, new viral DNA begins to be made, probably by circularisation using a rolling circle model.

Class 2: Single-stranded DNA viruses

Parvoviruses comprise the sole family in this group. They are small, with DNA of up to around 5 kilobases. Parvoviruses use the cellular DNA polymerases to make the viral genome double stranded, called the replicative form. Messenger RNAs are made using the appropriate DNA strand as the template and are translated into viral proteins.

Class 3: Double-stranded RNA viruses

This group includes the reoviruses and rotaviruses. All members have segmented genomes, and each RNA segment codes for a single polypeptide. Replication of viral

nucleic acid, transcription and translation occur solely in the cytoplasm without nuclear involvement at any stage. Each infectious virus carries its own RNA-dependent RNA polymerase, an enzyme unique to some RNA viruses and not found in uninfected cells. It enables the transcription of one strand (–) into mRNAs, which are subsequently translated into viral proteins. The transcription is thus asymmetric and conservative—that is, only mRNAs are formed and the parental duplex is not broken apart. Each mRNA is later encapsidated and copied once to form double-stranded molecules. Thus the replication of the double-stranded DNA and RNA viruses is very different.

Class 4: + single-stranded RNA viruses

This class comprises a large group of viruses containing RNA of the same polarity as mRNA. Because they code for all the proteins required during replication, the viral RNA extracted from the virions is infectious by itself. Poliovirus falls into this category and is used as an example. Macromolecular synthesis of viral components occurs entirely in the cytoplasm.

After entry of poliovirus into the cell, the viral RNA binds to ribosomes, acts as mRNA and is translated in its entirety into one large polypeptide. This is then proteolytically cleaved to give the products RNA polymerase and protease enzymes and new capsid proteins. Using the polymerase enzyme, –-stranded RNA is synthesised with the genomic RNA as the template, and a temporary double-stranded RNA is formed, called the replicative intermediate. When the – strands are ready, they can be used as templates to make more +-stranded RNA. This is required as genomic RNA for assembly into new virus particles and for transcription into more viral proteins.

At the same time as viral replication, host cell protein synthesis and RNA synthesis are inhibited. Initiation of translation of cellular mRNA requires the participation of a cap-binding protein at the 5′ end. Poliovirus induces the cleavage of this protein and thus halts the synthesis of cellular proteins. The RNA genome of poliovirus does not have such a cap, but the secondary structure of the mRNA forms an internal ribosomal entry site (IRES) so that it can attach to a ribosome.

Class 5: – single-stranded RNA viruses

Viruses of this group have single-stranded RNA of – polarity and must carry their own RNA transcriptase complex to be infectious, as the normal cellular enzymes are unable to replicate their RNA. Influenza virus is an example. It contains eight segments of –-stranded RNA, plus the RNA transcriptase complex within each virus particle.

After entry into the cell by receptor-mediated endocytosis, transcription to viral mRNA occurs in the nucleus.

Influenza virus is the only −-stranded RNA virus to replicate in the nucleus. To initiate transcription, a nucleotide sequence of about 10–13 bases, found at the 5′ end of the cellular mRNAs and already capped, is used. This is cleaved from cellular mRNAs by an endonuclease activity of the viral RNA transcriptase complex. Thus, all the viral mRNAs have a 5′-terminal segment of the host cell mRNA.

Once the mRNAs have been generated, they are translated into polypeptides. Unlike the transcription of mRNAs, the production of +-stranded RNAs, required as intermediates to make the progeny −-stranded RNAs, proceeds without the need for primers.

There is much trafficking of viral polypeptides in the cell; the haemagglutinin, neuraminidase and M_2 protein are inserted in the plasma membrane, and the M_1 protein below this point on the membrane, whereas the nucleocapsid assembles around the viral RNAs in the nucleus.

Class 6: Retroviruses

Viruses of this group are unique as they contain single-stranded + RNA (in the form of two identical subunits), yet they replicate via an integrated double-stranded DNA stage. Retroviruses are the only such family, and the virus particles contain a reverse transcriptase complex, with RNA-dependent DNA polymerase activity, from which the name *retrovirus* is derived. This enzyme is not found in uninfected cells.

After entry, synthesis of DNA complementary to the viral RNA occurs using the reverse transcriptase, originating at a primer binding site near the 5′ end of the viral genome. The primer is a specific transfer RNA (tRNA) and varies from one retrovirus to another (e.g., tRNAlys in HIV). In addition to RNA-dependent DNA polymerase activity, the reverse transcriptase complex has ribonuclease (RNase) H activity—that is, it is able to digest RNA from a DNA–RNA hybrid. The resulting single-stranded DNA is then made double stranded, using the reverse transcriptase as enzyme and starting from a purine-rich sequence. Thus, a linear double-stranded DNA form is produced, first found in the cytoplasm. The linear double-stranded DNA is able to circularise and is found in this form in the nucleus.

The next step is integration of the circular DNA into the host cell DNA. This is catalysed by an integrase enzyme carried by the virion. It is thought that the circular viral DNA is cleaved, leaving staggered ends, and the cellular DNA similarly, to allow insertion of the viral DNA into the cellular DNA; the viral DNA is now called a provirus. The site of insertion is not thought to be specific. The integrated state is a stable one and, as the DNA of the cell is replicated during cell growth, so the viral DNA is also replicated.

The replication cycle is completed using the normal cellular RNA polymerase II to synthesise viral RNA and

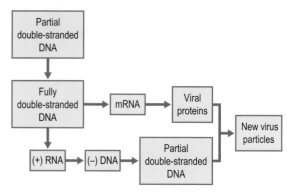

Fig. 7.2 Diagram of hepatitis B virus replication.

viral mRNAs, which are translated into polyproteins and processed into the final proteins found in the virus particle. A viral protease is responsible for many of these cleavages. The control of this stage is complex.

Class 7: Partial double-stranded DNA viruses

Hepadnaviruses are unique among the animal viruses in containing partial double-stranded DNA and replicating via an RNA intermediate, as shown in Fig. 7.2. One example of this group is hepatitis B virus.

The first stage in the replication cycle is the production, in the nucleus, of fully double-stranded DNA, followed by the synthesis of single-stranded positive-sense mRNA molecules encoding the individual viral proteins, plus a full-length RNA copy of the genome, known as the pre-genome, using the cellular DNA-dependent RNA polymerase. The mRNAs are transported into the cytoplasm and translated into the viral proteins, including the core protein, which encapsidates the pre-genomic RNA, together with newly synthesised viral RNA-dependent DNA polymerase (reverse transcriptase). Then, using this enzyme, a complementary negative strand of DNA is made, while the RNA is degraded. The DNA is next transcribed into positive-sense DNA and is found as partial double-stranded DNA in the new virus particles.

ASSEMBLY AND RELEASE

After synthesis of viral proteins and viral nucleic acid, there is a stage of assembly called morphogenesis. Generally the components that will constitute the new virions are produced in high quantities, and the assembly process is probably rather inefficient.

Morphogenesis may occur spontaneously once the capsid proteins have been made, the specificity depending on the amino acid sequence of the proteins. Thus the structural proteins of the viruses can form capsomeres by themselves, which then aggregate to form the procapsid, a structure without nucleic acid. Often there is proteolytic cleavage of a capsid protein to form the final virus particle. Details regarding the precise nature of the interaction between the nucleic acid and the structural proteins that make up the capsid are uncertain, despite extensive study. It is possible that the viral nucleic acid is inserted into the procapsid through a pore, or it might cause a structural reorientation of the procapsid, thereby becoming internalised. Alternatively, the capsomeres may accumulate around a condensed core of nucleic acid as the nucleic acid is being synthesised. Some evidence for specific viral components or cellular proteins, called scaffolding proteins, assisting the assembly process has been obtained.

Assembly is followed by release of virus particles, the productive phase of the infection. The release is either through cell lysis, as used by many nonenveloped viruses, or through budding, in most cases without cell death, as used by many enveloped viruses. In some cases, viruses can be transferred directly from the infected cell to neighbouring cells, thus avoiding any exposure to the extracellular environment or to the immune response of the host. The transfer could be through tight junctions or at sites of synaptic contact.

Budding can take place through the plasma membrane, thus releasing the virions from the cell (e.g., orthomyxoviruses and retroviruses), or through internal membranes, such as the inner nuclear membrane in the case of the herpesviruses, followed by fusion of the vesicles containing the viruses with the plasma membrane. Envelope glycoproteins specified by the virus are synthesised by essentially the same mechanism as cellular membrane glycoproteins. The viral proteins destined to become envelope proteins contain a sequence of 15–30 hydrophobic amino acids, known as the signal sequence. This sequence binds the growing polypeptide chain to a receptor on the cytoplasmic side of the rough endoplasmic reticulum and enables its passage through the membrane. Glycosylation occurs in the lumen of the rough endoplasmic reticulum, and the proteins are transported to the Golgi apparatus. There they are further glycosylated and acylated before transport to the plasma membrane, the direction probably determined by a sorting signal in the polypeptide sequence. The viral glycoproteins are very important in terms of antigenicity as the hydrophilic domains protrude from the surface of the cell, with the N terminus being farthest away, and change the surface structure significantly. They remain anchored in the membrane via a hydrophobic domain near the carboxyl (C) terminus. After insertion into the membrane, the viral glycoproteins accumulate together to form oligomers; at the same time the host cell glycoproteins move away. At the C terminus of the viral glycoproteins, there is frequently a short hydrophilic sequence that remains inside the cell and is assumed to interact with the internal components of the virus during assembly. Lipid rafts function as microdomains for the accumulation of many viral glycoproteins and may also initiate the actual budding sequence. It is not known how the nucleocapsids are directed to the assembly site. Once there, they are engulfed by the membrane; this process requires bending of the membrane, leading to its outward curvature. The bud is completed by the fusion of the two apposing membranes, and it finally separates from the plasma membrane of the host to become a new infectious virus. For retroviruses, budding occurs by hijacking a cellular pathway that normally creates vesicles that bud into late endosomal compartments called multivesicular bodies. These viruses then exit through the plasma membrane or via exosomes. During or shortly after budding, the viral protease enzyme cleaves at specific sites within precursor proteins to produce the proteins found in the mature virus particles.

Several thousand virus particles can be produced per infected cell, although this number varies considerably with virus type and host cell type. The budding viruses tend to be released slowly over several hours, whereas the lytic ones are released together. Only a few of the newly formed virus particles are infectious, as indicated by a high ratio of particles to infectious virions. Presumably, most do not have the correct complement of proteins, enzymes or viral nucleic acid or have been assembled incorrectly.

MICROSCOPY OF INFECTED CELLS

It is possible to observe effects on the host cell microscopically. First, there may be morphological changes called inclusion bodies in the infected cell, seen by altered staining characteristics. The inclusion bodies are nuclear or cytoplasmic and vary in their composition. They can consist of viral factories in which morphogenesis occurs, crystalline arrays of virus particles ready for release, overproduction of a particular viral protein or proteins, or some aberrant cellular structure, such as clumped chromatin. Virally encoded nonstructural proteins are likely to be involved in forming the matrix of these structures and in recruiting viral components to them. Some examples of inclusion bodies are shown in Fig. 7.3. Secondly, the cells may be killed by the viral infection. There are several possible reasons for this, including factors produced by the virus that induce apoptosis. It is likely that the accumulation of viral structural proteins is toxic for the cells, in some cases. In addition, some viruses, such as herpes simplex virus and the poxviruses, inhibit host cell macromolecular synthesis from an early stage in the replication cycle, leading to structural and functional damage. Plasma

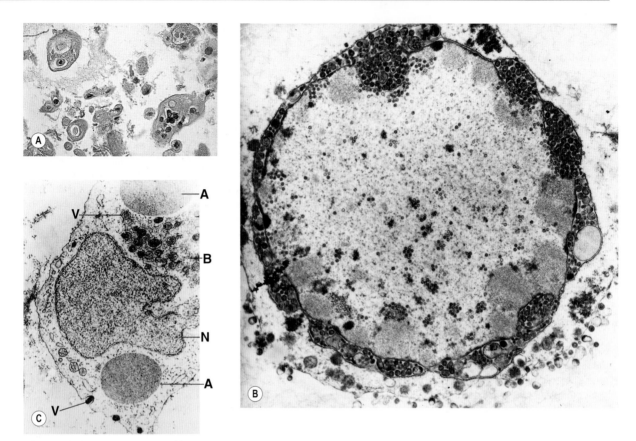

Fig. 7.3 Effects of viruses on cells. (A) Light microscopy of a skin lesion due to herpesvirus infection, showing cell fusion and intranuclear inclusions (Cowdry type A). ×60. (B) Electron micrograph of a cell infected with herpes simplex virus. Assembly of capsids within nucleus and enveloped virus between layers of nuclear membrane. ×9000. (C) Type A (accumulation of viral protein) and type B (virus factory) inclusions (identified as *A* and *B*, respectively) in the cytoplasm of a poxvirus-infected cell. *N*, the cell nucleus; *V*, virus. ×700.

membrane function and permeability change, and lysosomal membranes begin to break down, allowing leakage of the contents with degradative activity into the cytoplasm. There may also be marked effects on the cytoskeleton. These changes lead to a cytopathic effect, seen clearly in cell culture. It can take several forms, one of the most common being cell rounding and subsequent detachment from the solid surface (Fig. 7.4B). Another is the formation of a syncytium, whereby the membranes of adjacent infected cells fuse and a giant cell is formed containing many nuclei (Figs 7.3A and 7.4C). In some cases, the nuclei fuse to make hybrid cells, a property that has been exploited in monoclonal antibody production.

CHRONIC/PERSISTENT INFECTIONS

Some viruses are able to infect cells productively, but the cells are not killed by the replication process. Viruses that are released by budding frequently come into this category. The cell type used for the infection is critical, and, presumably, any inhibitory effect of the virus on the cellular metabolism does not take place. This type of interaction may lead to a chronic or persistent infection in which infected cells and viruses coexist over a long period of time. There will, however, be antigenic changes in the infected cells, often the insertion of viral glycoproteins in the plasma membrane. This in turn may lead to activation of host immune responses leading to cell death—for example, through the action of virus-specific cytotoxic T cells.

LATENCY

Latency represents a type of persistence whereby the virus is present in the form of its genome only and there is limited expression of viral genes. The genome is found either integrated into the host cell chromosome or as a circular nonintegrated episome. It is maintained throughout

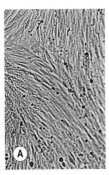 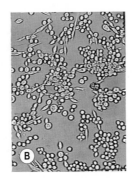 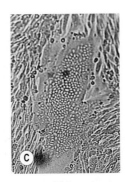

Fig. 7.4 Cytopathic effects. (A) Uninfected fibroblast cells. (B) Cell rounding due to herpes simplex virus. (C) Syncytium formation or cell fusion due to respiratory syncytial virus. All unstained. ×65.

cell division when the host cell replicates. Latent infections are more common with DNA viruses than RNA viruses, perhaps because no mechanisms exist to maintain RNA for long periods of time intracellularly. All herpesviruses are able to undergo latency, although the cellular site of latency differs among different viruses. Epstein–Barr virus persists in B lymphocytes as episomal viral DNA with limited transcription of viral genes, probably around 11 protein products being expressed. These ensure maintenance of the viral genome in dividing cells, prevent apoptosis of the host cells, and help to evade immune responses. For herpes simplex virus, latency occurs in neuronal cells with the viral genome being maintained in the nucleus as an episome. All the lytic genes are switched off, but one set of transcripts, the latency-associated transcripts (LATs), is abundantly expressed. The LATs can inhibit apoptosis and thus contribute to persistence of the virus. One clinical consequence of latency is that specific stimuli can trigger the reactivation of the virus from the latent state, such that the infection becomes productive with the appearance of new virions and the potential for causing clinical disease. The manifestations of such reactivated, or secondary, infections are often quite distinct from those of the original, or primary, infection, as they arise at anatomically distinct sites, and because by definition reactivated infections occur in a host whose immune system has prior knowledge of the pathogen and can therefore respond much more quickly, compared to the primary infection, which occurs in an immunologically naïve host.

TRANSFORMATION

In this type of virus–cell interaction, the virus infects the cell nonproductively and is found in the form of viral DNA, either integrated in the host cell DNA or unintegrated, or in both states. The properties of the cells are changed dramatically, a process called transformation. Transformed cells have similar properties to tumour cells, and a detailed study of the mechanism of viral transformation has led to increased understanding of the molecular basis of cancer. Only members of some virus families are able to transform cells. These include herpesviruses, adenoviruses, hepadnaviruses, papovaviruses and poxviruses of the DNA viruses and, of the RNA viruses, only retroviruses. The type of cell infected and the species are also important. It should be noted that transformation is a rare event: at most, only 1 in 10^5 cells infected by a particular virus will become transformed.

Some of the main properties of transformed cells that distinguish them from normal cells are listed below:

- loss of contact inhibition of growth
- can grow to high saturation density
- less requirement for serum factors
- indefinite number of cell divisions
- expression of viral antigens
- absence of fibronectin
- foetal antigens often present
- changes in agglutinability by plant lectins
- induction of tumours in experimental animals

All of the viruses that cause transformation in vitro have a similar interaction with the host cell. The initial stages are exactly as described above for the productive infections. There is attachment, entry, uncoating and, in most but not all cases, selected viral genes are expressed as proteins, giving the cell new antigenic properties. At this stage the viral nucleic acid becomes integrated in the host cell DNA, probably not at a specific site, or it circularises and is maintained in a nonintegrated episomal form in the nucleus. The association is a stable one, so that when the host cell DNA is replicated, the viral nucleic acid is also replicated and the number of viral genome copies per cell remains constant over many cell generations. Thus, transformation is a heritable alteration. Recent work in this area has concentrated on the molecular events surrounding transformation and in analysing the functions of the viral proteins found in transformed cells. Two examples of transforming viruses, one RNA and the other DNA, are described briefly below to illustrate the approaches taken. Both are associated with human tumours.

The first is human T lymphotropic or T cell leukaemia virus type I (HTLV-I), a retrovirus, which is found in CD4$^+$ T cells of patients with adult T cell leukaemia. It is able to transform CD4$^+$ lymphocytes in vitro with integration of the DNA provirus. Genetic analysis has revealed that the viral genome can code for several nonstructural proteins, including one of special interest called Tax, an oncoprotein of molecular weight 40 kDa. This protein, which has no cellular homologue, is able to activate transcription in the long terminal repeat of the integrated virus. Tax also affects the transcription of a remarkable number of cellular genes that are involved in cell cycle control and the cellular response to DNA damage. In short, it functions in a complex manner to promote cell proliferation, to accumulate DNA damage with the loss of genomic integrity, and to inhibit apoptosis. However, it is unlikely that Tax expression alone leads to the end-point of leukaemia, and further, so far unexplained,

molecular events occurring over a period of several years, are probably necessary.

The second example is human papillomavirus type 16 (HPV-16), found as integrated DNA in many cases of carcinoma of the cervix. In vitro, this virus is able to transform most types of human epithelial cells, including keratinocytes. The viral proteins responsible for transformation are the products of two genes, *E6* and *E7*, which are found in cervical tumour cells. The interaction between E6 and E7 oncoproteins and their cellular targets is required to maintain the malignant phenotype. Both proteins have multiple functions, but it is probably most important that E6 interacts with p53, and E7 with retinoblastoma protein, thereby inactivating them. As both p53 and retinoblastoma protein act as cellular growth-suppressing proteins, loss of their functions is likely to lead to transformation. In addition, integration of the viral genome normally involves the disruption of the *E2* gene, the product of which is required to stop transcription of the E6 and E7 promoters, and therefore the continued expression of the E6 and E7 proteins results. Further properties of the E6 and E7 proteins include the inhibition of apoptosis, overriding of cell cycle controls, chromosome destabilisation and, in vivo, various mechanisms to evade local immune responses.

RECOMMENDED READING

Cann, A. J. (2015). Ch. 4. (*Principles of molecular virology* (6th ed.). London: Academic Press, 105–135.

Flint, S. J., Racaniello, V., Rall, G. F., Skalka, A. M., & Enquist, L. W. (2015). *Principles of virology* (4th ed.). Washington: ASM Press.

Knipe, D. M., & Howley, P. M. (2014). Ch. 4-7. *Field's virology* (6th ed.), 87–189. Philadelphia: Lippincott Williams & Wilkins.

Marsh, M., & Helenius, A. (2006). Virus entry: open sesame. *Cell, 124*(4), 729–740.

PART 2

INFECTION AND IMMUNITY

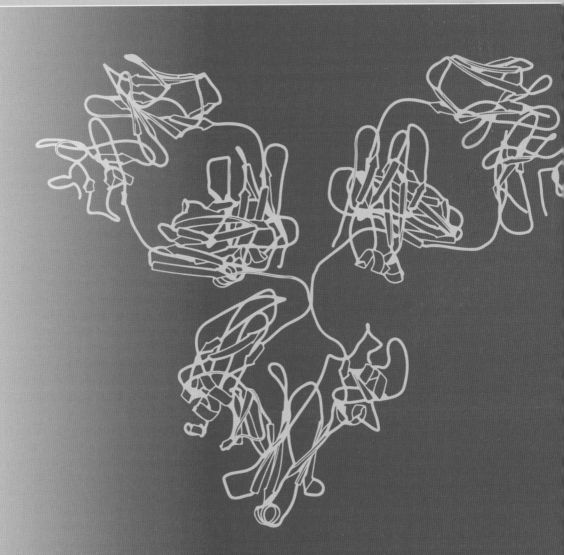

8 Innate and adaptive immunity

DAVID J. COUSINS

KEY POINTS

- The cells of the immune system are divided into lymphoid and myeloid lineages. The former include T lymphocytes and their subsets identified by CD markers, B lymphocytes and innate lymphoid cells (ILCs) including natural killer (NK) cells. The myeloid lineage includes neutrophils, eosinophils and basophils as well as monocytes/macrophages and dendritic cells.
- Innate immunity depends on physical, physiological and chemical barriers to infection, on the response to injury and on detection of pathogen-associated molecular patterns (PAMPs) by pattern recognition receptors (PRRs). Phagocytic cells and the enzyme cascade known as complement are key effectors responding to PAMPs and components of acute inflammation.
- Adaptive immunity depends on specific recognition of antigens, either directly by antibodies on the surface of B cells or through presentation of processed antigens in the context of MHC molecules by host cells to T cells. In contrast to innate immunity, on reexposure the responses are faster, more vigorous and more specific.
- Lymphocytes are activated by antigen and the appropriate combination of cytokines, signalling molecules secreted by other lymphocytes and by macrophages.
- Humoral adaptive immunity leads to antigen–antibody complexes that neutralise key aspects of microbial activity, either directly or through the activation of complement, opsonisation and directed cytotoxicity.
- Cell-mediated immunity generates cytotoxic T lymphocytes (CD8⁺), which directly kill cells containing intracellular pathogens, and helper T cells (CD4⁺), which secrete cytokines that stimulate other effector aspects of immunity.

INNATE AND ADAPTIVE IMMUNITY

The biosphere includes a few hundred different microbes that have been associated with human infections and many thousands more that have not. The majority of symptomatic infections (see Ch. 11) are of limited duration and leave little permanent damage. This is due largely to the immune system.

The immune system is split into two functional divisions. Innate immunity is the first line of defence against infectious agents, and most potential pathogens are checked before they establish an overt infection. If these defences are breached the adaptive immune system is called into play. Adaptive immunity produces a specific response to each infectious agent, and the effector mechanisms generated normally eradicate the offending material. Furthermore, the adaptive immune system remembers the infectious agent and can prevent it causing disease later (immunological memory).

THE IMMUNE SYSTEM

The immune system consists of a number of organs and several different cell types. Most cells of the immune system—tissue cells and white blood cells or leucocytes—develop from pluripotent stem cells in the bone marrow. These haemopoietic stem cells also give rise to red blood cells or erythrocytes. The production of leucocytes is through two main pathways of differentiation, the lymphoid and myeloid pathways (Fig. 8.1).

Lymphoid cells

The lymphoid lineage, which makes up around 20% of the white blood cell population in the blood, produces T lymphocytes and B lymphocytes and innate lymphoid cells (ILCs), including natural killer (NK) cells. Different lymphocyte cell types express different cell surface molecules; these distinguish different cell types and

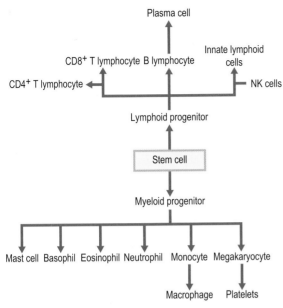

Fig. 8.1 Cells of the immune system. NK, natural killer.

Table 8.1	Major T lymphocyte markers	
Marker	Distribution	Proposed function
CD2	All T cells	Adherence to target cell
CD3	All T cells	Part of T cell antigen-receptor complex
CD4	Helper subset (Th)	MHC class II-restricted recognition
CD8	Cytotoxic subset (Tc)	MHC class I-restricted recognition
CD19	All B cells	Part of B cell receptor complex

CD, Cluster of differentiation; *MHC*, major histocompatibility complex.

identify cells at different stages of differentiation. The cell surface molecules have been named by the CD (cluster of differentiation) system and are identified using specific fluorescently labelled monoclonal antibodies. Some major lymphocyte markers are listed in Table 8.1.

Myeloid cells

The myeloid pathway gives rise to mononuclear phagocytes (monocytes, macrophages and dendritic cells) and granulocytes (basophils, eosinophils and neutrophils), as well as platelets and mast cells.

Mononuclear phagocytes

The common myeloid progenitor in the bone marrow gives rise to monocytes, which circulate in the blood and migrate into organs and tissues to become macrophages or dendritic cells. Monocytes are larger than lymphocytes and usually have a kidney-shaped nucleus. This actively phagocytic cell has a ruffled membrane and many cytoplasmic granules. These lysosomes contain enzymes and molecules that are involved in the killing of microorganisms. Mononuclear phagocytes adhere strongly to surfaces and have various cell membrane receptors to aid the binding and ingestion of foreign material.

Granulocytes

Granulocytes are short-lived cells (days) compared to long-lived macrophages (months or years). They are classified as neutrophils, eosinophils and basophils on the basis of their Giemsa staining patterns. The mature forms have a multilobed nucleus and many granules. Neutrophils constitute 60%–70% of the leucocytes in the blood, but also migrate into tissues in response to injury or infection.

Neutrophils. These are the most abundant circulating granulocyte. Their granules contain numerous microbicidal molecules, and the cells enter the tissues when a chemotactic factor is produced, as the result of infection or injury.

Eosinophils. Eosinophils are present in low numbers in a healthy individual (1%–2% of leucocytes), but their numbers rise in certain allergic conditions and parasitic infections. The granule contents can be released by the appropriate signal, and the cytotoxic molecules can then kill parasites.

Basophils. These cells are infrequent in the circulation (<0.2%) and have certain characteristics in common with tissue mast cells. Both cell types have receptors on their surface for the Fc portion of immunoglobulin (Ig) E, and cross-linking of this immunoglobulin by antigen leads to the release of various mediators that stimulate an inflammatory response.

INNATE IMMUNITY

The healthy individual is protected from potentially harmful microorganisms in the environment by a number of effective mechanisms that do not depend upon prior exposure to any particular microorganism. These innate defence mechanisms show broad specificity and are effective against a wide range of potentially infectious agents. The characteristics and constituents of innate and adaptive immunity are shown in Table 8.2.

FEATURES OF INNATE IMMUNITY

The components of the innate immune system recognise structures that are unique to microbes. These include complex lipids and carbohydrates such as peptidoglycan, lipopolysaccharides, lipoteichoic acid and mannose-containing oligosaccharides found in many microbial surface molecules (see Ch. 2). Other microbe-specific molecules include the double-stranded RNA found in replicating viruses and unmethylated CpG sequences in bacterial DNA. Therefore, the innate immune system is able to recognise non-self structures and react appropriately but does not recognise self structures, thus avoiding autoimmunity. The microbial products recognised by the innate immune system, known as pathogen-associated molecular patterns (PAMPs), are essential for survival of the microorganisms and cannot easily be discarded or mutated. Different classes of microorganism express different PAMPs that are recognised by different pattern recognition receptors (PRRs) on host cells (Table 8.3). One group of PRRs are the Toll-like receptors (TLRs), which are expressed on different cell types that are components of the innate immune system, including macrophages, dendritic cells, neutrophils, mucosal epithelial cells and endothelial cells. Recognition of microbial components by these receptors leads to a variety of outcomes, including cytokine release, inflammation and cell activation.

Innate defences act as the initial response to microbial challenge and can eliminate the microorganism from the host. However, many microbes have evolved strategies to overcome innate defences, and in this situation the more potent and specialised adaptive immune response is required to eliminate the pathogen. The innate immune system plays a critical role in the generation of an efficient and effective adaptive immune response. Cytokines produced by the innate immune system signal that infectious agents are present and influence the type of adaptive immune response that develops.

MECHANISMS OF INNATE IMMUNITY

Mechanical barriers and surface secretions

The intact skin and mucous membranes of the body provide a high degree of protection against pathogens; however, when the skin is damaged infection can be a serious problem. The skin is a resistant barrier because of its outer layer consisting mainly of keratin, which is indigestible by most microorganisms, and thus shields the epidermis from microorganisms and their toxins. The relatively dry

Table 8.2 Characteristics and determinants of innate and adaptive immunity

Innate immunity	Adaptive immunity
Broad specificity	Specific
No change with repeat exposure	Memory
Mechanical barriers	
Bactericidal substances	
Eubiotic microbiota	
Humoral	
Acute-phase proteins	Antibody
Interferons	
Lysozyme	
Complement	
Cell mediated	
Innate lymphoid cells/natural killer cells	T lymphocytes
Phagocytes	

Table 8.3 Examples of pathogen-associated molecular patterns (PAMPs) and pattern recognition receptors (PRRs) in innate immunity

PAMP	Source	PRR	Response
Sugars (mannose)	Microbial glycoproteins and glycolipids	Mannose receptors	Phagocytosis
		Mannose-binding protein	Complement activation
		Lectin-like receptors	Phagocytosis
N-formylmethionyl peptides	Bacterial protein synthesis	N-formylmethionyl peptides receptors	Chemotaxis and phagocyte activation
Phosphorylcholine	Microbial membranes	C-reactive protein	Complement activation
Lipoarabinomannan	Yeast cell wall	Toll-like receptor 2	
Lipoteichoic acid	Gram-positive bacterial cell wall	Toll-like receptor 2	Macrophage activation
Lipopolysaccharide	Gram-negative bacterial cell wall	Toll-like receptors 4 and 2	Cytokine production
Unmethylated CpG nucleotides	Bacterial DNA	Toll-like receptor 9	
dsRNA	Replicating viruses	Toll-like receptor 3	Type 1 interferon production

dsRNA, Double-stranded ribonucleic acid.

condition of the skin and the high concentration of salt in drying sweat are also inhibitory or lethal to many microorganisms. The sebaceous secretions and sweat of the skin contain bactericidal and fungicidal fatty acids, which constitute an effective protective mechanism against many potential pathogens.

The sticky mucus covering the respiratory tract acts as a trapping mechanism for inhaled particles. The action of cilia sweeps the secretions, containing the foreign material, towards the oropharynx so that they are swallowed and destroyed in the stomach. Nasal secretions and saliva contain mucopolysaccharides capable of blocking some viruses.

The washing action of tears and flushing of urine are effective in stopping invasion by microorganisms. The commensal microorganisms that make up the natural bacterial microbiota covering epithelial surfaces are also protective in a number of ways:

- Their very presence occupies a niche that cannot be used by a pathogen.
- They compete for nutrients.
- They produce by-products that can inhibit the growth of other organisms.

It is important not to disturb the relationship between the host and its indigenous microbiota (see Ch. 11).

Commensal organisms from the gut or bacteria normally present on the skin can cause problems if they gain access to an area that they do not normally populate. An example of this is urinary tract infection resulting from the introduction of *Escherichia coli*, a gut commensal, by means of a urinary catheter. Some commensal organisms possessing low virulence can cause infection because the innate defences are breached, for example by surgery or medical treatment, and are termed *opportunistic pathogens*.

Humoral defence mechanisms

A number of microbicidal substances are present in the tissue and body fluids. Some of these molecules are produced constitutively (e.g., lysozyme), and others are produced in response to infection (e.g., acute-phase proteins and interferon). These molecules all show the characteristics of innate immunity: there is no recognition specific to the microorganism and the response is not enhanced on reexposure to the same antigen.

Lysozyme

This is a basic protein of low molecular weight found in macrophages and neutrophils as well as in several tissue fluids, such as tears, saliva and mucus. It functions to damage bacterial cell walls by degrading peptidoglycan leading to lysis. The presence of layers external to peptidoglycan (e.g., the Gram-negative and mycobacterial outer membranes) protects against lysozyme in many cases. The action of other enzymes from phagocytes or of complement may remove this protection.

Basic polypeptides

A variety of basic proteins, derived from tissues and blood cells, have antibacterial properties. This group includes the basic proteins spermine and spermidine. Other toxic compounds include the arginine- and lysine-containing proteins protamine and histone. The bactericidal activity of basic polypeptides probably depends on their ability to react nonspecifically with acid polysaccharides at the bacterial cell surface.

Acute-phase proteins

The concentration of certain proteins found in blood rises dramatically during an infection; these are known as *acute-phase proteins* and monitoring them is often of diagnostic and prognostic value (see Ch. 63). Microbial products such as endotoxin can stimulate macrophages to release IL-1, which stimulates the liver to produce increased amounts of various acute-phase proteins. One well-characterised example is C-reactive protein; this binds to phosphorylcholine residues in the cell wall of certain microorganisms and activates the classical complement pathway. Also included in this group are α_1-antitrypsin, α_2-macroglobulin, fibrinogen and serum amyloid A protein, all of which act to limit the spread of the infectious agent or stimulate the host response.

Interferon

The observation that cell cultures infected with one virus resist infection by a second virus (viral interference) led to the identification of the family of antiviral agents known as *interferons*. A number of molecules have been identified; α- and β-interferons (see also Ch. 5) are part of innate immunity, and interferon-γ is produced by T cells as part of the adaptive immune response.

Complement

The existence of a heat-labile serum component with the ability to lyse red blood cells and destroy Gram-negative bacteria has been known since the 1930s. Complement is composed of a large number of different serum proteins present in low concentration in normal serum. These molecules are present in an inactive form but can be activated to form an enzyme cascade.

Approximately 30 proteins are involved in the complement system, some of which are enzymes, some are control molecules and others are structural proteins with no enzymatic activity. A number of the molecules involved are split into two components (a and b fragments) by the product of the previous step. There are three main pathways of complement activation, the classical, lectin and alternative that lead to the same physiological consequences:

- opsonisation
- cellular activation
- lysis.

The three pathways are initiated differently. Cleavage of C3 forms the connection between the pathways, and the binding of this molecule to a surface is the key process in complement activation.

The *classical pathway* is initiated by the binding of two or more of the globular domains of the C1q component of C1 to its ligand: immune complexes containing IgG or IgM and certain microorganisms and their products. This causes a conformational change in the C1 complex that leads to the autoactivation of C1r. The enzyme C1r then converts C1s into an active serine esterase that acts on the thioester-containing molecule C4 to produce C4a and a reactive C4b (Fig. 8.2). C4a is released, and some of the C4b becomes attached to a surface. C2 binds to the surface-bound C4b, becomes a substrate for the activated C1 complex, and is split into C2a and C2b. The C2b is released, leaving C4b2a—the classical pathway C3 convertase. This active enzyme then generates C3a and the unstable C3b from C3. A small amount of the C3b generated binds to the activating surface and acts as a focus for further complement activation. Activation of the classical pathway is regulated by C1 inhibitor and by a number of molecules that limit the production of the C3 convertase.

The *lectin pathway* is initiated by mannose-binding lectin (MBL) or mannose-associated serine proteases (MASPs) attaching to the surface of a microorganism. This leads to the production of C4b2a and the generation of C3b on the activating surface.

The *alternative pathway* is initiated by low-level intrinsic C3 hydrolysis to generate C3b. This molecule complexes, in the presence of Mg^{2+} ions, with factor B, which is then acted on by factor D to produce C3bBb. This is a C3 convertase, which is capable of splitting more C3 to C3b, some of which will become membrane bound.

The initial binding of C3b generated by either the classical or the alternative pathway leads to an amplification loop that results in the binding of many more C3b molecules to the same surface. Factor B binds to the surface-bound C3b to form C3bB, the substrate for factor D—a serine esterase—which is present in very low concentrations in an already active form. The cleavage of factor B results in the formation of the C3 convertase, C3bBb, which dissociates rapidly unless it is stabilised by the binding of properdin (P), forming the complex C3bBbP. This convertase can cleave many more C3 molecules, some of which become surface bound. This amplification loop is a positive feedback system that will cycle until all the C3 is used up unless it is regulated carefully.

Regulation

The nature of the surface to which the C3b is bound regulates the outcome. Self cell membranes contain a number of regulatory molecules that promote the binding of factor H rather than factor B to C3b. This results in the inhibition of the activation process. On non-self structures the C3b is protected, as regulatory proteins are not present, and factor B has a higher affinity for C3b than factor H at these sites.

Thus the surface of many microorganisms can stabilise the C3bBb by protecting it from factor H. In addition, another molecule, properdin, stabilises the complex. The deposition of a few molecules of C3b on to these surfaces is followed by the formation of the relatively stable C3bBbP complex. This C3 convertase will lead to more C3b deposition. Immune complexes composed of certain immunoglobulins (e.g., IgA and IgE) also function as protected sites for C3b and activate complement by the alternative pathway. Poor activation surfaces are made more susceptible to deposition by the presence of antibody that generates C3b by the classical pathway.

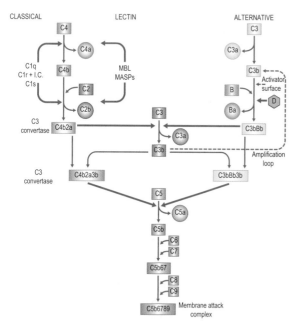

Fig. 8.2 Complement activation: classical and alternative pathways. Enzymatic reactions are indicated by thick *arrows*. *I.C.*, immune complex.

Membrane attack complex (MAC)

The next step after the formation of C3b is the cleavage of C5 (Fig. 8.3). The C5 convertases are generated from C4b2a of the classical and lectin pathways and C3bBb of the alternative pathway by the addition of another C3b molecule. These membrane-bound trimolecular complexes selectively bind C5 and cleave it to give fluid-phase C5a and membrane-bound C5b. The formation of the rest of the membrane attack complex is nonenzymatic. C6 binds to C5b, and this joint complex is released from the C5 convertase. The formation of C5b67 generates a hydrophobic complex that inserts into the lipid bilayer in the vicinity of the initial activation site. C8 and C9 bind to the membrane-inserted complex in sequence, resulting in the formation of a lytic polymeric complex containing up to 20 C9 monomers.

Functions

The complete insertion of the MAC into a cell will lead to membrane damage and lysis, probably by osmotic swelling. Some thin-walled pathogens, such as trypanosomes and malaria parasites, are killed by complement-mediated lysis. Some Gram-negative bacteria can be killed by complement in conjunction with lysozyme. However, complement-mediated lysis is of limited importance as a bactericidal mechanism compared with phagocyte destruction of bacteria. Phagocytic cells have receptors for certain complement components that facilitate the adherence of complement-coated particles. Therefore, complement is an opsonin, and in certain circumstances, this attachment may lead to phagocytosis. C3a and C5a are anaphylatoxins and trigger mast cells and basophils to release mediators of inflammation (see later in the chapter). They also stimulate neutrophils to produce reactive oxygen intermediates, and C5a acts directly on vascular endothelium to cause vasodilatation and increased vascular permeability.

Innate immune cells

Phagocytes

Microorganisms entering the tissue fluids or bloodstream are rapidly engulfed by neutrophils and mononuclear phagocytes. In the blood, the latter are known as *monocytes*, whereas in the tissues they differentiate into *macrophages*. These cells are actively phagocytic and contain digestive enzymes to degrade ingested material intracellularly within specialised vacuoles. They are also important sensor cells that link innate and adaptive immune mechanisms via the production of inflammatory mediators.

For phagocytic cells to be effective, they must be attracted to the site of infection. Once they have passed through the capillary walls they move through the tissues in response to a concentration gradient of molecules produced at the site of damage. These chemotactic factors include:

- cytokines and chemokines released from injured tissue
- factors from the blood (C5a)
- substances produced by neutrophils and mast cells (leukotrienes and histamine)
- bacterial products (formyl-methionine peptides).

During an inflammatory response, neutrophils move rapidly to the site of injury and are followed by monocytes that then differentiate into macrophages.

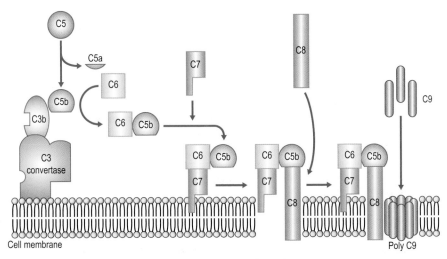

Fig. 8.3 Membrane attack complex.

Phagocytosis

Phagocytosis involves recognition and binding, ingestion and digestion. Phagocytes have receptors on their surface that mediate the attachment of particles coated with the correct ligand to facilitate binding. These include receptors for the Fc portion of certain immunoglobulin isotypes (see later in the chapter) and for components of the complement cascade. The presence of these molecules, or opsonins, on the particle surface markedly enhances the ingestion process. Whether mediated by specific receptors or not, the foreign particle is surrounded by the cell membrane, which then invaginates and produces an endosome or phagosome within the cell. The microbicidal machinery of the phagocyte is contained within organelles known as *lysosomes*. This compartmentalisation of potentially toxic molecules is necessary to protect the cell from self-destruction and produce an environment where the molecules can function efficiently. The phagosome and lysosome fuse to form a phagolysosome in which the ingested material is killed and digested by various enzyme systems.

Ingestion is accompanied by enhanced glycolysis and an increase in the synthesis of proteins and membrane phospholipids in the phagocyte. After phagocytosis, there is a respiratory burst consisting of a steep rise in oxygen consumption. This is accompanied by an increase in the activity of a number of enzymes and leads to the reduction of molecular oxygen to various highly reactive intermediates, such as the superoxide anion (O_2^-), hydrogen peroxide (H_2O_2), singlet oxygen ($O^\cdot$) and the hydroxyl radical ($OH^\cdot$). All of these chemical species have microbicidal activity. The superoxide anion is a free radical produced by the one-electron reduction of molecular oxygen; it is very reactive and highly damaging to animal cells, as well as to microorganisms. It is also the substrate for superoxide dismutase, which generates hydrogen peroxide for subsequent use in microbial killing. Myeloperoxidase uses hydrogen peroxide and halide ions, such as iodide or chloride, to produce at least two bactericidal systems. In one, halogenation (incorporation of iodine or chlorine) of the bacterial cell wall leads to death of the organism. In the second mechanism, myeloperoxidase and hydrogen peroxide damage the cell wall by converting amino acids into aldehydes that have antimicrobial activity.

Within phagocytes, there are several other mechanisms that can destroy ingested material. Some of these enzymes can damage membranes. For example, lysozyme and elastase attack peptidoglycan of the bacterial cell wall, and then hydrolases are responsible for the complete digestion of the killed organism. The cationic proteins of lysosomes bind to and damage bacterial cell walls and enveloped viruses, such as herpes simplex virus. The iron-binding protein lactoferrin has antimicrobial properties.

It complexes with iron, rendering it unavailable to bacteria that require iron for growth. The high acidity within phagolysosomes (pH 3.5–4.0) may have bactericidal effects, probably resulting from lactic acid production in glycolysis. In addition, many lysosomal enzymes, such as acid hydrolases, have acid pH optima. There are significant differences between macrophages and neutrophils in the killing of microorganisms. Although macrophage lysosomes contain a variety of enzymes, including lysozyme, they lack cationic proteins and lactoferrin. Tissue macrophages do not have myeloperoxidase but probably use catalase to generate the hydrogen peroxide system. Normal macrophages are less efficient killers of certain pathogens, such as fungi, than neutrophils. Once killed, most microorganisms are digested and solubilised by lysosomal enzymes.

Natural killer (NK) cells

NK cells recognise changes on virus-infected cells and destroy them by an extracellular killing mechanism. They express a variety of innate receptors that can recognise cellular stress and changes in the level of various major histocompatibility complex (MHC) class I molecules when cells are infected with certain viruses. If the NK cell binds to an uninfected host cell the presence of normal levels of MHC class I molecules leads to inhibition of the killing mechanisms. However, certain viruses, such as herpesviruses, evade the adaptive immune system by interfering with the production of MHC class I molecules. This leads to a reduced level of MHC class I molecules on the infected cell membrane, and therefore killing mechanisms are activated. NK cells have also been implicated in host defence against cancers by a mechanism similar to that used to combat virus infection.

Recently, several new types of innate cell that are related to NK cells have been discovered, termed *innate lymphoid cells* (ILCs). They are believed to reside in tissues and act as early sentinels of tissue damage and rapidly produce inflammatory mediators. They have been classified into three groups by the effector cytokine profile that they produce. ILC1s express IFNγ (and include classical NK cells), ILC2s express IL-5 and IL-13 and are believed to play a role in immunity to helminths, and ILC3s express IL-17 and function in antifungal immunity.

Eosinophils

Eosinophils are granulocytes with a characteristic bilobed nucleus and cytoplasmic granules. They are present in the blood of normal individuals at very low levels (<1%), but their numbers increase in patients with parasitic infections and allergies. Large parasites such as helminths cannot be internalised by phagocytes and therefore must be killed extracellularly. Eosinophils are not efficient phagocytic cells, although their granules contain an array of enzymes and toxic molecules active against parasitic worms. The release of these molecules must be controlled so that tissue damage is avoided. The eosinophils have specific receptors including Fc and complement receptors that bind the labelled target (i.e., antibody or complement-coated parasites). The granule contents are then released into the space between the cell and the parasite, thus targeting the toxic molecules onto the parasite membrane.

Inflammation

A number of the above factors and cell types are responsible for the process of acute inflammation. This is the reaction of the body to injury, such as invasion by an infectious agent, exposure to a noxious chemical or physical trauma. The signs of inflammation are redness, heat, swelling, pain and loss of function. The molecular and cellular events that occur during an inflammatory reaction are:

- vasodilatation
- increased vascular permeability
- cellular infiltration.

These changes are brought about mainly by chemical mediators (Table 8.4), which are widely distributed in a sequestered or inactive form throughout the body and are released or activated locally at the site of inflammation. After release, they tend to be inactivated rapidly, to ensure control of the inflammatory process.

There is increased blood supply to the affected area owing to the action of vasoactive amines, such as histamine and 5-hydroxytryptamine, and other mediators stored within mast cells. Other mediators, such as bradykinins and prostaglandins, are produced locally or released by platelets. The vasodilatation causes increased blood supply to the area, giving rise to redness and heat. The result is an increased supply of the molecules and cells that can combat the agent responsible for the initial trigger.

The same molecules, vasoactive amines, prostaglandins and kinins, increase vascular permeability, allowing plasma and plasma proteins to traverse the endothelial lining. The plasma proteins include immunoglobulins and molecules of the clotting and complement cascades. This leaking of fluid causes swelling (oedema), which in turn leads to increased tissue tension and pain. Some of the molecules themselves, for example prostaglandins and histamine, stimulate the pain responses directly. The inflammatory exudate has several important functions. Bacteria often produce tissue-damaging toxins that are diluted by the exudate. The presence of clotting factors results in the deposition of fibrin, creating a physical obstruction to the spread of bacteria. The exudate is drained continuously by the lymphatic vessels, and antigens, such as bacteria and their toxins, are carried to the draining lymph node where immune responses can be generated.

The production of chemotactic factors, including C5a, histamine, leukotrienes and molecules specific for certain cell types, attracts phagocytic cells to the site. The increased vascular permeability allows easier access for neutrophils and monocytes, and the vasodilatation means that more cells are in the vicinity. The neutrophils arrive first and begin to destroy or remove the offending agent. Mononuclear phagocytes arrive on the scene to finish off the removal of the residual debris and stimulate tissue repair.

The inflammatory process continues until the conditions responsible for its initiation have been resolved. In most circumstances, this occurs fairly rapidly, with an acute inflammatory reaction lasting for a matter of hours. If, however, the causative agent is not easily removed or is reintroduced continuously, chronic inflammation will ensue and the adaptive immune response will be initiated.

ADAPTIVE IMMUNITY

Microorganisms that overcome or circumvent the innate nonspecific defence mechanisms or are administered

Table 8.4 Mediators of inflammation

Mediator	Main source	Function
Histamine	Mast cells, basophils	Vasodilatation, increased vascular permeability, contraction of smooth muscle
Kinins (e.g., bradykinin)	Plasma	Vasodilatation, increased vascular permeability, contraction of smooth muscle, pain
Prostaglandins	Neutrophils, eosinophils, monocytes, platelets	Vasodilatation, increased vascular permeability, pain
Leukotrienes	Neutrophils, mast cells, basophils	Vasodilatation, increased vascular permeability, contraction of smooth muscle, induction of cell adherence and chemotaxis
Complement components (e.g., C3a, C5a)	Plasma	Cause mast cells to release inflammatory mediators; C5a is a chemotactic factor
Plasmin	Plasma	Breaks down fibrin, kinin formation
Cytokines	Lymphocytes, macrophages	Chemotactic factors, colony-stimulating factors, macrophage activation

deliberately (i.e., active immunisation) come up against the host's second line of defence: adaptive immunity. Adaptive immunity develops when specific molecules of the invading microorganism, termed *antigens,* come into contact with cells of the adaptive immune system (B and T lymphocytes) and initiate an immune response specific to the foreign material. An antigen is any substance capable of provoking a specific immune reaction in the host; however, antigens are usually large (>5000 Da) and the response is not to the entire molecule but to individual regions termed *epitopes*. Many antigens are protein molecules; however, peptides, polysaccharides and lipids can also be recognised by specific antigen receptors. The specific B cell antigen receptors are antibodies or immunoglobulins (Ig) and the T cell antigen receptors are called *T cell receptors* (TCRs). The cells that respond to a particular antigen are precommitted to respond to an individual epitope on the antigen. The adaptive response takes two forms, humoral and cell mediated, which usually develop in parallel. The part played by each depends on a number of factors, including the nature of the antigen, the route of entry and the individual who is infected. Humoral immunity depends on the appearance in the blood of antibodies produced by differentiated B cells termed *plasma cells*. Cell-mediated immunity depends mainly on the development of T cells that are specifically responsive to the inducing agent.

Specific immunity may be adaptive in two main ways:

1. induced by overt clinical infection or inapparent clinical infection
2. deliberate artificial immunisation.

This is active adaptive immunity, and contrasts with passive adaptive immunity, which is the transfer of preformed antibodies to a nonimmune individual by means of blood, serum components or lymphoid cells.

Actively adaptive immunity is long-lasting, although it may be circumvented by antigenic change in the infecting microorganism. Passively adaptive immunity provides only temporary protection. Passive immunity may be transferred to the foetus by the passage of maternal antibodies across the placenta.

ANTIBODIES

There are five distinct classes or isotypes of immunoglobulins: IgG, IgA, IgM, IgD and IgE. They differ from one another in terms of size, charge, carbohydrate content and function. All antibody molecules have the same basic four-chain structure composed of two light chains and two heavy chains (Fig. 8.4). The light chains (molecular weight 25,000 Da) are one of two types designated κ and λ, and

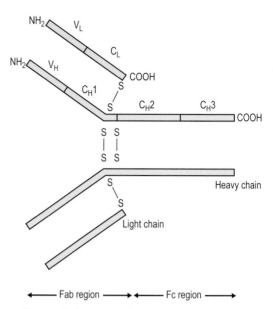

Fig. 8.4 Basic structure of an immunoglobulin molecule.

only one type is found in any one antibody molecule. The heavy chains vary in molecular weight from 50,000 to 70,000 Da, and it is these chains that determine the isotype. They are designated α, δ, ϵ, γ and μ for the respective classes of immunoglobulin. The individual chains are held together by disulphide bridges and noncovalent interactions. Individual light chains are comprised of two distinct immunoglobulin domains of approximately 110 amino acids. One end of the chain is identical in all members of the same type and is termed the *constant region of the light chain, C_L*. The other end shows considerable sequence variation and is known as the *variable region, V_L*. The heavy chains are also split into domains of approximately the same size, the number varying between the five types of heavy chain. One of these domains will show considerable sequence variation (V_H), whereas each of the others (C_H) are identical for the same domain of the same isotype. The tertiary structure generated by the combination of the V_L and V_H regions determines the antigen specificity. The variability in amino acid sequence in V_L and V_H regions is not found over their entire length but is restricted to short segments. These segments show considerable variation and are termed *hypervariable regions*. Hypervariable regions contain the residues that make direct contact with the antigen and are referred to as *complementarity determining regions*. In both light and heavy chains, there are three complementarity determining regions that, in combination, form the antigen binding site. The differences seen in the Fc region of the various heavy chains are responsible for the different biological activities of the antibody isotypes.

IgG

This is the major immunoglobulin of serum, making up 75% of the total and having a molecular weight of 150,000 Da in humans. Four subclasses are found in humans—IgG1, IgG2, IgG3 and IgG4—that differ in their relative concentrations, amino acid composition, number and position of interchain disulphide bonds, and biological function. IgG is the major antibody of the secondary response (see later in the chapter) and is found in both the serum and tissue fluids.

IgA

There are two subclasses of IgA: IgA1 and IgA2. In humans, most of the serum IgA occurs as a monomer, but in many other mammals it is found mostly as a dimer held together by a J chain. In the dimeric form, secretory IgA (sIgA) is the predominant antibody class in seromucous secretions such as saliva, tears, colostrum, and at mucosal-epithelial surfaces.

IgM

IgM is a pentamer of the basic unit with μ heavy chains and a single J chain. Because of its large size, this isotype is confined mainly to the intravascular pool and is the first antibody type to be produced during an immune response.

IgD

Many circulating B cells have IgD present on their surface, but IgD accounts for <1% of the circulating antibody. It is composed of the basic unit with δ heavy chains. The protein is very susceptible to proteolytic attack and therefore has a very short half-life in serum.

IgE

IgE is present in extremely low levels in serum. However, it is found on the surface of mast cells and basophils, which possess a receptor specific for the Fc part of this molecule (FcεR1).

Antibody diversity

An individual must have the capacity to produce an extremely large number of different antibodies to cope with the vast array of different antigens present in the environment. The antibody repertoire is the total number of antibody specificities in an individual and in humans is at least 10^{11}. This diversity is brought about through several processes.

1. Both heavy and light chain immunoglobulin gene loci contain multiple gene segments that are rearranged during B-cell development. In particular, the variable regions of light chains are produced by the joining of two separate gene segments, the *variable* (*V*) gene segment and the joining (J) segment in VJ recombination. The variable regions of heavy chains are even more complex including a further gene rearrangement in between V and J known as the diversity (D) segment in VDJ recombination.
2. Any light chain can join with any heavy chain to produce a different antigen specificity.
3. In mature B cells, further variation in antigen specificity is obtained via somatic hypermutation.

Mature antigenically naïve B cells express membrane-bound IgM. When first stimulated by antigen, some progeny will develop into plasma cells expressing secreted IgM, whereas others will switch to produce antibody of a different class such as IgG. However, the immunoglobulin produced will have the same variable domain and therefore bind to the same antigen.

Antibody function

The primary function of an antibody is to bind the antigen that induced its formation. Apart from cases where this results in direct neutralisation (e.g., inhibition of toxin activity or of microbial attachment), other effector functions must be generated. The binding of antigen is mediated by the Fab portion, and the Fc region controls the biological defence mechanisms. However, for every antibody of the same isotype, the heavy-chain constant domains are the same, and they therefore all perform the same functions.

T cell receptor

Unlike B cell antibodies, which recognise intact soluble or surface microbial antigens, T cells recognise specific peptide fragments associated with MHC molecules presented by antigen-presenting cells. The T cell antigen receptor is a heterodimer composed of an α and β or a γ and δ chain. Each chain contains a variable and constant domain, a transmembrane portion and cytoplasmic tail. The variable domains of the two chains fold to form an antigen-binding site. The majority of T cells use the α–β heterodimer in antigen recognition, and γ–δ T cells are prevalent in the gut mucosa. The T cell receptor is the molecule that is responsible for the recognition of specific MHC–antigen complexes and is different for every T cell. Genetic rearrangements of germline genes, similar to those seen in B cell immunoglobulins, produce functional T cell receptors. CD3 is present on all T cells and is noncovalently linked to the T cell receptor. The

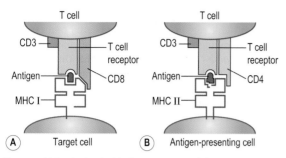

Fig. 8.5 Molecules involved in T cell recognition. (A) Antigen fragments that associate with class I molecules are recognised by T cells that have the CD8 molecule. (B) Antigen fragments that associate with MHC class II are recognised by T cells that have the CD4 molecule on their surface.

CD3 complex is involved in signal transduction, leading to cell activation, when a ligand binds to the T cell receptor. CD4 and CD8 are coreceptor molecules that are expressed on different subsets of T cells. CD4$^+$ve T cells recognise peptide in the context of MHC class II, and CD8$^+$ T cells recognise peptide bound to MHC class I (Fig. 8.5).

TISSUES INVOLVED IN ADAPTIVE IMMUNE REACTIONS

For the generation of an immune response, antigen must interact with and activate a number of different cells and these cells must interact with one another. The cells involved in immune responses are organised into tissues and organs collectively referred to as the *lymphoid system,* which comprises lymphocytes, epithelial and stromal cells. Lymphoid organs contain lymphocytes at various stages of development and are classified into primary and secondary lymphoid organs. The primary lymphoid organs are the major sites of lymphopoiesis. Here, lymphoid progenitor cells develop into mature lymphocytes by a process of proliferation and differentiation. In mammals, T lymphocytes develop in the thymus and B lymphocytes in the bone marrow and foetal liver. It is within the primary lymphoid organs that the lymphocytes acquire their repertoire of specific antigen receptors in order to cope with the antigenic challenges that the individual receives during its life. It is also within these tissues that self-reactive lymphocytes are eliminated to protect against autoimmune disease.

The secondary lymphoid organs create the environment in which lymphocytes can interact with one another and with antigen, and then disseminate the effector cells and molecules generated. Secondary lymphoid organs include lymph nodes, spleen and mucosa-associated lymphoid tissue (e.g., tonsils and Peyer's patches of the gut).

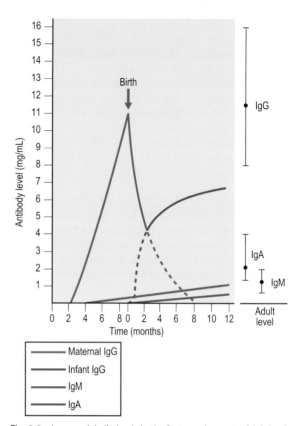

Fig. 8.6 Immunoglobulin levels in the foetus and neonate. Adult levels of the major isotypes are shown as normal ranges with mean serum levels.

DEVELOPMENT OF THE IMMUNE SYSTEM

In humans, lymphoid tissue appears first in the thymus at about 8 weeks of gestation. Peyer's patches are distinguishable by the fifth month, and immunoglobulin-secreting cells appear in the spleen and lymph nodes at about 20 weeks. From this time onwards, IgM and IgD are synthesised by the foetus (Fig. 8.6). At birth the infant has a blood concentration of IgG comparable to that of the maternal circulation, having received IgG (but not IgM) via the placenta. The rate of synthesis of IgM in the infant increases rapidly within the first few days of life but does not reach adult levels until about a year. Serum IgG does not reach adult levels until after the second year, and IgA takes even longer. From birth, there is a drop in the level of IgG due to the decay of maternal antibody, with the lowest levels of total IgG at around 3 months of age. This corresponds to an age of marked susceptibility to a number of infections. Cell-mediated immunity can be stimulated at birth, but these reactions may not be as powerful as in the adult.

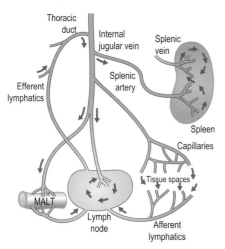

Fig. 8.7 Lymphocyte recirculation. *MALT,* mucosa-associated lymphoid tissue.

LYMPHOCYTE TRAFFICKING

Lymphocytes differentiate and mature in the primary lymphoid organs and then enter the blood lymphocyte pool. B cells are produced in the bone marrow and mature there before proceeding via the circulation to the secondary lymphoid organs. T cell precursors leave the bone marrow and mature in the thymus before migrating to the secondary lymphoid organs. Once in the secondary lymphoid tissues, lymphocytes move from one lymphoid organ to another through the blood and lymphatics (Fig. 8.7). One of the main advantages of this lymphocyte recirculation is that during the course of a natural infection the continual trafficking of lymphocytes enables many different lymphocytes to have access to the antigen. Only a very small number of the lymphocytes will recognise a particular antigen.

Pathogens can enter the body by many routes, but must be carried from the site of infection to the secondary lymphoid tissues. If the infection is in the tissues, antigen is carried in the lymphatics to the draining lymph node either in the fluid or by macrophages and dendritic cells. Blood-borne antigens are trapped in the spleen. The passage of lymphocytes through an area where antigen has been localised facilitates the induction of an immune response. Lymphocytes with appropriate receptors bind to the antigen and become activated. Once activated, the lymphocytes mature into effector cells. In the case of B lymphocytes, they become plasma cells and secrete antibody. T lymphocytes leave the secondary lymphoid tissue and return to the site of infection to destroy the infectious agent via direct cytotoxic activity (CD8$^+$ve cells) or by providing T-cell help to other effector cells (CD4$^+$ve cells).

The lymphocytes reactive to any particular antigen are only a small proportion of the total pool. Therefore, antigen binds to the small number of cells that can recognise it and selects them to proliferate and mature so that sufficient cells are formed to mount an adequate immune response. A cell that responds to an antigenic trigger and proliferates will give rise to cells with a genetically identical makeup (i.e., clones). This phenomenon is therefore known as *clonal selection.*

INITIATION OF ADAPTIVE RESPONSES

The first steps in the initiation of adaptive immune responses require the activation of the antigen-specific B cells or T cells. This process can be broadly classified into two categories based on the nature of the antigen, one that does not require T cell help (thymus independent) and the other that does (thymus dependent).

Thymus-independent antigens

A number of antigens will stimulate specific immunoglobulin production directly. These T-independent antigens are of two types: mitogens and certain large molecules. Mitogens are substances that cause cells, particularly lymphocytes, to undergo cell division (i.e., proliferation). Lipopolysaccharide (LPS) is an example of a B cell mitogen. Some large molecules with regularly repeating epitopes, for instance polymers of D-amino acids and simple sugars such as pneumococcal polysaccharide and dextran, can interact directly with the B cell surface immunoglobulin. They may also be held on the surface of specialised macrophages, in secondary lymphoid tissues, and the B cells interact with them there. The multiple repeats of the epitope interact with a large number of surface immunoglobulin molecules and a signal that is generated is sufficient to stimulate antibody production. The immune response generated tends to be similar on each exposure; that is, IgM is the main antibody and the response shows little memory.

Thymus–dependent antigens

Many antigens do not stimulate antibody production without the help of T lymphocytes. These antigens first bind to the B cell, which must then be exposed to T cell–derived cytokines before antibody can be produced. For the second activation signal (i.e., help) to be targeted effectively at the B cell, the T and B cells must be in close contact. However, T cells only recognise antigen that has been processed and presented in association with MHC class II. T-dependent responses rely on CD4$^+$ T cells known as T-follicular helper (Tfh) cells and their products (e.g., IL-4, IL-21) to control the antibody class, affinity

Table 8.5 Antigen-presenting cells in the lymph nodes		
Area	Antigen-presenting cell	Antigen
Subcapsular marginal sinus	Marginal zone macrophage	T-independent antigens
Follicles and B cell areas	Follicular dendritic cells	Antigen–antibody complexes
Medulla	Classical macrophages	Most antigens
T cell areas	Interdigitating/myeloid dendritic cells	Most antigens

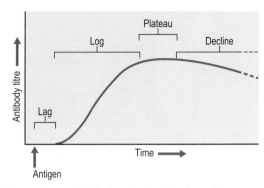

Fig. 8.8 Pattern of antibody production following antigen exposure.

and memory. All this happens within a germinal centre of a lymph node secondary follicle that has evolved to facilitate the necessary cellular and molecular interactions.

Antigen processing and presentation

The development of an antibody response to a T-dependent antigen requires that the antigen becomes associated with MHC class II molecules (i.e., processed) and expressed on the cell surface (i.e., presented) in a form that helper T cells can recognise.

All cells express MHC class I molecules, but class II molecules are confined to cells of the immune system, the antigen presenting cells (APCs). These cells present antigen to MHC class II–restricted T cells (CD4⁺), and therefore play a key role in the induction and development of immune responses. Within lymph nodes, different APCs are found in each of the main areas (Table 8.5). In primary responses to antigen the main professional APCs are macrophages and dendritic cells (DCs); however, in secondary responses, memory B cells can engulf specific antigen and present it to T cells via MHC class II.

T cell activation

The activation of resting CD4⁺ T cells requires two signals. The first is antigen in association with MHC class II molecules, and the second is the costimulatory signal. The second signal is delivered by the same APC that gave the first signal. The costimulatory signal is mediated by the interaction of a molecule on the APC engaging with its receptor on the T cell. The best characterised pairing is B7 (CD80) on the APC and CD28 on the T cell, although there are numerous other costimulatory molecules. When both of these signals are generated, biochemical changes occur within the T cell, leading to RNA and protein synthesis. The T cells progress through the cell cycle from the G_0 to the G_1 phase. The cells start to express IL-2 receptors and produce IL-2, a T cell growth factor that causes the expansion of the responsive T cell population and generation of a large number of antigen-specific CD4⁺ T cells.

The other main type of T lymphocyte is the CD8⁺ T cell. Antigen recognition by these cells is restricted by MHC class I molecules. Again, these cells require two signals to be activated: (1) antigen fragment in association with MHC class I and (2) the costimulatory signal. A cell that 'sees' both of these signals responds by clonal expansion and differentiation into a fully active effector T cell.

HUMORAL IMMUNITY – SYNTHESIS OF ANTIBODY

On exposure to antigen, antibody production follows a characteristic pattern (Fig. 8.8). There is a lag phase during which antibody cannot be detected. This is the time taken for the interactions described earlier to take place and for antibody to reach a level that can be measured. There is then an exponential rise in the antibody level or titre. This log phase is followed by a plateau with a constant level of antibody, when the amount produced equals the amount removed. The amount of antibody then declines, owing to the clearing of antigen–antibody complexes and the natural catabolism of the immunoglobulin.

If the response is to a T-dependent antigen, the B cells can switch to the production of another isotype; for example, in a primary response IgM gives way to IgG production. This process is under the control of T cells, as the class of antibody produced depends on signals from the T cell. At some point, again under the control of T cells, a proportion of the antigen-reactive cells develop into memory cells. These cells react if the epitope is encountered again.

There are a number of differences in the reaction profile on second and subsequent exposures to an antigen compared with the primary response (Fig. 8.9). There is a shortened lag and an extended plateau and decline. The level and affinity of antibody produced are much increased, and antibody is mostly of the IgG isotype. Some IgM is generated, but it will follow the same pattern as in the primary response.

CELL-MEDIATED IMMUNITY

Specific cell-mediated responses are mediated by the two different types of T lymphocyte, CD4$^+$ T-helper cells and CD8$^+$ cytotoxic T cells. As described earlier, CD4$^+$ T-helper cells bind antigen in the context of MHC class II and secrete effector cytokines when activated by professional APCs. T-helper cells and their effector cytokines orchestrate the process of cell-mediated immunity by providing instruction to other cell types of both the innate and adaptive immune systems. Specific T-helper cell phenotypes have been identified based on the effector cytokines that they produce (Table 8.6).

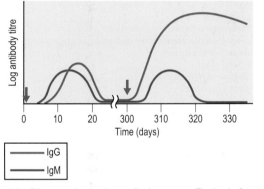

Fig. 8.9 Primary and secondary antibody response. The level of serum IgM and IgG detected with time after primary immunisation (day 0) and challenge (day 300) with the same antigen. Arrows indicate points of primary and secondary immunisation.

These T-helper cell subtypes differentiate in response to signals from APCs and develop to combat different types of pathogen. They secrete cytokines upon antigen-specific activation to recruit, activate and regulate various effector cells. Cytokines are biologically active molecules released by specific cells that elicit a particular response from other cells on which they act. A number of these regulatory molecules are shown in Table 8.7. The responses caused by these substances are varied and interrelated.

CD8$^+$ cytotoxic T cells (Tc cells) can recognise and kill cells infected with viruses and intracellular microbes via identification of antigenic peptides in the context of MHC class I, which is expressed by all cell types. When a target cell is recognised the CD8$^+$ cytotoxic T cell releases its granule contents in the direction of the target cell. The granules contain perforin and granzymes A, B and C. Perforin has homology to complement C9 and forms pores in the target cell membrane. These pores allow entry of the granzymes that are serine proteases and activate endogenous caspases and induce apoptosis of the target cell. Cyotoxic T cells can also kill target cells using the membrane protein FasL, which binds to the death receptor Fas on the target cell to induce apoptosis. NK cells use similar mechanisms to induce killing of target cells; however, the recognition mechanisms are different. NK cells use a variety of activating and inhibitory receptors to identify infected or stressed cells via altered expression of MHC molecules on the target cell. NK cells can also identify target cells because of their expression of CD16, which is a low affinity receptor for IgG. Hence, antibody-coated infected cells can be targeted via antibody-dependent cell-mediated cytotoxicity.

Table 8.6	T-helper cell subsets				
CD4$^+$ T cell subset	Inducing cytokines	Transcription factors	Effector cytokines	Target cells	Role in disease
Th1	IL-12 IFNγ	T-bet	IFNγ TNFα	Macrophage	Immunity to intracellular pathogens Autoimmune disease
Th2	IL-4	GATA3	IL-4 IL-5 IL-13	B cell Eosinophil Epithelial cell	Immunity to extracellular parasites Allergy, asthma
Th17	IL-23 IL-6 IL-1β TGFβ	RORγt	IL-17A IL-17F IL-22	Neutrophil	Immunity to extracellular microbes and fungi Inflammatory bowel disease
Treg	TGFβ IL-2	FOXP3	TGFβ IL-10	T-helper cell Many others	Immune suppression
Tfh	IL-6 IL-21 IL-27 IL-12	BCL6, IRF4, BATF	IL-4 IL-10 IL-21	B cell	B cell activation and isotype switching Induction of B cell memory

Table 8.7 Examples of some cytokines that are of importance in the immune system

Cytokine	Main source	Target	Main effects
IL-1	Macrophages Endothelial cells Some epithelial cells	T lymphocytes Tissue cells	Fever Inflammation T cell activation Macrophage activation Stimulates acute-phase protein production
IL-2	T lymphocytes	T lymphocytes NK cells B lymphocytes	T cell proliferation
IL-4	Th2/Tfh cells Mast cells	B lymphocytes T lymphocytes Mast cells	Stimulates proliferation, differentiation and class switch in B cells Differentiation and proliferation of T_H2 cells Mast cell growth
IL-8	Macrophages Endothelial cells	Neutrophils	Chemotaxis
IL-13	Th2 cells	Macrophages	Inhibits macrophage activation
IL-17	ILC2s Th17 cells ILC3s	Epithelial cells Epithelial cells Keratinocytes	Mucus production Chemokine release Neutrophil recruitment
TNF-α	Macrophages T lymphocytes	Macrophages Tissue cells	Fever Inflammation Macrophage activation Stimulates acute-phase protein production Kills certain tumour cells
Type I IFN (α and β)	Virus-infected cells	Tissue cells	Antiviral effect Induction of MHC class I Antiproliferative effects Activation of NK cells
IFNγ	Th1 cells ILC1/NK cells	Leucocytes and tissue cells	Macrophage activation Induction of MHC class I and II Antibody class switch Antiviral effect
GM-CSF	T lymphocytes Macrophages Endothelial cells Fibroblasts	Immature and committed progenitor cells in bone marrow	Stimulates growth and differentiation of myelomonocytic cells Macrophage activation

Many of the molecules detailed above act synergistically to produce their biological effects.

IL, Interleukin; *TNF*, tumour necrosis factor; *IFN*, interferon; *ILC*, innate lymphoid cell; *GM-CSF*, granulocyte–macrophage colony-stimulating factor; *NK*, natural killer; *MHC*, major histocompatibility complex.

Regulatory T cells

T-helper cells control the immune response by producing cytokines that direct other effector cell types. However, the effector response cannot continue indefinitely and an excessive response can cause tissue damage. Therefore, the immune system has numerous mechanisms in place to regulate or suppress responses. Regulatory T cells (Tregs) are $CD4^+$ antigen-specific cells that function to down-regulate immune response via several mechanisms including the secretion of the cytokines IL-10 and TGFβ.

RECOMMENDED READING

Abbas, A. K., & Janeway, C. A. (2000). Immunology: improving on nature in the twenty-first century. *Cell, 100*(1), 129–138.

Abbas, A. K., Lichtman, A. H., & Pillai, S. (2015). *Cellular and molecular immunology* (8th ed.). Philadelphia: Saunders.

Murphy, K., & Weaver, C. (2017). *Janeway's immunobiology* (9th ed.). London: Garland Science.

Websites

British Society for Immunology. Available at www.immunology.org.

Cytokines and Cells. Available at http://www.cells-talk.com.

9 Immunity in infection

DAVID J. COUSINS

KEY POINTS

- The immune response to microbes contributes both to the protection from as well as the damage (immunopathology) associated with infection.
- In viral infection, interferons provide a key innate defence and their overall effect is to inhibit viral replication.
- Antibodies act on extracellular viruses to prevent establishment of infection. In view of their intracellular replication, viruses are particularly targeted by cell-mediated immunity.
- Many of the symptoms and signs of virus infection reflect immune responses to viral antigens (immunopathology) rather than direct damage due to viral replication.
- Many viral infections induce a temporary immune suppression rendering the host susceptible to bacterial infection, whereas others such as HIV produce a more permanent effect.
- There are many vaccines that protect against viral infections. Smallpox has been eradicated by vaccination, and other eradications are feasible.
- In bacterial infection, phagocytosis and complement activation are key innate defences associated with acute inflammation.
- Antibodies are effective against the bacterial cell surface and extracellular virulence factors such as toxins. Cell-mediated immunity is essential for defence against intracellular bacteria.
- Parasites cause disease by diverse mechanisms including mechanical damage, physiological disturbance, tissue destruction and immunopathology.
- Some parasitic worm infestations are associated with raised levels of IgE and eosinophilia. These responses provide protection.
- Pathogens may evade immune responses by seclusion away from the immune system, by antigenic variation, by acquiring host-derived molecules or by immunosuppression.

IMMUNITY IN INFECTION

The host response to an invading pathogen depends on the characteristics of the infectious agent and where it is encountered. As discussed in the previous chapter the host uses a vast array of defence mechanisms that work in a concerted manner to eliminate the pathogen. The type of invading organism broadly determines the nature of the host response; the response to viral infection is quite different to the response to bacteria, which in turn is different to the response to larger parasites. In this chapter, we will describe the general characteristics of each class of infection. It is important to remember, however, that the precise response to a particular pathogen will have unique characteristics.

IMMUNOPATHOLOGY

Immunity was first recognised as a resistant state that followed infection. However, some forms of immune reaction can produce severe and occasionally fatal immunopathology. These are known as hypersensitivity reactions and result from an excessive or inappropriate response to an antigenic stimulus. The mechanisms underlying these deleterious reactions are those that normally eradicate foreign material, but for various reasons the response leads to a disease state. When considering each of the four hypersensitivity states it is important to remember this fact and consider the underlying defence mechanism and how it has given rise to the observed immunopathology. Various classifications of hypersensitivity reactions have been proposed; probably the most widely accepted is that of Coombs and Gell (Table 9.1).

THE RESPONSE TO VIRAL INFECTIONS

Interferons

At the time of the discovery of interferon in 1957, the term *interferon* (IFN) was used to identify a factor produced

Table 9.1 Coombs and Gell classification of hypersensitivity reactions

Hypersensitivity reaction	Mediators	Example diseases
Type I: Immediate, allergic	IgE Mast cells	Allergy/atopy Asthma Anaphylaxis
Type II: Cytotoxic, antibody dependent	IgG or IgM Complement Membrane attack complex (MAC)	Haemolytic anaemia Goodpasture's syndrome Grave's disease
Type III: Immune complex disease	IgG Neutrophils	Systemic lupus erythematosus (SLE) Acute proliferative glomerulonephritis Serum sickness
Type IV: Delayed, cell mediated	T cells	Multiple sclerosis Hashimoto's thyroiditis Mantoux test

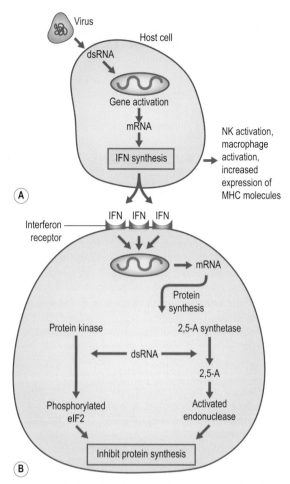

Fig. 9.1 Mechanisms of (A) induction of synthesis of interferon (IFN)α and IFNβ, and (B) inhibition of viral replication. *dsRNA*, double-stranded ribonucleic acid; *mRNA*, messenger RNA; *2,5-A*, 2′,5′-oligoadenylate; *MHC*, major histocompatibility complex; *NK*, natural killer cells; *eIF*, eukaryotic initiation factor.

by cells in response to viral infection that protected other cells of the same species from attack by a wide range of viruses. It is now clear that this activity is mediated by members of a family of regulatory proteins.

In humans, as in a number of other species, there are three classes of IFN:

1. Type I: The IFNα family (12 genes) and IFNβ (1 gene)
2. Type II: IFNγ (one gene)
3. Type III: The IFNλ family (three genes), also known as IL-28A, IL-28B and IL-29.

Type I IFNs can be produced by most cells in response to the presence of viruses and certain intracellular bacteria. Extracellular double-stranded viral RNA is detected by toll-like receptors (TLRs), whereas intracellular dsRNA is detected by RIG-I and MDA-5, all of which can induce type I IFN expression. IFNγ, which has an extensive role in the control of immune responses, is produced by activated T lymphocytes and innate lymphoid cells including natural killer (NK) cells (see Ch. 8).

IFNα and IFNβ share a common receptor composed of two chains (IFNAR1 and IFNAR2), whereas IFNγ binds to its own specific receptor, also composed of two chains (IFNGR1 and IFNGR2). The antiviral activity is mediated by the IFN released from a virus-infected cell binding to a neighbouring cell and inducing the synthesis of antiviral proteins (Fig. 9.1). IFNs can inhibit many stages of the virus life cycle—attachment and uncoating, early viral transcription, viral translation, protein synthesis and budding. Many new proteins can be detected in cells exposed to interferon, but major roles have been proposed for two enzymes that inhibit protein synthesis:

2′,5′-oligoadenylate synthetase (2,5-A synthetase) and a protein kinase (PKR). The activity of both of these enzymes is dependent on double-stranded RNA (dsRNA) provided by viral intermediates in the cell. PKR is responsible for the phosphorylation of the protein synthesis initiation factor eIF2 that leads to the inhibition of protein synthesis. The 2,5-A synthetase and forms 2′,5′-linked oligomers of adenosine from adenosine triphosphate (ATP). These oligomers activate a latent cellular endonuclease that degrades both viral and ribosomal RNA, with a resultant inhibition of protein synthesis. Apart from these well-characterised changes, many other changes occur in cells treated with interferons and some viral proteins can inhibit the interferon response. Type I IFNs are potent inhibitors of normal and malignant cell growth, and a number of clinical trials have shown that IFNα is active against some human cancers, especially those of haemopoietic origin.

Interferons are able to modify immune responses by:

1. altering the expression of cell surface molecules
2. altering the production and secretion of cellular proteins
3. enhancing or inhibiting effector cell functions.

One of the main ways in which interferons control immune responses is by the induction of major histocompatibility complex (MHC)-encoded molecules. Class I MHC genes are upregulated by all types of interferon, as is the production of β_2-microglobulin. IFNγ induces the expression of MHC class II antigens. In addition, interferons can induce or enhance the expression of Fc receptors and receptors for a number of cytokines. These activities increase the efficiency of antigen presentation and lead to a more effective immune response.

A number of immune effector cells act by killing infected target cells, and the cytotoxicity of macrophages, neutrophils, CD8+ T cells and NK cells is enhanced by interferons. NK cells are activated by interferons and able to destroy infected cells in an MHC unrestricted manner via the release of cytotoxic granules containing granzymes and perforin that penetrate the target cell and induce apoptosis. NK cells discriminate between healthy and infected cells via the expression of a variety of activating and inhibitory receptors. The activating receptors on NK cells can recognise stress-induced molecules on the surface of infected cells, whereas the inhibitory receptors recognise molecules that are present on healthy cells and stop NK cells from killing. Many viruses have evolved to down-regulate the expression of class I MHC molecules on the surface of infected cells in order to evade viral antigen presentation to CD8+ T cells. The inhibitory receptors on NK cells recognise this 'missing self' and the NK cell is activated to kill the infected cell. It is believed that the balance between the activating and inhibitory signals determines whether the NK cell kills the infected cell. Natural killing forms a first-line defence against viral attack, most importantly by herpesviruses, before the acquired immune response is generated. Natural killing is increased by interferons (both the number of effector cells and their killing potential), and therefore these two innate defence mechanisms appear to work together to protect the host from viral infection. These responses are rapid and help to protect the host until acquired responses develop.

Acquired immunity

The response to viral antigens is almost entirely T cell dependent. Immunodeficiencies involving T cells are always characterised by markedly enhanced susceptibility to viral infections; however, both T cell and antibody-mediated immunity are required to provide clearance and long-term immune protection from viral infection. The recognition of viral antigens is similar to that for all foreign material. B cells and immunoglobulin are able to combine with exposed epitopes, and T cells recognise processed viral fragments presented in the context of MHC molecules.

Dendritic cells and antigen-specific B cells can act as antigen-presenting cells (APCs) and thereby generate an immune response. B cells present antigen to T cells and in return are stimulated by growth and differentiation molecules. The uptake of an intact virion means that the B cell is able to present peptides derived from internal proteins to T cells (Fig. 9.2). Thus a B cell that is specific for a surface antigen can receive help from a T cell specific for another molecule as long as it is present within the

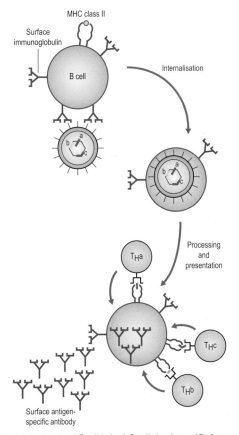

Fig. 9.2 Intrastructural T cell help. A B cell that is specific for a surface component of a virus binds the virus through its receptor, surface immunoglobulin. The virus contains three potential T cell epitopes (a, b and c) within its nucleocapsid. The entire virus can be internalised, and all viral polypeptides will be processed and fragments reexpressed in association with major histocompatibility (MHC) class II molecules (presentation) on the B cell surface.

same particle—intrastructural help. Exogenous virus proteins (i.e., those derived from an extracellular virus and taken into an APC) are presented in the context of MHC class II molecules and stimulate CD4$^+$ T-helper cells. Infected cells express virus-derived peptides in association with MHC class I molecules and stimulate CD8$^+$ cytotoxic T cells.

Humoral immunity

There are several ways in which antibody against viral components can protect the host. Antibodies cannot enter cells, and therefore are ineffective against latent viruses and those that spread directly from cell to cell. They do, however, bind to extracellular viral epitopes. These epitopes can be on intact virions or on the surface of infected cells. The binding of antibody to free virus can inhibit a number of processes essential to virus replication. Antibodies can block binding to the host cell membrane, and thus stop attachment and penetration. The immunoglobulins IgG and IgM have this important function in serum and body fluids, and IgA can neutralise viruses by a similar mechanism on mucosal surfaces. Antibody can also work at stages after penetration. Uncoating, with its release of viral nucleic acid into the cytoplasm, can be inhibited if the virion is covered by antibody.

Antibody can also cause aggregation of virus particles, thus limiting the spread of the infectious particles and forming a complex that is readily phagocytosed. Complement can aid in the neutralisation process by opsonising the virus or directly lysing enveloped viruses. In certain cases, complement alone can inactivate viruses. Some retroviruses have a protein that can act as a receptor for C1q, and other viruses have been reported to activate the alternative pathway. In some infections, viral proteins remain on the surface of the cell after entry or become associated with the cell membrane during replication. Antibodies against these molecules can cause cell lysis by the classical pathway, but an intact alternative pathway is necessary to amplify the initial triggering by the antibody-dependent pathway. In certain situations, antibody-mediated reactions are not always of benefit (see later in the chapter). Antibodies are also capable of modulating or stripping viral antigens from the cell surface, allowing the infected cell to avoid destruction by other effector mechanisms.

Viral infections, particularly those caused by enteroviruses, are frequent and severe when humoral immunity is impaired, as in certain inherited immunodeficiency states. In Bruton-type deficiencies, poliomyelitis may develop after vaccination with the live virus vaccine; meningoencephalitis, caused by echovirus and coxsackievirus, may also be seen. In many situations, viruses seem able to escape the humoral defence mechanisms. Some viruses become latent (e.g., herpesviruses) and are reactivated despite the presence of circulating antibody, as they can pass directly from cell to cell. Other escape mechanisms include antigenic variation in which the antigenic structure of the virus (e.g., influenza type A) changes so that antibodies formed to the previous strain are no longer effective.

In viral infections the efficiency of antibody depends largely on whether the virus passes through the bloodstream outside host cells to reach its target organ. Poliovirus crosses the intestinal wall, enters the bloodstream to cause a cell-free viraemia, and passes to the spinal cord and brain where it replicates. Small amounts of antibody in the blood can neutralise the virus before it reaches its target cells in the nervous system.

In comparison, in viral diseases such as influenza and the common cold the viruses do not pass through the bloodstream. These infections have a short incubation period, their target organ being at the site of entry into the body, namely the respiratory mucous membranes. In this type of infection a high level of antibody in the blood is relatively ineffective in comparison with its effect on blood-borne viruses. In this case the antibody must be present in the mucous secretions at the time of infection. There are very low levels of IgG or IgM in secretions, but IgA has been shown to be responsible for most of the neutralising activity present in nasal secretions against rhinoviruses and other respiratory-tract viruses.

One consequence of this is that conventional immunisation methods using killed virus or viral subunits, which produce high levels of circulating antibody, are unlikely to be effective against viruses that attack the mucous membranes. Some considerable effort is being directed at developing methods for stimulating local production of IgA in the mucous membranes themselves. Live virus vaccines are effective in this respect, and the intranasal administration of a live-attenuated influenza virus vaccine is an attempt to overcome this problem. The high degree of immunity provided by the oral polio vaccine is due in part to locally produced antibody in the gut neutralising the virus before it attaches to cell receptors to cause infection. The presence of IgA against polio has been demonstrated in faeces, duodenal fluid and saliva.

Humoral immunity does play a major protective role in polio and a number of other viral infections and is probably the predominant form of immunity responsible for protection from reinfection due to B cell memory. Passively administered antibody can protect against several human infections, including measles, hepatitis A and B, and chickenpox, if given before or very soon after exposure. Immunity to many viral infections is lifelong possibly because antibody levels are boosted by occasional reexposure to the virus.

Cell-mediated immunity

The destruction of virus-infected cells is an important mechanism in the eradication of virus from the host. The killing of an infected cell before progeny particles are released is an effective way of terminating a viral infection. For this process to occur the immune system must recognise the infected cell, and various types of effector cell have evolved to mediate these processes including NK cells described earlier and the cytotoxic T cell (Tc).

As viral proteins are synthesised within the cell some of these molecules are processed into small peptides. These endogenously produced antigen fragments become associated with MHC class I molecules, and this complex is then transported to the cell surface where it acts as the recognition unit for Tc cells. $CD8^+$ Tc cells have a receptor that binds to fragments of the virus sitting in the cleft of an MHC class I molecule. Some Tc cells are restricted in their recognition of antigen by MHC class II molecules and therefore are $CD4^+$. Once these Tc cells have bound to the infected cell they release cytotoxic granules that induce apoptosis (see Ch. 8). $CD4^+$ and $CD8^+$ T cells also produce various cytokines when stimulated by antigen, including molecules that are active in the elimination of virus (e.g., $IFN\gamma$ and $TNF\alpha$).

Many viruses, such as poliovirus and papillomavirus, replicate and produce fully infectious particles inside the cell. These viruses are liberated from the infected cell as it disintegrates. However, other viruses do not wait for the cell to die but are released by a process of budding through the cell membrane. During their replication, virus-encoded molecules (viral antigens) are inserted into the host cell membrane, and the nucleocapsid becomes associated with these molecules. The virus particle finally acquires an envelope as it is released. Such viruses include herpesviruses, alphaviruses, flaviviruses, retroviruses, hepadnaviruses, orthomyxoviruses and paramyxoviruses. Viral antigens often appear on the cell surface very early in the replicative cycle, many hours before progeny virus is liberated. These molecules, including those that are not incorporated into the released virion, can therefore act as signals indicating the presence of virus within a cell. If antibody binds to these cell surface viral antigens, the infected cell can be destroyed by antibody-dependent cell-mediated cytotoxicity (ADCC) caused by cells that express Fc receptors such as macrophages and neutrophils.

Induction of an immune response

The precise nature of the acquired immune reactions that are generated in response to infection depends to a great extent on the site of infection, type of virus, previous exposure to the agent and the genetic make-up of the host.

Both humoral and cell-mediated responses are produced to all infections. The virus or viral components entering the peripheral tissues, or being produced there, are carried to the draining lymph node either free in the lymph or in dendritic cells (DCs). Once in the secondary lymphoid tissues the free virus is taken up by macrophages and processed; viral peptides associate with MHC class II molecules and are transported to the cell surface. DCs that enter the lymph node present viral peptides, associated with MHC class II molecules, on their surface. A Th cell will bind to the peptide–MHC class II complex, expand clonally and produce helper factors (see previous chapter). The nature of the different cytokines produced determines the type and level of the response generated. B cells in the lymph node that bind antigen are stimulated into antibody production and antigen presentation. Other naïve T cells will enter the lymph node; if these cells have a TcR that interacts with an antigen fragment–MHC class I complex, they will respond to the growth factors present in the node and proliferate and mature into effector Tc cells. After a time, the products of the immune response leave the node to circulate round the body and localise at the site of infection. As the response progresses the pathogen is eliminated, the tissue repaired and memory cells generated. Finally, when all of the antigen has been eliminated, the immune response is terminated. In some instances, virus-induced immune responses may have immunopathological consequences.

IMMUNOPATHOLOGY

Viruses have evolved a multitude of mechanisms for exploiting weaknesses in the host immune system and subverting immune mechanisms. Some viruses are so successful in avoiding host defences that they persist in the host indefinitely, sometimes in a latent form without producing disease.

One of the most important strategies developed by viruses is to infect cells of the immune system itself. The effect of this is often to disable the normal functioning of the cell type that has been infected. Many common human viruses, including rubella, mumps, measles and herpes viruses, infect cells of the immune system, as does human immunodeficiency virus (HIV). The consequences of viral infection of cells of the immune system have been categorised in two ways:

1. Infections that cause temporary immune deficiency to unrelated antigens and sometimes to the antigens of the infecting virus. It is known that infection with influenza, rubella, measles and cytomegalovirus predisposes to bacterial and other infections. This is sometimes associated with depressed immunoglobulin

synthesis and interference with the antimicrobial functions of phagocytes.
2. Permanent depression of immunity to unrelated antigens and occasionally to antigens of the infecting virus. AIDS is an example of such a disease, where the patient becomes susceptible to otherwise harmless protozoa, bacteria, viruses and fungi.

Viruses have also developed other mechanisms to avoid the immune system. These include:

- antigenic variation
- release of antigens
- production of antigens at sites that are inaccessible to the immune system.

A microorganism can avoid the acquired immune response by periodically changing the structure of molecules that are recognised by the host immune system. The immune system selects the variants by not being able to mount an immune response against them before they are shed. The microorganism will only be able to change a component in a way that does not alter the functioning of the molecule. The molecules involved can be active enzymes, recognition molecules or structural proteins. HIV shows considerable variation in parts of the envelope glycoprotein within a given individual. The significance of antigenic variation is well illustrated by influenza viruses. Here, changes in the surface glycoproteins are linked to the occurrence of epidemics of infection (see Ch. 53). With influenza virus the infection is localised to the respiratory tract where the principal protection against reinfection is secretory IgA. The virus-specific IgA still present at the mucosal surface a few years after infection can protect against the original infecting virus but is insufficient to deal with an antigenic variant despite antigenic overlap. Thus IgA levels become a selective pressure, which will allow infection by the mutant, and antigenic drift occurs.

During the course of an infection, various antibodies are formed against different epitopes on a virus. These antibodies are of differing affinities and stimulate different effector functions. Antibodies against some of the epitopes will neutralise the virus, but other antibodies will be against unimportant epitopes or be of an ineffective isotype that may fail to neutralise the virus, and may actually aid in its infectivity by allowing uptake of virus–antibody complexes via Fc receptors or cause tissue damage through immune complex disease. Soluble antigens liberated from infected cells may 'mop up' free antibody so that it can no longer interact and destroy extracellular virus.

A number of infections continually shed virus into external secretions, such as saliva, milk or urine. As long as the infected cell forms virus only on the luminal surface of the mucosa, cells of the immune system and antibody will be unable to destroy the infected cell. IgA present in the secretions may neutralise the virus, but this class of antibody does not activate complement efficiently, so the cell will not be lysed. A similar situation applies to epidermal infections with wart virus. The infected cell is keratinised and about to be released from the surface of the body before any virus or viral antigens are produced. The infected cell is therefore isolated from the host's immune cells.

Susceptibility to infection is generally greater in the very young and very old because of a weaker immune response. However, the immunopathology tends to be less severe. In the very young, infections can spread rapidly and prove fatal without the clinical and pathological changes seen in adults. Latent infections are kept under control by the immune system, and in older people the infections show an increased incidence of activation (e.g., zoster, or shingles). Immunological immaturity makes the neonate highly susceptible to many viral infections. Maternally derived antibody provides passive protection for 3–6 months, after which time the infant is at risk of infection; respiratory and alimentary-tract infections are frequent.

Certain viral infections produce a milder disease in children than in adults (e.g., varicella, mumps, poliomyelitis and Epstein–Barr virus infections). Varicella often causes pneumonia in adults, and mumps may involve the testes and ovaries after puberty, giving rise to orchitis and oophoritis. Epstein–Barr virus is excreted in saliva, and in developing countries most individuals are infected early in life, usually asymptomatically. In developed countries where childhood infection is less common, first infection may be delayed to adolescence or early adulthood, when salivary exposure occurs during kissing. In this age group, Epstein–Barr virus infection gives rise to infectious mononucleosis.

Persistence of virus

Certain viruses give rise to a persistent infection, which is held in check as long as the immune system remains intact. Chickenpox is a persistent infection characterised by latency in that there is apparent recovery from the original infection but the virus can reappear later in life when a localised eruption, shingles, results. Other herpesviruses, cytomegalovirus and Epstein–Barr virus also persist after infection. If the carrier's immune system remains intact, there will be no evidence of disease. However, cytomegalovirus causes many problems in immunosuppressed patients. In other persistent infections, the immune system contributes to the pathology of the disease, often over a period of years. Thus, in subacute sclerosing panencephalitis, persistence of measles virus in neurones triggers their destruction by the host's immune system.

VACCINES

Natural infection with a virus is an extremely effective means of giving lifelong immunity from the disease. In most cases, where there is one virus type, this means that second attacks are extremely rare. The memory of the immune system ensures that, for these infections, a secondary response can be generated before the virus has time to cause the disease. The level of immunity needed to protect an individual depends on the incubation period of the virus and its life cycle. For viruses with very short incubation periods, a high level of protective immunity must be present before exposure to the infective agent. In the case of a virus with a long incubation period (10–20 days), the immune system has time to generate a protective response.

It is also important to consider the type of immune response that will be protective against different viruses. If antibody gives protection then steps must be taken to ensure that the material to be used for immunisation contains the correct epitopes. A denatured antigen will not generate antibodies that can combine with the native virus. Sometimes chemical treatment of the antigen may destroy important components. If T cell immunity is important, the vaccine must be in a form that will give rise to peptides in the correct compartment of the cell to produce antigen fragments in association with MHC-encoded products. It will have to associate with the MHC class II molecules to generate help and with MHC class I molecules to stimulate effector cell formation. For antibody production, T cell help is also required. Therefore, for an antibody response, a killed vaccine may be sufficient but, when T cell immunity is required, a live-attenuated vaccine is needed.

Vaccination has been responsible for the elimination of smallpox and for reducing the incidence of other viral diseases. It should be possible to control many viral diseases, but with some the problem is more difficult. New technologies and a better understanding of the immune system are helping with this task.

IMMUNITY IN BACTERIAL INFECTION

Modern medical science has managed to subdue many of the classical infectious diseases, but has helped to create new ones that result from interference with normal host defence mechanisms, consequent upon medical and surgical procedures such as chemotherapy, catheterisation, immunosuppression and irradiation.

When examining the relationship between bacteria and their host it is important to differentiate infection from disease. These issues are explored further in Ch. 11.

HOST DEFENCES

Few organisms can penetrate intact skin, and the various other innate defence mechanisms are extremely efficient at keeping bacteria at bay. When bacteria do gain access to the tissues, the ability of the host to limit damage and eliminate the microbe depends on the generation of an effective immune response against microbial antigens. In most cases, the host defences are directed against external components and secreted molecules. Antibodies may interfere with many important bacterial processes, and enzymes such as lysozyme may also contribute, but, ultimately, phagocytes are needed to destroy and remove the bacteria (Fig. 9.3). Where bacteria survive within phagocytes or other cells, cell-mediated responses are required.

Inflammation

Having successfully avoided the innate immune mechanisms that protect the individual (mechanical barriers, antibacterial substances and phagocytosis, described in Ch. 8), a bacterium starts to proliferate in the tissues. The presence of bacteria-specific molecules is recognised by pattern recognition receptors (e.g., TLRs, see Ch. 8), leading to cytokine release. These cytokines, along with tissue-damaging toxic bacterial products, trigger an inflammatory reaction. The resulting increase in vascular permeability leads to an exudation of serum proteins, including complement components, antibodies and clotting factors,

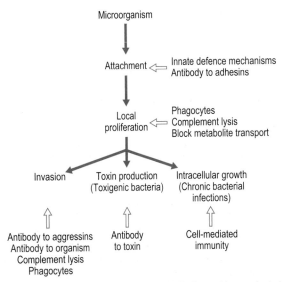

Fig. 9.3 Scheme showing the progress of infection and immunological defence mechanisms.

as well as phagocytic cells. The phagocytes are attracted to the site of inflammation by chemotactic factors including chemokines. Anaphylatoxins generated by complement activation further increase vascular permeability and encourage exudation of fluid and cells at the site of inflammation. Many of these mediators also cause vasodilatation, thereby increasing blood flow to the area.

Many types of microorganism (e.g., staphylococci and streptococci) are dealt with effectively by the phagocytes. The intensity and duration of the inflammatory process that is stimulated depend on the degree of success with which the microorganism initially establishes itself. This, in turn, depends on the extent of the injury, the amount of associated tissue damage and the number and type of microorganisms introduced. A localised abscess may arise at the site of infection.

If bacteria are not eliminated at the site of entry and continue to proliferate, they pass via the tissue fluids and lymphatics to the draining lymph node, where a specific acquired immune response is generated. The antibody and effector cells generated will leave the node to return to the area of infection to eliminate the bacteria. Some capsulated microorganisms, such as pneumococci, are able to resist phagocytosis and are not dealt with effectively until large amounts of antibody have been made. These 'mop up' the released capsular polysaccharide, and phagocytosis occurs. Other microorganisms produce exotoxins, and effective immunity to exotoxins requires the development of specific antibodies against the toxin (i.e., antitoxin).

The types of infection described above are usually referred to as *acute* infections, and contrast with the protracted or chronic infections usually induced by bacteria that have adapted to survive within the cells of the host. Included among these are tuberculosis and leprosy, brucella infections and listeriosis. In these infections, cell-mediated immunity plays a predominant part in the final elimination of the microorganism.

Humoral immunity

The attachment of a microorganism to an epithelial surface is a prerequisite for the development of an infectious process (see Ch. 11). A first line of defence by antibody could be to inhibit colonisation by stopping attachment. IgA can stop colonisation of the mucosal surface if it interferes with the attachment molecules (adhesins) present on the bacterial surface. IgA does not activate complement very efficiently; therefore, an inflammatory reaction is not stimulated. Damage to the gut wall during an inflammatory reaction would allow the entry of many potential pathogens into vulnerable tissues.

Many microorganisms owe their pathogenic abilities to the production of exotoxins. Among diseases dependent

on this type of mechanism are diphtheria, cholera, tetanus and botulism. Antibodies acquired by either immunisation or previous infection, or given passively as antiserum, are able to neutralise bacterial toxins.

The direct binding of antibody to a bacterium can interfere with bacterial function in numerous ways. Antibody can kill bacteria on its own or in conjunction with complement and phagocytes. To survive and multiply, bacteria must ingest nutrients and ions, antibodies that affect the activity of specific transport systems will deprive the bacteria of their energy supply and other essential chemicals. Some bacteria are invasive, moving into the tissues aided by enzymes that they produce. Invasion can also be inhibited by antibody that attaches to the flagella of the microorganism to affect its motility. Antibodies can agglutinate bacteria, and formation of the aggregate will impede spread of the organism.

In addition, the formation of an immune complex of bacteria and antibody will stimulate phagocytosis and complement activation. When a particle is coated with antibody, a large number of Fc portions are exposed to the outside. This increases the chance that the particle will be held in contact with the phagocyte long enough to stimulate phagocytosis. The interaction of multiple ligands increases the overall affinity of the binding, and if antibody and complement components are present on the same particle, the binding is even stronger.

The bacteria are internalised and attacked by the oxygen-dependent and oxygen-independent killing mechanisms within the phagocyte. Phagocytes are also responsible for the removal and digestion of bacteria that have been killed extracellularly. Bacteria are susceptible to the lytic action of complement, which may be activated by bacterial components. The presence of antibody on the bacterial cell surface further stimulates the activation of complement.

Cell-mediated immunity

Ultimately, all bacteria will be engulfed by a phagocyte, either to be killed or removed after extracellular killing. The host defence mechanisms of macrophages and monocytes can be enhanced by various activating stimuli recognised by pattern recognition receptors including the TLRs (see Ch. 8).

The immune system is also active in the production of macrophage-activating factors. In particular, cytokines produced by T lymphocytes are often required to potentiate bacterial clearance both by attracting phagocytes to the site of infection and by activating them. Th1 cells produce IFNγ in response to intracellular bacteria; Th17 cells produce IL-17 in response to extracellular bacteria (see Ch. 8).

EVASION

Once a microorganism becomes established in the tissues, having escaped the innate defence mechanisms, it can often make use of a number of evasion strategies that protect it from the immune reactions of the host. Pathogenic bacteria produce a rather ill-defined group of bacterial products called *aggressins* and *impedins*, possession of which is associated with virulence (see Ch. 10). If antibody to such substances is present, the pathogenicity of the microorganism is likely to be reduced.

Intracellular bacteria

Bacteria that can survive and replicate within phagocytic cells are at an advantage as they are protected from host defence mechanisms. Some microorganisms reside intracellularly only transiently, whereas others spend most of their life inside cells. An intracellular lifestyle demands potent evasion mechanisms to survive this hostile environment. Some bacteria, such as *Mycobacterium leprae,* have become so accustomed to their intracellular environment that they can no longer live in the extracellular space.

Listeria monocytogenes, the causative agent of listeriosis, can survive and multiply in normal macrophages, but is killed within macrophages activated by cytokines released from T cells. Listeriosis is most commonly seen in immunocompromised patients, pregnant women and neonates, in whom a lack of adequate T cell–derived macrophage-activating factors is probably the critical factor. *Salmonella* spp. and *Brucella* spp. can also survive intracellularly. Mycobacteria have a waxy cell wall that is very hydrophobic. This external surface is very resistant to lysosomal enzymes and persists for a long time even when the bacteria have been killed. In addition, these microorganisms have evolved other strategies to evade destruction. *M. tuberculosis* secretes molecules that inhibit lysosome/phagosome fusion, and *M. leprae* can escape from the phagosome and grow in the cytoplasm.

T lymphocytes represent the major host defence against intracellular pathogens. In many cases, the bacteria themselves do not directly harm the host: the pathogenesis is caused by the immune response. After invasion of the host, intracellular bacteria are taken up by macrophages, evade intracellular killing and multiply. During intracellular replication, some microbial molecules are processed and presented on the surface of the infected cell in association with MHC class II. This complex on the cell surface is recognised by specific $CD4^+$ Th1 cells, which are stimulated to release $IFN\gamma$ and $TNF\alpha$. These molecules in turn activate the macrophage so that the intracellular bacteria are killed. Peptides from intracellular bacteria can also be presented in MHC class I and attract $CD8^+$ CTLs that will kill the infected cell in a manner similar to the response to viral pathogens (see earlier in the chapter).

The accumulation of macrophages in response to bacteria can also cause the formation of a granuloma, which will prevent dissemination of the bacteria to other sites in the body. As conditions for the survival of the pathogen become less suitable, they stop replicating and die. Some intracellular bacteria infect cells that are unable to destroy them. In this situation, a more aggressive immune response may be needed to remove the pathogen and this can cause pathogenic damage unless kept under control (see later in the chapter).

IMMUNOPATHOLOGY

The immune response to an organism leads to some tissue damage through inflammation, lymph node swelling and cell infiltration. Sometimes the damage caused by the immune system is severe, leading to serious disease and death. Rheumatic fever can follow *Streptococcus pyogenes* throat infections and is believed to be due to antibodies formed against a streptococcal cell wall component cross-reacting with cardiac muscle or heart valve. Myocarditis develops a few weeks after the throat infection and can be re-stimulated if the patient is infected again with Lancefield group A streptococci.

Immune complex disease (type III hypersensitivity) is frequently associated with bacterial infection. Infective endocarditis caused by staphylococci and streptococci is associated with circulating complexes of antibody and bacterial antigen. Detection of these complexes can be helpful in diagnosis, but they may lead to joint and kidney lesions, vasculitis and skin rashes. Immune complexes may play a role in the pathogenesis of leprosy, typhoid fever and gonorrhoea.

Effects of endotoxin

Endotoxin interacts with cells and molecules of inflammation, immunity and haemostasis.

- Fever is induced by interleukin-1, produced by the liver in response to endotoxin, acting on the temperature-regulating hypothalamus.
- The action of lipopolysaccharide on platelets and activation of Hageman's factor causes disseminated intravascular coagulation with ensuing ischaemic tissue damage to various organs.
- Septic shock occurs during severe infections with Gram-negative organisms when bacteria or lipopolysaccharide enter the bloodstream.

- Endotoxin acts on neutrophils, platelets and complement to produce, both directly and through mast cell degranulation, vasoactive amines that cause hypotension.

Recognition of endotoxin through Toll-like receptor 4 (see p 86) causes macrophages to produce large quantities of potent cytokines such as interleukin-1, tumour necrosis factor and colony-stimulating factors. Endotoxin also causes polyclonal activation of B cells and can stimulate natural killer cells and other cell types to produce IFNγ.

Mycobacterial disease

Activated macrophages secrete a variety of biologically active molecules to counteract invading microbes, including:

- proteases
- tumour necrosis factor
- reactive oxygen intermediates that are harmful to the surrounding tissue.

Tissue destruction is an inevitable side effect of this important mechanism of resistance. In the acute phase of a response this is likely to be tolerated; however, in the case of resistant organisms such as mycobacteria, the process may become chronic and the tissue destruction extensive. Mycobacterial components are still able to stimulate a response after the bacterium has been killed, because they persist for a long time, adding to the tissue damage. Lysis of infected cells also occurs, which may result in microbial discharge from the granuloma into surrounding capillaries or alveoli, and hence facilitate dissemination to other parts of the body or to other individuals. Lysis of infected cells causes tissue destruction, and the severity of the effects depends on the tissue involved. *M. leprae* infects the Schwann cell, an irreplaceable component of the peripheral nervous system. Although the presence of *M. leprae* does not appear to affect the host cell, the presence of activated macrophages releasing toxic molecules or direct lysis by cytotoxic cells constitutes a major pathological mechanism in leprosy.

If the leprosy bacillus is released from a lysed non-phagocytic cell to be engulfed by an activated macrophage, the bacterium will be eliminated. Therefore, macrophage activation and target cell lysis can be beneficial as well as detrimental to the host.

The cell-mediated response that has the potential to eliminate these infections will give rise to type IV hypersensitivity reactions if the antigen is not removed efficiently. Chronic production of cytokines causes granuloma formation, which with time can lead to fibrosis and loss of organ function. This type of response is particularly prevalent in patients with tuberculosis.

Parasitic infections: pathogenesis and immunity

The term *parasitic diseases* refers to those caused by protozoa, worms (helminths) and arthropods (insects and arachnids). Such parasites affect many hundreds of millions of people and are responsible for many severe and debilitating diseases (see Chs 59 and 60). These infections are associated with a broad spectrum of effects. Some are due to the parasites themselves and others are a consequence of the host response to the invader. The nature and extent of the pathological effects are dependent upon the site and mode of infection, and also on the level of the parasite burden.

The development of protective immunity to such parasites is more complicated than that to bacteria and viruses because of the complicated life cycles of the parasites involved.

PATHOGENIC MECHANISMS

As with other infectious agents, the site occupied by a parasite is important. A host will survive with a large number of lung flukes, *Paragonimus* spp., in the lungs, but infection in the brain may cause far more serious effects. The severity of disease depends not only on the degree of infection but also on the physiological state of the host. A lowering of general health, due to malnutrition, for example, predisposes to more serious consequences following infection by parasites.

Mechanical tissue damage

Physical obstruction of anatomical sites leading to loss of function can be a major component of the diseases caused by parasites. The intestinal lumen can be blocked by worms such as *Ascaris lumbricoides* or tapeworms, and filarial parasites *(Wuchereria bancrofti* and *Brugia malayi)* can obstruct the flow of lymph through lymphatics.

Intestinal infection with the tapeworm *Taenia solium* is usually of little consequence, but the eggs may develop into larvae (cysticerci) in humans, causing cysticercosis. The cysticerci can be found in muscle, liver, eye or, most dangerously, the brain. Hydatid cysts, the larval stage of the dog tapeworm *(Echinococcus granulosus)* in humans, may reach volumes of 1–2 litres, and such masses can cause severe damage to an infected organ.

Physiological effects

Large numbers of *Giardia* spp. covering the walls of the small intestine can lead to malabsorption, especially of fats. Competition by parasites for essential nutrients leads to host deprivation. Thus depletion of vitamin B_{12} by the tapeworm *Diphyllobothrium latum* sometimes leads to pernicious anaemia. Other forms of anaemia result from blood loss, especially in hookworm infection, and from red blood cell destruction in malaria. Some parasites produce metabolites that may have profound effects on the host. *Trypanosoma cruzi* secretes a neurotoxin that affects the autonomic nervous system.

Tissue damage

The presence of parasites can result in the release of proteolytic enzymes that damage host tissues. Ulceration of the intestinal wall occurs in amoebic dysentery, and trophozoites (the active, motile forms of a protozoan parasite) can penetrate deep into the wall of the intestine to reach the blood and hence the liver, lungs and brain where secondary amoebic abscesses may occur. The skin damage caused by skin-penetrating helminths, such as *Strongyloides stercoralis* and hookworms, can also permit entry of other infectious agents.

The host reaction to parasites and their products can evoke immunological reactions that may lead to secondary damage to host tissues. This is seen in schistosomiasis, where the host response to parasite eggs in tissues leads to the formation of a granuloma with subsequent tissue destruction through fibrosis. Other types of immune reaction can be generated in various parasite infections (see later in the chapter).

IMMUNE DEFENCE MECHANISMS

The large size of parasites means that they display more antigens than do bacteria or viruses to the immune system. When the parasite has a complicated life cycle, some of these antigens may be specific to a particular stage of development. Parasites have evolved to be closely adapted to the host, and most parasitic infections are chronic and show a degree of host specificity. For example, the malaria parasites of humans, birds and rodents are confined to their own particular species. An exception to this is *Trichinella spiralis*, which is able to infect many animal species.

In the natural host there is no single defence mechanism that acts in isolation against a particular parasite. In turn the parasite will have evolved a number of strategies to evade elimination. In general terms, cell-mediated immune mechanisms are more effective against intracellular protozoa, whereas antibody, with the aid of effector cells, is involved in the destruction of extracellular targets. Again, because of the life cycles of some parasites, either cell-mediated or humoral immunity may be of greater importance at different states of their development.

Innate defences

Several of the innate or natural defence mechanisms that are active against bacteria and viruses are also effective against parasitic infections. The physical barrier of the skin protects against many parasites but is ineffective against those transmitted by a blood-feeding insect. In addition, other parasites, such as schistosomes, have evolved active mechanisms for penetrating intact skin.

Several nonspecific host defence mechanisms are involved in the control of parasitic infections. These include direct cellular responses by monocytes, macrophages and granulocytes, and by natural killer cells. Acquired immune reactions enhance the antiparasitic activity of these cells. For example, some *Leishmania* spp. are obligate parasites of mononuclear phagocytes and are completely dependent upon macrophages, where they survive in the phagolysosome. These parasites survive within nonstimulated resident macrophages, whereas they are destroyed in macrophages activated by IFNγ.

Complement is active against a number of parasites, including adult worms and active larvae of *T. spiralis* and schistosomula of *Schistosoma mansoni*. The spleen is thought to be active in the elimination of intracellular parasites, as filtering of infected erythrocytes is thought to remove intracellular plasmodium.

Macrophages

Macrophages play an important role in the elimination and control of parasitic protozoa and worms. They secrete interleukin (IL)-1, TNF and CSFs that affect not only T cells and antibody production but also granulocytes. Macrophages are also phagocytic cells and function as such in the elimination of parasites. Once internalised the parasite is killed by oxygen-dependent and -independent mechanisms and digested. Many of the molecules produced by macrophages are cytotoxic, and when produced in close proximity to a parasite will kill it. Specific antibodies, immunoglobulin (Ig) G and IgE, can mediate the attachment of the macrophage to the surface of parasites that are too large to internalise but are vulnerable to antibody-dependent cell-mediated cytotoxicity. Acting as APCs, they can aid elimination by helping in the initiation of an adaptive immune response.

In some parasitic infections the immune system is unable to eradicate the offending organism. The body reacts by trying to isolate the parasite within a granuloma. In this situation, there is chronic stimulation of those T cells specific for antigens on the parasite. The continual release of cytokines leads to macrophage accumulation, release of fibrogenic factors, stimulation of granuloma formation and, ultimately, fibrosis.

Granulocytes

Neutrophils and eosinophils are thought to play a role in the elimination of protozoa and worms. The smaller parasites can be phagocytosed by neutrophils and destroyed by both oxygen-dependent and -independent processes. Both cell types possess receptors for the Fc portion of immunoglobulin and for various complement components, so the presence of opsonins increases phagocytosis. Extracellular destruction of large parasites can occur by antibody-dependent cell-mediated cytotoxicity.

Eosinophilia and high levels of IgE are characteristics of many parasitic worm infections. It has been suggested that eosinophils are especially active against helminths, and IgE-dependent degranulation of mast cells has evolved to attract these cells to the site where the parasite is localised. The eosinophilia is dependent on IL-5 production by Th2 cells, which also causes an increase in their activation state. These effector cells are attracted to the site by chemotactic factors produced by mast cells (see later in the chapter). Once at the site they degranulate in response to perturbation of their cell membrane induced by antibodies and complement bound to the surface of the parasite. The toxic molecules are therefore released on to the surface of the target and cause its destruction.

Mast cells

The mediators stored and produced by mast cells play an important role in eliminating worm infections. Parasite antigens cause the IgE dependent release of mediators from mast cells; these molecules induce a local inflammatory response. Chemotactic factors are produced and attract eosinophils and neutrophils.

Acquired immunity

An individual with a parasitic infection mounts a specific response against the invading parasite. These immune reactions generate antibody and effector T cells directed against specific parasite antigens. Memory B and T cells are also produced. For a number of reasons, described later, much acquired immunity is ineffective in protecting the host against recurrent infection. However, in certain cases, such as amoebiasis and toxoplasmosis, immunity to reinfection is fairly complete. In schistosomiasis, the presence of surviving adult forms protects against further infections. However, this may be an effect of the parasite and not of the host.

Antibody

The specific immune response to parasites leads to the production of antibodies. Infection by protozoan parasites is associated with the production of IgG and IgM. With helminths, there is also synthesis of substantial amounts of IgE. IgA is produced in response to intestinal protozoa, such as *Entamoeba histolytica* and *Giardia lamblia*.

In addition to these specific T-dependent responses, a nonspecific hypergammaglobulinaemia is present in many parasitic infections. Much of this nonspecific antibody is the result of polyclonal B cell activation by released parasite antigens acting as mitogens. This response is ineffective at counteracting the parasite and can enhance the pathogenicity by causing the production of autoantibodies, and may actually lead to a diminished specific response due to B cell exhaustion.

There are a number of mechanisms by which specific antibodies can provide protection against and control parasitic infections (Table 9.2). As with viral and bacterial infections, antibodies are effective only against extracellular parasites and where parasite antigens are displayed on the surface of infected cells. The broad mechanisms of antibody function are similar to those described earlier in relation to viral and bacterial infection.

Antibody-dependent cell-mediated cytotoxicity has been shown to play a part in infections caused by a number of parasites, including *Tryp. cruzi*, *T. spiralis*, *S. mansoni* and filarial worms. The effector cells—macrophages, monocytes, neutrophils, eosinophils and natural killer cells—bind to the antibody-coated parasites by their Fc and complement receptors. In particular, major basic protein (MBP) from eosinophils damages the tegument of schistosomes and other worms, causing their death.

T cells

The importance of T cell–mediated immunity to parasites has been demonstrated extensively in murine models. CD4[+]

Table 9.2 Humoral defence mechanisms against parasite infections

Mechanism	Effect	Parasite
Neutralisation	Blocks attachment to host cell	Protozoa
	Acts to inhibit evasion mechanisms of intracellular organisms	Protozoa
	Binding to toxins or enzymes	Protozoa and worms
Physical interference	Obstructs orifices of parasite	Worms
	Agglutination	Protozoa
Opsonisation	Increases clearance by phagocytes	Protozoa
Cytotoxicity	Complement-mediated lysis	Protozoa and worms
	Antibody-dependent cell-mediated cytotoxicity	Protozoa and worms

T-helper cells act by providing help in antibody production, but they also secrete various cytokines that interact with other effector cells. CD8+ cells can be cytotoxic to the pathogen, but these cells also produce a variety of effector cytokines. In particular, the Th2 response has been shown to be critical in eradication of helminth parasites where IL-5 in particular drives the eosinophilia observed. Colony-stimulating factors (e.g., IL-3 and GM-CSF) are also produced by activated T cells. These molecules act on myeloid progenitors in the bone marrow, causing increased production of neutrophils, eosinophils and monocytes. They also increase the activity of these cells; the monocytosis and splenomegaly in malaria are caused by these T cell–derived molecules.

EVASION MECHANISMS

All animal pathogens, including parasitic protozoa and worms, have evolved effective mechanisms to avoid elimination by host defence systems (Table 9.3).

Seclusion

Many parasites inhabit cells or anatomical sites that are inaccessible to host defence mechanisms. Those that attempt to survive within cells avoid the effects of antibody but must possess mechanisms to avoid destruction if the cell involved is capable of destroying them. *Plasmodium* spp. inhabit erythrocytes, whereas toxoplasmas are less selective and infect nonphagocytic cells as well as

phagocytes. A number of different ways of avoiding destruction in macrophages have evolved. *Leishmania donovani* amastigotes are able to survive and metabolise in the acidic environment (pH 4–5) found in phagolysosomes, and *Tox. gondii* is able to inhibit the fusion of lysosomes with the parasite-containing phagosome.

L. major has a similar escape mechanism by attaching to a phagocyte complement receptor (CR1) that does not trigger the respiratory burst. Activation of the complement system by protozoan parasites seems to be a common mechanism for achieving attachment to target cells. *Tryp. cruzi* trypomastigotes can infect T cells of both the CD4 and CD8 subsets, and may be similar to retroviruses in using receptor molecules on the T cell surface for penetration.

The ability to resist complement destruction also appears to be important. For example, *L. tropica* is easily killed by complement and causes only a localised self-healing lesion in the skin, whereas a disseminating, often fatal, disease is seen with *L. donovani*, which is 10 times more resistant to complement killing. Large parasites such as helminths cannot infect individual cells; however, they can still achieve anatomical seclusion. *T. spiralis* larvae avoid the immune system by encysting in muscle; intestinal nematodes live in the lumen of the intestine.

Evasion

Parasites may avoid recognition by:

- antigenic variation
- acquiring host-derived molecules.

Trypanosomes have the capacity to express >100 different surface glycoproteins. By producing novel antigens throughout their lives, these parasites continuously evade the immune system. By the time the host has mounted a response against each new antigen, the parasite has changed again. Plasmodia pass through several discrete developmental stages, each with its own particular antigens. A similar situation is seen in certain helminths such as *T. spiralis*. As a result, each new stage of the life cycle is seen by the host as a 'new' infective challenge.

A number of parasites are known to adsorb host-derived molecules on to their surface. This is thought to mask their own antigens and enable them to evade immunological attack. Parasitic protozoa and worms also use devices to avoid immune destruction. Certain parasites retain a surface coat, or glycocalyx, that blocks direct exposure of their surface antigens.

Immunosuppression

Parasites are not always able to evade detection, and many have evolved mechanisms to suppress or divert immune

Table 9.3 Parasite escape mechanisms	
Escape mechanism	Organisms
Intracellular habitat	Malaria parasites, trypanosomes and *Leishmania* spp.
Encystment	*Toxoplasma gondii* and *Trypanosoma cruzi*
Resistance to microbicidal products of phagocytes	*Leishmania donovani*
Masking of antigens	Schistosomes
Variation of antigen	Trypanosomes and malaria parasites
Suppression of immune response	Most parasites (e.g., malaria parasites, *Trichinella spirolis* and *Schistosoma monsoni*)
Interference by antigens	Trypanosomes
Polyclonal activation	Trypanosomes
Sharing of antigens between parasite and host (molecular mimicry)	Schistosomes
Continuous turnover and release of surface antigens of parasite	Schistosomes

reactions. Some parasites produce or generate molecules that act against cells of the immune system. Thus the larvae of *T. spiralis* produce a molecule that is cytotoxic to lymphocytes. During many parasitic infections a large amount of antigenic material is released into the body fluids, and this may inhibit the response to or divert the response away from the parasite. High antigen concentrations can lead to tolerance by clonal exhaustion or clonal deletion. Many of these released molecules are polyclonal activators of T and B cells. This leads to the production of nonspecific antibody, impairment of B cell function and immunosuppression.

Schistosomes have a receptor for part of the antibody molecule. They also release several proteases that cleave antibody molecules and release products that prevent macrophage activation. A schistosome-derived inhibitory factor suppresses T-cell activity and may explain the inefficiency of cytotoxic T cells in damaging the parasite. Recent studies have also indicated that increased Treg activity may be induced in some parasitic infections.

IMMUNOPATHOLOGY

The immune response to parasites is aimed at eliminating the organisms, but many of the host reactions have pathological effects.

The IgE produced in parasitic worm infections can have severe effects on the host if it stimulates excessive mast cell degranulation. Anaphylactic shock can occur if a cyst ruptures and releases vast amounts of antigenic material into the circulation of a sensitised individual. Asthma-like symptoms occur in *Toxocara canis* infections when larvae of worms migrate through the lungs.

The polyclonal B cell activation seen with many parasitic infections can give rise to autoantibodies. In trypanosomiasis and malaria, antibodies against red blood cells, lymphocytes and deoxyribonucleic acid (DNA) have been detected. Host antigens incorporated into the parasite, as an immune evasion mechanism, may stimulate autoantibody production by giving rise to T cell help and overcoming tolerance. In Chagas' disease, about 20% of individuals develop progressive cardiomyopathy and neuropathy of the digestive tract that are believed to be autoimmune in nature. These effects are thought to result from cross-reactivity between antibody or T cells responsive to *Tryp. cruzi* and nerve ganglia.

Immune complex–mediated disease occurs in malaria, trypanosomiasis, schistosomiasis and onchocerciasis. The deposition of immune complexes in the kidney is responsible for the nephrotic syndrome of quartan malaria.

Enlargement of the spleen and liver in malaria, trypanosomiasis and visceral leishmaniasis is associated with increased numbers of macrophages and lymphocytes in these organs. The liver, renal and cardiopulmonary pathology of schistosomiasis is related to cell-mediated responses to the worm eggs. Symptoms similar to those seen in endotoxaemia induced by Gram-negative bacteria are found in the acute stages of malaria.

The nonspecific immunosuppression discussed earlier may explain why individuals with parasite infections are especially susceptible to bacterial and viral infections.

VACCINATION

No effective vaccine for humans has so far been developed against parasitic protozoa and worms, mainly because of the complex parasite life cycles and their sophisticated adaptive responses. However, successful vaccines have been developed for both protozoa and helminth animal parasites. As protection depends, in many cases, on both antibody and cell-mediated reactions, a vaccine must induce long-lived B and T cell immunity. Given the recent advances in animal vaccines, it must be hoped that vaccines against the globally important human parasites will be developed in the near future.

RECOMMENDED READING

Murphy, K., & Weaver, C. (2017). *Janeway's Immunobiology* (9th ed.). London: Garland Science.

Nash, A. A., Dalziel, R. G., & Fitzgerald, J. R. (2015). *Mims' Pathogenesis of Infectious Disease* (6th ed.). London: Academic Press.

Websites

All the Virology on the WWW. Available at www.virology.netDPDx

Laboratory Identification of Parasitic Diseases of Public Health Concern. Available at http://www.dpd.cdc.gov/dpdx/HTML/Para_Health.htm.

Todar's Online Textbook of Bacteriology. Available at http://www.textbookofbacteriology.net/index.html. (Accessed Nov 2017).

10 Bacterial pathogenicity

KARL G. WOOLDRIDGE

KEY POINTS

- Opportunist pathogens require a defect in host defence before they cause disease, whereas primary pathogens affect otherwise healthy individuals. The possession of virulence determinants generally differentiates pathogens from nonpathogens and, in turn, their number and potency separate opportunist from primary pathogens.
- Expression of virulence determinants is carefully regulated and may involve a form of chemical communication between bacteria known as quorum sensing.
- Adhesins are often involved the establishment of an infection. Bacterial adhesion may be mediated by fimbrial or nonfimbrial adhesins and generally involves interactions with host cell surface receptors or surface-associated proteins such as fibronectin.
- Invasive pathogens gain entry and spread either by subverting host uptake mechanisms or by tissue disruption. Once established, pathogens must deploy a variety of mechanisms to avoid host defences.
- Multiplication within host tissues requires specific mechanisms to gain essential nutrients such as iron. Many pathogens make siderophores that compete with the host's high-affinity iron transport and storage systems.
- Host damage may be direct, via the release of toxins, or indirect, via the effects of the host's innate and adaptive immune responses (immunopathology).
- Endotoxins and exotoxins are recognised. Endotoxin is synonymous with the lipopolysaccharide or lipooligosaccharide of Gram-negative bacteria, and sufficient amounts elicit a cascade of responses leading to endotoxic shock.
- Exotoxins are proteins that cause damage or dysfunction by signalling at host cell membranes (type I), by damaging membranes (type II) or by entering target cells and directly altering function (type III).

Pathogenicity, or the capacity to cause disease, is a relatively rare quality among microbes. It requires the attributes of transmissibility from one host or reservoir to a fresh host, survival in the new host, infectivity or the ability to breach the new host's defences, and virulence, a multifactorial that denotes the capacity of a pathogen to harm its host. Virulence (see Ch. 11) in the clinical sense is a manifestation of a complex parasite–host relationship in which the capacity of the organism to cause disease is considered in relation to the resistance of the host.

TYPES OF BACTERIAL PATHOGENS

Bacterial pathogens can be classified into two broad and overlapping groups, opportunists and primary pathogens, both with a broad spectrum of virulence capabilities. Some pathogens are capable of infecting a wide range of host species; such pathogens are referred to as zoonoses, whereas others are highly adapted to a single host or a closely related group of host species. Zoonotic and nonzoonotic pathogens can be either opportunist or primary pathogens, and organisms that exist as harmless commensals in one species may be pathogens in a second species.

Opportunistic pathogens

Opportunistic pathogens rarely cause disease in individuals with intact immunological and anatomical defences. Only when such defences are impaired or compromised, as a result of congenital or acquired disease, by the use of immunosuppressive therapy or surgical techniques, are these bacteria able to cause disease. Many opportunistic pathogens (e.g., coagulase-negative staphylococci) are part of the normal human microbiota, carried on the skin or mucosal surfaces where they cause no harm and indeed may have a beneficial effect by preventing colonisation by other potential pathogens. However, introduction of these organisms into anatomical sites where they are not normally found, or removal of competing bacteria by the use of broad-spectrum antibiotics, may allow their localised multiplication and subsequent development of disease.

Primary pathogens

Primary pathogens are capable of establishing infection and causing disease in previously healthy individuals with intact immunological defences; they may more readily cause disease in individuals with impaired defences.

The above classification is applicable to the vast majority of pathogens. However, there are exceptions and variations within both categories of bacterial pathogens. Different strains of any bacterial species can vary in their genetic make-up and virulence. For example, the majority of *Neisseria meningitidis* strains are harmless commensals and are best considered to be opportunistic bacteria; some hypervirulent clones of the organism, however, can cause disease in previously healthy individuals. Conversely, people vary in their genetic make-up and susceptibility to invading bacteria, including meningococci.

Zoonoses and nonzoonotic pathogens

Some pathogens are found in a variety of animals and may be transferred to humans coming into contact with animals directly or indirectly. Familiar examples include *Escherichia coli* O157, which are often found in association with cattle and other animals without causing apparent disease in these animals, but can cause gastrointestinal illness as well as serious complications such as haemolytic uremic syndrome (HUS) when it infects humans. By contrast, some pathogens are highly adapted to their host. For example, the pathogenic *Neisseria* species *N. meningitidis* and *N. gonorrhoeae* have only ever been isolated from human hosts and are not capable of infecting or initiating disease in other animals under normal conditions.

VIRULENCE DETERMINANTS

Both opportunistic and primary pathogens possess virulence determinants or aggressins that facilitate pathogenesis. Possession of a single virulence determinant is very rarely sufficient to allow the initiation of infection leading to pathology. Most pathogens possess several virulence determinants, all of which play some part at various stages of the disease process. It should be noted that many virulence determinants present in bacterial pathogens may also be present in commensal bacteria that rarely, if ever, cause disease. In addition, not all strains of a particular bacterial species are equally pathogenic. For example, although six separate serotypes of encapsulated *Haemophilus influenzae* are recognised, more serious systemic infection is almost exclusively associated with isolates of serotype b. Moreover, even within serotype b isolates, 80% of serious infections are caused by six of more than 100 clonal types.

Different strains of a pathogenic species, referred to as pathovars, may cause distinct types of infections, each associated with possession of a particular complement of virulence determinants. Different strains of *E. coli*, for example, cause several distinct gastrointestinal diseases, urinary tract infections, septicaemia, meningitis and a range of other minor infections (see Ch. 16).

Expression and analysis of virulence determinants

Many pathogens produce an impressive armoury of putative virulence determinants in vitro. However, relatively early in the study of pathogenesis, it was appreciated that a knowledge of the behaviour of the pathogen in vivo is crucial to an understanding of virulence.

Animal models have been used to compare the virulence of naturally occurring variants differing in the expression of a particular determinant and have provided much useful information. While some pathogens do not thrive or produce disease in typically available animal models, progress is being made in constructing better models by genetically manipulating the animals—for example, to express human receptors and other proteins important in human infection. Nevertheless, not all human clinical syndromes can be reproduced in animals, and extrapolation from animal studies to humans can be misleading. Furthermore, the possibility that observed differences in virulence may be due to additional cryptic phenotypic or genotypic variations cannot always be excluded. Molecular techniques have been used to construct isogenic mutants of bacteria that differ only in the particular determinant of interest, and these constructs have allowed more detailed analysis of the role of such components in pathogenesis. More recently, comparative analysis of bacterial genome sequences have revealed the extent of genetic variation, as well as genetic mobility among bacterial strains.

Most studies of bacterial virulence determinants are by necessity performed in model systems in vitro. However, growth conditions in vitro differ significantly from those found in tissues, and as the expression of many virulence determinants is influenced by environmental factors, it is essential that such studies use cultural conditions that mimic as closely as possible those found in the host and that, where possible, confirmatory evidence is obtained that the phenomena observed actually occur during human infection.

Genetic studies have shown that expression of several different virulence determinants in a single bacterium is sometimes regulated in a coordinated fashion. Iron limitation, the normal situation encountered in host tissues, is one environmental stimulus that coordinately increases the production of many bacterial proteins. Some of these proteins have a specific role in obtaining sufficient iron for the invading pathogen such as surface proteins involved in transporting iron from host molecules or bacterial iron-binding molecules called siderophores, while others play other roles in pathogenesis not directly associated with iron acquisition including diphtheria toxin of *Corynebacterium diphtheriae*. In other bacteria, such as *Staphylococcus aureus* and *Pseudomonas aeruginosa*, some virulence determinants are expressed exclusively or maximally during the stationary phase of growth. Expression of these factors is associated with the production of inducer molecules or pheromones in the bacterial culture that accumulate as the bacteria grow until a threshold level is reached and gene expression is triggered—a process known as quorum sensing. The ability to regulate production of virulence determinants may save energy in situations in which expression is not required (e.g., in the environment) and quorum sensing may be important in establishing a sufficiently large population of bacteria in tissue to guarantee survival of the infecting organism while not exposing the regulated virulence determinant to the immune system prematurely. It is also clear that most organisms express some proteins only when in direct contact with host cells.

Molecular studies have allowed mechanisms of transmission of virulence determinants to be investigated (see Ch. 6). Virulence determinants encoded by genomic DNA sequences, plasmids, bacteriophages and transposons have been reported. It is interesting that, in nature, these genetic elements can move between related organisms, transfer genes encoding virulence factors (e.g., toxins) horizontally and transform the recipient bacteria to more adapted or more virulent pathogens. Bacteria can exchange virulence genes by other mechanisms as well. For example, *Neisseria* recognise and take up DNA fragments that contain specific sequences (uptake sequences) and incorporate them into their own genomes. In this way they can either vary the structure of an existing gene or, in the process, acquire a new set of genes. Hundreds of genomes of bacterial pathogens have now been fully sequenced. The data reveal that several bacteria have acquired very large stretches of foreign DNA (often called pathogenicity islands) that contain virulence-related genes. This further demonstrates that the microbial population consists of a vibrant, kinetic and highly interactive community where bacteria evolve continuously, resulting in the emergence of new pathogens, or old pathogens with newly acquired capabilities.

Establishment of infection

Potential pathogens may enter the body by various routes, including the respiratory, gastrointestinal, urinary or genital tract. Alternatively, they may enter tissues directly through insect bites or by accidental or surgical trauma to the skin. Many opportunistic and several primary pathogens are carried as part of the normal human microbiota, which acts as a ready source of infection in the compromised host. For many primary pathogens, however, transmission to a new host and establishment of infection are more complex processes. Transmission of respiratory pathogens, such as *Bordetella pertussis*, may require direct contact with infectious material, as the organism cannot survive for any length of time in the environment. Sexually transmitted pathogens such as *Neisseria gonorrhoeae* and *Treponema pallidum* have evolved further along this route and require direct person-to-person mucosal contact for transmission. Humans are the only natural host for these pathogens, which die rapidly in the environment. The source of infection may be individuals with clinical disease or infected carriers, in whom symptoms may be absent or relatively mild, either because the disease process is at an early stage, or because of partial immunity or natural resistance to the pathogen.

For many gastrointestinal pathogens, such as *Salmonella*, *Shigella* and *Campylobacter* species, the primary source is environmental, and infection follows the ingestion of contaminated food or water. Many of these organisms also infect other animals, often without harmful effect, and these act as a reservoir of infection and source of environmental contamination (see Ch. 1).

Colonisation

For many pathogenic bacteria, the initial interaction with host tissues occurs at a mucosal surface, and colonisation—the establishment of a stable population of bacteria in the host—normally requires adhesion to that surface. This allows the establishment of a focus of infection, which may remain localised or may subsequently spread to other tissues. Adhesion is necessary to avoid innate host defence mechanisms such as peristalsis in the gut and the flushing action of mucus, saliva and urine, which removes nonadherent bacteria. For invasive bacteria, adhesion is an essential preliminary to penetration through tissues. Successful colonisation also requires that bacteria are able to acquire essential nutrients, such as iron, for growth.

Adhesion

Adhesion involves surface interactions among specific receptors on the mammalian cell membrane (normally carbohydrates, proteins or glycolipids) and ligands (usually proteins or glycoproteins) on the bacterial surface. The presence or absence of specific receptors on mammalian cells contributes significantly to tissue specificity of infecting pathogens. Non-specific surface properties of the bacterium, including surface charge and hydrophobicity, also contribute to the initial stages of the adhesion process. Several different mechanisms of bacterial adherence have evolved, all utilising specialised cell surface organelles or macromolecules that help to overcome the natural forces of repulsion that exist between the pathogen and its target cell (both are generally negatively charged).

Fimbrial adhesins

Electron microscopy of the surface of many Gram-negative and some Gram-positive bacteria reveals the presence of numerous thin, rigid, rodlike structures called fimbriae, or pili, that are easily distinguishable from the much thicker bacterial flagella (see Ch. 2). Fimbriae are involved in mediating attachment of some bacteria to mammalian cell surfaces. Different strains or species of bacteria may produce different types of fimbriae, which can be identified on the basis of antigenic composition, morphology and receptor specificity (Table 10.1). A broad division can be made between fimbriae, in which adherence in vitro is inhibited by D-mannose (mannose-sensitive fimbriae), and those unaffected by this treatment (mannose-resistant fimbriae).

The antigenic composition of fimbriae can be complex. For instance, two fimbrial antigens called colonisation factor antigen (CFA) I and II have been detected in enteropathogenic *E. coli* strains. CFA-II consists of three distinct fimbrial antigens designated as coli surface (CS) antigens 1, 2 and 3. Another *E. coli* strain, E8775, has been found to produce three other CS antigens, CS4, CS5 and CS6. Pyelonephritogenic *E. coli* isolates produce a group of adhesins called X-adhesins; two fimbrial types

designated S and M on the basis of receptor specificity have been identified in this group. The genes encoding a second type of fimbriae, the Chaperone Usher (CU) fimbriae, also found in *E. coli*, are found as multiple homologous, and often cryptic, variants, potentially with specificities for different carbohydrate receptors.

The evolutionary significance of such heterogeneity may be that the ability of an individual bacterium to express several different types of fimbriae allows different target receptors to be used at different anatomical sites of the infected host. In vitro, production of fimbriae is influenced by cultural conditions such as incubation temperature and medium composition, which may switch off the production of fimbriae or induce a phase change from one fimbrial type to another.

For some fimbriae the association with infection is clear. Thus the K88 fimbrial antigen is clearly associated with the ability of *E. coli* K88 to cause diarrhoea in pigs; pigs lacking the appropriate intestinal receptors are spared the enterotoxigenic effects of *E. coli* strains of this type. In many other instances the association between production of fimbriae and infection remains putative at present. Proteins making up fimbriae may be encoded either on the chromosome or on plasmids.

The structures of several fimbrial types have been studied in detail. Type 1 or common fimbriae, for example, consist of aggregates of a structural protein subunit called fimbrillin (or pilin) arranged in a regular helical array to produce a rigid rodlike structure 7 nm in diameter, with a central hole running along its length.

A highly conserved minor protein, located at both the tip and at intervals along the length of the fimbriae, mediates specific adhesion. Type 1 fimbriae bind specifically to D-mannose residues. Their role in vivo remains controversial; however, they may be involved in the pathogenesis of urinary tract infections.

Other Gram-negative bacteria, including those of the genera *Pseudomonas*, *Neisseria*, *Bacteroides* and *Vibrio*, produce fimbriae that share some homology, especially in the amino-terminal region of the fimbrillin subunits (the so-called *N*-methylphenylalanine fimbriae). These fimbriae have been shown to act as virulence determinants for *P. aeruginosa* and *N. gonorrhoeae*.

Nonfimbrial adhesins

Nonfimbrial adhesins include protein or polysaccharide structures that are exposed on the bacterial cell surface and/or secreted. Protein-based adhesins include the filamentous haemagglutinin of *B. pertussis*, a mannose-resistant haemagglutinin from *Salmonella enterica* serotype Typhimurium, and a fibrillar haemagglutinin from *Helicobacter pylori*. Outer membrane proteins are involved in the adherence of many, if not most, bacterial pathogens.

Table 10.1 Examples of fimbriae produced by Gram-negative pathogens

Designation	Bacterium
Common (type 1)[a]	Enterobacteriaceae Uropathogenic *Escherichia coli*
CFA I, CFA II (CS1, CS2, CS3), E8775 (CS4, CS5, CS6)	Enterotoxigenic *E. coli* from humans
K88 K99 F41	Enterotoxigenic *E. coli* from animals
Pap-G, Prs-G P fimbriae X-adhesins (S, M)	Uropathogenic *E. coli* Pyelonephritogenic *E. coli*
N-methylphenylalanine fimbriae	*Pseudomonas, Neisseria, Moraxella, Bacteroides, Vibrio* species

See text for abbreviations and explanation.
[a]Mannose-sensitive fimbriae.

Exopolysaccharides present on the surface of some Gram-positive bacteria are also involved in adhesion. For example, *Streptococcus mutans*, which is involved in the pathogenesis of dental caries, synthesises a homopolymer of glucose that anchors the bacterium to the tooth surface and contributes to the matrix of dental plaque. Actinomyces may adhere to other oral bacteria—a process called coaggregation in which multispecies biofilms are formed on host surfaces. Teichoic acid and surface proteins of coagulase-negative staphylococci mediate adherence of these bacteria to the surfaces of prosthetic devices and catheters, contributing to increasing numbers of hospital-acquired infections. Monospecific biofilms or biofilms consisting of multiple species can form at various anatomical sites; the formation of biofilms also hinders successful antibiotic treatment by restricting access of drugs to the bacteria, or efficient clearance of the pathogens by the immune system.

In addition to their primary role in motility, flagella act as adhesins in *Vibrio cholerae* and *Campylobacter jejuni*. Bacterial motility is also thought to be important in chemotaxis of these organisms towards intestinal cells and in penetration of these pathogens through the mucous layer during colonisation.

Binding to connective tissue proteins

Binding of pathogenic bacteria to a number of connective tissue proteins including laminin, vitronectin and collagen have been described. The best studied of these host proteins is fibronectin, a complex multifunctional glycoprotein found in plasma and associated with mucosal cell surfaces, where it promotes numerous adhesion-related functions. Many pathogenic bacteria bind fibronectin at the bacterial surface, and for some organisms fibronectin has been shown to act as the cell surface receptor for bacterial adhesion. In *Streptococcus pyogenes*, lipoteichoic acid mediates attachment of the bacterium to the amino terminus of the fibronectin molecule. Attachment of *S. aureus* to cell surfaces also involves the amino terminus of fibronectin, but the bacterial ligand appears to be protein in this instance. *T. pallidum* also binds fibronectin. The significance of the interaction with fibronectin in the pathogenesis of syphilis and many other bacterial diseases needs further clarification.

Consequences of adhesion

In addition to preventing loss of the pathogen from the host, adhesion induces structural and functional changes in mucosal cells, and these may contribute to disease. For example, adherence of enteropathogenic *E. coli* (EPEC) to epithelial cells induces rearrangements of the cell cytoskeleton causing loss of microvilli and localised accumulation of actin, without subsequent invasion of the host cell. In contrast, adherence of *H. pylori* to gastric epithelial cells causes enhanced production of the proinflammatory chemokine interleukin (IL)-8, which contributes to gastric pathology. In both cases, these changes involve the induction of intracellular signalling pathways triggered after binding of the bacteria to specific receptors on the epithelial cell surface. Adhesion of bacteria to mammalian cells may induce changes in gene expression in both bacterial and host cells that might favour either the bacterium or the host.

Invasion

Once attached to a mucosal surface, some bacteria exert their pathogenic effects without penetrating the tissues of the host: toxins, other aggressins and induction of intracellular signalling pathways mediate tissue damage at local or distant sites. For a number of pathogenic bacteria, however, adherence to the mucosal surface represents but the first stage of the invasion of tissues. Examples of organisms that are able to invade and survive within host cells include mycobacteria and members of the genera *Salmonella*, *Shigella*, *Escherichia*, *Yersinia*, *Legionella*, *Listeria*, *Campylobacter* and *Neisseria*. Some bacterial pathogens take this one step further and can only replicate within the cells of their hosts. Examples of these kinds of obligate intracellular pathogens include *Chlamydia* and *Rickettsia* species. Occupation of an intracellular niche confers the ability to avoid humoral host defence mechanisms and potentially provides a nutrient-rich environment that is devoid of competition from other bacteria. However, the survival of bacteria in professional phagocytes, such as macrophages or polymorphonuclear leucocytes, depends on subverting intracellular killing mechanisms that would normally result in microbial destruction (see later in the chapter). For some bacteria *(Neisseria meningitidis)*, penetration through or between epithelial cells allows dissemination from the initial site of entry to other body sites.

Uptake into host cells

The initial phase of cellular invasion involves penetration of the mammalian cell membrane; rather than eliciting mechanisms for host cell penetration themselves, many intracellular pathogens induce phagocytic processes in the host cell to gain access.

Shigellae invade colonic mucosal cells but rarely penetrate deeper into the host tissues. Inside the cell, they are surrounded by a membrane-bound vesicle derived from the host cell. Soon after entry, this vesicle is lysed by the action of a plasmid-encoded haemolysin (haemolysis is just one way of detecting a membrane-damaging toxin), and the bacteria are released into the cell cytoplasm. *Listeria monocytogenes* produces a heat shock protein with a similar function, termed listeriolysin. Once free in the cell cytoplasm, shigellae multiply rapidly, with subsequent inhibition of host cell protein synthesis. Several hours later the host cell dies, and bacteria spread to adjacent cells where the process of invasion is repeated.

Other bacteria remain within membrane-bound vesicles but modify these cellular compartments, preventing them from maturing and fusing with lysosomes. The pathogenic *Neisseria*, for example, elaborate a secreted toxin, immunoglobulin A protease, which, in addition to cleaving immunoglobulin A during colonisation of the mucosa (see later in the chapter), is also capable of cleaving a key endocytic vesicle protein, LAMP1, which is responsible for acidification of the endosome. Recently, immunoglobulin A protease has also been shown to traffic to the cell nucleus where it interacts with chromatin and modulates host cell gene expression. In this way the intracellular pathogen modifies the environment within the vesicle to favour its own survival. Some strains of salmonellae proceed through the superficial layers of the gut and invade deeper tissues, in particular cells of the reticuloendothelial system such as macrophages. Salmonellae also occupy a host-derived vesicle that does not lyse. In this case, several vesicles coalesce to form large intracellular vacuoles. These vacuoles traverse the cytoplasm to reach the opposite side of the cell and initiate spread to adjacent cells and deeper tissues. Although invasion of host cells is essentially a bacterium-directed but host-mediated process, the active participation of the bacterium and novel bacterial protein synthesis are still required.

Role of cell receptors

The availability of specific receptors defines the types of host cells that are involved. As a result, some pathogens can invade a wide range of cell types, whereas others have a more restricted invasive potential. Specific host receptors for some invasive pathogens have been identified. For example, *Legionella pneumophila* and *Mycobacterium tuberculosis* adhere to complement receptors on the surface of phagocytic cells. A specific receptor for *Yersinia pseudotuberculosis* belongs to a family of proteins termed integrins that form a network on the surface of host cells to which host proteins such as fibronectin can bind. Mimicry of the amino acid sequence (Arg-Gly-Asp) of fibronectin that mediates attachment to the integrins may represent a common mechanism of effecting intracellular entry. The ability to utilise integrins may not be restricted to intracellular bacteria. The filamentous haemagglutinin of *B. pertussis* may use the fibronectin integrin to mediate attachment in the respiratory tract. Some bacteria encode their own receptors. Enteropathogenic *E. coli*, for example,

produce a protein called Tir, which is secreted into the host cell cytoplasm, is translocated back across the host plasma membrane, where it is displayed on the surface and acts as a receptor for the bacterial adhesin Intimin (see later in the chapter) encoded by the *eae* gene (see Ch. 16).

A number of bacterial pathogens capable of crossing the blood–brain barrier, including *N. meningitidis*, *Haemophilus influenzae* and *Streptococcus pneumoniae*, as well as a number of neurotropic viruses and prions, have been shown to bind to the laminin receptor protein, suggesting that binding to this host receptor protein confers a neurotropism on these pathogens.

Survival and multiplication

To cause disease, most microorganisms must survive on an epithelial surface, within a lumen or within host tissues and, at some stage, multiply. Survival depends, to a large extent, on the organism's ability to avoid, evade or resist host defences. Multiplication depends on acquiring all of the nutrients necessary for growth; the most extensively studied nutritional challenge to pathogens is iron acquisition.

Avoidance of host defence mechanisms

Colonisation by bacterial pathogens, particularly of normally sterile areas of the body, results in the induction of specific and nonspecific humoral and cell-mediated immune responses designed to eradicate the organism from the site of infection. Products of the organism that are not normally found within sterile tissues of the host may be chemotactic for phagocytic cells that are attracted to the site. Moreover, complement components may directly damage the bacterium and release peptides chemotactic for phagocytic cells. Other humoral antibacterial factors include lysozyme and the iron chelators transferrin and lactoferrin. Lysozyme is active primarily against Gram-positive bacteria but potentiates the activity of complement against Gram-negative organisms. Transferrin and lactoferrin chelate iron in body fluids and reduce the amount of free iron to a level below that necessary for bacterial growth.

Pathogenic bacteria have evolved ways of avoiding or neutralising these highly efficient clearance systems. As most of the interactions between the bacterium and the immune effectors involve the bacterial surface, resistance to these effects is related to the molecular architecture of the bacterial surface layers.

Capsules

Many bacterial pathogens need to avoid phagocytosis; production of an extracellular capsule is the most common mechanism by which this is achieved. Virtually all the pathogens associated with meningitis and pneumonia, including *H. influenzae*, *N. meningitidis*, *E. coli* and *S. pneumoniae*, have polysaccharide capsules, and noncapsulate variants usually exhibit much reduced virulence. Most capsules are polysaccharides composed of sugar monomers that vary among different bacteria. Polysaccharide capsules reduce the susceptibility of bacterial pathogens to phagocytosis in a number of ways.

1. In the absence of specific antibody to the bacterium, the hydrophilic nature of the capsule may hinder interaction with phagocytes, a process that occurs more readily at hydrophobic surfaces. This may be overcome if the phagocyte is able to trap the bacterium against a surface, a process referred to as surface phagocytosis.
2. Capsules prevent efficient opsonisation of the bacterium by complement or specific antibody, events that promote interaction with phagocytic cells. Capsules may either prevent complement deposition completely or cause complement to be deposited at a distance from the bacterial membrane where it is unable to damage the organism.
3. Capsules tend to be weakly immunogenic and may mask more immunogenic surface components and reduce interactions with both complement and antibody. In some cases—for example serogroup B *N. meningitidis* and serotype K1 *E. coli*—the capsular polysaccharide may mimic host polysaccharide moieties (e.g., polysialic acid found on the surface of some neural tissues) and be seen as self-antigen.

Streptococcal M protein

The M protein present on the surface of *S. pyogenes* is not a capsule but functions in a similar manner to prevent complement deposition at the bacterial surface. The M protein binds both fibrinogen and fibrin, and deposition of this material on the streptococcal surface hinders the access of complement activated by the alternative pathway.

Meningococcal Factor H–binding protein

The complement system is a powerful weapon against bacterial pathogens but can potentially damage host cells as well. The host must, therefore, protect itself against the damaging activities of complement. The serum glycoprotein Factor H is a negative regulator of the complement system that protects host cells by binding to glycosaminoglycans present on the surface of host but not bacterial cells, from where it can downregulate the activity of complement and thus protect the host cell. *N. meningitidis* expresses a Factor H–binding protein on its surface, which recruits this complement regulator, thus affording similar protection to the bacterial pathogen.

Resistance to killing by phagocytic cells

Some pathogens not only survive within macrophages and other phagocytes but may actually multiply intracellularly. The normal sequence of events following phagocytosis involves fusion of the phagosome in which the bacterium is contained with lysosomal granules present in the cell cytoplasm. These granules contain enzymes and cationic peptides involved in oxygen-dependent and oxygen-independent bacterial killing mechanisms (see Ch. 8 on Cells/Phagocytes).

Different organisms use different strategies for survival (Table 10.2). *M. tuberculosis* is thought to resist intracellular killing by preventing phagosome–lysosome fusion; other bacteria are able to resist the action of such lysosomal components after fusion. Some organisms stimulate a normal respiratory burst but are intrinsically resistant to the effects of the potentially toxic oxygen radicals produced. Production of catalase by pathogens including *S. aureus* and *N. gonorrhoeae* is thought to protect these organisms from such toxic products. The smooth lipopolysaccharide of many bacterial pathogens is also thought to contribute to their resistance to the effects of bactericidal cationic peptides present in the phagolysosome.

Antigenic variation

Variation in surface antigen composition during the course of infection provides a mechanism of avoidance of specific immune responses directed at those antigens. This strategy is most highly developed in blood-borne parasitic protozoa, such as trypanosomes, but is also exhibited by bacteria. Pathogenic *Neisseria*, for example, are capable of changing surface antigens using three highly efficient mechanisms. These are mutation of individual amino acids, phase variation (switching genes on and off) and horizontal

Table 10.2 Some strategies adopted by bacteria to avoid intracellular killing

Species	Method
Mycobacterium tuberculosis	Prevents phagosome–lysosome fusion
Salmonella serotype Typhi	Fails to stimulate oxygen-dependent killing
Staphylococcus aureus	Produces catalase to negate effect of toxic oxygen radicals
Pathogenic *Neisseria* species	Inhibits phagosome–lysosome acidification

exchange of DNA. *N. meningitidis* can avoid the killing effect of antibodies against its major porin (PorA) by mutating amino acids and/or acquiring parts of or all of its *porA* gene from another meningococcal strain. The organism can switch off the expression of its capsule or several of its surface-exposed immunogenic proteins by shifts in the nucleotide sequence encoding them. The latter varies as a result of recombination or mutation during DNA replication.

Another mechanism of antigen variation in *Neisseria* is the genetic rearrangements demonstrated in the type IV pili. Usually only one complete pilin gene is expressed, while there may be several incomplete silent gene sequences present on the chromosome. Movement of the incomplete gene sequences, either from within the genome of the expressing strain or from DNA released by a coinfecting strain, to an expression locus results in the generation of a hybrid gene and the synthesis of a protein that may differ antigenically from the original.

The *Borrelia* species that cause relapsing fever use a similar strategy to generate antigenic variation in their outer surface proteins. Other bacteria show strain-specific antigenic variability. For example, group A streptococci produce up to 75 antigenically distinct serotypes of M protein. As well as proteins, other surface molecules are subject to phase (on/off) or antigenic variation. Production of capsular polysaccharide in *N. meningitidis* is subject to phase variation via the SiaD protein, which is involved in the biosynthesis of capsular polysaccharide. In *H. influenzae*, the lipopolysaccharide is antigenically variable via the phase-variable expression of genes encoding enzymes that modify the lipopolysaccharide.

The capacity for variation in surface antigens allows for longer survival of an individual organism in a host and means that antibody produced in response to infection by one strain of a pathogen may not protect against subsequent challenge with a different strain of that bacterium. This makes the variable antigens elusive targets for protective antibodies, and the development of vaccines based on inhibition of attachment or generation of opsonic or bactericidal antibodies is particularly difficult for these organisms.

Immunoglobulin A proteases

Several species of pathogenic bacteria that cause disease on mucosal surfaces produce a protease that specifically cleaves immunoglobulin A (IgA), the principal antibody type produced at these sites. These proteases are specific for human IgA isotype I. Nearly all of the pathogens causing meningitis possess an IgA protease and a polysaccharide capsule enabling them to persist on the mucosal surface and resist phagocytosis during the invasive phase of the disease.

Serum resistance

To survive in the bloodstream, bacteria must be able to resist lysis as a result of deposition of complement on the bacterial surface. In the Enterobacteriaceae, resistance is primarily due to the composition of the lipopolysaccharide, which is a major component of the bacterial outer membrane. Smooth colonial variants that possess polysaccharide 'O' side chains are more resistant than rough colonial variants that lack such side chains (see later in the chapter). The side chains sterically hinder deposition of complement components on the bacterial surface. Conversely, some O-chain polysaccharides activate complement by an alternative pathway leading to lysis of the bacterial cell. In *N. meningitidis* group B and *E. coli* K1, sialic acid capsules prevent efficient complement activation and, in *N. gonorrhoeae*, complement binds but forms an aberrant configuration in the bacterial outer membrane that is unable to effect lysis.

Iron acquisition

The concentration of free iron in blood, tissue fluids or bodily secretions is below that required for bacterial growth because it is sequestered inside cells (e.g., in red blood cells as haemoglobin) or bound (chelated) by high-affinity mammalian iron-binding proteins such as transferrin and lactoferrin. To multiply in body fluids or on mucous membranes bacterial pathogens have evolved efficient mechanisms for scavenging iron from mammalian iron-binding proteins. Bacteria such as *E. coli*, *Klebsiella pneumoniae* and some staphylococci produce extracellular iron chelators called siderophores for this purpose. Others, including *Campylobacter jejuni* and *N. meningitidis*, do not produce siderophores themselves, but are able to obtain iron from siderophores produced by other species or use host molecules such as noradrenalin, which has siderophore-like activity, as a source of iron. In an alternative strategy, pathogens including *N. meningitidis*, *Haemophilus parainfluenzae*, *H. influenzae* type b, *Staphylococcus epidermidis* and *S. aureus* have specific receptors for transferrin and/or lactoferrin on their surfaces and are able to bind these proteins and remove the bound iron directly from these host proteins. Production of siderophores, their cell surface receptors and receptors for transferrin, lactoferrin and other mammalian iron-binding proteins is iron regulated and occurs mainly under conditions of iron limitation.

Two other mechanisms of iron acquisition from mammalian iron chelators have been described. Some *Bacteroides* species remove iron by proteolytic cleavage of the chelator. In *L. monocytogenes*, reduction of the Fe^{3+} ion to Fe^{2+} reduces the affinity for the chelator sufficiently for it to be removed by the bacterium.

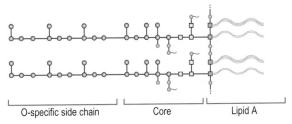

= various sugar residues
☐ = ketodeoxyoctonate (KDO)
▣ = glucosamine
~ = phosphoethanolamine
⌢ = fatty acid residues

Fig. 10.1 Diagrammatic representation of the structure of bacterial lipopolysaccharide. (From Rietschel, E. T., Galanos, C., & Lüderlitz, O. (1975). Structure, endotoxicity and immunogenicity of the lipid A component of bacterial lipopolysaccharide. In D. Schlessinger (Ed.) *Microbiology – 1975* (pp. 307-314). Washington, DC: American Society for Microbiology.)

Many bacteria express receptors for binding and/or internalising other mammalian iron-containing molecules, such as haem, haemoglobin and haemoglobin–haemopexin complexes. These mammalian molecules are located intracellularly, where they may be available to intracellular pathogens; they may also be released by bacterial haemolysins that lyse the red cells.

Damage or dysfunction

In order for an infection to become apparent there must be sufficient host damage or dysfunction for the individual to become symptomatic. It is particularly important to appreciate that there are generally two components to this: the direct effect of the organism and the host response. In many cases, this largely immune-mediated damage (immunopathology) can predominate. This may reflect an excessive innate response as in septic shock (see later in the chapter), or the adaptive response as in tuberculosis (see Ch. 27). The most obvious means by which bacteria cause host damage or dysfunction is by the production of toxins.

Toxins

In many bacterial infections, part or all the characteristic pathology of the disease is caused by toxins. Toxins may exert their pathogenic effects directly on a target cell or may interact with cells of the immune system, resulting in the release of immunological mediators (cytokines) that cause pathophysiological effects (see Chs 8 and 9). Such effects may not always lead to the death of the target cell but may selectively impair specific functions. Substances that have toxic physiological effects on target cells in vitro do not necessarily exert the same effects in vivo, but a number of toxins have been shown to be responsible for the typical clinical features of bacterial disease.

Two broad categories of toxin have been described: endotoxin, which is a component of the outer membrane of Gram-negative bacteria, and exotoxins, which are produced extracellularly by both Gram-negative and Gram-positive bacteria.

Endotoxin

Endotoxin, also called lipopolysaccharide or lipooligosaccharide, is a component of the outer membrane of Gram-negative bacteria and is released from the bacterial surface via outer membrane vesicles (blebs), which may be released from the bacterial cell surface, or by lysis and disintegration of the organism. Lipopolysaccharide is anchored into the bacterial outer membrane through a unique molecule termed lipid A (Fig. 10.1). Covalently linked to lipid A

is an eight-carbon sugar, ketodeoxyoctonate, in turn linked to the chain of sugar molecules (saccharides) that form the highly variable O antigen structures of Gram-negative bacteria. On bacteriological media, bacteria carrying lipopolysaccharide with O antigen form smooth colonies with hydrophilic surfaces; in contrast, those carrying lipopolysaccharide without the O antigen form rough colonies with hydrophobic surfaces.

The term *endotoxin* was originally introduced to describe the component of Gram-negative bacteria responsible for the pathophysiology of endotoxic shock, a syndrome with a high mortality rate, particularly in immunocompromised or otherwise debilitated individuals. Endotoxin activates complement via the alternative pathway, but most of the biological activity of the molecule is attributable to lipid A. Both endotoxin and lipid A are potent activators of macrophages, resulting in the induction of a range of cytokines involved in the regulation of immune and inflammatory responses (see Chs 8 and 9). Although endotoxin from Gram-negative organisms remains central to our understanding of septic shock, other structural and secreted components of bacteria that interact with pattern recognition receptors (Chs 8 and 9) can contribute to the pathogenesis of this clinical syndrome. Thus the multisystem effects, often involving complement, blood clotting factor and kinin activation together with extensive cytokine release, should not be seen as exclusive to Gram-negative infection.

Exotoxins

Exotoxins, in contrast to endotoxin, are diffusible proteins secreted into the external medium by the pathogen. Most pathogens secrete various protein molecules that facilitate adhesion to, or invasion of, the host. Many others cause damage to host cells. The damage may be physiological—for example, cholera toxin promotes electrolyte (and fluid) excretion from enterocytes without killing the cells—or pathological—where the toxin (e.g., diphtheria toxin) inhibits protein synthesis and induces cell death. Exotoxins vary in their molecular structure, biological function, mechanism of secretion and immunological properties. The list of bacterial exotoxins is vast and increasing; however, they are often classified by their mode of action on animal cells:

- Type I (membrane acting) toxins bind surface receptors and stimulate transmembrane signals, and include the super-antigenic toxins.
- Type II (membrane damaging) toxins directly affect membranes, forming pores or disrupting lipid bilayers.
- Type III (intracellular effector) toxins translocate an active enzymatic component into the cell and modify an intracellular target molecule.

Examples of exotoxins and their effects on target cells are shown in Table 10.3. Bacteria secrete toxins and other proteins using a number of distinct mechanisms that are understood to varying extents. Some of these systems are listed in Gram-negative bacteria as types I-VI, although this number does not reflect the total number of pathways that are known to mediate secretion of proteins across the bacterial envelope. Fig. 10.2 shows the basic components of the types I and V pathways, which are relatively well characterised. In type I, at least three proteins associated to form a channel spanning both membranes and the intervening periplasm through which large molecules (such as haemolysin of *E. coli*) are exported. In type V, however, a single precursor protein that consists of three domains is secreted sequentially across the inner and outer membranes. Although these latter proteins are called autotransporters, it is now known that both secretion steps require the activity of a number of additional cellular proteins. A typical example of an autotransporter is the IgA1 protease of *Neisseria* spp.

Enterotoxins cause symptoms of gastrointestinal disease, including diarrhoea, dysentery and vomiting. In some cases the disease is caused by ingestion of preformed toxin in food, but in most cases colonisation of the intestine is required before toxin is made.

Cholera toxin and heat-labile toxins of enterotoxigenic *E. coli* (ETEC) do not induce inflammatory changes in the intestinal mucosa but perturb the processes that regulate ion and water exchange across the intestinal epithelium (see Chs 16 and 21). In contrast, the enterotoxins of *Clostridium difficile, C. perfringens* type A and *Bacillus cereus* cause structural damage to epithelial cells, resulting in inflammation. Another gastrointestinal pathogen,

Table 10.3 Some effects of bacterial exotoxins

Toxic effect	Examples
Lethal action	
Effect on neuromuscular junction	*Clostridium botulinum* toxin A
Effect on voluntary muscle	Tetanus toxin
Damage to heart, lungs, kidneys etc.	Diphtheria toxin
Pyrogenic effect	
Increase in body temperature and polyclonal T cell activation	Super-antigenic exotoxins of *Staphylococcus aureus* and *Streptococcus pyogenes* (e.g., staphylococcal toxic shock syndrome toxin 1)
Action on gastrointestinal tract	
Secretion of water and electrolytes	Cholera and *Escherichia coli* enterotoxins
Pseudomembranous colitis	*Clostridium difficile* toxins A and B
Bacillary dysentery	Shigella toxin
Vomiting	*Staphylococcus aureus* enterotoxins A–E
Action on skin	
Necrosis	Clostridial toxins; staphylococcal α-toxin
Erythema	Diphtheria toxin; streptococcal erythrogenic toxin
Permeability of skin capillaries	Cholera enterotoxin; *E. coli* heat-labile toxin
Nikolsky sign[a]	*Staphylococcus aureus* epidermolytic toxin
Cytolytic effects	
Lysis of blood cells	*Staphylococcus aureus* α-, β- and δ-lysins; leucocidin Streptolysin O and S *Clostridium perfringens* α and θ toxins
Inhibition of metabolic activity	
Protein synthesis	Diphtheria toxin; shiga toxin

[a]Separation of epidermis from dermis.

enteropathogenic *E. coli* (EPEC), mediates damage by a process that involves secretion of a protein, Tir, directly across both bacterial membranes and the host cell membrane in a single step. Tir is subsequently inserted into the host cell membrane where it acts as a receptor for a bacterial adhesin, intimin. Binding of intimin to Tir results in phosphorylation of the latter protein, this in turn leads to a signalling cascade and cytoskeletal rearrangements within the host cell.

B. pertussis, the causative agent of whooping cough, produces various extracellular products, including a tracheal

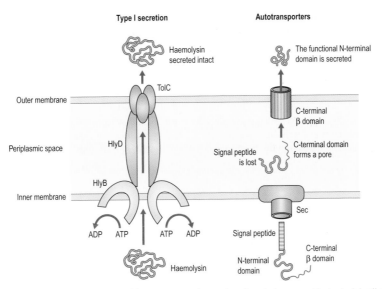

Fig. 10.2 Diagrammatic representation of type I and type V (autotransporter) secretion of exotoxins across the bacterial cell membrane. *ADP*, adenosine diphosphate; *ATP*, adenosine triphosphate; *Hly*, haemolysin; *Tol*, special receptor.

cytotoxin that inhibits the beating of cilia on tracheal epithelial cells, pertussis toxin, which exhibits several systemic effects, and an adenylate cyclase that interferes with phagocyte function.

Another group of toxins causes damage to subepithelial tissues following penetration and multiplication of the pathogen at the site of infection. Many of these toxins also inhibit or interfere with components of the host immune system. Membrane-damaging toxins such as staphylococcal α and β toxins, streptolysin O and streptolysin S, and *C. perfringens* α and θ toxins inhibit leucocyte chemotaxis at subcytolytic concentrations but cause necrosis and tissue damage at higher concentrations.

Systemic effects of toxins

Some toxins cause damage to internal organs following absorption from the focus of infection. Included in this category are the toxins causing diphtheria, tetanus and botulism, and those associated with streptococcal scarlet fever, staphylococcal toxic shock syndrome and haemolytic uremic syndrome associated with Shiga toxin–producing enteropathogens. The diphtheria toxin, which is encoded by a gene encoded by a bacteriophage, inhibits protein synthesis in mammalian cells. Tetanus toxin, in contrast, exerts its effect by preventing the release of inhibitory neurotransmitters whose function is to prevent overstimulation of motor neurons in the central nervous system, resulting in the convulsive muscle spasm characteristic of tetanus. Diphtheria and tetanus toxins represent the sole determinant of disease and are neutralised by specific antitoxin antibody. As a result, vaccination with toxoids (formalin- or genetically inactivated toxins) derived from these toxins is highly effective (see Ch. 68).

Botulism results from the ingestion of preformed toxin produced by *Clostridium botulinum* in food contaminated with this bacterium and is not a true infectious disease. The toxic activity is due to a family of serologically distinct polypeptide neurotoxins that prevent release of acetylcholine at neuromuscular junctions, resulting in the symptoms of flaccid paralysis. These toxins have been used clinically in treating squints and muscle spasm.

Other toxins cause disseminated multisystem organ damage. Such pathology is seen in staphylococcal toxic shock syndrome caused by certain strains of *S. aureus* that produce a toxin designated toxic shock syndrome toxin 1 (TSST-1). This toxin belongs to a group of functionally related proteins collectively referred to as superantigens, which include the staphylococcal enterotoxins, staphylococcal exfoliative toxin and streptococcal pyrogenic exotoxin A. These molecules are potent T cell mitogens whose reactivity with lymphocytes induces cytokine release; they may initiate tissue damage by mechanisms similar to those postulated to account for Gram-negative endotoxic shock (see earlier in the chapter).

Other extracellular aggressin

Many bacteria secrete a range of enzymes that may be involved in pathogenic processes.

Proteus spp. and some other bacteria that cause urinary tract infections produce ureases that break down urea in the urine; the release of ammonia may contribute to the pathology. The urease produced by the gastric and duodenal pathogen *H. pylori* is similarly implicated in the virulence of the organism as it acts to locally raise the pH and thus protect the organism from the highly acidic environment of the stomach. *L. pneumophila* produces a metalloprotease thought to contribute to the characteristic pathology seen in *Legionella* pneumonia.

Many other degradative enzymes, including mucinases, phospholipases, elastases, collagenases and hyaluronidases, are produced by pathogenic bacteria. Many nonpathogenic bacteria and opportunistic pathogens also produce such enzymes; in most cases their role in pathogenesis requires further clarification.

An understanding of the basic mechanisms of pathogenesis is important for the design of new or improved vaccines and appropriate therapies. Such knowledge is also invaluable in the analysis of new bacterial pathogens that are recognised from time to time. However, for some bacterial diseases—for example, syphilis—such approaches have still not defined the mechanisms of pathogenesis or the virulence determinants involved, and new strategies employed by such successful pathogens may yet be discovered.

RECOMMENDED READING

Hacker, J., & Hessemann, J. (Eds.). (2002). *Molecular infection biology: Interaction between microorganisms and cells.* New Jersey: Wiley-Blackwell.

Kadis, S., Montie, D. D., & Ajl, S. J. (Eds.). (2012). *Bacterial protein toxins* (Vol. 2A). Massachusetts: Academic Press.

Lamont, R. (Ed.). (2004). *Bacterial invasion of host cells (advances in molecular and cellular microbiology).* Cambridge: Cambridge University Press.

Locht, C., & Simonet, M. (Eds.). (2012). *Bacterial pathogenesis: Molecular and cellular mechanisms.* Poole: Caister Academic Press.

Nash, A. A., Dalziel, R. J., & Fitzgerald, J. R. (2015). *Mims' pathogenesis of infectious disease* (6th ed.). Massachusetts: Academic Press.

Salyers, A. A., & Whitt, D. D. (2011). *Bacterial pathogenesis: A molecular approach* (3rd ed.). Washington, DC: ASM Press.

11 The natural history of infection and the human microbiome

MICHAEL R. BARER

KEY POINTS

- Symptomatic infection is a rare outcome when human beings and microorganisms meet. Nonetheless, some organisms, known as obligate pathogens, must cause disease to survive; this applies to many viral pathogens. Many bacterial pathogens appear to derive little benefit from causing infection.
- Microorganisms that form short- or long-term associations with humans do so in a number of recognisable forms and stages, including entry/establishment, colonisation, commensalism, spread, survival and multiplication, damage and carriage. Where these associations lead to bacterial disease, the different stages are often associated with the virulence determinants described in Ch. 10.
- Infections can generally be recognised in one of four categories: toxin mediated, acute, subacute and chronic.
- The capacity of a particular microorganism to cause disease is known as its virulence. Where suitable

experimental models are available, we can recognise virulence quantitatively by the ability of a low number of organisms to produce infection or death in the host population. Such measurements can be useful in identifying virulence determinants and in developing vaccines.
- The total community of microbes associated with an individual is referred to as the individual's *microbiome*. A very substantial body of evidence now links the composition of the human microbiome to health and multiple disease states, notably nutritional status and diabetes.
- Microbiome analyses are achieved predominantly by nucleotide sequencing methods and produce community profiles characterised by organism lists and diversity indices. When a causal link is made between a particular microbial profile and human disease or dysfunction, then a dysbiosis is said to be in progress.

The purpose of this chapter is to link the basic properties of microorganisms with the patterns of infective disease experienced in public health and clinical practice, and with the tissue and organ pathology that can be observed. Although there are numerous exceptions to the general patterns described, the intention is to give an underlying structure that can be used to make sense of the many different types of organism and the diseases they cause. The term *natural history* is used in two senses here: first, to denote an overall biological consideration of the life cycle of the infective agent and how this intersects with the human host and, second, to consider the process of infection from the point of the encounter between the agent and the susceptible host through to its outcome.

While clinical practice is focused on infection and its prevention, the highly active research field of microbiomics has revealed numerous more subtle interactions between our microbiomes and human physiology. These interactions do not meet the criteria for infection, and, where the outcome is negative, the concept of dysbiosis is used to describe the relationship. Microbiomics certainly impinges on clinical practice, most obviously in *Clostridium difficile*–associated colitis, and the need to integrate this field into medicine will only increase.

MEETINGS BETWEEN HUMAN BEINGS AND MICROORGANISMS

The vast majority of microorganisms do not form stable associations with human beings. Clearly, pathogens must do so, at least temporarily. However, it is worth briefly considering how important this association is to the microorganism concerned. In some cases, humans constitute the only environment in which microorganisms can survive (i.e., they are obligate parasites of human beings). Thus humans are the reservoir and immediate source of the infections caused by this group (see Ch. 1). In other cases, colonisation or infection of human beings may be entirely incidental to the life cycle of the organism. These organisms may need to live in animals, as in the case of zoonoses, or in specific environmental reservoirs. Their life cycles in these habitats are critical to the epidemiology of the infections they cause. This biological perspective is difficult to avoid when considering the complex life cycles of parasitic protozoa and helminths, but such considerations are equally applicable to bacterial and viral pathogens.

In the previous chapter, a division was made between primary and opportunistic pathogens. Here this division is maintained but the primary group is further subdivided.

Obligate pathogens

These organisms have to cause disease in human beings in order to continue to survive and propagate. This is true for most viruses that cause human disease and for which humans are the only natural host. The major caveat to this is that the degree to which these agents cause symptomatic infections can vary over a very wide range. Thus asymptomatic infections with smallpox were virtually unknown, whereas they are very common with polio. This contributed substantially to the eradication of smallpox, as it was relatively straightforward to identify where transmission was taking place. Among bacterial pathogens, *Mycobacterium tuberculosis* is a prime example of an agent that has to cause symptomatic disease in order to survive and propagate. In some cases, pathogenicity reflects an early stage in the development of host–parasite relations, with pathogens evolving towards a more benign association with their host. Clearly, if a parasite kills all of its potential hosts then it has destroyed its own habitat. However, this does not always hold true. Some pathogens actually become more virulent as a means of increasing their potential to survive.

Accidental or incidental pathogens

This term applies to many bacterial pathogens. Causing disease confers no obvious biological advantage on the organism and indeed may be a dead end. There are two groups of bacterial pathogens for which this is probably the case. The first group have their natural habitat in humans but cause disease in only a small minority; these include the major pathogens of bacterial pharyngitis *(Streptococcus pyogenes)*, acute pneumonia *(Streptococcus pneumoniae)* and the principal agents of acute pyogenic meningitis *(Streptococcus pneumoniae, Neisseria meningitidis* and

Haemophilus influenzae type b). The second group have a habitat (or reservoir) in nature, but if they encounter a susceptible host in a particular way, infection may ensue. For example, the agent of cholera, *Vibrio cholerae,* lives in brackish water and causes human disease only when ingested. *Clostridium tetani,* the agent of tetanus, probably propagates in animal gastrointestinal tracts and infects wounds contaminated by soil containing animal excreta.

Pathogens in the environment

Whatever the method of acquisition, the organism must survive long enough to encounter a susceptible human host if it is going to cause human disease. The dynamics of pathogen survival in various environments are relevant to the control of infection. The capacities of different pathogens to survive and propagate in food and water are of particular concern, as is survival in aerosols and through desiccation and many other common environmental stresses. These properties provide the biological basis for the transmission of infection and many opportunities for improved control of specific pathogens.

STAGES OF INFECTION

Most infections can be broken down into a core series of steps:

- encounter
- entry and establishment
- spread
- survival and multiplication
- damage/dysfunction
- outcome.

It should be noted that the virulence determinants described in Ch. 10 were related to all but the first and last of these stages. Most pathogens can cause infection only via a limited set of routes (see earlier in the chapter). Thus *Vibrio cholerae* must be ingested; it cannot cause infection if rubbed on the skin. Human immunodeficiency virus (HIV) must gain access to circulating $CD4^+$ cells via a parenteral route, and so on. Some general points concerning the passage through alternative stages of infection are made in Fig. 11.1. Note that, although the simple direct pathway (A) reflects the norm for an exogenous infection, there are intermediates between this and (D), endogenous infection. A single organism may be capable of following multiple routes to infection. For example, *Staphylococcus aureus* may be introduced exogenously into a wound. Around 30% of individuals are colonised with this organism at any point in time but in only one-third of these (10%) does the organism appear to be a member of the normal microbiota. Both temporary

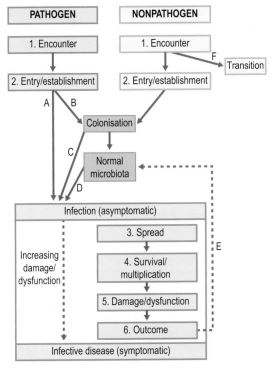

Fig. 11.1 Pathways to and stages of infection following encounter between a host and a microorganism. The blue sector includes the possible outcomes for a pathogen, the yellow, a nonpathogen, and the green, either of these. An organism detected in a diagnostic laboratory might reflect one or more of the stages identified, including transition. The possibility of transition from yellow to blue zones reflects the lack of a rigid division between pathogen and nonpathogen, and one aspect of opportunism. Detection in a diagnostic laboratory is most likely following colonisation or multiplication. Infection may become apparent because of many different pathways: (A) directly, without any colonisation phase; (B) many pathogens colonise first then proceed to infection either (C) after a brief period of colonisation or (D) after a sustained period in which they live as commensals as part of the normal microbiota (progression here is not inevitable). Note that infection becomes symptomatic only when the level of damage or dysfunction is sufficient. At the end of the symptomatic infection, a small number of pathogens may enter the normal microbiota (E), and the convalescent host is then described as a *carrier* for the organism concerned. (F), Some organisms may simply be passing through and form no stable association with the host.

and permanent relationships may provide for endogenous infections due to *Staph. aureus*.

Many opportunistic pathogens become part of the normal microbiota before they cause infection. They may be assisted in colonising a new host by interventions such as repeated use of antibiotics. This appears to be the case with *Pseudomonas aeruginosa,* which is resistant to most routinely used antibacterial agents, and is probably also the case for methicillin-resistant *Staph. aureus* (MRSA) and vancomycin-resistant enterococci (VRE). Most members of the normal microbiota appear to have very little capacity to cause disease. The number and identities

of readily culturable bacteria varies in different parts of the body (Table 11.1), and it is clear that a 'healthy' normal microbiota provides some protection against invading pathogens.

The survival of humankind to the present day reflects the fact that most untreated infections are not fatal. Indeed, many human genes, particularly those concerned with the immune response, clearly reflect the selection pressure provided by infection. Before the development of antibiotics and immunisation, at least 50% of deaths were attributable to infection (this is still the case in many resource-poor countries). Nevertheless, owing to our inherent and highly efficient defence mechanisms, many infections resolve without medical intervention. All doctors must have some skill in recognising those infections for which an intervention is unnecessary. This is particularly important in the case of antibiotic use because of the dangers of encouraging resistance.

PATHOLOGICAL PATTERNS ASSOCIATED WITH INFECTION

All of the foregoing reflects a set of proposed mechanisms that, by and large, fit and make sense of the available facts concerning the epidemiology and detailed pathogenesis of infection. In this section, the link to clinical practice is developed by describing the pattern of pathology directly observable in various infections. Most infections can be placed into one of four patterns:

1. Toxin mediated (mainly bacterial)
2. Acute (including acute viral syndromes and acute pyogenic bacterial infections)
3. Subacute (many virus and several atypical bacterial infections)
4. Chronic (chronic viral infections, chronic granulomatous bacterial, fungal and parasitic infections).

Simply by comparing the basic characteristics of a suspected infection against these four possibilities, the possible range of causal agents can be narrowed down substantially. Their features are summarised and exemplified from the perspective of bacterial infections in Table 11.2.

Toxin-mediated bacterial infections

This was the first recognised pathogenic mechanism in bacterial infection and resulted in early successful therapeutic and preventive measures. When a single toxin is responsible for most of the features of an infection, the dysfunction or damage is often distant from the site of bacterial multiplication, the disease may be reproduced by administration of the pure toxin alone and it can be prevented with

Table 11.1 Normal human microbiota[a]

Location[b]	Composition[c]	Abundance[d]
Dry skin (face, forearm)	Gram-positive anaerobes (e.g., propionibacteria)	10^2
Moist skin (axilla, groin)	Staphylococci (esp. coagulase negative); corynebacteria; Gram-negatives rare but more frequent after prolonged hospital stay	10^{6-7}
Oropharynx	Anaerobes; streptococci; *Neisseria*; *Candida*	10^9
Small intestine	Anaerobes, lactobacilli, Peptostreptococcus, Porphyromonas	10^{5-7}
Large intestine	Anaerobes, *Clostridium*, *Bacteroides*; enterobacteria; enterococci, *Candida*, protozoa	10^{9-11}
Vagina	Anaerobes, *Lactobacillus*; streptococci, *Candida*	10^{8-9}

[a]The term *microbiota* is preferred to 'flora', as the latter refers back to a period when bacteria were classified with plants.
[b]These are extremely broad. In practice, each microniche in the body constitutes a different environment colonised with different organisms; for example, the microbiota associated with the lumen and the mucosa of the gut are different.
[c]A very rough introductory guide. Note the predominance of anaerobes.
[d]Per square centimetre of surface or gram of fluid.

Table 11.2 Patterns in the presentation and pathology of bacterial infection

Pattern	Examples
Toxin-mediated disease	
Pathology often distant from site of bacterial growth	Diphtheria, tetanus
Protective immunity may be mediated by antitoxin antibodies alone	Staphylococcal food poisoning, cholera
Disease may be fully reproduced by administering the toxin alone	Pseudomembranous colitis
Acute pyogenic infection	
Generally rapid growing organisms	Streptococcal pharyngitis
Interaction with innate immune system and acute inflammation predominates	Staphylococcal abscess, bacterial meningitis, lobar pneumonia, acute cystitis
Where immune damage occurs, it is 'postinfective'	Poststreptococcal glomerulonephritis
Subacute infection	
No pattern to growth rate	Subacute bacterial endocarditis
Site of infection may be only partially accessible to the immune system	Atypical pneumonia
Immunopathology often in parallel with direct effects of organism	
Chronic (granulomatous)	
Bacterial growth rate often moderate or slow	Tuberculosis, brucellosis
Organisms often survive and grow intracellularly	
Immune damage occurs with infection – predominantly cell mediated	(Some fungal and parasitic infections have this pattern)

antibodies directed against the toxin. The clostridial diseases tetanus and botulism are toxin-mediated. In the latter case, as in several other forms of food poisoning, ingestion of only the toxin is required; so many cases of botulism are not strictly infections. Once the pathogen has grown and produced toxin, the onset of disease can be very rapid.

It is often possible to abolish the biological activity of toxins without affecting their immunogenicity. Such toxoids were among the first effective immunisations against bacterial infection. Diphtheria and tetanus toxoid vaccines have controlled these infections in the United Kingdom. In life-threatening toxin-mediated disease, the administration of pre-formed antibodies can be lifesaving. Antibiotics are not effective in treating established disease, but may prevent further toxin formation. In the special case of *Escherichia coli* O157 infections, however, some antibiotics actually stimulate further synthesis of toxin.

Acute pyogenic bacterial infections

Pyogenic means pus inducing. Pus is composed primarily of live and dead neutrophil polymorphs. The presence of pus generally reflects an acute inflammatory process and activation of the innate immune system. The inflammatory process may be localised, as in the formation of an abscess, or more disseminated through tissue planes. Anything more than a trivial acute pyogenic infection is usually accompanied by an increase in the blood neutrophil count. The acuteness of these infections is reflected in their rapid onset. Accordingly, the bacteria that cause them generally grow rapidly, producing visible colonies within 24 hours of inoculation. Medical intervention is most effective when given early in infection before the development of acquired immunity, which, when successful, terminates the illness. Serological evidence of acquired immunity cannot be used in the diagnosis of infection during its acute phase. Occasionally, immunopathology occurs after the causal organism is no longer detectable in the host; classic examples are post-streptococcal glomerulonephritis and rheumatic fever. Similarly, Guillain–Barré syndrome, a paralytic disease, sometimes follows acute *Campylobacter* infection.

Many bacteria that cause acute pyogenic infections also produce toxins. Thus there may be both acute pyogenic and toxin-mediated components to the damage and dysfunction that develops. This is particularly true of staphylococcal and streptococcal infections. The complex mixture of the pathogenic processes attributable to different virulence determinants can make the most severe of these infections very difficult to treat.

Subacute bacterial infections

These have a more insidious onset than acute infections and are accompanied by less prominent signs of acute inflammation. Classically, bacterial endocarditis was described as subacute, although this is no longer considered a suitable catch-all term for this type of infection. Because such diseases have a more protracted course, the adaptive immune response often contributes to damage. Hence, subacute forms of bacterial endocarditis are often accompanied by immune complex–mediated pathology, whereas *Mycoplasma pneumoniae* infection (a form of atypical pneumonia) may be accompanied by several different immunopathological reactions reflecting specific immune responses (see Ch. 35).

Chronic granulomatous bacterial infections

When bacterial infections persist over months or even years they tend to elicit a pathological entity known as a granuloma. Granulomas are a common form of localised cell-mediated immune response directed to antigens or other foreign bodies that appear to be refractory to elimination from tissues. An ordered accumulation of lymphocytes and macrophages occurs around a central focus in a manner that, to the experienced pathologist, can be more or less specific to the eliciting stimulus. Persisting bacterial infections, notably those due to mycobacteria (e.g., tuberculosis) and, to a lesser extent, *Brucella* spp., produce chronic granulomatous infections. The agents concerned are generally slow growing and have the capacity to survive inside host cells, notably macrophages. Cell-mediated immunopathology (delayed-type hypersensitivity; see Ch. 9) is a prominent feature of these infections.

Timing of key events in infection

As different infections proceed at different rates, the timing of the symptoms, their relation to immune responses and the ability to detect the causal agent all vary. The incubation period, the time between the encounter with the pathogen

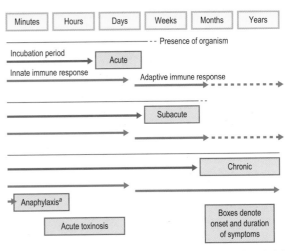

Fig. 11.2 Timescales for key events in infection. *a*Anaphylaxis is included for comparison and to illustrate the timescale when the adaptive immune response is primed against the antigen(s) concerned.

and the onset of symptoms, is an important practical consideration in understanding and managing infection. This is characteristic for different pathogens and can be vital in determining whether an individual is still at risk of developing disease after exposure to a particular agent. Incubation periods for the four patterns of infection discussed earlier are illustrated in Fig. 11.2, along with the time frames over which immune responses and presence of the pathogen are expected. A more dynamic view of individual infections is shown in Fig. 11.3, in which the additional concepts of recurrent, latent and reactivated infections are illustrated. Fig. 11.3 introduces the notion that the progression of an infection is related to the numbers of the pathogen. Although many other factors are involved, the concept is useful because it illustrates how, in some rapidly developing infections, the interval between the onset of symptoms and death may be short. The slope of increasing pathogen numbers clearly also reflects the balance between growth of the pathogen and the efforts of the immune system to resist. Accordingly, when the immune system is suppressed, progression may be exceptionally rapid and the response must be equally so.

VIRULENCE AND INFECTIVITY

By now it should be apparent that what makes a pathogen more or less virulent is, in most cases, extremely complex. Nonetheless, when infections can be studied in animal experimental systems, virulence can be seen as a quantifiable property. As the dose administered to a group of susceptible hosts is increased, the number acquiring infections also increases in a fairly well-defined

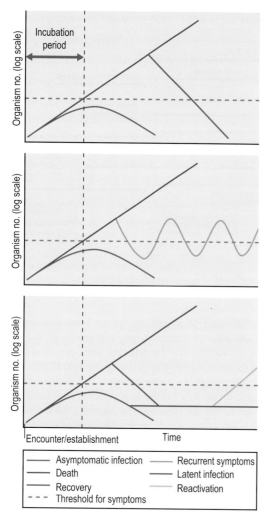

Fig. 11.3 legend (curves):
- Asymptomatic infection
- Death
- Recovery
- Threshold for symptoms
- Recurrent symptoms
- Latent infection
- Reactivation

Fig. 11.3 A model for incubation periods, progression and latency related to organism number.

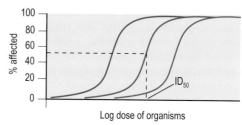

Fig. 11.4 Quantitative relationships between organism dose and outcome in experimental infection. The organism has been administered by a single route to a uniform host population. Note that the outcome (percentage affected, which could be percentage infected, percentage who died or many other endpoints) depends on the dose. This approach allows virulence to be compared between strains of a particular microorganism. A more virulent organism shifts the curve to the left *(blue curve)* and a less virulent organism to the right *(red curve)*. Lesser or greater host resistance would, respectively, have the same effect. The approach allows for the specific recognition of virulence determinants and the effects of immunisation. The dose required to produce the specified endpoint in 50% of the target population is often reproducible and can be used for statistical comparisons. The 50%-infected endpoint is known as the ID_{50}.

dose–response relationship (Fig. 11.4). Not only does recognition of this relationship help explain why, when a group of individuals is exposed to a pathogen only some get infected, it also provides a framework for understanding the effects of immunisation and immune deficiency, as well as a systematic basis for identifying individual traits that contribute to virulence and host resistance.

THE HUMAN MICROBIOME IN HEALTH AND DISEASE

In every other field of biology a close association between organisms is routinely analysed on the assumption that their interactions are directly linked to the overall function of the community that they inhabit. Partly because the application of this approach to microbial communities has been difficult and partly because our knowledge of mammalian physiology and function has been gained from studies that either ignore or deliberately exclude microbes, the contribution of the human microbiome to normal and abnormal physiology has largely been ignored. Yet there can be no doubt that human beings, and indeed all multicellular organisms, comprise complex ecosystems in which all exposed epithelia are colonised with enormous numbers of microbes. The notion that what we have regarded as our normal microbiota plays no part in our normal function must be naïve. As we have seen, microbes sense and respond to their environments, they produce and process bioactive compounds and they possess metabolic properties way beyond those encoded in the human genome. It would be truly astonishing if our microbiomes were just bystanders in human function.

Carl Woese's 16S work led to the development of bacterial community profiling techniques in the 1990s. The availability of high throughput sequencing technologies over the past 10 years has fuelled an explosion of microbiomic analyses in human, animal and other ecological studies. Many authorities now take the view that we should combine hosts and their microbiomes into superorganisms. The term recognises that the human genome and the genomes of all the microbes we carry (our metagenome) provide much greater insight into the determination of human function. In recognition of this, a global consortium has established the Human Microbiome Project. The analytical methods and some key examples of health and disease implications are outlined in the following sections.

Microbiomic methods and analyses

The primary aim is to determine the identities and relative abundances of all the microbes in a sample. For bacteria, archaea, protozoa and fungi, specific genes common to all can be targeted and amplified using 16S rRNA for the prokaryotes and 18S rRNA for the eukaryotes. Alternate targets may be used where greater discrimination between related organisms is required. For viruses, viral particles can be physically isolated (e.g., by filtration and centrifugation) and the DNA or RNA extracted and sequenced. Amplification can only be achieved with predefined viral groups. In all cases, bias may be introduced by the nucleic acid extraction method and by any amplification applied.

The sequences obtained are matched against previously identified microbial sequences. As noted in Ch. 3, the ability to identify will depend on the extent of the database for the target gene and the region sequenced. In practice, the sequences are separated into operational taxonomic units (OTUs), and, where possible, each is assigned to a named genus or species. In every sample, the most abundant organisms will be represented by many sequence reads. In order to detect less abundant organisms a greater depth of sequencing will be required, and as the number of sequence reads increases, so less and less abundant organisms are revealed. At present, most bacterial microbiomes are represented with several thousand reads, with the least abundant organisms representing fractions of a percent of the total population.

Inspection of the list of OTUs provides a community profile. The diversity of this community can be represented by indices that measure the number of different OTUs and the balance between them (known as evenness). These so-called *alpha diversity indices* can be compared between samples so that differences in diversity can be recognised and subjected to statistical analysis. Classically, an infection at an epithelial surface will lead to a collapse in diversity as the community is dominated by a single organism. At a more subtle level, more diverse communities appear to be associated with health and resilience, while less diverse communities may be associated with disease.

The difference between samples and communities can be displayed as beta diversity. This is generally achieved by a mathematical process known as principal component analysis, where an individual profile is represented as a single point on a two- or three-dimensional plot. The coordinates are determined by the features of all the samples that best discriminate between the analysed communities. The individual values can often be recognised as being determined by the relative abundance of large bacterial groups such as the Proteobacteria or Firmicutes. In this way, changes associated with clinical status can be recognised and potential causal links investigated.

The profiles and indices obtained this way can identify changes in the balance of communities and may identify specific bacterial species or groups as being strongly linked to disease. However, 16S-directed analyses do not discriminate signals from dead or live bacteria, nor do they recognise the functional activities resulting from the genes being expressed. The most sophisticated analyses in this field involve metagenomics, in which all the DNA sequences present in samples are directly analysed, metatranscriptomics, in which all the messenger RNA molecules present in a community are determined and, finally, metabolomics, in which the profile of key metabolites is assessed. While the analysis of these outputs requires very sophisticated bioinformatics, a straightforward 16S bacterial community profile can be produced from a sample DNA extract within hours. A standard analysis of 50–100 samples can be achieved in a single run on sequencers available in most large centres and the data processed in half a day. This brings sample analysis within striking distance of clinical application.

Examples of disordered physiology and diseases associated with microbiomic imbalances (dysbioses)

With recognition of the therapeutic and research opportunities presented by microbiomic studies, a feeding frenzy has developed in this area such that it is now possible to find studies claiming associations between microbial community structure and almost any human disease. Nonetheless, certain patterns are emerging that appear to be robust. In broad terms, the gut microbiome can affect human physiology either by altering the availability of nutrients for absorption or by interacting with cell and organ signalling processes or both. In the former case, both malnutrition and obesity can result, while in the latter, microbiome differences have been shown to associate with disordered patterns of development and with changes in established physiology.

In the area of nutrition, multiple studies link microbiomic features in stool with obesity, while a remarkable study associated kwashiorkor with microbiomic differences between twins discordant for this form of malnutrition. While metagenomic analyses in these investigations plausibly link the capacity of microbially encoded enzyme systems to harvest energy sources in the gut contents into forms that humans can use, it is also clear that there are signalling components to the relationship and inflammation-related signals feature prominently. The individuality of subjects' microbiome physiology has been emphasised in one remarkable study in which diametrically opposed glycaemic responses to glucose were observed between individuals while their faecal microbiomes provided the only significant association amongst the clinical metada.

Table 11.3 Some diseases with strong gut microbiome associations

Metabolic/gastrointestinal	Neurological	Immune mediated	Systemic
Obesity	Autism spectrum	Asthma	Nonalcoholic fatty liver disease
Undernutrition	Stress	Atopic dermatitis	Atherosclerosis
Type 2 diabetes	Stroke	Systemic lupus erythematosis	Type 1 diabetes
Clostridium difficile–associated diarrhoea			

In the area of signalling, it is particularly striking that the gut mucosa and mucosal immune system show disordered development in animals reared under sterile (germ-free) conditions. These observations raise major concerns over the use of broad-spectrum antibiotics in early life, and a substantial body of evidence now links antibiotic exposure to development of childhood asthma and a number of immunologically mediated conditions. Microbiomic involvement with systemic signalling raises endless possibilities for altered physiology—neurological development and function have been clearly implicated in this regard.

While the gut bacterial microbiome has been most extensively investigated, it should be emphasised that other epithelial interfaces and hollow organs have been investigated. In particular, the oral cavity, skin, lower respiratory tract and vagina all show distinct features relevant to health and susceptibility to infection. Moreover, it must be emphasised that non-bacterial components (archaea, fungi, protozoa, and viruses of both eukaryotic and prokaryotic cells) have yet to be subjected to analysis in many situations.

It must be concluded that microbiomics is an emerging discipline with potential to make major impacts on medicine, microbiology and infectious diseases. Some microbiomic disease associations are outlined in Table 11.3.

RECOMMENDED READING

Blaser, M. J. (2016). Antibiotic use and its consequences for the normal microbiome. *Science, 352*(6285), 544–545. doi:10.1126/science.aad9358.

Burnet, F. M. (1970). *Natural history of infectious diseases.* Cambridge: Cambridge University Press.

Ewald, P. W. (1996). *Evolution of infectious disease.* Oxford and New York: Oxford University Press.

Gilbert, J. A., Quinn, R. A., Debelius, J., Xu, Z. J. Z., Morton, J., Garg, N., … Knight, R. (2016). Microbiome-wide association studies link dynamic microbial consortia to disease. *Nature, 535*(7610), 94–103. doi:10.1038/nature18850.

Salyers, A. A., Wilson, B. A., & Whitt, D. D. (2011). *Bacterial pathogenesis: A molecular approach* (3rd ed.). Washington, DC: ASM Press.

Vehreschild, M., & Cornely, O. A. (2016). Fecal microbiota transfer 2.0. *Journal of Infectious Diseases, 214*(2), 169–170. doi:10.1093/infdis/jiv768.

Website

National Institutes of Health. The Human Microbiome Project. Available at http://commonfund.nih.gov/hmp/.

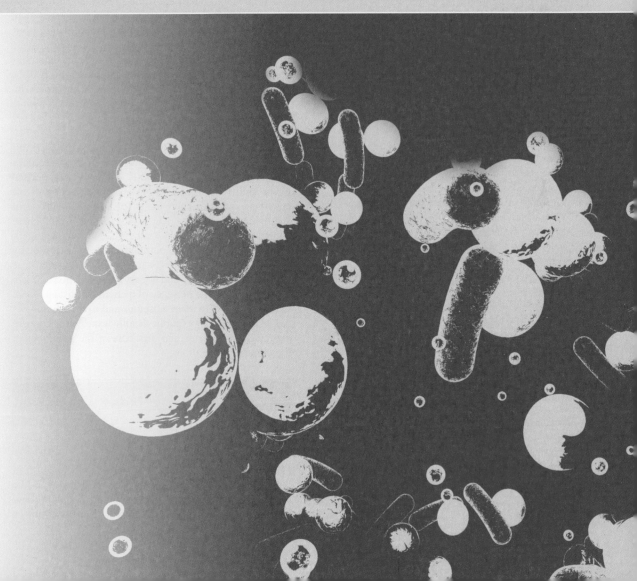

PART 3

BACTERIAL PATHOGENS AND ASSOCIATED DISEASES

12 *Staphylococcus*

Skin infections; osteomyelitis; bloodstream infection; food poisoning; foreign body infections; MRSA

HILARY HUMPHREYS

KEY POINTS

- Staphylococci are commonly found on the skin of healthy individuals. *Staphylococcus aureus* is present in the nose of 30% of healthy people but can cause infections where there is lowered host resistance (e.g., damaged skin).
- Many virulence factors have been described for *Staph. aureus*, but for most a specific role has not been determined. Exceptions include the enterotoxins, toxic shock syndrome toxin, the epidermolytic toxins and Panton-Valentine leukocidin (PVL).
- Staphylococci spread from colonised sites (e.g., skin) by hands, clothing, dust and desquamation from the skin.
- Meticillin-resistant *Staphylococcus aureus* (MRSA) is prevalent in many hospitals, is now present in the community and causes the same range of infections as meticillin-susceptible isolates.
- Flucloxacillin and related drugs are the agents of choice to treat meticillin-susceptible strains and vancomycin or teicoplanin for MRSA infections, but newer options include linezolid, daptomycin and newer cephalosporins.
- Coagulase-negative staphylococci (CoNS) (such as *Staph. epidermidis*) are major pathogens involving prosthetic implants such as intravascular lines or artificial joints; the pathogenesis involves biofilm production.
- Device removal is usually required for the successful treatment of infections caused by CoNS, as well as appropriate antibiotics, such as vancomycin or teicoplanin.

Sir Alexander Ogston, a Scottish surgeon, first showed in 1880 that a number of human pyogenic or pus-forming diseases were associated with a cluster-forming microorganism. He introduced the name *staphylococcus* (Greek: *staphyle*, bunch of grapes; *kokkos*, grain or berry), now used as the genus name for a group of facultatively anaerobic, catalase-positive, Gram-positive cocci. Staphylococci are resistant to dry conditions and high salt concentrations and are well suited to their ecological niche, which is the skin, but can survive for long periods in the environment. They may also be found as part of the normal microbiota of other sites such as the upper respiratory tract and are commonly carried by animals.

The major pathogen within the genus, *Staphylococcus aureus*, causes a wide range of major and minor infections in humans and animals (Table 12.1) and is characterised by its ability to clot blood plasma by the action of the enzyme coagulase. There are at least 30 other species of staphylococci, most of which lack this enzyme. These coagulase-negative staphylococci (CoNS) are skin commensals that can cause opportunistic infections especially associated with prostheses or foreign bodies (usually due to *Staph. epidermidis*), and urinary tract infections *(Staph. saprophyticus)*. The presence of meticillin-resistant *Staph. aureus* (MRSA) in many hospitals and in the community has become a major public health issue, with concern expressed by patients and members of the public about the clinical implications.

STAPHYLOCOCCUS AUREUS

DESCRIPTION

Staph. aureus is a Gram-positive coccus about 1 μm in diameter. The cocci are usually arranged in grape-like clusters. The organisms are nonsporing, nonmotile and usually non-capsulate. When grown on many types of

Table 12.1	Infections caused by *Staph. aureus*
Pyogenic infections	**Toxin-mediated infections**
Boils, carbuncles	Scalded skin syndrome
Surgical site (wound) infection	Pemphigus neonatorum
Abscesses, e.g., spinal	Toxic shock syndrome
Impetigo	Food poisoning
Mastitis	
Bloodstream infections	
Osteomyelitis	
Pneumonia, e.g., ventilator-associated	
Endocarditis	

Table 12.2	Some virulence factors of *Staph. aureus*
Virulence factor	**Activity**
Cell wall polymers	
Peptidoglycan	Inhibits inflammatory response; endotoxin-like activity
Teichoic acid	Phage adsorption; reservoir of bound divalent cations
Cell surface proteins	
Protein A	Reacts with Fc region of IgG
Clumping factor	Binds to fibrinogen
Fibronectin-binding protein	Binds to fibronectin
Exoproteins	
α-Lysin	Impairment of membrane
β-Lysin	permeability; cytotoxic effects
γ-Lysin	on phagocytic and tissue cells
δ-Lysin	
Panton–Valentine leucocidin	Dermo-necrotic and leucocidal
Epidermolytic toxins	Cause blistering of skin
Toxic shock syndrome toxin	Induces multisystem effects; superantigen effects
Enterotoxins	Induce vomiting and diarrhoea; superantigen effects
Coagulase	Converts fibrinogen to fibrin in plasma
Staphylokinase	Degrades fibrin
Lipase	Degrades lipid
Deoxyribonuclease	Degrades DNA

agar for 24 hours at 37°C, individual colonies are circular, 2–3 mm in diameter, with a smooth, shiny surface; colonies appear opaque and are often pigmented (golden-yellow, hence the *aureus*). The main distinctive diagnostic features of *Staph. aureus* are:

• Production of an extracellular enzyme, coagulase, which converts plasma fibrinogen into fibrin, aided by an activator present in plasma.
• Production of thermostable nucleases that break down DNA.
• Production of a surface-associated protein known as clumping factor or bound coagulase that reacts with fibrinogen.

Various automated systems are available that rapidly identify staphylococci. They are particularly useful for screening large numbers of strains.

PATHOGENESIS

Staph. aureus is present in the nose of 30% of healthy people and may be found on the skin. It causes infection most commonly at sites of lowered host resistance, such as damaged skin (e.g., surgical site infection) or mucous membranes (e.g., ventilator-associated pneumonia).

Virulence factors

Recent years have seen a greater understanding of the pathogenic interaction between the host and *Staph. aureus*. Most strains possess a large number of cell-associated and extracellular factors, some of which contribute to the ability of the organism to overcome the body's defences and to invade, survive in and colonise the tissues (Table 12.2). Although the role of each factor is not fully understood individually, it is likely that they are responsible for the establishment of infection, enabling the organism to bind to connective tissue, opposing destruction by the

bactericidal activities of humoral factors such as complement, and overcoming uptake and intracellular killing by phagocytes.

Neutrophils are important in the innate immune response against *Staph. aureus*. A multistep process results in the mobilisation of neutrophils from peripheral blood and/or the bone marrow in response to a variety of factors, and these neutrophils use a variety of mechanisms to kill the ingested bacteria. However, the interplay between the host and *Staph. aureus* is increasingly recognised as complex because the bacterium can colonise before invading, and both humoral and T cell responses play a role. These need to be explored further in advance of the development and use of any effective vaccine.

Staphylococcal toxins

Enterotoxins

Enterotoxins, types A–E, G, H, I and J, are commonly produced by up to 65% of strains of *Staph. aureus*, sometimes singly and sometimes in combination. These toxic proteins withstand exposure to 100°C for several minutes. When ingested as preformed toxins in contaminated food, microgram amounts of toxin can, within a few hours, induce the symptoms of staphylococcal food poisoning: nausea, vomiting and diarrhoea. However, enterotoxins, which are superantigens (see later in the chapter) probably also play a role in other serious staphylococcal infections—for example, bloodstream infection (BSI)—especially when accompanied by septic shock.

Toxic shock syndrome toxin (TSST)

This was discovered in the early 1980s as a result of epidemiological and microbiological investigations in the United States of toxic shock syndrome, a multisystem disease caused by staphylococcal TSST or enterotoxin, or both. A link was established with the use of highly absorbent tampons in menstruating women, although nonmenstrual cases are now as common. The absence of circulating antibodies to TSST is a factor in the pathogenesis of this syndrome.

TSST and the enterotoxins are now recognised as superantigens; that is, they are potent activators of T lymphocytes, resulting in the liberation of cytokines such as tumour necrosis factor, and they bind with high affinity to mononuclear cells. These characteristics partly explain the florid and multisystem nature of the clinical conditions associated with these toxins.

Epidermolytic toxins

Two kinds of epidermolytic toxins (types A and B) are commonly produced by strains that cause blistering diseases. These toxins induce intraepidermal blisters at the granular cell layer resulting in, for example, pemphigus neonatorum. The most dramatic manifestation of epidermolytic toxin is the scalded skin syndrome in small children, who lack neutralising antitoxin. Extensive areas of skin are affected, which, after the development of a painful rash, slough off; the skin surface resembles scalding (Fig. 12.1).

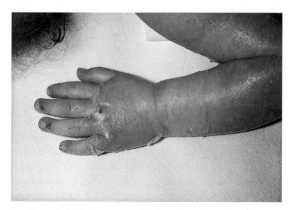

Fig. 12.1 Scalded skin syndrome (toxic epidermal necrolysis). (Courtesy Dr LG Millard, Queen's Medical Centre, Nottingham.)

Panton-Valentine leukocidin (PVL)

This toxin was recognised some decades back, but its potential contribution to the clinical manifestations and outcome have been described in the context of community-acquired infections. As the name suggests, PVL can adversely affect cells, resulting in leucopenia, but animal studies do not suggest high virulence. Nonetheless, epidemiological data in many countries reveal an association between necrotising pneumonia and some complicated skin and soft tissue infections (cSSTI) caused by PVL-positive strains of community-acquired MRSA (CA-MRSA).

EPIDEMIOLOGY

Sources and acquisition of infection

Infected lesions

Large numbers of staphylococci are disseminated in pus and dried exudate discharged from large infected wounds, burns and secondarily infected skin lesions, and in sputum coughed from the lung of patients with pneumonia. Direct contact is the most important mode of spread, but airborne dissemination may also occur. Cross-infection is an important method of spread of staphylococcal disease, particularly in hospitals, and scrupulous hand hygiene is essential in preventing spread. Food handlers may similarly introduce enterotoxin-producing food poisoning strains into food.

Healthy carriers

Staph. aureus grows harmlessly on the moist skin of the nostrils in about 30% of healthy persons, and the perineum is also commonly colonised. Organisms spread from these sites to the environment by hands, clothing, and dust consisting of skin squames and cloth fibres. Some carriers, called shedders, disseminate exceptionally large numbers of staphylococci.

During the first day or two of life most babies become colonised in the nose and skin by staphylococci, and transmission from babies to nursing mothers, who then develop mastitis, is well described.

Animals

Animals may disseminate *Staph. aureus* and cause human infection, for example, milk from a dairy cow with mastitis causing staphylococcal food poisoning. Also, livestock-associated MRSA causing human infection has been described, including where the background prevalence of MRSA is relatively low, for example, the Netherlands.

Environment

Although not spore forming, staphylococci may remain alive in a dormant state for several months when dried in pus, sputum, bedclothes or dust or on inanimate surfaces such as floors. Environmental reservoirs are therefore increasingly recognised as important in hospitals in contributing to endemic MRSA. Staphylococci are fairly readily killed by heat (e.g., moist heat at 65°C for 30 minutes), by exposure to light and by common disinfectants, hence the emphasis on regular and effective environmental decontamination in controlling MRSA.

The acquisition of *Staph. aureus* infection may be exogenous (from an external source such as the environment) and more theoretically preventable and endogenous (from a carriage site or minor lesion elsewhere in the patient's own body).

Meticillin–resistant *Staph. aureus* (MRSA)

MRSA produces a penicillin binding protein 2a, which is mediated through the *mecA* and other genes such as *mecC*. These genes, which include many mobile elements, are carried on the staphylococcal cassette chromosome mec (SCCmec) of which there are at least six different types recognised, and this results in resistance to almost all beta-lactam antibiotics. Generally, MRSA causes the same range of infections resulting in excess health-care costs, prolonged hospital stay and significant mortality. MRSA is endemic in hospitals globally, except in Scandinavia and in the Netherlands, although declining rates of MRSA BSI have been seen in recent years in the United Kingdom, France and other European countries. Vulnerable at-risk patients are those who have undergone major surgery and patients in the intensive care unit. Although 50%–60% of patients with MRSA are just colonised, that is, representing asymptomatic carriage, serious infections occur such as BSI, respiratory tract and bone/joint infections. These infections are then more difficult to treat than infections caused by meticillin-susceptible isolates, and MRSA can spread easily among patients in hospital.

CA-MRSA is increasing, especially in the United States, where 50% or more of *Staph. aureus* infections presenting to the emergency department may be meticillin-resistant. These occur often in otherwise healthy individuals with no recent health-care contact. PVL, alpha toxin and secreted proteases are implicated as particular virulence determinants. Community-acquired strains may cause the same range of infections as health care–associated strains such as BSI, but particularly cSSTI and severe pneumonia.

The control and prevention of MRSA involve the education of all health-care professionals and the public, fast and reliable detection in the laboratory, active surveillance, prompt patient isolation or cohorting when admitted to hospital, standard precautions and good professional practice by all health-care workers (including compliance with hand hygiene guidelines), effective hospital hygiene programmes and antibiotic stewardship programmes, for example, avoidance of the excess use of cephalosporins and fluoroquinolones. Such measures in Scandinavia and in the Netherlands, where an aggressive 'search and destroy' approach involving the extensive screening of all MRSA contacts is employed, have ensured low rates of health care–associated MRSA.

LABORATORY INVESTIGATION

One or more of the following specimens should be collected to confirm a diagnosis:

- Pus from abscesses, wounds, burns, etc. is much preferred to swabs.
- Sputum from patients with pneumonia (e.g., postinfluenzal) and bronchoscopic specimens (e.g., bronchoscopic lavage), are used in critically ill patients to diagnose ventilator-associated pneumonia.
- Faeces or vomit from patients with suspected food poisoning, or the remains of implicated foods.
- Blood from patients with suspected BSI such as septic shock, osteomyelitis or endocarditis.
- Midstream urine from patients with suspected cystitis or pyelonephritis.
- Anterior nasal, throat and perineal swabs (moistened in saline or sterile water) from suspected carriers; nasal swabs should be rubbed in turn over the anterior walls of both nostrils.

The characteristic clusters of Gram-positive cocci can often be demonstrated by microscopy, and the organisms cultured readily on blood agar and most other media within 24 hours or less. The tube or slide coagulase test, or the detection of DNase are performed to distinguish *Staph. aureus* from coagulase-negative species and antimicrobial susceptibility testing with cefoxitin to confirm MRSA using standard methods. Commercially available molecular methods using the polymerase chain reaction (PCR) have been developed to reduce the time to the detection of MRSA from 48 to 72 hours with culture to <12 hours to facilitate earlier preventative measures.

Typing

Most staphylococcal infections are sporadic, but the identification of an outbreak strain is an important aspect in the investigation of a source, particularly during outbreaks of MRSA. Originally, strains of *Staph. aureus* were differentiated into different phage types by observation of their pattern of susceptibility to lysis by a standard set of *Staph. aureus* bacteriophages (viruses that infect bacteria) but have been replaced by genotypic methods such as PCR and pulsed-field gel electrophoresis (PFGE). For local outbreak investigations, PFGE has been widely used but is technically demanding. Assessing the gene encoding the staphylococcal surface protein A (spa typing) is also used for typing MRSA, and finally, typing the *SCCmec* elements is used for the study of international evolution of MRSA. Increasingly, whole gene sequencing and microarray methods may be employed, which provide more in-depth detail on local variations as well as on emerging clones.

TREATMENT

Susceptibility to antibiotics

Staph. aureus and other staphylococci are inherently susceptible to many antimicrobial agents (Table 12.3). About 90% of strains found in hospitals are resistant to benzylpenicillin due to the production of the enzyme penicillinase, a β-lactamase that opens the β-lactam ring. Meticillin (previously used for laboratory testing and initially developed for therapy), oxacillin, cloxacillin and flucloxacillin, are stable to the enzyme. Cephalosporins and β-lactamase inhibitors are also stable to penicillinase (see Ch. 5).

Table 12.3 Antibiotics commonly used against staphylococci

Active agents	Agents lacking useful activity
Penicillins[a] (e.g., flucloxacillin)	Aztreonam
Cephalosporins (e.g., cefuroxime)	Polymyxins
Aminoglycosides[b] (e.g., gentamicin)	Mecillinam
Tetracyclines (e.g., doxycycline)	Nitroimidazoles
Macrolides (e.g., clarithromycin)	
Lincosamides (clindamycin)	
Glycopeptides (vancomycin and teicoplanin)	
Fluoroquinolones[c] (moxifloxacin)	
Rifampicin[b]	
Fusidic acid[b]	
Carbapenems (e.g., meropenem)	
Oxazolidinones (linezolid, tedizolid)	
Lipopeptide (daptomycin)	
Newer cephalosporins (ceftaroline, ceftobiprole)	

[a]Resistance common (see text).
[b]Not used alone but in combination.
[c]For categorisation of quinolones, see Table 5.3 and associated text.

MRSA strains are resistant to almost all β-lactam agents and often to other agents such as the aminoglycosides and fluoroquinolones. Glycopeptides (vancomycin or teicoplanin) are the agents of choice in the treatment of systemic infection with MRSA. Isolates of MRSA with reduced susceptibility or full resistance to glycopeptide antibiotics have been detected but are uncommon. These isolates have either thickened cell walls (reduced susceptibility) or the *vanA* gene (fully resistant) and can be difficult to detect in the routine diagnostic laboratory.

Choice of antibiotic for therapy

Pending receipt of susceptibility test results, the treatment of severe infections suspected to be caused by *Staph. aureus* should be flucloxacillin unless MRSA is endemic locally, in which case a glycopeptide such as vancomycin is indicated. Erythromycin, clindamycin or vancomycin (or teicoplanin) is indicated if the patient is allergic to penicillin. Fusidic acid and rifampicin are not used alone in serious infections because mutation to resistance arises readily. It is almost always necessary to remove an infected source, such as a central intravascular catheter or device, or to drain an abscess, for treatment to be effective.

Other agents that provide alternatives for the treatment of MRSA and can also be used to treat infections caused by isolates with reduced susceptibility to the glycopeptides, include linezolid, which can be administered parenterally or orally, co-trimoxazole, a tetracycline and daptomycin, which is bactericidal and is used to treat MRSA BSI. Recent years have seen the development of newer agents such as ceftaroline, ceftobiprole (both cephalosporins), tedizolid and telavancin, and the results from clinical trials show some promise, but their ultimate role in treatment remains unclear.

Life-threatening toxin-mediated disease, such as toxic shock syndrome, requires major medical support such as intravenous fluids to prevent multiorgan failure, often best provided in the intensive care unit (Fig. 12.2).

COAGULASE-NEGATIVE STAPHYLOCOCCI

Coagulase-negative staphylococci comprise a large group of related species commonly found on the surface of healthy persons, in whom they are rarely the cause of infection. *Staph. epidermidis* accounts for about 75% of all clinical isolates, probably reflecting its preponderance on the normal skin. Other important CoNS include *Staph. saprophyticus* (a cause of urinary infection in young women) and *Staph. lugdunensis* (may cause severe infections like *Staph. aureus*). The emergence of CoNS as major pathogens reflects the increased use of implants or medical devices

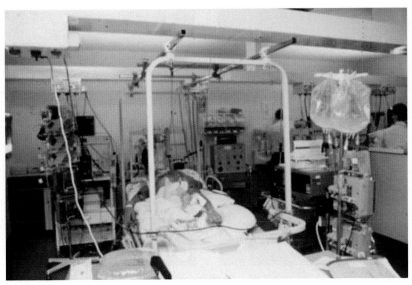

Fig. 12.2 Patients in the intensive care unit who require multiorgan support are at particular risk of MRSA.

such as intravascular lines and cannulae, cardiac valves, artificial joints, etc., and the increasing numbers of severely debilitated or immunocompromised patients in hospitals.

DESCRIPTION

Coagulase-negative staphylococci are morphologically similar to *Staph. aureus*, but they do not coagulate plasma and they lack clumping factor and deoxyribonuclease. Because *Staph. epidermidis* and other CoNS may contaminate clinical specimens, care has to be exercised in assessing its significance, especially from superficial sites. When isolated from sites such as blood or cerebrospinal fluid, further specimens should be obtained to confirm its clinical significance.

Coagulase-negative staphylococci are opportunistic pathogens that cause infection in debilitated or compromised patients, for example, premature neonates and oncology patients, often by colonising biomedical devices such as intravascular lines. They cause particular problems in:

- cardiac surgery (prosthetic valve endocarditis)
- neurosurgical patients with cerebrospinal fluid drains (meningitis)
- continuous ambulatory peritoneal dialysis (peritonitis)
- immunocompromised patients (e.g., bloodstream infection)
- intensive care units (multiple devices leading to septic shock)

PATHOGENESIS

Adherence to the prosthetic device by the production of an exopolysaccharide intercellular adhesion is a key step in the formation of a multilayered biofilm, essential for the pathogenesis of device-related *Staph. epidermidis* infection. A complex array of interrelated chemical messengers controls expression of polysaccharide and drives intercellular adhesion and biofilm formation. Physiological changes in the biofilm protect *Staph. epidermidis* from the host immune defence system, and restricted penetration, decreased growth rates and persistent bacterial cells as part of the biofilm often render antibiotic treatment unsuccessful (Fig. 12.3). Consequently, there is considerable interest in the development of antimicrobial-impregnated devices such as central intravascular catheters, the use of materials that are less prone to adherence by *Staph. epidermidis*, and antibiofilm therapeutic agents. Important factors in the pathogenesis of *Staph. saprophyticus* infection include a unique adhesion protein that allows it to adhere to uroepithelial cells in females during the reproductive years and the production of urease. Isolates of *Staph. lugdunensis* commonly produce thermostable DNase, lipase and haemolysins, not dissimilar to *Staph. aureus*.

TREATMENT

Device-associated infection usually requires the removal of the device or implants for successful management. The

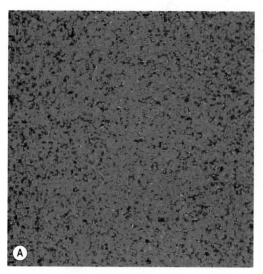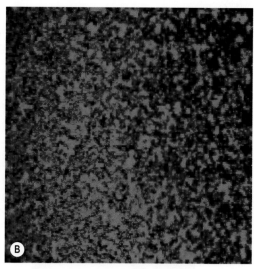

Fig. 12.3 Biofilm formed by *Staphylococcus aureus* after 24 hours of growth. Confocal microscopy images represent live *(green)* or dead *(red)* staining of untreated biofilm (A) and biofilm treated with 30% (v/v) ethanol (B). (Courtesy Dr Siobhan Hogan, the Royal College of Surgeons in Ireland.)

antibiotic treatment of CoNS infections is complicated because susceptibility is generally unpredictable. Strains resistant to penicillin, penicillinase-stable penicillins, gentamicin, erythromycin and chloramphenicol are common. If a strain is the cause of systemic infection, vancomycin or teicoplanin should be used. Rifampicin in combination with a glycopeptide is occasionally useful in treating central nervous system infections and with a fluoroquinolone such as ciprofloxacin in the management of device infections. Alternative agents such as daptomycin and linezolid may also have a role. Uncomplicated urinary tract infection caused by *Staph. saprophyticus* usually responds to trimethoprim.

RECOMMENDED READING

Ala'Aldeen, D., & Hiramatsu, K. (2004). *Staphylococcus aureus: Molecular and clinical aspects*. Chichester: Horwood Publishing.

Becker, K., Heilmann, C., & Peters, G. (2014). Coagulase-negative staphylococci. *Clinical Microbiology Reviews*, 27(4), 870–926. doi:10.1128/CMR.00109-13.

Brown, A. F., Leech, J. M., Rogers, T. R., & McLoughlin, R. M. (2014). *Staphylococcus aureus* colonization: modulation of host immune response and impact on human vaccine design. *Frontiers in Immunology*, 4, 1–20. doi:10.3389/fimmu.2013.00507.

DeLeo, F. R., Otto, M., Kreiswirth, B. N., & Chambers, H. F. (2010). Community-associated meticillin-resistant *Staphylococcus aureus*. *The Lancet*, 375(9725), 1557–1568. doi:10.1016/S0140-6736(09)61999-1.

Hogan, S., Stevens, N. T., Humphreys, H., O'Gara, J. P., & O'Neill, E. (2015). Current and future approaches to the prevention and treatment of staphylococcal medical device-related infections. *Current Pharmaceutical Design*, 21(1), 100–113.

Holmes, N. E., & Howden, B. P. (2014). What's new in the treatment of serious MRSA infection? *Current Opinion in Infectious Diseases*, 27(6), 471–478. doi:10.1097/QCO.0000000000000101.

Köck, R., Becker, K., Cookson, B., van Gemert-Pijnen, J. E., Harbarth, S., Kluytmans, J., Friedrich, A. W. (2014). Systematic literature analysis and review of targeted preventative measures to limit healthcare-associated infections by meticillin-resistant *Staphylococcus aureus*. *Eurosurveillance*, 19(29).

Price, J. R., Didelot, X., Crook, D. W., Llewelyn, M. J., & Paul, J. (2013). Whole genome sequencing in the prevention and control of *Staphylococcus aureus* infection. *Journal of Hospital Infection*, 83(1), 14–21. doi:10.1016/j.jhin.2012.10.003.

Websites

Centers for Disease Control and Prevention (CDC). Methicillin-resistant *Staphylococcus aureus* (MRSA). Retrieved from http://www.cdc.gov/mrsa/. (Accessed Jul 2017).

European Antimicrobial Resistance Surveillance Network (EARS-Net). https://ecdc.europa.eu/en. (Accessed Jul 2017).

Public Health England. MRSA. Available at https://www.gov.uk/search?q=MRSA. (Accessed Jul 2017).

13 *Streptococcus* and *Enterococcus*

Pharyngitis; scarlet fever; skin and soft tissue infections; streptococcal toxic shock syndrome; pneumonia; meningitis; urinary tract infections; rheumatic fever; poststreptococcal glomerulonephritis

MOGENS KILIAN

KEY POINTS

- *Streptococcus pyogenes* (group A streptococcus) is among the most prevalent of human bacterial pathogens.
- *Str. pyogenes* and *Str. dysgalactiae* subspecies *equisimilis* infections range from sore throat, scarlet fever and superficial skin infections to invasive soft tissue infections and septicaemia.
- *Str. pyogenes* and *Str. dysgalactiae* subspecies *equisimilis* produce several superantigenic extracellular toxins that are involved in the pathogenesis of the rash associated with scarlet fever and streptococcal toxic shock syndrome.
- Rheumatic fever and acute glomerulonephritis are potential immune-mediated sequelae of infections with *Str. pyogenes*.
- *Str. agalactiae* (group B streptococcus) causes neonatal septicaemia and meningitis.
- *Str. pneumoniae* is the principal cause of pneumonia, middle ear infections and meningitis and is one of the four most frequent causes of fatal infections worldwide.
- Commensal streptococci of the oral cavity and other streptococci and enterococci are among the most frequent causes of infective endocarditis.

Streptococci is the general term for a diverse collection of Gram-positive cocci that typically grow as chains or pairs (Greek: *streptos* = pliant or chain; *coccos* = a grain or berry) (Fig. 13.1). Virtually all of the streptococci that are important in human medicine and dentistry fall into the genera *Streptococcus* and *Enterococcus*. Occasional opportunistic infections are associated with other genera of streptococci, such as *Peptostreptococcus* (see Ch. 30) and *Abiotrophia* (nutritionally variant streptococci).

Streptococci are generally strong fermenters of carbohydrates, resulting in the production of lactic acid, a property responsible for the involvement of some oral streptococci in the decalcification of teeth, i.e., dental caries, and also are used in the dairy industry. Most are facultative anaerobes, although peptostreptococci are obligate anaerobes. Streptococci do not produce spores and are nonmotile. They are catalase negative.

CLASSIFICATION

The genus *Streptococcus* includes important pathogens and commensals of mucosal membranes of the upper respiratory tract and, for some species, the intestines. Members of the genus *Enterococcus* are intestinal commensal.

The genus *Streptococcus* includes more than 80 species. With few exceptions, the individual species are exclusively associated, as either pathogens or commensals, with humans or a particular animal species. The genus consists of six clusters of species, each of which is characterised by distinct pathogenic potential and other properties:

- The Pyogenic (pus generating) group includes most species that are overt human and animal pathogens.
- The Mitis group includes commensals of the human oral cavity and pharynx, although one of the species, *Streptococcus pneumoniae,* is also one of the most important human pathogens.
- The Anginosus group is part of the commensal microbiota of the oral cavity and pharynx and may cause infections often as part of a consortium of different species.
- The Salivarius group is part of the commensal microbiota of the oral cavity and pharynx.
- The Bovis group belongs in the colon.
- The Mutans group of streptococci colonises exclusively the tooth surfaces of humans and some animals; some species belonging to this cluster are involved in the development of dental caries.

Virtually all of the commensal species, including the enterococci, are opportunistic pathogens, primarily if they gain access to the bloodstream from the oral cavity or from the gut.

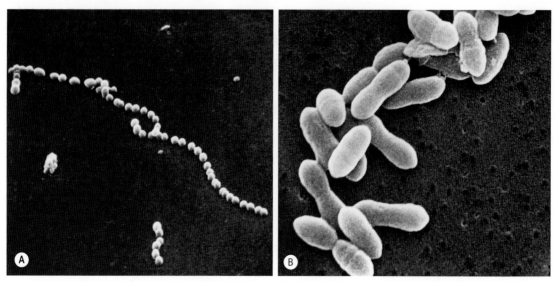

Fig. 13.1 Scanning electron micrograph of (A) *Str. pyogenes* showing typical chain formation (original magnification ×2000), and (B) *Str. pneumoniae* showing typical diplococcus formation (original magnification ×7000). (Courtesy A. P. Shelton, University Hospital, Nottingham.)

Haemolytic activity

Early attempts to distinguish between pathogenic and commensal streptococci recognised different types of reactions around colonies on blood agar plates. Colonies of streptococci belonging to the Pyogenic group are generally surrounded by a clear zone, usually several millimetres in diameter, caused by lysis of red blood cells in the agar medium induced by bacterial haemolysins. This is called β-haemolysis and constitutes the principal marker for potentially pathogenic streptococci in cultures of throat swabs or other clinical samples. Accordingly, the pyogenic streptococci are also referred to as haemolytic streptococci.

In contrast, most commensal streptococci give rise to a green discoloration around colonies on blood agar. This phenomenon is termed α-haemolysis, although not caused by haemolysis. The factor causing the green discoloration is hydrogen peroxide, which oxidizes haemoglobin to the green methaemoglobin.

Collectively, commensal streptococci are often called viridans streptococci, which refers to their α-haemolytic property (*viridis* = green). Not quite logically, this term also includes the few streptococci, such as those of the Salivarius and Mutans groups, that induce neither α- nor β-haemolysis. Moreover, in common usage, the term excludes *Str. pneumoniae*, although this species is also α-haemolytic.

Lancefield grouping

Historically, an important method of distinguishing between pyogenic streptococci has been the serological classification pioneered by the American bacteriologist Rebecca Lancefield, who detected different versions of the major cell wall polysaccharide among the pyogenic streptococci. The different forms of this polysaccharide can be distinguished with specific antibodies raised in rabbits. The polysaccharide is referred to as the group polysaccharide and identifies a number of different serological groups labelled by capital letters (Lancefield groups A, B, C, etc.). Among the pyogenic streptococci, some serological groups are identical to distinct species (Table 13.1).

STREPTOCOCCUS PYOGENES

This species, which consists of Lancefield group A streptococci, is among the most prevalent of human bacterial pathogens. It is associated exclusively with human infections. It causes a wide range of suppurative infections in the respiratory tract and skin, life-threatening soft tissue infections, and certain types of toxin-associated reactions. Some of these infections may, in addition, result in severe nonsuppurative sequelae due to adverse immunological reactions induced by the infecting streptococci. A similar spectrum of infections may be caused by the closely related *Str. dysgalactiae* subspecies *equisimilis* (group C and group G streptococci).

Some of the infections caused by *Str. pyogenes* resemble those caused by *Staphylococcus aureus,* but the clinical characteristics associated with these two groups of pyogenic cocci are often distinct. Similarities and differences can be explained by the virulence factors expressed by the two species.

PATHOGENESIS

Virulence factors

Strains of *Str. pyogenes* and *Str. dysgalactiae* subspecies *equisimilis* express a large arsenal of virulence factors involved in adherence, evasion of host immunity, and tissue damage (Fig. 13.2). Although some factors are expressed by all clinical isolates, others are variably present among strains of the two species. This variation is due to the horizontal transfer of virulence genes among strains, primarily by bacteriophages (transduction, see Ch. 14), and probably explains the temporal variations in the prevalence of severe infections and sequelae. It furthermore explains differences in the virulence of individual strains and, to some extent, the different clinical pictures that may be associated with infections due to *Str. pyogenes* and *Str. dysgalactiae* subspecies *equisimilis*. In some *Streptococcus* species pathogenic for animals the corresponding virulence factors are expressed in a form specifically adapted to interact with their particular host.

Adhesion

Interaction with host fibronectin, a matrix protein on eukaryotic cells, is considered the principal mechanism by which *Str. pyogenes* binds to epithelial cells of the pharynx and skin. The host fibronectin is recognised by the F protein, which is one of the many proteins expressed on the surface of *Str. pyogenes* (Fig. 13.2). The interaction between the streptococcal F protein and host cell fibronectin also mediates internalisation of the bacteria into host cells.

In addition to the F protein, surface-exposed lipoteichoic acid and M proteins appear to be involved in adherence to mucosal and skin epithelial cells.

M proteins

The ability of *Str. pyogenes* to resist phagocytosis by polymorphonuclear leucocytes is largely due to the

Table 13.1 *Streptococcus* species of clinical importance

Phylogenetic group	Species	Lancefield group	Type of haemolysis[a]
Pyogenic group	*Str. pyogenes*	A	β
	Str. agalactiae	B	β
	Str. dysgalactiae subsp. *equisimilis*	C, G, A	β
Mitis group	*Str. pneumoniae*	O	α
	Str. mitis	O	α
	Str. oralis	Not designated	α
	Str. sanguinis	H	α
Anginosus group	*Str. anginosus*	C, G, F, A	α or β
	Str. intermedius	C, F, NT	α or none
	Str. constellatus	C, F, NT	α, β or none
Bovis group	*Str. equinus* ('*Str. bovis*' is a later synonym)	D	α or none
Mutans group	*Str. mutans*	Not designated	None
	Str. sobrinus	Not designated	None

[a]On horse blood agar. Note that "α-haemolysis" is not haemolysis but green discoloration due to H_2O_2 production.

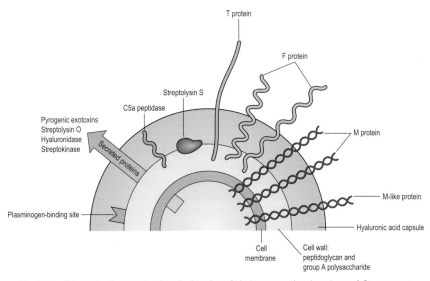

Fig. 13.2 Schematic diagram showing the location of virulence-associated products of *Str. pyogenes*.

cell-surface exposed M protein. The M protein is anchored in the cytoplasmic membrane, spans the entire cell wall, and protrudes from the cell surface as fibrils (Fig. 13.2). Some strains produce two different M proteins with antiphagocytic activity, and some an additional structurally related M-like protein. All of these proteins can bind various plasma proteins of the host, including fibrinogen, plasminogen, albumin, immunoglobulin (Ig) G, IgA, the proteinase inhibitor α_2-macroglobulin and some regulatory factors from the complement system (factor H and C4b-binding protein). As well as masking the bacterial surface with host proteins, some of these affinities are responsible for the ability of M proteins to resist phagocytosis. Thus, factor H can destabilise the important opsonin C3b when deposited on the bacterial surface. Likewise, the C4b-binding protein inhibits surface complement deposition by stimulating degradation of both C4b and C3b.

Str. pyogenes can release some of the M proteins with its own cysteine protease. If shed into the circulation, the M protein forms complexes with fibrinogen, which by indirect pathways induce the release of inflammatory mediators from neutrophils. This process plays an important role in the leakage of plasma into the tissues and lungs, and the ensuing low blood pressure seen in some invasive infections with *Str. pyogenes*.

Acquired resistance to infection by *Str. pyogenes* is the result of antibodies in secretions and plasma to the M protein molecule. However, as a result of genetic polymorphism in the gene encoding the M protein, the most distal part of the protein shows extensive variability among strains. As a consequence, individuals may suffer from recurrent *Str. pyogenes* infections with strains expressing different versions of the M protein. More than 150 different types of M protein have been identified by serological means and gene sequencing.

Capsule

Some strains of *Str. pyogenes* form a capsule composed of hyaluronic acid. Such strains grow as mucoid colonies on blood agar and are highly virulent in animal models. Although capsule production is rare among isolates from uncomplicated pharyngitis, a significant proportion of isolates from severe infections have a capsule. Like other bacterial capsules, the capsule has an antiphagocytic effect. The relative significance of the M protein and the capsule as antiphagocytic factors differs among strains.

The capsule is identical to the hyaluronic acid of the connective tissue of the host and is not immunogenic. In this way, the bacteria can partially disguise themselves with an immunological 'self' substance, but the M protein is still exposed on the surface.

C5a peptidase

The C5a peptidase, which is also found in most human pathogenic strains of *Str. agalactiae*, is present on the surface of all strains of *Str. pyogenes*. It specifically cleaves, and thereby inactivates, human C5a, one of the principal chemoattractants of phagocytic cells.

Streptolysins

Str. pyogenes produces two distinct haemolysins, termed *streptolysins O* (oxygen labile) and *S* (serum soluble), both of which lyse erythrocytes, polymorphonuclear leucocytes and platelets by forming pores in their cell membrane.

Streptolysin O belongs to a family of haemolysins found in many pathogenic bacteria. Intravenous injection into experimental animals causes death within seconds, as the result of an acute toxic action on the heart. Serum antibodies can be demonstrated after streptococcal infection, particularly after severe infections.

Streptolysin S is responsible for the β-haemolysis around colonies on blood agar plates. It can also induce the release of lysosomal contents with subsequent cell death after engulfment by phagocytes. In contrast to streptolysin O, it is not immunogenic.

Pyrogenic exotoxins

Most strains of *Str. pyogenes* produce one or more toxins that are called pyrogenic (fever generating) exotoxins because of their ability to induce fever. Three, designated SPE-A, SPE-B and SPE-C, have been characterised extensively, but there are several others. Purified SPE-A causes death when injected into rabbits and is the most toxic of the three, but SPE-B also causes myocardial necrosis and death in experimental animals.

The genes for SPE-A and SPE-C are transmitted between strains by bacteriophage (transduction), and stable production depends on lysogenic conversion in a manner analogous to toxin production by *Corynebacterium diphtheriae* (see Ch. 14). Even among strains that possess the genes, the quantity of toxin secreted varies dramatically.

SPE-A and SPE-C are also called erythrogenic toxins, as they are responsible for the rash observed in patients with scarlatina. They are genetically related to *Staph. aureus* enterotoxins and, like these, have superantigen activity. By cross-linking MHC class II molecules on antigen-presenting cells and the Vβ domain of the antigen receptor on a subset of T lymphocytes, these toxins cause comprehensive (antigen independent) activation of T lymphocytes. The result is massive release of proinflammatory cytokines such as interleukin (IL)-1 and IL-2, tumour necrosis factor (TNF)-α and interferon-γ. These cytokines may cause a variety of clinical signs, including inflammation, hypotensive shock and organ failure seen in some patients with severe streptococcal disease. The different clinical outcome in different individuals of infections with the same *Str. pyogenes* strain appears to be due to the fact that the toxins bind preferentially to certain major histocompatibility complex (MHC) class II tissue types.

Unlike SPE-A and SPE-C, all strains of *Str. pyogenes* produce SPE-B, which is a potent cysteine proteinase capable of cleaving many host proteins.

None of the pyrogenic exotoxins is associated unambiguously with any of the clinical syndromes caused by *Str. pyogenes*. However, most isolates from episodes of severe invasive disease and toxic shock–like syndrome produce SPE-A, and the protease SPE-B appears to be responsible for the extensive tissue destruction observed in many patients with severe invasive infections, including necrotising fasciitis.

Hyaluronidase

Str. pyogenes and several other pyogenic streptococci use a secreted hyaluronidase to degrade hyaluronic acid, the ground substance of host connective tissue. This property may facilitate the spread of infection along fascial planes. During infections, particularly those involving the skin, serum antibody titres to hyaluronidase show a significant rise.

Streptokinase

Streptokinase, also known as fibrinolysin, is another spreading factor. It is expressed by all strains of *Str. pyogenes* and cooperates with a surface-expressed plasminogen-binding site on the bacteria. Once host plasminogen is bound to the bacterial surface, it is activated to plasmin by streptokinase. Thus, in contrast to *Staph. aureus,* which aims at hiding behind a wall of coagulated plasma (fibrin), *Str. pyogenes* employs host plasmin to hinder the build-up of fibrin barriers. As a result, soft tissue infections due to *Str. pyogenes* are more diffuse, and often rapidly spreading, than the well-localised abscesses that typify staphylococcal infections.

Deoxyribonucleases (DNAases)

At least four distinct forms of DNAases are produced by *Str. pyogenes*. The enzymes hydrolyse nucleic acids and allow the bacteria to escape from the DNA net released from phagocytes (neutrophil extracellular traps).

CLINICAL FEATURES

Although a general decrease in the prevalence of serious infections with *Str. pyogenes* has occurred since the mid-19th century, regions of the world with low income and poor infrastructure continue to suffer a high burden of *Str. pyogenes* diseases with millions of deaths yearly. Resurgence in severe streptococcal infections and increased mortality due to streptococcal sepsis was observed in many industrialised countries in the 1980s and 1990s frequently associated with specific clones of the species.

The most common route of entry of *Str. pyogenes* is the upper respiratory tract, which is usually the primary site of infection and also serves as a focus for infections in other locations of the body. Spread from person to person is by respiratory droplets or by direct contact with infected wounds or sores on the skin. Not all individuals colonised by *Str. pyogenes* in the upper respiratory tract develop clinical signs of infection.

After an acute upper respiratory tract infection, the convalescent patient may carry the infecting streptococci for some weeks. Only a few healthy adults carry *Str. pyogenes* in the respiratory tract, but the carriage rate in young school children is just over 10%. It may be considerably higher before or during an epidemic.

Noninvasive streptococcal disease

The most common infections caused by *Str. pyogenes* are relatively mild and noninvasive infections of the upper respiratory tract (pharyngitis) and skin (impetigo). In the United States, >10 million cases of noninvasive *Str. pyogenes* infection are estimated to occur annually.

Pharyngitis

This is the most common infection caused by *Str. pyogenes*. Clinical signs such as abrupt onset of sore throat, fever, malaise and headache generally develop 2–4 days after exposure to the pathogen. The posterior pharynx is usually diffusely reddened, with enlarged tonsils that may show patches of grey-white exudate on their surface and, sometimes, accumulations of pus in the crypts. The local inflammation results in swelling of cervical lymph nodes. Occasionally, a peritonsillar abscess may develop (a condition known as quinsy); this is a very painful condition and potentially dangerous, as the pathogen may spread to neighbouring regions and to the bloodstream.

Despite the significant symptoms and clinical signs, differentiating streptococcal pharyngitis ('strep throat') from viral pharyngitis is impossible without microbiological or serological examination. Culture studies show that 20%–30% of cases of pharyngitis are associated with *Str. pyogenes* or *Str. dysgalactiae* subspecies *equisimilis*.

Scarlet fever

Pharyngitis caused by certain pyrogenic exotoxin-producing strains of *Str. pyogenes* may be associated with a diffuse

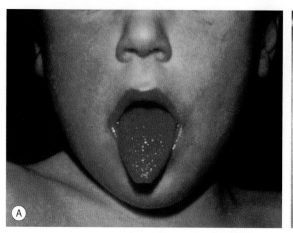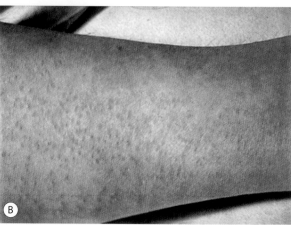

Fig. 13.3 The characteristic erythematous rash on (A) tongue and (B) skin associated with scarlet fever.

erythematous rash of the skin and mucous membranes (Fig. 13.3). The condition is known as scarlet fever or scarlatina. The rash develops within 1–2 days after the first symptoms of pharyngitis and initially appears on the upper chest, then spreading to the extremities. After an initial phase with a yellowish-white coating, the tongue becomes red and denuded ('strawberry tongue').

Between 1860 and 1870 the mean annual death rate from scarlet fever in England and Wales was close to 2500 per million of the population. Since then a steady decline in incidence has been observed. By the end of the 20th century, the number of scarlet fever cases in England and Wales had fallen below 25 per million, and death is now extremely rare.

Skin infections

Str. pyogenes may cause several types of skin infection, sometimes in association with *Staph. aureus*. The superficial and localised skin infection, known as impetigo or pyoderma, occurs mainly in children (Fig. 13.4). It primarily affects exposed areas on the face, arms or legs. The skin becomes colonised after contact with an infected person and the bacteria enter the skin through small defects. Initially, clear vesicles develop, which within a few days become pus filled. Secondary spread is often seen as a result of scratching.

Potentially more severe is the acute skin infection erysipelas (*erythros* = red; *pella* = skin), which occurs in the superficial layers of the skin (cellulitis) and involves the lymphatics. The infection is characterised by diffuse redness of the skin, and patients experience local pain, enlargement of regional lymph nodes and fever. Untreated, the infection may spread to the bloodstream, and was often fatal before antibiotics became available.

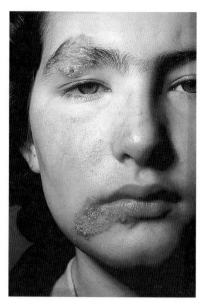

Fig. 13.4 Impetigo. (Courtesy Dr L. G. Millard, Queen's Medical Centre, Nottingham.)

Invasive soft tissue infections

Severe, sometimes life-threatening, *Str. pyogenes* infections may occur when the bacteria get into normally sterile parts of the body. The most severe forms of invasive infections are necrotising fasciitis, streptococcal toxic shock syndrome and puerperal fever, all of which are associated with bacteraemia.

Worldwide, rates of invasive infection increased from the mid-1980s to the early 1990s. In 2002, around 9000 cases of invasive *Str. pyogenes* infection occurred in the United

States. Although these infections may occur in previously healthy individuals, patients with chronic illnesses such as cancer and diabetes, and those on haemodialysis or receiving steroids, have a higher risk. Even with antibiotic treatment, death occurs in 10%–13% of all invasive cases: 45% of patients with toxic shock syndrome and 25% of patients with necrotising fasciitis.

Necrotising fasciitis

This infection progresses very rapidly, destroying fat and fascia. Although *Str. pyogenes* gains entry to these tissues through the skin after trauma, often of a minor nature, the skin itself may show only minimal signs of infection and may indeed be spared (Fig. 13.5). Systemic shock and general deterioration occur very quickly. The disease affects the fit young person with no obvious underlying pathology as well as the immunocompromised.

The clinical diagnosis may be difficult because *Staph. aureus* and anaerobes such as *Clostridium perfringens* can produce a similar clinical picture. Streptococci can be isolated from the blood, blister fluid and cultures of the infected area.

Streptococcal toxic shock syndrome

Patients with invasive and bacteraemic *Str. pyogenes* infections, and in particular necrotising fasciitis, may develop streptococcal toxic shock syndrome. The disease, which was first described in the late 1980s, is the result of the release of streptococcal toxins to the bloodstream. A striking feature of this acute fulminating disease is severe pain at the site of initial infection, usually the soft tissues. The additional clinical signs resemble those of staphylococcal toxic shock syndrome (see Ch. 12) and include fever, malaise, nausea, vomiting and diarrhoea, dizziness, confusion and a flat rash over large parts of the body. Without treatment, the disease progresses to shock and general organ failure.

Other suppurative infections

Historically, *Str. pyogenes* has been an important cause of puerperal sepsis. However, since the introduction of antibiotic therapy, this and other suppurative infections such as lymphangitis, pneumonia and meningitis are relatively rare.

Bacteraemia

Str. pyogenes is the second most common (after *Str. agalactiae*) of the pyogenic streptococci isolated from blood cultures. Bacteraemia is seen regularly in patients with necrotising fasciitis and toxic shock syndrome, but rarely as a complication to pharyngitis and local skin infections. Once in the blood, *Str. pyogenes* multiplies with incredible speed (doubling time 18 minutes), and the mortality rate approaches 40%. The potential complications include acute presentations of infective endocarditis leading to heart failure.

NONSUPPURATIVE SEQUELAE

Two serious diseases may develop as sequelae to *Str. pyogenes* infections:

1. Rheumatic fever, a potential sequela to pharyngitis (including scarlet fever)
2. Acute glomerulonephritis, which is primarily, but not exclusively, associated with skin infections.

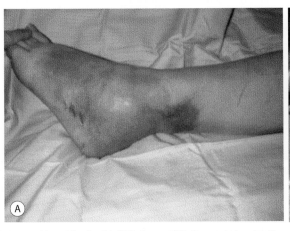 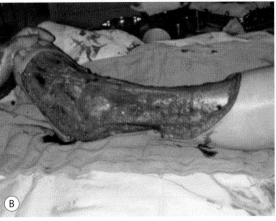

Fig. 13.5   Necrotising fasciitis (A) before and (B) after surgical exploration and debridement. (Courtesy Dr M Llewelyn, reproduced with permission from Elsevier.)

Both are caused by immune reactions induced by the streptococcal infection. The first clinical signs appear 1–5 weeks after the infection and at a time when the bacteria may have been eradicated by the immune system or as a result of antibiotic therapy.

Clinical correlations suggest that certain forms of psoriasis may also be triggered by *Str. pyogenes* throat infection. Preliminary evidence supports the hypothesis that some streptococcal superantigens cause disruption of immunological tolerance of a $CD8^+$ T cell subset that recognises cross-reactive epitopes on M proteins and skin keratin.

Rheumatic fever

This manifests as an inflammation of the joints (arthritis), heart (carditis), central nervous system (chorea), skin (erythema marginatum) and/or subcutaneous nodules. Polyarticular arthritis is the most common manifestation, whereas carditis is the most serious, as it leads to permanent damage, particularly of the heart valves.

Rheumatic fever is a major cause of acquired heart disease in young people throughout the world. The incidence of rheumatic heart disease worldwide ranges from 0.5 to 11 per 1000 of the population. New cases are relatively rare in most of Europe, but increased incidences have been observed among the aboriginal populations of Australia and New Zealand, and in Hawaii and Sri Lanka. Outbreaks of rheumatic fever have also been seen in the United States.

The disease is autoimmune in nature and is believed to result from the production of autoreactive (and poly-specific) antibodies and T lymphocytes induced by cross-reactive components of the bacteria and host tissues. Therefore, repeated episodes of *Str. pyogenes* infection increase the severity of the disease. The major antigens involved are myosin, tropomyosin, laminin and keratin in the human tissues, and the group A antigen (a polymer of *N*-acetylglucosamine) in the *Str. pyogenes* cell wall in addition to epitopes on some variants of surface M proteins.

Acute poststreptococcal glomerulonephritis

The clinical manifestations include:

- coffee-coloured urine caused by haematuria
- oedema of the face and extremities
- circulatory congestion caused by renal impairment.

Unlike rheumatic disease, outbreaks of poststreptococcal acute glomerulonephritis have continued to decline in most parts of the world. Regions that still exhibit a high incidence of this disease include Africa, the Caribbean, South America, New Zealand and Kuwait.

Poststreptococcal glomerulonephritis is usually referred to as an immune complex–mediated disease. However, the exact pathogenesis is not clear. Several mechanisms have been proposed, including:

- immune complex deposition in the glomeruli
- reaction of antibodies cross-reactive with streptococcal and glomerular antigens
- alterations of glomerular tissues by streptococcal products such as streptokinase
- direct complement activation by streptococcal components that have a direct affinity for glomerular tissues.

Disease is associated with a limited number of M types of *Str. pyogenes,* and there is evidence that particular variants of streptokinase are crucial nephritogenic factors.

Unlike rheumatic fever, there is a general absence of individual recurrences, suggesting that antibodies to nephritogenic factors protect against disease rather than the opposite.

STREPTOCOCCUS AGALACTIAE

Str. agalactiae is equivalent to Lancefield group B streptococci (GBS). Its primary human habitat is the colon. It may be carried in the throat, and, importantly, 10%–40% of women intermittently carry *Str. agalactiae* in the vagina.

Previously, *Str. agalactiae* was recognised primarily as a cause of bovine mastitis (*agalactia,* want of milk). However, since 1960 it has become the leading cause of neonatal infections in industrialised countries and is also an important cause of morbidity among peripartum women and nonpregnant adults with chronic medical conditions. Among β-haemolytic streptococci, *Str. agalactiae* is the most frequent isolate from blood cultures.

PATHOGENESIS

Virulence factors

Str. agalactiae produces several virulence factors, including haemolysins, capsule polysaccharide, C5a peptidase (only human pathogenic strains), hyaluronidase (not all strains), and various surface proteins that bind human IgA and serve as adhesins.

Ten different types of the capsular polysaccharide have been identified (Ia, Ib and II–IX). The serotype most frequently associated with neonatal infections is type III, whereas infections in adults are more evenly distributed over the different serotypes.

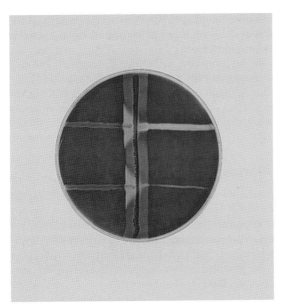

Fig. 13.6 Blood agar culture of strains of *Str. pyogenes* (group A) *(upper right)*, *Str. equisimilis* (group C) *(lower right)* and *Str. agalactiae* (group B) *(upper and lower left)* surrounding a vertical streak of *Staph. aureus*. The two *Str. agalactiae* strains show a positive CAMP reaction.

Among the haemolysins produced by *Str. agalactiae*, one, known as the CAMP factor (so-called because it was originally described by Christie, Atkins and Munch-Petersen), plays an important role in the recognition of this species in the laboratory. The CAMP factor lyses sheep or bovine red blood cells pretreated with the β-toxin of *Staph. aureus* (Fig. 13.6). Purified CAMP factor protein is fatal to rabbits when injected intravenously.

CLINICAL FEATURES

Infection in the neonate

Two different entities are recognised:

1. Early-onset disease, most cases of which present at or within 12 hours of birth
2. Late-onset disease, presenting >7 days and up to 3 months after birth.

Early-onset disease

This results from ascending spread of *Str. agalactiae* from the vagina into the amniotic fluid, which is then aspirated by the infant and results in septicaemia in the infant or the mother, or both. Infants borne by mothers carrying *Str. agalactiae* may also become colonised during passage through the vagina.

Depending on the site of initial contamination, neonates may be ill at birth or develop acute and fulminating illness a few hours or a day or two later. The clinical symptoms include lethargy, cyanosis and apnoea; when septicaemia progresses, shock ensues and death will occur if treatment is not instituted quickly. Meningitis and pulmonary infection may be associated.

As a result of improved recognition and prompt treatment of babies with symptoms, the fatality rate has been reduced to <10%. However, considerable morbidity persists among some survivors, especially those with meningitis.

Risk factors for neonatal colonisation and infection are:

- premature rupture of membranes
- prolonged labour
- premature delivery
- low birth weight
- intrapartum fever.

The immune status of the mother, and hence the level of maternal IgG antibodies in the infant, appears to be more important than the degree of colonisation of the mother's genital tract by *Str. agalactiae*.

It is possible that *Str. agalactiae* itself may cause premature rupture of membranes as a result of secretion of proteases and activation of local inflammation.

Late-onset disease

Purulent meningitis is the most common manifestation, but septic arthritis, osteomyelitis, conjunctivitis, sinusitis, otitis media, endocarditis and peritonitis also occur. The incidence of invasive infection is higher among pre-term infants than among those born at term.

The pathogenesis is distinct from that of early-onset disease. There is usually no history of obstetric complications and the disease is unrelated to vaginal colonisation in the mother. Many cases are acquired in hospital. Ward staff can be carriers of *Str. agalactiae*, and contamination of the baby may occur during nursing procedures, with subsequent baby-to-baby spread. Mastitis in the mother has also been described as a source of infection.

Infections in the adult

Ascending spread of *Str. agalactiae* leading to amniotic infection may result in abortion, chorioamnionitis, postpartum sepsis (endometritis) and other infections (e.g., pneumonia) in the postpartum period in young, previously healthy women.

Str. agalactiae is also a frequent cause of infection in certain risk groups of nonpregnant adults. Disease may manifest as sepsis, pneumonia, soft tissue infections such as cellulitis and arthritis, and urinary tract infections complicated by bacteraemia. The risk factors in these patients are diabetes mellitus, cirrhosis, renal failure, stroke and cancer. Older age, independent of underlying medical conditions, increases the risk of invasive *Str. agalactiae* infection.

OTHER PYOGENIC STREPTOCOCCI

Str. suis serotype 2 (group R streptococci) cause septicaemia and meningitis in pigs. They belong to a phylogenetic lineage separate from the other pyogenic streptococci. They occasionally infect people in contact with contaminated pork or infected pigs and may cause septicaemia, meningitis and respiratory tract infections. Abattoir workers, butchers and, to a lesser extent, those involved in domestic food preparation are at risk.

STREPTOCOCCUS PNEUMONIAE

Str. pneumoniae, commonly called the pneumococcus, is a member of the oropharyngeal microbiota of 5%–70% of the population, with the highest isolation rate in children during the winter months. In contrast to other streptococci, *Str. pneumoniae* generally occurs as characteristic diplococci (see Fig. 13.1B). Although closely related genetically to the commensal *Str. mitis* and *Str. oralis*, *Str. pneumoniae* is one of the four most frequent causes of fatal infections worldwide. It primarily causes disease of the airways and associated tissues (middle ear, paranasal sinuses, mastoids and lung parenchyma), but may spread to other sites, such as the meninges, joints, peritoneum, and endocardium.

Genetic plasticity is crucial to the success of *Str. pneumoniae* as a pathogen. Its frequent uptake of DNA from other strains of pneumococci and import of genes from related commensal streptococci facilitate its evasion of host immune factors. Gene transfer is by transformation and may result in new combinations of virulence factors including expression of a different capsular serotype. Experimental transfer of capsule genes in pneumococci was the basis of the original demonstration that DNA contains the genetic information in cells.

PATHOGENESIS

Virulence factors

Capsule

The capsular polysaccharide is a crucial virulence factor. The capsule is antiphagocytic, inhibiting complement deposition and phagocytosis where type-specific opsonic antibody is absent. A total of 95 different capsular serotypes has been identified.

The serotypes are designated by numbers, and those that are structurally related are grouped together (1, 2, 3, 4, 5, 6A, 6B, etc.). The different serotypes differ in virulence. Thus, about 90% of cases of bacteraemic pneumococcal pneumonia and meningitis are caused by some 23 serotypes.

IgA1 protease

Like the two other principal causes of bacterial meningitis (*Neisseria meningitidis* and *Haemophilus influenzae*), pneumococci produce an extracellular protease that specifically cleaves human IgA1 in the hinge region. This protease enables these pathogens to evade the protective functions of the principal immunoglobulin isotype of the upper respiratory tract.

Pneumolysin

Pneumococci produce an intracellular membrane-damaging toxin known as pneumolysin, which is released by autolysis. Pneumolysin inhibits:

- neutrophil chemotaxis
- phagocytosis and the respiratory burst
- lymphocyte proliferation and immunoglobulin synthesis.

In experimental models, it induces the features of lobar pneumonia and contributes to the mortality associated with this disease.

Autolysin

When activated, the pneumococcal autolysin breaks the peptide cross-linking of the cell wall peptidoglycan, leading to lysis of the bacteria. Autolysis enables the release of pneumolysin and, in addition, large amounts of cell wall fragments. The massive inflammatory response to these peptidoglycan fragments is an important component of the pathogenesis of pneumococcal pneumonia and meningitis.

CLINICAL FEATURES

Predisposing factors

Most *Str. pneumoniae* infections are associated with various predisposing conditions. Although occasional clustering of pneumococcal infections is recognised, person-to-person spread is uncommon.

Pneumonia results from aspiration of pneumococci contained in upper airway secretions into the lower respiratory tract, for example, when the normal mechanisms of mucus entrapment and expulsion by an intact glottic reflex and mucociliary escalator are impaired. This situation may arise in:

- disturbed consciousness in association with general anaesthesia, convulsions, alcoholism, epilepsy or head trauma
- respiratory viral infections, such as influenza
- chronic bronchitis and other forms of chronic bronchial sepsis.

Other predisposing disease states in which pneumococcal pneumonia may be the terminal event include:

- valvular and ischaemic heart disease
- chronic renal failure
- diabetes mellitus
- bronchogenic and metastatic malignancy
- advancing age.

Immune deficiencies that predispose to pneumococcal infection include:

- hypogammaglobulinaemia
- asplenia or hyposplenism
- malignancies such as multiple myeloma.

In these conditions, there is either a relative or absolute deficiency of opsonic antibody activity or an inability to induce a sufficient type-specific antibody response. Tuftsin, a naturally occurring tetrapeptide secreted by the spleen, also plays a role in combating pneumococcal sepsis; particularly at risk are those deficient in splenic activity:

- congenital asplenia
- traumatic removal
- functional impairment (e.g., homozygous sickle cell disease).

Human immunodeficiency virus (HIV) infection carries an increased risk of bacterial infections, including those caused by the pneumococcus, particularly in children.

Acute infections of the middle ear and paranasal sinuses occur in otherwise healthy children, but are usually preceded by a viral infection of the upper respiratory tract leading to local inflammation and swelling, and obstruction of the flow from these sites.

Pneumonia

Str. pneumoniae is the most frequent cause of pneumonia. The estimated annual incidence is 1–3 per 1000 of the population, with a 5% case fatality rate. Pneumococcal pneumonia follows aspiration with subsequent migration through the bronchial mucosa to involve the peribronchial lymphatics. The inflammatory reaction is focused primarily within the alveolus of a single lobule or lobe, although multilobar disease can also occur. Contiguous spread commonly results in inflammatory involvement of the pleura; this may progress to empyema.

Pericarditis is an uncommon but well recognised complication. Occasionally, lung necrosis and intrapulmonary abscess formation occur with the more virulent pneumococcal serotypes. Bacteraemia may complicate pneumococcal pneumonia in up to 15% of patients. This can result in metastatic involvement of the meninges, joints and, rarely, the endocardium. Some patients may have pneumonia, meningitis and infective endocarditis (Austrian syndrome).

The mortality rate from pneumococcal pneumonia in those admitted to hospital in the United Kingdom is approximately 15%. It is increased by age, underlying disease, bloodstream involvement, metastatic infection and certain types of pneumococci with large capsules (e.g., serotype 3).

Otitis media and sinusitis

Middle ear infections (otitis media) affect approximately half of all children between the ages of 6 months and 3 years; approximately one-third of cases are caused by *Str. pneumoniae*. Disease occurs after acquisition of a new strain to which there is no preexisting immunity. The prevalence is highest among children attending kindergarten or primary school, where there is a constant exchange of pneumococcal strains and emergence of new recombinant forms.

Meningitis

Str. pneumoniae is among the three leading causes of bacterial meningitis. It is assumed that invasion arises from the pharynx to the meninges via the bloodstream, as bacteraemia usually coexists. Meningitis may occasionally complicate pneumococcal infection at other sites, such as the lung and middle ear.

The incidence of pneumococcal meningitis is bimodal and affects children <3 years of age and adults of 45 years and above. The fatality rates are 20% and 30%, respectively, considerably higher than those associated with other types of bacterial meningitis.

Conjunctivitis

Pneumococci are among the most frequent causes of conjunctivitis. Cases throughout the world are caused primarily by a few epidemic clones that do not express capsular polysaccharide.

VIRIDANS STREPTOCOCCI

The viridans streptococci, and in particular the species of the Mitis and Salivarius groups, are dominant members of the resident microbiota of the oral cavity and pharynx in all age groups. They play an important role by inhibiting the colonisation of many pathogens, including pyogenic streptococci. This is achieved by two different mechanisms:

1. production of bacteriocins
2. production of hydrogen peroxide (also responsible for α-haemolysis).

Most strains secrete bacteriocins. Experimental implantation of strains of *Str. salivarius* with strong bacteriocin activity may prevent colonisation with *Str. pyogenes* in humans.

Mitis group

Str. mitis, Str. oralis and *Str. sanguinis,* among other viridans streptococci, colonise tooth surfaces as well as mucosal membranes. Because of their presence in the bacterial biofilms (dental plaque) on tooth surfaces, these species may enter the bloodstream during dental procedures such as tooth extraction or vigorous tooth cleaning, particularly when the gingival tissue is inflamed.

In healthy individuals, bacteria of such low virulence are cleared from the circulation within 1 hour. However, in patients with various predisposing conditions (Table 13.2), in particular heart valve damage due to poststreptococcal rheumatic fever, the circulating streptococci may settle in a niche protected from phagocytic cells. Local growth on the surface of heart valves eventually causes formation of vegetations, scarring and functional deficiency—a condition known as infective endocarditis. As

Table 13.2 Factors predisposing to infective endocarditis

Cardiac factors	Noncardiac factors
Rheumatic heart disease	Dental manipulations[a]
Atherosclerotic heart disease	Intravenous drug abuse
Congenital heart disease	Bacteraemia associated with
Cardiac surgery	intravenous cannulae and shunts
Prosthetic heart valves	Sepsis
Previous endocarditis	

[a]Procedures in which bleeding occurs.

the disease may progress over several months before diagnosis, patients sometimes have a subacute or chronic presentation. Infective endocarditis typically presents with intermittent fever and a new or changing heart murmur. Disruption of bacteria from the cardiac vegetations may cause embolic abscesses in various organs, including the brain. Until endocarditis due to skin staphylococci became more prevalent as a result of intravenous drug use and hospital-acquired infections, viridans streptococci were the most frequent causes of infective endocarditis.

Str. mitis and *Str. oralis* are increasingly recognised as causes of often fatal septicaemias in immunocompromised patients.

Mutans group

Str. mutans and *Str. sobrinus* exclusively colonise tooth enamel and do not occur until tooth eruption. Their proportions in the biofilm forming on tooth surfaces (dental plaque) are closely related to sugar consumption, and they are a major cause of dental caries because of their ability to produce large amounts of lactic acid even at pH values below 5.0 and to survive at low pH values. Like most other plaque streptococci, they may cause infective endocarditis.

Anginosus group

Str. anginosus, Str. intermedius and *Str. constellatus* are regular members of the commensal bacteria on tooth surfaces, in particular in the gingival crevices, and in the pharynx. They are often isolated from abscesses (notably in the brain and the abdominal cavity) and other opportunistic purulent infections. There is a particular association with appendicitis and postoperative infections.

Bovis group

Some of the species of this group are present in the human gut. Somewhat imprecisely, they are often referred to as group D streptococci—a characteristic that applies to enterococci too. They occasionally cause bacteraemia and infective endocarditis. These infections are often associated with colonic carcinoma (especially biotype I strains now renamed *Str. equinus*), which jeopardises the barrier function of the intestinal wall.

ENTEROCOCCUS SPECIES

As indicated by the name, members of the genus *Enterococcus* have their natural habitat in the human intestines. The species most commonly associated with human disease are *E. faecalis* and *E. faecium*. The diseases with which they are associated are:

- urinary tract infection
- infective endocarditis
- biliary tract infections
- suppurative abdominal lesions
- peritonitis.

E. faecalis and *E. faecium* are important causes of wound and urinary tract infection in hospital patients and may cause sporadic outbreaks. Bacteraemia carries a poor prognosis, as it often occurs in patients with major underlying pathology and in those who are immunocompromised. Bacteraemia associated with intravascular lines generally responds to line removal and antibiotics.

LABORATORY INVESTIGATION

Collection of specimens

The diagnosis of streptococcal infections is established by demonstrating the presence of the pathogen in throat or skin swabs, pus, blood cultures, cerebrospinal fluid (CSF), expectorates or urine according to the site of infection. In pneumococcal meningitis, the CSF is often macroscopically cloudy. The cell count is usually increased markedly and shows a predominance of polymorphonuclear leucocytes. Typical Gram-positive diplococci can commonly be demonstrated, sometimes in enormous numbers, by Gram-stain examination of a CSF deposit. The appearance is often typical, and a presumptive diagnosis can be made to allow appropriate therapy to be started before the identity of the organism is confirmed by culture.

Blood cultures are of value in patients with invasive streptococcal infections. This is also the case in patients with suspected pneumococcal pneumonia, particularly when this is severe, as up to 15% of patients are bacteraemic. Detection of bacteria by direct plating or microscopy of blood is not feasible owing to their low density.

Other body sites that may merit investigation according to the clinical presentation include joint and peritoneal fluids. Tympanocentesis provides the possibility of establishing the microbial cause of otitis media, but as most of these infections settle spontaneously, or with the assistance of a few days' antibiotic treatment, tympanocentesis is not usually necessary.

Cultivation and identification

Unlike staphylococci, streptococci lack the enzyme catalase, which releases oxygen from hydrogen peroxide. Catalase-negative Gram-positive cocci are therefore likely to be streptococci. The appearance of cocci in obvious chains (see Fig. 13.1) is another useful criterion, but the length of the chains varies with the species and conditions of growth. Optimal chain formation is seen in broth cultures. There may be marked variation in size and shape, particularly in older cultures or in direct smears from purulent exudates.

The primary cultivation medium for streptococci is blood agar, supplemented, whenever enterococci are suspected, with an agar medium (e.g., MacConkey medium) selective for enterobacteria. Streptococci of aetiological significance usually predominate in the culture even when the sample is taken from a site with a resident microbiota.

The pyogenic streptococci are detected initially by their β-haemolytic activity. The colonies are about 1 mm in diameter and, in contrast to those of staphylococci, lack pigment. Colonies of pneumococci are α-haemolytic, smooth, and may vary in size according to the amount of capsular polysaccharide produced; those of serotypes 3 and 37 are usually larger than the rest and have a watery or mucoid appearance. During prolonged incubation, autolysis of bacteria within the flat pneumococcal colonies results in a typical subsidence of the centre ('draughtsman colonies').

Species identification of pyogenic streptococci may be performed by MALDI-TOF combined with serological detection of group antigens by immune precipitation or coagglutination techniques. An additional test that is helpful in the presumptive identification of *Str. pyogenes* is the bacitracin sensitivity test. In contrast to most other streptococci, *Str. pyogenes* is uniformly sensitive and large inhibition zones are formed round bacitracin discs on blood agar. Likewise, *Str. agalactiae* can be identified presumptively by the CAMP reaction (see Fig. 13.6).

Pneumococci are distinguished from other α-haemolytic streptococci by their characteristic sensitivity to optochin (ethylhydrocupreine). Growth of pneumococci is inhibited around an optochin disc applied to an inoculated blood agar plate. With few exceptions, other α-haemolytic streptococci are not inhibited. In doubtful cases, the identity of pneumococci is confirmed by demonstrating bile solubility, autolysis or reactivity to a polyspecific antiserum ('omniserum') against capsular polysaccharides which, however, may be shared with commensal streptococci.

Other streptococci may also be identified by MALDI-TOF. However, some of the viridans streptococci are notoriously difficult to identify.

Enterococci and members of the Anginosus group are unique among the streptococci in their ability to grow on bile-containing media.

Antigen detection

Numerous commercial kits are available for the detection of *Str. pyogenes* directly in throat swabs without cultivation.

These diagnostic kits use specific antibodies to detect the group A antigen in the material on the swab. They allow practitioners to test whether a throat infection is caused by *Str. pyogenes* or a virus, but unfortunately do not rule out *Str. dysgalactiae* subspecies *equisimilis* (group C/G streptococci).

Antibody detection

Detection of antibodies against antigens of *Str. pyogenes* is an important means of establishing the diagnosis of poststreptococcal rheumatic fever and glomerulonephritis. In many cases, the initiating infection in the throat or on the skin is no longer present.

Immune responses vary depending on whether the original focus is the throat or skin. Antibodies against streptolysin O (the ASO test) are used to document antecedent streptococcal infection in the throat of patients with clinical signs of rheumatic fever. A significant increase in antibody titre appears 3–4 weeks after initial exposure to the microorganism. Detection of increased levels of serum antibodies to streptococcal hyaluronidase and DNAase B is also of diagnostic importance.

ASO estimation is unreliable in pyoderma-associated acute glomerulonephritis. A raised ASO titre is not observed in these patients, perhaps because lipids present in the skin inactivate the streptolysin O. Detection of antibodies against streptococcal DNAase B is recommended as a diagnostic tool in these patients.

Typing of streptococci

Strains of *Str. pyogenes* can be subdivided into serological types. The most comprehensive typing scheme is based on structural differences in the highly variable surface M protein. More than 150 different M types may be distinguished with type-specific antisera or by sequence differences in the gene *(emm)* encoding the M protein. An alternative typing scheme is based on the surface protein known as the T antigen.

Apart from serving epidemiological purposes, particular M types are associated with particular types of infection. Thus, certain M types are more commonly associated with skin infections than mucosal infections. Increases in the rate and severity of invasive *Str. pyogenes* infections (toxic shock syndrome and necrotising fasciitis) have been associated primarily with serotypes M-1 and M-3. Rheumatic fever is often, but not exclusively, associated with M serotypes 1, 3, 5, 6 and 18.

Pneumococci are typed on the basis of the differences in capsular polysaccharides, of which 95 have been described. The addition of India ink to a suspension of pneumococci shows the presence of the capsule as a clear halo around the organisms. Mixing a suspension of pneumococci with type-specific antisera increases the visibility of the capsule in the microscope and is the basis of the quellung reaction, or capsular swelling test. Serotyping of pneumococci is carried out mainly in reference laboratories.

Multilocus sequence typing (MLST) schemes based on allelic sequence profiles of seven housekeeping genes are available for several *Streptococcus* species and allow mapping of the global distribution of sequence types.

TREATMENT

Penicillin resistance has never been detected in *Str. pyogenes*. As a result, benzylpenicillin (penicillin G) or oral phenoxymethylpenicillin (penicillin V) are the drugs of choice for treatment of infections with *Str. pyogenes*. In cases of hypersensitivity to penicillin, erythromycin is usually the second choice for mild infections, but resistance occurs and is common in some countries. In severe infections, treatment with intravenous vancomycin is generally recommended.

Treatment for 3–5 days limits the effect of severe attacks of streptococcal infection and prevents suppurative complications such as otitis media, although the streptococci are eliminated from the infected area only if treatment is continued for 10 days.

Surgery is essential to remove damaged tissue in cases of necrotising fasciitis, as antibiotic penetration of the infected area is poor. Clindamycin is often added to penicillin because it inhibits protein synthesis, including production of exotoxin.

Most strains of *Str. agalactiae* are susceptible to penicillins, macrolides and glycopeptides.

Although streptococci are intrinsically resistant to aminoglycosides, these agents interact synergically with penicillins and the combination is often used in the treatment of streptococcal and enterococcal endocarditis.

Pneumococci and viridans streptococci may be resistant to penicillins owing to mutations in the target penicillin-binding proteins. These mutations have accumulated in strains of *Str. mitis*, and the altered genes have subsequently been transferred by genetic transformation to *Str. pneumoniae*. The incidence of penicillin resistance is quite variable geographically and reflects the local level of antibiotic usage.

Most pneumococcal infections with strains exhibiting intermediate-level resistance to penicillin (minimum inhibitory concentration 0.1–1 mg/L) respond to high-dose therapy; an exception is meningitis because of problems of penetration into the CSF. Penicillin resistance in pneumococci and other viridans streptococci is often linked to resistance to several other antibiotics. Resistance to erythromycin, tetracycline and chloramphenicol is not uncommon, and tolerance even to vancomycin has been reported.

The dose of penicillin necessary to treat susceptible pneumococcal infection is determined largely by pharmacological factors at the site of infection. For example, pneumococcal pneumonia responds to doses of penicillin as low as 0.3 g (0.5 mega-units) twice daily, whereas pneumococcal meningitis requires much higher doses. In patients unable to tolerate penicillin, erythromycin is the most widely used alternative agent for respiratory pneumococcal infections.

Unlike other streptococci, enterococci are intrinsically resistant to cephalosporins. Sensitivity to penicillins and other antibiotics varies widely, and clinical isolates must be tested for their susceptibility. Most isolates of *E. faecalis* are amoxicillin sensitive, whilst most *E. faecium* strains are resistant. Vancomycin resistance has been observed in enterococci, especially in *E. faecium* strains. Vancomycin-resistant enterococci (known as VRE) have become a widespread problem in many parts of the world. Anti-microbial agents with activity against VRE include the linezolid (an oxazolidinone).

PREVENTION AND CONTROL

Hygienic measures

Skin infections with *Str. pyogenes* are usually associated with poor hygiene and can, to a large extent, be prevented by standard hygienic measures. Late-onset neonatal infections with *Str. agalactiae* may also be prevented or significantly reduced by standard aseptic nursing procedures.

Likewise, hygiene is the most important preventive measure in relation to dental caries, which can be prevented largely by regular tooth-brushing with a fluoride-containing dentifrice combined with restricted consumption of fermentable carbohydrates, in particular sucrose.

CHEMOPROPHYLAXIS

Prophylactic use of antibiotics is relevant in some streptococcal infections. As the primary attack of rheumatic fever usually occurs during childhood, long-term penicillin prophylaxis until adulthood is recommended to reduce the risk of further attacks and further heart injury. This is not the case in patients with acute glomerulonephritis because of the lack of recurrences.

Two different approaches are used to prevent early-onset neonatal *Str. agalactiae* infections:

1. A risk-based strategy in which women of unknown colonisation status receive intrapartum antibiotic prophylaxis in case of: threatened delivery at <37 weeks' gestation; premature rupture of the membranes; intrapartum fever; previous delivery of a child who developed neonatal infection; or previous colonisation or urinary tract infection with *Str. agalactiae*
2. A screening-based approach in which all pregnant women at 35–37 weeks' gestation are screened for *Str. agalactiae* colonisation in vaginal and rectal specimens. All identified carriers are offered intrapartum chemoprophylaxis. This screening-based prophylaxis is used in the United States and in many European countries and has led to a significant decline in the incidence of early-onset neonatal infections due to *Str. agalactiae*. Intravenous or intramuscular penicillin is the agent of choice because its antimicrobial spectrum, narrower than that of ampicillin, reduces the likelihood of resistance developing in other bacteria and selection of other potential pathogens. Antimicrobial susceptibility testing of *Str. agalactiae* isolates is crucial for appropriate antibiotic prophylaxis selection for penicillin-allergic women because resistance to clindamycin, the most common agent used in this population, is increasing among isolates.

Patients at risk of developing infective endocarditis (see Table 13.2) should be given prophylactic antibiotics in association with dental procedures that lead to bleeding. The current international recommendations are amoxicillin 1 hour before dental treatment that normally involves bleeding such as tooth extraction or surgery or, in case of penicillin allergy, clindamycin. If the patient has been on long-term penicillin prophylaxis, the oral streptococci are likely to have reduced susceptibility to penicillins, and clindamycin or vancomycin is recommended as the alternative. In the United Kingdom, antibiotic prophylaxis is no longer recommended, but US and European guidelines recommend prophylaxis for high-risk patients and certain procedures. It is imperative that patients at risk maintain healthy periodontal conditions and that the amount of dental plaque is kept to a minimum.

VACCINES

Pyogenic streptococci

Attempts to develop a vaccine against *Str. pyogenes* infections have been hampered by two problems:

1. The considerable antigenic diversity of the M protein and other vaccine candidate antigens
2. The potential immunological cross-reactivity of many of the antigens with host tissue components.

Several strategies are currently being tested, including oral vaccination.

A vaccine against neonatal *Str. agalactiae* infection based on protein-conjugated type III capsular polysaccharide is being tested for use primarily in women of reproductive age. However, additional serotypes are increasingly prevalent.

Pneumococci

Before the widespread availability of effective antimicrobial drugs, the treatment of pneumococcal infections was based on the use of type-specific antiserum. This reduced the mortality rate associated with bacteraemic pneumococcal pneumonia, but not to the same extent that penicillin was subsequently shown to achieve. However, it indicated that type-specific antibody had a role in the control of pneumococcal disease and led to a variety of prototype vaccines. The vaccine that has been in use for many years contains a mixture of 23 polysaccharide serotypes chosen according to the prevalence of serotypes responsible for bacteraemic pneumococcal infection. It offers protection against 90% of isolates.

Like other vaccines based on pure polysaccharides, the immunogenicity of the multivalent vaccine is inadequate in those below 2 years of age and in those immunosuppressed as a result of malignancy, steroid therapy or other chronic disease. To overcome this problem, pneumococcal vaccines containing capsular polysaccharide coupled to a carrier protein are now available. These vaccines increase the immunogenicity of the polysaccharide by rendering the response dependent on T lymphocyte help. The current conjugate vaccines include 11–13 of the capsular polysaccharides and are now part of the childhood vaccination programme in many countries.

Immunisation is recommended for various groups at risk of pneumococcal disease, particularly those with congenital or surgical asplenia and those with hereditary haemoglobinopathies such as sickle cell disease, as pneumococcal infection can be fulminant in these patients. Vaccine efficacy is not complete, and many clinicians also prescribe oral phenoxymethylpenicillin as long-term chemoprophylaxis in this high-risk group. In some countries, including the United States and the United Kingdom, the vaccine is recommended for those over 65 years of age, with or without previous ill health, although there have been difficulties in establishing scientifically the efficacy in this group.

RECOMMENDED READING

Carapetis, J. R., Steer, A. C., Mulholland, E. K., & Weber, M. (2005). The global burden of group A streptococcal diseases. *The Lancet Infectious Diseases, 5*(11), 685–694.

Ferretti, J. J., Stevens, D. L., & Fischetti, V. A. (Eds). (2016). Streptococcus pyogenes: *Basic biology to clinical manifestations*. Oklahoma City (OK): University of Oklahoma Health Sciences Center. http://www.ncbi.nlm.nih.gov/books/NBK343616/.

Henriques-Normark, B., Blomberg, C., Dagerhamn, J., Bättig, P., & Normark, S. (2008). The rise and fall of bacterial clones: *Streptococcus pneumoniae. Nature Reviews. Microbiology, 6*(11), 827–837. doi:10.1038/nrmicro2011.

Marsh, P. D., Lewis, M. L. O., Rogers, H., Williams, D. W., & Wilson, M. (2016). *Marsh & Martin's oral microbiology* (6th ed.). Oxford: Elsevier.

Mitchell, T. J. (2003). The pathogenesis of streptococcal infections: From tooth decay to meningitis. *Nature Reviews. Microbiology, 1*(3), 219–230.

Reinert, R. R., Reinert, S., van der Linden, M., Al-Lahham, A., & Appelbaum, P. (2005). Antimicrobial susceptibility of *Streptococcus pneumoniae* in eight European countries from 2001 to 2003. *Antimicrobial Agents and Chemotherapy, 49*(7), 2903–2913.

Verani, J. R., McGee, L., Schrag, S. J., & Division of Bacterial Diseases, National Center for Immunization and Respiratory Diseases, Centers for Disease Control and Prevention (CDC). (2010). Prevention of perinatal group B streptococcal disease. Revised guidelines from CDC. *MMWR. Recommendations and Reports : Morbidity and Mortality Weekly Report, 59*(RR-10), 1–32.

Websites

Multi Locus Sequence Typing. Schemes for streptococci and several other pathogenic bacteria. Available at http://pubmlst.org/.

14 Coryneform bacteria, *Listeria* and *Erysipelothrix*

Diphtheria; listeriosis; erysipeloid

JIM McLAUCHLIN AND PHILIPPE RIEGEL

KEY POINTS

- The genus *Corynebacterium* includes *C. diphtheriae*, which causes the toxin-mediated infection diphtheria, but respiratory or cutaneous diphtheria is also caused by toxigenic strains of *C. ulcerans*. The infection diphtheria has largely been controlled by widespread use of a toxoid vaccine. *C. ulcerans* is now the predominant cause of United Kingdom toxigenic infection.
- Diphtheria toxin is encoded by a lysogenic bacteriophage and has cardiac and neurotoxic effects. Nontoxigenic strains are occasionally isolated from diverse infections.
- Other medically significant corynebacteria are part of the normal skin or mucosal flora and are opportunistic pathogens of hospital patients, particularly those with implanted medical devices.
- *Listeria* is a genus of environmental bacteria and includes *L. monocytogenes*, an important cause of disease in domestic animals, which also causes severe systemic disease in the immunosuppressed and elderly as well as the unborn or newly delivered.
- Listeriosis is transmitted predominantly by the consumption of contaminated ready-to-eat foods; the agent is able to grow in a variety of foods at refrigeration temperatures.
- *Erysipelothrix rhusiopathiae* causes economically important disease in domestic animals, notably pigs. Occasional human infections occur and present as a cellulitis.

CORYNEFORM BACTERIA

The term *coryneform* is used to describe aerobic, nonsporing and irregularly shaped Gram-positive rods. This morphology is typical of the genus *Corynebacterium* (name from Greek κορσψνη = club) but, according to this broad definition, includes environmental bacteria showing coccoid forms such as *Rhodococcus, Gordonia* and *Brevibacterium* species, and preferentially anaerobic bacteria of the genera *Actinomyces* (see Ch. 20), *Actinotignum (Actinobaculum)*, *Arcanobacterium* and *Propionibacterium*, which exhibit some branched forms.

CORYNEBACTERIUM DIPHTHERIAE AND C. ULCERANS

The major disease caused by *C. diphtheriae* is diphtheria, an infection of the local tissue mainly of the upper respiratory tract with the production of a toxin that causes systemic effects, notably in the heart and peripheral nerves. Diphtheria has virtually disappeared in developed countries following mass immunisation but is still endemic in many regions of the world. Skin infections are prevalent in some countries. Nontoxigenic strains have been associated with endocarditis, cutaneous abscess and osteoarthritis throughout the world.

C. ulcerans has been isolated from raw milk and can cause mastitis in cattle. In humans, it presents almost exclusively in cases of exudative pharyngitis, but occasional soft tissue infections occur. *C. ulcerans* can produce a toxin that is 95% identical to the diphtheria toxin, causing a diphtheria-like illness. It seems likely that many human infections are transmitted by dogs or cats.

Description

C. diphtheriae, like other members of the genus, are nonmotile, nonspore-forming, straight or slightly curved rods with tapered ends. They are Gram-positive, but easily decolourised, particularly in older cultures. Cells often contain metachromatic granules (polymetaphosphate), which stain bluish-purple with methylene blue. Snapping division produces groups of cells in angular and palisade arrangements that create a Chinese character effect. *C. diphtheriae* is aerobic and facultatively anaerobic, growing best on a blood- or serum-containing media at 35–37°C with or without carbon dioxide enrichment. On agar medium containing tellurite, colonies of *C. diphtheriae* are characteristically black or grey after 24–48 hours.

Four biovars of *C. diphtheriae* can be distinguished by biochemical features and cultural morphology: *gravis*, *intermedius*, *mitis* and *belfanti*. Bacilli of the *gravis* biotype are usually short, whereas those of biotype *mitis* are long and pleomorphic; biotype *intermedius* ranges from very long to short rods. In broth medium, *C. diphtheriae* biotype *gravis* forms a pellicle and a granular deposit, whereas *C. diphtheriae* biotype *mitis* produces a diffuse turbidity. The biotype *intermedius* forms no pellicle, but a fine granular deposit can be observed. The biotype *belfanti* is nitrate reductase test negative. The biotypes *gravis*, *intermedius* and *mitis* are genomically similar and can produce a diphtheria exotoxin, whereas bacteria of the biotype *belfanti* form a separate genetic clone and are rarely toxigenic.

Pathogenesis

The common mode of transmission of *C. diphtheriae* is droplet spread from a person with respiratory diphtheria or a carrier. Alternative modes of transmission are direct contact with cutaneous diphtheria lesions, infected secretions or infected animals *(C. ulcerans)* or consumption of unpasteurised dairy products *(C. ulcerans)*. Prolonged close contact with an infected person and intimate contact increases the likelihood of transmission.

To cause diphtheria, strains of *C. diphtheriae* or *C. ulcerans* must:

- invade, colonise and proliferate in local tissues
- be lysogenised by a specific β-phage, enabling it to produce toxin.

In the upper respiratory tract, diphtheria bacilli elicit an inflammatory exudate and cause necrosis of the cells of the faucial mucosa (Fig. 14.1). The diphtheria toxin possibly assists colonisation of the throat or skin by killing epithelial cells or neutrophils.

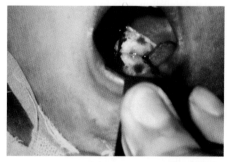

Fig. 14.1 Diphtheritic membrane on throat. (From Conlon, C., Snydman, D. (2000). *Mosby's Color Atlas and Text of Infectious Diseases.* Edinburgh: Mosby Elsevier. Courtesy Nigel Day.)

The organisms do not penetrate deeply into the mucosal tissue and bacteraemia does not usually occur. The exotoxin is produced locally and spread by the bloodstream to distant organs, with a special affinity for heart muscle, the peripheral nervous system and the adrenal glands.

Diphtheria bacilli can colonise the throats of people who have been immunised against diphtheria or who have become immune as a result of natural exposure, but usually no pseudomembrane develops.

The diphtheria toxin is a heat-stable polypeptide, composed of two fragments: A (active) and B (binding). The toxin binds to a specific receptor on susceptible cells and enters by receptor-mediated endocytosis. The A subunit is cleaved and released from the B subunit as it inserts and passes through the lysosomal membrane into the cytoplasm. Fragment A catalyses the transfer of adenosine diphosphate (ADP)-ribose from nicotinamide adenine dinucleotide (NAD) to the eukaryotic elongation factor 2, which inhibits the function of the latter in protein synthesis. Inhibition of protein synthesis is probably responsible for both the necrotic and neurotoxic effects of the toxin. Production of toxin by lysogenised bacilli is enhanced considerably when the bacteria are grown in low iron conditions. Other factors such as osmolarity, amino acid concentrations and pH have a role.

Nontoxigenic strains of *C. diphtheriae* and *C. ulcerans* may cause pharyngitis and cutaneous abscesses. Systemic disease, including endocarditis, septic arthritis and osteomyelitis, has also been reported. *C. diphtheriae* biotype *belfanti* may be involved in the processus of a chronic atrophic rhinitis named ozena. The virulence factors of these nontoxigenic strains remain unknown. Conversion of a nontoxigenic strain to a toxigenic strain by phage infection can occur in human populations.

Clinical features

The incubation period of diphtheria is 2–5 days, with a range of 1–10 days. At first, patients present with malaise, sore throat and moderate fever. A thick, adherent grey pseudomembrane is present on one or both tonsils or adjacent pharynx. In nasopharyngeal infection, the pseudomembrane may involve nasal mucosa, the pharyngeal wall and the soft palate. In this form, oedema involving the cervical lymph glands may occur in the anterior tissues of the neck, a condition known as bullneck diphtheria.

Laryngeal involvement leads to obstruction of the larynx and lower airways. Organisms multiply within the membranes and toxaemia is prominent. The patient is gravely ill, with a weak pulse, restlessness and confusion. Laryngeal diphtheria is characterised by gradually increasing hoarseness and stridor and most commonly occurs as an extension of pharyngeal involvement in children. Intoxication takes the form of myocarditis and peripheral neuritis and may be associated with thrombocytopenia. Visual disturbance, difficulty in swallowing and paralysis of the arms and legs also occur but usually resolve spontaneously. Complete heart block may result from myocarditis. Death is most commonly due to congestive heart failure and cardiac arrhythmias.

Cutaneous diphtheria occurs mostly in tropical countries. The lesion is usually characterised by an ulcer covered by a necrotic pseudomembrane and may involve any area of the skin. Although the organism usually produces toxin, systemic toxic manifestations are uncommon.

Diagnosis

A revision of the England and Wales guidance for the control and management of diphtheria was published in 2015. This revision was prompted by developments in local epidemiology, including the increasing number of *C. ulcerans* cases, the introduction of routine real-time PCR (qPCR) testing of potentially toxigenic corynebacteria

isolates by the national reference laboratory and the identification of circulating nontoxigenic toxin gene bearing (NTTB) *C. diphtheriae* strains in England.

The diagnosis is made on clinical grounds, supported by a history of diphtheria among contacts, lack of prior immunisation or travel in countries where diphtheria is endemic. Cases can be classified according to clinical and laboratory criteria as possible, probable or confirmed cases of toxigenic infection.

The role of the laboratory is to confirm the diagnosis by recovery of *C. diphtheriae* in culture followed by appropriate tests for detection of toxin production (Fig. 14.2). The clinician should inform the laboratory of the presumptive diagnosis of diphtheria because isolation of *C. diphtheriae* requires special media. Material for culture should be obtained on a swab from the inflamed areas surrounding the pseudomembranes.

Direct microscopy of a smear is a sensitive but not a specific test because *C. diphtheriae* is morphologically similar to other coryneforms. The recommended media

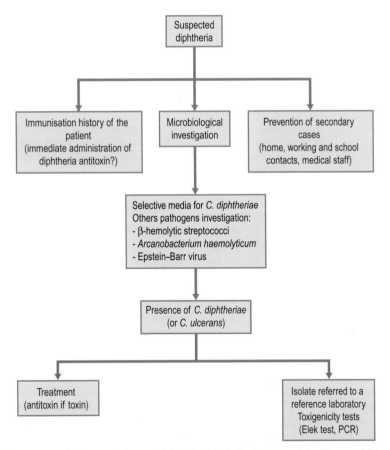

Fig. 14.2 Algorithm for the management of a suspected case of diphtheria. *Note:* Antitoxin treatment should not await laboratory confirmation, which may take several days. (Algorithm courtesy Dr A. Efstratiou, Central Public Health Laboratory, London.)

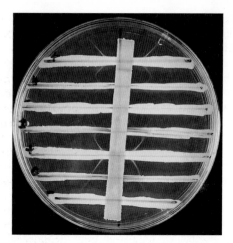

Fig. 14.3 Elek plate for the detection of *C. diphtheriae* toxin production. Cultures are streaked horizontally, then overlaid with an antitoxin-impregnated strip. Toxin and antitoxin diffuse into the culture during incubation, and precipitin lines develop where toxin and antitoxin are present in a critical ratio. Positive reactions in test cultures are indicated by precipitin lines that arc with those produced by positive controls. The *C. diphtheriae* cultures are (top to bottom): National Collection of Type Cultures (NCTC) strain 10648 (positive control); test culture (positive); NCTC 10356 (negative control); NCTC 3984 (weak positive control); NCTC 10648 (positive control); test culture (negative); NCTC 10356 (negative control). (Courtesy Dr A Efstratiou, Health Protection Agency, London.)

include blood agar and a selective medium containing tellurite and cysteine. Identification is based on carbohydrate fermentation reactions and enzymatic activities. Commercial kits such as the API Coryne strip provide a reliable identification. MALDI-TOF is also a reliable tool for rapid diagnosis of potentially toxigenic *Corynebacterium* species.

Toxigenicity testing is essential. Production of diphtheria toxin is demonstrated by the agar immunoprecipitation test (Elek test; Fig. 14.3) or by the tissue culture cytotoxicity assay, which has replaced the virulence test in guinea pigs. The toxin gene can be detected by the polymerase chain reaction (PCR), which is now the most appropriate test for toxicity when available. This test shows excellent correlation with guinea pig virulence, although there is the rare possibility of strains harbouring the *tox* gene but unable to express it. These latter strains are named nontoxigenic toxin gene bearing *C. diphtheriae* and *C. ulcerans* (NTTB).

The confirmation of identification, and the determination of toxigenicity requires submission of the isolate to the national reference laboratory.

The detection of the *tox* gene by PCR directly from clinical specimens is feasible but has to be validated in terms of sensitivity and specificity. All biotypes are potentially toxigenic, although the biotype *belfanti* is rarely

toxigenic. Multilocus sequence typing provides high-resolution data appropriate for the epidemiological investigation of diphtheria.

Measurement of antibodies to diphtheria toxin in serum collected before administration of antitoxin may support the diagnosis when cultures are negative. An algorithm for the management of suspect cases of diphtheria is given in the guidance for the control and management of diphtheria which was published in 2015.

Treatment

Diphtheria antitoxin should only be used for confirmed or probable cases of diphtheria in a hospital setting. Diphtheria antitoxin should be given to classic respiratory cases without waiting for laboratory confirmation as antitoxin neutralises only circulating toxin that rapidly diffuses from the local lesions and soon becomes irreversibly bound to tissue cells. In most cutaneous infections, large-scale toxin absorption is unlikely, and therefore the risk of giving antitoxin is usually considered to be substantially greater than any benefit.

Treatment with parenteral penicillin or macrolides eradicates the organism and terminates toxin production. *C. diphtheriae* and *C. ulcerans* are universally sensitive to penicillins, but some strains are resistant to erythromycin, tetracyclines and rifampicin. Macrolides may be preferred to penicillin for elimination of the bacilli from the throat, particularly in treatment of persistent carriers.

Antibiotic treatment should continue for 14 days based on local antimicrobial susceptibility testing.

Patients should be placed in strict isolation, nursed by staff whose immunisation history is documented and have daily platelet counts and electrocardiography.

Epidemiology

Diphtheria has virtually disappeared in developed countries following mass immunisation in the 1940s but is still endemic in many regions of the world, and some countries have experienced outbreaks of diphtheria at the end of the 20th century. About 50,000 cases of diphtheria occurred in the newly independent states of the former Soviet Union during 1990–1996, leading to infection in short-term visitors from Western Europe. In the United States, only 45 cases were reported during 1980–1995. In 2002, one case of diphtheria was reported in the United States, but more toxigenic strains were referred to North American reference laboratories. In 2014, 7321 cases of diphtheria were reported worldwide to the World Health Organization, with 35 of them from European countries, but many more cases are likely to go unreported. The surveillance data in England and Wales show that between 1986 and 2013, 2662 *C. diphtheriae* isolates were received at the PHE, of which 68 (2.6%) were toxigenic. Both *C. diphtheriae* and *C. ulcerans* are causes of diphtheria in the United Kingdom. Until the early 1990s, toxigenic infections were more commonly caused by *C. diphtheriae* than *C. ulcerans*, whereas since the 1990s, *C. ulcerans* has been the predominant cause of UK toxigenic infection. The species cannot be linked to the clinical presentation. Since the start of laboratory surveillance in 1986, the clinical presentation in over 85% of toxigenic infections has been non-classical respiratory diphtheria for both *C. diphtheriae* (59 of 68 isolates; 86.8%) and *C. ulcerans* (59 of 66 isolates; 89.4%).

Both *C. ulcerans* and *C. diphtheriae* have resulted in severe or fatal disease in the United Kingdom, with six deaths between 1986 and 2013, four of which were caused by *C. ulcerans*. Nontoxigenic strains capable of causing mild disease continue to circulate throughout the world. In European countries, carriage rates of nontoxigenic strains ranged from 0 in Ireland to 4 per 1000 in Turkey. An increase in laboratory reports in the United Kingdom of nontoxigenic *C. diphtheriae* was observed from 58 in 1992, peaking at 294 in 2000 before falling to 39 in 2009, and remaining around 30–60 isolates per year since then.

Acquired immunity to diphtheria is due primarily to toxin-neutralising antibody (antitoxin). Passive immunity in utero is acquired transplacentally and can last for 1 or 2 years after birth. Active immunity can probably be produced by a mild or subclinical infection in infants who retain some maternal immunity. Unimmunised children under 15 years old are most likely to contract diphtheria. The disease is also found among adults whose immunisation was neglected. The mortality rate is highest among young children and in people aged over 40 years. Skin infections caused by *C. diphtheriae* may result in early development of natural immunity against the disease.

The Schick test, an intradermal injection of stabilised diphtheria toxin, was formerly used to determine individual susceptibility to the toxin. Absence of a reaction indicates immunity. Tissue culture neutralisation tests, enzyme-linked immunosorbent assay (ELISA) and passive haemagglutination assay to measure serum antitoxin levels are now preferred. For epidemiological purposes the minimum protective level is considered to be 0.01 international units (IU) of diphtheria antitoxin per milliliter in a serum sample. A level of 0.1 IU/mL is desirable for individual protection.

C. diphtheriae persists longer in skin lesions than in the tonsils or nose, and cutaneous diphtheria appears to be more contagious than respiratory diphtheria. Untreated people who are infected with the diphtheria bacillus can be contagious for up to 2 weeks but seldom for >4 weeks. If treated with appropriate antibiotics, the contagious period can be limited to <4 days. *C. diphtheriae* can survive in the environment in dust and on dry vomitus for several months, and transmission via vomitus has been documented. Animal-to-human transmission and foodborne transmission by consumption of contaminated foods such as raw milk have been described but are very rare.

Control

High population immunity achieved through mass immunisation (at least 95% coverage in children and at least 90% coverage in adults) is the most effective measure to control epidemic diphtheria. Immunisation with diphtheria toxoid was first introduced in 1923. Large-scale immunisation programmes introduced in the 1940s reduced the incidence of diphtheria dramatically, although the disease was not eradicated completely. Immunisation schedules are discussed in Ch. 70.

Prevention of secondary cases by the rapid investigation of close contacts is essential. These investigations should include ascertainment of the immunisation histories of all home and school contacts. Primary courses of immunisation or a booster are given if necessary.

OTHER MEDICALLY IMPORTANT CORYNEBACTERIA

The nondiphtheria corynebacteria (diphtheroids) are diverse and comprise strictly aerobic bacteria usually isolated from the environment as well as facultative or preferentially anaerobic bacteria, which are commensals of the skin and mucous membranes. The principal species involved and the main clinical syndromes associated with infection are shown in Table 14.1.

Corynebacterium pseudotuberculosis

C. pseudotuberculosis is primarily an animal pathogen and rarely infects humans. It causes caseous lymphadenitis in sheep and goats and abscesses or ulcerative lymphangitis in horses. Human infections occur mainly in patients with animal contact. Infection usually presents as a subacute or chronic granulomatous lymphadenitis involving the axillary or cervical nodes, but pneumonias have been described. Some strains are lysogenised by bacteriophages of *C. diphtheriae* and thus produce diphtheria toxin, but no clinical cases of diphtheria-like disease have been attributed to *C. pseudotuberculosis*. Treatment requires prolonged antibiotic therapy with erythromycin, penicillins or tetracycline, and surgical drainage or excision.

Corynebacterium jeikeium

C. jeikeium (formerly CDC coryneform group JK) is part of the normal skin flora, particularly in inguinal, axillary and rectal areas. Colonisation by antibiotic-resistant strains

Table 14.1 Habitat and disease associations of corynebacteria

Organism	Major habitat	Disease association
Corynebacterium diphtheriae	Throat, skin	Diphtheria (toxigenic strains), wound infections, bacteraemia, endocarditis
C. ulcerans	Human throat and skin Animals: raw milk, dogs, cats	human: diphtheria (toxigenic strains), pharyngitis and wound infection Cattle: mastitis
C. pseudotuberculosis	Sheep, horses, goats	Human: lymphadenitis Animals: abscesses and abortion
C. jeikeium	Skin	Bacteraemia, endocarditis; infection of foreign bodies and CSF shunts
C. urealyticum	Skin, urinary tract	Urinary tract infection, pyelonephritis, endocarditis
C. amycolatum	Humans and animals	Human: bacteraemia, endocarditis, peritonitis and wound infection Cattle: mastitis
C. glucuronolyticum	Urinary tract of humans and animals	Urogenital tract infection
C. minutissimum	Skin, urinary tract	Erythrasma, bacteraemia
C. striatum	Respiratory tract, skin	Respiratory tract infection, wound infection, bacteraemia
C. pseudodiphtheriticum	Respiratory tract	Respiratory tract infection, endocarditis
C. kroppenstedtii	Unknown	Breast abscess, granulomatous mastitis
Arcanobacterium haemolyticum	Throat	Pharyngitis, skin ulcers, endocarditis
Rhodococcus equi	Animals, soil	Pulmonary infection and soft tissue infection in immunodeficient patients

are unusual in healthy individuals but is common in hospitalised patients, particularly those who are neutropenic or receiving antibiotics. Most infections are associated with skin damaged by wounds or invasive devices. Such infections include:

- prosthetic valve endocarditis
- bacteraemia associated with infected long-term intravenous cannulae
- peritonitis in patients on peritoneal dialysis
- bacteraemia and local infection following insertion of an epicardial pacemaker
- central nervous system infection in patients with ventriculoperitoneal or atrial shunts for hydrocephalus.

Most infections occur in patients in hospital for prolonged periods and who have received broad-spectrum antimicrobial therapy. Spread is through environmental contamination, the hands of ward staff or autoinfection.

Treatment

Most isolates of *C. jeikeium* recovered from infections are highly resistant to penicillins and cephalosporins in vitro. Systemic amoxicillin, gentamicin, rifampicin or ciprofloxacin can be used if the isolate is susceptible, but the penicillins are incompletely bactericidal unless they are combined with aminoglycosides. Resistance to aminoglycosides and macrolides has been reported in >60% of isolates and resistance to fluoroquinolones is variable. Glycopeptides are the drugs of choice for treating serious infections. *C. jeikeium* is sensitive to glycopeptides

and these antibiotics are bactericidal. Combinations of vancomycin with gentamicin have been used to treat infective endocarditis. Peritonitis secondary to peritoneal dialysis and meningitis related to shunts can be treated with intraperitoneal or intrathecal vancomycin, respectively.

Corynebacterium urealyticum

C. urealyticum (formerly CDC coryneform group D-2) is a frequent skin coloniser, mainly in hospital patients. The groin, abdominal wall and axilla are most frequently colonised. This microorganism is associated with urinary tract infections, particularly with alkaline-encrusted cystitis and pyelitis related to its strong urease production. Infection is a consequence of the use of broad-spectrum antibiotics for patients with underlying conditions that predispose to urinary tract infection. The organism may also cause pyelonephritis and is an infrequent cause of endocarditis, osteomyelitis or soft tissue infection. Like *C. jeikeium*, *C. urealyticum* is usually highly resistant to most antimicrobial agents, except glycopeptides. Vancomycin, tetracyclines, erythromycin and norfloxacin have proven effective in treatment. Prolonged treatment with appropriate antibiotics, acidification of the urine and removal of crusts is essential for proper management of encrusted cystitis.

Corynebacterium amycolatum

C. amycolatum is a human skin commensal similar to other corynebacteria but lacks cell wall mycolic acids. Its biochemical characteristics are variable, and it is often misidentified. Strains isolated from hospital patients may be multiresistant to antibiotics except glycopeptides. *C. amycolatum* has been reported as causing bacteraemia, endocarditis, peritonitis and wound infection.

Corynebacterium glucuronolyticum

C. glucuronolyticum (syn. *C. seminale*) is most commonly isolated from men with prostatitis and urethritis, but can be also isolated from the female genital tract. It is commonly isolated from semen, especially in sexually experienced individuals. It exhibits strong β-glucuronidase activity, and some strains produce urease. It is usually sensitive to antibiotics, although tetracyclines and macrolides are the most effective in vitro.

Corynebacterium minutissimum

C. minutissimum is believed to be the cause of erythrasma, a relatively common and localised infection of the stratum corneum that produces reddish-brown scaly patches in intertriginous sites. Lesions usually involve the groin, toeweb and axillae, and they fluoresce coral red when examined by Wood's light. The organism can be cultured from skin scrapings, but the diagnosis is usually based on clinical aspects and the characteristic fluorescence. More serious infections have been described, including bacteraemia and breast abscess. Some infections attributed to *C. minutissimum* may have been caused by *C. amycolatum*. *C. minutissimum* is sensitive to penicillins; susceptibility to erythromycin is variable.

Corynebacterium striatum

This species is part of the normal flora of the nose and skin. It is a rare cause of pulmonary infection, particularly in patients with chronic obstructive airway disease or those who are intubated. Transmission to mechanically ventilated patients in an intensive care unit has been documented. It has also been isolated from blood, catheter tips, wounds, leg ulcers, peritoneal fluid, urine, semen, vaginal exudate and placental tissues. *C. striatum* is sensitive to penicillins and glycopeptides; susceptibility to aminoglycosides, ciprofloxacin, erythromycin and rifampicin is variable. Many isolates are resistant to cephalosporins.

Corynebacterium pseudodiphtheriticum

C. pseudodiphtheriticum is a commensal of the human nasopharynx. It is occasionally associated with respiratory tract infections, including tracheobronchitis, necrotising tracheitis, pneumonia and lung abscess. Most isolates come from patients with endotracheal tubes or chronic obstructive pulmonary disease. It has also been reported to cause endocarditis in patients with prosthetic valves or preexisting valvular damage. *C. pseudodiphtheriticum* is usually susceptible to most antibiotics except erythromycin.

Corynebacterium kroppenstedtii

C. kroppenstedtii was first described in 1998, after isolation of a single strain from human sputum. Later, when an association was found between corynebacterial infection and granulomatous mastitis, most of the corynebacteria were identified as *C. kroppenstedtii*. Isolation of the species requires Tween-supplemented media and prolonged incubation. *C. kroppenstedtii* is sensitive to many antibiotics including penicillins. Treatment of granulomatous mastitis is usually based on steroids, but addition of antibiotics such as tetracyclines is appropriate.

Arcanobacterium haemolyticum

A. haemolyticum is phylogenetically related to *Actinomyces* spp. (see Ch. 20). It causes pharyngitis and chronic skin ulcers. Cases of cellulitis, osteomyelitis, brain abscesses and endocarditis have rarely been described. The species produces at least two extracellular toxins, phospholipase D and a haemolysin.

Most patients are young adults who present with sore throat; some have membranous exudates and peritonsillar abscesses. The organism is rarely found in healthy individuals, but occurs in about 2% of symptomatic 15–25-year-olds with pharyngitis. Infection cannot be differentiated from streptococcal pharyngitis on clinical findings alone. *A. haemolyticum* is often isolated in association with streptococci of the *Streptococcus anginosus* group. A scarlatiniform rash occurs in half of the patients with pharyngitis, perhaps caused by a toxin genetically related to the erythrogenic toxin of *Str. pyogenes*. Erythromycin or other macrolides seem to be effective in treatment. *A. haemolyticum* is sensitive to penicillin, but treatment failure has been documented.

Rhodococcus equi

R. equi is a pathogen of horses, pigs and cattle. It is a rare cause of severe pulmonary infections in patients with the acquired immune deficiency syndrome, neoplastic diseases or renal transplants. Most infections develop insidiously, with fever and respiratory symptoms difficult to distinguish from mycobacterial infection. Infections are often recurrent and refractory to treatment and may be associated with pleural effusion and bacteraemia. The diagnosis is usually established from bronchoscopy specimens, pleural fluid cultures or blood cultures.

R. equi is usually sensitive to tetracyclines, macrolides, rifampicin, imipenem and vancomycin, but resistance to penicillins has been reported. Treatment includes surgical drainage when feasible and prolonged therapy with an antibiotic combination such as erythromycin and rifampicin or imipenem and vancomycin, established by in vitro tests.

Other *Corynebacterium* species and coryneform bacteria

- *C. accolens* is usually recovered from respiratory specimens.
- *C. afermentans* ssp. *lipophilum* and CDC coryneform groups G *(C. tuberculostearicum)* and F-1 may be isolated from a variety of sources, including blood, wound, semen and urine.
- *C. argentoratense, C. propinquum, C. matruchotii* and *C. durum* have been isolated from the throat, but no pathogenic role has been demonstrated.
- *C. aurimucosum* (syn. *C. nigricans*) exhibits black-pigmented colonies. It has been isolated from genital specimens of women with complications of pregnancy.
- *C. bovis* is commonly isolated from bovine mastitis but is rarely encountered in human infection.
- *C. macginleyi* strains have been isolated from the eye, often in association with infection.
- *C. xerosis* has been confused with *C. amycolatum* and is very rare.
- *Rothia dentocariosa* is commonly isolated from respiratory tract specimens and has been associated with endocarditis and brain abscess.
- *Turicella otitidis* and *C. auris* have been isolated from ears of healthy patients and those with ear infections, but their implications in these infections remain controversial.
- Several species of *Arthrobacter* and *Actinotignum* *(Actinobaculum)* have been recovered from patients with urinary tract infections.

LISTERIA

Organisms of the genus *Listeria* are nonsporing Gram-positive bacilli. The genus contains 17 species *(L. monocytogenes, L. aquatica, L. booriae, L. cornellensis, L. fleischmannii, L. floridensis, L. grandensis, L. grayi, L. innocua, L. ivanovii, L. marthii, L. newyorkensis, L. riparia, L. rocourtiae, L. seeligeri, L. weihenstephanensis, L. welshimeri),* but almost all cases of human listeriosis are caused by *L. monocytogenes*. The disease chiefly affects the immunosuppressed and elderly as well as, to a lesser extent, pregnant women and unborn or newly delivered infants. Listeriosis is transmitted predominantly by the consumption of contaminated food. The majority of animal listeriosis is also due to *L. monocytogenes*, but *L. ivanovii* is associated with about 10% of infections in sheep.

Listeria spp. grow well on a wide variety of nonselective laboratory media, and isolates of *L. monocytogenes* exhibit β-haemolysis on blood agar. These bacteria are nonmotile at 37°C, but exhibit characteristic tumbling motility when tested at 25°C.

LISTERIA MONOCYTOGENES

Description

L. monocytogenes is genetically similar to other *Listeria* species but can be differentiated by phenotypic or genotypic tests. This species can be subdivided by a variety of phenotypic and now almost exclusively genotypic methods including whole genome sequencing, and this is invaluable for identification of outbreaks and public health control.

The properties of the organism favour food as an agent in transmission of listeriosis since the bacterium is widespread in the environment, able to colonise places where food is produced and grows in a wide range of foods having relatively high water activities (a_w >0.95) and over a wide range of temperatures (<0–45°C). Growth at refrigeration temperatures is relatively slow, with a maximum doubling time of about 1–2 days at 4°C. Multiplication in food is restricted to the pH range 5–9. *L. monocytogenes* is not sufficiently heat resistant to survive pasteurisation.

Pathogenesis

L. monocytogenes is an intracellular parasite, and it is in this environment that the pathogen gains protection and evades some of the host's defences. However, the host has a number of strategies to deal with such parasites. Nonspecific mechanisms of resistance are important as first lines of defence once the mucous membranes have been breached. Human neutrophils and nonactivated macrophages can phagocytose and kill the bacteria. Protective immunity in humans probably depends on T lymphocytes, with antibodies playing little or no role.

L. monocytogenes enters phagocytic and nonphagocytic cells and listerial surface proteins of the internalin family (reminiscent of the M protein of *Str. pyogenes*) are involved with subverting mammalian cytoskeletal structures and generating contractile forces that result in engulfment of the bacterium. InlA is involved with crossing the intestinal and maternofetal barrier and interacts with the mammalian cell surface protein E-cadherin. InlB promotes entry of *L. monocytogenes* into epithelial, endothelial, hepatocyte and fibroblast cells and interacts with the hepatocyte growth factor receptor. After internalisation, *L. monocytogenes* becomes encapsulated in a membrane-bound compartment. In the phagocyte, most cells in the phagocytic vacuole are probably killed. However, those surviving in the phagocytic vacuole, and those in the membrane-bound compartment of nonprofessional phagocytes, mediate the dissolution of the vacuole membrane by means of a haemolysin (listeriolysin O), and in addition, possibly, the action of a phospholipase C.

In the host cell cytoplasm, where bacterial growth occurs, the organism becomes surrounded by polymerised host cell actin. The ability to polymerise actin preferentially on the older pole of the listeria cell with a surface protein (ActA) subverts the host cell's cytoskeleton and confers intracellular motility to the bacterium. The resulting comet tail-like structure pushes the bacterium into an adjacent mammalian cell (with the assistance of the InlC protein), where it again becomes encapsulated in a vacuole. A listerial lecithinase is involved with dissolution of these membranes; the haemolysin may also contribute in this process. Intracellular growth and movement in the newly invaded cell are then repeated. The genes associated with virulence in *L. monocytogenes* occur as homologous in *L. ivanovii* and *L. seeligeri*.

Clinical aspects of infection

L. monocytogenes principally causes intrauterine infection, meningitis and septicaemia. The incubation period varies widely between individuals from 1 to 90 days, with an average for intrauterine infection of around 30 days. Infections of other organs occur as does cutaneous and ocular infection.

Infection in pregnancy and the neonate

Listeriosis in pregnancy is classified by foetal gestation at onset, as this correlates best with the clinical features, microbiology and prognosis. Maternal listeriosis occurs throughout gestation but is rarely recognised before 20 weeks of pregnancy. The mother is usually previously well with a normal pregnancy. Pregnant women often have a series of mild symptoms (chills, fever, back pain, sore throat and headache, sometimes with conjunctivitis, diarrhoea or drowsiness) but may be asymptomatic until the delivery of an infected infant. Symptomatic women may have positive blood cultures. Cultures from high vaginal swabs, stool and midstream urine samples, together with pre- or postnatal antibody tests, are not helpful in diagnosis. With the onset of fever, foetal movements are reduced, and premature labour occurs within about 1 week. There may be a transient fever during labour, and the amniotic fluid is often discoloured or stained with meconium.

Culture of the amniotic fluid, placenta or high vaginal swab after delivery invariably yields a heavy growth of *L. monocytogenes*. Fever resolves soon after birth, and the vagina is usually culture negative after about 1 month. Maternal infection without infection of the fetus can occur and even progress to placental infection without ill effects for the fetus. Repeated pregnancy-associated infections are exceedingly rare, and an association between *Listeria* carriage and habitual abortion has not been substantiated.

Although the outcome of infection for the mother is benign, the outcome for the infant is more variable. Abortion, stillbirth and early-onset neonatal disease are common, depending on the gestation at infection. Neonatal listeriosis is divided into disease of early and late onset. Early onset neonatal listeriosis is predominantly a septicaemic illness, contracted in utero and babies are ill either at birth or within 1 day. In contrast, late neonatal infection is predominantly meningitic and may be associated with hospital cross-infection acquired from contact with an early onset neonatal case and babies are ill between 3 and 18 days after delivery (two-thirds between 5 and 12 days after delivery). The main characteristics of these two forms are summarised in Table 14.2. Early-onset disease represents a spectrum of mild to severe infection, which can be correlated with the microbiological findings. Those neonates who die from infection usually do so within a few days of birth and have pneumonia, hepatosplenomegaly, petechiae, abscesses in the liver or brain, peritonitis and enterocolitis.

In late-onset neonatal disease the cerebrospinal fluid (CSF) protein content is almost always raised and the glucose level reduced. The total number of white cells is increased, but the counts are variable; neutrophils usually predominate, but lymphocytes or monocytes may be the main cell type. In about 50% of Gram films, bacteria, which may resemble rods or cocci, are seen.

Adult and juvenile infection

Adult infection is now the most common manifestation of the disease in Northern Europe and North America. In adults and juveniles the main syndromes are bacteraemia and central nervous system infection. There was a dramatic increase in the incidence of listerial bacteraemia in patients over 60 years of age in Northern Europe at the start of the twenty-first century; the rate in this group increased almost four-fold in England and Wales between 1990 and 2016. Most cases occur in immunosuppressed patients, including those receiving steroid or cytotoxic therapy or with malignant neoplasms. Autoimmune disease, diabetes, alcohol-related disease and immunosuppressive treatments are all risk factors for listerial infection. However, about one-third of patients with meningitis and around 10% with primary bacteraemia are apparently immunocompetent.

Table 14.2 Characteristics of neonatal infection with *L. monocytogenes*

	Type of infection	
	Early	Late
Typical onset after delivery	Within 1 day	5–12 days
Maternal factors[a]	Common	Rare
Source of infection	Intrauterine infection acquired haematogenously from mother	Hospital-acquired from early-onset case, postnatal environment or maternally acquired during delivery
Signs/symptoms	Disseminated infection Cardiopulmonary distress Central nervous system signs Vomiting and diarrhoea Hepatosplenomegaly Skin rash	Meningitis Irritability Poor appetite Fever
Laboratory findings	Leucocytosis or leucopenia Thrombocytopenia Mottling on chest radiography Increased fibrinogen	Leucocytosis; occasional radiographic changes CSF: total protein and white cell count raised; glucose level lowered
Sites of isolation	Blood, superficial sites and amniotic fluid; less commonly gastric aspirate, CSF and HVS	Commonly CSF; rarely blood
Mortality rate	30%–60%	10%–12%

CSF, Cerebrospinal fluid; *HVS*, high vaginal swab.
[a]Obstetric problems; low birth weight; maternal fever; abnormal amniotic fluid.

Listeriosis in children older than 1 month is very rare, except in those with underlying disease.

Meningitis

The clinical presentation is the same in all groups, but progression is more rapid in immunocompromised subjects. A peripheral blood leucocytosis occurs, and the CSF white blood cell count is raised. The CSF glucose level is low and the protein level is raised; a very high protein concentration may be a poor prognostic indicator. Gram stains of the CSF are often negative, and the clinical features of infection are such that it is not possible to tell listerial meningitis from meningococcal or pneumococcal infection. However, *L. monocytogenes* can be isolated from blood cultures in most cases.

In the rare cases of encephalitis, cerebritis or cerebral abscesses, the CSF may be normal, but the white blood cell count is often raised mildly and the protein level is slightly increased, with a low glucose concentration. The Gram film and culture are usually negative. Blood cultures are the main source of the organism in many of these patients.

Bacteraemia

Primary bacteraemia is more common in men than in women and occurs most often in patients >60 years of age as well as those with haematological malignancy. As compared to patients with central nervous system infections, those with listerial bacteraemia present more often with gastrointestinal symptoms, particularly cases with gastric malignancies, or those receiving treatment to reduce stomach acid secretion.

Gastroenteritis

Foodborne outbreaks of acute gastroenteritis with fever have been described. The foods associated with these outbreaks have been diverse but heavily contaminated by the bacterium. Symptoms develop in 1–2 days. Large numbers of *L. monocytogenes* are present in the stool, and a few patients develop serious systemic infection. The ability to cause gastroenteritis may be specific to certain strains.

Other infections

Rarer manifestations of listeriosis include arthritis, hepatitis, endophthalmitis, pneumonia, endocarditis, peritonitis in patients on continuous ambulatory peritoneal dialysis and cutaneous or ocular lesions acquired as occupational zoonoses.

Epidemiology
Incidence

Most Western countries report infection rates of 1–10 cases per million of the population per year. Pregnancy and neonatal disease account for about 10% of cases. Among these, 15%–25% of infections lead to abortion and stillbirth, and about 70% are neonatal infections. In about 5% of maternal infections, bacteraemia occurs and the fetus is not affected.

The incidence of infection increases with age so that the mean age of adult infections is >55 years. Men are more commonly infected than women over the age of 40 years. Immunosuppression is a major risk factor for both the epidemic and sporadic forms of listeriosis and probably accounts for the increasing incidence with age. The peak incidence of human disease usually occurs in July, August or September. Most cases are apparently sporadic, and the patients live in urban areas without exposure to animals.

L. monocytogenes, like other *Listeria* species, has been isolated from numerous environmental sites, including soil, sewage, water and decaying plant material, where this bacterium can survive for >2 years. Although the true home of *Listeria* is probably in the environment, these organisms are also found in excreta of apparently healthy animals, including humans. Up to 5% of healthy adults may have the organism in their faeces. Faecal carriage in humans probably reflects consumption of contaminated foods and is likely to be transitory.

Numerous types of raw, processed, cooked and ready-to-eat foods contain *L. monocytogenes*, usually at low levels of contamination. The tolerance of the bacterium to sodium chloride and sodium nitrite, and the ability to multiply (albeit slowly) at refrigeration temperatures makes *L. monocytogenes* of particular concern as a postprocessing contaminant in long-shelf-life refrigerated foods. Even when present at high levels in foods, spoilage or taints are not generally produced. The widespread distribution of *L. monocytogenes* and the ability to survive on dry and moist surfaces favour postprocessing contamination of foods from both raw product and factory sites.

Transmission

Most cases are sporadic, and in only a few is a specific route of infection identified. The consumption of contaminated foods is the principal route of transmission. Microbiological and epidemiological evidence supports an association with many food types (dairy, meat, vegetable, fish and shellfish as well as complex foods such as sandwiches) in both sporadic and epidemic listeriosis. Foods associated with transmission often show the following common features:

- able to support the multiplication of *L. monocytogenes* (relatively high water activity and near-neutral pH)
- relatively heavily contaminated with the implicated strain
- processed with an extended (refrigerated) shelf life
- ready to eat and consumed without further cooking

The food type currently most commonly associated with transmission in the United Kingdom is preprepared sandwiches served in hospitals.

Outbreaks of human listeriosis involving more than 100 individuals have occurred, some lasting for several years. This is likely to represent a long-term colonisation of a single site in the food manufacturing environment as well as the long incubation periods shown by some patients. Sites of contamination within food processing facilities involved in human infection have included equipment, plant and machinery (shelving, conveyor belts, slicing machines), condensates and drains. *L. monocytogenes* survives well in moist environments with organic material, and it is from such sites that contamination of food occurs during processing. Epidemiological typing is invaluable for the identification of common-source foodborne outbreaks and for tracking the bacterium in the food chain.

Listeriosis transmitted by direct contact with the environment, infected animals or animal material is relatively rare. Papular or pustular cutaneous lesions have been described, usually on the arms and hands of farmers or veterinarians 1–4 days after attending bovine abortions. Infection is invariably mild and usually resolves without antimicrobial therapy, although serious systemic involvement has been described. Conjunctivitis in poultry workers has also been reported.

Hospital cross-infection between newborn infants occurs. Typically, an apparently healthy baby (rarely more than one) develops late-onset listeriosis typically 5–12 days after delivery in a hospital in which an infant with congenital listeriosis was born shortly before. The same strain of *L. monocytogenes* is isolated from both infants and the mother of the early-onset case, but not from the mother of the late-onset case. The cases are usually delivered or nursed in the same or adjacent delivery suites or neonatal units, and consequently, staff and equipment (particularly respiratory resuscitation equipment) are common to both. There is little evidence of cross-infection or person-to-person transmission outside the neonatal period.

Laboratory acquired infection (conjunctivitis) has been reported and in the United Kingdom, pregnant women are advised not to manipulate live cultures of *Listeria*.

Diagnosis and treatment

Conventional culture of blood and or CSF remain the mainstays of diagnosis, although Gram-staining of surface swabs and of meconium-stained amniotic fluid has been reported to have a very high predictive value for neonatal listeriosis during outbreaks. PCR-based procedures for amplification of *L. monocytogenes*-specific DNA sequences from serum and CSF have been reported.

L. monocytogenes is susceptible to a wide range of antibiotics in vitro, including ampicillin, penicillin, meropenem, vancomycin, tetracyclines, chloramphenicol, aminoglycosides and co-trimoxazole. There is little agreement about the best treatment, but many patients have been treated successfully with ampicillin or penicillin with or without an aminoglycoside. Cephalosporins are ineffective and chloramphenicol is not recommended for treatment of listeria infections.

No significant change in the antimicrobial susceptibility of *L. monocytogenes* has been recognised over the past 40 years, and resistance to any of the agents recommended for therapy is unlikely.

Prognosis

The mortality rate in late neonatal disease is about 10%. In contrast, the mortality rate in early disease is 30%–60%, and about 20%–40% of survivors develop sequelae such as lung disease, hydrocephalus or other neurological defects. Early use of appropriate antibiotics during pregnancy may improve neonatal survival.

The mortality rate in both adult meningitis and bacteraemia is about 20%–50%. Amongst patients with meningitis, mortality is significantly lower in patients <60 years of age; however, the death rates are similar in these age groups in patients with bacteraemia. Between 25%

and 75% of patients surviving central nervous system infection suffer sequelae such as hemiplegia and other neurological defects.

ERYSIPELOTHRIX

Erysipelothrix is a genus of aerobic, nonsporing, nonmotile, Gram-positive bacilli. The genus comprises at least four species: *E. rhusiopathiae*, *E. inopinata*, *E. larvae* and *E. tonsillarum*. *E. rhusiopathiae* causes economically important disease in domestic animals, notably pigs. Human infections from *E. rhusiopathiae* are rare but present as a localised cutaneous infection (erysipeloid), which occasionally becomes diffuse and may lead to bacteraemia and endocarditis. Infection is most often associated with close animal contact and usually occurs in such occupational groups as butchers, abattoir workers, veterinarians, farmers and fish handlers.

The organism is cultured most often from biopsies, aspirates or blood. The bacilli are short (1–2 μm) but may produce long filamentous forms resembling lactobacilli. Growth is improved by incubation in 5%–10% carbon dioxide. Colonies on blood agar are α-haemolytic.

Penicillin and other β-lactam antibiotics are effective. Erythromycin and clindamycin offer suitable alternatives, but *E. rhusiopathiae* is resistant to vancomycin.

RECOMMENDED READING

Allerberger, F., & Wagner, M. (2010). Listeriosis: a resurgent foodborne infection. *Clinical Microbiology and Infection, 16*(1), 16–23. doi: 10.1111/j.1469-0691.2009.03109.x.

Bernard, K. (2012). The genus *Corynebacterium* and other medically relevant coryneform-like bacteria. *Journal of Clinical Microbiology, 50*(10), 3152–3158. doi:10.1128/JCM.00796-12.

Both, L., Collins, S., de Zoysa, A., White, J., Mandal, S., & Efstratiou, A. (2015). Molecular and epidemiological review of toxigenic diphtheria infections in England between 2007 and 2013. *Journal of Clinical Microbiology, 53*(2), 567–572. doi:10.1128/JCM.03398-14.

Brooke, C. J., & Riley, T. V. (1999). *Erysipelothrix rhusiopathiae*: biology, epidemiology and clinical manifestations of an occupational pathogen. *Journal of Medical Microbiology, 48*(9), 789–799.

Cossart, P., & Toledo-Arana, A. (2008). *Listeria monocytogenes*, a unique model in infection biology: an overview. *Microbes and Infection, 10*(9), 1041–1050. doi:10.1016/j.micinf.2008.07.043.

Denny, J., & McLauchlin, J. (2008). Human *Listeria monocytogenes* infections in Europe: an opportunity for improved European surveillance. *Euro Surveillance, 13*(3), pii: 8082.

Efstratiou, A., Engler, K. H., Mazurova, I. K., Glushkevich, T., Vuopio-Varkila, J., & Popovic, T. (2000). Current approaches to the laboratory diagnosis of diphtheria. *The Journal of Infectious Diseases, 181*(Suppl. 1), S138–S145.

Farber, J. M., & Peterkin, P. I. (1991). *Listeria monocytogenes*, a food-borne pathogen. *Microbiological Reviews, 55*(3), 476–511.

Lianou, A., & Sofos, J. N. (2007). A review of the incidence and transmission of *Listeria monocytogenes* in ready-to-eat products in

retail and food service environments. *Journal of Food Protection, 70*(9), 2172–2198.

Low, J. C., & Donachie, W. (1997). A review of *Listeria monocytogenes* and listeriosis. *The Veterinary Journal, 153*(1), 9–29.

Robson, J. M., McDougall, R., Van Der Valk, S., Waite, S. D., & Sullivan, J. J. (1998). *Erysipelothrix rhusiopathiae*: an uncommon but ever present zoonosis. *Pathology, 30*(4), 391–394. doi:10.1080/00313029800169686.

Swaminathan, B., & Gerner-Smidt, P. (2007). The epidemiology of human listeriosis. *Microbes and Infection, 9*(10), 1236–1243.

Wagner, K. S., White, J. M., Crowcroft, N. S., De Martin, S., Mann, G., & Efstratiou, A. (2010). Diphtheria in the United Kingdom 1986–2008: the increasing role of *Corynebacterium ulcerans*. *Epidemiology and Infection, 138*(11), 1519–1530. doi:10.1017/S0950268810001895.

Zakikhany, K., Neal, S., & Efstratiou, A. (2014). Emergence and molecular characterisation of non-toxigenic tox gene-bearing *Corynebacterium diphtheriae* biovar *mitis* in the United Kingdom, 2003–2012. *Euro Surveillance, 19*(22).

Websites

Public Health England. Diphtheria Guidelines Working Group. Public health control and management of diphtheria (in England and Wales): 2015 Guidelines. Retrieved from https://www.gov.uk/government/publications/diphtheria-public-health-control-and-management-in-england-and-wales. (Accessed Oct 2017).

15 *Bacillus*

Anthrax; food poisoning

IAN A. COOPER, PAUL RUSSELL AND JOANNE E. THWAITE

> ## KEY POINTS
>
> - Bacteria belonging to the *Bacillus* genus are common environmental Gram-positive bacilli.
> - *Bacillus anthracis* causes cutaneous, inhalational, gastrointestinal and injectional anthrax.
> - The principal virulence factors of *B. anthracis* are the toxin complex and the polypeptide capsule.
> - Nonspecific symptoms can make inhalational and gastrointestinal anthrax difficult to diagnose and therefore difficult to treat effectively.
> - *B. anthracis* Sterne strain (toxin-negative) is used as an animal vaccine.
> - Several recombinant protein vaccines for anthrax are in development.
> - *Bacillus cereus* commonly causes food poisoning.
> - *B. cereus* strains with anthrax toxin genes can cause an 'anthrax-like' disease.

The family Bacillaceae consists of rod-shaped bacteria that form endospores; there are two main subdivisions: the anaerobic spore-forming bacteria of the genus *Clostridium,* and the aerobic or facultatively anaerobic spore-forming bacteria of the genus *Bacillus. Bacillus* species are ubiquitous in the environment and are frequently isolated in laboratories as contaminants of media or specimens. The *Bacillus* genus encompasses many medically, industrially and scientifically important species, including *B. anthracis, B. cereus, B. subtilis* and *B. thuringiensis. B. anthracis,* the cause of anthrax, is the most clinically important pathogen of the group. The organism holds a crucial place in the history of medical microbiology.

- Robert Koch's work on anthrax showed that a causative organism of a disease could be isolated from the blood of infected animals, artificially grown in pure culture and then used to reproduce the disease in animals. This led to the development of current methods of isolation and identification of bacteria, and to the formulation of *Koch's postulates* (see Ch. 1).
- Louis Pasteur showed that animals could be actively immunised by infecting them with cultures of *B. anthracis* that had been attenuated by growing them at 43°C.

Although naturally occurring cases of anthrax are rare in the industrialised nations, the cases of anthrax in the United States caused by the deliberate contamination of mail with *B. anthracis* spores is a reminder of the potential for this pathogen to be used as a biological weapon.

B. cereus is typically associated with episodes of food poisoning, especially when reheating cooked rice. An atypical strain of *B. cereus* has been implicated as the causative agent of an 'anthrax-like' disease in humans. Other species of *Bacillus* are occasionally incriminated as human pathogens, usually in people who are immunocompromised.

BACILLUS ANTHRACIS

DESCRIPTION

B. anthracis is a large (4–8 × 1–1.5 μm) nonmotile, spore-forming bacillus. The spores, which form readily when the bacterium is grown on certain artificial media, are oval, refractile and central in position. The temperature range for growth is 12–45°C (optimum 35°C); it grows on all standard media as typical colonies with 'ground-glass' surface appearance and a wavy margin with small projections, the so-called medusa head appearance. Table 15.1 lists some of the differences between *B. anthracis* and other important members of the genus *Bacillus.*

Genome sequences of multiple strains of *B. anthracis* have been determined. In addition to the chromosome, wild-type strains harbour two plasmids termed *pXO1* and *pXO2,* encoding the toxin and capsule, respectively. Most of the chromosomal genes of *B. anthracis* are also found

Table 15.1 Distinguishing properties of some important *Bacillus* species

Property	*B. anthracis*	*B. cereus*[a]	*B. subtilis*
Colony size	Large	Large	Small
Motility	−	+	+
Capsule	+	−	−
Mouse pathogenicity	+++	+	−
Gamma phage susceptibility	+	−	−
Anaerobic growth	+	+	−
Optimal growth temperature (°C)	35	30	37

[a]Atypical strains may cause an anthrax-like disease.

in *B. cereus*. A plasmid similar to pXO1 has been found in some *B. cereus* strains (see later in the chapter).

PATHOGENESIS

Anthrax is a *zoonosis*—a disease of animals transmissible secondarily to humans. Humans are relatively resistant to infection with *B. anthracis*. In humans, naturally acquired anthrax infection arises most commonly when a person comes into contact with infected animals or contaminated animal products. The disease is usually a consequence of the exposure of a susceptible host to spores of *B. anthracis*. Spores are not found in host tissues but appear on exposure of the vegetative cells to oxygen in the air. During naturally occurring disease, formation of spores occurs when the vegetative cells in infected blood and other body fluids or tissues from a corpse are exposed to air.

B. anthracis spores introduced into the body by abrasion, inhalation, injection or ingestion germinate, and the resulting vegetative cells grow and produce the toxins, which result in cell death and oedema. Spores can also be phagocytosed by macrophages and transported from the site of infection to regional lymph nodes, where they germinate and vegetative bacteria multiply causing disease.

Virulence factors

The pathogenicity of *B. anthracis* depends primarily on two major virulence factors:

1. The poly-D-glutamic acid capsule
2. The toxin complex comprising three proteins: the protective antigen (PA), edema factor (EF) and lethal factor (LF).

The *B. anthracis* capsule is composed of a high molecular weight polypeptide (poly-D-glutamic acid) capsule whose biosynthesis is encoded by the *capBCADE* operon located on the pXO2 plasmid. The capsule appears to enhance the virulence of *B. anthracis* by inhibiting the phagocytosis

of vegetative cells in the extracellular environment of the lymphatic system and bloodstream. It is mainly the action of the toxin that mediates damage to the host. The three components of the tripartite toxin combine to form two binary toxins, the oedema toxin and lethal toxin, formed by association of PA with EF and LF, respectively. In each case, PA binds to host cells and forms a pore, which facilitates the entry of the associated oedema or lethal factor to the cell cytosol (Fig. 15.1).

The oedema toxin is thought to be responsible for the characteristic localised swelling associated with cutaneous anthrax. EF is a calmodulin-dependent adenylate cyclase that catalyses the production of intracellular cyclic adenosine monophosphate (cAMP) from host adenosine triphosphate (ATP), inducing interleukin (IL)-6 and inhibiting tumour necrosis factor (TNF)-α in monocytes. In addition to disrupting cytokine responses, the oedema toxin may also increase host susceptibility to infection by impairing neutrophil function. However, it is the lethal toxin that is believed to play the major role in damage to the host and death. LF is a zinc metalloprotease that inactivates mitogen-activated protein kinase kinase (MAPKK), particularly in macrophages. The lethal toxin stimulates macrophages to produce IL-1β and TNF-α. During infection, IL-1β accumulates within macrophages and TNF-α is released. As the concentration of lethal toxin increases later in the infection process, macrophage lysis produces a sudden release of IL-1β, causing shock and death.

Thus the pathogenesis of anthrax is related to the sensitivity of macrophages to:

- the antiphagocytic activity of the capsule
- the adenylate cyclase activity of the oedema toxin
- the metalloprotease activity of the lethal toxin.

CLINICAL FEATURES

The three classical clinical manifestations of anthrax, which are based on the route of infection, are cutaneous,

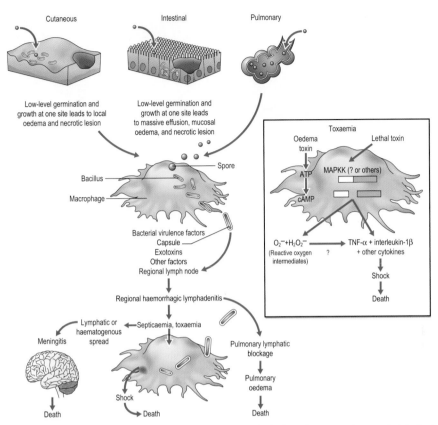

Fig. 15.1 Pathophysiology of anthrax. *Bacillus anthracis* spores reach a primary site in the subcutaneous layer, gastrointestinal mucosa or alveolar spaces. For cutaneous and gastrointestinal anthrax, low-level germination occurs at the primary site, leading to local oedema and necrosis. Endospores are phagocytosed by macrophages and germinate. Macrophages containing bacilli detach and migrate to the regional lymph node. Vegetative anthrax bacilli grow in the lymph node, creating regional haemorrhagic lymphadenitis. Bacteria spread through the blood and lymph and multiply, causing severe septicaemia. High levels of exotoxins are produced that are responsible for overt symptoms and death. In a small number of cases, systemic anthrax can lead to meningeal involvement by means of lymphatic or haematogenous spread. In cases of pulmonary anthrax, peribronchial haemorrhagic lymphadenitis blocks pulmonary lymphatic drainage, leading to pulmonary oedema. Death results from septicaemia, toxaemia or pulmonary complications and can occur 1–7 days after exposure. The inset describes the effects of anthrax exotoxins on macrophages. See "Virulence factors" for explanation. *ATP*, adenosine triphosphate; *cAMP*, cyclic adenosine monophosphate; *IL*, interleukin; *MAPKK*, mitogen-activated protein kinase kinase; *TNF*, tumour necrosis factor. (Reproduced with permission from Dixon et al 1999. © Massachusetts Medical Society, USA.)

gastrointestinal and inhalational anthrax. All these forms can lead to bacteraemia and anthrax meningitis. With the spate of anthrax cases in heroin users across Europe since 2009, a further novel clinical manifestation of the disease, termed *injectional anthrax,* has been described.

Cutaneous anthrax

The primary lesion is often described as a *malignant pustule* because of its characteristic appearance (Fig. 15.2). Coagulation necrosis of the centre of the pustule results in the formation of a dark-coloured *eschar* that is later surrounded by a ring of vesicles containing serous fluid and an area of oedema and induration, which may become extensive. In patients with severe toxic signs and widespread oedema, the prognosis is poor.

Inhalational anthrax

This is a consequence of the inhalation of spores, and is the most acute form of the disease and is associated with a high mortality rate. The infectious human dose by the airborne route is in the range of 25,000 to 55,000 spores. Although sometimes incorrectly referred to as pneumonic anthrax, the disease does not develop as a bronchopneumonia.

The high mortality rate of inhalational anthrax is attributed to the intense inflammation, haemorrhage and septicaemia that result from the multiplication of organisms within macrophages in the bronchi and subsequent spread from the lungs to the lymphatics and bloodstream. The production of toxins and the considerable bacterial load, up to 10^8 colony forming units/mL of blood, which

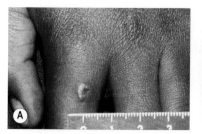
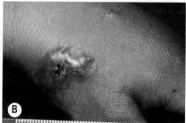
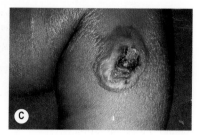

Fig. 15.2   Stages in the development and resolution of cutaneous anthrax lesions. (A) As first seen. (B) On day 2 or 3. (C) On day 6. (Images kindly provided by Dr Peter Turnbull.)

rapidly occur in the terminal septicaemic phase, result in increased vascular permeability and hypotension similar to endotoxic shock.

In the past, cases of anthrax, including the inhalational form of the disease, were reported in persons working in industries handling animal skins, hides and wool, giving rise to the name of *Woolsorter's disease*. In the United Kingdom, anthrax from this source was minimised by the close control of imported wool and fleeces and by the disinfection of suspect materials. An accident at a former Soviet Union biological weapons factory in the 1980s resulted in the release of spores into the air. In the town of Sverdlovsk, located downwind of the factory, 79 cases of human inhalation anthrax were recorded, some up to 6 weeks after exposure; even with antibiotic therapy, there were 68 deaths. In 2001, letters contaminated with *B. anthracis* spores, which were sent through the US postal system, resulted in 22 reported cases of anthrax of which there were five fatalities. Of the 22 cases, 11 were confirmed to be inhalational anthrax. Without a specific notification of an anthrax outbreak, diagnosis of an inhalational case can be very difficult—evidence of widening of the mediastinum due to lymphaden-opathy is indicative of a probable inhalational anthrax infection.

Gastrointestinal anthrax

Gastrointestinal anthrax occurs when *B. anthracis* is ingested, for example, through consumption of contaminated meat. Infection can occur in the upper (throat and oesophagus) or lower parts of the gastrointestinal tract (stomach and intestines). The incubation period, before symptoms appear, for the gastrointestinal forms of the disease is typically 1–7 days. Symptoms can be nonspecific such as fever and chills, sore throat, stomach pain and diarrhoea but may progress to haemorrhagic diarrhoea, bloody vomiting and swollen abdomen. Successful treatment and outcome is reliant on early diagnosis—without intervention, the mortality of gastrointestinal anthrax is >50%.

Injectional anthrax

The injectional form of anthrax has recently been described in European countries, in persons injecting heroin contaminated with *B. anthracis* spores. Injectional anthrax, due to the mode of entry, can rapidly disseminate throughout the body. Initial symptoms may be similar to those of cutaneous anthrax, but there may also be the occurrence of marked soft tissue infection beneath the skin, such as in the muscle, and around the injection site in the form of an abscess/cellulitis. Diagnosis can be more difficult because common bacterial species of the skin microbiota can also cause infections at injection sites—redness or swelling at an injection site of a drug user does not necessarily mean that they have contracted injectional anthrax.

Meningitis

Haemorrhagic meningitis may complicate any form of anthrax infection, when the bacteraemia spreads across the blood-brain barrier to the central nervous system (CNS). A striking pathological sign of anthrax meningitis is termed the *Cardinal's cap*, characterised by dark-red extensive haemorrhaging beneath the lining of the skull.

Naturally occurring infections of animals

All mammals are susceptible to anthrax, although, in general, carnivores are relatively resistant to the disease. Herbivores are highly susceptible, and omnivores show an intermediate level of resistance. Disease in wild herbivores or domesticated animals follows the ingestion of spores along with coarse vegetation or soil particles. These abrasive particles probably contribute to trauma of the mouth or intestinal tract, allowing entry of the spores into the host. More rarely, infection occurs after the inhalation of dust into the respiratory tract and, as in human disease, through skin abrasions leading to malignant pustules.

Although cases of anthrax are usually localised and sporadic, there may be large outbreaks of disease in wild or domesticated livestock. In the United Kingdom, the disease is occasionally found in livestock, chiefly cattle. Disease in pigs is atypical, appearing as a chronic disease with few fatalities. Sudden death in any herbivore should be treated with suspicion and a veterinary officer summoned to examine the carcass, without a postmortem examination. A blood slide should be taken for Gram or McFadyean's polychrome methylene blue staining. Under the Anthrax Order (1991), an animal, if found to be positive, must remain on the farm/premises and be disposed of on site by incineration or by such other method as the Divisional Veterinary Officer may approve. Deep burial in quicklime is an alternative method of disposal, but the spores remain viable for many years and may subsequently contaminate pasture and infect grazing animals. Very large numbers of bacilli are present in the terminal stages of disease in animals, and thus these highly infectious animals serve as a source of anthrax both by direct spread to another beast and by contamination of the environment.

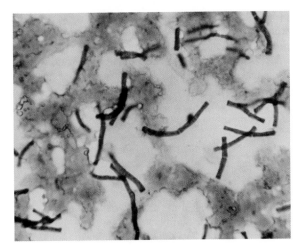

Fig. 15.3 Guinea pig spleen imprint showing typical anthrax bacilli.

Human infections in the United Kingdom (since the 1980s)

During the period 1981–2001 there were 14 human cases of anthrax in the United Kingdom, all of which were the cutaneous form of the disease. However, in recent years, there have been two fatal cases of inhalational anthrax reported in the United Kingdom (Scotland 2006 and London 2008), where the cause of the infection was attributed to the making and playing of traditional African animal hide drums contaminated with *B. anthracis* spores. The first case of drug-associated (heroin) injectional anthrax was recorded in Norway in 2000, and two subsequent European outbreaks followed. The first outbreak, recorded between December 2009 and February 2010, resulted in 52 confirmed cases, with 17 fatalities in the United Kingdom. Further injectional anthrax cases, again attributed to contaminated heroin, were reported in the United Kingdom in 2012 and 2013. DNA sequence analysis of 60 *B. anthracis* isolates from the European outbreaks suggests two distinct contamination events; however, the origin and point of spore introduction is unknown.

Animal models of disease

Various animals, including mice, guinea pigs, rabbits and nonhuman primates, have been used as models of human anthrax. Several strains of mice are highly susceptible to anthrax, but the response between infecting dose and morbidity is not always clear. To resolve this problem, a partially attenuated strain of *B. anthracis* is used in a mouse strain that is deficient in complement C5 (e.g., A/J strain).

Guinea pigs are extremely susceptible to anthrax, both by injection and by inhalation. After subcutaneous

challenge, the animal usually dies within 2–3 days, showing a marked inflammatory lesion at the site of inoculation and extensive gelatinous oedema in the subcutaneous tissues. Large numbers of the bacilli are present in the local lesion and are profusely present in the heart, blood and capillaries of the internal organs. Bacilli are especially numerous in the spleen (Fig. 15.3), which is enlarged and soft, giving rise to the description *splenic fever* in the ox and the German name for the organism—*Milzbrandbazillus* (spleen-destroying bacillus). Mice, guinea pigs and rabbits offer models of human inhalational anthrax that, although limited by their differing physiology to the human respiratory tract, are useful for some pathogenesis studies and initial medical countermeasure efficacy studies.

Studies in nonhuman primates have provided significant insight into the pathogenesis of inhalational anthrax and offer a relevant animal model for the evaluation of medical countermeasures for human inhalational anthrax; the estimation of the infectious dose in humans is based largely on nonhuman primate studies. Small particles of <5 μm containing spores are deposited on the alveolar walls and taken up by phagocytes. These phagocytes migrate to the draining lymph nodes, which become inflamed and enlarged. Surprisingly, ungerminated spores in phagocytes can remain in these lymph nodes for at least 100 days after exposure.

LABORATORY INVESTIGATION

Clinical specimens

The fully developed malignant pustule (associated with cutaneous and some cases of injectional anthrax) may be difficult to swab, and the central necrotic area gives a poor yield. Fluid aspirated from the surrounding vesicles, when present, is more likely to yield anthrax bacilli. Specimens should be taken before antibiotic therapy has been instituted. In laboratories unfamiliar with the disease, additional precautions for staff safety need to be organised.

Gram stain may show typical large Gram-positive bacilli, and culture on blood agar yields nonhaemolytic colonies. Colony morphology is typically large, flat, greyish, 'ground-glass' colonies with the characteristic 'medusa head' appearance. Staining of films from these colonies shows long chains of Gram-positive bacilli, some containing spores. Demonstration of nonmotility, gelatin liquefaction, growth in straight chains and enhanced growth aerobically, as seen in the characteristic inverted fir tree appearance in a gelatin stab, will generally identify *B. anthracis*. The US Food and Drug Administration (FDA) has approved a diagnostic method for the differentiation of *B. anthracis* vegetative cells from other *Bacillus* species based on the susceptibility of *B. anthracis* to gamma phage.

Serological diagnosis by enzyme-linked immunosorbent assay (ELISA) may be of value retrospectively, but is seldom used diagnostically. For the rapid identification of bacteria and diagnosis of disease, the polymerase chain reaction (PCR) should be used. As *B. anthracis* possesses a number of unique genes, the selection of suitable gene targets is not problematic. Toxin production can be demonstrated by immunological or gene probe methods in reference laboratories.

Environmental samples

It may be necessary to isolate *B. anthracis* from potentially contaminated material such as animal hair, hides or soil. The heat treatment of aqueous extracts of these materials at 60°C for 1 hour kills all except spore-forming bacteria and fungi. However, the isolation of *B. anthracis* may still prove difficult because of the presence of competing bacterial flora and/or materials that may inhibit its growth. For some soil types, selective agars have been developed that allow preferential growth of *B. anthracis*.

TREATMENT

B. anthracis is susceptible in vitro to a wide range of antimicrobial agents and many have been used successfully for the treatment of anthrax in humans. For cutaneous anthrax, penicillin remains the drug of choice, as β-lactamase–producing strains of *B. anthracis* are rare. Most strains are also sensitive to macrolides, aminoglycosides, tetracyclines and chloramphenicol. For inhalational anthrax, ciprofloxacin (or a similar fluoroquinolone) is recommended prophylactically or as early treatment for those considered at greatest risk of inhalational exposure

following a large-scale release of anthrax spores in a deliberate attack.

The efficacy of antibiotics for the treatment of anthrax is dependent largely on the time at which therapy commences. Treatment with antibiotics is generally ineffective when septicaemic disease has developed, and, in the later stages of disease, the general principles applied to the management of any patient in shock are more important than antimicrobial therapy. As septicaemia develops rapidly in both intestinal and inhalational anthrax, these forms of the disease can be especially difficult to treat. In 2012, the FDA approved the first monoclonal antibody (raxibacumab) through the animal efficacy rule or "Animal Rule" for the treatment of human inhalational anthrax. Raxibacumab is a recombinant human monoclonal antibody and received approval for the treatment of adult and paediatric inhalational anthrax cases, in conjunction with antibiotics, as well as use as a prophylactic in the absence of other suitable therapeutics. In March 2015, a polyclonal immunoglobulin G (IgG) (Anthrasil), prepared from the plasma of persons immunised against anthrax, received FDA approval for treating inhalational anthrax in conjunction with antibiotics. It has been common practice to isolate patients with anthrax because of its highly infectious reputation; however, human-to-human spread is extremely rare.

EPIDEMIOLOGY AND CONTROL

Human infections generally occur in countries where the disease is common in animals including those in Asia, Africa and Southern and Eastern Europe and the southern and Central Americas. Cases continue to occur sporadically in many other countries. When the disease is established in livestock and pasture becomes heavily contaminated with spores, an enzootic focus is created. Occasionally the disease may erupt in large numbers of domestic animals, with associated human cases. In this situation, anthrax is epizootic. Areas in which anthrax used to be enzootic, such as much of Europe, have been able to control the disease by controlling livestock and animal feeds (especially bone meal) and by strict regulations on the importation of animal hides, although outbreaks do still occur.

The ability of the bacterium to persist in the soil is a consequence of the formation of spores that are able to survive for long periods in the environment. An indication of the robustness of the spores is their ability to survive exposure to chemical disinfectants and heat. For example, the spores will resist dry heat at 140°C for 1–3 hours and boiling or steam at 100°C for 5–10 minutes. Autoclaving at 121°C (15 lb/in^2) destroys them in 15 minutes.

Heavy contamination of soil exists in enzootic foci in many parts of the world, and spores may be recovered many years after the last known case. Artificial contamination of Gruinard Island off the northwest coast of Scotland occurred in 1942–1943 because of tests of a biological warfare bomb containing live *B. anthracis* spores. Even in 1979, spores could still be detected in a 3-hectare area of the island. In the 1980s, the area was decontaminated by burning the vegetation and spraying with 5% formaldehyde in seawater. By 1987, the ground was declared anthrax-free and, after reseeding, sheep were able to graze safely. In enzootic areas, disinfection of soil is not a practical control measure and pastures known to be heavily contaminated should not be used for grazing animals. Control in animals depends on:

- early diagnosis
- isolation and incineration of infected animals
- use of vaccines.

In countries in which the disease is relatively rare in animals, contamination from/by imported materials is the most common form of human infection. Anthrax is a recognised industrial hazard that, in the United Kingdom, is notifiable to Consultants in Communicable Disease Control and to the Health and Safety Executive. There is control on the importation of animal hides and hair, which are disinfected if considered infected. In general, the infectivity of *B. anthracis* for humans is not of a high order. Workers at risk of exposure in the leather or wool industries, where spores could be widely distributed in large numbers in the dust and air, and veterinarians may be offered routine immunisation and antibiotic prophylaxis if exposed to a known risk.

Immunisation

Live-attenuated bacilli were first used by Louis Pasteur in May 1881, when he confounded professional scepticism in a famous public demonstration of the efficacy of a live vaccine at a farm at Pouilly-le-Fort in France. The 25 sheep that were vaccinated with heat-attenuated live bacilli and then inoculated with material containing virulent *B. anthracis* resisted infection, whereas 22 of 25 sheep acting as controls succumbed within 48 hours. Thousands of sheep, cattle and horses were subsequently vaccinated, and the mortality rate among domesticated animals fell dramatically. Later, in 1937, the Sterne strain of *B. anthracis* (34F2), which lacks the pXO2 plasmid encoding the capsule, was adopted for the immunisation of animals. This vaccine is still in use today. Prior to its introduction, anthrax was one of the leading causes of uncontrolled mortality in cattle, sheep, goats, horses and pigs worldwide.

Live-attenuated anthrax vaccines are generally not considered to be sufficiently safe for human use, and alternative vaccines based on the components of the anthrax

toxin have been developed. The currently licensed human vaccines are based on an alum precipitate of culture supernatant fluid. Predominantly, they contain PA, but there are also traces of LF and EF, which might account for the transient side effects experienced by some vaccinees.

New recombinant PA vaccine preparations free of toxin components may give better immunity and fewer adverse reactions; several types are in clinical trials.

BACILLUS CEREUS

DESCRIPTION

B. cereus is a large Gram-positive bacillus that resembles *B. anthracis*, except that it is motile, β-haemolytic, resistant to gamma phage and lacks the poly-D-glutamic acid capsule. Like other members of the genus, it is a saprophyte and is found in soil, water and vegetation. *B. cereus* closely resembles *B. anthracis* in culture, forming large grey irregular colonies described as *anthracoid*. Large inocula injected into laboratory animals may cause death but without the haemorrhagic appearance of anthrax. Blood smears do not show the characteristic pink capsule with McFadyean's polychrome methylene blue stain.

PATHOGENESIS

B. cereus is most commonly associated with food poisoning but the organism can also cause posttraumatic ophthalmitis, which requires rapid, aggressive management locally.

Atypical *B. cereus* strains capable of causing a disease that resembles anthrax have been described; four of these strains were associated with respiratory infections and two with cutaneous infections. Sequence analysis of the *B. cereus* strains, which caused disease resembling inhalational anthrax, revealed that whilst they were genetically distinct, they possessed either a plasmid similar to pXO1 or genes that encode the anthrax toxin complex.

Further isolates have been analysed from primates that died from an anthrax-like disease. PCR and sequence analysis suggests the presence of both pXO1 and pXO2 plasmids; however, the strains differ from *B. anthracis* in that they are motile and resistant to gamma phage, and some strains were resistant to penicillin G. These strains have been named *B. cereus* biovar *anthracis* and provide the first description of nonanthracis strains causing anthrax-like disease in animals. These strains have important environmental, veterinary and scientific considerations as to their origin, evolution and distribution. In 2016, agencies of the US government, specifically the

Centers for Disease Control and Prevention and Department for Health and Human Services, made an interim ruling to add to the select agent list (Tier 1) *B. cereus* biovar *anthracis* strains—an action taken to regulate *B. cereus* biovar *anthracis* to prevent potential misuse of this agent.

Food poisoning

Spores of *B. cereus* are particularly heat resistant, and most strains produce toxins. The organism is widespread in the environment and is found in most raw foods, especially cereal grains such as rice. Enormous numbers of organisms (up to 10^{10} organisms/g) may be found in contaminated food (commonly lightly cooked Chinese dishes), leading to two types of food poisoning:

1. Cases in which vomiting, occurring within 6 hours of ingestion, is the main symptom. It is caused by preformed toxin, which is a low molecular weight, heat- and acid-stable peptide (cereulide) that can withstand intestinal proteolytic enzymes.
2. A diarrhoeal form of food poisoning, occurring 8–24 hours after ingestion, similar to enteritis caused by *Escherichia coli* or *Salmonella enterica* serotypes. This is caused by three enterotoxins (haemolysin BL, nonhaemolytic enterotoxin and cytotoxin K), which, like the *Clostridium perfringens* enterotoxin, are heat labile and formed in the intestine.

LABORATORY INVESTIGATION

In the case of food poisoning, laboratory confirmation can be made if samples such as the vomit or faeces from an infected patient or suspect food are available for testing. High numbers of *B. cereus,* often exceeding 10^8 organisms per gram of sample, are sufficient to make the diagnosis in the absence of other food-poisoning bacteria. Large, facultatively anaerobic Gram-positive bacilli that produce anthracoid colonies on blood agar after overnight incubation at 37°C are almost certain to be *B. cereus*. Food reference laboratories are able to confirm identification and type, if necessary. Immunoassays are available for the detection of diarrhoeal enterotoxin.

Methods for the laboratory identification of *B. cereus* strains that cause an inhalation anthrax-like disease are based on culture and DNA sequencing.

TREATMENT

Both the emetic and diarrhoeal syndromes associated with *B. cereus* are short lived, and no specific treatment is needed. Most sufferers, even those with underlying conditions, seldom come to any harm. Acute symptoms last <24 hours, and recovery on a reduced diet and fluids is rapid. In comparison, human cases of inhalation anthrax-like disease caused by *B. cereus* can be fatal. However, it is likely that antibiotic regimens for the treatment of anthrax would be equally effective for the treatment of disease caused by atypical strains of *B. cereus*.

CONTROL

Food poisoning caused by *B. cereus* is easily prevented by proper cooling and storage of food. Ideally, all dishes should be freshly prepared and eaten. Rice, in particular, should not be stored for long periods at temperatures in excess of 10°C.

OTHER *BACILLUS* SPECIES

B. subtilis, B. pumilus and *B. licheniformis* have been implicated in causing food poisoning similar to that of *B. cereus*. Although very rare, toxigenic strains of *B. licheniformis* and *B. pumilus* have been reported. There is also one report of an emetic *B. subtilis* strain (B174). Some *Bacillus* strains produce antibacterial peptides, such as the antibiotic Bacitracin, which may facilitate growth in the intestinal tract. *Bacillus polymyxa* is the source of the antibiotic polymyxin.

B. cereus, B. subtilis and, rarely, other members of the genus may be found in wounds and tissues of immunocompromised or burned patients. There is a single instance in which *B. pumilus* has been reported to be responsible for cutaneous lesions similar to those caused by *B. anthracis*. Opportunist pathogens are also common contaminants of specimens and laboratory media, which can make clinical interpretation of microbiological results challenging. When found in numbers in normally sterile sites, such as blood or cerebrospinal fluid, these otherwise insignificant pathogens require specific treatment. Most strains produce abundant β-lactamase, which differs from the enzyme found in staphylococci.

STERILISATION TEST BACILLI

Geobacillus stearothermophilus, formerly *Bacillus stearothermophilus,* was, until the discovery of archaebacteria in hot springs, the most heat-resistant organism known. Spores withstand 121°C for up to 12 minutes, and this has made the organism ideal for testing autoclaves that run on a time–temperature cycle designed to ensure the destruction of spores. Strips containing *G. stearothermophilus* are included with the material being autoclaved and are subsequently examined by culture for surviving spores. The organism grows only at raised temperatures, typically between 50°C and 60°C; there is hardly any growth below 40°C. *Bacillus globigii* (now recognised as *Bacillus atrophaeus*) is a red-pigmented variant of *B. subtilis*. It has been used to test ethylene oxide sterilisers,

and *B. pumilus* has been used to test the efficacy of ionising radiation.

Chapter 15 is Crown Copyright © 2019, Published by Elsevier Ltd. This is an open access article under the Open Government Licence (OGL) (http://www.nationalarchives.gov.uk/doc/open-government-licence/version/3/).

RECOMMENDED READING

Beyer, W., & Turnbull, P. C. B. (2009). Anthrax in animals. *Molecular Aspects of Medicine, 30*(6), 481–489. doi:10.1016/j.mam.2009.08.004.

Brézillon, C., Haustant, M., Dupke, S., Corre, J. P., Lander, A., Franz, T., ... Goossens, P. L. (2015). Capsules, toxins and AtxA as virulence factors of emerging *Bacillus cereus* biovar *anthracis*. *PLoS Neglected Tropical Diseases, 9*(4), e0003455. doi:10.1371/journal.pntd.0003455.

Ceuppens, S., Boon, N., & Uyttendaele, M. (2013). Diversity of *Bacillus cereus* group strains is reflected in their broad range of pathogenicity and diverse ecological lifestyles. *FEMS Microbiology Ecology, 84*(3), 433–450. doi:10.1111/1574-6941.12110.

Driks, A. (2009). The *Bacillus anthracis* spore. *Molecular Aspects of Medicine, 30*(6), 368–373. doi:10.1016/j.mam.2009.08.001.

Friebe, S., van der Goot, F. G., & Burgi, J. (2016). The ins and outs of anthrax toxin. *Toxins, 8*(3), 69. doi:10.3390/toxins8030069.

Goossens, P. L. (2009). Animal models of human anthrax: The quest for the Holy Grail. *Molecular Aspects of Medicine, 30*(6), 467–480. doi:10.1016/j.mam.2009.07.005.

Hoffmaster, A. R., Ravel, J., Rasko, D. A., Chapman, G. D., Chute, M. D., Marston, C. K., ... Fraser, C. M. (2004). Identification of anthrax toxin genes in *Bacillus cereus* associated with an illness resembling inhalation anthrax. *Proceedings of the National Academy of Sciences of the USA, 101*(22), 8449–8454.

Hugh-Jones, M., & Blackburn, J. (2009). The ecology of *Bacillus anthracis*. *Molecular Aspects of Medicine, 30*(6), 356–367. doi:10.1016/j.mam.2009.08.003.

Logan, N. A. (2012). *Bacillus* and relatives in foodborne illness. *Journal of Applied Microbiology, 112*(3), 417–429. doi:10.1111/j.1365-2672.2011.05204.x.

Rao, S. S., Mohan, K. V. K., & Atreya, C. D. (2010). Detection technologies for *Bacillus anthracis*: Prospects and challenges. *Journal of Microbiological Methods, 82*(1), 1–10. doi:10.1016/j.mimet.2010.04.005.

Websites

Federal Bureau of Investigation (FBI): Anthrax links. Available at https://www.fbi.gov/history/famous-cases/amerithrax-or-anthrax-investigation.

UK Government: Zoonoses reports. Available at https://www.gov.uk/search?q=zoonoses+report.

UK National Archives: Zoonoses reports. Available at http://webarchive.nationalarchives.gov.uk/20110317185228/http://www.defra.gov.uk/foodfarm/farmanimal/diseases/atoz/zoonoses/reports.htm.

US Food and Drug Administration (FDA): FDA approves raxibacumab to treat inhalational anthrax. Available at https://wayback.archive-it.org/7993/20170111193902/https://www.fda.gov/NewsEvents/Newsroom/PressAnnouncements/ucm332341.htm.

16 *Escherichia coli* and *Shigella*

Extraintestinal infections; gastrointestinal infections; travellers' diarrhoea; haemolytic uraemic syndrome; antimicrobial resistance

CLAIRE JENKINS

KEY POINTS

- *Escherichia coli* may be a gut commensal or possess pathogenic mechanisms that enable them to cause extraintestinal or gastrointestinal infection in humans.
- Many pathogenicity factors described in *E. coli* are encoded on mobile genetic elements, such as bacteriophage, plasmids or clustered in chromosomal regions called pathogenicity islands.
- *E. coli* are distinguished from *Shigella* based on clinical, biochemical and serological characteristics but are pylogenetically the same species.
- *E. coli* are associated with both gastrointestinal and extraintestinal infections including urinary tract infection (UTI), bacteraemia, abdominal or pelvic infection, surgical site infections, meningitis abscesses and wound infections.
- The development of commercially available PCR assays targeting specific virulence genes has improved the detection of diarrhoeagenic *E. coli* and *Shigella*.
- Shiga toxin-producing *E. coli* are zoonotic, cause outbreaks of foodborne disease and are an important cause of acute renal failure in young children.
- Other diarrheagenic *E. coli* and *Shigella* are commonly associated with travellers' diarrhoea.
- Recent outbreaks of *Shigella flexneri* and *S. sonnei* in industrialised countries have been associated with transmission in men who have sex with men.
- Antibiotic treatment is appropriate in urinary infection and sepsis, but most enteric infections are managed conservatively.
- Nosocomial ExPEC expressing extended-spectrum β-lactamases (ESBLs) are an increasing problem.

CLASSIFICATION

The genus *Escherichia* belongs to the Enterobacteriaceae family and currently includes the species *E. coli, E. fergusonii, E. albertii, E. hermanii, E. vulneris* and *E. blattae*. Strains of *E. coli* and related Gram-negative bacteria predominate among the aerobic commensal microbiota in the gut of humans and animals. These bacteria are present wherever there is faecal contamination, a phenomenon that is exploited by public health microbiologists as an indicator of faecal pollution of water sources, drinking water and food. The species encompasses a variety of strains, which may be commensal or possess combinations of pathogenic mechanisms that enable them to cause extraintestinal or gastrointestinal infection in humans.

Shigella species are distinguished from *E. coli* based on clinical, biochemical and serological characteristics. However, DNA–DNA recombination studies and, more recently, whole genome sequencing (WGS) analyses show that *E. coli* and *Shigella* spp. form a single genetic group and share many characteristics. There are four species: *S. sonnei, S. flexneri, S. boydii* and *S. dysenteriae*. Clinically, *E. coli* and *Shigella* spp. are the most important members of the genus.

In recent times, the clonal diversity of *E. coli* and *Shigella* spp. has been explored by large-scale multilocus sequence typing (MLST) studies. These studies indicated that recombination events had a major influence on evolutionary relationships in *E. coli*. WGS data of multiple strains has confirmed the important contribution of horizontal gene transfer, demonstrating that the core genome of *E. coli* comprises approximately 2200 genes, but each strain has a large accessory genome that renders the total gene pool across the species effectively infinite. Pathotypes of *E. coli*, such as extraintestinal *E. coli*, enteropathogenic *E. coli*, enterotoxigenic *E. coli*, enteroinvasive *E. coli*, enteroaggregative *E. coli*, enterohaemorrahgic *E. coli* and *Shigella* spp. show multiple independent origins and parallel evolution.

LABORATORY INVESTIGATION

Strains of *E. coli* grow well in the laboratory on a wide range of selective and nonselective media, and the majority (>90%) ferment lactose, producing large red colonies on MacConkey agar. They grow over a wide range of temperature (15–45°C). Certain strains are haemolytic when grown on blood agar. Selective media are used to recover *E. coli* and *Shigella* from specimens containing complex microbiota, such as faecal specimens. Classically, these media contain substrates selectively used by one or a few species and facilitate distinction between colonies of pathogenic and nonpathogenic strains. For example, detection of *Shigella* from faeces relies on the use of differential and selective media, such as deoxycholate agar (DCA) and xylose-lysine deoxycholate (XLD).

E. coli can be differentiated from other enteric Gram-negative bacteria by the ability to utilise certain sugars and by a range of other biochemical reactions. Several such assays are available commercially (e.g., API 20E and API 20NE from BioMerieux), and more automated identification systems based on the same approach are used in larger microbiology laboratories. Typically, isolates are identified by comparison of their biochemical profile with a reference database that contains the percentages of positive results for each substrate/species pair. There are limitations to this approach; isolates that are rare, atypical, biochemically inactive or closely related to other species may be misidentified. MALDI-TOF-MS (see Ch. 3) has been implemented in many clinical microbiology laboratories. This approach has been used for the rapid identification of *E. coli* associated with extraintestinal infections and has facilitated early administration of appropriate antibiotic treatment. In contrast, *Shigella* spp. are identified as *E. coli* by commercial MALDI-TOF-MS systems. Therefore, lactose-negative colonies isolated from

a faecal sample from a patient with diarrhoeal illness, identified as *E. coli* by MALDI-TOF-MS, require additional biochemical and serological testing for definitive identification (Table 16.1). Differentiation of *E. coli* pathotypes, such as Shiga toxin–producing *E. coli* (STEC) O157, is currently not feasible in routine MALDI-TOF-MS analyses with commercial databases.

The distinction between strains of *Shigella* spp. and *E. coli* depends on a combination of diagnostic tests including motility, lysine and ornithine decarboxylase activity, indole production and the utilisation of lactose, mannitol and ortho-nitrophenyl-β-galactoside (ONPG). Despite being difficult to differentiate, *Shigella* spp. are generally less active biochemically than *E. coli*, react with a limited set of antisera and harbour a combination of pathogenicity genes located on a plasmid (pINV) shared only with the enteroinvasive *E. coli* (EIEC) group (see Table 16.1). EIEC possess biochemical characteristics of both *Shigella* spp. and *E. coli* and represent an evolutionary intermediate form between the two. EIEC are notoriously difficult to identify, and confirmation of the identification requires serological typing.

The development of rapid, commercially available PCR assays targeting specific virulence genes has improved the detection of diarrheagenic *E. coli* and *Shigella*. Target genes are typically associated with either adherence to the gut mucosa, toxin production or invasion of the host (see Table 16.2). These genotypic methods are important in differentiating between diarrheagenic *E. coli* and commensal strains or rapidly detecting strains associated with life-threatening disease, such as the STEC group, associated with haemolytic uraemic syndrome.

TYPING

Traditionally, *E. coli* and *Shigella* are characterised by serotyping. For *E. coli*, serotyping is based on the somatic

Table 16.1 Key tests to determine the biochemical and serological differences between *E. coli* and *Shigella*						
	E. coli	EIEC	*S. sonnei*	*S. flexneri*	*S. boydii*	*S. dysenteriae*
Motility	+	+/–	–	–	–	–
Lactose	+	+/–	–[a]	–	–	–
Mannitol	+	+	+	+	+	–
ONPG	+	+/–	+	–	–	–[b]
Indole	+	+/–	–	+/–	+/–	+/–
Lysine decarboxylase	+	+/–	–	–	–	–
Ornithine decarboxylase	+	+/–	+	–	–	–
Sonnei agglutination	–	–	+	–	–	–
Polyflex agglutination	–	–	–	+	+	–
ipaH gene	–	+	+	+	+	+

EIEC, Enteroinvasive *E. coli*; ONPG, ortho-nitrophenyl-β-galactoside.
[a]Late lactose fermenter.
[b]*S. dysenteriae* serotype 1 is ONPG positive.

Table 16.2 Commercial PCR assays target specific virulence genes that identify the diarrheagenic *E. coli* groups

Diarrheagenic *E. coli* groups	PCR target gene	Location	Function
EPEC	Intimin *(eae)* gene	Chromosome	Intimate attachment to the host gut mucosa
ETEC	Heat-labile (LT) and heat-stable toxin (ST)	Plasmid	Enterotoxin
EAEC	Aggregative adherence regulator (aggR)	Plasmid	Regulates the expression of aggregative adherence fimbriae
STEC	Shiga toxins 1 (stx1) and 2 (stx2)	Bacteriophage	Enterotoxins
EIEC and *Shigella*	Invasion plasmid antigen H (ipaH)	Plasmid but may also have multiple copies on the chromosome	E3 ubiquitin ligase

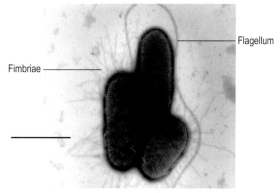

Fig. 16.1 Electron micrograph of *E. coli* showing flagellum and fimbriae *(arrows). Bar* = 0.5 µm.

Table 16.3 Common serogroups of diarrheagenic *E. coli*

Pathogenic group	Common serogroups
Enteropathogenic *E. coli* (EPEC)	O26, O55, O111, O114, O119, O125, O126, O127, O128, O142
Enterotoxigenic *E. coli* (ETEC)	O6, O8, O15, O25, O27, O63, O78, O115, O143, O153, O159, O167
Enteroinvasive *E. coli* (EIEC)	O28, O29, O121, O124, O136, O143, O153, O159, O167
Shiga toxin–producing *E. coli* (STEC)	O26, O55, O103, O111, O145, O157[a]
Enteroaggregative *E. coli* (EAEC)	O3, O44, O92, O104

[a]Other serogroups are far less common than O157 in human disease.

LPS O, flagella H and capsular (K) antigens, as detected in agglutination assays with specific rabbit antibodies. Strains of *E. coli* express lipopolysaccharide (LPS) O antigens and flagellar H antigens. Some strains express fimbriae (Fig. 16.1), and certain strains, especially those associated with extraintestinal infections, may produce a polysaccharide capsule. In contrast, the shigellae are nonmotile, noncapsulate and do not to express fimbriae. Many strains of *Shigella* spp. share lipopolysaccharide (LPS) antigens with strains of *E. coli*, with the exception of *S. sonnei*, where the antigen (when expressed) is shared with *Pleisomonas shigelloides*. Serotyping is important because of the high epidemiological and medical significance of serotype characterisation for strains of *Shigella* and *E. coli* (see Table 16.3).

Strains are serotyped (*E. coli, S. dysenteriae, S. boydii* and *S. flexneri*) or phage typed (STEC O157 and *S. sonnei*) to facilitate outbreak investigations and identify emerging clones associated with antimicrobial resistance or severe disease. Phage typing is a rapid and cost-effective typing approach to typing during outbreak investigations. However, it is a low-level discriminatory method requiring a specific skill set, and few laboratories now report phage typing data.

For *E. coli*, >200 different O-antigens have been described, and others continue to emerge. More than 50 H antigens have been identified. Because certain strains of *E. coli* cease to express flagella during growth in vitro, strains may need to be grown in semisolid agar (Craigie tubes) to induce flagella expression. The term K antigen was formerly used collectively for surface or capsular antigens that prevent flagella-specific antibodies from binding to the somatic antigens. In modern usage, K antigen refers to the acidic polysaccharide capsular antigens. Currently, there are 15 established *S. flexneri* serotypes. The scheme differentiates isolates serologically based on the expression of the major type specific somatic antigen (I–VI) and common group factor antigens (3;4 and 7;8). *S. boydii* and *S. dysenteriae* are composed of 20 and 15 recognised serotypes, respectively. Many strains previously identified as *S. boydii* serotype 13 found not to harbour the *ipaH* gene (characteristic of *Shigella* spp. and EIEC) and to be more active biochemically than *Shigella* species have been reclassified as *Escherichia albertii*.

If a higher level of discrimination is required, there are a variety of molecular typing methods available including pulsed-field gel electrophoresis (PFGE), multilocus variable number tandem repeat (VNTR) analysis (MLVA) and, more recently, whole genome sequencing (WGS). Recently, WGS has been used to investigate outbreaks at the local level and to monitor global transmission.

CLINICAL SYNDROMES ASSOCIATED WITH EXTRAINTESTINAL *E. COLI*

E. coli are associated with both gastrointestinal and extraintestinal infections including urinary tract infection (UTI), bacteraemia, abdominal or pelvic infection, surgical site infections, meningitis and various abscesses including wound infections.

E. coli infections account for approximately 80% of all UTIs, causing cystitis in the bladder and acute pyelonephritis in the kidneys. Most urinary tract infections are thought to be caused by organisms originating from the patient's own faecal microbiota. UTIs occur more frequently in women than in men because the shorter, wider, female urethra appears to be less effective in preventing access of the bacteria to the bladder. The high incidence in pregnant women can be attributed to impairment of urine flow due partly to hormonal changes and partly to pressure on the urinary tract. Other causes of urinary stagnation that may predispose to urinary tract infection include urethral obstruction, urinary stones, congenital malformations and neurological disorders, all of which occur in both sexes. In men, prostatic enlargement is the most common predisposing factor. Catheterisation and cystoscopy may introduce bacteria into the bladder and therefore carry a risk of infection.

Bacteraemia is a major complication of infection by *E. coli* as it can lead to severe sepsis with acute organ failure and septic shock. In recent years, *E. coli* bacteraemia has increased, and in the United Kingdom the species now accounts for >30% of bacteraemia in those >75 years. The primary source of bacteraemia is UTIs. Other classic sources of blood infections include the digestive tract, implicating both specific intestinal pathogens and opportunistic enteric bacteria, which can translocate from the intestinal lumen to blood in hosts with underlying conditions.

Certain types of *E. coli* can cause meningitis (neonatal meningitis *E. coli*, or NMEC) in the newborns. Fatality rates can approach 40%, and survivors usually suffer from severe neurological sequelae.

PATHOGENESIS

Extraintestinal pathogenic *E. coli* (ExPEC) are facultative pathogens that belong to the normal gut microbiota of a certain fraction of the healthy population, where they live as commensals. Infections occur through microbial colonisation of normally sterile sites. The balance between host defences and virulence factors is a key factor that determines commensalism or disease. Each anatomic site presents specific defences against infection, and bacteria must therefore express specific virulence factors to counter these defences.

Many strains express haemolysin(s), and, in general, strains of *E. coli* isolated from human extraintestinal infections are more likely to be haemolytic than strains isolated from the faeces of healthy humans. Haemolysin production is an important pathogenic mechanism for releasing essential ferric ions bound to haemoglobin, and the expression of certain haemolysins has been shown to be regulated by iron availability. Strains of *E. coli* can express siderophores, such as enterobactin, which remove ferric ions from mammalian iron transport proteins such as transferrin and lactoferrin. Some strains also express the siderophore, aerobactin; this may be plasmid encoded. The ability of strains of *E. coli* to acquire ferric ions is a recognised pathogenic mechanism. Expression of the aerobactin-mediated iron-uptake system is a common feature of strains isolated from patients with septicaemia, pyelonephritis and lower urinary tract infection. Some strains may also utilise siderophores produced by certain species of fungi (e.g., ferrichrome, coprogen, rhodotorulic acid) to acquire iron from environmental sources.

The ability to colonise extraintestinal sites and establish infection requires a mechanism for attachment to the host mucosa. In urinary tract infections, attachment is mediated primarily by type 1 pili binding to proteins called uroplakins that coat the uroepithelium. Other fimbrial adhesins include P-fimbriae and S-fimbriae. Afimbrial adhesins, such as AfaE, also play a role. Crosstalk between P fimbriae, type 1 pili and other adhesion clusters prevents coexpression of multiple surface structures. *E. coli* associated with causing meningitis also utilise type 1 pili to bind to the CD48 positive endothelial cells of the blood–brain barrier.

Survival in the blood is facilitated by an antiphagocytic polysialic acid capsule and manipulation of the classical complement pathway by the bacterial outer-membrane protein A (OmpA). Invasion of macrophages and monocytes prevents apoptosis and chemokine release, providing a niche for replication before dissemination back into the blood. A lambdoid phage that encodes an O acetyltransferase acetylates the O antigen to provide phase variation and diversity to the capsule, thus hiding the bacteria from host defences. The K1 capsule, which is found in approximately 80% of *E. coli* isolates causing neonatal meningitis, also has a role in invasion by preventing phagolysosomal fusion and thus allowing delivery of live bacteria across the blood–brain barrier. In the central nervous system the bacterium can induce oedema, inflammation and neural damage.

GASTROINTESTINAL DISEASE

Commensal bacteria in the gut represent an important barrier against infection as colonisation by harmless bacteria protects the host from invading pathogens. In contrast, enteric pathogens modulate inflammation, leading to host responses that facilitate their survival and restrain other commensal microbiota. Certain pathotypes of *E. coli* cause gastrointestinal disease ranging in severity from mild, self-limiting diarrhoea to haemorrhagic colitis and the associated, potentially life-threatening haemolytic uraemic syndrome. Such strains fall into at least five groups:

1. Enteropathogenic *E. coli* (EPEC) cause infantile diarrhoea most commonly where hygiene standards are low.
2. Enterotoxigenic *E. coli* (ETEC) cause community-acquired diarrhoeal disease in areas of poor sanitation and are a common cause of travellers' diarrhoea.
3. Enteroaggregative *E. coli* (EAEC) cause acute and chronic diarrhoeal disease in developing countries and are a common cause of travellers' diarrhoea.
4. Shiga toxin–producing *E. coli* (STEC) cause symptoms ranging from mild to bloody diarrhoea, haemorrhagic colitis and haemolytic uraemic syndrome.
5. Enteroinvasive *E. coli* (EIEC) cause dysentery.

Many pathogenicity factors described in *E. coli* are encoded on mobile genetic elements such as bacteriophage, plasmids or clustered in chromosomal regions called pathogenicity islands (PAIs). The mechanisms by which the *E. coli* and *Shigella* spp. cause disease are described later in the chapter.

Enteropathogenic *E. coli* (EPEC)

EPEC were associated with morbidity and mortality in infants with diarrhoea in the 1940s and 50s and remain a current global cause of diarrhoea in infants <2 years. It is most common in developing countries where mortality rates are high. Clinical manifestations include profuse persistent diarrhoea, vomiting and fever, all of which contribute to severe dehydration, which can be life threatening in very young and/or malnourished children.

Initially, strains of *E. coli* belonging to the EPEC group were defined by serotype (see Table 16.3) and then by their localised adherence (LA) pattern on HEp-2 cells. Currently, EPEC are defined as having the intimin or *eae* (for *E. coli* attaching and effacing) gene, encoding a 97 kDa bacterial outer-membrane protein involved in cellular attachment. The *eae* is encoded on a PAI, called the locus of enterocyte effacement (LEE), which encodes a number of proteins associated with a Type III secretion system. During infection, the bacterium intimately attaches to the host gut mucosa, disrupting the apical cytoskeleton of the epithelial cells lining the gut mucosa, effacing the microvilli and forming pedestal-like structures. Symptoms of diarrhoea are not toxin mediated and are caused by the cellular changes in the host's gut mucosa, for example, destruction of the microvilli, resulting in the reduction in the absorptive capacity of the intestinal epithelium.

Certain strains of EPEC also carry an adherence factor (EAF) plasmid encoding a cluster of 14 genes coding for the expression and assembly of the bundle-forming pilus (BFP) and are known as typical (tEPEC) or classical EPEC. Transmission of tEPEC is human to human or from food or water contaminated by human faeces. EPEC without the EAF plasmid are designated atypical EPEC (aEPEC). Epidemiological studies show they are more common than tEPEC and are associated with a varied animal reservoir, including domesticated and wild animals.

Historically, EPEC was identified at diagnostic laboratories by serotyping (see Table 16.3) or by the fluorescent actin staining (FAS) test. This approach has now been replaced by PCR targeting the *eae* gene (see Table 16.2).

Enterotoxigenic *E. coli* (ETEC)

ETEC are one of the top four etiologic agents of severe diarrhoea in infants <5 years of age in developing countries and are responsible for approximately 280 million cases in this age group and 840 million cases in total. ETEC are a common cause of travellers' diarrhoea. The illness caused by ETEC has a short incubation period and symptoms of watery diarrhoea, similar to *Vibrio cholerae* infection. Like tEPEC, transmission of ETEC is human to human or from food or water contaminated by human faeces.

ETEC are defined by the presence of plasmid-encoded heat-labile (LT) and heat-stable (ST) toxins and the expression of fimbrial antigens, also plasmid encoded. The fimbrial antigens were known previously as colonisation factor antigens (CFAs) but are now referred to as coli surface (CS) antigens suffixed with a number—for example, CS2 (although CFA/I are still referred to as such). More than 25 different CS antigens are known. ETEC cause disease by adhering to the host gut mucosa via CS antigens (and possible other colonising factors) and producing either one or both of the LT/ST enterotoxins.

Serotyping has limited use in identifying strains of *E. coli* belonging to the ETEC group as there are a large number of associated serotypes (at least 78 O antigens and 34 H antigens), and common serotypes change over time. ETEC can be detected by PCR targeting the genes encoding LT and ST in isolated colonies or directly from faecal specimens (see Table 16.2).

Enteroaggregative *E. coli* (EAEC)

EAEC has been highlighted as a common bacterial cause of diarrhoea in studies in the United States and in Europe and is an emerging cause of travellers' diarrhoea. It makes a significant contribution to morbidity in children <2 years of age in developing countries and has been associated with causing diarrhoea in HIV-infected patients. Symptoms include persistent watery, mucoid, secretory diarrhoea with low-grade fever that may continue for >10 days. Transmission of EAEC is similar to that of ETEC and tEPEC, via food and water contaminated with human faeces or person-to-person spread. There is little or no evidence to suggest EAEC has a significant animal reservoir.

Historically, EAEC were characterised by the production of an aggregative adherence (AA) or stacked-brick pattern of bacterial cells attached to HEp-2 cells. Certain EAEC harbour a plasmid, designated pAA, encoding a number of putative virulence factors including AggR (involved in the regulation of many of the virulence genes involved in both the aggregation and toxin production stages of EAEC pathogenesis) and are known as typical EAEC. Atypical strains also adhere to HEp-2 cells in a stacked-brick formation but do not have the pAA plasmid. Recent studies suggest that the *aggR* gene also regulates chromosomally encoded genes located on the Aai operon, involved in Type VI secretion.

Current evidence suggests that the mechanism of pathogenesis involves adherence of the bacteria to the host gut mucosa by fimbrial and afimbrial adhesins. To date, five types of aggregative adherence fimbriae have been described (AAFI–V) all encoded on pAA and regulated by AggR. This is followed by the production of enterotoxins and cytotoxins, including a cytoskeleton-altering plasmid-encoded toxin (Pet), SHet, a toxin also produced by *Shigella flexneri*, heat-stable enterotoxin (EAST-1) and Pic, a mucinase, both encoded by many other pathogens. Mucosal inflammation induced by both the pathogen and the host's own immune system.

EAEC strains are phenotypically and genetically diverse, and therefore comprehensive diagnostic assays based on biochemical, serological or molecular approaches all have limitations. The gold standard method for the identification of EAEC is the HEp-2 adherence assay with the characteristic aggregative or stacked-brick adherence pattern, but this is technically demanding and unsuitable as a routine diagnostic tool, and PCR targeting *aggR* is the most commonly used detection method (see Table 16.2).

Shiga toxin–producing *E. coli* (STEC)

First reported in 1983, STEC (also known as verocytotoxin-producing *E. coli* [VTEC]) are responsible for gastrointestinal illnesses, including severe abdominal pain and bloody diarrhoea, that can develop into haemolytic–uremic syndrome (HUS) between 4 and 15 days after the onset of diarrhoea. HUS is specifically associated with haemolytic anaemia and acute renal failure requiring long-term dialysis treatment and can be fatal. STEC is the most common aetiologic agent of infectious HUS in children and is an emerging pathogen in industrialised countries. The number of cases of STEC O157 in England and Wales between 1996 and 2015 is shown in Fig. 16.2.

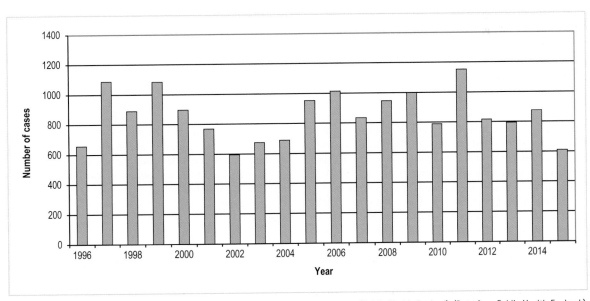

Fig. 16.2 Number of cases of STEC O157 in England and Wales between 1996 and 2015 (Public Health England). (Data from Public Health England.)

STEC are defined by the production of two phage-encoded Shiga toxins, Stx1 (identical to Stx1 of *S. dysenteriae* serotype 1) and Stx2. Both toxin types have a number of variants, and Stx2, specifically the Stx2a subtype, is most commonly associated with HUS. Stx, circulating via the bloodstream, is thought to cause vascular damage in the colon and kidneys, specifically by adhering to cell surface globotriaosylceramide (gb3) and the induction of apoptosis. Many STEC associated with causing severe bloody diarrhoea or HUS also have the LEE PAI, and adhere to the host gut mucosa in a similar way to EPEC.

More recently, Stx-positive/LEE negative strains causing HUS were found to harbour the *aggR* gene, previously associated with the EAEC group. In 2011, over 4000 previously healthy people from 16 different countries were associated with an outbreak of foodborne illness caused by an EAEC Shiga toxin–producing strain identified as *E. coli* serotype O104:H4. Over 900 cases developed HUS and >50 people died. This highly pathogenic hybrid pathogen carried virulence genes found in both typical EAEC strains (*aggA*, *aggR*, *set1*, *pic* and *aap*) and STEC (*stx*2a). STEC negative for both the LEE and *aggR* have also been associated with HUS, and it is likely that other, as yet unknown, attachment mechanisms exist.

The infectious dose of STEC is low (10–100 organisms), and transmission is via contaminated food or water; direct contact with animals, especially ruminants; indirect contact with a contaminated environment or person to person. A number of large outbreaks have occurred in the United Kingdom associated with the consumption of contaminated beef and dairy products, direct contact with calves and lambs at petting farms and, more recently, consumption of contaminated raw vegetables and salad leaves.

Microbiological diagnosis of HUS is difficult as the onset of severe symptoms often occurs several days after the diarrhoeal prodrome, when patients no longer have detectable levels of STEC in their stools. The recommended diagnostic method is the detection of *stx* directly from faecal specimens using PCR and the subsequent culture and identification of *stx*-positive colonies. The most common STEC serotype in the United Kingdom, STEC O157:H7, does not ferment sorbitol (as opposed to most other *E. coli* strains) and can be clearly identified as colourless, sorbitol nonfermenting colonies on sorbitol Mac-Conkey agar containing cefixime and tellurite (CT-SMAC). HUS can be caused by other serogroups of Stx-producing *E. coli* (e.g., O26, O55, O103, O111 and O145) that (unlike STEC O157:H7) do not have specific biochemical characteristics that aid identification, and this further complicates the bacterial diagnosis of HUS. Immunomagnetic separation techniques, involving magnetic beads coated in antibodies to the most commonly detected serogroups, may facilitate detection when STEC is present in the faecal specimen at low levels.

Enteroinvasive *E. coli* (EIEC)

EIEC has similar pathogenic, biochemical and genetic properties to *Shigella*. EIEC infections occur most commonly in developing countries and are associated with travellers recently returned from these regions. Like *Shigella*, EIEC is transmitted mainly through contaminated water and food or direct person-to-person spread. Again, like *Shigella*, symptoms include dysentery with faecal blood, mucus and leukocytes, although volunteer studies indicate that the infectious dose is higher.

The major virulence factor is a 220 kb plasmid, designated the invasion plasmid (pINV). The pathogenic mechanism of EIEC is virtually identical to that of *Shigella* (see later in the chapter).

Differential diagnosis from *Shigella* is difficult even using the PCR approach as the *ipaH* gene, the target for detecting *Shigella* on the pINV plasmid, is also carried by EIEC. EIEC and *Shigella* can only be clearly differentiated by the keratoconjunctivitis or Sereny test (now rarely used) or by extended biochemical tests and serotyping (see Table 16.1).

SHIGELLA

Symptoms of shigellosis are mild watery diarrhoea or more severe inflammatory bacillary dysentery, characterised by fever, abdominal cramps, and blood and mucus in stools. Dysentery caused by *S. sonnei* usually causes a milder illness than the other three *Shigella* spp. *S. dysenteriae* serotype 1 produces Stx1 and has been associated with HUS similar to the syndrome caused by STEC. A large proportion of all diarrhoeal episodes, an estimated 167 million worldwide, including over a million deaths annually, are attributed to *Shigella*, with the greatest burden occurring in developing countries in children <5 years.

The incubation period is usually between 2 and 3 days but may be as long as 8 days. The onset of symptoms is usually sudden, and frequently the initial symptom is abdominal pain. This is followed by the onset of watery diarrhoea, and in all but the mildest cases this is accompanied by fever, headache and malaise. The symptoms typically last about 4 days but may continue for 14 days or more. Postinfectious complications may include reactive arthritis and irritable bowel syndrome.

The shigellae are facultative intracellular pathogens derived from *E. coli* by a combination of gene loss and acquisition. Deletions are associated with the loss of metabolic pathways (e.g., *cadA*) no longer required for an intracellular lifestyle and antivirulence factors (e.g., *nadA* and *nadB*) that would suppress pathogenicity. Acquired genes are associated with bacterial invasion and intracellular survival (e.g., *virB* and *mxiE*), iron acquisition (e.g., *iuc* and *fuc*) and toxin production (e.g., *set1A* and *set1B*) encoded on the invasion plasmid pINV and the chromosomally located *Shigella* pathogenicity islands (SHIs) SHI-1 and SHI-2, SHI-O and SRL.

Pathogenesis by *Shigella* involves four steps:

1. Bacteria invade epithelial M cells in the large intestine and translocate to the submucosa
2. On reaching the submucosa, they are engulfed by macrophages where they survive and multiply
3. Eventually they induce apoptosis and release of cytokines that result in a breakdown of the integrity of the epithelium
4. On escaping from the macrophage, bacilli invade the basolateral aspect of epithelial cells and traverse the cytoplasm of the invaded cell, and newly invade neighbouring cells by causing polymerisation of host actin at one pole of the bacterial cell. This provides the propulsive force required for directed motility and produces the actin tails recognisable by fluorescence microscopy.

Diarrhoea results from the breakdown of the integrity of the colonic epithelium and subsequent reduction in its capacity to reabsorb fluid and the action enterotoxins (ShET1 and ShET2) in the jejunum.

S. dysenteriae and *S. boydii* are rare compared to *S. flexneri* and *S. sonnei*. *S. flexneri* is the most commonly isolated species and is endemic in developing countries. Historically, in industrialised countries, *S. flexneri* was isolated mainly in travellers returning from high-risk countries where standards of hygiene are low. The recent increase in domestically acquired *S. flexneri* infection in the United Kingdom is associated with transmission between men who have sex with men (MSM) (see Fig. 16.3). *S. sonnei* are the most common species isolated in industrialised countries, traditionally linked to outbreaks in nurseries and schools. Like *S. flexneri*, more recently *S. sonnei* has also been linked to transmission in MSM.

TREATMENT

The treatment of gastrointestinal disease focuses on the early administration of fluid and electrolytes as the single most important factor. Antimicrobial drugs play a minor role, although they may be used to limit severity and duration of symptoms in the very young and very old. Despite the potentially serious consequences of STEC infection, the use of antimicrobials that induce the bacterial SOS response (e.g., fluoroquinolones) is contraindicated; these drugs have been shown to increase expression of Stx, and the administration of antibiotics in the United Kingdom is contraindicated.

Uncomplicated cystitis usually responds to empirical treatment with oral antimicrobial agents, such as trimethoprim or nitrofurantoin, but more serious infections and infections not responding to first-line antimicrobials require specific antimicrobial therapy based on laboratory results.

Bacterial meningitis is a medical emergency, and vigorous early treatment with cefotaxime and gentamicin is recommended.

Many strains of *E. coli* isolates from blood cultures commonly express resistance to antimicrobial agents, and treatment should be guided by laboratory tests of sensitivity where possible. ExPEC expressing extended-spectrum β-lactamases (ESBLs) are an increasing problem. ESBLs are enzymes produced by certain bacteria that are able to hydrolyse and inactivate extended-spectrum cephalosporins; these include ceftazidime, ceftriaxone and cefotaxime. Many outbreaks of ESBL-producing *E. coli* have been reported in ICUs and, due largely to plasmid dissemination, may involve unrelated strains of the same

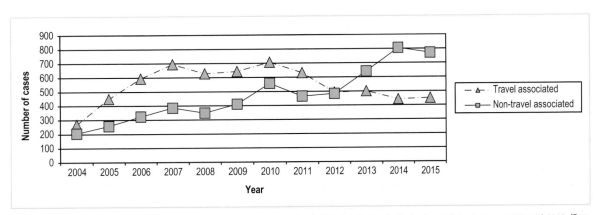

Fig. 16.3 Number of cases of travel-associated versus non–travel-associated *Shigella* infection in England and Wales between 2004 and 2015. (Data from Public Health England.)

species and different Gram-negative species. Risk factors for infection by ESBL-producing Enterobacteriaceae included increased length of hospital stay, admission to the ICU or preexisting comorbidities and prior use of third-generation cephalosporins.

CONTROL

The spread of *E. coli* and *Shigella* spp. in hospitals and nurseries is mainly from patient to patient. It can be prevented only by very strict hygiene. Infected patients, and recently admitted patients suspected of being infected, may be isolated by barrier nursing techniques to prevent spread. In some cases, outbreaks can be terminated only by closing the ward or nursery, and following a deep-cleaning protocol before reopening.

Transmission of diarrheagenic *E. coli* and *Shigella* spp. can occur by person-to-person spread or via food and/or water contaminated by human or animal faeces. There are increased risks associated with travel to regions where hygiene standards are low. The provision of safe supplies of water together with education in hygienic practice in the handling and production of food, particularly that given to young children, is essential. Travellers to countries with poor hygiene, especially in the tropics, should select eating places with care and, if possible, should consume only hot food and drinks and bottled water. Self-peeled fruits are probably safe, but salads should be avoided. Unheated milk should also be considered unsafe.

STEC infections are acquired most frequently from meat, unpasteurised milk and direct contact with animals. Foodborne infections should be avoided by normal food hygiene, with particular attention to processing and handling cooked meat products separately from raw meat, and the thorough cooking of raw meats, especially if minced.

Strategies for the control of STEC and *Shigella* in the public health setting include the sanitary disposal of faeces, handwashing, hygiene measures and the isolation/exclusion of infected cases. Where information indicates a point source, efforts aim to minimise ongoing exposure. Guidelines for the management of *Shigella* and STEC infection in the United Kingdom recommend exclusion of cases of *S. sonnei* from school or work until 48 hours after the first normal stool, and clinical surveillance for both cases and contacts. However, cases and contacts in risk groups (including children aged 5 and under, food handlers and care workers) of STEC, *S. dysenteriae*, *S. flexneri* and *S. boydii* should be screened microbiologically for clearance (defined in the United Kingdom as two negative stool samples not <48 hours apart).

Vaccination

Vaccination constitutes a major challenge for the control of *E. coli* and *Shigella* infections, and few vaccines exist. An ETEC vaccine, rCTB-CF, is available consisting of a combination of recombinant cholera toxin B subunit and formalin-inactivated ETEC cells. A safe effective vaccine for *Shigella* is greatly sought after because oral rehydration therapy is less effective against this pathogen than against other toxin-producing gastrointestinal pathogens such as *Vibrio cholerae* and enterotoxigenic *E. coli*. More importantly, there are limited therapeutic options because of increasing resistance to antimicrobials. The genus *Shigella* comprises a wide range of serotypes, but studies have shown that a vaccine covering *S. sonnei* and *S. flexneri* serotypes 2a, 3a and 6 would provide protection against >65% of *Shigella* infections. Vaccines targeting the variable LPS antigens include polysaccharide conjugates and synthetic conjugates. An alternative strategy is to target the conserved antigens, such as the major outer membrane proteins and the invasion plasmid antigens.

RECOMMENDED READING

Adams, N. L., Byrne, L., Smith, G. A., Elson, R., Harris, J. P., Salmon, R., ... Jenkins, C. (2016). Shiga toxin-producing *Escherichia coli* O157, England and Wales, 1983-2012. *Emerging Infectious Diseases, 22*(4), 590–597.

Barichello, T., Fagundes, G. D., Generoso, J. S., Elias, S. G., Simões, L. R., & Teixeira, A. L. (2013). Pathophysiology of neonatal acute bacterial meningitis. *Journal of Medical Microbiology, 62*(Pt. 12), 1781–1789. doi:10.1099/jmm.0.059840-0.

Barry, E. M., Pasetti, M. F., Sztein, M. B., Fasano, A., Kotloff, K. L., & Levine, M. M. (2013). Progress and pitfalls in Shigella vaccine research. *Nature Reviews. Gastroenterology & Hepatology, 10*(4), 245–255. doi:10.1038/nrgastro.2013.12.

Byrne, L., Jenkins, C., Launders, N., Elson, R., & Adak, G. K. (2015). The epidemiology, microbiology and clinical impact of Shiga toxin-producing *Escherichia coli* in England, 2009-2012.

Epidemiology and Infection, 143(16), 3475–3487. doi:10.1017/S0950268815000746.

Croxen, M. A. & Finlay, B. B. (2010). Molecular mechanisms of *Escherichia coli* pathogenicity. *Nature Reviews. Microbiology, 8*(1), 26–38. doi:10.1038/nrmicro2265.

Croxen, M. A., Law, R. J., Scholz, R., Keeney, K. M., Wlodarska, M., & Finlay, B. B. (2013). Recent advances in understanding enteric pathogenic *Escherichia coli*. *Clinical Microbiology Review, 26*(4), 822–880. doi:10.1128/CMR.00022-13.

Dale, A. P. & Woodford, N. (2015). Extra-intestinal pathogenic *Escherichia coli* (ExPEC): disease, carriage and clones. *The Journal of Infection, 71*(6), 615–626. doi:10.1016/j.jinf.2015.09.009.

Fleckenstein, J. M., Munson, G. M., & Rasko, D. A. (2013). Enterotoxigenic *Escherichia coli*: orchestrated host engagement. *Gut Microbes, 4*(5), 392–396. doi:10.4161/gmic.25861.

Hazen, T. H., Sahl, J. W., Fraser, C. M., Donnenberg, M. S., Scheutz, F., & Rasko, D. A. (2013). Refining the pathovar paradigm via phylogenomics of the attaching and effacing *Escherichia coli*. *Proceedings of the National Academy of Sciences in the United States of America, 110*(31), 12810–12875. doi:10.1073/pnas.1306836110.

Holt, K. E., Baker, S., Weill, F. X., Holmes, E. C., Kitchen, A., Yu, J., ... Thomson, N. R. (2012). *Shigella sonnei* genome sequencing and phylogenetic analysis indicate recent global dissemination from Europe. *Nature Genetics, 44*(9), 1056–1059. doi:10.1038/ng.2369.

Lai, Y., Rosenshine, I., Leong, J. M., & Frankel, G. (2013). Intimate host attachment: enteropathogenic and enterohaemorrhagic *Escherichia coli*. *Cellular Microbiology, 15*(11), 1796–1808. doi:10.1111/cmi.12179.

Launders, N., Byrne, L., Jenkins, C., Harker, K., Charlett, A., & Adak, G. K. (2016). Disease severity of Shiga toxin-producing *E. coli* O157 and factors influencing the development of typical haemolytic uraemic syndrome: a retrospective cohort study, 2009-2012. *British Medical Journal Open, 6*(1), e009933. doi:10.1136/bmjopen-2015-009933.

Nataro, J. P., Mai, V., Johnson, J., Blackwelder, W. C., Heimer, R., Tirrell, S., ... Hirshon, J. M. (2006). Diarrheagenic *Escherichia coli* infection in Baltimore, Maryland, and New Haven, Connecticut. *Clinical Infectious Diseases, 43*(4), 402–407.

Niyogi, S. K. (2005). Shigellosis. *Journal of Microbiology, 43*(2), 133–143.

O'Leary, J., Corcoran, D., & Lucey, B. (2009). Comparison of the EntericBio multiplex PCR system with routine culture for detection of bacterial enteric pathogens. *Journal Clinical Microbiology, 47*(11), 3449–3453. doi:10.1128/JCM.01026-09.

Parsot, C. (2005). *Shigella* spp. and enteroinvasive *Escherichia coli* pathogenicity factors. *FEMS Microbiology Letters, 252*(1), 11–18.

Peng, J., Yang, J., & Jin, Q. (2009). The molecular evolutionary history of *Shigella* spp. and enteroinvasive *Escherichia coli*. *Infection, Genetics and Evolution, 9*(1), 147–152. doi:10.1016/j.meegid.2008.10.003.

Ronald, A. (2003). The etiology of urinary tract infection: traditional and emerging pathogens. *Disease-A-Month, 49*(2), 71–82.

Schroeder, G. N. & Hilbi, H. (2008). Molecular pathogenesis of *Shigella* spp.: controlling host cell signaling, invasion, and death by type III secretion. *Clinical Microbiology Reviews, 21*(1), 134–156. doi:10.1128/CMR.00032-07.

Shah, N., DuPont, H. L., & Ramsey, D. J. (2009). Global etiology of travelers' diarrhoea: systematic review from 1973 to the present. *The American Journal of Tropical Medicine and Hygiene, 80*(4), 609–614.

Simms, I., Field, N., Jenkins, C., Childs, T., Gilbart, V. L., Dallman, T. J., ... Hughes, G. (2015). Intensified shigellosis epidemic associated with sexual transmission in men who have sex with men – *Shigella flexneri* and *S. sonnei* in England, 2004 to end of February 2015. *Eurosurveillance, 20*(15).

Working Group of the former PHLS Advisory Committee on Gastrointestinal Infections. (2011). Preventing person-to-person spread following gastrointestinal infections: guidelines for public health physicians and environmental health officers. *California Department of Public Health (CDPH), 7*(4), 362.

Yang, J., Nie, H., Chen, L., Zhang, X., Yang, F., Xu, X., ... Jin, Q. (2007). Revisiting the molecular evolutionary history of *Shigella* spp. *Journal of Molecular Evolution, 64*(1), 71–79.

Websites

Centers for Disease Control and Prevention. *E. coli (Escherichia coli)*. Available at http://www.cdc.gov/ecoli/.

Centers for Disease Control and Prevention. *Shigella* – Shigellosis. Available at http://www.cdc.gov/shigella/index.html.

European Union Reference Laboratory VTEC. Laboratory methods for VTEC detection and typing. Available at http://www.iss.it/vtec/index.php?lang=2&anno=2016&tipo=3.

Preventing person-to-person spread following gastrointestinal infections: guidelines for public health physicians and environmental health officers. Retrieved from http://webarchive.nationalarchives.gov.uk/+/http://www.hpa.org.uk/cdph/issues/CDPHvol7/No4/guidelines2_4_04.pdf. (Accessed Mar 2013).

Public Health England. *Escherichia coli (E. coli)*: guidance, data and analysis. Available at https://www.gov.uk/government/collections/escherichia-coli-e-coli-guidance-data-and-analysis.

Public Health England. Vero cytotoxin-producing *Escherichia coli* (VTEC): guidance, data and analysis. Available at https://www.gov.uk/government/collections/vero-cytotoxin-producing-escherichia-coli-vtec-guidance-data-and-analysis.

Public Health England. Shigella: guidance, data and analysis. Available at https://www.gov.uk/government/collections/shigella-guidance-data-and-analysis.

Public Health England. UK Standards for Microbiology Investigations B 30: Investigation of faecal specimens for enteric pathogens. Available at www.hpa.org.uk/ProductsServices/MicrobiologyPathology/UKStandardsForMicrobiologyInvestigations/TermsOfUseForSMIs/AccessToUKSMIs/SMIBacteriology/smiB30InvestigationofFaecalSpecimensforEnteric/.

Public Health England. STEC Operational Guidelines. Retrieved from http://webarchive.nationalarchives.gov.uk/20140714084352/http://www.hpa.org.uk/webc/HPAwebFile/HPAweb_C/1279889252950.

17 *Salmonella*

Enteric fever; gastrointestinal infection; food poisoning

CLAIRE JENKINS

KEY POINTS

- There are >2600 different antigenic types of *Salmonella*; 99% of those pathogenic to humans belong to *S. enterica* subspecies *enterica*.
- Most serotypes of *S. enterica* cause foodborne gastroenteritis and have animal reservoirs.
- *S. enterica* serotypes Typhi and Paratyphi cause typhoid fever.
- Typhoid and other serious systemic *Salmonella* infections are treated with ciprofloxacin, azithromycin or ceftriaxone.
- Antibiotics are contraindicated in the management of *Salmonella* gastroenteritis unless invasive complications are suspected.
- Clean water, sanitation and hygienic handling of food prevent disease.

DESCRIPTION

Salmonellae are typical members of the Enterobacteriaceae: facultatively anaerobic Gram-negative bacilli able to grow on a wide range of relatively simple media and distinguished from other members of the family by their biochemical characteristics and antigenic structure. The genus *Salmonella* consists of two species; *Salmonella enterica* and *S. bongori*. There are six subspecies of *S. enterica* differentiated by biochemical variations, namely subspecies *enterica* (I), *salamae* (II), *arizonae* (IIIa), *diarizonae* (IIIb), *houtenae* (IV) and *indica* (VI) (Fig. 17.1). There are over 2600 different antigenic types of *Salmonella*. They were originally classified as separate species, but it is now accepted that they represent serotypes (serovars) of *Salmonella enterica*. The nomenclature is often abbreviated, so that *S. enterica* subsp. *enterica* serovar Enteritidis is designated *Salmonella* Enteritidis (*S.* Enteritidis).

HOST RANGE

Subspecies I, *S. enterica* subsp. *enterica* cause 99% of human and animal infections. Members of this group are widely distributed in nature, and all vertebrates appear capable of harbouring these bacteria in their gut. The two main pathologies associated with *S. enterica* are gastroenteritis and typhoidal disease (Fig. 17.1). The typhoidal salmonellae, *S.* Typhi, *S.* Paratyphi A, B and C, all belong to subspecies *enterica*. They are host restricted and only found in humans, rarely undergo recombination events, exhibit convergent evolution driven by genome degradation and are monophyletic. The host generalist serovars, such as *S.* Typhimurium and *S.* Enteritidis, show a wide host range and can be isolated from many different animal species. Host-adapted serovars are those that are adapted to a specific animal reservoir but can infect humans, and include Cholerae-suis (pigs), Dublin (cattle), Gallinarum-pullorum (poultry), Abortus-equi (horses) and Abortus-ovis (sheep).

PATHOGENESIS

In the small bowel, salmonellae cross the intestinal mucous layer and adhere to intestinal epithelial cells using a variety of adhesins including type I fimbriae, curli fimbriae, Pef fimbriae, and Std fimbriae (Fig. 17.2). Following attachment to the host gut mucosa, the bacteria penetrate the intestinal epithelial cells in a complex process that morphologically resembles phagocytosis. Virulence genes involved in invasion and required for intracellular survival are encoded on five pathogenicity islands, SPI1–SPI5. The invasion of the host epithelial cells by *Salmonella* is mediated by T3SS1 effectors (SipA, SipC, SopB, SopE, SopE2) that trigger the rapid appearance of membrane ruffles on the surface of the host cell and subsequent formation of spacious phagosomes or vacuoles.

Following invasion, the bacteria remain within a modified phagosome known as the *Salmonella*-containing

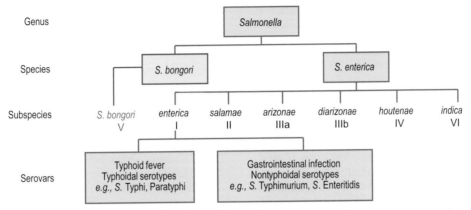

Fig. 17.1 Classification of *Salmonella* species and subspecies.

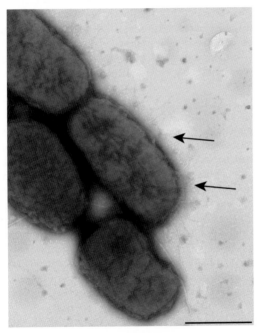

Fig. 17.2 Electron micrograph of *S. Enteritidis*. *Arrows* indicate fimbriae. Bar = 0.5 μm. (From Zuckerman, A. J. (2004) *Principles and Practice of Clinical Virology* (5th ed.). Chichester: John Wiley & Sons Ltd.)

vacuole (SCV), where their survival and replication are controlled by the downregulation of T3SS1 and upregulation of T3SS2 (SseF, SseG, SifA and SseJ). Once inside the host cell, these effectors are capable of altering host cellular functions such as cytoskeletal architecture, membrane trafficking, signal transduction, and cytokine gene expression that result in bacterial intracellular survival and colonisation. The SCVs cross the basolateral membrane and release the bacteria into the submucosa where they are internalised within phagocytes and are disseminated

through the lymph and the bloodstream. All of the clinical manifestations of infection with *Salmonella* begin after ileal penetration, where inflammation of the ileal mucosa results in the efflux of water and electrolytes, resulting in diarrhoea.

CLINICAL SYNDROMES

Although salmonellae can cause a wide spectrum of clinical illness, there are four major syndromes, each with its own diagnostic and therapeutic problems:

- enteric fever
- gastroenteritis
- bacteraemia with or without metastatic infection
- asymptomatic carrier state

Although uncommon, infection with *Salmonella* can result in sequelae, including reactive arthritis (Reiter's syndrome) irritable bowel syndrome, inflammatory bowel disease and Guillain–Barré syndrome.

Enteric fever

Enteric fever is caused by strains of *S.* Typhi or *S.* Paratyphi A, B or C. The clinical features tend to be most severe with *S.* Typhi (typhoid fever). After penetration of the ileal mucosa the organisms pass via the lymphatics to the mesenteric lymph nodes. They multiply and invade the bloodstream via the thoracic duct. The liver, gallbladder, spleen, kidney and bone marrow become infected during this primary bacteraemic phase in the first 7–10 days of the incubation period. After multiplication in these organs, bacilli pass into the blood, causing a second and more acute bacteraemia, the onset of which approximately coincides with that of fever and other signs of clinical illness. From the gallbladder, a secondary invasion of the intestine takes place. Peyer's patches and other gut lymphoid tissues become involved in an inflammatory reaction followed by necrosis, sloughing and the formation of characteristic typhoid ulcers.

Onset

The interval between ingestion of the organisms and the onset of illness varies with the size of the infecting dose. It can be as short as 3 days or as long as 50 days but is usually about 2 weeks. The onset is usually insidious. Early symptoms are often vague: a dry cough and epistaxis associated with anorexia, a dull continuous headache, abdominal tenderness and discomfort are among the most common symptoms. Diarrhoea is uncommon, and early in the illness many patients complain of constipation.

Progression

In the untreated case the temperature shows a stepladder rise over the first week of the illness, remains high for 7–10 days, and then falls during the third or fourth week. Physical signs include a relative bradycardia at the height of the fever, hepatomegaly, splenomegaly and often a rash of rose spots. These are slightly raised, discrete, irregular, blanching, pink macules, 2–4 mm in diameter, most often found on the front of the chest. They appear in crops of up to a dozen at a time and fade after 3–4 days, leaving no scar. They are characteristic of, but not specific for, enteric fever.

Relapse

Apparent recovery can be followed by relapse in 5%–10% of untreated cases. Relapse is usually shorter and of milder character than the initial illness but can be severe and may be fatal. Severe intestinal haemorrhage and intestinal perforation are serious complications that can occur at any stage of the illness.

Morbidity and mortality

Classic typhoid fever is a serious infection that, when untreated, has a mortality rate approaching 20%. It is notoriously unpredictable in its presentation and course. Mild and asymptomatic infections are not uncommon. In endemic areas, and particularly where it co-exists with schistosomiasis, chronic infection can present with fever lasting many months, accompanied by chronic bacteraemia. Occasionally, diarrhoea may dominate the picture from the outset, particularly in paratyphoid infections, which sometimes present as typical gastroenteritis, no different from that caused by most *S. enterica* serotypes.

Gastroenteritis and food poisoning

Acute gastroenteritis is characterised by vomiting, abdominal pain, fever and diarrhoea, often accompanied by headache, malaise and nausea. The incubation period is usually 8–48 hours, the onset abrupt, and the clinical course short and self-limiting. Symptoms vary from the passage of two or three loose stools, which may be disregarded by the sufferer, to a severe and prostrating illness with the frequent passage of watery, green, offensive stools, fever, shivering, abdominal pain and, in the most severe cases, dehydration leading to hypotension, cramps and renal failure. Vomiting is rarely a prominent feature of the illness.

Severe infections occur most often in the very young and the elderly, although mild subclinical infections also occur in these age groups. Infections with certain serotypes in those already ill or debilitated from other causes are likely to be more severe and life threatening. In most cases the acute stage is over within 2–3 days, although it may be more prolonged. Persistent or high fever suggests bacteraemia, possibly with metastatic infection.

Bacteraemia and metastatic disease

Bacteraemia is a constant feature of enteric fever caused by strains of *S.* Typhi and Paratyphi A and C. Rarely, complications of infection with nontyphoidal salmonellae (NTS) can occur. Transient bacteraemia occurs in up to 4% of cases of acute gastroenteritis, but in most cases the organisms are cleared from the bloodstream without ill effect. Occasionally, dissemination of the bacilli throughout the body results in the establishment of one or more localised foci of persisting infection, especially where preexisting abnormality makes a tissue or organ vulnerable. Atherosclerotic plaques within large arteries, damaged heart valves, joint prostheses and other implants are all susceptible to metastatic infection.

Osteomyelitis is most often found in long bones, costochondral junctions and the spine. Multiple bony sites may be affected, and sickle cell anaemia is an important predisposing factor. Suppurative arthritis can occur either as an extension of contiguous osteomyelitis or as a primary infection.

Meningitis is a particularly serious complication of infection in neonates and very young children. Abscess formation can occur in almost any organ or tissue. Even in the absence of obvious tissue damage, the ability of salmonellae to enter and survive within macrophages and other cells, particularly in the liver and biliary tree, but also in bone marrow and the kidney, leads occasionally to persistent infection and the chronic carrier state.

Risk factors predisposing the host to NTS infection include immunosuppression, decreased gastric acidity, recent use of antibiotics, changes in the intestinal micro-biota, hemoglobinopathies and extremes of age. *Salmonella* and HIV coinfections have been reported, and HIV-positive patients are more frequently infected with NTS than with *S.* Typhi.

The prolonged carrier state

Most people infected with *Salmonella* continue to excrete the organism in their stools for days or weeks after complete clinical recovery, but approximately 2%–5% of typhoid patients fail to fully clear the infection within 1 year of recovery, instead progressing to a state of carriage. The basic requirements for establishment of long-term extraintestinal infection are likely to involve successful breach of the intestinal epithelial barrier, evasion of early innate immune-mediated killing and localisation to the biliary tract and gallbladder. The long duration of the carrier state enables the enteric fever bacilli to survive in the community in non-epidemic times and to persist in small and relatively isolated communities. Age, sex and gallbladder abnormalities are important determinants of the frequency of carriage, at least of *S.* Typhi. The risk of becoming a chronic carrier following an acute infection increases with age, is greater for women than for men, and is particularly associated with cholelithiasis and cholecystitis.

Asymptomatic carriage of NTS is thought to occur infrequently (0.15% in healthy adults, 3.9% in children) and is reported most commonly in the context of transplant patients, the elderly, HIV+ individuals and those with malaria coinfection. However, there are numerous well-documented cases of otherwise healthy carriers of NTS. The possibility for long-term human carriage of NTS is particularly important in Sub-Saharan Africa, where recent reports have indicated the emergence of invasive NTS (iNTS) exhibiting numerous characteristics classically associated with typhoidal serovars. For instance, phylo-genetic analysis based on whole genome sequences of such iNTS isolates has indicated genomic degradation representing potential host adaptation.

Infective dose

For human infections, the number of bacteria that must be ingested in order to cause infection is uncertain and varies with the serotype. The accepted dictum that large inocula of these bacteria are required for induction of human illness is based largely on volunteer studies. In most of these, the median infective dose for most serotypes, including Typhi, has varied from 10^6 to 10^9 viable organisms. However, investigation of outbreaks suggests that in natural infection the infective dose might be <1000 viable organisms.

LABORATORY INVESTIGATION

The salmonellae grow well on a wide range of laboratory media. Selective media containing substrates used to facilitate distinction between colonies of pathogenic and nonpathogenic enteric bacteria are used to recover *Salmonella* from specimens from nonsterile sites. For example, detection of *Salmonella* from faeces relies on the use of differential and selective media such as deoxycholate agar (DCA) and xylose-lysine deoxycholate (XLD). Enrichment media, such as tetrathionate or selenite broth, are also useful to detect small numbers of salmonellae in faeces, foods or environmental samples. Suspect colonies are characterised further by their ability to utilise certain sugars and by a range of other biochemical reactions. Several such assays are available commercially (e.g., API 20E and API 20NE from BioMerieux), and more automated identification systems based on the same approach are used in larger microbiology laboratories. MALDI-TOF can identify *Salmonella* to the genus level; however, current protocols are unable to distinguish the different serovars, including the typhoidal serovars. An alternative to MALDI-TOF is separation and detection of bacterial proteins by high-performance liquid chromatography mass spectrom-etry (LC-MS). Recent studies have demonstrated that serovar level identification of *Salmonella* is possible by LC-MS but that it is slower than MALDI-TOF analysis.

PCR assays for the detection of gastrointestinal patho-gens, including *Salmonella* spp., directly from faecal specimens have been implemented in a number of local laboratories, although culture methods are just as sensitive because of the enrichment step. PCRs targeting genes specific for subspecies 1 and 3 and the typhoidal serovars have been described.

Enteric fever
Blood culture

Bone marrow culture is the most reliable method for the diagnosis of enteric fever. The organisms may also be recovered from the bloodstream at any stage of the illness but are most commonly found during the first 7–10 days and during relapses.

Stool and urine culture

Specimens of faeces and urine should be submitted for examination, although the isolation of *Salmonella* from these specimens may indicate merely that the patient is a carrier. In typhoid fever, patients' stools may contain *Salmonella* from the second week and urine cultures from the third week of the infection. In *S.* Paratyphi B infections the clinical course may be much shorter than in typhoid; diarrhoea may occur early, and stool cultures are often positive in the first week of the illness.

Serological tests

Infections with both invasive serotypes may induce specific serum antibodies to *Salmonella* surface antigens, and serological tests have been applied to the routine diagnosis of infection with *S.* Typhi and *S.* Paratyphi A, B and C. The Widal agglutination test, formerly used for the detection of specific O, H and Vi antigens, has been largely replaced by sensitive and specific methods, such as enzyme-linked immunosorbent assay (ELISA) and immunoblotting.

The Widal test is unable to differentiate carriers from individuals with a history of prior infection. In 1934, Arthur Felix identified the Vi antigen and showed that antibody responses to Vi disappeared from the majority of patients recovering from acute typhoid fever but that anti-Vi antigen responses persisted in the blood of chronic carriers. Since then, various modified diagnostic techniques targeting Vi antigen have been developed to increase the specificity and sensitivity of the test. Despite improvements in specificity, there remains ambiguity associated with the use of the test in endemic settings. Novel approaches include identification of antibody responses to antigens uniquely expressed by *S.* Typhi during the carrier state and the identification of other host-associated peripheral blood biomarkers specific to the chronic carrier state.

Serotyping and phage typing

Typical strains of *S. enterica* express two sets of antigens, which are readily demonstrable by serotyping. Long-chain lipopolysaccharide (LPS) comprises heat-stable polysaccharide commonly known as the somatic or O antigens. These molecules are located in the outer membrane and are anchored into the cell wall by antigenically conserved lipid A and LPS-core regions. The long-chain LPS molecules exhibit considerable variation in sugar composition and degree of polysaccharide branching, and this structural heterogeneity is responsible for the large number of serotypes. Salmonellae are usually highly motile when growing in laboratory media, and flagellar protein subunits contain the epitopes that form the basis of the flagella-based serotyping scheme generally known as the H antigens (Fig. 17.3). In most strains of *S. enterica* the flagella exhibit the property of diphasic variation, whereby one of two genetically distinct flagellar structures are expressed. When one flagellar structure is expressed it contains *phase 1* antigens, whereas when the other set is operative, *phase 2* antigens are synthesised.

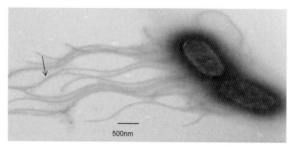

Fig. 17.3 Electron micrograph of *S.* Typhi. *Arrow* indicates the flagella that carry the H antigens. Bar = 500 nm.

Certain serotypes of *S. enterica* express a surface polysaccharide, of which the Vi (virulence) antigen of *S.* Typhi is the most important example. As the polysaccharide may encapsulate the entire bacterium, antibodies designed to recognise the LPS antigens may be prevented from binding; this can occasionally make detection of the O antigens difficult. The Vi antigen is a surface-associated capsular polysaccharide produced by *S.* Typhi, *S.* Dublin and *S.* Paratyphi C. Although not required for colonisation, the Vi capsule is thought to enhance systemic virulence by increasing bacterial resistance to complement and phagocytic killing.

The various O antigens of salmonellae are numbered with Arabic numerals. The flagellar antigens of phase 1 are designated by lowercase letters and those of phase 2 by a mixture of lowercase letters and Arabic numerals. The antigenic structure of any serotype of *Salmonella* is thus expressed as an antigenic formula, which has three parts, describing the O antigens the phase 1 H antigens and the phase 2 H antigens, in that order. The three parts are separated by colons, and the component antigens in each part by commas; for example, the distinctive antigenic formula of *S.* Enteritidis is 1, 9, 12: g, m: 1, 7.

The original Kauffmann–White scheme, which elegantly catalogued salmonellae (but named them as individual species), placed them into some 30 groups on the basis of shared O antigens and further subdivided the groups into clusters with H antigens in common. Some salmonellae, such as *S.* Typhi (9, 12, [Vi]: d), express only one flagellar phase. Some of the most common serotypes are shown in Table 17.1.

Historically, phage typing schemes have proved useful for discriminating within strains of *S. enterica* serotypes Typhimurium, Virchow, Enteritidis and Typhi but are rarely used now.

Molecular typing

There are a number of issues with the serotyping approach; specifically, the expense and expertise required to produce

Table 17.1 Antigenic structure of some representative salmonellae

Serotype	O antigens	H antigens Phase 1	Phase 2
Typhi	9, 12, [Vi]	d	–
Paratyphi B	1, 4, 5, 12	b	1, 2
Typhimurium	1, 4, 5, 12	i	1, 2
Enteritidis	1, 9, 12	g, m	1, 7
Virchow	6, 7	r	1, 2
Kedougou	1, 13, 23	i	1, w
Hadar	6, 8	Z10	e, n, x
Heidelberg	1, 4, 5, 12	r	1, 2
Infantis	6, 7, 14	r	1, 5
Newport	6, 8, 20	e, h	1, 2
Panama	1, 9, 12	l, v	1, 5
Dublin	1, 9, 12	g, p	–

the antisera and that serotyping does not reflect the genetic relatedness between serovars nor does it provide an evolutionary perspective. In 2012, Achtman and colleagues proposed a sequenced-based approach, multilocus sequence typing (MLST), based on the sequences of multiple housekeeping genes. Isolates that possess identical alleles for the seven gene fragments analysed are assigned a common sequence type (ST), and related STs from clonal complexes are termed e-Burst Groups (eBGs). ST and eBGs strongly correlate with serovar, and so this approach facilitates backward compatibility with historical data. Alternative molecular typing methods have been described previously, including pulsed-field gel electrophoresis, ribotyping, repetitive extragenic palindromic sequence-based PCR (rep-PCR) and a combined PCR- and sequencing-based approach that directly targets O and H antigen-encoding genes.

Advances in whole genome sequencing (WGS) methodologies have resulted in the ability to perform high-throughput sequencing of bacterial genomes at low cost, making WGS an economically viable alternative to traditional typing methods for public health surveillance and outbreak detection. WGS has begun to streamline laboratory testing of salmonellae into a single microbiological workflow, supplanting phenotypic, serological and other less robust genotypic typing schemes. For example, WGS bioinformatics pipelines can accurately predict antimicrobial susceptibility patterns, determine serotype and provide multiple virulence profiles for a single strain. It is possible to derive *Salmonella* serotypes from the genome data with reference to either the MLST scheme described by Achtman and colleagues or with the use of the SEQSERO program, recently developed by Deng and colleagues. SEQSERO quickly extracts both O- and H-antigen types from genomic data, quickly predicting serotype with high accuracy when compared with traditional serotyping data. WGS also provides the opportunity to resolve bacterial strains to the single nucleotide resolution needed for identifying cases linked to a common source of infection and has been used to identify outbreak clusters of *Salmonella* in outbreaks associated with eggs (*S.* Enteritidis PT14b), black pepper (*S.* Montivideo), tomato (*S.* Newport), cucumber (*S.* Newport), watermelon (*S.* Newport) and peanut butter (*S.* Tennessee).

TREATMENT

Enteric fever

The introduction of chloramphenicol in 1948 transformed a life-threatening illness of several weeks' duration associated with a mortality rate of >20% into a short-lasting febrile illness with a mortality rate of <2%. The problem of bone marrow toxicity and the emergence of plasmid-mediated chloramphenicol resistance in many parts of the world prompted the search for alternative agents. Amoxicillin and co-trimoxazole are as effective as chloramphenicol and are used widely. However, simultaneous resistance to these drugs has become increasingly common in strains of *S.* Typhi in several endemic areas, and imported multiresistant typhoid is being encountered worldwide. Currently, the first line of therapy in uncomplicated cases in the presence of multidrug resistance is 5–7 days of a fluoroquinolone given at high doses. The alternative therapy includes azithromycin or third-generation cephalosporins. Quinolones remain the best choice for patients in areas where isolates with decreased susceptibility to ciprofloxacin are uncommon, such as Africa, South America and Central America, but should be avoided in many parts of Asia, where the incidence of quinolone resistance is high. The advantages of treating with azithromycin are a prolonged intracellular concentration, oral route of administration and safety in paediatric patients. Cefixime is also safe and effective in paediatric patients. Ceftriaxone is the first line of treatment in the presence of quinolone resistance or decreased susceptibility to ciprofloxacin, while cefixime or azithromycin are used as alternatives. Azithromycin and carbapenems are treatment options in cases of full resistance to ciprofloxacin and cephalosporins, and tigecycline has emerged as an option in ceftriaxone-resistant isolates.

Gastroenteritis

Management of gastroenteritis includes replacement of fluids and electrolytes and control of nausea, vomiting and pain. Drugs to control the hypermotility of the gut are contraindicated; they may give symptomatic relief for a while but can transform a trivial gastroenteritis into a life-threatening bacteraemia by paralysing the bowel. Antibiotics have no part to play in the management in most cases. Randomized, placebo-controlled, double-blind studies have failed to show any benefit from any antibiotic on the duration and severity of the diarrhoea or the duration of fever; some antibiotics seemed to prolong the carrier state.

Therapy should be considered in patients with invasive disease risk, such as neonates, adults >50 years, immunosuppressed patients, and patients with vascular abnormalities or prosthetic valves, grafts or joints. In these cases, a fluoroquinolone is the first-line therapy, and azithromycin, cephalosporins, co-trimoxazole, or ampicillin are alternatives.

The number of multidrug-resistant NTS has increased in many countries since the 1990 report of the multidrug-resistant *S.* Typhimurium DT104 strain that spread around the globe. A European survey from 2000 to 2004 on 135,000 isolates reported NTS resistance among 57%–66%, including multidrug resistance in 15%–18% and resistance to nalidixic acid in 14%–20% during the same period. African and Asian countries report increased numbers of strains resistant to ciprofloxacin and to the cephalosporins. The latter is associated with the production of extended spectrum beta-lactamases.

Salmonella bacteraemia

In bacteraemia, a third-generation cephalosporin or intravenous fluoroquinolone is recommended for 7–14 days. Uncomplicated bacteraemia should be treated for 10–14 days. A careful search for focal metastatic disease should be undertaken, especially when relapse follows cessation of treatment. Surgical drainage of metastatic abscesses may be required, with surgical intervention if heart valves or large vessels are affected.

In *Salmonella* meningitis in infancy, treatment with cefotaxime and ceftriaxone is recommended. Both drugs penetrate into the cerebrospinal fluid reasonably well and are highly active against most salmonellae. Resistance to any of the drugs used to treat invasive infection may occur, so treatment should be supported by susceptibility testing whenever possible.

Chronic asymptomatic carriers

Treatment of the NTS carrier state is not recommended because antibiotic treatment is not superior to placebo for eradication of intestinal carriage in asymptomatic adults. When the patient has chronic cholecystitis or gallstones, antibiotics alone are most unlikely to eradicate the infection. Cholecystectomy together with appropriate antibiotic treatment results in cure in about 90% of cases but has

significant risk, not least from metastatic infection from dissemination of the organisms during surgery.

In the absence of biliary disease, chronic carriage treatment has been tried with 3 months of amoxicillin or co-trimoxazole or 1 month of ciprofloxacin. However, the increasing development of multidrug-resistant strains, decreasing susceptibility to fluoroquinolones and development of beta-lactam resistance complicate the treatment regimens of carriers.

The chronic human carrier is the principal reservoir of enteric fever salmonellae, but even in the developing world, direct person-to-person spread by asymptomatic carriers is uncommon. Typhoid Mary, who is reputed to have caused many infections by her cooking, was an exception. Good personal hygiene, adequate sanitation and a reliable supply of potable water are the real safeguards against enteric fever. Prolonged carriage of other *S. enterica* serotypes is of even less public health importance and rarely justifies exclusion from any employment or intrusive efforts to eradicate the infection.

EPIDEMIOLOGY

Incidence of enteric fever

Historically, strains of *S.* Typhi have been the major cause of typhoidal illness; however, in certain parts of the world, such as south-central Asia and Southeast Asia, the predominant cause of enteric fever is *S.* Paratyphi A. In 2000, an estimated 21.7 million cases of typhoid fever occurred, with 217,000 deaths. In parts of Sub-Saharan Africa, strains of *S.* Enteritidis and *S.* Typhimurium are major causes of bloodstream infections. In England and Wales, *S.* Typhi and *S.* Paratyphi account for most systemic infections (Fig. 17.4). Cases of enteric fever in endemic areas are generally more frequent in infants, preschool-age and school-aged children than in adults. The highest incidence has been documented in impoverished, overcrowded areas with poor access to sanitation, such as the urban slum areas of North Jakarta (Indonesia), Kolkata (India) and Karachi (Pakistan), with annual incidence rates of blood culture–confirmed enteric fever ranging from 180 to 494/100,000 among 5–15-year-olds and 140–573/100,000 among those 2–4 years old.

Gastroenteritis and *Salmonella* food poisoning

Worldwide, *Salmonella* is one of the most prevalent causes of foodborne illness. Globally, the annual incidence of foodborne salmonellosis is conservatively estimated at 80.3 million cases, but other estimates range from 200 million to 1.3 billion cases. In the United States, it was estimated that nontyphoidal *Salmonella* spp. are responsible

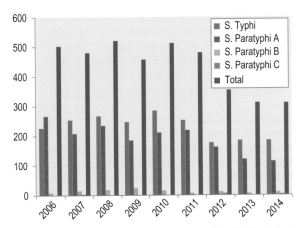

Fig. 17.4 Human cases of *S.* Typhi and *S.* Paratyphi identified in England and Wales from 2006 to 2014. (Public Health England.)

for 1 million cases of domestically acquired foodborne illness annually. The estimated NTS-associated illnesses incidence in Europe is 690 per 100,000 inhabitants per year. This incidence varies among regions from 240 per 100,000 in Western Europe to 2390 per 100,000 person-years in Central Europe. In the United States the Foodborne Diseases Active Surveillance Network (FoodNet) found that NTS infections were the most commonly reported (17.6 cases per 100,000 inhabitants), and the incidence has not declined since 1996, when the surveillance was initiated. FoodNet data from 1996 to 2005 report that NTS infections have been the leading cause of death (39%) among foodborne bacterial pathogens, with highest mortality among adults >65 years and highest incidence among children <5 years of age (69.5 infections per 100,000 children).

Childhood infections were associated with day-care centre attendance and contact with cats or reptiles. FoodNet reported an incidence of invasive salmonellosis of 0.9 cases per 100,000 inhabitants, with the highest risk among infants (7.8 cases per 100,000 inhabitants).

Source attribution

No other zoonosis is as complex in its epidemiology and control as salmonellosis. Transmission to humans can occur by consumption of food animal products, nonanimal food products, contaminated water or contact with animals. Farm animals are the major reservoir for NTS in industrialised countries. NTS are naturally found in chickens, ducklings, sheep, goats, pigs, reptiles, amphibians, birds, pet rodents, dogs, cats and a variety of wild animals. NTS pet transmission to humans easily occurs by contact with animal faeces.

The carcasses or products (cooked meats, eggs, milk) of naturally infected domestic animals are the most common sources of food poisoning. Poultry (particularly hens), ducks and turkeys, and their eggs, are the most significant reservoirs of food poisoning salmonellae globally. In the United States between 1985 and 2002 contamination of eggs was identified as the source of 53% of all cases of *Salmonella* reported to the Centers for Disease Control and Prevention (CDC). The incidence of salmonellosis in each country in the European Union correlates significantly with the presence of *Salmonella enterica* serotype Enteritidis in laying hens, suggesting this is the primary source of infection across Europe. Since 1998 there has been a steady decline in the numbers of salmonellas causing intestinal infection in England and Wales, largely because of vaccination of broiler flocks and restrictions of the importation of eggs from abroad.

Pigs share the honours with poultry in much of Northern Europe, whereas beef cattle are important sources in the United States. Rats and mice are commonly infected with food-poisoning salmonellae and may contaminate human food with their faeces.

Food poisoning may occasionally be caused by food contaminated by a human case or carrier, and the more sophisticated the manipulation of the food, the greater the chance of contamination.

Outbreaks

Frequent factors associated with outbreaks of salmonellosis include raw ingredients in contact with contaminated animal or people, improper storage or incomplete cooking of food products. In a Canadian study, almost a third (30%) of *Salmonella* foodborne outbreaks between 1976 and 2005 were associated with fresh vegetables and fruit (produce) and 15% with poultry meat. In the United States between 1998 and 2002, most foodborne outbreaks linked to *Salmonella* were associated with complex multiingredient foods and eggs. In England and Wales, most salmonellosis outbreaks were linked to poultry meat (21%), with fresh vegetables and fruit (produce) accounting for only 5%.

In recent years in England and Wales, there has been a reduction in outbreaks attributed to *Salmonella* spp. The decline in *S.* Enteritidis PT4 outbreaks (commonly associated with the consumption of contaminated hen eggs) clearly indicates the effect of successful intervention measures, such as improved biosecurity and vaccination of UK poultry flocks introduced in the late 1990s. This interpretation is supported by similar trends in salmonellosis post introduction of similar control measures in other countries.

In contrast, outbreaks attributed to *S.* Enteritidis non-PT4 across Europe are increasing (mainly PT1 and PT14b), with the majority of these associated with eggs or egg dishes linked to food service establishments. This resurgence is associated with substantive changes in market supply, with the sourcing of eggs from other egg producers in member states where there is a lack of vaccination of layer flocks against *Salmonella* or controlled assurance, and this continues to be a public health concern.

Surveillance

Several online networks (see Websites section later in the chapter) have been established to enable the rapid exchange of information relating to outbreaks of disease. The CDC curates the International Molecular Subtyping Network for Foodborne Disease Surveillance, dubbed PulseNet. This site presents the six regional networks and different protocols for the molecular subtyping of *Salmonella*. The website, supported by the World Health Organization, contains phenotypic and epidemiological information from the Global Salm-Surv *Salmonella* surveillance programme, including information on the major *Salmonella* serovars identified globally as well as antimicrobial resistance. The European Centre for Disease Prevention and Control (ECDC) performs *Salmonella* surveillance in all EU member states.

PREVENTION AND CONTROL

Enteric fever

The most important measures for enteric infection prevention are provision of safe water access, safe food handling practices, sanitation measures, public education and vaccination. Enteric fever is a public health problem only where the wide public availability of wholesome drinking water and the provision of adequate means for the proper disposal of human excreta do not exist. Chlorination of water sources suspected to be contaminated is recommended during enteric fever outbreaks. The improvement in safe water and sanitation, the primary goal for prevention, is difficult to achieve in developing countries.

Nontyphoidal Salmonella

For NTS, measures to limit the number of infections from animals may include proper hand washing after being in contact with animals in general and contact avoidance with all animals, especially amphibians known to be 90% colonised with *Salmonella* spp.

To reduce the incidence of food poisoning, whether due to salmonellae or to other bacteria, two basic precepts must be observed:

1. Raw foodstuffs of animal origin, which are always potentially contaminated, must never have direct or indirect contact with cooked foods.
2. Foodstuff thought to be contaminated should be treated or held under temperature conditions that prevent the organisms from growing.

Cooked foods should be served and eaten immediately after cooking and while still hot or cooled rapidly and held at refrigerator temperature until eaten so that at least the inoculum eaten by any individual is small. It is often found that the food incriminated in an outbreak had been cooked several hours or even a day or two before and then left at room temperature before being reheated immediately before serving. This procedure ensures that salmonellae that survived the initial cooking or gained access to the food from contaminated kitchen surfaces or implements had excellent opportunities to multiply in the interval before being warmed up for consumption. Health education, particularly of food handlers, is a most important and continuing requirement.

Vaccination

Heat-killed, phenol-preserved whole-cell vaccines have been used for many years in countries with a high endemic level of typhoid fever. The parenteral Vi vaccine was licensed in 1990, and it is based on a capsular polysaccharide antigen of *S.* Typhi. This vaccine, widely used in developing and industrialised countries, is licensed for adults and children >2 years. Vi vaccine is safe in immunocompromised hosts and administrated in a single parenteral dose with a booster recommended every 2 years. To improve capsular polysaccharide immunogenicity it has been covalently linked to recombinant *Pseudomonas aeruginosa* exoprotein A (Vi-rEPA). The conjugated vaccine produces a T-cell dependent response and induces immunological memory that may result in prolonged protection (see Chs 9 and 68). Vi capsular polysaccharide-based vaccines, however, are unlikely to provide effective protection against *S.* Paratyphi, since they lack the Vi antigen.

Alternatively, an oral live-attenuated typhoid vaccine is used. The currently approved oral live attenuated *S.* Typhi Ty21a vaccine was derived from the wild-type Ty2 *S.* Typhi strain after chemical mutagenesis. Oral administration mimics the infection route that the wild-type strain would take and it induces not only humoral and cellular immune responses at the mucosal level but also systemically. This vaccine is well tolerated, and the duration of protection is at least 5 years, at which time a booster is recommended. Side effects are mild, infrequent and limited to gastrointestinal discomfort or fever. However, the administration of live-attenuated *Salmonella* vaccines to immunosuppressed individuals, including HIV-infected individuals, is not recommended. Other disadvantages of this vaccine include the need for multiple doses, cold-chain dependence and poor immunogenicity in younger children.

The World Health Organization recommends vaccination to travellers. Travellers to endemic areas, where incidence of typhoid fever is high and standards of hygiene are poor, should be offered immunisation, especially if they intend to visit rural areas.

RECOMMENDED READING

Ao, T. T., Feasey, N. A., Gordon, M. A., Keddy, K. H., Angulo, F. J., & Crump, J. A. (2015). Global burden of invasive nontyphoidal *Salmonella* disease, 2010. *Emerging Infectious Diseases, 21*(6), 941–949. doi:10.3201/eid2106.140999.

Bell, R. L., Jarvis, K. G., Ottesen, A. R., McFarland, M. A., & Brown, E. W. (2016). Recent and emerging innovations in *Salmonella* detection: a food and environmental perspective. *Microbial Biotechnology, 9*(3), 279–292. doi:10.1111/1751-7915.12359.

Crump, J. A., & Mintz, E. D. (2010). Global trends in typhoid and paratyphoid Fever. *Clinical Infectious Diseases, 50*(2), 241–246. doi:10.1086/649541.

Gunn, J. S., Marshall, J. M., Baker, S., Dongol, S., Charles, R. C., & Ryan, E. T. (2014). *Salmonella* chronic carriage: epidemiology, diagnosis and gallbladder persistence. *Trends in Microbiology, 22*(11), 648–655. doi:10.1016/j.tim.2014.06.007.

Langridge, G. C., Fookes, M., Connor, T. R., Feltwell, T., Feasey, N., Parsons, B. N., ... Thomson, N. R. (2015). Patterns of genome evolution that have accompanied host adaptation in *Salmonella*. *Proceedings of the National Academy of Sciences of the United States of America, 112*(3), 863–868. doi:10.1073/pnas.1416707112.

Majowicz, S. E., Musto, J., Scallan, E., Angulo, F. J., Kirk, M., O'Brien, S. J., ... International Collaboration on Enteric Disease 'Burden of Illness' Studies. (2010). The global burden of nontyphoidal *Salmonella* gastroenteritis. *Clinical Infectious Diseases, 50*(6), 882–889. doi:10.1086/650733.

Michael, G. B., & Schwarz, S. (2016). Antimicrobial resistance in zoonotic nontyphoidal *Salmonella*: an alarming trend? *Clinical Microbiology and Infection, 22*(12), 968–974. doi:10.1016/j.cmi.2016.07.033.

Raffatellu, M., Wilson, R. P., Winter, S. E., & Bäumler, A. J. (2008). Clinical pathogenesis of typhoid fever. *Journal of Infection in Developing Countries, 2*(4), 260–266.

Sánchez-Vargas, F. M., Abu-El-Haija, M. A., & Gómez-Duarte, O. G. (2011). Salmonella infections: an update on epidemiology, management, and prevention. *Travel Medicine and Infectious Disease, 9*(6), 263–277. doi:10.1016/j.tmaid.2011.11.001.

Wain, J., House, D., Parkhill, J., Parry, C., & Dougan, G. (2002). Unlocking the genome of the human typhoid bacillus. *The Lancet Infectious Diseases, 2*(3), 163–170.

Wain, J., Hendriksen, R. S., Mikoleit, M. L., Keddy, K. H., & Ochiai, R. L. (2015). Typhoid fever. *Lancet, 385*(9973), 1136–1145. doi:10.1016/S0140-6736(13)62708-7.

Websites

Centers for Disease Control and Prevention. *Salmonella*. Available at http://www.cdc.gov/salmonella/.

European Centre for Disease Preventiona dn Control. Available at http://ecdc.europa.eu/en/Pages/home.aspx.

Public Health England. *Salmonella*: guidance, data and analysis. Available at https://www.gov.uk/government/collections/salmonella-guidance-data-and-analysis.

Public Health England. Typhoid and paratyphoid: guidance, data and analysis. Available at https://www.gov.uk/government/collections/typhoid-and-paratyphoid-guidance-data-and-analysis.

PulseNet International. Available at http://www.pulsenetinternational.org.

SeqSero 1.0. *Salmonella* serotyping by whole genome sequencing. Available at http://www.denglab.info/SeqSero.

Warwick Medical School. EnteroBase. Available at https://enterobase.warwick.ac.uk/.

Wellcome Trust Sanger Institute. *Salmonella*. Available at http://www.sanger.ac.uk/resources/downloads/bacteria/salmonella.html.

World Health Organization. Global Foodborne Infections Network (GFN). Available at http://www.who.int/salmsurv/en/.

18 *Klebsiella, Enterobacter, Proteus* and other enterobacteria

Urinary tract infection; bacteraemia; pneumonia; antimicrobial resistance

MICHAEL R. BARER AND ANDREW SWANN

KEY POINTS

- Many of these genera are notable as reservoirs of transmissible antimicrobial resistance and are significant causes of hospital-acquired infection.
- *Klebsiella* spp. cause urinary tract infections and, less frequently, biliary sepsis, liver abscess, bacteraemia and pneumonia.
- *Enterobacter* spp. have many features in common with *Klebsiella* spp.
- *Hafnia alvei* is closely related to *Enterobacter* spp. and is an opportunistic pathogen.
- *Serratia* spp. are opportunistic pathogens causing respiratory and wound infections, meningitis and bacteraemia.
- Strains of *Proteus, Providentia* and *Morganella* are closely related. They are regularly isolated from urinary tract infections.
- Antibiotic susceptibilities of these genera are unpredictable, and treatment should be guided by laboratory results.

The genera described in this chapter conform to the general definition of the Enterobacteriaceae in that they are aerobic or facultatively anaerobic, ferment glucose and produce catalase but not oxidase. Together with organisms of the genera *Salmonella* (Ch. 17), *Shigella, Escherichia* (Ch. 16) and *Yersinia* (Ch. 19), they are commonly referred to as Enterobacteriaceae. Lactose-fermenting genera of the enterobacteria are sometimes referred to as coliforms.

Species of clinical interest are listed alphabetically in Table 18.1, along with common synonyms.

KLEBSIELLA

CLASSIFICATION

The name *Klebsiella aerogenes* was originally used for the nonmotile, capsulate, gas-producing strains commonly found in human faeces and in water; certain biochemically atypical *Klebsiella* strains isolated from the respiratory tract of humans and animals were designated *K. pneumoniae*. The name *K. pneumoniae* is now used for the species as a whole, and the former *K. aerogenes* is referred to as *K. pneumoniae* subspecies *aerogenes*. The atypical respiratory strains are included in the subspecies *ozaenae, pneumoniae* and *rhinoscleromatis* (Table 18.1). A further species, *K. oxytoca,* is encountered occasionally in clinical specimens.

DESCRIPTION

Klebsielleae are nonmotile, capsulate Gram-negative rods about 1–2 μm long. They are facultative anaerobes, but growth under strictly anaerobic conditions is poor. They may survive drying for months and remain viable for many weeks at room temperature. Species can be differentiated by simple biochemical tests. Capsular material is produced in greater amounts on media rich in carbohydrate. In these conditions the growth on agar is luxuriant, greyish white and extremely mucoid (Fig. 18.1). The polysaccharides of the different capsular types are complex acid polysaccharides and resemble the K-antigens of *Escherichia coli* (see Ch. 16).

About 80 capsular (K) antigens are presently recognised. Types K1, K2, K3, K5 and K21 are of particular significance in human disease, and the prevalence of these types

Table 18.1 Principal genera and species of Enterobacteriaceae of clinical interest

Genus	Species	Synonyms
Citrobacter	Cit. amalonaticus	Levinea amalonatica
	Cit. freundii	
	Cit. koseri	C. diversus, L. amalonatica
Cronobacter	C. sakazakii	
Edwardsiella	E. tarda	E. anguillimortifera
Enterobacter	Ent. aerogenes	K. mobilis
	Ent. cloacae	
	Ent. agglomerans	Erwinia herbicola
Escherichia[a]		
Hafnia	H. alvei	Ent. alvei, Ent. hafniae
Klebsiella	K. oxytoca	
	K. pneumoniae	
	ssp. aerogenes	K. aerogenes
	ssp. ozaenae	K. ozaenae
	ssp. pneumoniae	K. pneumoniae
	ssp. rhinoscleromatis	K. rhinoscleromatis
Morganella	M. morganii	Pr. morganii
Proteus	Pr. mirabilis	
	Pr. vulgaris	
Providencia	Prov. alcalifaciens	
	Prov. rettgeri	Pr. rettgeri
	Prov. stuartii	
Salmonella[a]		
Serratia	S. liquefaciens	Ent. liquefaciens
	S. marcescens	
	S. odorifera	
Shigella[a]		
Yersinia[a]		

[a]See appropriate chapter.

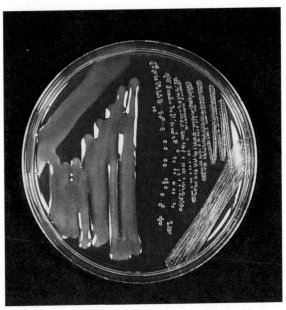

Fig. 18.1 Mucoid *(left)* and nonmucoid *(right)* variants of *Klebsiella* species on carbohydrate-rich medium. (Courtesy George Sharp and Richard Edwards, Queen's Medical Centre, Nottingham.)

limits the usefulness of capsular serotyping as an epidemiological tool.

Strains express long-chain lipopolysaccharide (somatic or O antigens), and 12 O-types are recognised, although somatic antigen typing can be hampered by capsular polysaccharide layers. Certain O-antigens are identical to or related to *E. coli* O-antigens. It is therefore possible to divide *Klebsiella* strains into a small number of groups that may be further subdivided into capsular types, but this is of little practical value in classification.

There is some association between antigenic structure, biochemical activities and habitat. Members of capsular types 1–6 occur most frequently in the human respiratory tract. Considerable overlap occurs with capsular antigens of unrelated organisms; capsular type 2, for example, is immunologically similar to the type 2 pneumococcus.

Capsular swelling (specific antibody-mediated differentiation of capsule types), bacteriocin and phage typing methods have been used in the past, but these phenotypic approaches have now been replaced by MLST and whole

genome sequencing. Some authors divide *K. pneumoniae* strains into classical and hypervirulent (HV) biotypes. The former are commonly associated with antibiotic resistance and hospital-acquired infections while the latter are less frequently resistant but are associated with aggressive community-acquired infections including liver abscesses. HV strains were first reported in Taiwan but are now well recognised in Southeast Asia and sporadically elsewhere.

PATHOGENESIS

Klebsiella spp. are primarily a cause of infections involving the urinary tract but may also cause soft tissue infections, endocarditis, central nervous system infections, and cases of severe bronchopneumonia, sometimes with chronic destructive lesions and multiple abscess formation in the lungs (Friedländer's pneumonia) and liver. In many cases there is also bacteraemia, and the mortality rate is high.

Colonisation of the respiratory tract is very common in hospital patients receiving antibiotics, but its clinical significance is often difficult to assess. Some debilitated patients develop bronchopneumonia in which a *Klebsiella* spp. appears to be the primary infecting agent.

The *ozaenae* and *rhinoscleromatis* subspecies of *K. pneumoniae* take their names from the diseases with which they are associated. Rhinoscleroma is a chronic upper respiratory tract disease that occurs in many parts of the world, where it is associated with prolonged exposure to crowded and unhygienic conditions. The lesions occur in the nose, larynx, throat and, to a lesser extent, trachea and consist of granulomatous infiltrations of the submucosa. Ozaena (atrophic rhinitis) is an uncommon chronic disease of the nasal mucosa, in which *K. pneumoniae* ssp. *ozaenae* is of disputed significance.

Pathogenic mechanisms

Expression of a polysaccharide capsule is a major pathogenic mechanism providing strains with protection against opsonisation and the action of serum complement; so-called hypercapsule production is associated with HV strains. Adhesion to host tissues has been attributed to the expression of a range of fimbrial and nonfimbrial adhesins. In common with other members of the Entero-bacteriaceae, *Klebsiella* expresses type 1 fimbriae that exhibit mannose-sensitive haemagglutination and probably play a role in adhesion to the human host. Strains may also express type 3 fimbriae, which may be used to adhere to material in the environment. Additional fimbrial structures (type 6 and KPF-28) and non-fimbrial adhesins have been described. Adhesins CF29K and CS31A are plasmid-encoded and enable strains to adhere to cultured human intestinal cell lines. Such strains may also be invasive, a process that involves an outer membrane protein, OmpX.

In common with many enteric bacteria, *Klebsiella* expresses an enterobactin-mediated iron-sequestering system that uses ferric siderophore receptors anti-genically related to those expressed by strains of *E. coli*. Less frequently, strains of *Klebsiella* may also express various combinations of aerobactin, yersiniabactin or salmochelin. The importance of iron in infections with *Klebsiella* can be illustrated by the fact that strains are particularly virulent in patients with iron-overload conditions such as thalassaemia. Infections are also particularly associated with diabetes, liver disease and solid organ transplantation.

TREATMENT

Clinical isolates of *Klebsiella* characteristically produce a chromosomally encoded β-lactamase that renders them resistant to ampicillin and amoxicillin, but combinations of these drugs with β-lactamase inhibitors such as clavulanic acid are often effective. Third-generation cephalosporins may be effective, but ESBLs are found with increasing frequency. The relationship between possession of multiple genes encoding β-lactamases and phenotypic resistance appears complex, and well-standardised

susceptibility testing is currently considered a better guide to therapy than detection of specific mechanisms. Carbapenemases expressing *K. pneumoniae* were first detected in 1996, and such strains are now widespread, and it appears that *Klebsiella* has been significant in disseminating multiple varieties of this group of enzymes.

Klebsiella infection of the urinary tract often responds to trimethoprim, nitrofurantoin, co-amoxiclav or oral cephalosporins. Pneumonia and other serious infections may respond to co-amoxiclav, but agents such as piperacillin-tazobactam or carbapenems are frequently required.

ENTEROBACTER

DESCRIPTION

Enterobacter species have many features in common with those of the genus *Klebsiella* but are readily distinguished by their motility, although nonmotile variants occur occasionally. *Ent. cloacae* is clinically the most important species. *Ent. agglomerans*, an anaerogenic, yellow-pigmented organism, formerly known as *Erwinia herbicola*, is also encountered occasionally. Strains of *Ent. amnigenus* and *Ent. asburiae* have also been isolated from human infections.

The colonies of *Enterobacter* strains may be slightly mucoid. In general, their fermentative activity is more limited than that of typical *Klebsiella*.

PATHOGENESIS

The normal habitat of *Enterobacter* spp. is probably soil and water, but the organisms are occasionally found in human faeces and the respiratory tract. Infection of hospital patients, notably of the urinary tract, occurs. *Enterobacter* spp. are also an important cause of bacteraemia but much less so than *Klebsiella* spp.

The pathogenic mechanisms are poorly understood. In common with certain strains of *Klebsiella*, they express type 1 and type 3 fimbriae. Most strains also express an aerobactin-mediated iron-uptake system, which is generally associated with extraintestinal human bacterial pathogens. Strains may produce a haemolysin resembling the α-haemolysin produced by strains of *E. coli*. Very rarely, strains hybridize with gene probes for verocytotoxin 1 (see Ch. 16).

An outer membrane protein, termed *OmpX*, may be a pathogenic factor for strains of *Ent. cloacae*. This protein appears to reduce production of porins, leading to decreased sensitivity to β-lactam antibiotics, and might play a role in host cell invasion.

TREATMENT

Enterobacter strains produce a chromosomal β-lactamase with cephalosporinase activity and are nearly always highly resistant to penicillins and many cephalosporins. Many are also resistant to tetracyclines, chloramphenicol and streptomycin, although most are sensitive to other aminoglycosides, including gentamicin. Most strains are susceptible to fluoroquinolones, co-trimoxazole and carbapenems. *Enterobacter* strains differ from *Serratia* strains in being sensitive to the polymyxins.

CRONOBACTER

DESCRIPTION

Cronobacter sakazakii is one of several related species and subspecies of *Cronobacter* formerly included with the genus *Enterobacter*. Strains can be detected by 16S-23S rRNA gene sequencing.

PATHOGENESIS

C. sakazakii is an emerging pathogen associated with powdered milk, causing necrotising enterocolitis, sepsis and meningitis in infants. In England, Wales and Northern Ireland, 72 cases of bacteraemia were identified in 2004, declining to 28 in 2013. The mechanisms by which disease is caused appear to include adhesion to the host tissues, multiplication within host tissues and possibly toxins.

TREATMENT AND CONTROL

Disease usually responds to treatment with ampicillin and gentamicin. Infections associated with powdered milk can be prevented by irradiation or other means of disinfection.

HAFNIA

DESCRIPTION

Hafnia alvei was also formerly placed in the genus *Enterobacter*. At present the genus contains only one species.

Strains of *H. alvei* are motile, noncapsulate, Gram-negative rods that grow well on general laboratory media at 30–37°C and can be differentiated by biotyping. There is an antigenic scheme for *H. alvei* that includes many serotypes, and strains can be characterised further by phage typing.

PATHOGENESIS

Strains are found in the faeces of humans and other animals and also in sewage, soil, water and dairy products. *H. alvei* is encountered in blood, urine or wounds of hospital patients as an opportunist pathogen. Strains express mannose-resistant and mannose-sensitive haemagglutination indicating expression of type-1 fimbriae. A siderophore-mediated high-affinity iron uptake mechanism has been described, and the bacteria can utilize siderophores expressed by strains of *E. coli*. Some strains can cause attaching and effacing lesions of intestinal cells, as described for strains of enteropathogenic *E. coli* (EPEC; see Ch. 16).

TREATMENT

Strains are usually sensitive to carbapenems, chloramphenicol, quinolones, aminoglycosides and trimethoprim but resistant to penicillins.

SERRATIA

DESCRIPTION

Although numerous *Serratia* species have been described, *S. marcescens* is the one most commonly encountered in clinical specimens. Several others, including *S. liquefaciens* (formerly known as *Ent. liquefaciens*) and *S. odorifera*, are sometimes isolated.

Serratia spp. are motile Gram-negative rods that grow well on laboratory media at 30–37°C and utilise most carbohydrates with the production of acid and gas. They vary considerably in size, ranging from small coccobacilli to rods indistinguishable from other enterobacteria. Capsules are not normally formed, except on a well-aerated medium poor in nitrogen and phosphate. Certain strains of *S. marcescens* produce red-pigmented colonies on agar. The pigment, prodigiosin, is formed only in the presence of oxygen and at a suitable temperature, which is not necessarily the same as that for optimal growth. Certain organisms unrelated to *S. marcescens,* including an actinomycete and certain

Gram-negative rods isolated from seawater, also form prodigiosin.

PATHOGENESIS

S. marcescens and other *Serratia* species are widely distributed in nature, but faecal carriage is uncommon in the general human population. Pigmented strains may cause concern by giving rise to red colours in food or by simulating the appearance of blood in the sputum or faeces. Pigmented and nonpigmented strains are found occasionally in the human respiratory tract and in faeces. Most infections occur in hospital patients; they include infections of the urinary and respiratory tracts, meningitis, wound infections, bacteraemia and endocarditis. Some strains become established endemically in hospitals and may cause outbreaks of infection. *Serratia* spp. can multiply at ambient temperatures in fluids containing minimal nutrients, and outbreaks have followed the introduction of the organisms directly into the bloodstream in contaminated transfusion fluids. Only a small proportion of the strains responsible for infection are pigmented.

Pathogenic mechanisms

Serratia spp. may express a range of fimbriae including those exhibiting mannose-sensitive and mannose-resistant haemagglutination, although the tissue specificity of these adhesins is unknown. Some strains express cell surface components, causing them to be highly hydrophobic, and this may be involved in adhesion to eukaryotic cell surfaces. The expression of long-chain LPS has been described as a pathogenic mechanism for *S. marcescens*. A 56-kDa protease, which may be involved in host tissue damage, has been detected in virulent strains of *S. marcescens*. An iron-regulated haemolysin has been described, but a role for this toxin in the pathogenesis of disease has not been demonstrated. *Serratia* spp. also expresses an enterobactin-mediated high-affinity iron-uptake system, and some may acquire ferric ions mediated by aerobactin. Toxins resembling *E. coli* verocytotoxin and heat-labile toxin have been described.

TREATMENT

Serratia strains are commonly resistant to cephalosporins. Resistance to ampicillin and gentamicin is variable, but many strains destroy these antibiotics enzymatically. An aminoglycoside, such as gentamicin, is usually the most reliable first-line choice. Fluoroquinolones or carbapenems may be useful in recalcitrant cases.

PROTEUS AND RELATED GENERA

CLASSIFICATION

The history of the genera *Proteus, Providencia* and *Morganella* is inextricably linked, and they are best considered together.

There has been much debate over the taxonomy of this group, with successive proposals to combine and separate the genera *Proteus* and *Providencia*. The organisms once known as biotypes A and B of *Proteus inconstans* are now regarded as separate species of the genus *Providencia*: *Prov. alcalifaciens* and *Prov. stuartii*. Similarly, *Proteus rettgeri* is now known as *Prov. rettgeri*, even though it resembles *Proteus* spp. rather than other organisms of the genus *Providencia* in producing urease. The former *Pr. morganii* has been allocated to a new genus, *Morganella*, and is known as *Morganella morganii*. This leaves only *Pr. vulgaris* and *Pr. mirabilis* in the genus *Proteus*.

DESCRIPTION

There is considerable morphological variation, but in agar-grown cultures the microscopical appearance is much like that of other coliform bacteria. Strains of *Proteus* spp. can be differentiated from *Morganella* spp. and *Providencia* spp. by their ability to swarm on suitable agar media; the swarming characteristically takes place in a discontinuous manner, with each period of outward progress followed by a stationary period (Fig. 18.2). Various methods have been devised to inhibit swarming, mainly to avoid interference with the isolation of other organisms.

The various species are differentiated by standard biochemical tests and MALDI. Swarming in *Pr. mirabilis* is a complex multicellular phenomenon. Strains exhibit the Dienes phenomenon (the mutual inhibition of swarming), and this forms the basis for a precise method of differentiation among such strains. Test organisms are inoculated on to the surface of an agar plate, and those that show no line of demarcation in areas where the swarming growths meet are regarded as identical.

PATHOGENESIS

Pr. mirabilis is a prominent cause of urinary tract infection and of bacteraemia. Other strains of *Proteus* and *Providencia* are usually isolated from hospital patients, especially in elderly men following surgery or instrumentation. Bacteraemia generally occurs only in patients with serious

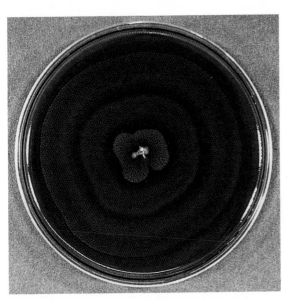

Fig. 18.2 Swarming growth of *Pr. mirabilis* inoculated centrally onto a blood agar plate and incubated overnight at 37°C. (Courtesy George Sharp and Richard Edwards, Queen's Medical Centre, Nottingham.)

underlying conditions or as a complication of urinary tract surgery, but outbreaks of bacteraemia, often with meningitis, may occur among the newborn in hospitals. A variety of other infections, usually of surgical wounds or bedsores, occur in hospitals and are usually considered to originate from the gut microbiota.

M. morganii is uncommon in human disease but occasionally causes infections in hospital patients.

Pathogenic mechanisms

These bacteria are characteristically highly motile, and chemotaxis may play a part in pathogenesis. Strains of *Proteus* spp. express mannose-resistant haemagglutination and may also produce calcium-dependent and calcium-independent haemolysins in addition to a range of proteases such as an IgAase. *M. morganii* exhibits mannose-sensitive haemagglutination and expresses phenolate and hydroxamate siderophores for high-affinity iron uptake.

Proteus spp. and other urease-producing organisms create alkaline conditions in the urine and may provoke the formation of calculi (stones) in the urinary tract.

TREATMENT

Most strains of *Pr. mirabilis* do not produce β-lactamase; they are consequently sensitive to ampicillin and most other β-lactam antibiotics. *Pr. vulgaris* strains are usually resistant to penicillins and many cephalosporins,

although they may be sensitive to β-lactamase–stable derivatives such as cefotaxime. All strains are resistant to polymyxins and tetracyclines. *Proteus* and *Providencia* strains are inherently sensitive to aminoglycosides, but enzymic or nonenzymic resistance mechanisms are now common.

Pr. mirabilis urinary tract infections usually respond to ampicillin or trimethoprim, but nitrofurantoin is not effective. Treatment of infection associated with renal stones is often unsuccessful. Serious infection with other *Proteus, Providencia* or *Morganella* strains can often be treated with an aminoglycoside or a cephalosporin such as cefotaxime. However, susceptibility is unpredictable and treatment should be guided by laboratory findings.

CITROBACTER

DESCRIPTION

The genus *Citrobacter* was first proposed for a group of lactose-negative or late lactose-fermenting Gram-negative bacilli that share certain somatic antigens with salmonellae and were also known as the Ballerup-Bethesda group. These organisms are now known as *Citrobacter freundii*. Other species included in the genus are *Cit. koseri* (formerly known as *Cit. diversus*) and *Cit. amalonaticus*. They grow well on ordinary media and are unpigmented. Mucoid forms sometimes occur.

Serotyping schemes based on the LPS antigens have been developed for *Cit. freundii* and *Cit. koseri*. Antigen–antibody cross-reactions between strains of *Citrobacter* spp. and strains of *Salmonella* and *E. coli* have been described. For example, certain strains of *Cit. freundii* share LPS epitopes with *E. coli* expressing O157 antigens.

PATHOGENESIS

Citrobacter spp. are often found in human faeces and may be isolated from a variety of clinical specimens. They do not often give rise to serious infections but may cause bacteraemia.

Cit. koseri occasionally causes neonatal meningitis; in this condition there is a high mortality rate, and the formation of cerebral abscesses is common.

Pathogenic mechanisms expressed by strains of *Citrobacter* spp. are poorly understood. Strains of *Cit. koseri* express type 1 (mannose-sensitive) fimbriae, and occasional strains produce a form of *E. coli*, verocytotoxin type 2.

TREATMENT

Cit. freundii is usually sensitive to aminoglycosides, fluoroquinolones and chloramphenicol; sensitivity to ampicillin, tetracycline and cephalosporins varies. Resistance to aminoglycosides occurs frequently among *Cit. koseri* strains. Choice of treatment should be based on laboratory tests of susceptibility.

EDWARDSIELLA

Edwardsiella tarda, E. hoshinae and *E. ictaluri* belong to a group of Enterobacteriaceae with distinctive properties, originally described as the Asakusa group. Members of the genus are small, motile, facultatively anaerobic Gram-negative rods and grow optimally at 37°C. Strains are biochemically inactive compared with other members of the Enterobacteriaceae but will utilise glucose. They grow well on ordinary media but produce only small colonies 0.5–1 mm in diameter after 24 hours.

Edwardsiella spp. are principally associated with freshwater environments and can be isolated from healthy amphibians, reptiles and fish. *E. tarda* is most frequently associated with human disease. Two biotypes of *E. tarda* exist in nature, with most human infections caused by biotype 2. Wound infection is most common, but meningitis and septicaemia have been reported. This bacterium is rarely found in the faeces of healthy people, but a higher isolation rate has been found in patients with diarrhoea. Some strains produce a heat-stable toxin causing fluid accumulation in the infant mouse test developed for detecting *E. coli* heat-stable toxin I.

OTHER GENERA

Various other Gram-negative bacilli, more or less related to those described in this chapter, surface occasionally in clinical specimens, usually from seriously ill, immunologically vulnerable patients. Identification is best left to specialist reference laboratories. Where a pathogenic role is suspected, priority should be given to the often unpredictable antimicrobial susceptibility pattern of the isolate so that appropriate treatment can be started quickly.

19 *Pasteurella, Yersinia* and *Francisella*

Plague; tularaemia; mesenteric adenitis; pasteurellosis

PETRA OYSTON

KEY POINTS

- *Pasteurella, Yersinia* and *Francisella* all contain pathogenic species that cause zoonotic infections in humans.
- *Pasteurella multocida* is usually transmitted to humans by bites and scratches of infected animals, often cats.
- *Yersinia pestis* can be transmitted by fleas to cause bubonic plague or by inhalation of infectious aerosols to cause pneumonic plague.
- *Y. pseudotuberculosis* and *Y. enterocolitica* are acquired by ingestion of contaminated food to cause yersiniosis, a gastroenteritis.
- *Francisella tularensis* can be transmitted to humans by direct contact with infected animals, via insect or arthropod vectors, or through inhalation of infectious aerosols to cause the febrile disease tularaemia.
- All the above respond to antibiotic therapy, but for plague and tularaemia, a delay in initiation reduces efficacy significantly.
- No licensed vaccines are available for prophylaxis of any of these diseases.

HISTORICAL PERSPECTIVE

The genus *Pasteurella* was named in honour of Louis Pasteur who discovered *Pasteurella multocida* to be the cause of fowl cholera in 1880. One of Pasteur's protégés, Alexandre Yersin, and a Japanese researcher Kitasato Shibasaburo, identified the aetiological agent of bubonic plague in 1894 during an outbreak in Hong Kong. Yersin named the organism *Pasteurella pestis* in honour of his old mentor, but it was subsequently renamed *Yersinia pestis* after Yersin himself in 1970: the contribution of Shibasaburo is often overlooked in this story of discovery. Subsequently, the bacterial agent behind an outbreak of a plague-like disease in rodents, initially named *Bacterium tularensis* after its geographical source in Tulare County, California, was added to the genus *Pasteurella*. This organism was renamed as *Francisella tularensis* in 1919, in honour of Edward Francis who pioneered much of the early work on *F. tularensis*. Therefore this chapter summarises three genera that are now known to be genetically distinct but shared a genus previously. The bacteria in the three genera share some commonalities—namely, they are Gram-negative coccobacilli, and there are animal pathogens in all three genera capable of causing severe disease in humans. However, as this chapter will reveal, each genus has its own distinct features, particularly with regard to the diseases caused.

PASTEURELLA

P. multocida is an opportunistic pathogen, and nearly all human cases have a history of contact with animals that are the primary host. Other species of *Pasteurella* (*dagmatis, pneumotropica, bettyae, haemolytica* and *caballi*) only rarely cause disease in humans, and some species have never been isolated from humans. In some cases the low virulence strains are associated with underlying morbidities, such as immunosuppression due to HIV. This section will therefore focus on the major pathogen of the genus, *P. multocida*.

Description

P. multocida organisms are aerobic and facultatively anaerobic coccobacilli, although they are often pleomorphic in culture. They are Gram-negative, nonmotile, nonspore forming and capsulate in culture at the optimal growth temperature of 37°C. In smears of blood or tissue stained with methylene blue they show bipolar staining. *P. multocida* does not grow on MacConkey's medium. *Pasteurella* grow best in media containing blood and, in contrast to *Yersinia,* they are oxidase-positive. Sugars are fermented without gas production. Five capsular antigens A, B, D, E and F (C is not valid) and at least 11 somatic lipopolysaccharide (LPS) antigens have been identified. The expression of the capsule is affected by cultural conditions and is lost in rough strains, which also fail to express smooth type O antigens. The organisms are killed in a few minutes at 55°C and by 0.5% phenol in 15 minutes. They may survive and remain virulent in dried blood for about 3 weeks and in culture or infected tissues for many months if kept frozen.

Pathogenesis

The name *P. multocida* means, literally, killer of many species, reflecting that it is virulent to many species of animals and birds, causing fowl cholera and haemorrhagic septicaemia, which are usually fatal. It also causes respiratory infections and contributes to the pathogenesis of atrophic rhinitis in pigs. Carriage of the organism is usually asymptomatic, but stress may provoke fatal systemic infection. Focusing on human infections, most arise following animal bites and scratches, particularly from cats, although colonisation of the oropharynx is common in people working with animals, and this can in turn give rise to an invasive infection in individuals with underlying pathologies such as cirrhosis of the liver or bronchiectasis. Infection is aggressive, often resulting in soft tissue infections at the site of bites or scratches. These are very pyogenic, with rapidly spreading cellulitis leading to septicaemia, liver and brain abscesses, arthritis. A purulent secretion occurs in approximately half the wounds, but lymphadenopathy and fever only occur in 20% of cases. Maternal infection can result in chorioamnionitis and neonatal sepsis. Hospital admission is recommended in cases of sepsis, involvement of joint and tendon, immunocompromised, severe cellulitis and infections refractory to oral therapy. Hands are especially prone to complicated infections because of the numerous joints, tendons and small compartments. Septicaemia caused by *Pasteurella* has a mortality rate of 40%.

Laboratory investigation

Approximately 2% of attendances at accident and emergency departments in the United Kingdom are due to infections of bites and scratches. Nearly 60% of cat bites are infected with *P. multocida,* often growing in the presence of anaerobic species. A history of animal bite or scratch prior to presentation of discharging wounds or sepsis should alert clinicians to the possibility of *Pasteurella* infection. Diagnosis depends on culturing the bacterium from blood cultures or established wound infections. The organism can be differentiated from other Gram-negative bacilli by its high sensitivity to penicillin, which aids identification.

Treatment

The best prevention of *Pasteurella* infection is avoidance of animal bites and scratches and prompt cleaning of wounds to prevent infection from becoming established. Prophylactic antibiotics are not normally recommended. Erythromycin, clindamycin and flucloxacillin should not be used for either prophylaxis or therapy of *Pasteurella* infections as there are numerous reports of breakthrough infections with these drugs, and resistance is reported for the majority of isolates.

Treatment of established infections must be aggressive. First, the wound should be debrided; inadequate debridement can result in failure of antibiotic therapy. Where deep wounds make debridement difficult, irrigation with saline may help. Pus must be drained and affected joints washed out. Delayed closure of bite wounds improves outcome, as does elevation and immobilisation of severely affected limbs. If infection is advanced and severe, amputation may be required.

Following debridement, combination therapy is advised. Recommended combinations are co-amoxiclav/ciprofloxacin or imipenem/clindamycin. Ciprofloxacin/linezolid has been shown to be an effective combination in penicillin-allergic patients. However, deep infections may not respond to antibiotic therapy, and where damage is severe, amputation may be necessary. Superficial soft tissue infections require 10 days of therapy, but more difficult and severe infections, such as osteomyelitis, can require 6–8 weeks of therapy. Even after resolution of infection, severe tissue damage can result in permanent impaired function.

Epidemiology

P. multocida is carried in the nasopharyngeal region of many species of wild and domestic animals. In human infections following animal bites, the organism passes directly to the person in the animal's saliva. As stated above, cat bites are particularly hazardous. People may also become infected through breathing droplets generated by the coughing of animals suffering from respiratory infection. Infection may be occupationally related (e.g., farmers, veterinarians and postmen), but most infections are caused by companion animals.

The disease in farm animals can be prevented by vaccination with preparations derived from killed capsule bacteria.

YERSINIA

The genus *Yersinia* sits within the Enterobacteriaceae. Three species of *Yersinia* are pathogenic for humans: *Y. pestis, Yersinia pseudotubercuilosis* and *Yersinia enterocolitica*. Genomic comparisons revealed that *Y. pestis* is actually a clone that evolved from *Y. pseudotuberculosis* 1500–20,000 years ago. However, because of the severity of the disease this clone causes and its historical importance, it retains species designation.

YERSINIOSIS

Description

Yersiniosis is caused by the enteropathogens *Y. pseudotuberculosis* and *Y. enterocolitica*. Both are Gram-negative coccobacilli capable of growing on most laboratory media. They are motile at 22–28°C, but not at 37°C, which distinguishes them from other motile Enterobacteriaceae. Both species grow poorly at 37°C compared to ambient temperature, and both can grow at 4°C, albeit slowly. *Y. enterocolitica* generally grows more quickly than *Y. pseudotuberculosis*. Many biochemical tests are temperature-dependent for their outcome. Both species are antigenically complex: *Y. enterocolitica* expresses at least 54 different O antigens and 19 H factors, whilst *Y. pseudotuberculosis* has eight major O serotypes, several of which can be separated into subtypes.

Pathogenesis

Yersiniosis is an acute self-limiting gastroenteritis. Less commonly, it can result in acute mesenteric lymphadenitis, and even more rarely terminal ileitis. Generally, infection is self-limiting. Diarrhoea can be minimal or absent, although diarrhoea caused by *Y. enterocolitica* is bloody in up to half of cases. Both pathogens are zoonotic: *Y. enterocolitica* infects domestic animals, particularly pigs, whereas *Y. pseudotuberculosis* infects a range of wild animals and birds, and as such it is more rarely identified in human infections. *Y. enterocolitica* infections are usually associated with the consumption of undercooked contaminated pork meat, while transmission of *Y. pseudotuberculosis* to humans is probably due to environmental contamination by animal excreta; outbreaks have been reported following consumption of contaminated lettuce, raw vegetables and milk, for example.

Infection is best prevented by standard food hygiene precautions, particularly avoiding eating undercooked or raw meat, especially by younger children. Pasteurisation of milk effectively destroys the organism as does chlorination of water. However, as noted above, these bacteria grow at 4°C; thus extended refrigerated storage of high-risk products should be avoided as contamination will increase with time.

Y. pseudotuberculosis strains can express a superantigenic toxin causing Far East scarlet-like fever—a childhood disease with rash, arthralgia and polyarthritis most commonly seen in eastern Russia, Korea and Japan. There is also epidemiological evidence linking *Y. pseudotuberculosis* with Kawasaki disease in children. There are other rare immunological complications associated with enteric yersiniosis, providing further incentive to identify this cause of a self-limiting gastric infection.

Laboratory investigation

Differential diagnosis is difficult, and diarrhoea with abdominal pain and fever can result in a misdiagnosis of appendicitis. Diagnosis is normally by culture and serology. For *Y. pseudotuberculosis,* infection is confirmed by isolation of the organism in culture from normally sterile sites such as blood, local lesions or mesenteric nodes, particularly the ileocaecal nodes. It is rarely isolated from faeces. *Y. enterocolitica* can be isolated from blood, lymph nodes or other tissues as well as from faeces. Identity can be confirmed by MALDI-TOF and by biochemical and motility test, but serology is also commonly used.

Treatment

Most cases of yersiniosis are a self-limiting enteritis, so antibiotics are not indicated. However, more serious presentations, including scarlet-like fever, need antibiotic therapy. Therapy with cefotaxime, ceftriaxone or ciprofloxacin is often recommended for sepsis. Of note is the differential susceptibility to penicillins; *Y. enterocolitica* is resistant while *Y. pseudotuberculosis* is usually susceptible.

Epidemiology

Yersiniosis is the third most common cause of diarrhoea in Scandinavian countries and New Zealand. Infection seems 10-fold less common in the United Kingdom than the United States. Some of these differences reflect differences in diet, whilst some are due to different virulence of strains from different geographical sources.

Y. enterocolitica has been isolated from abscesses, from blood and infected wounds and from the intestinal contents of apparently healthy animals of many species throughout the world. Pigs carry pathogenic serotypes quite frequently, cattle, sheep and goats less so. Human disease usually results from ingestion of contaminated food or from contact with the environment. Raw pork, milk and drinking water have been implicated as sources. Person-to-person transmission also occurs. Blood transfusion is a significant hazard as the organism can grow in refrigerated blood from donors with 'silent' bacteraemia. Flies are believed to play a role in transmission by contaminating food, and infection has been demonstrated in fleas and lice. However, enteric infection is the usual route of transmission, and preventive measures are those appropriate for foodborne disease. Infection is most common in children <5 years of age.

Many animal species are infected with *Y. pseudotuber-culosis*, but there is little proof of direct transmission to humans. Most human infections probably result from the ingestion of contaminated water, vegetables or other food. Serotypes seems to differ geographically; about 90% of all human cases in Australia, Europe and North America are attributed to strains of serotype I, followed by serotypes II and III, whereas in Japan serotypes IV and V predominate.

Y. PESTIS AND PLAGUE

Plague has been a scourge of mankind for centuries, and outbreaks continue to the present day. Although antibiotics are available, resistance is emerging in this dangerous pathogen. As such, innovative approaches to the design and development of new therapeutic compounds are in progress. Currently there is no licensed vaccine available for prevention of plague in the United States or Western Europe, although both live-attenuated strains and killed whole cell extracts have been used historically. Live strains are still approved for human use in some parts of the world, such as the former Soviet Union, but poor safety profiles render them unacceptable to many countries. The development of safe, effective next-generation vaccines, including the recombinant subunit vaccine currently in clinical trials, is a research priority.

Plague

Plague occurs principally in three clinical forms in humans: bubonic, septicaemic and pneumonic plague, with bubonic plague, arising following the bite of an infected flea, being the best-known form of the disease. Symptoms of bubonic plague include fever, chills, headache and notably a painful bubo (swollen lymph node). Local bacterial proliferation at the site of the bite can result in the development of an abscess or ulcer at the site of infection. Fever and malaise develop 2–6 days after infection, but the bubo can take longer to develop and may not generally be visible later in infection if the infected lymph node is deeper in the body. The bubo is described as being exquisitely painful. In addition to the bubo, patients develop a significant bacteraemia later in infection. Those patients with blood colony counts >100 bacteria per mL have higher fatality rates than those with lower counts. Untreated, the case fatality rate is 40%–60%, but where therapy is used this can be reduced to around 14%.

Occasionally, in about 10%–25% of cases, plague infection by flea transmission fails to result in the development of the diagnostic bubo, but a significant bacteraemia still occurs, which is known as primary septicaemic plague. Symptoms of septicaemic plague are very non-specific, resembling those of most Gram-negative septicaemic infections. Patients develop fever, chills, headache and malaise; however, there is nothing specific except patient history that may indicate plague. Difficulties in diagnosis result in delays in initiating antibiotic therapy, and thus mortality rates are higher than for bubonic plague; untreated septicaemic plague is almost always fatal.

Pneumonic plague is highly acute, with an incubation period of 1–3 days, after which there is sudden onset of flulike symptoms including fever, chills, headache, generalised body pains, weakness and chest discomfort. A cough develops with sputum production, which may be bloody, and increasing chest pain and difficulty in breathing. The aerosols produced by this coughing contain large numbers of plague bacilli, which can infect susceptible contacts. Prognosis is poor and diagnosis difficult, and this form of the infection is usually fatal unless antibiotic therapy commences within 24 hours of exposure. For this reason, prophylactic therapy of contacts is recommended, to be initiated prior to symptoms developing.

For all the presentations of plague, death occurs as a result of shock, probably due to endotoxin. This results in disseminated intravascular coagulation, multiple organ failure and respiratory distress syndrome. Disseminated intravascular coagulation can lead to thrombi depositing in small blood vessels, and thus the extremities such as fingers and toes often turn black. In addition to potential complications of meningitis and pneumonia, there may be generalised lymphadenopathy and abscess formation on the liver and spleen.

Description

Y. pestis is the causative agent of plague. It is an ovoid coccobacillus, although it will produce unusual filamentous forms if grown under stressful conditions. Although it will produce a capsule at 37°C, the small size of the rod makes this hard to see in Indian ink films and is best observed by immunofluorescence. The organism grows well on rich media, including blood agar, although growth is slow and can take over 48 hours to produce isolated colonies. Growth is better at ambient temperature than 37°C, with an optimum around 28°C. The organism is nonmotile, oxidase negative, catalase positive, does not ferment lactose and is indole negative. As a dangerous pathogen, it must be handled under appropriate containment, and it is a notifiable disease. It can be inactivated by heat or chemical disinfectants.

Laboratory investigation

Definitive laboratory diagnosis of *Y. pestis* infection is based on isolation of the pathogen from clinical specimens or by the demonstration of a diagnostic change in antibody titre in paired serum samples. *Y. pestis* will grow on most routine laboratory media, such as brain–heart infusion, sheep blood or MacConkey agars. Incubation for 2 days at 37°C will produce visible opaque colonies with irregular edges. Cultures are definitively identified as *Y. pestis* by specific phage lysis or by MALDI-TOF. Automated bacteriological test systems frequently misidentify *Y. pestis*. Polymerase Chain Reaction (PCR) tests have been evaluated but are not used routinely in clinical settings for diagnosis of plague.

Even if *Y. pestis* cannot be isolated, plague can be confirmed by serological responses to the capsular protein, designated F1-antigen. Passive haemagglutination and F1-antigen haemagglutination-inhibition tests are available and confirmatory. Enzyme-linked immunosorbent assay (ELISA) for IgG and IgM antibodies are also useful in laboratory diagnosis in early phases of infection; seroconversion usually occurs at 1–2 weeks post exposure. Direct detection of the capsular F1-antigen has also been used for diagnosis. Rapid tests based on a monoclonal antibody against F1-antigen, including an antigen capture ELISA and a dipstick format, have been developed and used successfully in the field. Both F1-antigen and antibodies against it should be assayed for simultaneously, as patients will be positive for one while negative for the other.

Treatment

If plague is suspected, antibiotic treatment must be started immediately without waiting for laboratory confirmation, and patients must be placed in isolation to reduce the risk of spread in the event of pneumonic plague developing. In the past, streptomycin has been the drug of choice for treatment of plague, particularly the pneumonic form. Gentamicin is another aminoglycoside that has been used to treat plague and is generally considered as effective as streptomycin whilst being more readily available. Because of the toxicity of streptomycin, patients are usually moved onto another antibiotic, usually tetracycline, 3 days after their temperature has returned to normal. Tetracycline is bacteriostatic but effective in treatment of uncomplicated plague. In cases of plague meningitis, chloramphenicol is the drug of choice because of its tissue penetration. Fluoroquinolones such as ciprofloxacin, gatifloxacin and moxifloxacin have been shown to be therapeutic in

laboratory animals, but so far this class of antibiotic has rarely been used to treat human plague, although ciprofloxacin does appear effective, and ciprofloxacin is now included in CDC guidelines. The fluoroquinolone antibiotic levofloxacin was approved by the FDA for the therapy or prophylaxis of plague infections, based on efficacy in African Green monkeys. Other classes of antibiotics, such as penicillins, cephalosporins and macrolides, have been shown to be ineffective in treatment of plague. It should be stressed that, even with effective antibiotics, late initiation of therapy reduced the effectiveness of the antibiotics. Antibiotic-resistant strains are rare but have been isolated from clinical samples.

Persons in contact with pneumonic plague patients or handling infectious body fluids should receive prophylactic antibiotic therapy within 6 days of assumed exposure to reduce the risk of their developing disease. Suggested drugs such as doxycycline, ciprofloxacin, chloramphenicol and co-trimoxazole have been used for such individuals.

Without treatment, bubonic plague has a mortality rate of 50%–90%, and septicaemic and pneumonic plague are almost always fatal. Timely diagnosis and initiation of therapy can reduce bubonic plague fatalities to 5%–20% and pneumonic plague to 50% mortality. The earlier antibiotic therapy can be started the better the prognosis, and diagnosis of pneumonic and septicaemic plague is often too late for therapy to be effective.

There is no licensed vaccine available. A subunit vaccine is in clinical trials. Historically, live-attenuated and killed whole cell vaccines have been used, and although they are partially protective, they are not used routinely because of safety concerns.

Epidemiology

Plague is a zoonotic disease primarily affecting rodents. Infection circulates in rodent populations in the environment, transmitted among animals by fleas. Humans are accidental hosts, with most infections occurring following the bite of an infected flea when in close contact with infected rodents. Occasionally, infection arises, usually in hunters, during handling and skinning of dead animals. Domestic animals, notably cats, are also susceptible to plague and can transmit the infection to humans. Dogs are relatively resistant to plague, and thus unlikely to directly transmit plague to human contacts, but they can import infected fleas into the home. Susceptible livestock can also pose a threat to humans, whether due to proximity and handling of sick animals, as occurred in Ecuador where an outbreak was linked to infected guinea pigs, or through consumption, as occurred in Libya following consumption of infected goats and camel meat. As would be expected, the distribution of naturally arising plague infections in humans mirrors the distribution of sylvatic plague.

FRANCISELLA

Description

The taxonomy of the genus *Francisella* is complex, and new molecular information results in increasing levels of complexity, so that there are now subspecies that are then separated further into biovars or clades. Additionally, the ongoing isolation of new environmental and fish pathogenic strains means the picture is likely to only increase in complexity in the future. Three species are currently recognised: *Francisella tularensis*, *Francisella philomiragia* and *Francisella novicida*. Of these, *F. tularensis* is the most significant human pathogen. There are at present three accepted subspecies of *F. tularensis*: subspecies *tularensis* (sometimes known as Type A), subspecies *holarctica* (sometimes known as Type B) and subspecies *mediasiatica*. Subspecies vary in their geographical distribution and virulence in humans.

F. tularensis is a small (0.2–0.5 µm × 0.7–1.0 µm) Gram-negative coccobacillus that is nonmotile and an obligate aerobe. For growth, it needs an enriched medium such as cysteine glucose blood agar, and it requires 2–4 days' incubation to produce colonies.

Pathogenesis

F. tularensis is able to infect a wide range of hosts including humans to cause tularaemia. An intracellular pathogen, it is one of the most highly infectious bacteria known, with an infectious dose in humans as low as 10 bacteria by the inhalational route.

Tularaemia in humans can occur in several forms depending on the route of infection. Although tularaemia can be a severely debilitating and even fatal disease, especially when caused by virulent strains, many cases of disease caused by lower virulence strains go undiagnosed because of the nonspecific nature of the symptoms. The incubation period is normally 3–5 days (range 1–21 days), and patients develop flu-like symptoms, which may be protracted and relapsing if untreated.

Infection through the skin results in ulceroglandular tularaemia; where no ulcer is reported, this is termed *glandular tularaemia*. These forms of tularaemia are the most common presentations of the disease and can arise following the bite of an infected vector or through direct contact with the flesh of an infected animal. A lesion develops at the site of infection, often a single papule that develops into an ulcer surrounded by a zone of inflammation. The ulcer is relatively painless and heals within

a week. Within 3–5 days following infection, the patient develops fever, chills, malaise, headaches and a sore throat. The local draining lymph nodes become enlarged and painful, like a bubo, which takes a significant time to resolve.

Less commonly, infection can occur through the conjunctiva, which is termed *oculoglandular tularaemia*. Ingestion of infected meat can result in *oropharyngeal or gastrointestinal tularaemia*. Any of the above infections may disseminate and progress to systemic disease without the appearance of swollen lymph nodes or ulcers. This is termed *typhoidal tularaemia*. Severe complications may also occur, such as septic shock. However, of greatest concern is infection through inhalation, which results in respiratory or pneumonic tularaemia. Symptoms can be variable and depend on the virulence of the strain involved. Infection with the most highly virulent strains can have a case fatality rate of up to 30% if untreated, but antibiotic therapy reduces this to approximately 2%. Presentation can range from a mild pneumonia to an acute infection with high fever, malaise, chills, cough and delirium.

Laboratory investigation

Diagnosis of tularaemia is difficult because of the nonspecific nature of most of the symptoms, particularly if the ulcer has already healed. Most cases of tularaemia are diagnosed on the basis of clinical picture and serology. A range of serological tests for the detection of antibodies against *F. tularensis* are commercially available. The antibody response peaks at 4–6 weeks but can be detected from 2 weeks.

The organism is fastidious but can grow in routine laboratory media, albeit slowly. Because of the infection risk posed to laboratory personnel, the ordering physician should clearly indicate if tularaemia is suspected. In addition, such notification will increase the likelihood of a positive identification as the culture conditions can be tailored to improve recovery of the organism. PCR and ELISA can be used to positively identify the bacteria, both following isolation and in specimens. Such direct detection of the pathogen is useful in patients who are serologically negative, for example, in the early days of infection.

Treatment

Historically, aminoglycosides have been the drugs of choice for the treatment of tularaemia, but are rarely used now, and gentamicin is a suitable alternative aminoglycoside, but because of the requirement for parenteral dosing and monitoring of serum levels, aminoglycosides are now only used for the most serious cases. Doxycycline is effective in the treatment of tularaemia, but the tetracyclines have been associated with high relapse rates on withdrawal. Chloramphenicol is usually reserved for the treatment of meningitis. Ciprofloxacin has been shown to be highly effective in oral therapy of tularaemia and can be considered the current drug of choice for uncomplicated tularaemia. Supportive care should be provided as appropriate; some patients may require intensive care with respiratory support should sepsis develop. Suppurating nodes should be drained.

There is no licensed vaccine available for prophylaxis, although a live-attenuated strain has been used extensively and shown to be effective in preventing infection.

Epidemiology

F. tularensis is mainly isolated in the northern hemisphere, most frequently in Scandinavia, North America, Japan and Russia (100–400 cases/year), but has never been isolated in the United Kingdom. It circulates in populations of small rodents, rabbits and hares, and outbreaks in human populations frequently mirror outbreaks of disease occurring in wild animals. A wide range of arthropod vectors have been implicated in the transmission of the disease. Rural populations and especially those individuals who spend periods of time in endemic areas such as farmers, hunters, walkers and forest workers are most at risk of contracting tularaemia. Outbreaks have also been associated with contaminated water supplies and can involve large numbers of cases; there appears to be a link between subspecies *holarctica* and water but not for subspecies *tularensis*.

Very little is known about the ecology of *F. novicida*, although there is a link with infection from brackish water, and new species of *Francisella*-like organisms are being isolated from fish, indicating that the pathogenic *Francisella* may have derived from an aquatic ancestor. Comparative genomics of the multiple genome sequences that are becoming available for different species and subspecies is helping cast light on the evolution of the pathogenic *Francisella*. However, there are many questions still unanswered about the environmental niches occupied by *Francisella*.

Chapter 19 is Crown Copyright © 2019, Published by Elsevier Ltd. This is an open access article under the Open Government Licence (OGL) (http://www.nationalarchives.gov.uk/doc/open-government-licence/version/3/).

RECOMMENDED READING

Dennis, D. T., & Campbell, G. L. (2005). Plague and other yersinia infections. In D. L. Kasper, E. Braunwald, A. S. Fauci, S. L. Hauser, D. L. Longo, & J. L. Jameson (Eds.), *Harrison's principles of internal medicine* (16th ed., pp. 921–929). New York: McGraw-Hill.

Dennis, D. T., Inglesby, T. V., Henderson, D. A., Bartlett, J. G., Ascher, M. S., Eitzen, E., ... Working Group on Civilian Biodefense. (2001). Tularemia as a biological weapon: medical and public health management. *Journal of the American Medical Association, 285*(21), 2763–2773.

Matyas, B. T., Nieder, H. S., & Telford, S. R. (2007). Pneumonic tularemia on Martha's Vineyard: clinical, epidemiologic, and ecological characteristics. *Annals of the New York Academy of Sciences, 1105*, 351–377.

McNally, A., Thomson, N. R., Reuter, S., & Wren, B. W. (2016). Add, stir and reduce: *Yersinia* spp. as model bacteria for pathogen evolution. *Nature Reviews. Microbiology, 14*(3), 177–190.

Wilson, B. A., & Ho, M. (2013). *Pasteurella multocida*: from zoonosis to cellular microbiology. *Clinical Microbiology Reviews, 26*(3), 631–655.

20 *Campylobacter* and *Helicobacter*

Enteritis; polyneuropathy; gastritis; peptic ulcer disease; gastric cancer

JULIAN M. KETLEY AND ARNOUD H. M. VAN VLIET

KEY POINTS

- *Campylobacter jejuni*, a foodborne pathogen generally associated with faecal contamination of food or water, is a common cause of bacterial enteritis.
- This flagellate, spiral and toxigenic micro-aerobe is capable of invading host cells.
- The generally self-limiting clinical presentation includes acute abdominal pain followed by diarrhoea with blood and leucocytes; antibiotic treatment is required only in severe cases.

- *Helicobacter pylori* is a flagellated spiral micro-aerobe causing peptic ulcer and gastritis. Infection is a risk factor for gastric cancer.
- It produces a cell-damaging toxin and a system that alters host cell signal transduction pathways.
- The transmission route is unclear. Colonisation and disease rates are falling in industrialised countries.
- Treatment is by eradication of *H. pylori* using a combination of antibiotics and proton pump inhibitors.

Campylobacter and *Helicobacter* are phylogenetically related, spirally shaped, flagellate bacteria. Both genera can be found in most mammals, with specific species associated with human disease. They are adapted to colonise mucous membranes and penetrate mucus with particular facility. In most industrialised countries, *Campylobacter jejuni* is the most frequently identified cause of acute infective diarrhoea, causing much morbidity and economic loss. Life-long colonisation of the stomach with *Helicobacter pylori* is essentially the cause of 'idiopathic' peptic ulceration, and a notable risk factor for the development of gastric cancer.

CAMPYLOBACTER

Campylobacters were first isolated in 1906 from aborting sheep in the United Kingdom. Originally thought to be vibrios, they were later placed in their own genus with *C. foetus* as the type species. The discovery that *C. jejuni* and *C. coli* commonly cause acute enteritis in humans was not made until the late 1970s.

Several other species, such as *C. upsaliensis, C. lari* and the closely related bacterium *Arcobacter butzleri,* are occasionally associated with diarrhoea, mainly in children in developing countries. *C. foetus* is a major cause of abortion in sheep and cattle worldwide. It is a rare cause of human foetal infection and abortion and infrequently causes bacteraemia in patients with immune deficiency. Several other species of *Campylobacter,* notably *C. concisus* and *C. rectus,* are associated with periodontal disease, with *C. concisus* also implicated in gastroenteritis and inflammatory bowel disease, although a causal link or mechanism has not yet been established.

CAMPYLOBACTER JEJUNI AND C. COLI

Description

C. jejuni and *C. coli* are small spiral Gram-negative rods with a single flagellum at one or both poles (Fig. 20.1); this endows the bacteria with rapid darting motility. They are sensitive to oxygen and superoxides, yet oxygen and increased carbon dioxide concentrations are essential for growth, so micro-aerobic conditions must be provided for the cultivation of these capnophiles. They are often called thermophilic campylobacters because they grow best at 37–42°C. Campylobacters are inactive in many conventional biochemical tests, including metabolism of sugars, but they are strongly oxidase- and catalase-positive. Under laboratory conditions, they are easily destroyed by heat and other physical and chemical agents. Campylobacters undergo coccal transformation under adverse conditions, a change controversially associated with a viable, nonculturable state.

Campylobacters readily take up naked DNA from their surroundings, which can be incorporated into the genome and contributes, with phase variation through hypermutable sequence tracts, to making them genetically diverse. *C. jejuni* and *C. coli* are closely related and phenotypically similar, but can be differentiated by polymerase chain reaction (PCR) tests. Colorimetric assays for arylsulfatase activity may be inconclusive, and their use is not recommended.

A capsular polysaccharide, not the lipooligosaccharide, forms the major antigen for the Penner serotyping system. Bacteriophages able to infect campylobacters are also used in strain typing. Genetic fingerprinting methods, such as multilocus sequence typing (see Chs 3 and 64), and, more recently, whole genome sequencing-based approaches, are available alternatives to more classical methods used in source attribution and epidemiological studies.

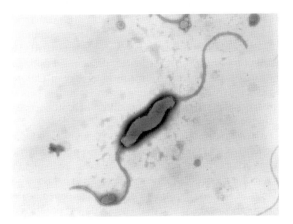

Fig. 20.1 Electron micrograph of *C. jejuni* showing single unsheathed bipolar flagellum (original magnification ×11,500). (Photomicrograph by Dr A. L. Curry and D. M. Jones, Manchester Public Health Laboratory.)

Pathogenesis

C. jejuni accounts for 80%–90% of human Campylobacter infections in most parts of the world. Infection is acquired by ingestion of as few as 500–800 organisms. The bacteria are protected from gastric acid in the stomach by the food matrix associated with transmission. The jejunum and ileum are the first sites to become colonised, and the infection extends distally to affect the terminal ileum and, usually, the colon and rectum. The organisms invade host cells, and symptoms are usually evident within 7 days. In well-developed infections, mesenteric lymph nodes are enlarged, fleshy and inflamed, and there may be transient bacteraemia. Histological examination of the mucosa shows an acute neutrophil response, oedema and, sometimes, superficial ulceration. These mucosal changes are indistinguishable from those seen in salmonella, shigella or yersinia infections.

Understanding of the mechanisms by which campylobacters cause enteric disease is limited. Colonisation of the intestine requires factors such as chemotactic motility, iron-uptake systems and several potential adhesins (Fig. 20.2). Both *C. jejuni* and *C. coli* produce at least one toxin, cytolethal distending toxin, that blocks the cell cycle of host cells, but its precise role in virulence is unclear. Campylobacters can also invade host cells and may translocate across the epithelium by a paracellular route. The Campylobacter invasion antigens (Cia) are among several virulence factors that are secreted from the bacteria by the flagellar secretion system. Epithelial damage and associated inflammatory responses are likely to be due to host cell damage as well as interaction with bacteria

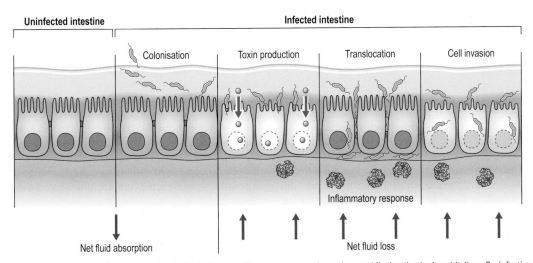

Fig. 20.2 The pathogenesis of *C. jejuni* and *C. coli*. Net fluid absorption occurs across the undamaged ileal and colonic epithelium. On infection of the host intestine, campylobacters use chemotactic motility to reach the mucous layer and colonise the epithelial surface. Campylobacters translocate directly across the cell layer, invade host cells and produce a cytotoxin. Cell damage disrupts the integrity of the mucosal cell layer and stimulates an inflammatory response. Disruption of the absorptive function of the epithelium and, possibly, stimulation of secretion lead to diarrhoeal disease.

entering the submucosa. Therefore, clinical symptoms are influenced by the extent of the associated cellular immune response, and diarrhoea is likely to result from disruption of the intestinal mucosa due to cell invasion, the production of toxin(s) and inflammation.

Analysis of the genome sequences of many *C. jejuni* strains has revealed the existence of many genes responsible for the production of various glycans, as well as the presence of short hypervariable sequences. These so-called hypermutable 'homopolymeric tracts' can act as a genetic on/off switch and many are present in genes responsible for glycan biosynthesis. The amount of the genome invested in glycan biosynthesis indicates an important role for glycans in campylobacters. The genes responsible for glycosylation of the lipooligosaccharide, capsule and flagellum are highly variable, suggesting a role in avoidance of host immune responses, bacteriophage infection or adaptation to other environmental changes. In contrast, genes involved in general protein glycosylation are highly conserved and correspond to those found in eukaryotes. Disruption of glycosylation pathways in *C. jejuni* affects host cell invasion and intestinal colonisation. Extensive glycosylation may reflect molecular mimicry of host epitopes as part of a strategy to avoid host immune responses.

Immune response

Specific humoral antibodies appear within 10 days of onset, peak in 2–4 weeks, and then decline rapidly. Most of the antibody is in the form of immunoglobulin (Ig) G, but healthy persons exposed to repeated infection show a progressive increase in IgA, which provides substantial immunity. Mild clinical symptoms, such as mild watery diarrhoea or even asymptomatic colonisation, may reflect increased levels of immunity and/or development of tolerance from repeated infections.

Epidemiology
Incidence

Campylobacter enteritis is the most common form of acute infective diarrhoea in most developed countries. In the United Kingdom, laboratory reports indicate an annual incidence of about 1 per 1000 population, but the true figure is probably much higher. The European Food Safety Authority estimated that the annual incidence was between 2 and 20 million cases in 27 member countries of the European Union. The disease occurs among all age groups (especially young adults), shows a pronounced summer peak and is often associated with travel.

In developing countries, infection is hyperendemic, and children are repeatedly exposed to infection from an early age. By the time they are 2–3 years old, children have developed substantial immunity that lasts into adulthood.

The maintenance of immunity probably depends on continuous exposure to infection.

Sources and transmission

C. jejuni and *C. coli* are found in a wide variety of animal hosts, notably birds, an adaptation that is reflected in their high optimum growth temperature, which mimics the avian body temperature. Fig. 20.3 summarises the principal sources and routes of transmission to human beings. There is a constant shedding of the bacteria from wild birds and other animals into the surface water of lakes, rivers and streams, in which campylobacters can survive for many weeks at low temperatures. Farm animals are often infected from such sources and flies have been implicated in spread. Pigs can be infected with *C. coli*, but pork meat is not considered a risk factor for *C. coli*. Cattle are commonly infected, and raw milk often becomes contaminated. The distribution of raw or inadequately pasteurised milk and untreated water has caused major outbreaks of Campylobacter enteritis, some affecting several thousand people. Direct contact with infected animals or their products can also give rise to infection.

At least 60% and occasionally as high as 90% of chickens sold in shops are contaminated with campylobacters, and contaminated broiler chickens are thought to account for about 50% of human infections in industrialised countries. Red meats are less often contaminated.

Properly cooked poultry and meats do not pose a risk, but cross-contamination to other foods, such as bread and salads, probably accounts for many infections. Unlike salmonellae, campylobacters do not multiply in food, so explosive food-poisoning outbreaks are rare. Most infections are sporadic or confined to one household; the spread of infection between individuals is of minor importance. In recent years, undercooked chicken liver pâté has become a source of human infection, and is now a major source of *C. jejuni* outbreaks associated with eating out and catering.

Molecular typing has shown that there are differences between *C. jejuni* and *C. coli* isolates in their capability to infect animal and avian hosts. There are lineages that have a strong association with specific hosts such as starlings, while others are considered to be more 'generalist', being capable of colonising a diverse range of hosts. The latter types are more commonly associated with human disease.

Clinical features

The typical features of Campylobacter enteritis are shown in Fig. 20.4. The average incubation period is 3 days, with a range of 1–7 days. The illness may start with abdominal pain and diarrhoea, or there may be an

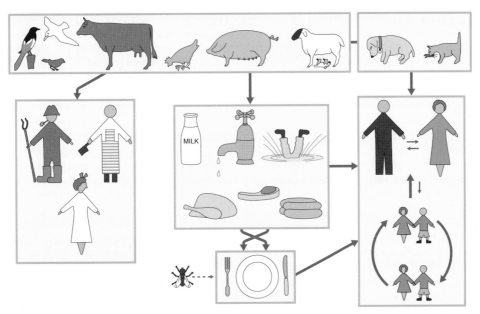

Fig. 20.3 Sources and transmission of C. jejuni and C. coli. Top boxes: animal reservoirs and sources of infection (the sheep has just given birth to a dead campylobacter-infected lamb and puppy or kitten with campylobacter diarrhoea). Left-hand box: transmission by direct occupational contact (farmer, butcher, poultry processor). Right-hand box: transmission by direct domestic contact (infected companion animals; intra-familial spread, mainly from children). Central box: indirect transmission through consumption of untreated water, raw milk, raw or undercooked meat and poultry, food cross-contaminated from raw meats and poultry; possible transmission from flies. (From document VPH/CDD/FOS/84.1 by permission of the World Health Organization, which retains the copyright.)

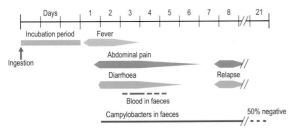

Fig. 20.4 Typical course of untreated campylobacter enteritis of average severity. There is considerable variation among individual patients.

influenza-like prodrome of fever and generalised aching, sometimes with rigors and sweating. Abdominal pain and diarrhoea are the main symptoms. Nausea is common, but vomiting is less pronounced. Severe watery diarrhoea may lead to prostration. Leucocytes are almost always present in the faeces, and frank blood may be apparent. Symptoms usually resolve within a few days, but excretion of bacteria may continue for several weeks. Prolonged carriage occurs only in patients with immunodeficiency. Campylobacter enteritis cannot be distinguished clinically from salmonella or shigella infection, but abdominal pain tends to be more severe in Campylobacter infection. Indeed, a common reason for patients with Campylobacter enteritis to be admitted to hospital is suspected acute appendicitis.

Occasionally, illness starts with symptoms of colitis without preceding ileitis, which can make it difficult to distinguish from acute ulcerative colitis. In developing countries, infection often presents as milder diarrhoea and asymptomatic colonisation is common. Clinical differences are mostly due to host immune status, the development of tolerance, or variation in strain virulence.

Complications

Two conditions may arise 1–2 weeks after the onset of illness:

1. Reactive (aseptic) arthritis, typically affecting the ankles, knees and wrists, affects 1%–2% of patients. It may be incapacitating, but is ultimately self-limiting.
2. Guillain–Barré syndrome, an autoimmune peripheral polyneuropathy, affects around 1 in 1000 infected individuals per year; it may cause serious and potentially fatal paralysis lasting for several months. It is thought that antibodies to lipooligosaccharide epitopes, present in a significant proportion of strains, cross-react with epitopes of myelin in nerve sheaths, causing demyelination. Other factors are likely to modulate the generation of the autoimmune response following infection.

Laboratory investigation

Faecal specimens should be refrigerated pending delivery to the laboratory. Specimens sent by post should be placed in an appropriate transport medium.

Microscopy

The motility and morphology of campylobacters are sufficiently characteristic for a rapid presumptive diagnosis to be made by direct microscopy of fresh faeces, in either wet preparations or stained smears. This is occasionally useful, but is not done routinely.

Culture

Isolation of campylobacters from faeces requires some form of selective culture to inhibit competing faecal flora. Charcoal-based blood-free agar containing bile acids, cefoperazone or other selective antimicrobial agents is widely used. Plates are incubated in closed jars or specialised incubators with the oxygen tension lowered to 5%–15% and carbon dioxide raised to 5%–10%. Incubation at 42–43°C gives added selectivity against other faecal flora and more rapid growth of *C. jejuni* and *C. coli,* but may exclude other *Campylobacter* species. Plates are incubated for 48 hours. Colonies are typically flat with a tendency to spread on moist agar.

Serology

Serology can be useful in patients presenting with aseptic arthritis or Guillain–Barré syndrome occurring after diarrhoea that was not investigated. Group-specific complement fixation tests and enzyme-linked immunosorbent assay (ELISA) can detect recent infection with *C. jejuni* or *C. coli.*

Treatment

Campylobacteriosis is usually self-limiting, and patients seldom require more than fluid and electrolyte replacement. Antimicrobial treatment should be reserved for patients with severe or complicated infections. Erythromycin is effective if given early in the disease. Ciprofloxacin and other fluoroquinolones are also effective, but resistance rates are rising.

Control

The wide distribution of campylobacters in nature precludes any possibility of reducing the reservoir of infection. Efforts are mostly directed to interrupting transmission and reducing numbers of *Campylobacter* in poultry, although more recently there have been public information campaigns, such as in the United Kingdom where the Food Standards Agency highlighted the cross-contamination risks of the common practice of washing whole chicken carcasses. The purification of water and the heat treatment of milk are obvious and basic measures. The control of colonisation in broiler chickens merits high priority, but the means to achieve this are beset with difficulty. Terminal γ-irradiation or chemical washes of carcasses can eliminate campylobacters and other pathogens, but public acceptability is a problem. Newer approaches include the 'double-bagging' of chickens, where the bird is packaged in an oven-ready roast-in bag to avoid direct consumer contact with the meat prior to cooking.

HELICOBACTER

Remarkably, *H. pylori*, which colonises roughly half of the world's population, remained undiscovered until 1982 when Warren and Marshall in Western Australia overturned the dogma that bacteria could not colonise the stomach. The discovery revolutionised the treatment of duodenal and gastric ulcers and earned them a Nobel Prize in 2005.

Over 20 species of *Helicobacter* are now officially recognised, with more awaiting formal recognition. One group, the gastric helicobacters, colonise the stomachs of animals—the monkey, cat, dog, ferret and cheetah each harbour their own species. The enterohepatic group colonise the intestines and liver of a wide range of animals, mostly rodents, and enteric *Helicobacter* species have been linked to the development of inflammatory bowel disease in humans. *H. cinaedi* and *H. fennelliae* are associated with proctitis in homosexual men.

Less common helicobacters, originally named *H. heilmannii*, are found in the human stomach and are associated with gastritis, ulcers and malignancy. Molecular studies suggest transmission from an animal source. The bacteria are more tightly spiralled than *H. pylori,* with up to 12 sheathed polar flagella. They belong to two groups: one closely related to a pathogenic gastric helicobacter of pigs, and the other to canine and feline helicobacters.

HELICOBACTER PYLORI

Description

H. pylori is a Gram-negative, spirally shaped bacterium. It is strictly micro-aerophilic and capnophilic, requires carbon dioxide and a rich growth media, but it has a tuft of sheathed unipolar flagella, unlike the unsheathed flagella of campylobacters (Fig. 20.5; cf. Fig. 20.1). It is biochemically inactive in most conventional tests, but produces an

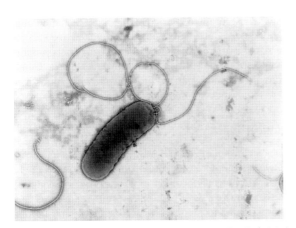

Fig. 20.5 *H. pylori* showing multiple sheathed unipolar flagella (original magnification ×11,500). (Photomicrograph by Dr A. L. Curry and D. M. Jones, Manchester Public Health Laboratory.)

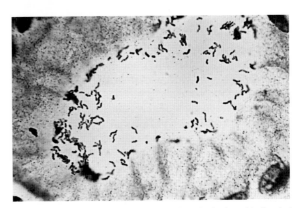

Fig. 20.6 Section of gastric mucosa showing colonisation with *H. pylori* (Warthin–Starry silver stain; original magnification ×1400). (Photomicrograph by Mr G. H. Green, Worcester Royal Infirmary.)

exceptionally powerful urease, almost 100 times more active than that of *Proteus vulgaris,* which is vital to its survival in the stomach. When exposed to adverse conditions, *H. pylori* undergoes coccal transformation more rapidly than *C. jejuni* and is more fragile, a point of importance when referring samples to a laboratory.

Antigens and strain typing

Although various antigens are expressed by *H. pylori,* serotyping is of limited practical value. However, its genetic diversity can be exploited by molecular typing based on DNA analysis. Like campylobacters, *H. pylori* exhibits considerable genetic diversity arising from natural competence, a high mutation rate and frequent recombination events. Consequently, a host can be colonised by a population of closely related variants analogous to the 'quasi-species' observed with certain viruses.

Pathogenesis

H. pylori is highly adapted and lives only on gastric mucosa. Colonisation ceases abruptly where gastric mucosa ends, for example, in areas of intestinal metaplasia in the stomach. Conversely, areas of gastric metaplasia elsewhere in the gut, notably the duodenum, may become colonised with *H. pylori,* thus setting the scene for ulceration.

The gastric antrum is the most favoured site, but other parts of the stomach may be colonised, especially in patients taking an acid-lowering drug such as an H_2 antagonist or proton pump inhibitor, or in subjects with a natural lower acid output. The bacteria are noninvasive, being present in the mucus overlying the mucosa. Although gastric acid is potentially destructive to *H. pylori,* protection is provided by its powerful urease, which acts on the urea passing through

the gastric mucosa to generate ammonia, and this may neutralise acid around the bacteria. Colonisation often extends into gastric glands (Fig. 20.6). Where they are numerous, the underlying mucosa usually shows a superficial gastritis of the type known as chronic active or type B gastritis (not to be confused with type A atrophic autoimmune gastritis of pernicious anaemia). This is characterised by infiltration with chronic inflammatory cells and polymorphonuclear leucocytes. Mucus-secreting foveolar cells often show damage where the bacteria are numerous.

Virulence factors

All isolates of *H. pylori* produce a vacuolating toxin (VacA) of variable activity, while >60% of isolates produce a cytotoxin (CagA). As well as providing acid protection, urease may also promote colonisation in other ways, such as contributing to urea-dependent chemotactic motility towards the gastric epithelium. In addition, host factors strongly influence the outcome of infection, such as polymorphisms in genes involved in proinflammatory responses.

The *cagA* gene is a marker for strains that confer an increased risk of both peptic ulceration and gastric malignancy, although other factors play a role, as strains lacking the toxin can still cause gastritis. The gene forms part of a pathogenicity island, which also encodes a secretion system capable of injecting bacterial macromolecules, including CagA and peptidoglycan fragments, into host cells. The injected CagA protein is phosphorylated by a host kinase and subsequently interacts with various signal transduction pathways to affect epithelial cell morphology and behaviour. Peptidoglycan binds to the intracellular NOD1 receptor and contributes to the initiation or continuation of a proinflammatory immune response. An anti-apoptotic effect may aid bacterial persistence on the gastric epithelium.

The vacuolating toxin has been associated with pore formation in host cell membranes, the loosening of the tight junctions between epithelial cells (thus affecting mucosal barrier permeability), and specific immune suppression. The *vacA* gene, present in all *H. pylori* strains, exhibits a high degree of allelic variation in different regions of the gene, leading to differences in activity. Each allele encodes different VacA types associated with an increased risk of certain patterns of gastroduodenal disease.

In addition to VacA and CagA, *H. pylori* expresses adhesin proteins that allow reversible adhesion to host receptors mostly present in inflamed tissue, including sialyl-Lewis X and the ABO blood group antigens. The combination of *H. pylori* genotypes and host genetic polymorphisms influences the risks associated with *H. pylori* infection.

Epidemiology

Humans appear to be the sole reservoir and source of *H. pylori*. Infection is presumed to be by the oral–oral or, possibly, faecal–oral route and has been suggested to be mostly intrafamilial. Volunteer studies indicate that the adult infectious dose is relatively high, but infections resulting from lower doses may resolve quickly, whereas higher doses lead to persistent infection.

Infection rates are strongly related to poor living conditions and overcrowding during childhood. There is a steady rise in seropositivity with increasing age (about 50% infected by the age of 60 years in industrialised countries). In developed nations, progressively fewer children are becoming colonised, but most children in developing countries are infected by the time they reach puberty. High rates of infection correlate broadly with high rates of gastric cancer. The so-called African enigma, in which high seropositivity is associated with low gastric cancer risk, may be due to intestinal helminth infection driving the local immune response towards a protective T helper cell 2 (Th2), rather than the deleterious Th1 response.

Inmates of psychiatric units and orphanages and professional staff carrying out endoscopy examinations show higher than average infection rates. Nosocomial infection from inadequately disinfected endoscopes has also occurred.

The course of infection

After an incubation period of a few days, patients suffer a mild attack of acute achlorhydric gastritis with symptoms of abdominal pain, nausea, flatulence and bad breath. Colonisation results in the formation of mucosa-associated lymphoid tissue (MALT) and infiltration of polymorphonuclear leucocytes, together producing the active gastritis. Symptoms last for about 2 weeks, but hypochlorhydria

may persist for up to a year. Despite a substantial humoral antibody response, infection and chronic active gastritis persist, but after several decades, there may be a progression to atrophic gastritis and intestinal metaplasia. Conditions are then inhospitable for *H. pylori*, which disappears or is much reduced in number.

Clinical features

The outcome of infection by *H. pylori* reflects an interaction between strain virulence, proinflammatory host genotypes and environmental factors. Despite the presence of chronic active gastritis, most infections are symptomless, and endoscopic appearances of the stomach are normal. However, in some infected persons the chronic active gastritis forms a launch pad for more serious clinical outcomes, such as gastric and duodenal ulcers, nonulcer dyspepsia and gastric malignancies.

Peptic ulceration

H. pylori is actively involved in the pathogenesis of peptic ulceration unrelated to nonsteroidal antiinflammatory agents or the Zollinger–Ellison syndrome. Infection is virtually a prerequisite for ulceration, and elimination of *H. pylori* allows healing of ulcers without recurrence. Recurrent ulceration is almost always associated with recrudescence of infection.

The topographical pattern of gastritis is a predictor of clinical outcome. In antral predominant gastritis, hyperacidity induced by *H. pylori* via increased gastrin production promotes duodenal gastric metaplasia and this leads to colonisation of the duodenum, inflammation and finally ulceration. With corpus-predominant gastritis or pangastritis, host interactions lead to the suppression of acid production and destruction of parietal cells. Consequently, duodenal ulceration is not evident, although hypoacidity can lead to epithelial changes and gastric gland atrophy that increase the risk of gastric ulceration.

Nonulcer dyspepsia

Some cases of nonulcer dyspepsia are associated with *H. pylori*, as eradication has a small but significant effect on dyspepsia and prevents the development of peptic ulcers in some patients. Although currently there is no way of identifying such patients, a 'test and treat' strategy is justified on economic grounds.

Gastric cancer

Atrophic gastritis resulting from longstanding infection with *H. pylori* is associated with an increased risk of developing gastric cancer. In addition, gastric MALT lymphoma is strongly associated with *H. pylori* infection, and in most cases complete regression has been observed after eradication of the infection.

Other disease

H. pylori infection has been associated statistically with several conditions outside the digestive tract, including coronary heart disease, iron deficiency anaemia and cot death. Although these are of great potential importance, the links remain unproven because of possible confounding factors. Epidemiological data link eradication of *H. pylori* infection with development of oesophageal cancer, allergy and asthma.

Laboratory investigation

Noninvasive tests are used for initial screening. Definitive tests of infection depend on finding *H. pylori* in specimens of gastric mucosa obtained by biopsy.

Noninvasive tests

Serology Serological tests, mostly based on ELISA or latex agglutination, detect antibodies to *H. pylori* or its products and are used to screen patients with dyspepsia. They are less useful for screening children and are unreliable for excluding infection in elderly patients, or as a test for cure in patients who have received treatment (owing to variable persistence of antibody). The accuracy of rapid bedside tests of whole blood is poor.

Urea breath test This test detects bacterial urease activity in the stomach by measuring the output of carbon dioxide resulting from the splitting of carbon-13 or carbon-14 labeled urea into carbon dioxide and ammonia; infected patients give high readings. The test has excellent sensitivity and specificity, but carbon-14 is weakly radioactive, so it is not used in children. A mass spectrometer is needed to assay nonradioactive carbon-13. The urea breath test cannot be used during or directly after antibiotic therapy.

Faecal antigen test Stool antigen tests that detect *H. pylori* antigens in faeces are available. Tests based on the use of monoclonal antibodies are more accurate than polyclonal antibody tests and have the potential to supplant serology for routine screening.

Polymerase chain reaction (PCR) DNA probes for the direct detection of *H. pylori* in gastric juice, faeces, dental plaque and water supplies have been developed. Some can also detect genes expressing antibiotic resistance and presence of the *cagA* pathogenicity island. Newer versions can detect *H. pylori* within a few hours. Present methods are unsuitable for general use because clinical samples may contain compounds that inhibit the reaction.

Invasive tests

Collection of specimens Ideally, patients for endoscopy should not have received antibiotics or proton pump inhibitors for 1 month before the test. Mucosal biopsy specimens are taken from the gastric antrum within 5 cm of the pylorus, and preferably also from the body of the stomach. For maximum sensitivity, duplicate specimens are taken: one for histopathology (placed in fixative); the other for culture (placed in the neck of a sterile bottle made humid by adding a tiny amount of normal saline). Specimens for culture must be processed as soon as possible, certainly on the same day, or placed in transport medium.

Biopsy urease test This is a simple and cheap test that can be performed at the bedside. A biopsy specimen is placed into a small quantity of urea solution with a dye such as phenol red, which detects alkalinity resulting from the formation of ammonia. Most infected patients (70%) give a positive result within 2 hours, and 90% after 24 hours. Newer tests have faster reaction times, and a test with monoclonal antibody promises higher sensitivity and specificity.

Histopathology and microscopy Histopathology provides a permanent record of the nature and grading of a patient's gastritis as well as detecting *H. pylori*. Organisms can be seen in sections stained with haematoxylin and eosin, but more specific stains make the task easier (see Fig. 20.6). The bacteria can also be seen in smears of biopsy material stained with Gram stain. Fluorescein-based molecular probes under development are potentially able to detect *H. pylori* and its virulence factors.

Culture Culture is no more sensitive than skilled microscopy of histological sections but has several advantages: isolates can be tested for antimicrobial resistance and typed for epidemiological studies; information about the presence of virulence factors can inform clinical outcome.

Rich growth media (commonly including lysed or whole animal blood or complement-inactivated serum), selective agars and incubation conditions similar to those used for campylobacters are used for primary isolation (see Ch. 20). Sensitivity is increased if a nonselective medium is used in parallel. High humidity is essential. Plates are left undisturbed for 3 days and incubated for a week before being discarded as negative. *H. pylori* forms discrete domed colonies, unlike the effuse colonies of *C. jejuni* and *C. coli*.

Treatment

Elimination of *H. pylori* infection is not always necessary and is associated with an increase in prevalence of other inflammatory diseases and oesophageal cancer. Two unequivocal indications for treatment are:

- peptic ulcer disease
- gastric MALT lymphoma.

Possible indications are:

- patients with nonulcer dyspepsia refractory to conventional treatment
- patients with a family history of gastric carcinoma.

In vitro, *H. pylori* is sensitive to most β-lactam antibiotics, macrolides, tetracyclines and nitroimidazoles, but resistant to trimethoprim. In practice, the choice of antibiotic is dependent on stability in acid, activity against very slow growing organisms, and diffusion into the gastric mucus layer; this mainly limits treatment to four main antibiotics: amoxicillin, clarithromycin, tetracycline and metronidazole. It is also sensitive to bismuth subcitrate or subsalicylate and partially sensitive to the acid-lowering proton pump inhibitors omeprazole and lansoprazole.

To eradicate *H. pylori* infection, at least two antimicrobial agents must be given in combination with an acid-lowering agent (triple therapy), as monotherapy rapidly leads to antibiotic resistance. A popular regimen is a 1-week course of the macrolide clarithromycin, plus amoxicillin and omeprazole (or lansoprazole). These regimens eliminate *H. pylori* in about 90% of patients. Alternative therapies usually contain tetracycline; use of metronidazole is now avoided because of its mutagenic properties and the high prevalence of resistance (>50% in many industrialised nations). Similar regimens are used with children but eradication rates are generally lower than those in adults.

Recrudescence of infection demands a repeat biopsy with culture and sensitivity testing of the infecting strain. Treatment failure may result from poor compliance or antibiotic resistance, which is common for metronidazole and clarithromycin, but still rare for tetracycline and amoxicillin. Some fluoroquinolones are active against *H. pylori*, and changes in treatment regimen may improve compliance and eradication rates.

Control

Social deprivation is the dominant factor governing the prevalence of *H. pylori* infection. In Western society, social advancement has brought about a reduction of infection, and peptic ulcer disease is on the decline. However, this is far from the case in developing countries, where a cheap and effective vaccine would be valuable, particularly for the prevention of gastric cancer.

RECOMMENDED READING

Blaser, M. J., & Atherton, J. C. (2004). *Helicobacter pylori:* Biology and disease. *Journal of Clinical Investigation, 113*(3), 321–333. doi:10.1172/JCI200420925.

Gerrits, M. M., van Vliet, A. H., Kuipers, E. J., & Kusters, J. G. (2006). *Helicobacter pylori* and antimicrobial resistance: Molecular mechanisms and clinical implications. *Lancet Infectious Diseases, 6*(11), 699–709. doi:: http://dx.doi.org/10.1016/S1473-3099(06)70627-2.

Gilbreath, J. J., Cody, W. L., Merrell, D. S., & Hendrixson, D. R. (2011). Change is good: Variations in common biological mechanisms in the epsilonproteobacterial genera *Campylobacter* and *Helicobacter*. *Microbiology and Molecular Biology Reviews, 75*(1), 84–132. doi:10.1128/MMBR.00035-10.

Janssen, R., Krogfelt, K. A., Cawthraw, S. A., van Pelt, W., Wagenaar, J. A., & Owen, R. J. (2008). Host-pathogen interactions in *Campylobacter* infections: The host perspective. *Clinical Microbiology Reviews, 21*(3), 505–518. doi:10.1128/CMR.00055-07.

Sheppard, S. K., & Meric, G. E. (Eds.). (2014). *Campylobacter ecology and evolution*. Norfolk: Caister Academic Press.

Kusters, J. G., van Vliet, A. H., & Kuipers, E. J. (2006). Pathogenesis of *Helicobacter pylori* infection. *Clinical Microbiology Reviews, 19*(3), 449–490. doi:10.1128/CMR.00054-05.

Nachamkin, I., Szymanski, C. M., & Blaser, M. J. (Eds.). (2008). *Campylobacter* (3rd ed.). Washington: ASM Press.

Young, K. T., Davis, L. M., & Dirita, V. J. (2007). *Campylobacter jejuni*. *Nature Reviews. Microbiology, 5*(9), 665–679.

Websites

American College of Gastroenterology. Treatment of Helicobacter pylori infection. Available at http://gi.org/guideline/treatment-of-helicobacter-pylori-infection/. (Accessed Oct 2017).

British Society of Gastroenterology. Helicobacter pylori. Available at http://www.bsg.org.uk/patients/general/helicobacter-pylori.html. (Accessed Oct 2017).

Centers for Disease Control and Prevention. *Foodborne Illness A-Z:* Campylobacter. Available at https://www.cdc.gov/campylobacter/. (Accessed Oct 2017).

Public Health England. Campylobacter. Available at https://www.gov.uk/government/collections/campylobacter-guidance-data-and-analysis. (Accessed Oct 2017).

The Helicobacter Foundation. http://www.helico.com. (Accessed Oct 2017).

World Health Organization. Campylobacter. Available at http://www.who.int/mediacentre/factsheets/fs255/en/. (Accessed Oct 2017).

21 Vibrio, Mobiluncus, Gardnerella and Spirillum

Cholera; vaginosis; rat bite fever

MICHAEL R. BARER

KEY POINTS

- *Vibrio cholerae* belonging to serogroups O1 and O139 are the causative agents of epidemic cholera.
- Cholera toxin is the key virulence determinant, causing extensive loss of water and electrolytes in the form of rice-water stools; death from cholera can be prevented with rehydration therapy.
- *V. parahaemolyticus* is a major cause of diarrhoea in Japan and Southeast Asia; infection is associated with the consumption of seafood.
- Infection with *V. vulnificus* may result in rapid-onset and fatal septicaemia, particularly in people with conditions of iron overload, and is associated with the consumption of seafood.
- Although *Mobiluncus* spp. and *Gardnerella vaginalis* are associated with bacterial vaginosis their culture is no longer essential to diagnosis. Shifts in the local microbiome are considered more significant.
- *Spirillum minus* causes rat bite fever.

VIBRIO

The *Vibrio* genus includes more than 30 species commonly found in aquatic environments. Some cause disease in human beings as well as in marine vertebrates and invertebrates. The most important pathogens of man are *Vibrio cholerae, V. parahaemolyticus* and *V. vulnificus*, but various other species are occasionally implicated as opportunist pathogens. Historically, vibrios have been associated almost exclusively with epidemic and pandemic cholera caused by a particular antigenic form of *V. cholerae*.

DESCRIPTION

Vibrios are short Gram-negative rods, which are often curved and actively motile by a single polar flagellum (Fig. 21.1). Nearly all produce the enzyme oxidase and give a positive indole reaction. The genus can be divided into nonhalophilic vibrios, including *V. cholerae* and other species that are able to grow in media without added salt, and halophilic species such as *V. parahaemolyticus* and *V. vulnificus* that require salt for growth. Vibrios grow readily on ordinary media provided that their requirements for electrolytes are met, and grow best when abundant oxygen is present. Most grow at 30°C but some of the halophilic species grow poorly at 37°C, whereas *V. cholerae, V. parahaemolyticus* and *V. alginolyticus* grow at 42°C.

Vibrios have a low tolerance to acid and prefer alkaline conditions (growth range pH 6.8–10.2, optimum pH 7.4–9.6).

VIBRIO CHOLERAE

Description

Strains of *V. cholerae* can be differentiated by their lipopolysaccharide O-antigens into some 200 different serogroups. Epidemic cholera is associated with the O1 and O139 antigens. Other serogroups are collectively known as "non-O1, non-O139 *V. cholerae*" and correspond to strains formerly known as *nonagglutinable vibrios* or *noncholera vibrios*. Some of these strains can cause diarrhoea in man. All strains of *V. cholerae* share the same flagellar (H) antigen.

Strains of *V. cholerae* O1 may be further subdivided on the basis of their O antigens into the subtypes *Inaba* and *Ogawa*; some strains possess determinants of both of these subtypes and are known as subtype *Hikojima*.

Two biotypes of *V. cholerae* O1 are described, classical and El Tor. The El Tor variant produces haemolysin-lysing sheep erythrocytes and has been dominant since the beginning of the seventh pandemic in 1961; the classical biotype, which was responsible for most of the earlier pandemics, appears to have become extinct in the 1980s.

V. cholerae is unusual amongst the Proteobacteria in possessing two circular chromosomes (~3 and 1 Mb), the

221

bacillary dysentery. Anuria develops, muscle cramps occur, and the patient quickly becomes weak and lethargic with loss of skin turgor, low blood pressure, and an absent or thready pulse. There are, however, all grades of severity, and milder cases cannot be distinguished clinically from other secretory diarrhoeas. Symptomless infections are common.

Pathogenic mechanisms

Cholera is a noninvasive and essentially toxin-mediated disease. While many contributions to virulence have been described, cholera toxin (CT) and the toxin coregulated pilus (TCP) are of overriding importance. Both regulation of virulence factor expression and quorum sensing appear to play roles in *V. cholerae* virulence.

V. cholerae is acid sensitive, and relatively high doses are said to be required for sufficient numbers to pass the gastric barrier. However, conditions reducing stomach acid, including early *H. pylori* infection and drugs suppressing acid production, increase susceptibility.

The alkaline environment of the small intestine promotes replication and vibrios show chemotaxis toward epithelial cells, facilitated by active motility and the production of mucinase and other proteolytic enzymes. Once the organism has penetrated the mucous layer it adheres to the enterocyte surface. TCP is the major adhesin; it also promotes cell–cell association leading to the production of microcolonies.

Once adherent, the bacteria produce CT, an A+5B subunit enterotoxin. The five B subunits (11.6 Kd) and single A subunit (27.2 Kd) are virtually identical to the heat-labile toxin (LT) of enterotoxigenic *E. coli* (ETEC). The A subunit is made up of two peptides (A_1 and A_2) linked by a single disulphide bridge. The B subunit binds to sugar residues of ganglioside GM_1 on the cells lining the villi and crypts of the small intestine. The CT-GM_1 complex is endocytosed and trafficked to the Golgi apparatus and endoplasmic reticulum where the A_1 subunit is released and ADP ribosylates the G protein component of adenyl cyclase rendering it permanently active. The resultant intracellular increase in cyclic AMP produces hypersecretion of Cl^- ions which, with the balancing outflow of Na^+ ions, leads to a massive net outflow of water across enterocytes leading to a serious loss of water and electrolytes that in severe cases may be fatal within 12 to 24 hours. Although the Na^+-linked mechanisms for water uptake are overwhelmed, the glucose and amino acid–linked uptake mechanisms are not and this provides the basis for life-saving oral rehydration therapy.

Non-01, non-0139 V. cholerae

These strains of *V. cholerae* cause mild, sometimes bloody diarrhoea, often accompanied by abdominal cramps.

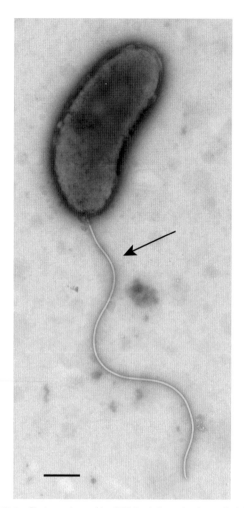

Fig. 21.1 Electron micrograph of *Vibrio cholerae* showing typical short rod morphology with a single polar flagellum. Bar = 2 μm.

larger of which appears ancestral and the smaller perhaps acquired more recently. Horizontal gene transfer, including bacteriophage integration, has been critical to the development of this pathogen, the origin of the O139 serotype and the emergence of antibiotic resistance.

Pathogenesis
Clinical manifestations

Cholera is characterized by the sudden onset of effortless vomiting and profuse watery diarrhoea. Although vomiting is a common feature, the rapid dehydration and hypovolaemic shock, which may cause death in 12 to 24 h, are related mainly to the profuse, watery, colourless stools with flecks of mucus and a distinctive fishy odour—*rice-water stools*—which contain little protein and are very different from the mucopurulent blood-stained stools of

Symptoms may occasionally be severe, in which case the disease resembles cholera. Wound infections may occur in patients exposed to aquatic environments, and bacteraemia and meningitis have been reported. They may elaborate a wide range of virulence factors, including enterotoxins, cytotoxins, haemolysins and colonizing factors. A few produce cholera toxin.

Laboratory investigation

Stool specimens are inoculated into alkaline peptone water, in which vibrios grow rapidly and accumulate on the surface. After incubation for 3 to 6 hours, a loopful from the surface is inoculated onto a suitable solid medium such as thiosulphate–citrate–bile salts–sucrose (TCBS) agar. On this medium *V. cholerae* forms yellow sucrose-fermenting colonies, which are tested for the enzyme oxidase and for agglutination with rabbit antibodies specific for the O1 lipopolysaccharide antigens before biochemical or MALDI confirmation.

Immunological stool dipstick tests are available for cholera and appear to have some value especially in resource limited settings.

Epidemiology

V. cholerae O1

The natural habitat for this global pathogen is in semisaline (brackish) waters where it can associate in biofilms with zooplankton and chitinous surfaces.

A series of six pandemics, originating in the Bengal Basin, ravaged the world in the 19th and 20th centuries.

Subsequently, cholera was contained within the endemic foci and surrounding areas of India and Bangladesh until 1961, when a seventh pandemic due to the El Tor biotype of *V. cholerae* O1, originally isolated from pilgrims at the quarantine station known as El Tor, began to supplant the classic biotype in India. By 1973 the El Tor biotype had entirely displaced the classic biotype in Bangladesh and spread to Indonesia, the Far East and Africa. In 1991 it reached South America, where the first epidemic in that subcontinent of the 20th century occurred in Peru. In the following decade more than 1 million cases were reported (Fig. 21.2). In 2010, several months after a catastrophic earthquake, a new outbreak began in Haiti; it was apparently initiated by asymptomatic infections in United Nations security forces from Nepal. The outbreak produced cases in several other nations in the region and illustrated the potential importance of asymptomatic individuals in dissemination and the significance of fragile public health infrastructures in facilitating the over 0.5 million cases that ensued.

Infection is generally spread by contaminated water or foods such as uncooked seafood or vegetables. The source of the contamination is usually the faeces of carriers or patients with cholera, but contamination may occur from natural aquatic reservoirs, too. Cholera is characteristically an infection of crowded communities with poor standards of hygiene and shared communal water supplies such as tanks, ponds, canals, or rivers used for bathing, washing, and household use. Outbreaks occur either as explosive epidemics, usually in nonendemic areas, or as protracted epidemic waves in endemic areas. The seasonal incidence is fairly consistent in different endemic regions, although

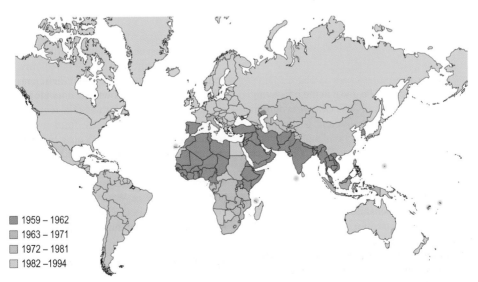

- ■ 1959 – 1962
- ■ 1963 – 1971
- ■ 1972 – 1981
- ■ 1982 –1994

Fig. 21.2 Areas reporting indigenous cholera to the World Health Organization 1959–1994. (Redrawn from data in Public Health Laboratory Service, *Communicable Disease Report Review* 1:R48–R50, 1991; WHO, *Weekly Epidemiological Record* 70:201–208, 1995.)

the climatic conditions during epidemic waves may be distinctive for each region. For example, in Bangladesh the cholera season (November to February) follows the monsoon rains and ends with the onset of the hot dry months. In Calcutta the main epidemic wave (May to July) rises to its peak in the hot dry season and ends with the onset of the monsoon, but extends inland to neighbouring states during the rainy season. Resultant changes in local salinity and the densities of lytic cholera bacteriophages appear influential in determining these seasonal patterns.

Spread of infection is facilitated by the high ratio of symptomless carriers to clinical cases, which can be as high as 100 to 1, and was recognised as a particular feature of El Tor infections prior to the extinction of the classic biotype.

V. cholerae O139

This strain emerged in the 1990s and closely resembles *V. cholerae* O1 El Tor biochemically and physiologically, and may eventually attain the status of a subtype (*Bengal*). The disease is indistinguishable from that caused by O1 strains and is confined to the subcontinent.

Other non-O1, non-O139 V. cholerae serogroups

Such strains occur widely in aquatic environments, and many infections are associated with exposure to saline environments or consumption of seafood. They appear to survive and multiply in a wide range of foods, and it is likely that foodborne outbreaks occur as with other enteric pathogens. There has been strong recent interest in the impact of climate change on the incidence of enteric, wound, and systemic infections due to these and other vibrios.

Treatment

In cholera absolute priority must be given to the life-saving replacement of fluid and electrolytes. Oral rehydration therapy, ideally with a rice-based solution, is often sufficient, but severe cases may require intravenous rehydration. The World Health Organization (WHO) promotes the use of oral rehydration therapy in all cases of severe diarrhoea, including that due to *V. cholerae*.

Single-dose azithromycin has become the antimicrobial treatment of choice where sensitivities and availability permit; doxycycline and ciprofloxacin are also used. Antimicrobials reduce the period of excretion of *V. cholerae* in the stools of patients with cholera and may help reduce transmission. Tetracycline-resistant strains began to appear in the 1970s and were soon followed by the appearance of strains resistant to a wide range of antimicrobials.

Control

Public health measures used in the control of any disease spread by faecal contamination are of value in the control of cholera. Most important are the provision of safe drinking water supplies and the proper disposal of human faeces.

Although cholera can be life threatening it is easily prevented and treated. Cholera among travellers is rare, and few infections are reported from industrialized countries.

Vaccines

The immune response to cholera is directed against the bacterium rather than the toxin. It is specific for a given serotype. Infection with the classic biotype is followed by almost complete immunity for several years, but infection with the El Tor biotype confers little or no immunity. It is not surprising, therefore, that the development of effective vaccines has proved difficult.

Traditional whole-cell vaccines are not very effective and are no longer recommended for travellers. Oral vaccines that combine purified B subunit and killed whole cells are now widely available and appear to be safe and moderately protective. A live attenuated vaccine strain CVD 103-HgR, based on a deletion of the CT A_2 subunit first produced in the 1990s, has recently been reformulated and appears to be highly protective (~90%).

VIBRIO PARAHAEMOLYTICUS

Description

V. parahaemolyticus is a halophilic vibrio and does not grow in the absence of sodium chloride. This property is conveniently demonstrated by inoculating the organism onto cystine–lactose–electrolyte-deficient (CLED) agar, which supports the growth of nonhalophilic vibrios but not halophilic species. Strains of *V. parahaemolyticus* from clinical specimens generally form green, non–sucrose-fermenting colonies on TCBS agar, but sucrose-fermenting strains are found in estuarine and coastal waters.

Strains associated with gastroenteritis usually express a thermostable haemolysin that causes β-haemolysis of human red cells in Wagatsuma agar, a special medium containing mannitol. This haemolysis is known as the Kanagawa phenomenon.

Pathogenesis

V. parahaemolyticus can cause explosive diarrhoea, but symptoms usually abate after 3 days. Other symptoms include abdominal pain, nausea and vomiting; there may be blood in the stools. A few extraintestinal infections have been reported, particularly from wounds.

Kanagawa-positive strains cause diarrhoea in volunteers. In contrast, volunteers have ingested 10^{10} cells of Kanagawa-negative strains without ill effects. Kanagawa-positive strains also adhere to human intestinal cells, whereas Kanagawa-negative strains do not. The heat-stable haemolysin disrupts the cytoskeleton of cell membranes and causes fluid accumulation in the rabbit ileal-loop toxin test. *V. parahaemolyticus* also produces a thermo-labile haemolysin that causes morphological changes in tissue culture cells resembling those caused by cholera toxin and the heat-labile enterotoxin of *E. coli*.

Most strains from seafood and the environment are Kanagawa negative, although positive colonies can usually be found if a sufficient number are tested. It is likely that a few Kanagawa-positive strains multiply selectively in the human intestine as infection develops and predominate in the stools of patients with diarrhoea.

Laboratory investigation

The faeces of patients with a history of recent consumption of seafood may be examined by the methods used for *V. cholerae*. In the examination of seafood and sea or estuarine waters for halophilic species, including *V. parahaemolyticus*, enrichment culture in alkaline peptone water containing 1% sodium chloride is used. Around 13 O types (somatic antigens) and 71 K types (capsular antigens) are recognized; serotype O3:K6 has been detected widely in India, Asia, Africa and Latin America.

Epidemiology

V. parahaemolyticus is a common cause of diarrhoea in Japan and Southeast Asia. It also causes illness associated with seafood in many other countries, including the United States and the United Kingdom. The organisms are common in fish and shellfish and in the waters from which they are harvested. Infections occur more frequently in warmer months when the organisms are most prevalent in the aquatic environment. There is a particular risk associated with the consumption of raw seafood prepared and eaten in Japanese-style restaurants.

Extraintestinal infections are always associated with exposure to the aquatic environment or handling of contaminated seafood.

Treatment and control

Patients with diarrhoea generally require only fluid replacement therapy. Infection can be avoided by normal food hygiene procedures and by refrigeration of seafood to reduce the possibility of bacterial multiplication. For wound infections and septicaemia, the most effective antimicrobial agents include tetracyclines, ciprofloxacin, ceftazidime and gentamicin.

VIBRIO VULNIFICUS

This halophilic species differs from other vibrios by utilizing lactose. There are three biotypes of *V. vulnificus* based on physiological, biochemical and serological properties. Biotype 1 is the predominant human pathogen. Biotype 2 infects eels, and biotype 3 causes human wound infections.

Pathogenesis

There are three distinct clinical syndromes:

Rapid onset of fulminating septicaemia followed by the appearance of cutaneous lesions. More than 50% of those with primary septicaemia die. The condition is invariably associated with the consumption of raw shellfish. It is thought that the organisms enter the bloodstream by way of the portal vein or the intestinal lymph system. Elderly males with liver function defects due to alcohol abuse and people with iron-overload conditions are particularly susceptible, but any deficiency in the immune system may be a contributing factor.

A rapidly progressing cellulitis following contamination of a wound sustained during exposure to salt water. Infections of this kind occur in otherwise healthy persons as well as in the debilitated and are characterized by wound oedema, erythema and necrosis, which progresses to septicaemia only occasionally. The infection can be rapidly fatal.

Acute diarrhoea following the consumption of shellfish. This is less common; victims generally have mildly debilitating underlying conditions. Death is rare.

Pathogenic mechanisms

Strains of *V. vulnificus* are acid tolerant, surviving in stomach acid by breaking down amino acids to produce amines and CO_2. A capsular polysaccharide and long-chain lipopolysaccharide enable pathogenic strains to resist phagocytosis and the killing effects of human serum complement. Two siderophores, a catechol (vulnibactin) and a hydroxamate, have been reported indicating the presence of high-affinity iron-uptake systems; however, many strains are unable to obtain ferric ions bound to human transferrin. Patients with iron overload disorders such as haemochromatosis are highly susceptible; high levels of free serum iron are thought to facilitate the rapid septicaemia observed in patients infected with this organism.

Several toxins may contribute to tissue damage. They include a metalloprotease, a collagenase, a mucinase and a cytotoxin. A vascular permeability factor has also been described. Strains of *V. vulnificus* express El Tor haemolysin and thermo-labile haemolysin, but a role in pathogenesis has not been demonstrated.

Epidemiology

Infections occur most frequently in areas where the water temperature remains high throughout the year, such as the mid-Atlantic and Gulf coast states of the United States. They are much more common during the warmer months of the year when *V. vulnificus* is most abundant. Wound infections are associated with injuries sustained in the aquatic environment, whereas septicaemic infections are associated with the consumption of raw shellfish.

Treatment

V. vulnificus wound infections and primary septicaemia require early antimicrobial treatment to reduce morbidity and mortality from the illness and to prevent complications. The most effective antimicrobial agents include tetracyclines, fluoroquinolones such as ciprofloxacin, ceftazidime and gentamicin. Because of the high case fatality rates, it is particularly important for clinicians to suspect *V. vulnificus* wound or bloodstream infections in persons with shellfish or warm seawater exposure and a history of chronic liver disease or conditions of iron overload.

VIBRIO ALGINOLYTICUS

Description

V. alginolyticus is a halophilic organism formerly regarded as biotype 2 of *V. parahaemolyticus*. It fails to grow on CLED agar but grows in the presence of 10% sodium chloride. It forms large, yellow (sucrose-fermenting) colonies on TCBS. There is pronounced swarming on nonselective solid media.

Pathogenesis

This organism causes wound and ear infections. Clinical features include mild cellulitis and a seropurulent exudate. The pathogenic mechanisms are not fully understood although genetic homology among *V. alginolyticus, V. cholerae* and *V. parahaemolyticus* has been shown.

Epidemiology

This organism is widely distributed in seawater and seafood and is probably the most common vibrio found in these sources in the United Kingdom. It occurs in large numbers throughout the year. Infections are invariably associated with exposure to seawater. Strains appear to be sensitive to ciprofloxacin.

OTHER VIBRIOS

- *Photobacterium damsela* is a halophilic marine vibrio found in tropical and semitropical aquatic environments. It is associated with severe infections of wounds acquired in warm coastal areas.
- *Vibrio fluvialis* is easily confused with *Aeromonas hydrophila*, but can be differentiated by growth on media containing 6% sodium chloride. Patients experience diarrhoea, abdominal pain, fever and dehydration. Low numbers of *V. fluvialis* can be isolated from fish and shellfish, and from warm seawater. It seems likely that infection is from contaminated seafood. Strains of *V. fluvialis* express El Tor haemolysin, and a vacuolating toxin acting on HeLa cells, but the role of these in pathogenesis has not been demonstrated.
- *Vibrio hollisae* is associated with bacteraemia and diarrhoea, especially in warm coastal areas such as the Gulf of Mexico. Infections are strongly associated with the consumption of raw seafood. The organism is difficult to isolate because it grows poorly on TCBS agar. Strains of *V. hollisae* exhibit gene sequences homologous with those encoding the thermo-stable haemolysin of *V. parahaemolyticus*.
- *Vibrio mimicus* is a nonhalophilic vibrio named for its similarity to *V. cholerae* and occurrence in similar environments. Most isolates are from the stools of patients who develop gastroenteritis after consumption of raw oysters, although a few cases of otitis media have also been reported. In vitro, strains of *V. mimicus* express thermo-stable direct haemolysin, El Tor haemolysin, and thermo-labile haemolysin.
- *Vibrio furnissii* is most commonly isolated from stool samples. It has occasionally been implicated in gastroenteritis.

Other aquatic organisms that are probably related to vibrios include *Aeromonas* spp. and *Plesiomonas shigelloides*. *Aeromonas* spp., notably *A. hydrophila*, have been implicated in diarrhoea and occasionally cause more serious infection in compromised individuals. *A. salmonicida* is an economically important pathogen of fish. *P. shigelloides* is an organism of uncertain taxonomic status that sometimes causes waterborne outbreaks of diarrhoea in warm countries.

MOBILUNCUS

The name *Mobiluncus* was first proposed for a group of curved, motile, Gram-variable, anaerobic bacteria isolated from the vagina of women with bacterial vaginosis. Its taxonomic position is uncertain. Studies of 16S RNA suggest that the genus is most closely related to *Actinomyces*.

DESCRIPTION

There are two subspecies: *M. curtisii* and *M. mulieris*; *M. curtisii* can be divided further into two subspecies: *M. curtisii* ssp. *curtisii* and *M. curtisii* ssp. *holmesii*. *M. curtisii* is short rod (mean length 1.5 μm) and Gram-variable, whereas *M. mulieris* is longer (mean length 3.0 μm) and gram-negative. Both have multiple flagella originating from the concave aspect of the cells. Cell wall studies have revealed no outer membrane, but both species are thought to be Gram-negative.

PATHOGENESIS

Bacterial vaginosis

Mobiluncus spp. are isolated from 97% of women with bacterial vaginosis (nonspecific vaginitis) and are rarely found in the vagina of healthy women. Bacterial vaginosis appears to be a polymicrobial infection, with certain organisms playing a key role, especially when they overgrow the lactobacilli of the normal microbiota, raising the vaginal pH above 4.5. The condition is characterized by the presence of a thin, homogeneous vaginal discharge with a characteristic "rotten fish" smell. This becomes more pronounced on alkalization and can be evoked by placing a drop of potassium hydroxide solution on the fresh exudate on a slide or the speculum used for the vaginal examination. The characteristic smell is ascribed to amines produced by one or more of the bacterial species that form the complex microbial microbiota of the vagina.

Mobiluncus are frequently found in association with *Gardnerella vaginalis* (see upcoming discussion) and with other organisms that may also be of aetiological importance. It appears that both the combination of species and their relative numbers are of importance in the development of the syndrome. The organisms may be isolated from the urethra of male consorts of infected women but do not persist in men once condom use is implemented.

Mobiluncus spp. are occasionally isolated from extragenital sites, especially from breast abscesses. A fatal case of bacteraemia caused by *M. curtisii* has been reported.

Pathogenic mechanisms

The mechanisms that allow *Mobiluncus* spp. to cause disease are poorly understood. They express pili and are able to obtain iron from lactoferrin, but the role of these in the pathogenesis of disease is speculative. Strains of *Mobiluncus* spp. express a relatively thermo-stable toxin that is cytotoxic for Vero (African green monkey) cells, but a role in pathogenesis has not been demonstrated. Primates can be infected experimentally, and animal studies may help to elucidate the pathogenesis of vaginitis.

LABORATORY INVESTIGATION

Microscopy of fresh unstained vaginal exudate reveals epithelial cells covered with adherent bacteria (*clue cells*). *Mobiluncus* spp. can be grown in Columbia blood broth and peptone–starch–dextrose broth containing 10% horse serum. The organisms are essentially anaerobic but grow slowly in 5% oxygen in nitrogen. They do not produce oxidase or catalase but ferment sugars.

A multiplex PCR comprising primers for both *Mobiluncus* spp. and *G. vaginalis* has been applied to cases of bacterial vaginosis.

TREATMENT

Treatment of bacterial vaginosis aims to restore the normal vaginal microbiota by eliminating *Mobiluncus* and other organisms that may be involved. Oral or intravaginal metronidazole and clindamycin have been successfully used. Although *M. mulieris* is more susceptible than *M. curtisii* to metronidazole, treatment with this drug appears to eliminate all *Mobiluncus* spp. in patients with vaginosis.

GARDNERELLA

Gardnerella vaginalis (formerly *Corynebacterium vaginale* or *Haemophilus vaginalis*) is commonly isolated together with *Mobiluncus* spp. in bacterial vaginosis. It has been implicated in cases of cervical cancer and infections of the urinary tract, but because the organism is frequently present in the vagina of asymptomatic patients its role in disease is equivocal.

DESCRIPTION

G. vaginalis is a nonmotile, nonsporing, microaerophilic coccobaccilus. It is Gram-variable, but because the cell wall contains lipopolysaccharide it appears to be Gram-negative.

LABORATORY INVESTIGATION

G. vaginalis grows on various media such as Columbia agar containing colistin and nalidixic acid as selective agents. Plates are incubated at 35°C to 37°C in 5% to 10% carbon dioxide for 2 to 3 days. On media containing human erythrocytes, the organism produces zones of β-haemolysis. *G. vaginalis* does not produce oxidase or catalase, but ferments starch and hydrolyses hippurate, and these properties provide a means of presumptive identification. Genes encoding the 60 kDa heat-shock protein chaperonin *Cpn* 60 can be used to detect *G. vaginalis* by PCR.

PATHOGENESIS

Whether *G. vaginalis* can cause disease in isolation is unclear. The organisms may simply flourish in the vaginal environment provided by other bacteria. Infections with *G. vaginalis* are associated with proteolysis yielding nitrous products such as cadaverines and putrescines, which contribute to the characteristic odour resulting from these infections. The ability to lyse human red cells offers a mechanism for acquiring metabolic iron and may aid multiplication. Similarly, *G. vaginalis* can acquire ferric ions from human lactoferrin. Strains produce various mucinases such as sialidase and proline dipeptidase, which are thought to damage the vaginal mucosa as part of the pathogenic process. Patients infected with *G. vaginalis* produce IgA antibodies to the haemolysin.

TREATMENT

For the treatment of bacterial vaginosis, see previous section *Mobiluncus*.

SPIRILLUM MINUS

The organism commonly known as *Spirillum minus* is of uncertain taxonomic position since a type-strain for this taxon has not been identified. Along with *Streptobacillus moniliformis* (see Ch. 31) it is one of the causes of rat bite fever in humans.

DESCRIPTION

S. minus is a spiral Gram-negative organism about 2 to 5 μm in length and 0.2 μm in diameter. Longer forms of up to 10 μm may be observed. The regular short coils have a wavelength of 0.8 to 1 μm. The organisms are very actively motile, showing darting movements like those of a vibrio. The movement is due to polar flagella, which vary in number from one to seven at each pole. The organisms can be demonstrated in fresh specimens by dark-ground illumination or by staining with Giemsa or Leishman stain. The organism has not been reliably cultivated on artificial media, and many of its properties are unknown. It can be cultured in vivo by intraperitoneal injection into guinea pigs or mice.

LABORATORY INVESTIGATION

In rat bite fever, *S. minus* may be demonstrated in the local lesion, in the regional lymph glands, or in the blood by direct microscopy or by animal inoculation. In theory, *S. minus* DNA may be amplified by broad range bacterial 16S rRNA gene primers.

PATHOGENESIS

S. minus is transmitted to humans by animal bite; human-to-human transmission has not been recorded. The clinical syndrome of rat bite fever begins with an acute onset of fever and chills 1 to 4 weeks after the bite, although infection without fever may occur. The bite usually heals before the onset of symptoms but it often reulcerates. Local lymphadenopathy and lymphangitis develop with the onset of fever and systemic disease. A generalized rash with large brown to purple macules is usually observed, but some patients present with urticarial lesions. A roseolar rash may spread from the area of the original bite. Fever usually declines within 1 week before returning again after a few days; the fever may then recur in an episodic fashion for months or even years.

Endocarditis, meningitis, hepatitis, nephritis and myocarditis are rare complications. In most untreated cases, symptoms resolve within 2 months, after six to eight episodes of fever, and fewer than 6.5% of untreated cases are fatal.

EPIDEMIOLOGY

S. minus occurs naturally in wild rats and other rodents, causing bacteraemia. Human rat bite fever occurs mainly in Africa, Japan (where it is known as *sodoku*) and the Far East. There have been a few reports from Europe and the United States. The disease is prevalent in laboratory workers who handle rats, and in children who live in rat-infested homes.

TREATMENT

Infections respond to treatment with penicillin, erythromycin and tetracyclines. In the rare case of endocarditis, the addition of an aminoglycoside may be of value.

RECOMMENDED READING

Baker-Austin, C., Trinanes, J. A., Taylor, N. G. H., *et al.* (2013). Emerging Vibrio risk at high latitudes in response to ocean warming. *Nature Climate Change*, *3*(1), 73–77. doi:10.1038/nclimate1628.

Chen, W. H., Cohen, M. B., Kirkpatrick, B. D., *et al.* (2016). Single-dose live oral cholera vaccine CVD 103-HgR protects against human experimental infection with *Vibrio cholerae* O1 El Tor. *Clinical Infectious Diseases*, *62*(11), 1329–1335. doi:10.1093/cid/ciw145.

Dendle, C., Woolley, I. J., & Korman, T. M. (2006). Rat-bite fever septic arthritis: illustrative case and literature review. *European Journal of Clinical Microbiology & Infectious Diseases: Official Publication of the European Society of Clinical Microbiology*, *25*(12), 791–797. doi:10.1007/s10096-006-0224-x.

Letchumanan, V., Chan, K. G., & Lee, L. H. (2014). *Vibrio parahaemolyticus*: a review on the pathogenesis, prevalence, and advance molecular identification techniques. *Frontiers in Microbiology*, *5*, 13. doi:10.3389/fmicb.2014.00705.

Maraki, S., Christidou, A., Anastasaki, M., *et al.* (2016). Non-O1, non-O139 *Vibrio cholerae* bacteremic skin and soft tissue infections. *Infectious Diseases*, *48*(3), 171–176. doi:10.3109/23744235.2015.1104720.

Nelson, E. J., Harris, J. B., Morris, J. G., *et al.* (2009). Cholera transmission: the host, pathogen and bacteriophage dynamic. *Nature Reviews. Microbiology*, *7*(10), 693–702. doi:10.1038/nrmicro2204.

Sack, D. A., Sack, R. B., Nair, G. B., *et al.* (2004). Cholera. *Lancet*, *363*, 223–233.

Safa, A., Nair, G. B., & Kong, R. Y. (2010). Evolution of new variants of Vibrio cholerae O1. *Trends in Microbiology*, *18*, 46–54.

Vezzulli, L., Colwell, R. R., & Pruzzo, C. (2013). Ocean warming and spread of pathogenic vibrios in the aquatic environment. *Microbial Ecology*, *65*(4), 817–825. doi:10.1007/s00248-012-0163-2.

Websites

Centers for Disease Control and Prevention: Vibrio vulnificus. http://www.cdc.gov/nczved/divisions/dfbmd/diseases/vibriov/.

Centers for Disease Control and Prevention: Vibrio parahaemolyticus. http://www.cdc.gov/nczved/divisions/dfbmd/diseases/vibriop/.

Health Protection Agency: Cholera. http://www.hpa.org.uk/infections/topics_az/cholera/menu.htm.

Todar's Online Textbook of Bacteriology: Vibrio cholerae and Asiatic Cholera. http://textbookofbacteriology.net/cholera.html.

22 Pseudomonads and nonfermenters

Opportunist infection; cystic fibrosis; melioidosis

CRAIG WINSTANLEY

KEY POINTS

- Pseudomonads are Gram-negative, aerobic, saprophytic and innately resistant bacteria causing opportunist infections in humans, animals, plants and insects. The most important pseudomonad species responsible for human infections is *Pseudomonas aeruginosa*.
- *Ps. aeruginosa* is an important cause of hospital-acquired infections, especially in intensive care units and in neutropenic patients. Infections range from topical to systemic and may be trivial or life threatening.
- *Ps. aeruginosa* causes a range of other opportunistic infections, including infections of patients with burns or wounds, and eye infections associated with contact lens use.
- *Ps. aeruginosa* is a major cause of chronic debilitating and life-threatening respiratory infections in individuals with cystic fibrosis. During these long-term infections, *Ps. aeruginosa* undergoes specific adaptations, such as conversion to a mucoid phenotype and increased antibiotic resistance.
- Other Gram-negative glucose nonfermenters associated with opportunistic infections and antimicrobial resistance include bacteria in the genera *Acinetobacter*, *Achromobacter*, *Burkholderia* and *Stenotrophomonas*.
- *Burkholderia pseudomallei* is the causative agent of melioidosis, a serious tropical infection of humans and animals endemic in Southeast Asia and northern Australia.
- The *Burkholderia cepacia* complex causes life-threatening pulmonary infections in individuals with cystic fibrosis or chronic granulomatous disease.

In wine there is truth, in beer there is strength, in water there are pseudomonads!

(Adaptation of German proverb)

The term *pseudomonads* describes a large diverse group of aerobic, nonfermentative, Gram-negative bacilli, originally contained within the genus *Pseudomonas*. Presently, the group comprises >100 species. Most are saprophytes found widely in aquatic environments, including rivers and ponds, in the rhizosphere of plants, and in a variety of other moist environments. The group includes important pathogens for humans, animals, plants and insects.

Historically, the genus *Pseudomonas* has been used as a taxonomic dumping ground for novel species, often with diverse phenotypic characteristics. However, comprehensive analyses of the group have led to revised classifications, and many pseudomonads of clinical interest have been allocated to new genera including *Burkholderia*, *Brevundimonas*, *Delftia*, *Ralstonia*, *Pandoraea* and *Stenotrophomonas*. Other important Gram-negative glucose nonfermenters associated with opportunistic infections include bacteria in the genera *Acinetobacter* and *Achromobacter* (see Table 22.1).

Pseudomonas aeruginosa is the species most commonly associated with human disease, but *Burkholderia pseudomallei* has long been recognised as an important pathogen in tropical countries. Members of the *Burkholderia cepacia* complex are important pathogens in immunocompromised patients, particularly in individuals with cystic fibrosis or chronic granulomatous disease. *Stenotrophomonas maltophilia* also infects immunocompromised patients, with a mortality rate reaching 60% in patients with haematological malignancies. *Achromobacter* spp. cause a range of infections, including bacteraemia and infections of cystic fibrosis patients. Several other pseudomonads are occasionally isolated from clinical specimens as true opportunistic pathogens; these include *Ps. fluorescens*, *Ps. putida*, *Ps. stutzeri* and various glucose nonfermenters. In immunocompromised patients, it is important to distinguish whether culture of these bacteria reflects invasive infection rather than transitory colonisation.

Table 22.1 The principal genera and species of pseudomonads and other nonfermenters of clinical interest

Genus	Species
Pseudomonas	Ps. aeruginosa
	Ps. fluorescens
	debridement, putida
	debridement, stutzeri
	debridement, mendocina
Burkholderia	B. pseudomallei
	B. mallei
	B. cepacia complex
	B. gladioli
Delftia	D. acidovorans
Comamonas	C. testosteroni
Stenotrophomonas	Sten. maltophilia
Ralstonia	R. pickettii
Brevundimonas	Brev. diminuta
Pandoraea	P. apista
Achromobacter	Ach. xylosoxidans
Acinetobacter	A. baumannii

There are several reasons for the preeminence of *Ps. aeruginosa* as an opportunistic human pathogen:

- its large genome, which facilitates adaptability
- its innate resistance to many antibiotics and disinfectants
- its armoury of putative virulence factors
- an increasing supply of patients compromised by age, underlying disease or immunosuppressive therapy

The *Ps. aeruginosa* genome is unusually large (5.5–7.0 Mb), a feature shared by other Gram-negative opportunistic pathogens. With the advent of new sequencing technologies, studies using comparative genomics, and related approaches such as transcriptomics, proteomics and metabolomics, are providing valuable insights into the versatility, virulence and resistance of these important pathogens.

PSEUDOMONAS AERUGINOSA

DESCRIPTION

Ps. aeruginosa is a nonsporing, noncapsulate, nonfastidious Gram-negative bacillus; it is usually motile by virtue of one or two polar flagella. It is a strict aerobe but can grow anaerobically if nitrate is available as a terminal electron acceptor. The organism grows readily on a wide variety of culture media, over a wide temperature range, and emits a sweet grape-like odour that is easily recognised. Most strains produce diffusible pigments; typically, the colony and surrounding medium is greenish-blue due to production of a soluble blue phenazine pigment, *pyocyanin*, and the yellow-green fluorescent pigment *pyoverdine*; additional pigments include *pyorubrin* (red) and *melanin* (brown). Some isolates (10%–15%) produce pigment only when grown on pigment-enhancing media. Individual colonies vary from dwarf (small colony variants) to large mucoid types; most commonly, they are relatively large and flat with an irregular surface, a translucent edge and an oblong shape with the long axis parallel to the line of inoculum.

Ps. aeruginosa differs from members of the Enterobacteriaceae by deriving energy from carbohydrates by an oxidative rather than a fermentative metabolism. The species is inactive in carbohydrate fermentation tests, and only glucose is utilised. However, all strains give a rapid positive oxidase reaction (within 30 seconds), and this is a useful preliminary test for nonpigmented isolates.

Typing of *Ps. aeruginosa* isolates for epidemiological purposes originally relied on serotyping, susceptibility to phages and bacteriocin production. These techniques were superseded by molecular typing methods, including DNA fingerprinting by pulsed-field gel electrophoresis (PFGE) or multilocus sequence typing (MLST), but the accessibility and affordability of whole genome sequencing allows us an even greater level of resolution.

PATHOGENESIS

Ps. aeruginosa is pathogenic for a wide range of animal, plant and insect hosts. In humans, it can infect almost any anatomical surface or organ, causing an expanding spectrum of infections with variable morbidity and mortality. Community infections are uncommon and usually mild, but in hospital and other health-care settings, *Ps. aeruginosa* infections are more common, more varied, more severe and often associated with antimicrobial resistance.

Community infections

Infections such as otitis externa and varicose ulcers are often chronic but not disabling. In contrast, corneal infections, in particular keratitis associated with use of contact lenses, can be rapidly destructive. Recreational and occupational factors associated with *Ps. aeruginosa* infections include the relatively mild whirlpool or Jacuzzi rash (an acute self-limiting folliculitis) and serious industrial eye injuries, which may lead to panophthalmitis.

Hospital infections

Infections in hospital or other health-care settings can be localised, as in catheter-related urinary tract infection, infected ulcers, bedsores, burns and eye infections. However, in vulnerable patients compromised by age or diseases such as leukaemia, acquired immune deficiency syndrome (AIDS), and chemotherapy-induced neutropenia, *Ps. aeruginosa* infections often become bacteraemic, and the organism may be cultured from various organs postmortem. *Ps. aeruginosa* bacteraemia or necrotising pneumonia, though uncommon, is associated with a high mortality rate in neutropenic patients. Patients in critical care units are at particular risk; *Ps. aeruginosa* is the second most common cause of ventilator-associated pneumonia. Bacteraemic infections are uniquely characterised by the black necrotic skin lesions known as *ecthyma gangrenosum*.

Cystic fibrosis

The lungs of individuals with cystic fibrosis are particularly susceptible to life-threatening chronic infections caused by *Ps. aeruginosa*. Initial pulmonary infection with typical non-mucoid forms of *Ps. aeruginosa* occurs in early childhood and is often asymptomatic. This is followed by the emergence of mucoid alginate-producing variants, which grow within protective bacterial biofilms or microcolonies, and are associated with a damaging inflammatory response (Fig. 22.1). Subsequent repeated and debilitating episodes of pulmonary exacerbation are the main cause of morbidity and mortality. Once transition to the mucoid phenotype has occurred, eradication of *Ps. aeruginosa* is seldom if ever achieved. Using genomics and other approaches, there has been considerable progress in our understanding of how *Ps. aeruginosa* populations evolve to adapt to the cystic fibrosis lung environment, including

the accumulation of mutations associated with not only mucoidy but also loss of certain virulence factors, enhanced antibiotic resistance and increased mutation rates (hypermutability). However, it has also become apparent that infecting populations of *Ps. aeruginosa* can be highly diverse, such that two identical looking colonies from the same patient sputum sample may differ significantly in important phenotypes, such as resistance to antibiotics.

This has important implications clinically because diagnostic laboratories will often analyse and report resistance data derived from single isolates, which may not be representative of diverse bacterial populations. *Ps. aeruginosa* is also an important cause of chronic lung infections in patients with (non-cystic fibrosis) bronchiectasis or chronic obstructive pulmonary disease, and the bacteria undergo similar adaptations to those seen in cystic fibrosis.

Virulence factors

Most isolates of *Ps. aeruginosa* exhibit an armoury of cell-associated and extracellular virulence factors that can initiate or maintain infection. However, it is worth noting that virulence factors important in acute infections may not be required in chronic infections, and that most identified virulence factors have been characterised using animal models of acute infection. *Ps. aeruginosa* secretes an array of virulence factors, including exotoxin A and various cytotoxic proteases, elastases, phospholipases and rhamnolipids, as well as hydrogen cyanide and the toxic pigment pyocyanin. The intracellular action of exotoxin A is similar to that of diphtheria toxin fragment A. Pyoverdine (formerly known as fluorescein) provides *Ps. aeruginosa* with a potent bacterial siderophore to compete with mammalian iron-binding proteins such as transferrin. In association with pyocyanin, this also explains the characteristic blue-green pus of *Pseudomonas*-infected wounds.

Ps. aeruginosa exhibits highly evolved sensory systems, including quorum sensing, that allow regulation and coordinated expression of multiple virulence factors. Indeed, the cell density–dependent quorum sensing system regulates the production of many of the identified secreted virulence factors produced by *Ps. aeruginosa*. The pathogen also produces a Type III secretion system that allows injection of toxin or damaging effector proteins directly into the cytoplasm of host cells. Notably, strains of *Ps. aeruginosa* generally only secrete either exotoxin S or exotoxin U via their Type III secretion system. Indeed, phylogenetic analyses based on whole genome sequence comparisons suggest that the vast majority of *Ps. aeruginosa* isolates fall into two major subgroups: Group I is associated with an ability to invade host cells and production of exotoxin S, and Group II is associated with cytotoxicity and production of exotoxin U. This suggests

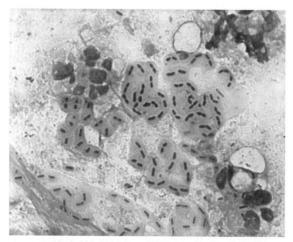

Fig. 22.1 Gram-stained sputum from patient harbouring mucoid *Ps. aeruginosa*. Note spawnlike microcolony and adjacent phagocytes. (Original magnification ×400.)

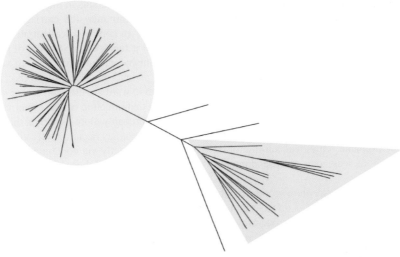

Fig. 22.2 Phylogenetic tree of *Ps. aeruginosa* based on comparisons of whole genome sequence data. The two major groups are highlighted: Group I *(blue)*; Group II *(pink)*.

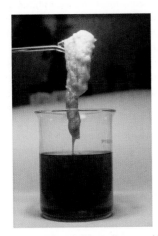

Fig. 22.3 Alcohol extraction of alginate from mucoid *Ps. aeruginosa*.

that *Ps. aeruginosa* can be subdivided into two distinct major pathotypes (see Fig. 22.2).

Virulence factors that are important in chronic infections are less well understood. However, it is clear that biofilm formation is important. The alginate-like exopolysaccharide, composed of D-mannuronic acid and L-guluronic acid, which is responsible for the mucoid colonial phenotype (Fig. 22.3), is implicated in this process.

LABORATORY INVESTIGATION

Material should be cultured on a selective medium that enhances the production of pyocyanin to aid detection. A selective medium containing acetamide as the sole carbon and nitrogen source may be used for enrichment from water or soil. About 10%–15% of isolates do not produce detectable pigment even on suitable media; in such cases, a positive oxidase test provides rapid presumptive evidence of the identity. Presumptive identification of isolates exhibiting atypical phenotypic features can be made with an appropriate commercial multitest system. It should be noted that isolates from cystic fibrosis patients can exhibit extensive variations in colonial morphology. Species identification can also be achieved based on a series of growth and biochemical tests (API-20NE kits) or by MALDI-TOF MS. Various reliable polymerase chain reaction (PCR) assays are also available. Although PCR-based detection directly applied to patient samples is possible, these approaches are not used routinely.

TREATMENT

Treatment of *Ps. aeruginosa* infection remains challenging. Most isolates are intrinsically resistant to commonly used antimicrobial agents. This problem is exacerbated because strains can acquire additional resistance either via mobile genetic elements or because of mutations occurring during the infection process, typically leading to changes such as the upregulation of efflux pumps or the enhanced production of antibiotic-inactivating enzymes. Indeed, specific multidrug-resistant clones (such as ST235) are increasingly common in hospitals worldwide.

Aminoglycosides (gentamicin, amikacin and tobramycin) and β-lactam compounds (piperacillin, ticarcillin, ceftazidime and carbapenems) are often used, alone or in combination. Combinations provide the potential for antibacterial synergy and reduced antibiotic resistance, but there is little evidence of clinical superiority. Fluoroquinolones such as ciprofloxacin exhibit good activity against *Ps. aeruginosa* and penetrate well into most tissues, but resistance may develop. Unlike most antipseudomonal agents, ciprofloxacin can be given orally. Monotherapy with extended-spectrum β-lactams (e.g., ceftazidime or carbapenems) may be effective but should be avoided in the treatment of chronic infections. In patients presenting with acute febrile neutropenia, empirical antimicrobial therapy should include at least one antipseudomonal antibiotic.

Polymyxins, though nephrotoxic, show good activity against *Ps. aeruginosa*, and resistance is unusual though not unheard of. Interest in these agents has been revived as a treatment of last resort for multiresistant *Ps. aeruginosa*, especially in patients with cystic fibrosis. Aerosolised delivery of colistin (polymyxin E) or tobramycin directly into the lungs has proved safe and clinically effective in the management of *Ps. aeruginosa* lung infection in individuals with cystic fibrosis.

Given the dangers posed by antimicrobial resistance, the threat of untreatable infections and the paucity of new antibiotics, there has been considerable interest in the development of novel therapeutic agents, such as agents targeting biofilms or virulence factors. In particular, there are a number of agents with activity against the *Ps. aeruginosa* quorum sensing system. Phage therapy has also been proposed as an alternative strategy, especially in the context of infections of burn patients. However, at present, antibiotics remain the first line of therapeutic attack.

EPIDEMIOLOGY

The ability of *Ps. aeruginosa* to persist and multiply in moist environments and equipment including sinks, drains, flower vases, hydrotherapy pools, ponds, rivers, humidifiers, washing machines and even distilled water is of particular importance in infection control. Consumption of salad vegetables contaminated with *Ps. aeruginosa* is a potential risk for immunocompromised patients in intensive care units. The organism is resistant to, and may multiply in, many disinfectants and antiseptics commonly used in hospitals. It can be a troublesome contaminant in pharmaceutical preparations and may cause eye infections following the faulty chemical sterilisation of contact lenses.

Ps. aeruginosa has relatively low intrinsic virulence but accounts for approximately 10% of all hospital-acquired infections. Such infections usually originate from exogenous sources, but some patients suffer endogenous infection, particularly of the urinary tract. Healthy carriers usually harbour strains in the gastrointestinal tract, but in the open community the carriage rate seldom exceeds 10%–15%. In contrast, acquisition of *Ps. aeruginosa* in a hospital is rapid, and up to 30% of patients may excrete the organisms within a few days of admission.

Burn patients are especially at risk; the presence of the organism in ward air, dust and eschar shed from the burns suggests that infection can be airborne. However, contact spread is probably more important than the airborne route. Transmission may occur directly via the hands of medical staff, or indirectly via contaminated apparatus. Severely burned patients and those with chest injuries who require artificial ventilation are highly susceptible to *Ps. aeruginosa*; pulmonary infection frequently precedes bacteraemia, which is often fatal. Intensive care equipment can be difficult to clean, and infection can undoubtedly be spread by this source.

Severe eye infections caused by *Ps. aeruginosa*, in particular, keratitis, may result from contaminated contact lenses, industrial eye injuries or the introduction of contaminated medicaments during ophthalmic procedures. Extremely painful ear infections acquired under the hyperbaric conditions of deep-sea diving operations have been reported.

The warm, moist and aerated conditions under which *Ps. aeruginosa* thrives are ideally met in poorly maintained recreational hot tubs or whirlpools. Ear infections and an irritating folliculitis (Fig. 22.4) may be acquired from such sources.

Epidemics of gastrointestinal infection can occur in newborn and young infants in maternity units and paediatric wards and may result from contaminated milk feeds. Other important *Ps. aeruginosa* infections in infants include bacteraemia and meningitis.

Although most cystic fibrosis patients acquire their *Ps. aeruginosa* strain from the environment, a number of specialist transmissible clones, such as the UK Liverpool

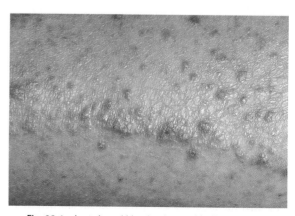

Fig. 22.4 Jacuzzi or whirlpool rash caused by *Ps. aeruginosa*.

Epidemic Strain, have been identified. Such clones transmit from patient to patient and can be associated with greater morbidity. Hence, they require additional cross-infection control measures.

CONTROL

Prevention is easier than cure; once *Ps. aeruginosa* has gained access to a niche in the hospital environment, particularly in hospital water supplies, or has established infection, it is notoriously difficult to eradicate. Three guidelines to control infection are offered in the knowledge that it is not always easy to put them into practice:

1. Patients at a high risk of acquiring infection with *Ps. aeruginosa* (e.g., a patient being evaluated for organ transplantation) should not be admitted to a ward where cases of *Ps. aeruginosa* infection are present.
2. Antimicrobial and other therapeutic substances and solutions must be free from *Ps. aeruginosa*. Particular danger exists when multidose ointments, creams or eye drops are used to treat several individuals over a period. Contamination of a sterile preparation can easily occur between uses, and *Ps. aeruginosa* readily multiplies at a range of temperatures in many medicaments. Contamination of medicinal products is also a hazard with other related pathogens, including the *Burkholderia cepacia* complex and *Ps. fluorescens*.
3. It is important to ensure that devices such as catheters and nebulisers are kept clear from *Ps. aeruginosa*, which readily forms highly resistant biofilms on surfaces.
4. In hospital units, episodes of cross-infection due to a single strain may occur as sporadic infections in individual patients over a period of months or years. For this reason, it is advantageous to identify highly transmissible epidemic strains by fingerprinting all clinically relevant isolates with a suitable typing system.

BURKHOLDERIA

Although most of the presently >30 known *Burkholderia* species are saprophytes, *B. pseudomallei*, *B. mallei* and the *B. cepacia* complex are important human or animal pathogens.

BURKHOLDERIA PSEUDOMALLEI

The environmental saprophyte *B. pseudomallei* causes melioidosis, a life-threatening tropical infection of humans and animals in Southeast Asia and Northern Australia. In endemic areas the organism is found in soil and surface water, particularly rice paddy fields and monsoon drains. Isolation rates are highest during the rainy season and in still rather than flowing water.

The incidence of melioidosis is increasing; it has emerged in South America, and the acquisition of *B. pseudomallei* in individuals with cystic fibrosis has been reported after recreational visits to Southeast Asia. As laboratory facilities can be limited in the rural tropics, published cases may represent only the tip of the iceberg. In northeastern Thailand, *B. pseudomallei* is responsible for up to 20% of community-acquired bacteraemias, and the species is the most common cause of fatal community-acquired pneumonia in Northern Australia.

A closely related species, *B. mallei*, causes glanders, a potentially fatal infectious disease of horses, mules and donkeys. Laboratory-acquired infection with either organism is a serious risk (hazard category 3), and both are regarded as potential bioterrorism agents.

MELIOIDOSIS

Human infection is acquired mainly percutaneously through skin abrasions or by inhalation of contaminated particles, especially during monsoon rains. Melioidosis commonly presents as pyrexia. The clinical manifestations are protean and range from dormant subclinical infection, diagnosed by the presence of specific antibodies, to acute pneumonia or chronic pulmonary infection that may resemble tuberculosis and other conditions, leading to a fulminating bacteraemia with a mortality rate of 80%–90%. The organism can survive intracellularly within the reticuloendothelial system, and this may account for latency and the emergence of symptoms resembling other infections many years after exposure. Suppurative parotitis is a characteristic presentation of melioidosis in children.

Laboratory investigation

B. pseudomallei can be difficult to identify in laboratories with little experience of the organism. The organism may be seen, usually in very small numbers, as small, bipolar-stained Gram-negative bacilli in exudates and can be cultured on appropriate media from sputum, urine, pus or blood, producing wrinkled or mucoid colonies after several days of growth. Fresh cultures emit a characteristic pungent odour of putrefaction. The organism is oxidase positive and motile but does not produce diffusible pigments. Formal identification by gas liquid chromatography and 16S rDNA sequencing should be confirmed by a reference laboratory.

Enzyme-linked immunosorbent assay (ELISA) for a conserved *B. pseudomallei* lipopolysaccharide antigen allows identification of specific antibodies in the evaluation of pyrexia of unknown origin. However, where melioidosis is endemic, a high rate of seropositivity due to childhood exposure to *B. pseudomallei* or subclinical exposure to the less virulent *B. thailandensis* limits this form of diagnosis. In some cases, serological diagnosis may require the use of the patient's own isolate as the reference strain.

Treatment

Accurate and early diagnosis, including culture of *B. pseudomallei*, and appropriate antibiotic therapy are key to successful management. The optimum treatment of severe melioidosis is unclear. Intravenous ceftazidime, followed by a combination of co-trimoxazole and doxycycline, is emerging as the treatment of choice. Imipenem or meropenem have sometimes been effective when treatment with ceftazidime has proved unsuccessful. Prolonged treatment is necessary to avoid relapse.

BURKHOLDERIA CEPACIA COMPLEX

B. cepacia, the cause of soft rot of onions, is also an important human pathogen causing life-threatening respiratory infection in immunocompromised patients, particularly those treated in intensive care or with chronic granulomatous disease. In cystic fibrosis, anxiety over *B. cepacia* is based on the innate multiresistance of the organism to antibiotics, its transmissibility by social contact, and the risk of cepacia syndrome, an acute, fatal necrotising pneumonia, sometimes accompanied by bacteraemia.

The *B. cepacia* complex comprises 17 phenotypically similar but genetically distinct species (genomovars). With few exceptions, all have been isolated from cystic fibrosis patients. The species with the most medical relevance are *B. cenocepacia, B. multivorans, B. dolosa,* and *B. gladioli*. Around 90% of human infections are caused by *B. multivorans* and *B. cenocepacia*.

In cystic fibrosis, accurate identification is vital for the implementation of optimal treatment regimens and infection control procedures to reduce patient-to-patient spread and in the management of patients selected for lung transplantation. Laboratory identification from clinical specimens and from environmental sites is challenging as most commercially available multitest kits may misidentify *Ps. aeruginosa, Achromobacter xylosoxidans, Stenotrophomonas maltophilia, Acinetobacter baumanni* and various other species as *B. cepacia* complex. Use of selective media is essential, and presumptive phenotypic identification should be confirmed by molecular identification, such as PCR assays and sequencing of the *recA* gene.

B. cepacia complex isolates produce several putative virulence determinants, including proteases, catalases, haemolysin, exopolysaccharide, cable pili and other adhesins. In vitro, the lipid A of these bacteria stimulates proinflammatory cytokines 10-fold more than *Ps. aeruginosa* lipid A.

The organisms are intrinsically resistant to most antibiotics, including polymyxins. Some are susceptible to ceftazidime, trimethoprim, tetracycline and chloramphenicol. The carbapenem meropenem appears to be the most active agent. Unfortunately, human infections are usually intractable to therapy unless combinations of three or four antibiotics are used. Strict infection control measures, including segregation, are necessary to limit the spread of highly transmissible strains.

GLUCOSE NONFERMENTERS

The heterogeneous group of aerobic Gram-negative bacilli commonly referred to as glucose non-fermenters is taxonomically distinct from the carbohydrate-fermenting Enterobacteriaceae and the oxidative pseudomonads. Their clinical relevance is based on their role as opportunistic pathogens in hospital-acquired infections and their intrinsic resistance to many antimicrobial agents. They grow easily on common culture media, but unequivocal identification may be difficult as most species are relatively inert in the biochemical tests used in identification of Gram-negative bacteria. Susceptibility to antibiotics is very variable, and treatment should be based on the results of laboratory tests.

- *Acinetobacter* species are saprophytes found in soil, water and sewage and occasionally as commensals of moist areas of human skin. The organisms survive well in the hospital environment and now account for around 10% of nosocomial infections in intensive care units in Europe. Serious infections, including meningitis, osteomyelitis, wound infections (including war wounds), pneumonia and bacteraemia, are most commonly associated with *A. baumannii*. Patients in intensive care units are at particular risk. Isolates are often inherently resistant to many antimicrobial agents, including β-lactam agents (other than carbapenems), aminoglycosides and fluoroquinolones.
- *Stenotrophomonas maltophilia* is an emerging opportunistic pathogen that is resistant to most commonly used antimicrobials but remarkable for its sensitivity to cotrimoxazole.
- *Alcaligenes* and *Achromobacter* species are saprophytes found in moist environments, including those in hospital wards, and are associated with a range of

hospital-acquired opportunistic infections, including bacteraemia and ear discharges.

- *Eikenella corrodens* is a commensal of mucosal surfaces. It may cause a range of infections, in particular, endocarditis, meningitis, pneumonia, and infections of wounds and various soft tissues.
- *Chryseobacterium* (formerly *Flavobacterium*) *meningosepticum* is a saprophyte whose natural

habitat is soil and moist environments, including nebulisers; it may cause opportunistic nosocomial infections, particularly in infants. As the name suggests, this species is associated with meningitis and has been responsible for high mortality in epidemic outbreaks.

RECOMMENDED READING

Brooke, J. S. (2012). *Stenotrophomonas maltophilia:* an emerging global opportunistic pathogen. *Clinical Microbiology Reviews, 25*(1), 2–41. doi:10.1128/CMR.00019-11.

Fothergill, J. L., James, C. E., & Winstanley, C. (2012). Novel therapeutic strategies to counter *Pseudomonas aeruginosa* infections. *Expert Reviews of Anti-Infective Therapy, 10*(2), 219–235. doi:10.1586/eri.11.168.

Freschi, L., Jeukens, J., Kukavica-Ibrulj, I., Boyle, B., Dupont, M. J., Laroche, J., ... Levesque, R. C. (2015). Clinical utilization of genomics data produced by the international *Pseudomonas aeruginosa* consortium. *Frontiers in Microbiology, 6*, 1036. doi:10.3389/fmicb.2015.01036.

Lipuma, J. J. (2010). The changing microbial epidemiology in cystic fibrosis. *Clinical Microbiology Reviews, 23*(2), 299–323. doi:10.1128/CMR.00068-09.

Mahenthiralingam, E., Urban, T. A., & Goldberg, J. B. (2005). The multifarious, multireplicon *Burkholderia cepacia* complex. *Nature Reviews. Microbiology, 3*(2), 144–156.

McConnell, M. J., Actis, L., & Pachon, J. (2013). *Acinetobacter baumannii:* human infections, factor contributing to pathogenesis and animal models. *FEMS Microbiology Reviews, 37*(2), 130–155. doi:10.1111/j.1574-6976.2012.00344.x.

Pendleton, J. N., Gorman, S. P., & Gilmore, B. F. (2013). Clinical relevance of the ESKAPE pathogens. *Expert Review of Anti-infective Therapy, 11*(3), 297–308. doi:10.1586/eri.13.12.

Silby, M. W., Winstanley, C., Godfrey, S. A. C., Levy, S. B., & Jackson, R. W. (2011). *Pseudomonas* genomes: diverse and adaptable. *FEMS Microbiology Reviews, 35*(4), 652–680. doi:10.1111/j.1574-6976.2011.00269.x.

Wiersinga, W. J., Currie, B. J., & Peacock, S. J. (2012). Melioidosis. *The New England Journal of Medicine, 367*(11), 1035–1044. doi:10.1056/NEJMra1204699.

Winstanley, C., O'Brien, S., & Brockhurst, M. A. (2016). *Pseudomonas aeruginosa* evolutionary adaptation and diversification in cystic fibrosis chronic lung infections. *Trends in Microbiology, 24*(5), 327–337. doi:10.1016/j.tim.2016.01.008.

Websites

International *Burkholderia cepacia* Working Group. Available at http://ibcwg.org/.

Pseudomonas Genome Database. Available at http://pseudomonas.com/.

Public Health England. Pseudomonas. Available at https://www.gov.uk/government/collections/pseudomonas-aeruginosa-guidance-data-and-analysis.

UK Cystic Fibrosis Trust. Consensus documents. Available at https://www.cysticfibrosis.org.uk/the-work-we-do/clinical-care/consensus-documents. (Accessed Jul 2017).

23 *Haemophilus*

Respiratory infections; meningitis; chancroid

MARY P. E. SLACK

KEY POINTS

- Most strains of *Haemophilus influenzae* are noncapsulate (nontypeable), but some strains possess a polysaccharide capsule (types a–f).
- *H. influenzae* type b (Hib) is a major human pathogen that causes invasive infections including meningitis and epiglottitis.
- Nontypeable strains (NTHi) cause 90% of noninvasive respiratory infections including otitis media in children and acute exacerbations of chronic obstructive pulmonary disease (COPD) in adults.
- Following the introduction of Hib conjugate vaccine, the number of invasive *H. influenzae* infections declined dramatically; the majority of invasive infections are now caused by NTHi.
- Fifteen to twenty percent of *H. influenzae* strains are ampicillin resistant (β-lactamase-mediated); ceftriaxone is the treatment of choice for invasive disease.
- Conjugate Hib vaccine is routinely offered to infants at 2, 3, 4 and 12 months in the United Kingdom.
- *H. ducreyi* causes chancroid, sexually transmitted genital ulcers in Africa and Southeast Asia but rarely in the United Kingdom. Single-dose therapy with azithromycin or ceftriaxone is effective.
- Chancroid lesions may facilitate the transmission of HIV.

DESCRIPTION

Haemophili are small, pleomorphic, nonmotile Gram-negative rods or coccobacilli with occasional longer, filamentous forms (Fig. 23.1). They are aerobic and facultatively anaerobic, and addition of 5%–10% carbon dioxide to the incubation atmosphere may enhance growth. *Haemophilus* spp. require one or both of two growth factors: X factor and V factor. The differential requirements for X and V factors are important criteria for defining species of *Haemophilus*. X factor (haemin) is required for the synthesis of cytochrome *c* and other iron-containing respiratory enzymes. V factor (nicotinamide adenine dinucleotide [NAD]) is essential for oxidation-reduction processes in cell metabolism. Growth factor dependence forms an important step in identification of *Haemophilus* spp.

H. influenzae is the major human pathogen in the genus. Some strains of *H. influenzae* produce a polysaccharide capsule, which is demonstrable by capsule stains and a Quellung reaction (swelling of the capsule) with type-specific antisera. There are six capsular types, designated a–f, which can be identified by a polymerase chain reaction (PCR) method. The most important is type b, which has a capsule composed of polyribosyl ribitol phosphate (PRP). Non-capsulated strains are designated non-typeable *H. influenzae* (NTHi).

H. influenzae is associated with a variety of invasive infections such as meningitis, epiglottitis, pneumonia and septic arthritis and localised disease of the respiratory tract including bronchitis and otitis media. Other haemophili of medical importance include *H. ducreyi,* the causative organism of chancroid, and *H. parainfluenzae.*

H. haemolyticus is another species that requires both X factor and V factor. It is frequently isolated from the respiratory tract, where it is a commensal organism. Microbiologists used to rely on the production of zones of β-haemolysis on horse blood agar to differentiate *H. haemolyticus* from NTHi, but recent studies have shown that 10%–40% of strains of *H. haemolyticus* are non-haemolytic. MALDI-TOF can differentiate *H. haemolyticus* from NTHi.

Two related organisms, *H. aphrophilus* and *H. paraphrophilus,* are now combined as a single species within the genus *Aggregatibacter* as *A. aphrophilus*; like *H. parainfluenzae,* they occasionally cause infective endocarditis and other miscellaneous conditions.

H. ducreyi is responsible for a sexually transmitted infection, chancroid (see later in the chapter).

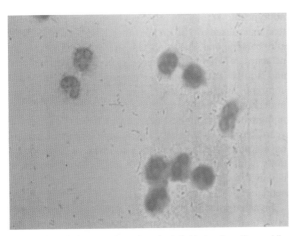

Fig. 23.1 Gram stain of cerebrospinal fluid showing *Haemophilus influenzae*: Gram-negative pleomorphic coccobacilli.

EPIDEMIOLOGY

During the influenza pandemic of 1889–1892, Pfeiffer noted the constant presence of large numbers of small bacilli in the sputum of patients affected with the disease and he suggested that the bacillus was the causative agent. Although the true aetiological agent of influenza was shown in 1933 to be a virus, it remains possible that secondary infection with *H. influenzae* contributed to the high mortality rate seen in the 1889–1892 and 1918–1919 influenza pandemics.

H. influenzae is an obligate parasite of human mucous membranes; it is not found in any other animal species. It colonises the throat and nasopharynx, and, to a lesser extent, the conjunctivae and genital tract. NTHi are present in the nasopharynx or throat of 25%–80% of healthy people; capsulate strains (about half of which are capsular type b) are present in 5%–10%. *H. influenzae* type b is an important cause of serious systemic infection in children throughout the world. Meningitis is more common in winter months, in families of low socio-economic status and in household contacts of a case. The disease is usually seen in the youngest member of a family and uncommonly in children who have no siblings. Household contacts of patients with invasive disease have an increased risk of acquiring infection if they are <5 years of age. The risk for children <2 years of age is 600- to 800-fold higher than the age-adjusted risk for the general population.

Outbreaks of infection have been described in close communities such as nursery schools. Contact with a case in a day-care centre or nursery has also been associated with increased attack rates in children <2 years of age, although the calculated risk is lower than that seen in household contacts.

Very high incidence rates have been reported in certain populations of Australian Aborigines, American Indians and the Inuit. In these racial groups the peak incidence of infection occurs at a younger age. By contrast, very low rates have been reported in Hong Kong Chinese. It is possible that socioeconomic considerations are important in determining such racial differences, but host genetic factors may also play a role. Immunosuppression, whether iatrogenic or associated with malignancies (especially Hodgkin's disease), asplenia or agammaglobulinaemia, also predispose to invasive disease. There is seasonal variation, with most cases occurring during the winter months.

The mortality rate associated with *H. influenzae* meningitis is around 5%. Neurological sequelae, including intellectual impairment, seizures and profound or severe hearing loss, may be present in 10%–20% of survivors.

TRANSMISSION

H. influenzae is transmitted by aerosols of respiratory secretions or by direct contact with contaminated material. Prior infection with respiratory viruses predisposes to nasopharyngeal colonisation by mechanisms including obstruction to outflow of respiratory secretions, suppression of mucociliary clearance and depression of local immunity. Contiguous spread (usually of NTHi) may result in noninvasive mucosal infections, including otitis media and acute sinusitis.

The species is associated with two types of infections, which are quite distinct in their epidemiological profiles: invasive infections and noninvasive infections (Table 23.1).

CLINICAL FEATURES OF *HAEMOPHILUS INFLUENZAE* INFECTION

Invasive infections

In the pre-Hib vaccine era, invasive infections, notably meningitis and epiglottitis, were mainly caused by Hib and resulted from invasion of the bloodstream. Other invasive infections, including septic arthritis, osteomyelitis, pneumonia and cellulitis or bacteraemia without a clearly defined focus of infection may also be caused by *H. influenzae* type b.

Hib infections are unusual in the first 2 months of life but are otherwise seen mainly in early childhood, in children <2 years of age. Acute epiglottitis has a peak incidence between 2 and 4 years of age. The incidence of invasive disease in children has been reduced dramatically in countries where a conjugate Hib vaccine has been introduced, and consequently the epidemiology is changing (see later in the chapter).

Table 23.1 Clinical spectrum of *Haemophilus influenzae* infections

Type of infection	Age group	Strains
Invasive	90% children <4 years[a]	90% *H. influenzae* type b[a] 10% NTHi 1% types e and f
Neonatal and maternal	Neonates; pregnant and parturient women	>90% NTHi
Noninvasive respiratory	Children and adults	>90% NTHi

[a]Percentages observed before the introduction of Hib conjugate vaccine; since the introduction of routine vaccination, the epidemiology has changed (see text).

The polysaccharide PRP capsule is the major virulence factor for Hib. When the organism invades the bloodstream, the capsule enables the organisms to evade phagocytosis and complement-mediated lysis in the nonimmune host. The rarity of infections in the first 2 months of life correlates with the presence of maternal capsular antibodies and the occurrence of infection in early infancy with the absence of such antibodies. As the prevalence and mean level of capsular antibodies in the population rise, *H. influenzae* type b infections become less common.

What determines whether acquisition of type b organisms in a susceptible host results in asymptomatic carriage and the stimulation of protective antibodies or the induction of invasive disease is unclear. However, animal experiments suggest that when invasion occurs, the organism penetrates the submucosa of the nasopharynx and establishes systemic infection through the bloodstream.

The type b capsular polysaccharide facilitates all phases of the invasion process. Other virulence factors that may be involved include:

- fimbriae, which assist attachment to epithelial cells
- immunoglobulin A (Ig A) proteases, which are also involved in colonisation
- outer membrane proteins and lipopolysaccharide, which may contribute to invasion at several stages

Initiation of invasive infection may be potentiated by intercurrent viral infection. Host genetic factors and immunosuppression may also play a role. It is unclear whether it is exposure to *H. influenzae* type b, or some other organism (e.g., *Escherichia coli* K100) possessing cross-reacting antigens, that usually stimulates natural protective antibody production.

Since the introduction of routine infant immunisation with conjugate Hib vaccine, invasive disease caused by nontypeable strains (NTHi) has become more common than that caused by Hib in the United Kingdom. Meningitis and bacteraemia due to NTHi are sometimes seen in neonates. NTHi infections may also occur in older children and adults. Pneumonia and bacteraemia are the most common manifestations, often in patients with an underlying disease, notably chronic lung disease or malignancy. The highest rates occur in adults aged >60 years, and the case fatality rate is high. Pregnant women have an increased susceptibility to invasive NTHi infections, which are associated with miscarriage, premature labour and postpartum infection in the mother and the neonate.

Invasive infections due to *H. influenzae* of serotypes other than b (principally types a, e and f) are uncommon. The spectrum of disease is similar to that seen with type b.

Noninvasive disease

H. influenzae produces a variety of mucosal infections, which are often associated with some underlying physiological or anatomical abnormality. Noninvasive infections are usually caused by NTHi. The most common are:

- otitis media
- sinusitis
- conjunctivitis
- acute exacerbations of chronic obstructive pulmonary disease (COPD)
- pneumonia

Acute sinusitis and otitis media are usually initiated by viral infections, which predispose to secondary infection with potentially pathogenic components of the resident microbial flora, notably *Streptococcus pneumoniae*, *Moraxella catarrhalis* and NTHi. The mechanisms may involve:

- obstruction to the outflow of respiratory secretions
- decreased clearance of microorganisms via normal mucociliary mechanisms
- depression of local immunity
- formation of biofilms within which bacteria can exist in a polymicrobial community and which protect the organisms from antibacterial therapy

Acute exacerbations of COPD are similarly initiated by acute viral infections. Respiratory viruses compromise an already impaired mucociliary clearance mechanism in patients with chronic lung disease and allow bacterial colonisation of the lower respiratory tract. In this situation, NTHi is a key pathogen, triggering inflammation and further damaging pulmonary function by a direct toxic effect on cilia. NTHi colonisation of the lower respiratory tract also causes inflammation in cases of bronchiectasis, cystic fibrosis, interstitial lung disease and pneumonia.

DIAGNOSIS

Gram-stained smears of cerebrospinal fluid, pus, sputum or aspirates from joints, middle ears or sinuses can provide a rapid presumptive identification. Haemophili tend to stain poorly, and dilute carbol fuchsin is a better counterstain than neutral red or safranin.

The viability of *H. influenzae* in clinical specimens declines with time, particularly at 4°C. Specimens should therefore be transported to the laboratory and cultured without delay. Ordinary blood agar contains X and V factors but growth of *H. influenzae*, which requires both factors, is poor. Growth is enhanced if the medium is supplemented with NAD. Streaking an organism that excretes this substance (e.g., *Staphylococcus aureus*) across the surface of the agar stimulates growth in its vicinity (satellitism). Heating blood agar for a few minutes at 70–80°C until it turns brown (chocolate agar) greatly enhances the growth of *H. influenzae*. This process removes serum NADase, which limits the amount of V factor, and also liberates extra X and V factors from the red cells into the medium. X factor is heat stable, but heating of media at 120°C for several minutes destroys V factor. Chocolate agar can be used without further supplementation for specimens obtained from sites that would normally be expected to be sterile. Plates should be incubated in an aerobic atmosphere enriched with 5%–10% carbon dioxide.

Anaerobic growth considerably reduces the haemin requirement of X-dependent species. *A. aphrophilus* has a requirement for carbon dioxide, but this character may be lost on subculture. *H. influenzae* does not require a carbon dioxide–enriched atmosphere but often grows better in such conditions.

Specimens of expectorated sputum inevitably become contaminated by upper respiratory flora, commonly including *H. influenzae,* and the finding of the organism in such specimens does not necessarily signify involvement in disease. Support for the significance of *H. influenzae* is provided if, in a purulent sample, the organism is present as the predominant isolate or in a viable count of over 10^6 colony-forming units per mL. Addition of bacitracin (10 international units/mL) facilitates the selective isolation of *H. influenzae* from mixed cultures of respiratory organisms. Obtaining bronchial secretions by bronchoalveolar lavage reduces the problem of contamination with commensal organisms.

The temptation to obtain throat swabs in patients with suspected acute epiglottitis should be resisted, as attempts

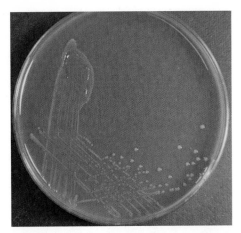

Fig. 23.2 Culture of *H. influenzae* on chocolate agar.

to obtain the sample may precipitate complete airway obstruction. Blood culture is indicated for patients with suspected invasive disease and is usually positive in those with acute epiglottitis.

Identification

H. influenzae grows poorly on blood agar. On chocolate agar the colonies are smooth, grey or colourless (Fig. 23.2), with a characteristic seminal odour. Confirmation of the identity depends on demonstrating a requirement for one or both of the growth factors, X and V:

- *H. influenzae* requires both X and V factors.
- *H. parainfluenzae* requires V factor alone.
- *A. aphrophilus (H. aphrophilus)* and *H. ducreyi* require X factor alone.

The culture is plated on nutrient agar that is deficient in both X and V factor, and paper discs containing X factor, V factor and X + V factor are placed on the surface of the agar. After overnight incubation, growth is observed around the discs supplying the necessary growth factors (Fig. 23.3).

DNA sequencing is increasingly being used for identification and typing of *Haemophilus* spp., and MALDI-TOF is a valuable tool for identification in a clinical microbiology laboratory. The capsular type of *H. influenzae* isolates can be determined by slide agglutination with type-specific antisera or by PCR-based capsular genotyping. NTHi strains cannot be typed by conventional type-specific antiserum agglutination. PCR-based techniques can differentiate between typeable (capsulated) and nontypeable strains by detection of the *cap* locus that encodes the polysaccharide capsule. Serological capsule typing is prone to misinterpretation, and molecular typing is the preferred method for typing *H. influenzae*.

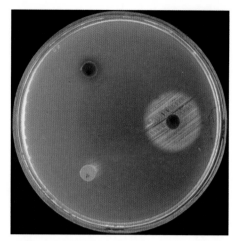

Fig. 23.3 Determination of the growth factor requirement of *H. influenzae*. Growth around the disc containing both X and V factors *(right-hand disc)*, but not around discs of the individual factors *(left-hand discs)*, indicates that the organism is *H. influenzae* (see text).

Antigen detection

The detection of type b polysaccharide antigen in body fluids or pus is useful, particularly in patients who received antibiotics before specimens were obtained. A rapid latex agglutination test with rabbit antibody to type b antigen is used most commonly.

In the absence of confirmatory cultures, the results should be regarded with caution as some serotypes of *Streptococcus pneumoniae* and *E. coli* may share similar antigens.

Antimicrobial susceptibility tests

Accurate determination of the antimicrobial susceptibility of *H. influenzae* requires careful standardisation of the methodology. Disc tests are less reliable for detecting enzyme-mediated ampicillin (β-lactamase) and chloramphenicol (chloramphenicol acetyltransferase) resistance than microbiological or biochemical techniques that demonstrate antibiotic inactivation.

TREATMENT

H. influenzae is usually susceptible to ampicillin (or amoxicillin), chloramphenicol and tetracyclines. Among cephalosporins, compounds such as cefuroxime, cefotaxime and ceftriaxone are highly active. Other antibiotics active against *H. influenzae* include amoxicillin-clavulanic acid, ciprofloxacin, azithromycin and clarithromycin.

Ceftriaxone (or a related cephalosporin such as cefotaxime) is the antibiotic of first choice for the treatment of meningitis and acute epiglottitis. It is bactericidal for *H. influenzae*, achieves good concentrations in the meninges and cerebral tissues and is highly effective.

β-Lactamase–mediated resistance to ampicillin is now encountered in up to 15% of type b strains and about 20% of invasive NTHi isolates in the United Kingdom. Occasional strains are resistant to ampicillin through alterations in penicillin binding protein 3 (β-lactamase negative, ampicillin resistant, BLNAR), and a few strains demonstrate both mechanisms of resistance (β-lactamase positive, amoxicillin-clavulanic acid resistant, BLPACR). For these reasons, ampicillin should not be used as a single agent in meningitis when *H. influenzae* is a possibility and the results of susceptibility tests are not available. Resistance to chloramphenicol may also be encountered, but in most parts of the world this remains uncommon.

Antibiotic therapy is only one component of the clinical management of patients with *Haemophilus* meningitis and full supportive care is required to achieve the most favourable outcome. Skilled medical and nursing care is also vital in the management of acute epiglottitis, where maintenance of a patent airway is crucial.

For the treatment of less serious respiratory infections, such as otitis media, sinusitis and acute exacerbations of chronic obstructive pulmonary disease (COPD) oral antibiotics such as amoxicillin, amoxicillin-clavulanic acid and clarithromycin are all effective.

CONTROL

H. influenzae type b disease in the United Kingdom

Before the introduction of conjugate Hib vaccine into the infant immunisation schedule in 1992, approximately 1500 cases of invasive Hib disease, including 900 cases of meningitis, occurred in the United Kingdom every year, with 60 deaths. Immunisation rates have remained high (about 93%), and between 1992 and 1999 *H. influenzae* type b disease in children <5 years old fell by 95% (Fig. 23.4). In 1998, only 21 cases of invasive Hib disease in children <5 years were reported in England and Wales. From 1999 there was a small but gradual increase in the number of cases, most notably in fully immunised children born in 2000 and 2001, but also in older children and adults. In 2003, children over 6 months and under 4 years of age were offered a booster dose of Hib vaccine, and in 2006 a routine booster dose of Hib vaccine, given at 12 months of age in combination with meningococcus group C conjugate vaccine, was incorporated into the UK infant immunisation schedule. These campaigns have had a marked effect on the incidence of invasive Hib disease, most dramatically in 1- to 4-year-olds but also in older children and adults. Hib conjugate vaccines reduce

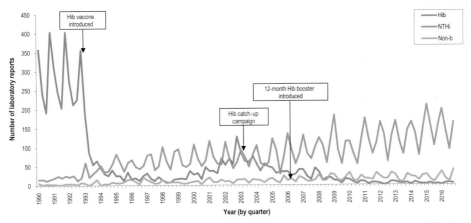

Fig. 23.4 Cases of invasive *Haemophilus influenzae* infections by serotype per quarter: England and Wales, 1990–2016. (Data from Public Health England.)

nasopharyngeal carriage of type b strains of *H. influenzae*, thereby interrupting transmission of the organism to susceptible hosts. This phenomenon of indirect protection of unimmunised individuals is known as herd protection. Hib conjugate vaccine has no effect on the carriage rate of NTHi or other capsular types of *H. influenzae*.

Active immunisation

Early *Haemophilus* vaccines consisting of purified type b capsular polysaccharide were poorly immunogenic in children <2 years old and in patients with immune deficiency. Conjugate vaccines in which the polysaccharide is covalently coupled to proteins such as tetanus toxoid, a nontoxic variant of diphtheria toxin, *Neisseria meningitidis* outer membrane protein or diphtheria toxoid produce a lasting anamnestic response, which is not age-related and may be effective in high-risk patients who respond poorly to polysaccharide vaccine alone. In the United Kingdom, *H. influenzae* type b vaccine is offered routinely to infants at 2, 3 and 4 months of age as part of a pentavalent diphtheria, tetanus, pertussis, polio, Hib vaccine (see Ch. 70). A Hib booster dose (in combination with meningococcus C vaccine), given at 12 months of age, was introduced in 2006. The booster dose of Hib vaccine given in the second year of life is crucial for sustaining immunity against Hib, to prevent declining Hib antibodies and waning herd protection.

Conjugate Hib vaccine is recommended for children and adults with splenic dysfunction because they are at increased risk of invasive Hib infection.

Prophylaxis

Rifampicin (20 mg/kg [maximum 600 mg] for children >3 months and adults; 10 mg/kg for infants <3 months)

given orally once daily for 4 days eradicates carriage of *H. influenzae* type b and prevents secondary infection in household and nursery contacts.

In countries where Hib vaccine is routinely administered to infants, invasive *H. influenzae* isolates are nearly always NTHi but need to be confirmed by serotyping.

For confirmed cases of invasive Hib infection, chemoprophylaxis should be offered to any vulnerable contacts in the household, that is, children aged <10 years and immunosuppressed or asplenic individuals of any age. Any unvaccinated or partially vaccinated children under 10 years of age should be appropriately immunised against Hib.

OTHER HAEMOPHILI

H. ducreyi is the cause of chancroid, a sexually transmitted infection, most prevalent in tropical regions, particularly Africa and Southeast Asia. Chancroid has declined in importance in most countries where it was previously endemic, but *H. ducreyi* has recently been established as a cause of chronic skin ulcers in some South Pacific Islands. Patients present with painful penile ulcers (soft sore or soft chancre) and inguinal lymphadenitis. Typical small Gram-negative bacilli can be seen in material from the ulcers or in pus from lymph node aspirates. It is likely that the lesions of chancroid have facilitated the transmission of human immunodeficiency virus (HIV) in some tropical countries. *H. ducreyi* is an extremely fastidious organism requiring specialised culture media. A multiplex PCR has been developed for the simultaneous amplification of DNA targets from *H. ducreyi*, *Treponema pallidum* and herpes simplex virus types 1 and 2.

Susceptibility to antimicrobial agents varies geographically. Many strains are β-lactamase producers, and resistance to tetracycline and co-trimoxazole is common.

Chancroid may be treated with azithromycin, ceftriaxone, ciprofloxacin or erythromycin. Azithromycin and ceftriaxone have the advantage of single-dose therapy. Strains with intermediate resistance to ciprofloxacin or erythromycin have been reported. Treatment failures are much more likely in patients with concurrent HIV infection. Oral ciprofloxacin for 3 days or erythromycin for 7 days is recommended for HIV-positive individuals. The use of condoms dramatically reduces the transmission of *H. ducreyi*. All sexual partners should be identified by contact tracing and treated.

An unrelated Gram-negative rod, *Calymmatobacterium granulomatis,* causes a somewhat similar sexually transmitted disease, granuloma inguinale or donovanosis, in parts of the tropics. Intracellular organisms, known as Donovan bodies (not to be confused with the Leishman–Donovan bodies of leishmaniasis), can be demonstrated in the stained smears from the lesions. Tetracyclines are usually used in treatment.

HACEK GROUP

The HACEK group, consisting of the *Haemophilus* spp. (including *H. parainfluenzae*), *Aggregatibacter aphrophilus* (formerly *H. aphrophilus* and *H. paraphrophilus*), *Aggregatibacter actinomycetemcomitans* (formerly *Actinobacillus actinomycetemcomitans*), *Cardiobacterium* spp., *Eikenella corrodens* and *Kingella* spp., is implicated in 1%–3% of cases of infective endocarditis, often related to poor dental hygiene. They also cause dental infections, lung abscess and brain abscess. All of the HACEK group of organisms are small fastidious Gram-negative coccobacilli and are commensals of the oropharyngeal/respiratory tract. Endocarditis is usually treated successfully with a combination of ampicillin and gentamicin.

RECOMMENDED READING

Coker, T. R., Chan, L. S., Newberry, S. J., Limbos, M. A., Suttorp, M. J., Shekelle, P. G., & Takata, G. S. (2010). Diagnosis, microbial epidemiology, and antibiotic treatment of acute otitis media in children: a systematic review. *Journal of the American Medical Association, 304*(19), 2161–2169. doi:10.1001/jama.2010.1651.

Gkentzi, D., Collins, S., Ramsay, M. E., Slack, M. P., & Ladhani, S. (2013). Revised recommendations for the prevention of secondary cases of *Haemophilus influenzae* type b (Hib) disease. *Journal of Infection, 67*(5), 486–489. doi: http://dx.doi.org/10.1016/j.jinf.2013.06.013.

Kim, K. S. (2010). Acute bacterial meningitis in infants and children. *The Lancet Infectious Diseases, 10*(1), 32–42. doi:10.1016/S1473-3099(09)70306-8.

Ladhani, S. N. (2012). Two decades of experience with the *Haemophilus influenzae* serotype b conjugate vaccine in the United Kingdom. *Clinical Therapeutics, 34*(2), 385–399. doi:10.1016/j.clinthera.2011.11.027.

Lewis, D. A. (2014). Epidemiology, clinical features, diagnosis and treatment of *Haemophilus ducreyi* - a disappearing pathogen? *Expert Reviews in Anti-Infective Therapy, 12*(6), 687–696. doi:10.1586/14787210.2014.892414.

O'Farrell, N., & Lazaro, N. (2014). UK National Guidelines for the management of chancroid. *International Journal of STD and AIDS, 25*(14), 975–983. doi:10.1177/0956462414542988.

Tristram, S., Jacobs, M. R., & Appelbaum, P. C. (2007). Antimicrobial resistance in *Haemophilus influenzae. Clinical Microbiology Reviews, 20*(2), 368–389. doi:10.1128/CMR.00040-06.

Ulanova, M., & Tsang, R. S. W. (2009). Invasive *Haemophilus influenzae* disease: changing epidemiology and host-parasite interactions in the 21st century. *Infection, Genetics and Evolution, 9*(4), 594–605. doi:10.1016/j.meegid.2009.03.001.

Van Eldere, J., Slack, M. P. E., Ladhani, S., & Cripps, A. W. (2014). Non-typeable *Haemophilus influenzae*, an under-recognised pathogen. *The Lancet Infectious Diseases, 14*(12), 1281–1292. doi:10.1016/S1473-3099(14)70734-0.

Watt, J. P., Wolfson, L. J., O'Brien, K. L., Henkle, E., Deloria-Knoll, M., McCall, N., ... Hib and Pneumococcal Global Burden of Disease Study Team. (2009). Burden of disease caused by *Haemophilus influenzae* type b in children younger than 5 years: global estimates. *The Lancet, 374*(9693), 903911. doi:10.1016/S0140-6736(09)61203-4.

Websites

UK Department of Health. *Haemophilus influenzae* type b (Hib), *H. influenzae* meningitis notifiable (except in Scotland). Available at https://www.gov.uk/government/publications/haemophilus-influenzae-type-hib-the-green-book-chapter-16. (Access Apr 2013).

24 *Bordetella*

Bordetella pertussis; whooping cough

NORMAN K. FRY AND GAYATRI AMIRTHALINGAM

KEY POINTS

- Whooping cough (pertussis) is caused by *Bordetella pertussis*.
- Pertussis is an exclusively human disease (most severe in infants) and has no known animal or environmental reservoir.
- Typical symptoms comprise paroxysmal cough, with vomiting and whooping, which can last for several weeks or even months.
- Milder symptoms in older children/adults make clinical diagnosis difficult.
- Laboratory confirmation can be achieved by isolation of the organism, detection of its DNA by PCR or detection of specific antibodies, such as anti-pertussis toxin IgG, in sera or oral fluid.
- Treatment for diagnosed cases is unlikely to affect the clinical course of the illness, but may limit ongoing transmission.
- Vaccination is safe and effective and remains the best control method available.
- Immunity from natural *B. pertussis* infection or vaccination is not lifelong.
- Waning protection following immunisation with acellular vaccines is generally considered to be more rapid than that from whole-cell vaccines.

Bordetella are small Gram-negative coccobacilli, aerobic (except for one species, *B. petrii*), non–acid-fast, nonsporing, slow-growing and fastidious in their growth requirements. Twelve of the sixteen members of the genus are capable of infecting humans, but by far the most significant human pathogen is *B. pertussis,* which remains one of the most common causes of morbidity and mortality in infants from a disease that is potentially preventable through vaccination.

DESCRIPTION

The genus *Bordetella* belongs to the ß-subclass of Proteobacteria in the family Alcaligenaceae. The three species, *B. pertussis, B. parapertussis* and *B. bronchiseptica,* were the first to be described and are sometimes referred to as the 'classical' *Bordetella* species. The classical species were originally classified in the genus *Haemophilus*. However, *Bordetella* growth is not dependent on either of the nutritional factors X and V (see Ch. 23), and *B. parapertussis* and *B. bronchiseptica* do not require blood for their growth. There are currently 14 species within the genus *Bordetella* that appear in the list of prokaryotic names with standing in nomenclature (http://www.bacterio.net/): *B. avium, B. bronchialis, B. bronchiseptica, B. flabilis, B. hinzii, B. holmesii, B. muralis, B. parapertussis, B. pertussis, B. petrii, B. sputigena, B. trematum, B. tumbae* and *B. tumulicola*. There are two additional species in the literature, '*B. ansorpii*', which still awaits formal description, and the recently described *B. pseudohinzii* sp. nov.

Bordetella pertussis

This is the most fastidious of the bordetellae and produces toxic products. In standard methods for culture, these are absorbed by culture media containing charcoal, starch or a high concentration of blood, as in the original Bordet–Gengou medium, in order to achieve successful growth. *B. pertussis* is a strict aerobe, with an optimal growth temperature of 35–36°C. Even under these conditions, it can take up to 3–4 days for visible colonies to appear. Subculture reveals no growth on nutrient agar.

Typical *B. pertussis* colonies are small, greyish, convex, smooth, and have an entire edge and a pearl-like lustre (metallic appearance), which is most pronounced in young colonies.

B. pertussis reacts strongly with homologous antiserum demonstrating agglutination using polyclonal rabbit antisera containing antibodies directed against the somatic lipopolysaccharide (LPS), or "O" antigens. *B. pertussis* can be further divided into serotypes (or fimbrial types) by agglutination with specific antisera. The organism produces three major agglutinogens (agglutinogen 1, fimbrial antigen 2 and fimbrial antigen 3). Agglutinogen 1 is common to all strains and is thus often left out of serotype notation; the three serotypes pathogenic to humans are serotype 1,2 (Fim2), serotype 1,3 (Fim3) and, more rarely, serotype 1,2,3 (Fim2,3). The fimbrial antigens are important in immunity to infection and are included as components in some acellular vaccine formulations.

Bordetella parapertussis

This organism is readily distinguished from *B. pertussis* by its ability to grow on nutrient agar, and the production of a brown diffusible pigment on tyrosine agar after 2 days (Table 24.1). It also grows more rapidly than *B. pertussis* on charcoal–blood agar and demonstrates agglutination with *B. parapertussis* antiserum.

B. parapertussis usually causes less severe illness than *B. pertussis* in humans, and is uncommon compared to *B. pertussis* in most countries. It also causes chronic pneumonia in sheep.

Bordetella bronchiseptica

Colonies of this species are visible on nutrient agar after overnight incubation; it differs from the other species by also being motile and giving a positive reaction in the urease test and by reducing nitrate (Table 24.1). *B. bronchiseptica* will not produce a brown pigment on tyrosine agar, but will hydrolyse the tyrosine causing a clearing of the agar. *B. bronchiseptica* is a common respiratory pathogen of animals, including horses, dogs, pigs, rabbits, cats and rodents. Although rarely encountered in human infections, it can cause respiratory disease, pneumonia and bacteraemia, and can cause persistent infections in those with underlying conditions, such as cystic fibrosis patients.

Bordetella avium and Bordetella hinzii

Both of these species cause respiratory infection in poultry, but reports of infection in humans are very rare.

Table 24.1 Differential properties of *Bordetella* species

Characteristic	Species							
	B. pertussis	*B. bronchiseptica*	*B. parapertussis*	*B. avium*	*B. hinzii*	*B. holmesii*	*B. trematum*	*B. petrii*
Year of description	1906	1912	1937	1984	1995	1995	1996	2001
Host range	Human	Broad range e.g., dogs, pigs, horses, rabbits, Human	Human, sheep	Birds (Human)	Birds (Human)	Human	Human	Environmental Human
Site(s) of isolation	RT	RT	RT	RT	RT	RT, blood	Wounds, ear	Mouth
Motility	−	+	−	+	+	−	+	−
Growth (days)	3–4	1	1–2	1	2	2–3	1	2
Growth on MacConkey's	−	+	+	+	+	+/−	+	+
Brown pigment	−	−	+	−	−	+	−	−
Oxidase	+	+	−	+	+	−	−	+
Urease	−	+	+	−	−	−	−	−
Nitrate reduction	−	+	−	−	−	−	+/−	−
G+C content (mol%)	67.7–68.9	68.2–69.5	68.1–69.0	61.6–62.6	65.0–67.0	61.5–62.3	64.0–65.0	63.3–64.3

Adapted from Gerlach, G., von Wintziingerode, F., Middendorf, B., & Gross, R. (2001). Evolutionary trends in the genus *Bordetella*. *Microbes and Infection*, 3(1), 61–72; Parton, R. (1998). Bordetella. In L. Collier, A. Balows, & M. Sussman (Eds.), *Topley & Wilson's Microbiology and Microbial Infections* (pp. 901–918). London: Arnold; von Wintzingerode, F., Schatte, A., Siddiqui, R. A., Rösick, U., Göbel, U. B., & Gross, R. (2001). *Bordetella petrii* sp. nov., isolated from an anaerobic bioreactor, and emended description of the genus *Bordetella*. *International Journal of Systematic and Evolutionary Microbiology*. 51(4), 1257–1265; von Wintzingerode, F., Gerlach, G., Schneider, B., & Gross, R. (2002). Phylogenetic relationships and virulence evolution in the genus *Bordetella*. *Current Topics in Microbiology and Immunology*. 264(1), 177–199, by Neal, S. (2004). Genotypic diversity and epidemiological typing of *Bordetella pertussis*. PhD thesis, University of Glasgow. RT, respiratory tract.

Bordetella holmesii

This species can be isolated from the respiratory tract and sputum from humans and was first described following isolation from the blood of patients with underlying disorders (e.g., asplenic patients) and cases of septicaemia, mainly in young adults. It is also notable for carrying ca. 8–10 copies of the insertion element IS*481*, which is also used as a target to detect *B. pertussis* by PCR due to its high copy number in this species ($n = 50$–238).

Bordetella trematum

This species is typically isolated from infections (e.g., skin, ear) and wounds in humans including ulcers. It has also been reported from a fatal case of bacteraemia with septic shock.

Bordetella petrii

This species was unusual in being isolated originally from an anaerobic, dechlorinating bioreactor culture enriched from river sediment. Subsequently, clinical isolates have been found in patients with chronic respiratory infection and bone or joint infections.

Bordetella bronchialis, Bordetella flabilis and Bordetella sputigena

These three recently described environmental species of *Bordetella* have all been isolated from the respiratory specimens of cystic fibrosis patients.

Bordetella muralis, Bordetella tumulicola and Bordetella tumbae

These three species were isolated from the plaster wall surface of mural paintings inside the stone chamber of a tumulus in Asuka village, Nara Prefecture, Japan.

'Bordetella ansorpii'

This species still awaits formal description, and there are only two reports of isolates from clinical cases in the literature, one from an epidermal cyst and the other from the blood of a patient with acute myeloid leukaemia.

Bordetella pseudohinzii

To date, this recently described species appears to be restricted to causing infections in (laboratory) mice and is thus a potential confounder of the use of such animal models in pulmonary research.

PATHOGENESIS

The mechanism of infection and the development of disease by *B. pertussis* can be divided into four stages: (1) attachment, (2) evasion of host defences, (3) local damage and (4) systemic manifestations. *B. pertussis* is well equipped to evade the host's defences with a number of virulence factors, which perform an important role in colonisation and immunomodulation (Fig. 24.1). In the initial preventable stage of the infection the ciliated epithelium of the bronchi and trachea is colonised with bacteria whose agglutinogens (including fimbriae) play a vital and type-specific role in attachment (see Fig. 24.1).

CLINICAL FEATURES

Pertussis (severe cough) has been recognised as a clinical entity for several centuries. Typically, an infant or child suffers many bouts of paroxysmal coughing each day. During these bouts, with no pause for air intake, the tongue protrudes fully and fluids stream from the eyes, nose and mouth, and the face becomes cyanotic. With a massive inspiratory effort, air is sucked through the narrowed glottis, producing a long high-pitched whoop—hence the term *whooping cough*. Such attacks often terminate with vomiting. Between the attacks, the patient does not usually appear ill.

If a characteristic attack is witnessed, a diagnosis of pertussis is usually made on clinical grounds alone. However, the illness is often mild and atypical, especially in:

- older children and adults
- younger children who have been incompletely immunised.

In these cases, the laboratory has a vital role in diagnosis because similar coughing may be caused by a variety of other microorganisms and such illness is generally mild and of short duration. With genuine pertussis, the illness is likely to persist for months rather than weeks and the clinical course of the illness is unlikely to be affected by antibiotic treatment. Although one attack usually confers long-lasting immunity, this does not necessarily preclude subsequent infection.

Animal models of pertussis infection

A number of animal models have been used to study pertussis infection including mice, rabbits, guinea pigs and newborn piglets. However, although many aspects of the disease have been reproduced in these models, none adequately represents the full spectrum of the

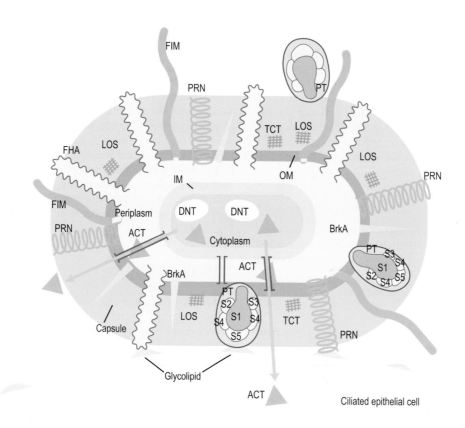

Fig. 24.1 *Bordetella pertussis* antigens. Redrawn from Crowcroft, N. S., Pebody, R. G. (2006). Recent developments in pertussis. Lancet. *367*(9526): 1926-36. IM, inner membrane; OM, outer membrane; S1–5, subunits 1–5.

Antigen	Function
Agglutinogens including fimbriae (FIM)	Attachment to ciliated respiratory epithelium possibly important for type-specific immunity
Filamentous haemagglutinin (FHA)	Adhesion and immunomodulation
Pertactin (PRN)	Adhesion. Important immunogen
Pertussis toxin (PT)	Attachment of *B. pertussis* to ciliated respiratory cells. Important immunogen
	Activates cyclic adenosine phosphate (cAMP), histamine sensitising factor (HSF), lymphocytosis promoting factor (LPF), islet-activating protein (IAP), interferes with leucocyte function, haemolytic
Adenylate cyclase toxin (ACT)	Activates cAMP, interferes with leucocyte function, haemolytic
Dermonecrotic toxin (DNT) or heat-labile toxin	Unknown role in vivo. Dermal necrosis and vasoconstriction in vitro
Tracheal cytotoxin (TCT)	Ciliostasis, inhibition of DNA synthesis, kills ciliated epithelial cells
Lipooligosaccharide (LOS)	Causes fever
BrkA (Bordetella resistance to killing genetic locus, frame A	Outer membrane protein that mediates adherence and resists complement

disease in humans. Several studies have been performed on nonhuman primate species including macaques, Cebus monkeys and chimpanzees. More recently, a baboon model has been developed, which is the first to encompass the full spectrum of human disease including coughing and transmission. This model is an exciting development and is being utilised to examine pertussis pathogenesis and host responses to infection and vaccination.

Human challenge studies allow the prospect of studying the natural course of disease and immune responses to infection. Pertussis presents unique considerations to human challenge studies due to its highly contagious nature and transmission route. Appropriate containment facilities and study design are advisable in order to prevent onward transmission to contacts. Treatment with antibiotics, to ensure clearance prior to discharge, and appropriate follow-up procedures are also required.

LABORATORY INVESTIGATION

Laboratory confirmation of a clinical diagnosis can be useful for management of cases and clusters and provides valuable information at a national level to inform vaccination policy.

Bacterial culture

Bacterial culture has the highest specificity of the available tests and the additional advantage that the isolate can be referred to a reference laboratory for phenotypic and genotypic testing and archiving, providing valuable microbial epidemiological information.

The organism can be readily recovered from the nasopharynx. A nasopharyngeal or pernasal swab (NPS/PNS) is recommended, or if hospitalised, a nasopharyngeal aspirate (NPA) is preferred. Commensal microorganisms that may overgrow *B. pertussis* can be suppressed by the addition of cephalexin (30 mg/L) to the charcoal–blood agar plate. The swab tip is directed downwards towards the midline, passing gently along the floor of the nose for ca. 5 cm (depending on the patient's age) until stopped by the posterior wall of the nasopharynx. A culture plate should be inoculated as soon as possible after withdrawal of the swab; the swab may be placed in transport medium (e.g., Regan-Lowe) for transfer to a laboratory, but should still ideally be inoculated within 24 hours.

In the laboratory, the inoculum is spread to give separate colonies, and the plate incubated for ≥7 days before being discarded as negative. Because of the prolonged incubation, the medium should have a good depth (6–7 mm) and plates may be incubated in a suitable secondary container with an open jar of sterile water to reduce drying in the incubator or hot room.

Detection of bacterial DNA

Specimens (NPS/PNS/NPA) for direct detection by nucleic acid detection methods (typically PCR) should ideally be taken as close to onset as possible and preferably within the first 3 weeks of cough onset. In a community setting and/or if a NPS/PNS is not available, a throat swab may be used. PCR is more sensitive than culture, and real-time formats can offer a same-day result within hours. The likelihood of successful detection using PCR decreases with duration of cough and is affected by age and vaccination status of the patient but, because of its high sensitivity, can be useful up to several weeks post-onset of cough.

Many PCR assays for Bordetella have been described in the scientific literature or are available commercially. Targets for *B. pertussis, B. parapertussis* and *B. bronchiseptica* include the insertion elements (e.g., IS*481*, IS*1001*, IS*1002*), because of their presence in multiple copies. Single copy targets, for example, the genes for the pertussis toxin (PT) promoter (*ptxP*), PT, recombinase A, filamentous haemagglutinin and porin, are typically less sensitive than the IS targets, but are often used in combination to allow definitive species identification.

Detection of Bordetella antibody

When an individual has been symptomatic with a cough for >2 weeks, investigation of sera or oral fluid for specific IgG antibodies to *B. pertussis* can be useful in seeking laboratory confirmation of pertussis infection. These investigations are particularly useful in the diagnosis of cases in adolescents and adults who tend to present late in the course of the illness. However, care must be taken in interpretation. Amongst the various serological antibody tests, determination of titres to anti-PT IgG is the most widely used, and reporting in international units allows comparison between sites and countries. Recommendations for both thresholds and interpretation exist. Whilst seropositive results (above a designated threshold) can be helpful to support a clinical diagnosis, seronegative results cannot be used to exclude pertussis infection because the sensitivity of the assay is <100% (typically estimated to be ca. 80%). The serological response in infants/young children may differ from that of older children/adults, and results can also be confounded by prior infection or vaccination with a vaccine containing *B. pertussis* components. In practice, the vast majority of such serological investigations comprise a single sample from the patient at one point in time (i.e., >2 weeks after cough onset); however, further sampling from the same patient may be informative to determine a rise or fall in antibody level. The use of a combination of laboratory methods can also be useful in the investigation of clusters.

Risk factors

A number of risk factors have been shown to be associated with poor outcome/fatality in pertussis infection including significantly lower birth weight, younger gestational age, younger age at time of cough onset and higher peak white blood cell (WBC) and lymphocyte counts. This highlights the importance of early recognition of infection, particularly in young infants, and treatment with appropriate antibiotic and supportive therapy.

EPIDEMIOLOGY

Source and transmission of infection

Pertussis is highly contagious, with up to 90% of susceptible household contacts developing disease.

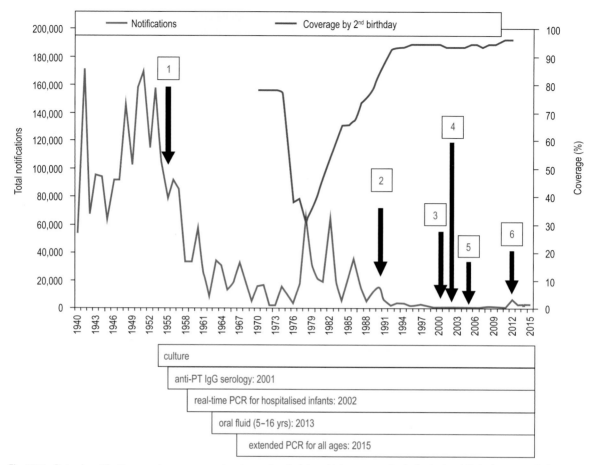

Fig. 24.2 Pertussis notifications, vaccine coverage, major changes to schedule and laboratory testing in England and Wales (1940–2015). Changes to vaccination policy are indicated by numbers in boxes: (1) 1957: routine infant diphtheria tetanus whole-cell pertussis vaccination (DTwP) was introduced and the course completed by 6 months of age; (2) 1990: the 'accelerated' infant DTwP schedule was introduced (given at 2, 3 and 4 months); (3) 2000/2001: there was temporary use of both three- and five-component diphtheria tetanus acellular pertussis vaccine (DTaP); (4) 2001: the preschool DTaP booster was introduced for children aged between 3½ and 5 years; (5) 2004: the five-component DTaP was used for the primary course at 2, 3 and 4 months; (6) 2012: the maternal immunisation programme was introduced. In order to monitor pertussis infection in England and Wales, an enhanced surveillance of laboratory-confirmed pertussis was introduced in 1994. Major changes to laboratory testing services are indicated below the graph.

The transmission dynamics of pertussis remain poorly understood, although a number of studies that have investigated the routes of transmission in young infants have suggested siblings and adults in the household, particularly the mother, are important sources of infection. However, in up to one-third of cases, the source remains unknown and this may either reflect transmission from contacts outside the household, or from asymptomatic transmission, or from cases with mild or atypical disease. Fig. 24.2 illustrates how variations in the rates of uptake of pertussis vaccine in England and Wales have affected the incidence of pertussis more than the steady improvement in the general health of the population that continued throughout the period. After the gradual introduction of pertussis vaccination during the 1950s, there was a steady reduction in the size of epidemics until the 1970s. Unfounded fear of brain damage caused a loss of faith in the vaccine, and three large epidemics occurred before the slow restoration of confidence in the vaccine began to take effect.

Incidence and mortality

Pertussis infection occurs worldwide, affects all ages and is a major cause of death in malnourished populations. In 2013, the World Health Organization (WHO) estimated that pertussis was still causing ca. 63,000 deaths in children under 5 years of age. Although pertussis remains a major cause of death in low-income countries, the burden of disease has substantially declined following the introduction of routine immunisation programmes. However, more recently, some high-income countries with long-standing vaccination programmes have reported increases in disease rates and a shift in the distribution of pertussis cases to older age groups. This may reflect changes in the sensitivity of surveillance systems with the availability of newer diagnostics, or a genuine increase in disease rates in older age groups due to waning immunity following natural infection or vaccination.

In the 2015 WHO Pertussis Position paper, a review of the epidemiology of pertussis in 19 high- and middle-income countries concluded that there was no evidence of widespread resurgence of pertussis, but that rates of disease had increased in the United Kingdom, United States, Australia and Portugal. The change from whole-cell to acellular pertussis vaccines in their routine immunisation programmes has been proposed as a contributory factor to the resurgences observed in these countries.

Rates of pertussis disease and case fatality rates continue to be highest in young infants <3 months of age, before protection is conferred through active immunisation.

The disease occurs in epidemic waves at ca. 4-yearly intervals—the time needed to build up a new susceptible population after the 'herd' immunity produced by an epidemic. Fig. 24.2 shows the pattern for England and Wales up to 2015, since when the situation has remained unchanged. The maintenance of a 4-year cycle is thought to result from the interaction of various factors, such as the degree of immunity produced by high vaccination rates, and the levels of natural immunity that follow either large epidemics or a high background incidence of endemic pertussis in interepidemic intervals.

Epidemiological typing

Epidemiological strain typing can assist outbreak investigation and provide useful surveillance data. Genotyping of *B. pertussis* presents problems due to its monomorphic nature. To date, methods for genotyping have included pulsed-field gel electrophoresis (PFGE), multilocus variable-number tandem-repeat analysis (MLVA), multi-antigen sequence typing (MAST), and whole genome sequencing (WGS). Whole genome sequencing and single nucleotide polymorphism analysis can be considered the gold standard for epidemiological typing, but it is important to also relate genotype to phenotypic expression, particularly of vaccine antigen genes.

Treatment and control

Most antibiotics have little or no clinical effect when the infection is well established. Treatment is primarily aimed at eliminating *B. pertussis* and thereby preventing ongoing transmission, although studies have only demonstrated efficacy in preventing spread if administered within 7–14 days of onset of illness. The drug of choice is a macrolide such as azithromycin, clarithromycin or erythromycin. Because of the side effects associated with erythromycin, newer macrolides such as azithromycin and clarithromycin are often preferred and have been demonstrated to be as effective as erythromycin in eradicating *B. pertussis* from the nasopharynx. Antibiotics are also recommended for prophylaxis of contacts of suspected or confirmed cases. However, a UK review of the use of erythromycin in the management of persons exposed to pertussis reported little effect in preventing secondary transmission, which was limited to close prolonged household contact. Consequently, in the United Kingdom, chemoprophylaxis with macrolides is recommended in household or health-care settings where individuals at high risk of severe disease such as young infants (or at risk of transmitting to a high-risk group such as health-care workers or women in late pregnancy) are present. Although not demonstrated, efficacy of newer macrolides would be expected to be comparable given their biological effects.

Vaccination

Vaccination remains the most effective population control strategy for pertussis. Two types of pertussis vaccines are available: whole-cell (wP) vaccines based on killed whole *B. pertussis* organisms and acellular (aP) vaccines based on one or more purified components of the following pertussis antigens: pertussis toxin (PT), pertactin (PRN), filamentous haemagglutinin (FHA) and FIM types 2 and 3. Whole-cell vaccines were introduced into routine immunisation programmes in many high-income countries in the 1950s but were replaced with aP vaccines from the 1980s. Because of the heterogeneity of wP and aP vaccines, comparisons of efficacy and effectiveness are challenging. Also, given the potential difficulty in clinical diagnosis described above, estimates of vaccine efficacy require accurate laboratory confirmation using well-validated methods. For example, one study in the United Kingdom found an efficacy of 93% against pertussis confirmed by bacterial culture, compared with only 82% for cases diagnosed solely on clinical criteria. A systematic review of the efficacy of pertussis vaccines reported a pooled efficacy of wP vaccines against pertussis disease in children of 78%, but this varied significantly among vaccines from 46%–92%. A randomised controlled trial comparing three-component and five-component aP-containing vaccines with wP vaccine concluded that the efficacies of the wP and the aP vaccines were similar against culture-confirmed pertussis. Recent studies have suggested that aP vaccines may be less effective than the highest efficacy wP vaccines and that multicomponent aP vaccines are more effective than one-component and two-component aP vaccines. A number of studies have investigated the duration of protection following wP and aP vaccines, with increasing evidence that protection following booster doses of aP vaccines wanes faster in individuals primed with aP compared with wP vaccines.

In response to an increase in infant disease and deaths in some high- and middle-income countries, a range of supplementary immunisation activities have been introduced, including the inclusion of adolescent booster doses, cocooning (offering vaccine to all household contacts of a newborn infant) and, most recently, vaccination of pregnant women. Although adolescent boosters have demonstrated an impact in this target group, there is limited evidence of indirect protection to infants. Cocooning may have some impact in preventing infant disease; however, this strategy is resource intensive and is likely to be less cost-effective than a strategy to vaccinate pregnant women. Based on the evidence from the United Kingdom, vaccination of pregnant women has been demonstrated to be safe and highly effective in preventing disease in young infants from birth. Consequently, the WHO has concluded that this is likely to be the most cost-effective additional strategy for preventing infant disease and countries experiencing high rates of infant disease despite high coverage of their childhood programme should consider this supplementary activity. Vaccination of pregnant women has now been implemented in a number of countries including the United Kingdom, United States, Australia, Argentina, Spain and Belgium.

Safety of pertussis vaccine

Vaccination with wP vaccines is associated with minor local and systemic reactions such as erythema and local swelling. As local reactions increase with age and number of wP immunisations, to reduce the reactogenicity in older children, booster doses with aP vaccines are recommended.

Historical concerns regarding wP vaccines potentially causing neurological sequelae suggested by the National Childhood Encephalopathy Study in the United Kingdom have not subsequently been confirmed in a number of follow-up studies.

RECOMMENDED READING

Amirthalingam, G., Gupta, S., & Campbell, H. (2013). Pertussis immunisation and control in England and Wales, 1957 to 2012: A historical review. *Eurosurveillance, 18*(38), pii: 20587.

Bart, M. J., Harris, S. R., Advani, A., Arakawa, Y., Bottero, D., Bouchez, V., ... Mooi, F. R. (2014). Global population structure and evolution of *Bordetella pertussis* and their relationship with vaccination. *mBio, 5*(2), e01074. doi:10.1128/mBio.01074-14.

Carbonetti, N. H. (2016). *Bordetella pertussis*: New concepts in pathogenesis and treatment. *Current Opinion in Infectious Diseases, 29*(3), 287–294. doi:10.1097/QCO.0000000000000264.

Gerlach, G., von Wintzingerode, F., Middendorf, B., & Gross, R. (2001). Evolutionary trends in the genus *Bordetella*. *Microbes and Infection, 3*(1), 61–72.

Guiso, N., & Wirsing von König, C. H. (2016). Surveillance of pertussis: Methods and implementation. *Expert Review of Anti-infective Therapy, 14*(7), 657–667. doi:10.1080/14787210.2016.1190272.

Kilgore, P. E., Salim, A. M., Zervos, M. J., & Schmitt, H.-J. (2016). Pertussis: Microbiology, disease, treatment, and prevention. *Clinical Microbiology Reviews, 29*(3), 449–486. doi:10.1128/CMR.00083-15.

Parton, R. (1998). Bordetella. In L. Collier, A. Balows, & M. Sussman (Eds.), *Topley & Wilson's Microbiology and Microbial Infections* (pp. 901–918). London: Arnold.

Sealey, K. L., Belcher, T., & Preston, A. (2016). *Bordetella pertussis* epidemiology and evolution in the light of pertussis resurgence. *Infection, Genetics and Evolution, 40*, 136–143. doi:10.1016/j.meegid.2016.02.032.

Winter, K., Zipprich, J., Harriman, K., Murray, E. L., Gornbein, J., Hammer, S. J., ... Cherry, J. D. (2015). Risk factors associated with infant deaths from pertussis: A case-control study. *Clinical Infectious Diseases, 61*(7), 1099–1106. doi:10.1093/cid/civ472.

von Wintzingerode, F., Schattke, A., Siddiqui, R. A., Rösick, U., Göbel, U. B., & Gross, R. (2001). *Bordetella petrii* sp. nov., isolated from an anaerobic bioreactor, and emended description of the genus *Bordetella. International Journal of Systematic and Evolutionary Microbiology, 51*(4), 1257–1265.

von Wintzingerode, F., Gerlach, G., Schneider, B., & Gross, R. (2002). Phylogenetic relationships and virulence evolution in the genus *Bordetella. Current Topics in Microbiology and Immunology, 264*(1), 177–199.

World Health Organization. (2015). Pertussis vaccines: WHO position paper - August 2015. *Weekly Epidemiological Record, 90*(35), 433–458. Available at http://www.who.int/wer/2015/wer9035.pdf?ua=1. (Accessed Nov 2017).

Websites

Public Health England. (2016). Guidelines for the Public Health Management of Pertussis in England. Available at https://www.gov.uk/government/uploads/system/uploads/attachment_data/file/541694/Guidelines_for_the_Public_Health_Management_of_Pertussis_in_England.pdf. (Accessed Nov 2017).

Public Health England. Pertussis: guidance, data and analysis. Available at https://www.gov.uk/government/collections/pertussis-guidance-data-and-analysis. (Accessed Nov 2017).

25 *Legionella*

Legionnaires' disease; legionellosis; Pontiac fever

NORMAN K. FRY

KEY POINTS

- Legionellae inhabit freshwater, soil and manmade water systems. The genus includes *Legionella pneumophila*, which is a major cause of a potentially fatal form of pneumonia known as Legionnaires' disease, and a self-limiting influenza-like illness called Pontiac fever.
- Sixteen serogroups of *L. pneumophila* are recognised, but most human infection is caused by serogroup 1.
- Legionnaires' disease is usually diagnosed by detecting soluble antigen in urine; demonstrating the presence of the organism or its DNA in lower respiratory tract specimens; or legionella antibodies in serum of patients.
- The treatment of choice is currently the newer macrolides and fluoroquinolones (e.g., azithromycin and levofloxacin) to which legionellae are sensitive.
- Epidemiological typing of *L pneumophila* isolates (or genomic DNA) can support or refute links between clinical and environmental isolates (or specimens), which can help inform investigations and allow control measures to be initiated to prevent further cases.
- Suppression of biofilm in water systems using a range of measures including heat, biocides, avoidance of certain materials and limiting available nutrients, together with control of any potential aerosol generation, is essential to control the risk of disease.

The *Legionella* genus belongs to the family Legionellaceae within the γ-Proteobacteria and are Gram-negative rods whose natural habitat is fresh water. Legionellae can also be found in manmade water habitats, soil, potting mixes and composts. More than 58 species have been described, and many more await formal description. Amongst them, the most important pathogen is *Legionella pneumophila*,

and this species has been divided into three subspecies: *L. pneumophila* subsp. *pneumophila, L. pneumophila* subsp. *fraseri* and *L. pneumophila* subsp. *pasculleii*.

At least 29 of the 58 (50%) *Legionella* species have been associated with human disease (Table 25.1), but all species should be regarded as potentially pathogenic. Most infections are caused by *L. pneumophila* belonging to serogroup 1 (sg1). *L. pneumophila* strains possessing a virulence-associated epitope recognized by the monoclonal antibody (mAb) 3/1 (initially designated mAb 2) are positively associated with outbreaks and cause the majority of community- and travel-associated cases.

Infection caused by other species is rare; of these, *L. longbeachae* is a predominant cause of Legionnaires' disease in some parts of the world, particularly in Australasia, and may be increasing, or more increasingly recognised, in Europe. Cases of *L. longbeachae* infection are strongly associated with exposure to potting mixes and composts.

Infection is typically acquired accidentally via inhalation of aerosols containing *Legionella* species due to some failure to control a manmade water system. Aspiration of water containing legionellae can also cause infection, but this is rare. The traditional dogma that the disease is not transmissible from person to person has been challenged recently; however, in this particular case a combination of severe symptoms and close contact by a family member/carer likely contributed to this unusual event and such cases are likely to remain rare.

Legionellae give rise to two main clinical syndromes:

1. Legionnaires' disease (LD), a severe (and sometimes fatal) form of pneumonia that can progress rapidly to a multisystem illness unless recognised promptly and treated with appropriate antibiotics
2. Pontiac fever (PF), an acute, nonpneumonic self-limiting influenza-like illness.

Other manifestations include coinfection with other microorganisms such as *Streptococcus pneumoniae* and

Table 25.1 Legionella species

Species	No. serogroups	Associated with human disease	Autofluorescence under ultraviolet light
L. anisa		Y	Y (blue-white)
L. beliardensis			
L. birminghamensis		Y	
L. bozemanae	2	Y	Y (blue-white)
L. brunensis			
L. busanensis			
L. cardiaca		Y	
L. cherrii			Y (blue-white)
L. cincinnatiensis			
L. drancourtii			
L. dresdenensis			
L. drozanskii			
L. dumoffii		Y	Y (blue-white)
L. erythra		Y	Y (red)
L. fairfieldensis			
L. fallonii		Y	
L. feeleii	2	Y	
L. geestiana			
L. gormanii		Y	Y (blue-white)
L. gratiana			Y (blue-white)
L. gresilensis			
L. hackeliae	2	Y	
L. impletisoli			
L. israelensis			
L. jamestowniensis			
L. jordanis		Y	
L. lansingensis		Y	
L. londiniensis		Y	
L. longbeachae	2	Y	
L. lytica			Y (blue-white)
L. maceachernii		Y	
L. massiliensis			
L. micdadei		Y	
L. moravica			
L. nagasakiensis		Y	
L. nautarum			
L. norrlandica			
L. oakridgensis		Y	
L. parisiensis		Y	Y (blue-white)
L. pneumophila	16	Y	
L. quateirensis			
L. quinlivanii	2		
L. rowbothamii			Y (blue-white)
L. rubrilucens		Y	Y (red)
L. sainthelensi	2	Y	
L. santicrucis			
L. shakespearei			
L. spiritensis	2		
L. steelei		Y	
L. steigerwaltii			Y (blue-white)
L. taurinensis			Y (red)
L. tucsonensis		Y	Y (blue-white)
L. wadsworthii		Y	
L. waltersii		Y	
L. worsleiensis		Y	
L. yabuuchiae			

Haemophilus influenzae, cavity lung disease, extrapulmonary disease, nonpulmonary disease and late sequelae. Legionellae have rarely been associated with infections such as endocarditis (usually with prosthetic valve) or wounds (e.g., sternal-wound infection). Often the source is not identified, but such infections tend to be nosocomial and associated with those in known risk groups such as immunocompromised patients.

DESCRIPTION

Depending on the age of the culture legionellae are ca. 2–20 μm long by 0.3–0.9 μm wide; fresh cultures produce coccobacilli about 2–6 μm long, whereas older cultures may produce filamentous forms up to 20 μm long. *L. pneumophila* usually has only limited motility, and some strains are completely nonmotile. The bacterium has one or two polar flagellae, the expression of which may depend on temperature. In contrast to other aquatic bacteria, *L. pneumophila* requires iron salts and the amino acid L-cysteine to grow.

In clinical specimens (e.g., sputum or lung) or in environmental specimens such as water deposits, legionellae typically appear as short rods or coccobacilli. Legionellae are Gram-negative bacteria, but stain poorly in the Gram procedure if neutral red or safranin is used as the counterstain. Dieterle's silver impregnation method is an alternative means of staining legionellae. More sensitive and specific methods of identifying legionellae include antibody-coupled fluorescent dyes and immunoperoxidase staining.

PATHOGENESIS

The pathogenesis of legionellosis is principally due to the ability of *L. pneumophila* to invade and multiply within the alveolar macrophages of the human host leading to inflammation of the lungs and pneumonia. Similarities between this process and that of infection and intracellular replication of amoebae by legionellae in nature are well documented. Many factors capable of promoting intracellular infection and virulence have been identified. These include surface structures that enhance infection such as lipopolysaccharide, flagellae, type IV pili, the major outer membrane protein (MOMP), the heat-shock protein (Hsp60) and the macrophage infectivity potentiator protein (Mip). Two protein secretion systems are also essential for intracellular infection, the type II and type IV sections systems, also known as T2S and Dot/Icm (defective in organelle trafficking/intracellular multiplication), respectively.

Clinical presentation

LD presents with a range of nonspecific clinical manifestations and symptoms that can include fever, diarrhoea and confusion; fever with multisystem disease including renal failure; hospital-acquired pneumonia; community-acquired pneumonia; pneumonia with extrapulmonary features; and severe fulminant disease.

Legionnaires' disease

Susceptibility to infection and disease is associated with a number of risk factors—smoking, older age, chronic cardiovascular or respiratory disease, diabetes, alcohol misuse, cancer (especially profound monocytopenia as seen in hairy cell leukaemia), immunosuppression and other preexisting medical conditions. The incubation period of LD is typically from 2 to 10 days (median 6–7 days), but may rarely be shorter or longer. The mortality rate typically ranges from 8% to 12%, but can be higher in those with additional risk factors (as discussed earlier in the chapter) and those cases that are nosocomial, or have a delay in diagnosis and treatment. The case-fatality rate in nosocomial cases is higher and ranges from 15%–34%.

Pontiac fever

Pontiac fever (PF) is a mild, self-limiting, nonpneumonic, nonfatal form of legionellosis that has also been associated with exposure to aerosols containing *Legionella*. PF has a much shorter incubation period than LD (usually 24–48 hours, but ranging from 5 to 66 hours) with a duration of 2–5 days and is more common in younger people. PF is usually only identified when cases occur as part of an outbreak because of its mild symptoms and a lack of consensus on diagnostic criteria and case definition.

Models of legionella infection

Several models have been employed to reveal some of the mechanisms of legionella infection.

Guinea pigs infected by inhalation of a *L. pneumophila*–containing aerosol demonstrate some of the clinical and histological features of Legionnaires' disease in humans. Immunocompetent mice inoculated intratracheally have been used as a model of *L. pneumophila* lung infection to evaluate the role of cellular and humoral immunity in regulating intrapulmonary growth of the bacteria. Various nonmammalian models for investigating bacterial pathogens have also been used to study aspects of legionella infection, multiplication and host interactions, including the free-living soil nematode *Caenorhabditis elegans*; the Greater wax moth (*Galleria mellonella*) larvae and the soil-dwelling amoeba *Dictyostelium discoideum,* best known for its remarkable life cycle, consisting of both a unicellular and multicellular phase. Other studies have reported on the use of *in vitro* proliferation assays using, for example, *Acanthamoeba polyphaga,* THP-1 human and J774 murine macrophage cell lines to screen for potential human pathogenicity factors.

LABORATORY INVESTIGATION

The lack of distinctive clinical features of LD necessitates laboratory investigation to obtain confirmation of the diagnosis. The tests used are listed in Table 25.2.

Culture of legionella

Culture remains the gold standard amongst the available methods as all legionella (except those requiring co-culture with amoebae) can be recovered on artificial media. Cultures are made on buffered charcoal yeast extract (BCYE) medium with and without the antibiotics cefamandole, polymyxin and anisomycin (BMPA) medium, added to suppress other respiratory tract flora. Specificity of culture of legionella is ca. 100% and sensitivity is estimated to be in the order of 11%–65%.

To reduce overgrowth of legionella by other organisms, clinical (and environmental) specimens may be treated with acid, heat or dilution, or a combination of all three. Legionella colonies typically take from 48 to 72 hours to appear on BCYE agar. Inoculated plates are examined daily and are usually kept for 10 days of incubation before reporting as negative for culture. Some of the less common non–*L. pneumophila* species may take longer to grow,

may prefer a lower temperature (e.g., 30°C), and show improved growth in an atmosphere of 5% CO_2. These cultures should be incubated for at least 14 days. Typical colonies have a 'cut glass' appearance by plate microscopy, and some species can be differentiated into groups by the property of autofluorescence (blue-white or red) under longwave ultraviolet light (Table 25.1). Presumptive legionella colonies can be Gram stained and subcultured on to blood agar and/or a medium lacking cysteine (BCY–Cys) to show that they will *not* grow on these media.

Serological characterisation of strains can be performed using a commercially available fluorescent-conjugated mAb, which binds to an outer membrane protein of *L. pneumophila.*

L. pneumophila serogroup specificity is conferred by the lipopolysaccharide structure, and some serogroups can be further subdivided into mAb subgroups, which can be useful in screening isolates in epidemiological investigations prior to analysis using genotypic methods. *L. pneumophila* sg 1 can be divided into nine such mAb subgroups (Philadelphia, Allentown/France, Benidorm, Knoxville, OLDA, Oxford, Heysham, Camperdown and Bellingham). Definitive identification to the species level of non–*L. pneumophila* species is best achieved using genotypic methods, of which sequencing of the macrophage infectivity potentiator gene (*mip*) is one of the most widely used.

Detection and epidemiological typing of legionella nucleic acid in clinical specimens

There are now many published polymerase chain reaction (PCR) assays and several commercial kits for the detection of *Legionella* spp., especially those more commonly associated with human infection including *L. pneumophila.* PCR and sequencing protocols are also available that allow genotyping of *L. pneumophila* in clinical material, using the seven-gene sequence–based typing scheme (http://bioinformatics.phe.org.uk/legionella/legionella_sbt/php/sbt_homepage.php).

Such methodologies are more rapid than waiting for the appearance of colonies by culture and can provide valuable typing data even when culture is unsuccessful.

Detection of legionella antigen in urine

The legionella urinary antigen (UAG) test is the most widely used test for the diagnosis of legionella infection. There are a number of commercial enzyme-linked immunosorbent assay (ELISA) tests available that are generally considered to be more sensitive than the more rapid immunochromatographic (ICT) assays. Whilst most assays claim to be specific for *L. pneumophila* sg 1, this likely reflects the lack of availability of urine from culture-confirmed cases of other serogroups required for more

Table 25.2 Laboratory diagnostic tests and specimens for confirmation of legionella infection

Nature of test	Test	Appropriate specimen
Detection of whole organism	DFA	Recommended: Lower respiratory tract specimens (sputum, BAL, bronchial aspirates, tracheal aspirates etc.) or other clinical material (post-mortem specimens; e.g., lung biopsies) Less suitable: pleural fluid
Detection of viable organism	Culture	
Detection of specific DNA	PCR	
Detection of soluble antigen	ELISA	Urine
	ICT	
Detection of antibody	IFA	Serum
	ELISA	

ELISA, Enzyme-linked immunosorbent assay; *ICT*, immunochromatographic test; *IFA*, indirect fluorescent antibody test; *PCR*, polymerase chain reaction. *BAL*, bronchoalveolar lavage; *DFA*, direct fluorescent antibody test.

complete verification and validation. The sensitivity of UAG tests for *L. pneumophila* sg 1 compared to culture-confirmed cases ranges from 71% to 92%. Legionella antigenuria is detectable very early in infection (typically 2–3 days post-onset of clinical symptoms). In most cases, antigenuria ends after 10–14 days, but can persist for a much longer period of time. It has been suggested that legionellosis due to non–*L. pneumophila* may be greatly underreported because of the over reliance on UAG testing.

Detection of legionella by direct fluorescent antibody testing

Direct testing of respiratory specimens by direct fluorescent antibody (DFA) using commercially available fluorescent-conjugated mAb is a rapid method for detection of *L. pneumophila* antigen from all serogroups and can be performed on fixed histology specimens. Reported sensitivity ranges from 22% to 70%.

Detection of legionella antibody in human sera

The indirect fluorescence antibody (IFA) test is the most commonly used method for serological diagnosis, and there are commercially available kits in this and the ELISA format. Although IFA/ELISA can yield acceptable sensitivity and specificity for *L. pneumophila* sg 1, the delay in the development of a measurable antibody response constitutes a major drawback in the diagnosis of patients in the acute phase.

TREATMENT

Although erythromycin continues to be an effective agent against *Legionella* spp., the treatment of choice has changed to the newer macrolides and fluoroquinolones (e.g., azithromycin and levofloxacin).

Susceptibility testing of clinical isolates is rarely justified. Resistance is rarely reported, the methodology is technically demanding and, by its nature, results take several days. As the likelihood of person-to-person transmission remains extremely low, antibiotic usage is unlikely to contribute to the development of resistance in other patients.

EPIDEMIOLOGY

In 1976, a large outbreak of pneumonia resulting in many unexplained deaths occurred at the 58th convention of the American Legion at the Bellevue Stratford Hotel in Philadelphia, USA. Joseph McDade, a specialist in rickettsia at the Centers for Disease Control and Prevention (CDC), Atlanta, USA, along with his team, finally discovered the aetiological agent, the so-called Legionnaires' disease bacterium, by inoculating guinea pigs with clinical material from patients. This bacterium was later formally named as *Legionella pneumophila*.

LD can occur both sporadically and in large outbreaks. In Europe, most cases (ca. 80%) are community-acquired and sporadic. LD demonstrates a seasonal pattern, with reported cases peaking in late summer to early autumn. The incidence of LD appears to be positively associated with certain climate changes, for example, increased precipitation. Available evidence also supports the increased survival of *L. pneumophila* in aerosols at high relative humidity. Legionellae can infect, multiply and survive within protozoan hosts (e.g., *Acanthamoeba*), and the bacteria are protected from adverse environmental conditions, such as desiccation and disinfectants, by persisting in amoebic cysts.

Sources of sporadic cases of infection are rarely investigated and identified, but many systems have been demonstrated to act as potential sources of *Legionella*. The vast majority of travel-associated and nosocomial cases are linked to contaminated water systems, for example, showers, baths, spa pools, respiratory therapy and air conditioning equipment, food display misters and humidifiers, whilst community cases are predominantly linked to contaminated aerosols from wet cooling systems such as cooling towers. A large community outbreak of LD in France linked to industrial cooling towers challenged the accepted view concerning how far bacteria in contaminated aerosols can be spread; in this case the distance was reported to be at least 6 km.

Recent travel history is also associated with LD, especially with overnight stays in hotel accommodation. A combination of unoccupied rooms, water systems with stagnation and inadequate control measures can combine to result in *Legionella* growth and subsequent risk of infection. Cruise ships are another potential source of legionella for similar reasons and have also been associated with clusters of cases and outbreaks of LD.

CONTROL

Prevention is best achieved by vigilant control, proper risk assessment and maintenance of water systems and potential aerosol sources. The prevention of the formation and accumulation of biofilm is perhaps the most important control measure against *Legionella* proliferation, since, once established, it is extremely difficult to eliminate. Increased risk factors that contribute to biofilm formation include presence of nutrients, scale, corrosion, water temperature, stagnation and/or low flow. In low-nutrient environments, legionellae enter a slow metabolic nonreplicative state, which can make them difficult to recover and more resistant to biocides.

Those with health and safety responsibilities for others must comply with their legal duties in relation to *Legionella*. To assist in this process the Health and Safety Executive (HSE), the national independent watchdog for work-related health, safety and illness, which acts in the public interest to reduce work-related death and serious injury across Great Britain's workplaces, produces information and guidance, for example, Legionnaires' disease: the control of legionella bacteria in water systems (L8, 4th edition). This document lists the precautions that should be taken, including:

- avoiding water temperatures between 20°C and 45°C and conditions that favour the growth of legionella bacteria and other microorganisms
- avoiding water stagnation that may encourage the growth of biofilm
- avoiding the use of materials that harbour bacteria and other microorganisms, or provide nutrients for microbial growth
- controlling the release of water spray
- maintaining the cleanliness of the system and water in it
- using water treatment techniques
- taking action to ensure the correct and safe operation and maintenance of the water system.

Investigation of legionella outbreaks, or single nosocomial cases, is important in order to identify possible sources of legionella-containing aerosols in order that control and eradication measures can be deployed. Definitive epidemiological typing of *L. pneumophila* isolates (or genomic DNA from PCR-positive specimens) is a prerequisite to support or refute epidemiology links between clinical and environmental isolates and can inform incident investigation. Once the source has been identified, legionellae may be eradicated from a water source typically using a combination of the measures listed previously.

Notification, public health action and travel-associated cases

Legionnaires' disease is a notifiable disease in England and Wales. Consequently, health-care professionals are required to inform the local health protection teams (HPTs) of any suspected cases. It is also recommended that relevant clinical specimens from patients with suspected LD be sent to the Public Health England National Reference Laboratory at Colindale, London to allow confirmation and further investigation including molecular typing. Public Health England collects data on notifiable diseases including LD, which assists in tracking and identifying clusters and in preventing and controlling outbreaks whilst monitoring trends in disease occurrence over time. According to certain criteria, and to assist in the investigation of cases, clusters and outbreaks, an outbreak control team (OCT) may be formed. By their nature, these teams can involve representatives from a number of agencies, including public and environmental health, hospitals, food water and environmental laboratories, infection control teams, estates, port authorities and communications.

The European Surveillance Scheme is managed by the European Centre for Disease Prevention and Control (ECDC), which monitors trends and detects clusters and outbreaks of travel-associated Legionnaires' disease across Europe. This scheme contributes to the evaluation and monitoring of control and prevention programmes in collaboration with European Union Member States. Further information about the European Legionnaires' Disease Surveillance Network (ELDSNet) is available at http://ecdc.europa.eu/en/healthtopics/legionnaires_disease/ELDSNet/Pages/index.aspx.

RECOMMENDED READING

Correia, A. M., Ferreira, J. S., Borges, V., Nunes, A., Gomes, B., Capucho, R., ... Gomes, J. P. (2016). Probable person-to-person transmission of Legionnaires' disease. *New England Journal of Medicine, 374*(5), 497–498. doi:10.1056/NEJMc1505356.

Cunha, B. A., Burillo, A., & Bouza, E. (2016). Legionnaires' disease. *The Lancet, 387*(10016), 376–385. doi: http://dx.doi.org/10.1016/S0140-6736(15)60078-2.

Khodr, A., Kay, E., Gomez-Valero, L., Ginevra, C., Doublet, P., Buchrieser, C., & Jarraud, S. (2016). Molecular epidemiology, phylogeny and evolution of *Legionella. Infection, Genetics and Evolution, 43*, 108–122. doi:10.1016/j.meegid.2016.04.033.

Mercante, J. W., & Winchell, J. M. (2015). Current and emerging *Legionella* diagnostics for laboratory and outbreak investigations. *Clinical Microbiology Reviews, 28*(1), 95–133. doi:10.1128/CMR.00029-14.

Phin, N., Parry-Ford, F., Harrison, T., Stagg, H. R., Zhang, N., Kumar, K., ... Abubakar, I. (2014). Epidemiology and clinical management of Legionnaires' disease. *The Lancet Infectious Diseases, 14*(10), 1011–1021. doi:10.1016/S1473-3099(14)70713-3.

Websites

Centers for Disease Control and Prevention. *Legionella* (Legionnaires' Disease and Pontiac Fever). Available at https://www.cdc.gov/legionella/index.html. (Accessed Nov 2017).

Health and Safety Exectutive. Legionella and Legionnaires' disease. Available at http://www.hse.gov.uk/legionnaires/. (Accessed Nov 2017).

Public Health England. Legionnaires' disease: guidance, data and analysis. Available at https://www.gov.uk/government/collections/legionnaires-disease-guidance-data-and-analysis. (Accessed Nov 2017).

26 *Neisseria* and *Moraxella*

Meningitis; septicaemia; gonorrhoea; respiratory infections

LUKE R. GREEN AND CHRISTOPHER D. BAYLISS

KEY POINTS

- *Neisseria meningitidis* (meningococcus) and *N. gonorrhoeae* (gonococcus) are obligate human parasites.
- *N. meningitidis* lives commensally in the nasopharynx, is transmitted via aerosols and close contact (e.g., prolonged kissing), and causes disease that can rapidly progress from fever and mild malaise to meningitis, septicaemia or septicaemic shock (circulatory failure, multiorgan dysfunction and coagulopathy).
- Treatment is by intravenous administration of penicillin or ceftriaxone. Prophylactic antibiotics (e.g., rifampicin or ciprofloxacin) can be given to contacts to eradicate carriage and control outbreaks.
- Of the 13 serogroups, groups A, B, C, W, X and Y cause >90% of cases. Group B is most prevalent in the developed world. Vaccines are available against A, C, W and Y and for some group B strains.
- *N. gonorrhoeae* causes the sexually transmitted disease gonorrhoea. Asymptomatic carriage in women is common, but the organism may give rise to acute salpingitis, which may be followed by pelvic inflammatory disease and a high probability of sterility if inadequately treated.
- In the United Kingdom, cephalosporins such as ceftriaxone are the drugs of choice. Use of antibiotics is limited in some countries by a high prevalence of resistance.
- Early diagnosis, effective treatment and contact tracing are key to preventing the spread of disease. There is no effective vaccine to prevent gonorrhoea.
- *Moraxella catarrhalis* is an upper respiratory tract commensal that causes lower respiratory tract infections and otitis media.

The genus *Neisseria* contains two species of clinical significance: *N. meningitidis* (meningococcus) and *N. gonorrhoeae* (gonococcus). They are Gram-negative diplococci and obligate human pathogens, typically found inside polymorphonuclear pus cells of the inflammatory exudate. Although similar in terms of morphological and cultural characteristics, they are associated with entirely different diseases:

- *N. meningitidis* causes a range of diseases embraced by the term *invasive meningococcal disease*. Most common are purulent meningitis (variously called epidemic cerebrospinal meningitis, cerebrospinal fever or, because of the purpuric rash that is sometimes present, spotted fever) and an acute septicaemic illness with a petechial rash in the presence or absence of meningitis. About one-third of cases of meningococcal disease present as septicaemia; meningitis (with or without septicaemia) accounts for most others.
- *N. gonorrhoeae* causes the sexually transmitted disease gonorrhoea, which most commonly presents as a purulent infection of the mucous membrane of the urethra in men and the cervix uteri in women. In the newborn the gonococcus may give rise to a purulent conjunctivitis and in young girls a vulvovaginitis. Disseminated gonococcal infection, which is recognised by a rash and evidence of blood spread, may also occur, more commonly in women.

Other members of the *Neisseria* genus are common commensals of the upper respiratory tract (which is also the reservoir of the meningococcus and, occasionally, the gonococcus) and are of low pathogenicity in the immunocompetent host. Commensal species include *N. lactamica*, *N. cinerea*, *N. subflava* (of which there are several biovars), *N. sicca*, *N. polysaccharea*, *N. mucosa* and *N. flavescens*. Several other commensal species, including *N. elongata*, *N. weaveri* and *N. bacilliformis*, are unusual in being rod shaped.

Moraxellae are non-fermentative organisms that may be coccoid or rod shaped. There is still uncertainty as to their taxonomic position. Some strains resemble *Acinetobacter* spp. and other glucose nonfermenters. The most important member of the group, *Moraxella catarrhalis* (formerly known as *Branhamella catarrhalis*), is a common commensal of the upper respiratory tract and an opportunistic pathogen associated with otitis media in children and exacerbations of chronic obstructive pulmonary disease in adults.

NEISSERIA

DESCRIPTION

N. meningitidis and *N. gonorrhoeae* are morphologically and culturally very similar. They are Gram-negative oval cocci occurring in pairs with the apposed surfaces flat or slightly concave (bean shaped) and with the axis of the pair parallel and not in line as in the pneumococcus. In pus from inflammatory exudates, such as the cerebrospinal fluid (CSF) or urethral discharge, many diplococci are found in a small proportion of the polymorphonuclear cells. This is more marked with the gonococcus than with the meningococcus. Extracellular cocci also occur, and there may be considerable variation in their size and intensity of staining.

Nonpathogenic neisseriae grow on ordinary nutrient media, but meningococci and gonococci require the addition of heated blood (or ascitic fluid) and incubation at 35–37°C, in a moist atmosphere containing 5%–10% carbon dioxide. Growth is rather slow (more so with the gonococcus) but, grey, glistening, slightly convex colonies of 0.5–1.0 mm in diameter appear in 8–24 hours. After incubation for a further 24 hours, the colonies are much larger, and the gonococcus, in particular, tends to have a slightly roughened surface and a crenated margin.

Colonies of meningococci and gonococci react quickly in the test for cytochrome oxidase; nonpathogenic neisseriae react more slowly. Species identification depends on carbohydrate utilisation reactions. *N. gonorrhoeae* produces acid from glucose, but not maltose, whilst *N. meningitidis* produces acid from both. The commensal species, *N. lactamica* and *N. sicca*, utilise lactose or sucrose, respectively. Neither of these carbohydrates is utilised by the pathogenic *Neisseria*. Commercial kits that rapidly detect preformed enzymes, such as aminopeptidases and β-galactosidase, are commonly used for identification.

Genome analysis

Genome sequence analysis shows that *N. meningitidis* and *N. gonorrhoeae* are very similar, although each species has several hundred unique genes, which may explain their differing interactions with the host. The genomes are between 2.1 and 2.5 million bp in length, encoding between 2000 and 2700 open reading frames and having a 51%–53% GC content. Importantly, these species have evolved highly efficient ways of varying their genes and antigens, thus undermining host defence mechanisms. Diversity is generated in a number of ways, including natural transformation with DNA from other cells of the same or related species and by a range of recombination and mutation-based systems, including phase variation (reversibly switching genes on and off) and antigenic variation of expressed antigens using information from silent genetic loci. Among the key antigenically variable antigens is the PilE protein, which is the predominant constituent of the pilus, a multifunctional appendage associated with attachment to mucosal surfaces. Antigenic variation is the result of genetic recombination between the PilE expression locus *(pilE)* and one or more silent allelic loci *(pilS)*.

NEISSERIA MENINGITIDIS

CLASSIFICATION

Classical typing

Meningococci are divisible into 13 serogroups, based on antigenic differences in their capsular polysaccharides, but only six of these have significant pathogenic potential. Over 90% of worldwide invasive disease is caused by strains from serogroups A, B, C, W, X and Y. The serogroup is usually determined by a slide agglutination test with absorbed group-specific antisera but can now be identified by PCR.

Meningococcal serotypes and serosubtypes are determined by specific monoclonal antibodies raised against the antigenically hypervariable outer membrane proteins (porins) PorA and PorB. Strain identities are designated by their serogroup (e.g., B), serotype (e.g., 15) and serosubtype (e.g., P1.16). As a result of genetic variation in the antigens used for typing, and incomplete coverage of typing reagents, nontypeable strains are often isolated. In these cases, the corresponding porin genes can be sequenced and classified. Immunotyping, based on antigenic variation of lipooligosaccharides, is sometimes carried out.

Whole genome sequence typing

Whole genome sequencing (WGS), multilocus sequence typing (MLST) and multilocus enzyme electrophoresis (MLEE) are able to distinguish numerous genotypes of meningococci. As WGS becomes more affordable, gene-by-gene comparative analysis is increasingly used to type meningococci. Diagnosed cases are referred to the

Meningococcal Reference Unit for WGS analysis before contiguous sequences or de novo assembled draft genomes are uploaded to the Bacterial Isolate Genomic Sequence database (BIGSdb) within *Neisseria* PubMLST (pubmlst.org/neisseria/), a repository for typing information on isolates of this genus. BIGSdb allows investigation of sequence variation across multiple loci including the 1605 core genome MLST or the traditional seven genes used in MLST. Use of these methods has established that meningococcal populations are genetically highly diverse but can be structured into sequence types (ST), clonal complexes (cc; alternatively called lineages and consisting of groups of related STs) and higher order clades. These analyses have demonstrated that *N. meningitidis* and *N. gonorrhoeae* are genetically similar, with divergence occurring relatively recently due to a change in ecological niche from the nasopharynx to the urogenital tract.

A few hypervirulent lineages are associated with the majority of disease worldwide. For example, cc32 and cc11 (formerly electrophoretic types ET-5 and ET-37) were the dominant serogroup B and C clonal types, respectively, responsible for causing disease in the United Kingdom and the rest of Europe in the 1980s. The dominant strain types change over time, and an increase in the incidence of disease may coincide with the introduction of a new clonal complex into a particular community.

PATHOGENESIS

The natural habitat of the meningococcus is the human nasopharynx, and transmission is largely via close contact. Acquisition may be transient, lead to asymptomatic colonisation (carriage) or result in invasive disease. The carrier:case ratio varies in different outbreaks and with the strain and population surveyed. Around 5%–10% of general populations are normally carriers of meningococci, but in some populations (e.g., university students and army cadets) carriage rates are typically higher, ranging from 20% to 50% or more. In communities experiencing outbreaks of invasive meningococcal disease the carriage rate of the epidemic strain may also be high. The incidence of meningococcal disease increases when:

- meningococcal strains of high virulence are encountered
- factors that increase meningococcal transmission are present
- susceptible individuals who lack bactericidal antibodies to the current strains are present in the population

Some studies show that a sharp increase in the carrier rate of pathogenic groups of meningococci precedes the occurrence of clinical cases. Bacterial, environmental and host factors are probably all equally important in the development of disease.

Bacterial factors

Some meningococcal strains are more capable than others to cause invasive disease, although the basis for this is still unclear. Surface structures subject to phase or antigenic variation, such as capsular polysaccharide, outer membrane proteins and lipooligosaccharide are major virulence components. The capsule protects the meningococcus from phagocytic killing, opsonisation and complement-mediated bactericidal killing in the blood. Outer membrane and pilus proteins act as adhesins, facilitating attachment to host cells, while lipooligosaccharide is a key mediator of the pathogenesis of fulminant sepsis and meningitis.

Environmental factors

Environmental risk factors for carriage and disease include overcrowding, respiratory viral infections, including influenza, and damage to the upper respiratory tract caused by very low humidity, dust or trauma. Meningococcal infections tend to peak during the winter months in countries with temperate climates but in the dry season in countries in Sub-Saharan Africa. Household contacts of a case are 500–800 times more likely to develop meningococcal infection than the general population.

Host factors

For largely unknown reasons, some individuals are more susceptible to infection than others, and some do worse than others. The absence of bactericidal antibody in the blood is believed to be the factor most closely related to susceptibility to clinical infection. The disappearance of antibody acquired from the mother increases the risk for infants and young children. Similarly, congenital and acquired antibody deficiencies also increase risk, as does asplenia. Group-specific (anticapsular) antibody is protective, and this is the basis of the success of vaccination against meningococcal disease. Antibodies to immunogenic and surface-exposed outer membrane proteins also protect, but the range of antigens involved and the role of non-specific defence mechanisms in preventing clinical disease are ill understood. The complement system is important, as shown by the recurrent attacks of meningococcal infections in those with defects in the pathway. A genetic basis of susceptibility, severity and outcome of meningococcal disease is far from clear, but studies suggest that genetic polymorphisms in key regulators of complement activation, surfactant proteins and several other proteins may increase risk.

PATHOPHYSIOLOGY

During meningococcal septicaemia there are signs and symptoms of circulatory failure, multiorgan dysfunction and coagulopathy. There is increased vascular permeability and vasodilatation that result in capillary leak syndrome with peripheral oedema. Loss of intravascular fluid and plasma proteins results in hypovolaemia and reduced venous return, and hence reduced cardiac output, hypotension and reduced perfusion of vital organs. Systemic hypoxia, acidosis, and gross electrolyte and metabolic impairment eventually culminate in multiorgan dysfunction. At the molecular level, the underlying pathophysiology of meningococcal sepsis is complex and involves numerous interactive cascades, including cytokine, chemokine, host cell receptors and coagulation and complement components.

Meningococcal lipooligosaccharide, or more specifically its lipid A moiety, is thought to be primarily responsible for septic shock, extensive tissue damage and multiorgan dysfunction by stimulating the release of inflammatory mediators including tumour necrosis factor-α and a series of interleukins, other cytokines and major intravascular cascade systems. Levels of circulating lipooligosaccharide exceeding 700 ng/L are associated with fulminant septic shock, disseminated intravascular coagulation and a high fatality rate.

CLINICAL MANIFESTATIONS

Meningococci are able to cause a wide range of clinical symptoms and syndromes varying in severity from a transient, mild malaise with fever to meningitis or acute meningococcal septicaemia. It is critical to remember that the clinical picture can progress from one end of the spectrum (i.e., mild symptoms) to the other (i.e., severe disease) within a very short time frame and that death can occur within hours of the appearance of symptoms.

Bacteraemia with or without sepsis, meningococcal septicaemia with or without meningitis, meningoencephalitis, chronic meningococcaemia, pneumonia, septic arthritis, pericarditis, myocarditis, endocarditis, conjunctivitis, panophthalmitis, genitourinary tract infection, pelvic infection, peritonitis and proctitis are among the diseases caused by meningococci. Meningitis and/or septicaemia are by far the most common presentations of disease. It is important to note that the spectrum of clinical manifestations can alter during the course of disease.

A significant number of the patients who recover end up with permanent neurological sequelae, including intellectual impairment, cranial nerve deficits and deafness due to auditory nerve damage. The mortality rate from meningococcal disease varies between 5% and 70%, depending on a number of factors including the severity of disease, the speed with which it develops, the organs involved, the age and immune status of the patient, the socioeconomic status, the standard of health care and the speed with which the disease is diagnosed and antibiotics administered.

LABORATORY INVESTIGATION

In any suspected meningococcal infection, blood culture must be undertaken; if meningitis is suspected, a lumbar puncture should be performed as soon as possible, unless there are signs of raised intracranial pressure. Typically, the CSF will contain high numbers of white blood cells, high protein levels and reduced glucose levels. Microscopic examination of the stained centrifuged deposit should be performed without delay; the presence of Gram-negative diplococci will enable urgent antibiotic therapy to be started. The CSF is also cultured on heated blood (chocolate) agar and on blood agar. In the absence of visible meningococci, glucose broth may be added to the remaining sediment of the centrifuged deposit to facilitate the isolation of very sparse organisms. Cultures are incubated overnight at 37°C in an atmosphere of 5%–10% carbon dioxide. As many patients receive penicillin before admission to hospital, lumbar puncture yields more positive cultures than blood.

A rapidly positive oxidase test on any Gram-negative diplococci that are grown is strong evidence that the isolates are pathogenic *Neisseria*. Sugar utilisation tests or commercial kits are used to further differentiate species. Direct slide agglutination with specific antisera may be carried out on suspensions of colonies picked from solid medium.

Growth of the meningococcus from a normally sterile site, such as CSF or blood, is definitive evidence of disease. Rapid PCR (polymerase chain reaction) tests are useful and may be positive when early antibiotic treatment has prevented successful culture. Meningococcal capsular polysaccharide may be detected in CSF by latex agglutination.

Where facilities exist, isolates should be sent to a reference laboratory for further procedures that provide important epidemiological information. Meningococcal disease is a notifiable disease in England and Wales, with a requirement for all diagnosed cases of meningococcal infection to be referred to the Meningococcal Reference Unit.

Meningococci may be found in genital sites, and it is important to identify these organisms accurately and differentiate them from gonococci.

TREATMENT

Treatment should begin at the point of first contact as soon as meningococcal disease is suspected, even before the patient is transferred to hospital or investigated. Intravenous penicillin, cefotaxime or ceftriaxone are the drugs of choice. Although these agents do not cross uninflamed meninges well, they readily pass into CSF when inflammation is present. Chloramphenicol is effective, but risks of blood dyscrasia have limited its use.

In the absence of organisms in the Gram-stained CSF deposit, it is wise to give therapy with cefotaxime or ceftriaxone, which cover *Haemophilus influenzae* and *Streptococcus pneumoniae*, the other two principal causes of meningitis in childhood after the neonatal period.

Most clinical isolates of meningococci are presently sensitive to benzylpenicillin. However, meningococci of reduced susceptibility to penicillin have been reported, and it is important that accurate sensitivity testing is carried out on all isolates from clinical disease. At the end of a course of therapy with penicillin, eradicative treatment with rifampicin or ciprofloxacin should be given because penicillin does not eradicate meningococci from the nasopharynx, and a patient returning home as a carrier may infect others. This probably does not apply to ceftriaxone and cefotaxime, which also eradicate throat carriage.

The mortality rate in septicaemic illness may range from 14% up to 50% in some outbreaks. The rate in meningitis is about 2%–7%. Bad prognostic signs are:

- the presence of coma on admission to hospital
- a rapidly coalescing purpuric rash (Fig. 26.1)
- signs of shock

Occasionally, in the most fulminating forms of septicaemia, there may not be time for the rash to develop before death. In such cases, meningococci are isolated from the blood in life or post mortem, and haemorrhagic adrenals are seen at autopsy, these being characteristic of the Waterhouse–Friderichsen syndrome.

EPIDEMIOLOGY

Incidence rates of invasive meningococcal disease are highest in infants of <1 year and toddlers of 1–4 years (20–45 and 5–17 cases, respectively, per 100,000 in the United Kingdom between 2005 and 2015), with 30%–50% of cases occurring in the first 4 years of life. While the peak prevalence of disease is in the first year, there is a smaller peak in adolescence (Fig. 26.2) and a growing proportion of cases in people >65 years. The increase in immunity observed with increasing age is likely due to asymptomatic carriage, often for many months, of virulent or avirulent meningococci or other neisseriae. Meningococcal infections occur worldwide and are notifiable in most countries. *N. meningitidis* is the only bacterium capable of generating epidemic outbreaks of meningitis. These

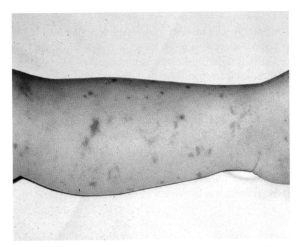

Fig. 26.1 Early purpuric rash of meningococcal septicaemia. Obtained with permission from Meningitis Research Foundation.

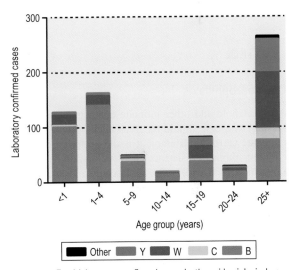

Fig. 26.2 Total laboratory confirmed cases in the epidemiological year 2014/2015. Serogroup B, orange; C, yellow; W, blue; Y, green; Other, black. Data obtained from Public Health England.

occur every 5–15 years in Sub-Saharan Africa; endemic disease or localised outbreaks are seen in the rest of the world.

- Serogroup A disease (ST-5 or ST-7 complexes) is most prevalent in Sub-Saharan Africa (the African meningitis belt) and the Middle East, where tens of thousands of cases are reported each year. Recent introduction of an effective vaccine is beginning to prevent epidemics by serogroup A strains in this region.

- Serogroup B strains are dominant among pathogenic meningococci in most industrialised countries and are a major cause of sporadic or endemic disease. Prolonged outbreaks in several countries have caused significant morbidity and mortality.
- Serogroup C strains (especially ST-11 complexes) have caused epidemics (e.g., China, Africa, Brazil) and more localised outbreaks in North America and Europe. Effective vaccination has reduced the incidence of serogroup C disease in many countries.
- Serogroup W strains have been associated with outbreaks following the pilgrimage to Mecca (the Hajj) and are a significant cause of disease in parts of the African meningitis belt. Since 2009, serogroup W cases in the United Kingdom have accelerated year on year due to expansion of a hypervirulent ST-11 strain.
- Serogroup Y (ST-23 and related sequence types) has caused increased rates of disease in the United States and South America, and serogroup X has been responsible for localised outbreaks in parts of the African meningitis belt.

CONTROL

Chemoprophylaxis

All household and other intimate contacts (e.g., mouth kissing) of a case should be given chemoprophylaxis to eliminate carriage. Rifampicin is the preferred drug for children, although resistance can develop rapidly. Ciprofloxacin is used widely for adolescents and adults as a single oral dose. While chemoprophylaxis is effective in contacts and in limited outbreak settings, the development of antibiotic resistance, availability of drugs, and the large size of some outbreaks mean that the prevention of disease by vaccination is often the best control strategy.

Vaccination

Resistance to meningococcal infection is closely associated with the possession of bactericidal antibodies that may be maternal in origin or actively produced in response to carriage. Vaccines containing the native, unconjugated, group-specific capsular polysaccharide of meningococci of groups A, C, W and Y have been available since the 1970s and are good immunogens in children >2 years. However, polysaccharide vaccines do not induce immunological memory, and protection is limited to 3–5 years. Also, they have no effect on nasopharyngeal carriage and thus do not generate herd immunity.

Despite their limitations, meningococcal polysaccharide vaccines were used extensively to help control epidemics of serogroup A disease in countries of the African meningitis belt. However, the development of protein-conjugated vaccines has changed the outlook for prevention. These vaccines are immunogenic in young children, induce immunological memory and decrease nasopharyngeal carriage. In the United Kingdom, introduction of a conjugate vaccine against serogroup C meningococci into the routine childhood immunisation programme has led to significant reductions in serogroup C disease. This is partly the result of herd immunity effects, which protect unvaccinated individuals.

A low-cost serogroup A specific conjugate vaccine has been introduced widely across the meningitis belt in Sub-Saharan Africa. Since the introduction of MenAfriVac, the incidence of disease has declined greatly, dropping as low as 2.5 per 100,000 population in some areas.

Quadrivalent conjugate vaccines offering protection against serogroups A, C, W and Y are available and have recently been introduced into the United Kingdom national immunisation programme to reduce the increasing incidence of serogroup W disease.

The development of a vaccine to protect against serogroup B disease has been much harder to achieve. The group B capsular polysaccharide is a poor immunogen that does not induce a protective IgG response. Consequently, strategies have focused on noncapsular antigens such as outer membrane proteins, vesicles and lipooligosaccharides. Initially, these approaches were limited by the diversity of major outer membrane structures. Recently, however, genome sequence analysis (reverse vaccinology) or sequential protein extraction and immunisation were used to identify novel, conserved surface proteins capable of eliciting protective immunity. Two new MenB vaccines (Bexsero and Trumenba) have been licensed for use and, in September 2015, Bexsero was added to the UK national immunisation schedule for infants.

NEISSERIA GONORRHOEAE

The name 'gonorrhoea' derives from the Greek words *gonos* (seed) and *rhoia* (flow) and described a condition in which semen flowed from the male organ without erection. It became apparent that gonorrhoea was associated with sexual promiscuity, one of the diseases celebrated by being named after the Roman goddess of love, Venus. Indeed, gonorrhoea is a classical venereal disease, being spread almost exclusively by sexual contact, having a short incubation period and being relatively easy to diagnose and treat. In the United Kingdom the highest infection rates are seen in men aged 20–24 years and women aged 16–19 years.

Gonococci are as antigenically heterogeneous as meningococci; many of the major cell surface antigens are shared between both species, with the exception of the capsule, which is not encoded by the gonococcus. Classically, strains are characterised by auxotyping, which recognises requirements for specific nutrients, such as arginine, proline, hypoxanthine and uracil. Panels of monoclonal antibodies that recognise specific proteins are also used to divide strains into various serovars. Epidemiological typing makes use of both methods as well as newer molecular techniques, such as MLST and WGS.

PATHOGENESIS

N. gonorrhoeae is exclusively a human pathogen. It is never found as a normal commensal, but a proportion of those infected, particularly women, may remain asymptomatic. These individuals may develop systemic or ascending infection at a later stage.

Gonorrhoeal infection is generally limited to superficial mucosal surfaces lined with columnar epithelium. The areas most frequently involved are the cervix, urethra, rectum, pharynx and conjunctiva. Squamous epithelium, which lines the adult vagina, is not susceptible to infection by the gonococcus. However, the prepubertal vaginal epithelium, which has not been keratinised under the influence of oestrogen, may be infected. Hence, gonorrhoea in young girls may present as vulvovaginitis.

The most common clinical presentation is acute urethritis in the male a few days after unprotected vaginal or anal sexual intercourse. Dysuria and a purulent penile discharge make most sufferers seek treatment rapidly. A few men have relatively minor symptoms, which may disappear rapidly. Truly asymptomatic infection is rare in the active male. However, up to 5% may carry the organism without apparent distress, and this is more common with certain types of gonococci. Rectal and pharyngeal infection is less often symptomatic and may be discovered only after tracing contacts.

Endocervical infection is the most common form of uncomplicated gonorrhoea in women. Such infections are usually characterised by vaginal discharge and sometimes by dysuria. The cervical os may be erythematous and friable, with a purulent exudate. In women with vaginal infection, only half may have symptoms of discharge and dysuria. Most seek attention because of their partner's symptoms, or as part of contact tracing or screening of high-risk individuals. Local complications include abscesses in Bartholin's and Skene's glands. Rectal infections (proctitis) with *N. gonorrhoeae* occur in about one-third of women with cervical infection and are rarely symptomatic. In contrast, gonococcal proctitis in homosexual men is often symptomatic.

Asymptomatic carriage in women is common, especially in the endocervical canal. At menstruation or after instrumentation, particularly termination of pregnancy,

gonococci ascend to the fallopian tubes to give rise to acute salpingitis, which may be followed by pelvic inflammatory disease and a high probability of sterility if treated inadequately. Peritoneal spread occurs occasionally and may produce a perihepatic inflammation (Fitz-Hugh–Curtis syndrome). Some lineages of *N. gonorrhoeae* spread more widely and give rise to disseminated gonococcal infection.

Disseminated infection is seen more commonly in women, who may present with painful joints, fever and a few septic skin lesions on their extremities. The diagnosis of a venereal disease may not be obvious, and isolation of gonococci from joint fluid, blood culture and skin aspirates requires particular care. The organisms are invariably present in the cervix, but in many cases antibiotics have been given before the diagnosis is considered. Rarely, disseminated gonococcal infection may present as endocarditis or meningitis.

Babies born to infected women may suffer ophthalmia neonatorum, in which the eyes are coated with gonococci as the baby passes down the birth canal. A severe purulent eye discharge with periorbital oedema occurs within a few days of birth. If untreated, ophthalmia leads rapidly to blindness. It may be prevented in areas of high prevalence by the instillation of 1% aqueous silver nitrate in the eyes of newborn babies. Alternatively, topical erythromycin can be used; this has the advantage of being active against chlamydia and is less toxic than silver nitrate.

Vulvovaginitis in prepubertal girls occurs either in conditions of poor hygiene or by sexual abuse; it should always be investigated carefully and the child put in touch with social services and other professionals capable of dealing with this difficult condition.

LABORATORY INVESTIGATION

Cultivation of *N. gonorrhoeae* from sites with few commensals, such as the male urethra, rarely presents any problems, and Gram staining of a smear is usually 95% sensitive. *N. gonorrhoeae* is intolerant of drying and temperature changes; it readily undergoes autolysis. It is a fastidious microbe, requiring humidity, 5%–7% carbon dioxide and complex media for growth. Ideally, exudate is taken directly from the patient on to appropriate preheated, freshly prepared solid media and immediately placed in a carbon dioxide incubator. This is usually possible only in specialised clinics with sufficient patient numbers to justify the expense. Where there is likely to be any delay, transport media must be used to carry the material on swabs.

The combination of oxidase-positive colonies and Gram-negative diplococci provides a presumptive diagnosis. The use of gonococcal-specific antibodies and carbohydrate utilisation tests, with or without the detection of preformed enzymes, will give full speciation of the organism. DNA probes have also been used to detect gonococci in urethral and cervical specimens. PCR-based methods are available in some specialised laboratories.

TREATMENT

The susceptibility of isolates of *N. gonorrhoeae* to commonly used antibiotics varies so much that regular testing is essential.

Penicillin, especially in slow-release intramuscular forms such as procaine penicillin, remains the preferred therapy in many parts of the world. Small decreases in susceptibility can be overcome by increasing the size of the single dose. However, by the 1970s the dose of penicillin required to cure simple acute gonorrhoea in men in some parts of the world had reached an impossibly large injection.

Strains of *N. gonorrhoeae* that are completely resistant to penicillins are now common throughout the world, although the prevalence varies from country to country. These strains possess the gene coding for the TEM-type β-lactamase commonly found in *Escherichia coli*.

Ceftriaxone or cefixime are recommended as first-line therapy in the United Kingdom, but these drugs are expensive and may not be affordable in developing countries. Alternatives to cephalosporins and penicillin include fluoroquinolones (e.g., ciprofloxacin), azithromycin, tetracyclines, co-amoxiclav and spectinomycin. Use of these antibiotics is often limited in places where inappropriate use has led to a high prevalence of resistance. Dual therapy with azithromycin is recommended by Public Health England to delay the emergence of ceftriaxone resistance; however, a recent outbreak of azithromycin-resistant gonorrhoea in the United Kingdom has led to concerns that gonorrhoea may become untreatable. Resistance, or reduced susceptibility, to most of the commonly used antibiotics is increasing in the United Kingdom (Table 26.1).

Single-dose therapy appears adequate for uncomplicated cases of acute genital gonorrhoea in men and women. There are obvious advantages to this approach in obtaining complete compliance and stopping the chain of infection. In disseminated gonococcal disease and any complicated infection, treatment for 7–10 days is necessary.

EPIDEMIOLOGY AND CONTROL

Acute gonorrhoea is usually easily diagnosed and treated, and was well controlled in much of the world until the 1960s. The remarkable changes in travel, migration, sexual licence and availability of oral contraceptives rapidly

Table 26.1 Resistance to antimicrobial agents among isolates of *N. gonorrhoeae* in the United Kingdom

Antimicrobials	Percentage resistant (95% confidence intervals)	
	2013	2014
Ceftriaxone	0.2 (0.1–0.5)	0.0 (-)
Azithromycin	1.6 (1.1–2.3)	1.0 (0.6–1.6)
Cefixime (MIC ≥0.125 mg/L)	5.1 (4.2–6.3)	1.4 (0.9–2.1)
Cefixime (MIC ≥0.25 mg/L)	1.3 (0.8–1.9)	0.1 (0.0–0.5)
Ciprofloxacin	29.3 (27.2–31.5)	37.3 (34.9–39.7)
Penicillin	18.4 (16.6–20.2)	22.6 (20.6–24.8)
Tetracycline	77.8 (75.7–79.6)	82.8 (80.9–84.6)
Spectinomycin	0.0 (-)	0.0 (-)

Data from the Gonococcal resistance to antimicrobials surveillance programme (GRASP), Public Health England, 2014.

reversed this process so that there was an increase in gonorrhoea and nonspecific genital infection (caused mainly by chlamydiae; see Ch. 34) every year until scares about the acquired immune deficiency syndrome in the 1980s temporarily halted the rise. Barrier methods of contraception, condoms in particular, greatly reduce the rate of transmission.

The keys to control of gonorrhoea are:

- rapid diagnosis
- use of effective antibiotics
- tracing, examination and treatment of contacts

Unfortunately, in many places, inappropriate self-medication has contributed to widespread antimicrobial resistance. Inability to treat contacts ensures the spread of the disease and reinfections.

There is no effective vaccine to prevent gonorrhoea. The organism is noncapsulated, and its immunogenic outer membrane proteins are antigenically variable. These, and lack of suitable animal models, have hampered vaccine development.

MORAXELLA

Moraxellae are Gram-negative, asaccharolytic, oxidase-positive, catalase-positive short rods, coccobacilli or, in the case of *M. catarrhalis*, diplococci. They are commensals of mucosal surfaces and occasionally give rise to opportunistic infections. *M. lacunata* is occasionally encountered as a cause of angular blepharoconjunctivitis.

The related genus *Kingella* contains organisms that differ from the moraxellae in being catalase negative, glucose-fermenting coccobacilli. In common with some other Gram-negative rods, such as *Cardiobacterium hominis* and *Eikenella corrodens*, *Kingella* species (usually *K. kingae*) are sometimes found in endocarditis. They have also been implicated in joint infections.

MORAXELLA CATARRHALIS

PATHOGENESIS

M. catarrhalis is a respiratory tract commensal and, as with other members of the upper respiratory tract flora such as the pneumococcus and *H. influenzae,* it can gain access to the lower respiratory tract in patients with chronic chest disease or compromised host defences. *M. catarrhalis* is commonly isolated from sputum, and a pathogenic role is suspected only when the sputum contains large numbers of pus cells and Gram-negative diplococci, and when culture yields a heavy growth of *M. catarrhalis* in the absence of other recognised respiratory pathogens. In addition to causing chest infection itself, *M. catarrhalis* may protect other respiratory pathogens from the action of penicillin or ampicillin by producing β-lactamase.

M. catarrhalis is also a cause of otitis media and sinusitis in children. In acute otitis media the organism is present in 15%–20% of cultures of middle ear fluid, presumably migrating from the nasopharynx to the middle ear via the eustachian tube.

LABORATORY INVESTIGATION

Sputum is examined by Gram film. In true infections, large numbers of Gram-negative diplococci may be seen dispersed between the pus cells. Sputum is cultured on media suitable for the isolation of other potential respiratory pathogens (e.g., blood agar and chocolate agar) and incubated in 5% carbon dioxide overnight. In situations in which it is held to be pathogenic, *M. catarrhalis* is predominant in culture.

M. catarrhalis produces rough, circular, convex colonies that can be lifted off intact with a wire loop from agar culture medium. Colonies are oxidase positive. In common with other moraxellae, they do not ferment sugars and are easily differentiated from neisseriae by the tributyrin test. Growth on nutrient agar at 22°C has been suggested as a differential characteristic, but clinically significant isolates of *M. catarrhalis* may not grow in these conditions. Tests for deoxyribonuclease and for butyrate esterase are positive. Around 90% of strains are β-lactamase positive.

TREATMENT

M. catarrhalis is sensitive to amoxicillin, combined with clavulanic acid (co-amoxiclav) in the case of β-lactamase–producing strains, and also to cephalosporins, tetracyclines, macrolides and fluoroquinolones. No vaccine is currently available, although several are in development.

RECOMMENDED READING

Ala'Aldeen, D. A. A., & Turner, D. P. J. (2006). *Neisseria meningitidis.* Ch. 14. In S. Gillespie & P. Hawkey (Eds.), *Principles and practice of clinical bacteriology* (2nd ed.). Chichester: John Wiley. doi:10.1002/9780470017968.ch14.

Barker, R. M., Shakespeare, R. M., Mortimore, A. J., Allen, N. A., Solomon, C. L., & Stuart, J. M. (1999). Practical guidelines for responding to an outbreak of meningococcal disease among university students based on experience in Southampton. *Communicable Disease and Public Health, 2*(3), 168–173.

Bignell, C. (2009). European (IUSTI/WHO) guideline on the diagnosis and treatment of gonorrhoea in adults. *International Journal of STD and AIDS, 20*(7), 453–457. doi:10.1258/ijsa.2009.009160.

Hart, C. A., & Thomson, A. P. J. (2006). Meningococcal disease and its management in children. *British Medical Journal, 333*(7570), 685–690.

Health Protection Agency Meningococcus and Haemophilus Forum. (2012). *Guidance for public health management of meningococcal disease in the UK.* London: Public Health England. Available at https://www.gov.uk/government/uploads/system/uploads/attachment_data/file/322008/Guidance_for_management_of_meningococcal_disease_pdf.pdf. (Accessed Jul 2017).

Murphy, T. F., & Parameswaran, G. I. (2009). *Moraxella catarrhalis,* a human respiratory tract pathogen. *Clinical Infectious Diseases, 49*(1), 124–131. doi:10.1086/599375.

Pollard, A. J., Feavers, I., & Cohn, A. (2016). Prevention of meningococcal disease through vaccination. Chapter 7. In I. Feavers, A. J. Pollard, & M. Sadarangani (Eds.), *Handbook of meningococcal disease management* (1st ed.). Cham: Springer International Publishing. doi:10.1007/978-3-319-28119-3_7.

Public Health England. (2015). Gonococcal resistance to antimicrobials surveillance programme 2014 report: *Surveillance of antimicrobial resistance in* Neisseria gonorrhoeae. London: Public Health England. Available at https://www.gov.uk/government/uploads/system/uploads/attachment_data/file/476582/GRASP_2014_report_final_111115.pdf. (Accessed Jul 2017).

Stephens, D. S., Greenwood, B., & Brandtzaeg, P. (2007). Epidemic meningitis, meningococcaemia, and *Neisseria meningitidis. Lancet, 369*(9580), 2196–2210.

Website

Meningococcal disease: guidance, data and analysis. Available at https://www.gov.uk/government/collections/meningococcal-disease-guidance-data-and-analysis. (Accessed Jul 2017).

27 *Mycobacterium*

Tuberculosis; leprosy and opportunistic infections

MICHAEL R. BARER

KEY POINTS

- The mycobacteria include the major global pathogens of tuberculosis and leprosy.
- Approximately one-quarter of humanity is estimated to be infected with the tubercle bacillus and this is associated with roughly 100 million new infections, 10 million new cases of disease and 1.5 million deaths annually. Leprosy has been brought under control with the 10 million cases reported in 1985 reduced to under 200,000 in 2014.
- The mycobacteria are characterised by their bilaminar cell envelope containing 50–90 carbon chain length mycolic acids covalently linked to a peptidoglycan-arabinogalactan macromolecular complex. This confers their acid-fast staining properties and resistance to many antimicrobial agents.
- Most of the nearly 200 named mycobacterial species are environmental saprophytes, although some occasionally cause disease, notably in the immunosuppressed. *Mycobacterium tuberculosis* and *M. leprae* are obligate pathogens.
- Tuberculosis is a chronic granulomatous infection.
- Most infected individuals (~90%) control the infection and do not develop symptomatic disease, but remain latently infected. The majority of infected individuals who become symptomatic do so within 2 years of infection, but the remainder are at risk of reactivation, particularly if they become immunocompromised.
- The lung is the usual site of initial infection and disease, but nonpulmonary disease is common, rising to ~50% in some populations. Only pulmonary disease is associated with transmission via patient-generated aerosols.
- Diagnosis of disease is predominantly made by clinical and chest X-ray examination and definitively confirmed by detecting *M. tuberculosis* by acid-fast staining, culture and nucleic acid amplification techniques.
- Detection of cell-mediated immunity to *M. tuberculosis* by interferon gamma release assay (IGRA) tests or tuberculin skin testing does not clearly distinguish between active and latent infection.
- Antituberculous therapy employs different agents (notably rifampicin and isoniazid) from most other bacterial infections and currently requires at least 6 months.
- Drug resistance is a major problem in some regions and is increasing worldwide.
- Bacillus Calmette-Guérin (BCG) is an attenuated live vaccine; its protective efficacy varies greatly between geographical regions and its overall impact on tuberculosis control is limited.
- In leprosy, the nerves and skin are the principal sites of disease, resulting in deformities and visible lesions. *M. leprae* has never been cultivated in vitro.
- Transmission is probably by the aerogenous route rather than by touch.
- Tuberculoid leprosy is characterised by excessive granuloma formation in the presence of a very small (paucibacillary) bacterial load, whereas lepromatous leprosy is characterised by a huge (multibacillary) bacterial load and little or no immune reactivity.
- Diagnosis is by clinical examination, microscopic detection or PCR of bacilli in skin or nasal smears and biopsies. Multidrug treatment regimens are highly effective and BCG vaccination appears to offer some degree of protection.

The genus *Mycobacterium* (fungus-bacterium) alludes to the mould-like pellicles formed when isolates are grown in liquid media. The pellicle reflects their extremely hydrophobic lipid-rich, waxy cell walls. Mycobacteria show varying degrees of acid-fastness, or resistance to decolourisation by a dilute mineral acid (or acid with alcohol) after staining with carbolfuchsin or auramine.

The mainly saprophytic nontuberculous mycobacteria (NTM), also previously known as mycobacteria other than tuberculosis (MOT) or atypical mycobacteria, include some important opportunistic pathogens (see Ch. 28). In contrast, the major global diseases of tuberculosis and leprosy are caused by obligate pathogens.

THE *MYCOBACTERIUM TUBERCULOSIS* COMPLEX (MTBC)

This refers to a group of genetically very closely related variants of what is strictly speaking a single species. All cause tuberculosis, a chronic granulomatous disease affecting humans and many other mammals. Three variants are of overriding importance in clinical disease affecting humans:

- *M. tuberculosis,* the predominant cause of human tuberculosis
- *M. bovis,* the principal cause of tuberculosis in cattle and many other mammals, and occasionally infecting humans
- *M. africanum,* which is an intermediate form between the human and bovine types. It causes

human tuberculosis and is found mainly in equatorial Africa. Type 1 is more common in West Africa and has several features in common with *M. bovis;* type 2 is mainly of east African origin and more closely resembles *M. tuberculosis.*

Horizontal gene transfer amongst the progenitors of the MTBC appears to have ceased many millennia ago, thus variation within the complex predominantly reflects accumulation of mutations and gene loss mainly attributable to single nucleotide polymorphisms and large sequence polymorphisms. The current view of the MTBC lineage is outlined in Fig. 27.1. Key points to note include the significance of the RD9 deletion separating the major agents of disease affecting humans from *M. africanum* and animal adapted strains, and the recent acquisition of the RD1 deletion as a result of the in vitro propagation of *M. bovis* at the beginning of the 20th century by Calmette and Guérin to produce BCG (see later in the chapter). The modern *M. tuberculosis* variant, which arose from the TbD1 deletion, has given rise to five further variants, which, together with the ancestral lineage strains, are known as the six global lineages.

DESCRIPTION

Tubercle bacilli are nonmotile, nonsporing, noncapsulate, straight or slightly curved rods about 3×0.3 µm in size. In sputum and other clinical specimens, they may occur singly or in small clumps, and in liquid cultures, they often grow as twisted rope-like colonies termed *serpentine*

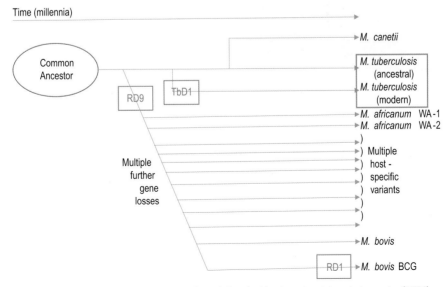

Fig. 27.1 Origins and genetic deletions differentiating the *Mycobacterium tuberculosis* complex (MTBC).

cords (Fig. 27.2). They are able to grow on a wide range of enriched culture media, but Löwenstein–Jensen (LJ) medium has been the most widely used in clinical practice. This is an egg–glycerol-based medium to which malachite green dye is added to inhibit the growth of some contaminating bacteria and to provide a contrasting colour against which colonies of mycobacteria are easily seen. Strains of *M. bovis* grow poorly, or not at all, on standard LJ medium but grow much better on media containing sodium pyruvate in place of glycerol. The Middlebrook series of agar-based media and broths are also widely used with various supplements albumin are also used.

On subculture, human tubercle bacilli usually produce visible growth on LJ medium in 2–4 weeks, although on primary isolation from clinical material colonies may take up to 8 weeks to appear. Colonies are of an off-white (buff) colour and (except for the very rarely encountered *M. canetti*, which has smooth colonies) usually have a dry breadcrumb-like appearance. Growth is characteristically heaped up and luxuriant or 'eugonic', in contrast to the small, flat 'dysgonic' colonies of *M. bovis*.

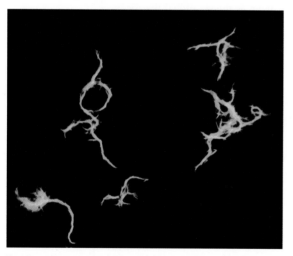

Fig. 27.2   Fluorescently stained microcolonies of *M. tuberculosis* showing 'serpentine cord' formation.

The optimal growth temperature of tubercle bacilli is 35–37°C, but they fail to grow at 25°C or 41°C. Most other mycobacteria grow at one or the other, or both, of these temperatures.

All mycobacteria are obligate aerobes, but *M. bovis* grows better in conditions of reduced oxygen tension. Thus, when incorporated in soft agar media, *M. tuberculosis* grows on the surface, whereas *M. bovis* grows as a band a few millimetres below the surface. This provides a useful differentiating test. Various other differential characteristics of human tubercle bacilli are shown in Table 27.1.

Tubercle bacilli survive in milk and other organic materials and on pasture land, so long as they are not exposed to ultraviolet light, to which they are very sensitive. They are also heat sensitive and are destroyed by pasteurisation. Mycobacteria are susceptible to alcohol, formaldehyde, glutaraldehyde and, to a lesser extent, hypochlorites and phenolic disinfectants. They are considerably more resistant than other bacteria to acids, alkalis and quaternary ammonium compounds.

PATHOGENESIS

In achieving chronic infections lasting many years, *M. tuberculosis* must resist immune elimination by both innate and adaptive immune responses. Early replication appears to take place within alveolar macrophages within which the organism prevents phagosome–lysosome fusion. The process of host sensitisation through presentation of bacterial antigens is delayed, and, probably after small numbers have been disseminated to multiple body sites, direct spread is halted by the formation of granulomas in immune competent individuals, largely mediated by CD4+ T lymphocytes. In the majority, this contains the infection unless they become immunocompromised. In a minority, the granulomas become necrotic and produce cavities that enable further transmission. In this way, the tubercle bacillus manipulates the host immune response such that can survive in the long term. Two patterns of disease are widely recognised: primary and secondary. The former

Table 27.1 Some differential characteristics of the principal tubercle bacilli causing human disease				
Species	Atmospheric preference	Nitratase	TCH	Pyrazinamide
M. tuberculosis	Aerobic	Positive	Resistant[a]	Sensitive
M. bovis	Micro-aerophilic	Negative	Sensitive	Resistant
M. bovis BCG	Aerobic	Negative	Sensitive	Resistant
M. africanum I	Micro-aerophilic	Negative	Sensitive	Sensitive
M. africanum II	Micro-aerophilic	Positive	Sensitive	Sensitive

TCH, Thiophen-2-carboxylic acid hydrazide.
[a]Strains from southern India may be sensitive.

predominates in childhood and, where disseminated, is associated with a poor cell-mediated immune response, while the latter is driven by a hypersensitive tissue destructive response.

Primary tuberculosis

Inhaled bacilli are engulfed by alveolar macrophages and replicate to form the initial lesion. Some bacilli are carried in phagocytic cells to the hilar lymph nodes where additional foci of infection develop. The initial focus of infection together with the enlarged hilar lymph nodes forms the primary complex. In addition, bacilli are seeded by further lymphatic and haematogenous dissemination in many organs and tissues, including other parts of the lung. When the bacilli enter the mouth, as when drinking milk containing *M. bovis,* the primary complexes involve the tonsil and cervical nodes (scrofula; Fig. 27.3) or the intestine, often the ileocaecal region, and the mesenteric lymph nodes.

During infection, antigens of *M. tuberculosis* are processed by antigen-presenting cells, and presented to antigen-specific T lymphocytes, which in turn activate macrophages through IL-12–dependent interferon-γ release. In due course, this leads to formation of a compact cluster, or granuloma, around the foci of infection (Fig. 27.4). In mature granulomas, some of these macrophages transform into epithelioid cells, so named because they resemble epithelial cells, while others fuse to form multinucleate Langhans giant cells. The centre of the granuloma contains a mixture of necrotic tissue and dead macrophages and, because of its cheese-like appearance and consistency, is referred to as caseation.

Activated human macrophages inhibit the replication of the tubercle bacilli, but their ability to kill ingested bacilli is limited. The centre of the granuloma is both anoxic and acidic, conditions that lead to growth arrest of the bacilli but not their elimination. Granuloma formation is usually sufficient to limit the primary infection: the lesions become quiescent and surrounding fibroblasts produce dense scar tissue, which may become calcified.

In a minority of cases infection progresses, possibly due to ineffective granuloma formation, and gives rise to the serious manifestations of primary disease, including progressive local lesions (particularly in infants; Table 27.2), meningitis, pleurisy and disease of the kidneys,

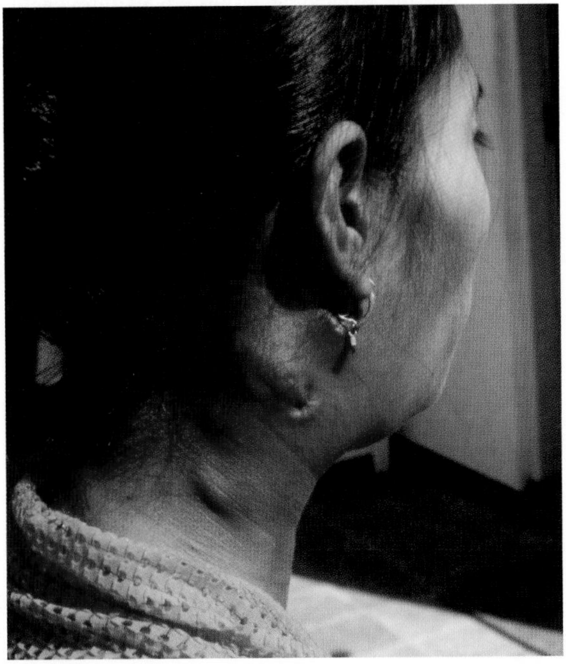

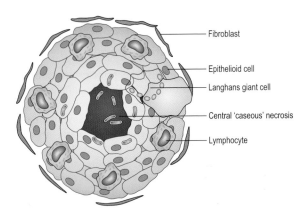

Fig. 27.4 The granuloma of primary tuberculosis.

- Fibroblast
- Epithelioid cell
- Langhans giant cell
- Central 'caseous' necrosis
- Lymphocyte

Table 27.2 Stages of primary tuberculosis in childhood

Stage	Time (from onset)	Characteristics
1	3–8 weeks	Primary complex develops and tuberculin conversion occurs
2	2–6 months	Progressive healing of primary complex Possibility of pleural effusion
3	6–12 months	Possibility of miliary or meningeal tuberculosis
4	1–3 years	Possibility of bone or joint tuberculosis
5	3–5 years or more	Possibility of genitourinary or chronic skin tuberculosis

Adapted from Miller, F. J. W. (1982). *Tuberculosis in Children.* Edinburgh: Churchill Livingstone.

Fig. 27.3 Tuberculous cervical lymphadenitis (scrofula) with sinus formation in an Indonesian woman.

spine (Pott's disease) and other bones and joints. If a focus ruptures into a blood vessel, bacilli are disseminated throughout the body with the formation of numerous granulomata. This, from the millet seed-like appearance of the lesions, is known as miliary tuberculosis.

Tuberculin reactivity

In otherwise healthy individuals, 6–8 weeks after the initial infection, the phenomenon of tuberculin conversion occurs. This delayed type hypersensitivity, reflecting, as we know now, expansion of antigen-specific T cells, was discovered by Robert Koch while attempting to develop a remedy for tuberculosis based on old tuberculin—a heat-concentrated filtrate of a broth in which tubercle bacilli had been grown. Although Koch's tuberculin proved unsuccessful as a therapeutic agent, it formed the basis of the tuberculin skin test. Though still widely used and valuable, this test does not clearly distinguish between sensitisation due to infection and that due to BCG vaccination; it is being replaced by interferon gamma release assays (IGRAs) (see later in the chapter).

Latent and asymptomatic tuberculosis

In most infected individuals, the primary infection is asymptomatic and no disease arises. Nonetheless, live bacilli remain and disease can be reactivated at any time in later life. It has been assumed that the asymptomatic state reflects complete quiescence of the early lesions, but recent evidence from positron emission tomography (PET) scanning shows this not to be the case in some individuals, and live bacilli have been recovered from their airways. This raises the alarming possibility that asymptomatic individuals may nonetheless be infectious. Moreover, it is now widely accepted that the distinction between latent and active disease is artificial and that disease in individuals may be at any point on a spectrum between quiescent infection and actively progressing disease.

Because 25%–30% of humanity is infected by *M. tuberculosis,* and this provides a reservoir of infection that makes elimination of disease very challenging, there is much current effort focused on differentiating those individuals in whom disease is most likely to progress from those in whom it will remain quiescent. The IGRA tests provide some advance over skin testing in this regard, but transcriptional profiling of the cells in peripheral blood shows promise that discriminatory biomarkers may be identified in the future.

While immunological control is central to latent or asymptomatic infection, there is less clarity concerning the physiological state of the remaining bacteria. A variety of in vitro models provoke a state of dormancy

(a reversible state of metabolic shutdown) in which the bacilli become tolerant to the lethal action of antibiotics. While evidence that any one of these models represents the bacillary populations present in human infection, these studies show adaptation of the tubercle bacillus to multiple environments. The description of *M. tuberculosis*–encoded resuscitation promoting factors and the recognition of bacilli in human and animal infections dependent on these and other growth stimulating factors provides evidence that at least one of these populations is relevant to human infection. It is likely that both immune surveillance and bacterial dormancy contribute to latent or asymptomatic disease.

Postprimary tuberculosis

Progressive and symptomatic pathology in the postprimary pattern of tuberculosis (TB) (Table 27.3) may reflect reactivation of infected foci or new exogenous infection in a latently infected or BCG vaccinated individual leads to postprimary TB. For unknown reasons, pulmonary disease tends to develop in the upper lobes. The same process of granuloma formation occurs, but the necrotic element of the reaction causes extensive tissue destruction and the formation of large areas of caseation. Proteases liberated by activated macrophages soften and liquefy the caseous material, and an excess of tumour necrosis factor (TNF) and other immunological mediators causes the wasting and fevers characteristic of the disease.

Eventually the expanding lesion erodes through the wall of a bronchus, the liquefied contents are discharged and a well-aerated cavity is formed. The atmosphere of the lung, with a high carbon dioxide level, is ideal for supporting the growth of the bacilli, and huge numbers of these are found in the cavity walls. For this reason, closure of the cavities by collapsing the lung, either by artificial pneumothorax or by excising large portions of the chest wall, was a standard treatment for tuberculosis in the pre-chemotherapy era.

Table 27.3 Main differences between primary and postprimary tuberculosis in nonimmunocompromised patients

Characteristic	Primary	Postprimary
Local lesion	Small	Large
Lymphatic involvement	Yes	Minimal
Cavity formation	Rare	Frequent
Tuberculin reactivity	Negative (initially)	Positive
Infectivity[a]	Uncommon	Usual
Site	Any part of lung	Apical region
Local spread	Uncommon	Frequent

[a]Pulmonary cases.

Once the cavity is formed, large numbers of bacilli gain access to the sputum, and the patient becomes an open or infectious case. This is a good example of the transmissibility of a pathogen being dependent on the host's immune response to infection. Surprisingly, about 20% of cases of open cavitating tuberculosis in the pretherapy era resolved without treatment.

In postprimary tuberculosis, dissemination of bacilli to lymph nodes and other organs is unusual. Instead, spread of infection occurs through the bronchial tree so that secondary lesions develop in the lower lobes of the lung and, occasionally, in the trachea, larynx and mouth. Bacilli in swallowed sputum cause intestinal lesions. Secondary lesions may also develop in the bladder and epididymis in cases of renal tuberculosis. Postprimary cutaneous tuberculosis (lupus vulgaris) usually affects the face and neck. Some cases of cutaneous tuberculosis are secondary to sinus formation between tuberculous lymph nodes and the skin (scrofuloderma) and other structures including bones and joints (Fig. 27.5).

Immunocompromised individuals

People with congenital or acquired immunodeficiency, particularly those receiving therapeutic antibodies directed against TNF, are at a much higher risk of developing tuberculosis due to reactivation of latent disease or following infection or reinfection. HIV infection is a major predisposing factor to active tuberculosis worldwide (see later in the chapter). As a result, even when tuberculosis is treated effectively in HIV-positive patients, the mortality rate from other AIDS-related conditions is high, with many dying within 2 years. Cavity formation is less prominent, and diffuse infiltrates may develop in any part of the lung. In contrast to postprimary disease in nonimmunocompromised individuals, lymphatic and haematogenous dissemination are common. Sometimes there are numerous minute lesions teeming with tubercle bacilli throughout the body—a rapidly fatal condition termed *cryptic disseminated tuberculosis*. The interval between infection and development of disease is considerably shortened in immunocompromised persons.

The tuberculin test and other immunological tests

Although Robert Koch's attempts to use old tuberculin as a remedy for tuberculosis failed, an Austrian physician, Clemens von Pirquet, used the Koch phenomenon as an indication of bacterial 'allergy' resulting from previous infection. Individuals with active tuberculosis were usually tuberculin positive, but many of those with disseminated and rapidly progressive disease were negative. This led to the widespread but erroneous belief that tuberculin reactivity is an indicator of protective immunity to tuberculosis.

Modern tuberculin testing is achieved with a purified protein derivative (PPD) from *M. tuberculosis* culture. Intradermal testing takes several forms including the Mantoux, Heaf and tine methods with dosage defined in international units (IU).

The tuberculin test does not distinguish between active disease, quiescent infection and past BCG vaccination and, in some regions, sensitisation by environmental mycobacteria. The last two of these problems have been overcome by the IGRA tests. Knowledge of the genome sequences of *M. tuberculosis* and BCG enabled recognition of the RD1 deletion in the latter. IGRA tests employ key antigens located within this region to detect sensitised lymphocytes in peripheral blood.

LABORATORY INVESTIGATION

Clinical disease due to *M. tuberculosis* is definitively diagnosed by specific detection of the organism in clinical specimens. Many cases are nonetheless presumptively diagnosed and treated without this information based on clinical features, radiology and sometimes tissue pathology; response to therapy may also contribute.

Specimens

The most usual specimen for diagnosis of pulmonary tuberculosis is sputum but, if none is produced, bronchial

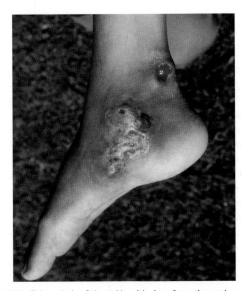

Fig. 27.5 Tuberculosis of the ankle with sinus formation and overlying involvement of the skin.

washings, brushings or biopsies and early-morning gastric aspirates (to harvest any bacilli swallowed overnight) may be examined. Tissue biopsies are homogenised by grinding for microscopy and culture. Cerebrospinal fluid, pleural fluid, urine and other fluids are centrifuged and the deposits examined.

Direct and rapid assessment

Microscopy: Use is made of the acid-fast property of mycobacteria to detect them in sputum and other clinical material. Auramine-based acid-fast staining of heat-fixed smears is widely used as fluorescence microscopy can be used with a ×40 objective to rapidly screen many fields of view. Ziehl–Neelsen (ZN) staining requires oil immersion microscopy but this is more readily available in resource-poor settings. Where scanty bacilli are detected in an auramine stain, restaining with ZN may increase confidence in the specificity of the result. Although nontuberculosis mycobacteria (NTM) often show different morphology from the tubercle bacillus the distinction is not certain by microscopy.

PCR: Nearly 30 years of experience in detecting *M. tuberculosis* by PCR has finally led to development of PCR methods as good as and more sensitive than smear microscopy. In particular, the Xpert MTB-RIF system offers the major advantage of a cassette design in which DNA extraction and highly specific PCR are effected on a homogenised sputum sample. Moreover, inclusion of testing for polymorphisms responsible for the majority of rifampicin resistance presents a major advantage in early detection of multidrug-resistant (MDR) organisms (see later in the chapter). Multiple commercial nucleic acid detection methods are available. The best are all comparable to the Xpert system in sensitivity and specificity but require a separate DNA extraction step. The World Health Organization (WHO) recommends the Xpert system, particularly where MDR is common, but its relative expense and requirement for dedicated equipment remain a barrier to its universal adoption.

Culture-based methods

As sputum and certain other specimens frequently contain many bacteria and fungi that would rapidly overgrow any mycobacteria on the culture media, these must be destroyed. Decontamination methods make use of the relatively high resistance of mycobacteria to acids, alkalis and certain disinfectants. Sodium hydroxide is applied for times varying between laboratories (5–20 minutes), neutralised with buffer or acid and bacilli pelleted by centrifugation. Due to variable levels of lipid inclusions, mycobacteria may pellet very slowly and at least 20 minutes at 3000 x g is recommended. The deposit is used to inoculate liquid and/or solid media. When combined with automated growth detection the time to detection in liquid media can be as little as 4 days, while it would be unusual to see colonies on solid media in <10; Middlebrook 7H9 medium is the basis for the former, and LJ predominates amongst the latter. Specimens such as cerebrospinal fluid and tissue biopsies, which are unlikely to be contaminated, are inoculated directly on to culture media.

Inoculated media are incubated at 35–37°C; where NTM infection is suspected, incubation of solid media at lower and higher temperatures is desirable (see Ch. 28). Incubation of liquid media for 4 weeks and solid media for 12 weeks is generally recommended. Positive cultures are sampled and tested for acid-fast bacilli. Definitive identification in well-resourced areas is now generally achieved by genetic methods and may be by whole genome sequencing (WGS). Where these methods are not available, presumptive identification from solid medium is achieved by recognising slow growth (>7 days), lack of yellow pigmentation, failure to grow outside 35–37°C or on media containing p-nitrobenzoic acid (also used in liquid media).

Strain typing for epidemiology

Restriction length polymorphism (RFLP) analysis provided the first reliable method based on digestion of genomic DNA and probe-based detection of the insertion sequence IS6110 (1–20 copies depending on the strain). PCR-based methods need less starting DNA and include spoligotyping and variable number tandem repeat-mycobacterial interspersed repetitive units (VNTR-MIRU) and MLST methods (see Ch. 3). However, the availability of low-cost DNA sequencing has replaced these methods with WGS in many regions.

Drug susceptibility testing

Phenotypic methods based on growth inhibition on LJ or Middlebrook media are widely used and have been well standardised but may fail or take several weeks to achieve. WGS allows rapid detection of polymorphisms linked to drug resistance. In some cases (e.g., isoniazid and rifampicin resistance), this linkage is strong and highly predictive of the phenotypic result. In both cases, however, there remains uncertainty regarding the response to therapy.

TREATMENT

The central dogma of antituberculous therapy is inclusion of at least two drugs that the infecting organism is sensitive to at the commencement of therapy. The rationale for this is that at this time the bacillary load may be very high indeed (e.g., 10^{12}). With spontaneous mutation rates for individual resistance to isoniazid or rifampicin in the region of $10^{-7/8}$ it is certain that some resistant mutant cells are present, but even more unlikely ($10^{-14/16}$) that any bacilli doubly resistant are there. Use of a single effective agent has the potential to select out resistant bacilli, a problem that emerged in the early days of tuberculosis therapy. Inclusion of four drugs in the initial standard regimen has eliminated this problem, but poor compliance or failure to adhere to this approach has underpinned the emergence of the drug-resistance problem we now face.

The need for multiple drugs to treat tuberculosis is not exclusively linked to managing the problem of resistance. It is clear that the organism occupies many different environments (e.g., intra- and extracellular) and can be found to express multiple physiological states (e.g., growing, nongrowing and dormant). As antituberculous therapies developed it was recognised that different drugs made somewhat distinct contributions to a successful outcome. Drugs have been classified into sterilising, bactericidal and bacteriostatic groups (Table 27.4) based largely on the grounds of animal and clinical studies. These labels provide a framework that is often used in discussion but do not identify a formally recognised scientific description of their action.

The current World Health Organization recommendations are that all new patients with tuberculosis, irrespective of site or severity of disease, and in the absence of evidence of drug resistance, should receive a 6-month course of therapy, consisting of a 2-month intensive phase of rifampicin, isoniazid, pyrazinamide and ethambutol, followed by a 4-month phase of rifampicin and isoniazid. Ideally, the drugs are given daily, but they may be given thrice weekly during the continuation phase or throughout, provided all doses are given under careful supervision and that the patient is not HIV seropositive.

Multidrug-resistant strains are defined as those resistant to isoniazid and rifampicin, with or without resistance to additional drugs. Extensively drug-resistant tuberculosis (XDR-TB) is defined as resistance to, at least, isoniazid, rifampicin, any fluoroquinolone and any injectable agent. It is estimated annually that around 0.5 million of the 8–9 million new cases of tuberculosis are MDR or XDR. Treatment of drug-resistant tuberculosis is highly specialised and involves use of second-line and new antituberculous agents (Table 27.5). Indeed, it is recommended that all tuberculosis treatment should be delivered by specialist clinical services, and international TB control groups will not provide second-line drugs to clinical services that do not meet their standards. The use of directly observed therapy short (DOTS) course, where intake of medicines is observed by clinical staff, has been widely adopted, especially where compliance is likely to be poor.

Drugs other than those identified as first-line agents are referred to as second-line agents and as agents required

Table 27.4 Traditional classification of the in vivo activity of antituberculosis drugs

Sterilising	Bactericidal	Bacteriostatic
Rifampicin	Isoniazid	Ethionamide
Pyrazinamide	Streptomycin	Prothionamide
	Ethambutol[a]	Thiacetazone
	Quinolones	p-Aminosalicylic acid
	Macrolides	Cycloserine

[a]In early stages of therapy.

Table 27.5 Second-line antituberculosis agents and those used in the treatment of MDR/XDR tuberculosis infections

Oral second-line (bacteriostatic)	p-Aminosalicylic acid (PAS)
	Cycloserine
	Terizidone
	Ethionamide
	Prothionamide
Injectable second-line	Capreomycin
	Amikacin
	Streptomycin
	Kanamycin
Fluoroquinolones	Levofloxacin
	Ofloxacin
	Moxifloxacin
Agents used in MDR/XDR cases	Clofazimine
	Linezolid
	Meropenem
	Thioacetazone
	Clarithromycin
	Bedaquiline
	Delamanid

to treat MDR/XDR infections. Drugs other than first-line agents may be required if patients suffer toxicity either directly or due to interactions with other drugs (e.g., those needed for HIV treatment). These agents are summarised in Table 27.5. Several new drugs and regimens are being investigated to combat drug-resistant tuberculosis and to shorten therapy. Progress is painfully slow due to the time taken to evaluate, but two new drugs, bedaquiline and delamanid, have been introduced.

In well-resourced settings, contacts of newly diagnosed cases of tuberculosis are investigated for evidence of infection. If they appear latently infected based on tuberculin or IGRA and lack of other signs/symptoms they may be offered prophylactic treatment. In the United Kingdom, this is predominantly isoniazid + rifampicin for 3 months or isoniazid for 6 months. If they are contacts of MDR cases, they are monitored and ideally, if disease becomes active, an isolate is obtained and therapy based on its resistance pattern.

EPIDEMIOLOGY

In 2016 WHO estimated 10.4 million new cases. Six countries, India, China, Indonesia, Nigeria, Pakistan and South Africa, accounted for 60% of the cases. Approximately 10% of cases were in children and 11% in those co-infected with HIV.

In the 1950s, Riley and Wells showed, by extracting tuberculosis ward air to guinea pig colonies, that the infection is transmitted by patient-generated aerosols. Acid-fast sputum smear-positive patients are responsible for the majority of transmissions, although recent direct measurements on patient aerosols suggest that their bacterial content is not accurately predicted by sputum analysis. Most transmission of the disease occurs within households or other environments where individuals are close together for long periods.

Tuberculosis is a disease of poverty, and country infection rates can be directly linked to the gross domestic product (GDP). In wealthy settings, the annual rates are below 3 per 100,000, while they rise to anywhere between 50 and 500 per 100,000 in resource-poor settings. Migration and infections acquired from periods of residency in countries associated with these high rates bring the overall rate to around 10 per 100,000 in countries such as England.

As noted previously, the lifetime risk of infected individuals for symptomatic tuberculosis is around 10% but if they acquire HIV this rises to 10% per annum if they are not on effective antiretroviral therapy.

Bovine tuberculosis is spread from animal to animal, and sometimes to human attendants, in moist cough spray or through unpasteurised milk. Various nondomestic animal reservoirs are recognised in different countries (e.g., badgers, deer, possums). The bovine infection is highly prevalent in the United Kingdom, necessitating the slaughter of ~30,000 from tuberculin-positive herds per annum under current regulations. Human infection is rare in the United Kingdom, probably controlled by milk pasteurisation and the slaughter programme. Occupational exposure to goats and seals has resulted in a few cases of tuberculosis due to *M. caprae* and *M. pinnipedii,* respectively.

CONTROL

The modern approach to tuberculosis control is targeted to early detection and treatment of active infectious cases and the selective treatment of those with latent/asymptomatic infection where the risk of progression to active infection exceeds the risk of adverse reaction to prophylactic chemotherapy.

Active case finding involves a deliberate search, often on a house-to-house basis or in workplaces, for suspects

with a chronic cough of a month or more in duration. Merely waiting for patients with symptoms to seek medical attention is much less effective, even when supported by education programmes. Regular chest examination by mass miniature radiography detects <15% of individuals with tuberculosis, and its use is now restricted to certain high-risk situations.

The most important factors affecting the incidence of tuberculosis are socioeconomic ones, particularly those leading to a reduction of overcrowding in homes and workplaces. In resource-poor countries, it is estimated that each patient with open tuberculosis infects about 20 contacts annually, whereas in Europe the corresponding figure is two or three.

Vaccination

BCG is a living attenuated vaccine derived from a strain of *M. bovis* by repeated subculture between the years 1908 and 1921. This species was selected rather than *M. tuberculosis,* as the vaccine was initially intended for veterinary use. Although originally administered orally, BCG is now given by intracutaneous injection.

The protective efficacy of BCG varies enormously from country to country (Table 27.6). Early trials in the United Kingdom indicated that administration of BCG to schoolchildren afforded 78% protection, but a major trial in south India involving individuals of all ages found no protection. Several explanations have been advanced for this difference, the most likely one being prior exposure of the human population to environmental mycobacteria, which, in some regions, confer some protection, but in others induce inappropriate immune reactions that antagonise protection. For this reason, neonatal vaccination is recommended.

When BCG vaccination is introduced into a region, it has an immediate impact on the incidence of the serious

Table 27.6 Variations in the protective efficacy of BCG vaccinations in nine major trials

Country or population	Age range of vaccinees (years)	Protection (%)
North American Indian	0–20	80
United Kingdom	14–15	78
Chicago, Illinois, USA	Neonates	75
Puerto Rico	1–27	31
South India (Bangalore)	All ages	30
Georgia and Alabama, USA	>5	14
Georgia, USA	6–17	0
Illinois, USA	Young adults	0
South India (Chingleput)	All ages	0[a]

[a]Some protection demonstrated in those vaccinated neonatally on 15-year follow-up.

but noninfectious forms of childhood tuberculosis such as meningitis, but has little impact on the annual infection rate in the community as the smear-positive source cases arise mostly from among the older, unvaccinated, tuberculin-positive members of the community. Vaccination has not therefore proved to be an effective control measure.

Being a living vaccine, serious infections and even disseminated disease may occur in immunocompromised persons. Thus, BCG should never be given to persons known to be HIV-positive. Many attempts are currently being made to develop alternative vaccines.

MYCOBACTERIUM LEPRAE

Leprosy is a particularly tragic affliction, as the nature of the infection often causes severe disfigurement and deformity, which, throughout history, have led to social ostracism or even total banishment from society of those suffering from the disease. The disease was long endemic in the British Isles; Robert the Bruce of Scotland was one of its victims. The last British patient to acquire the disease in this country died in the Shetland Islands in 1798. In Norway, the disease persisted into the 20th century; Armauer Hansen first described the causative organism in that country in 1873. Surprisingly, leprosy and a closely related mycobacterium have recently been detected in squirrels in the United Kingdom.

The current situation is cause for optimism as the number of registered patients on treatment declined from >10 million in 1982 to 514,718 in 2003 and 175,554 in 2014. The decline has been slower in recent years, but this may reflect a higher case detection rate. Leprosy has been eliminated from 119 out of the 122 countries in which the disease was regarded as a public health problem in 1985, and, in stark contrast to tuberculosis, resistance to therapy has not proved to be a barrier to treatment. The World Health Organization has therefore adopted a 'final push' strategy with the goal of eliminating this disease.

Leprosy is often cited as a disease of great antiquity but literary and skeletal evidence of this very characteristic disease go back no further than 500 BC. Biblical leprosy was almost certainly not the same as the disease that now bears this name. This raises the intriguing question of the ancestry of this bacillus, which has no widespread animal reservoirs. Natural environmental reservoirs for a progenitor of *M. leprae*, such as amoebae, have been postulated but not convincingly demonstrated.

DESCRIPTION

M. leprae has never convincingly been cultivated in vitro; this has been attributed to a loss or disruption of many of the genes required for metabolism. The genome of *M. leprae* is smaller than that of cultivable mycobacteria, and about half of its genes are defective counterparts of functional ones found in other mycobacteria. In the 1970s, it was shown that armadillos experimentally infected with *M. leprae* often developed extensive disease, with up to 10^{10} bacilli in each gram of diseased tissue. This animal has therefore provided sufficient bacilli for research projects and for the production of a skin test reagent, leprosin-A. Limited replication, yielding 10^6 bacilli after 6–8 months, also occurs in the mouse footpad, and this has been used for testing the sensitivity of bacilli to antileprosy drugs.

Leprosy bacilli resemble tubercle bacilli in their general morphology, but they are not so strongly acid-fast. In clinical material from lepromatous patients, the bacilli are typically found within macrophages in dense clumps. A characteristic surface lipid, phenolic glycolipid-1 (PGL-1), has been extracted from *M. leprae*, and its unique carbohydrate antigenic determinant has been synthesised. A rapid detection assay has been developed for this antigen.

PATHOGENESIS

The principal target cell for the leprosy bacillus is the Schwann cell. The resulting nerve damage is responsible for the main clinical features of leprosy: anaesthesia and muscle paralysis. Repeated injuries to, and infection of, the anaesthetic extremities leads to their gradual destruction (Fig. 27.6). Infiltration of the skin and cutaneous nerves by bacilli leads to the formation of visible lesions, often with pigmentary changes.

The first sign of leprosy is a nonspecific or indeterminate skin lesion, which often heals spontaneously. If the

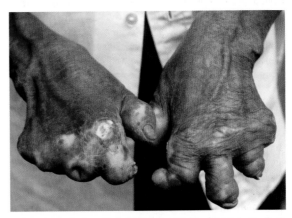

Fig. 27.6 Borderline tuberculoid leprosy. Trophic changes in the hands secondary to nerve damage, vasculitis and anaesthesia.

Table 27.7 Characteristics of the five points on the spectrum of leprosy

Characteristic	TT	BT	BB	BL	LL
Bacilli seen in skin	−	±	+	++	+++
Bacilli in nasal secretions	−	−	−	+	+++
Granuloma formation	+++	++	+	−	−
Reaction to lepromin	+++	+	±	−	−
Antibodies to *M. leprae*	±	±	+	++	+++
Main phagocytic cell	Mature epithelioid	Immature epithelioid	Immature epithelioid	Macrophage	Macrophage
In vitro correlates of CMI	+++/++	+	+	−	−
Type 1 reactions	−	+	+	+	−
Type 2 reactions	−	−	±	++	+++

CMI, Cell-mediated immunity. See text for other abbreviations.

disease progresses, its clinical manifestation is determined by the specific immune responsiveness of the patient to the bacillus, and there is a distinct immunological spectrum of the disease (Table 27.7). The points on the spectrum are:

- hyper-reactive tuberculoid (TT) leprosy, with small numbers of localised skin lesions containing so few bacilli that they are not seen on microscopy and an inappropriately intense granulomatous response that often damages major nerve trunks
- anergic lepromatous (LL) leprosy, in which the skin lesions are numerous or confluent and contain huge numbers of bacilli, usually seen as clusters or globi within monocytes. Cooler parts of the body, such as the ear lobes, are particularly heavily infiltrated by bacilli (see Fig. 27.7). There is no histological evidence of an immune response.
- intermediate forms classified as borderline tuberculoid (BT), mid-borderline (BB) or borderline lepromatous (BL).

Destruction of the nasal bones may lead to collapse of the nose (Fig. 27.8). In addition, large numbers of leprosy bacilli are discharged in nasal secretions in multibacillary disease. The eye is frequently damaged by direct bacillary invasion, uveitis or corneal infection secondary to paralysis of the eyelids (Fig. 27.9). Blindness is a common and tragic complication of untreated leprosy.

Additional tissue damage in leprosy is caused by immune reactions resulting from delayed hypersensitivity (Jopling type 1 reactions) or a vasculitis associated with the deposition of antigen–antibody complexes (Jopling type 2 reactions, erythema nodosum leprosum) (Table 27.8). The former, which occurs in borderline cases (BT, BB and BL), may rapidly cause severe and permanent nerve damage and requires urgent treatment with antiinflammatory agents and, sometimes, surgical decompression of a greatly swollen

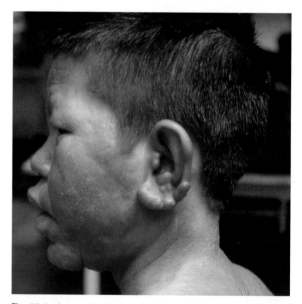

Fig. 27.7 Lepromatous leprosy. Nodular swelling of face, enlargement of ear lobes and loss of eyebrows.

nerve. The latter occurs at the multibacillary pole of the spectrum (BL and LL) and is principally due to deposition of antigen–antibody complexes.

LABORATORY INVESTIGATION

The clinical diagnosis may be confirmed by histological examination of skin biopsies and by the detection of acid-fast bacilli in nasal discharges, scrapings from the nasal mucosa and slit-skin smears. The latter are prepared by making superficial incisions in the skin, scraping out some tissue fluid and cells and making smears on glass

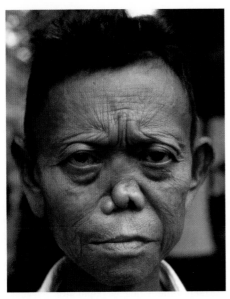

Fig. 27.8 Treated lepromatous leprosy. The nodularity of the skin has resolved on treatment, but the absence of eyebrows and the nasal collapse remain.

Table 27.8 Main characteristics of the reactions in leprosy

Characteristic	Type 1 (reversal reaction)	Type 2 (erythema nodosum leprosum)
Immunological basis	Cell mediated	Vasculitis with antigen–antibody complex deposition
Type of patient	BT, BB, BL	BL, LL
Systemic disturbance	No (or mild)	Yes
Haematological changes	No	Yes
Proteinuria	No	Frequently
Relation to therapy	Usually within first 6 months	Rare during first 6 months

See text for explanation of abbreviations.

slides. Smears are obtained from obvious lesions, the ear lobes and apparently unaffected skin. Secretions and skin smears are stained by the ZN method, and the number of bacilli seen in each high-power field may be recorded as the bacillary index. However, for usual practical purposes, patients with clinically active leprosy but in whom no bacilli are seen on slit-skin smear examination are described as having paucibacillary disease, and those who are positive at any site are described as having multibacillary disease. This is an important distinction for the selection of treatment (see later in the chapter).

It is widely assumed, but unproven, that leprosy bacilli that stain strongly and evenly are viable, whereas those that stain weakly and irregularly are dead. The percentage of the former gives the morphological index, which declines during chemotherapy. An increase in the morphological index is a useful indication of noncompliance of the patient and the emergence of drug resistance. Where facilities exist, PCR may be used to detect *M. leprae* in clinical specimens.

TREATMENT

Multidrug therapy based on dapsone, rifampicin and clofazimine is highly effective. The choice of regimen is determined by whether the patient has paucibacillary or multibacillary disease (Table 27.9). Clofazimine causes skin discolouration, particularly in fair-skinned people. If this results in the patient refusing the drug, a combination of rifampicin, ofloxacin and minocycline, administered monthly for 24 months for multibacillary disease, may be used instead. A single dose of rifampicin (600 mg), ofloxacin (400 mg) and minocycline (100 mg) has been advocated for the treatment of adults with single-lesion paucibacillary leprosy, although some authorities consider this to be inadequate.

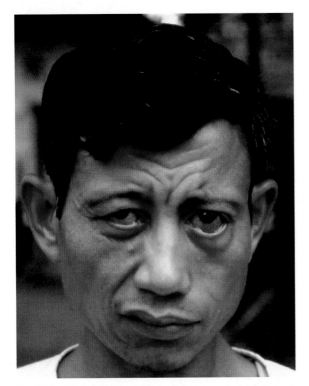

Fig. 27.9 Tuberculoid leprosy. The only feature on presentation was paralysis of the left facial nerve, resulting in loss of the left nasolabial fold and an inability to close the eye, predisposing to corneal damage.

Table 27.9 WHO recommendations for multidrug therapy of leprosy

Type of leprosy	Drug	Dose (mg)	Frequency	Total duration (months)
Paucibacillary	Rifampicin	600	Monthly, supervised	6
	Dapsone	100	Daily, unsupervised	
Multibacillary	Rifampicin	600	Monthly, supervised	12
	Dapsone	100	Daily, unsupervised	
	Clofazimine	300 and 50	Monthly, supervised	
			Daily, unsupervised	

The treatment of leprosy demands far more than the administration of antimicrobial agents. It is often necessary to:

- correct deformities
- prevent blindness and further damage to anaesthetic extremities
- treat reactions with antiinflammatory drugs
- attend to the patient's social, psychological and spiritual welfare.

EPIDEMIOLOGY

Once thought to be restricted to humans, leprosy has been reported in chimpanzees and sooty mangabey monkeys in Africa, and in free-living armadillos in Louisiana, USA. It was also thought that leprosy was transmitted by skin-to-skin contact, but it now appears more likely that the bacilli are disseminated from the nasal secretions of patients with lepromatous leprosy. In addition, the blood of patients with lepromatous leprosy contains enough bacilli to render transmission by blood-sucking insects a definite, though unproven, possibility.

As in the case of tuberculosis, transmission of bacilli from patients with multibacillary leprosy to their contacts occurs readily, but only a minority of those infected develop overt disease. The infectivity of patients with paucibacillary leprosy is much lower. Leprosy often commences during childhood or early adult life but, as the incubation period is usually 3–5 years, it is rare in children aged <5 years.

As with the use of tuberculin, skin testing reagents have been studied in leprosy. Lepromins and leprosins have been used in epidemiological studies. These reagents do not precisely detect infected or exposed individuals but they had some value is population surveys when prevalence of the disease was higher.

CONTROL

The most effective control measure in leprosy, as in tuberculosis, is the early detection and treatment of infectious cases. This requires that patients should attend for therapy as soon as signs of the disease appear. Unfortunately, owing to the stigma associated with the disease, many patients delay seeking treatment until they have infected many contacts and developed irreversible disfigurement and handicap. Women, in particular, are likely to conceal their disease.

No living attenuated vaccines have been prepared for *M. leprae,* but BCG vaccine seems to protect against leprosy in regions where it protects against tuberculosis, strongly suggesting that protection is induced by common mycobacterial antigens.

RECOMMENDED READING

Casali, N., Nikolayevskyy, V., Balabanova, Y., Harris, S. R., Ignatyeva, O., Kontsevaya, I., ... Drobniewski, F. (2014). Evolution and transmission of drug-resistant tuberculosis in a Russian population. *Nature Genetics*, *46*(3), 279–286. doi:10.1038/ng.2878.

Cole, S. T., Brosch, R., Parkhill, J., Garnier, T., Churcher, C., Harris, D., ... Barrell, B. G. (1998). Deciphering the biology of *Mycobacterium tuberculosis* from the complete genome sequence. *Nature*, *393*(6685), 537–544.

Galagan, J. E. (2014). Genomic insights into tuberculosis. *Nature Reviews. Genetics*, *15*(5), 307–320. doi:10.1038/nrg3664.

Houben, R., & Dodd, P. J. (2016). The global burden of latent tuberculosis infection: a re-estimation using mathematical modelling. *PLoS Medicine*, *13*(10), e1002152. doi:10.1371/journal.pmed.1002152.

Takiff, H. E., & Feo, O. (2015). Clinical value of whole-genome sequencing of *Mycobacterium tuberculosis*. *Lancet Infect Dis*, *15*(9), 1077–1090. doi:10.1016/s1473-3099(15)00071-7.

Wallis, R. S., Maeurer, M., Mwaba, P., Chakaya, J., Rustomjee, R., Migliori, G. B., ... Zumla, A. (2016). Tuberculosis-advances in development of new drugs, treatment regimens, host-directed therapies, and biomarkers. *Lancet Infect Dis*, *16*(4), e34–e46. doi:10.1016/S1473-3099(16)00070-0.

White, C., & Franco-Paredes, C. (2015). Leprosy in the 21st century. *Clinical Microbiology Reviews*, *28*(1), 80–94. doi:10.1128/cmr.00079-13.

Websites

Centers for Disease Control and Prevention. Tuberculosis (TB). Available at: http://www.cdc.gov/tb/.

International Federation of Anti-Leprosy Associations. Available at: http://www.ilep.org.uk/.

International Leprosy Association. Available at: http://www.leprosy-ila.org/.

International Union Against Tuberculosis and Lung Disease. Available at: http://www.theunion.org/.

List of Prokaryotic Names with Standing in Nomenclature. Available at: http://www.bacterio.cict.fr/.

WHO Tuberculosis: http://www.who.int/tb/en/.

Nontuberculous mycobacteria, *Actinomyces, Nocardia* and *Tropheryma*

Opportunist disease; actinomycosis; nocardiasis; Whipple's disease

MICHAEL R. BARER

KEY POINTS

- Nontuberculous mycobacteria (NTM) are predominantly opportunistic pathogens. They are of increasing importance in industrialised nations, accounting for over 50% of clinical mycobacterial isolates in some regions.
- The reservoir and immediate source of infection is predominantly environmental.
- Presentations include localised lymphadenitis, postinoculation (injection or trauma) skin lesions, tuberculosis-like pulmonary lesions, solitary nonpulmonary lesions and disseminated disease.
- Lymphadenitis occurs in otherwise healthy young children (<6 years of age) and in the immunosuppressed.
- Individuals with preexisting lung disease (e.g., cystic fibrosis and bronchiectasis) are susceptible to chronic pulmonary infection.
- Skin diseases include swimming pool granuloma (*Mycobacterium marinum*), Buruli ulcer *(M. ulcerans)* and postinoculation abscesses caused by various rapid growers.
- Diagnosis is supported by culture and identification, which is predominantly by PCR-based methods or whole genome sequencing. Repeated detection in the face of progressive disease assists in distinguishing pathogenic association from contamination or colonisation.
- Therapy of NTM infection depends on the causative organism and is largely empirical as few clinical trials have been conducted and drug susceptibility tests have not been validated.
- Several species of *Actinomyces* cause chronic lesions characterised by multiple abscesses, granulomata,

tissue destruction, extensive fibrosis and sinus formation.
- More than half of human cases occur in the cervicofacial region and often involve the jaw. Other cases occur in the thorax, abdomen and pelvis.
- Diagnosis is supported by detection of the characteristic 'sulphur granules' in clinical material and by culture of the organism. Treatment is usually by prolonged penicillin-based regimens.
- Many species of *Nocardia* have been described but only a few, notably *N. asteroides,* cause human disease. Lung involvement in immunocompromised individuals predominates. Secondary abscesses, notably in the brain, occur in about one-third of patients.
- Postinoculation cutaneous infections (primary cutaneous nocardiasis) may result in fungating tumour-like masses termed *mycetomas.*
- *Tropheryma whippelii,* the cause of Whipple's disease, was one of the first bacterial pathogens identified by 16S rRNA studies. It has now been cultured in fibroblasts, and its genome has been sequenced.
- Whipple's disease is a rare multisystem disease with prominent infection of the intestinal epithelium commonly associated with weight loss, diarrhoea and joint symptoms. It can be treated with doxycyclin and hydroxychloroquine.
- *T. whippelii* can be detected by PCR in faeces, saliva and other samples. Detection has been associated with asymptomatic carriage, Whipple's disease, endocarditis and encephalitis and with acute gastroenteritis, pneumonia and bacteraemia.

NONTUBERCULOUS MYCOBACTERIA

In addition to the tubercle and leprosy bacilli there are >150 recognised species of mycobacteria in the *List of Prokaryotic Names with Standing in Nomenclature* that normally exist as saprophytes of soil and water. Termed *environmental* (or nontuberculous) *mycobacteria,* some of these species occasionally cause opportunist disease in animals and humans. Those species described here are well-recognised opportunistic pathogens but many other species have been considered to cause disease. Mycobacterial species into slow and rapid growers depending on their ability to produce visible colonies on solid media in <7 days on subculture. In addition, phenotypic identification is assisted by their pigment formation, which divides them into photochromogens, which develop yellow or orange pigmentation in (or after exposure to) light, scotochromogens, which become pigmented in the dark, and nonchromogens. Traditionally, mycobacterial species were characterised by a range of physical and biochemical properties but molecular methods including 16S rRNA-directed analyses, whole genome sequencing and, most recently, MALDI analysis allow rapid and definitive identification.

DESCRIPTION

The photochromogens include the commonly elongated and beaded *M. kansasii* (Fig. 28.1), and *M. simiae,* both of which can cause pulmonary infection. *M. marinum* causes a warty skin infection known as swimming pool granuloma or fish tank granuloma. It grows best at 33°C and microscopically resembles *M. kansasii.*

Slowly growing scotochromogens include *M. gordonae, M. scrofulaceum* and *M. szulgai.* Nonchromogens include

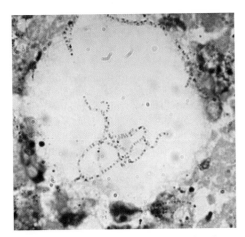

Fig. 28.1 *Mycobacterium kansasii* in sputum, showing elongated and beaded appearance. (Courtesy Professor John Stanford.)

the important opportunistic pathogens in the *M. avium* complex (MAC). This group consists of *M. avium avium* (the avian tubercle bacillus), a pathogen of birds and also a cause of lymphadenitis in pigs as well as occasional disease in various other wild and domestic animals, and *M. avium intracellulare,* principally a human pathogen but also a cause of disease in animals including pigs. Many isolates formerly included in this species are now identified as *M. avium hominissuis,* although this term has not been formally published. Also of note are:

- *M. avium paratuberculosis,* the cause of chronic hypertrophic enteritis or Johne's disease of cattle. There have been claims, which remain to be substantiated, that it is a cause of Crohn's disease in humans. It produces little or no mycobactin, a lipid-soluble iron-binding compound essential for growth, and this substance must be added to media used for cultivation.
- *M. avium sylvaticum,* a cause of tuberculosis in wood pigeons. Like *M. avium paratuberculosis,* it needs mycobactin for growth.
- *M. avium lepraemurium,* the cause of a leprosy-like disease of rats, mice and cats.
- *M. chimaera* was formerly recognised as part of the MAC. It is found in many water supplies and has recently emerged as an important cause of infections acquired during cardiopulmonary bypass.

Both *M. avium hominissuis* and *M. avium intracellulare* are causative agents of lymphadenitis and pulmonary disease. They are also a cause of disseminated disease in profoundly immunosuppressed patients, notably in those with the acquired immunodeficiency syndrome (AIDS). Clinical isolates can be typed by RFLP and MIRU-VNTR but whole genome sequencing is now preferred.

Other nonchromogens include:

1. *M. ulcerans* is a very slowly growing species that grows in vitro only at 31–34°C. Colonies are nonpigmented or a pale lemon-yellow colour. *M. ulcerans* is the cause of Buruli ulcer; unlike other mycobacterial pathogens, it produces a toxin that causes tissue necrosis and is involved in the pathogenesis of the disease. *M. shinshuense,* a very rare cause of skin ulcers in Japan and China, is a variant of *M. ulcerans.*
2. *M. xenopi,* originally isolated from a *Xenopus* toad, is a thermophile that grows well at 45°C. It is principally responsible for pulmonary lesions in humans. Most reported cases have been from London and South East England and northern France. Two phylogenetically similar species, *M. celatum* and *M. branderi,* have been described.

3. *M. malmoense* is a cause of pulmonary disease and lymphadenitis. It grows very slowly, often taking as long as 10 weeks to appear on primary culture, and is therefore likely to be missed if cultures are discarded earlier. For unknown reasons, disease due to this pathogen is prevalent in several European countries.

4. *M. terrae* (the radish bacillus), *M. nonchromogenicum* and *M. triviale* are sometimes grouped as the *M. terrae* complex. They are very rare causes of pulmonary disease and, in the case of *M. terrae,* infections of injuries acquired while farming or gardening.

5. *M. haemophilum,* characterised by its growth requirement for haem or other sources of iron, is a rare cause of granulomatous or ulcerative skin lesions in xenograft recipients and other immunocompromised individuals, and of lymphadenitis in otherwise healthy children.

6. *M. genavense* is a very slow growing organism occasionally isolated from patients infected with HIV or with other causes of immunosuppression, from pet and zoo birds and, rarely, other animals.

Rapid growers

Four rapidly growing nonchromogenic species are well-recognised human pathogens: *M. chelonae, M. abscessus, M. fortuitum* and *M. peregrinum. M. abscessus* and the closely related *M. abscessus* subsp. *massiliense* have recently emerged as important pathogens in patients with cystic fibrosis and other chronic lung diseases; the others all occasionally cause pulmonary or disseminated disease but are principally responsible for postinjection abscesses and wound infections, including corneal ulcers.

Most of the many other rapidly growing species are pigmented, and, although disease due to them is exceedingly rare, they frequently contaminate clinical specimens. They are found on the genitalia and gain access to urine samples, although, contrary to a common belief, *M. smegmatis* is rarely found in this site. *M. flavescens,* which grows more slowly than other members of this group grow and is therefore sometimes classified as a slow grower, is an occasional cause of postinjection abscesses.

PATHOGENESIS

Compared with tubercle bacilli, environmental mycobacteria are of low virulence and, although human beings are in regular contact with these organisms and therefore

Table 28.1 Principal types of opportunist mycobacterial disease in humans, and the usual causative agents

Disease	Usual causative agent
Lymphadenopathy	*M. avium complex*
Skin lesions	*M. scrofulaceum*
Posttraumatic abscesses	*M. chelonae*
	M. abscessus
	M. fortuitum
	M. peregrinum
Swimming pool granuloma	*M. marinum*
Buruli ulcer	*M. ulcerans*
Pulmonary disease and solitary	*M. avium complex*
nonpulmonary lesions	*M. abscessus*
	M. kansasii
	M. xenopi
	M. malmoense
Disseminated disease	
AIDS related	*M. avium complex*
	M. genavense
Non-AIDS related	*M. avium complex*
	M. chelonae
	M. abscessus

frequently infected, overt disease is uncommon except in those who are profoundly immunosuppressed. Five main types of opportunist mycobacterial disease have been described in humans (Table 28.1):

1. Localised lymphadenitis
2. Skin lesions following traumatic inoculation of bacteria
3. Tuberculosis-like pulmonary lesions
4. Tuberculosis-like nonpulmonary lesions
5. Disseminated disease.

Lymphadenitis

This is caused by a number of different species that vary in relative frequency from region to region. The *M. avium* complex is the predominant cause worldwide. Earlier reports claimed a high incidence of *M. scrofulaceum,* but these strains were probably misidentified members of the *M. avium* complex. In most cases, a single node, usually tonsillar or preauricular, is involved, and most patients are children aged <5 years (Fig. 28.2). Unless contraindicated by the risk of nerve damage, excision of the node, usually performed for diagnostic purposes, is almost always curative. This disease was very rare where children were vaccinated with BCG (Bacille Calmette–Guérin) neonatally, but the incidence increased considerably in countries where such vaccination was terminated. Lymphadenitis occasionally occurs as part of a more disseminated infection, particularly in individuals with AIDS.

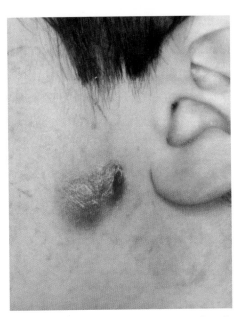

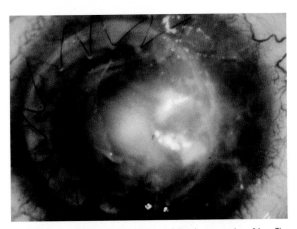

Fig. 28.3 Keratitis due to *M. chelonae* following corneal grafting. The cornea shows a characteristic 'cracked windscreen' appearance. (From Khooshabeh, R., Grange, J. M., Yates, M. D., McCartney, A. C. E., Casey, T. A. (1994). A case report of *Mycobacterium chelonae* keratitis and a review of mycobacterial infections of the eye and orbit. *Tubercle and Lung Disease*, 75(5), 377–382, with permission from Elsevier.)

Fig. 28.2 Preauricular lymphadenitis due to an environmental mycobacterium in a child. (Courtesy Professor Ali Zumla, University College London.)

Skin lesions

Three main types have been described: postinjection (and posttraumatic) abscesses, swimming pool granuloma and Buruli ulcer.

Postinjection and posttraumatic abscesses

These are usually caused by the rapidly growing pathogens *M. abscessus*, *M. chelonae*, *M. fortuitum* and, less frequently, *M. peregrinum* and *M. flavescens*. Abscesses occur sporadically, particularly in the tropics, or in small epidemics when these bacteria contaminate batches of injectable materials. Abscesses develop within a week or so, or for up to a year or more, after the injection. They are painful, may become quite large—up to 8 or 10 cm in diameter—and may persist for many months. Treatment is by drainage with curettage or total excision. Chemotherapy is not required unless there is local spread of disease or multiple abscesses, as may occur in insulin-injecting diabetics.

More serious lesions, also usually due to these rapidly growing pathogens, have followed surgery, particularly procedures involving insertion of prostheses such as heart valves, and corneal infections have followed ocular injuries or surgery (Fig. 28.3). Infections by *M. terrae* have occurred in farmers and others who have been injured while working with soil.

Swimming pool granuloma

This is also known as fish tank granuloma and, occasionally, fish fancier's finger, and is caused by *M. marinum*. Those affected are mostly users of swimming pools, keepers of tropical fish and others involved in aquatic hobbies. The bacilli enter scratches and abrasions and cause warty lesions similar to those seen in skin tuberculosis. The lesions, which usually occur on the knees and elbows of swimmers and on the hands of aquarium keepers, are usually localised, although secondary lesions sometimes appear along the line of the dermal lymphatics. This is termed *sporotrichoid spread* as a similar phenomenon occurs in the fungus infection sporotrichosis (see Ch. 58). A few cases of disseminated disease have occurred in immunosuppressed patients, including those treated with systemic steroids.

Buruli ulcer

This disease, caused by *M. ulcerans*, was first described in Australia, although the name is derived from the Buruli district of Uganda where a large outbreak was investigated extensively in the 1960s. Buruli ulcer has been reported in over 30 countries including Ghana, Nigeria, Congo Kinshasa, Côte d'Ivoire, Togo, Mexico, Malaysia, Papua New Guinea and Australia, and is limited to certain localities, characteristically low-lying areas subject to periodic flooding. *M. shinshuense*, a rare cause of similar lesions in Japan and China, is a variant of *M. ulcerans*. There is strong though indirect evidence that *M. ulcerans* is introduced from the environment into the human dermis

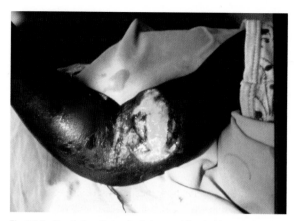

Fig. 28.4 Buruli ulcer. Undermined ulcer overlying the biceps and swelling of the surrounding tissues. (Courtesy Dr Alan Knell, Wellcome Tropical Institute.)

by minor injuries, particularly by spiky grasses and, possibly, by biting insects. It is becoming a major public health problem in central and western equatorial Africa, where the number and severity of cases has increased; in some areas, its incidence exceeds that of tuberculosis and leprosy. The risk of the disease is higher in those infected with HIV, in whom the disease may be more aggressive, but this is not the sole cause of the increase.

The first manifestation of the disease is a hard cutaneous nodule, which may be itchy. The nodule enlarges and develops central softening and fluctuation owing to necrosis of the subcutaneous adipose tissue caused by an exotoxin, which also has immunosuppressive properties. The overlying skin becomes anoxic and breaks down, the liquefied necrotic contents of the lesion are discharged, and one or more ulcers with deeply undermined edges are thereby formed (Fig. 28.4). At this stage, the lesion is teeming with acid-fast bacilli and there is no histological immunological evidence of an active cell-mediated immune response. During this anergic stage, the lesion may progress to an enormous size, sometimes involving an entire limb or a major part of the trunk.

For unknown reasons, the anergic phase may eventually give way to an immunoreactive phase when a granulomatous response develops in the lesion, the acid-fast bacilli disappear and immune reactivity to antigens of *M. ulcerans* is detectable. Healing then occurs but the patient is often left with considerable disfigurement and disability caused by extensive scarring and contractures.

Pulmonary disease

This is seen most frequently in middle-aged or elderly men with lung damage caused by smoking or exposure to industrial dusts. It also occurs in individuals with congenital or acquired immune deficiencies, malignant disease and cystic fibrosis, but a substantial minority of cases occur in persons with no apparent underlying localised or generalised disorder. The disease may be caused by many species, although the most frequent are the *M. avium* complex and *M. kansasii*. Other causative organisms in the United Kingdom are *M. xenopi* and *M. malmoense,* with the former being more common in the south of the country and the latter in the north.

Localised nonpulmonary disease

Localised nonpulmonary lesions resembling those seen in tuberculosis are uncommon. Disease involving the meninges, bone (including the spine) and joints, kidney and male genitalia has been described. Mycobacterial peritonitis is a serious complication of peritoneal dialysis.

Disseminated disease

In the 1980s and early 1990s, up to a half of all persons dying from AIDS in the United States had disseminated mycobacterial disease, almost always due to the *M. avium* complex. This AIDS-related disease was also common in Europe but not in Africa. The introduction of highly active antiretroviral therapy (see Ch. 52) has led to a substantial decline in the incidence of this disease in developed nations.

The source of the causative organisms is uncertain. Some consider that disease is due to reactivation of dormant foci of infection acquired in childhood, whereas others argue that it results from recent infection from the environment; these explanations are not mutually exclusive. Acid-fast bacilli are readily isolated from bone marrow aspirates, intestinal biopsies, blood and faeces. A few cases of AIDS-related disseminated disease have been caused by other species, including *M. genavense.*

Disseminated disease occurs occasionally in individuals with other congenital or acquired causes of immunosuppression, including renal transplantation. Again, the *M. avium* complex is the usual cause, but disseminated disease due to other infections, notably *M. chelonae,* has occurred in recipients of renal transplants and in other immunocompromised patients (Fig. 28.5).

LABORATORY INVESTIGATION

Most environmental mycobacteria can be detected microscopically and cultured on media suitable for *M. tuberculosis* (see Ch. 27). Great care must be taken to differentiate true disease from transient colonisation or superinfection. In particular, there are no clinical or

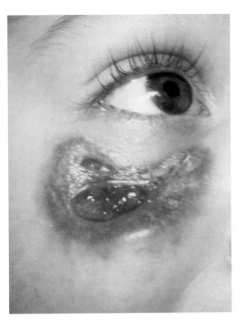

Fig. 28.5 Skin ulcer on the face due to disseminated *M. chelonae* in an immunocompromised child. (Courtesy Dr Kurt Schopfer.)

radiological characteristics that reliably differentiate pulmonary disease caused by opportunist mycobacteria from tuberculosis, and the diagnosis is therefore made by isolation and identification of the pathogen. As a rule, a diagnosis of opportunist mycobacterial disease may be made when a heavy growth of the pathogen is repeatedly isolated from the sputum of a patient with compatible clinical and radiological features, and in whom other causes of these features have been carefully excluded. Fibreoptic bronchoscopy is a useful aid to diagnosis, as lesions may be directly biopsied.

Identification is usually undertaken by specialist reference laboratories. Phenotypic identification has largely been abandoned in favour of genetic methods. Several commercial systems are available, but the trend is towards whole genome sequencing; MALDI identification is also possible.

TREATMENT

Most slowly growing environmental mycobacteria are resistant to many antituberculosis drugs in vitro, although infections often respond to various combinations of these drugs. Few controlled trials of therapy for pulmonary disease caused by the *M. avium* complex and other slowly growing species, including *M. xenopi*, *M. kansasii* and *M. malmoense*, have been conducted, but the available data indicate that a 2-year regimen of rifampicin and ethambutol with addition of either clarithromycin or ciprofloxacin, or both if there is no clinical response after one year, is highly effective.

Similar drug regimens based on a macrolide (clarithromycin or azithromycin) and ethambutol are effective against AIDS-associated disease caused by the *M. avium* complex. There is, however, evidence that reduction of the viral load by use of antiretroviral agents contributes more to remission of such disease than does antibacterial therapy.

Pulmonary and nonpulmonary disease due to the rapidly growing species *M. abscessus*, *M. chelonae*, *M. fortuitum* and *M. peregrinum* have been treated successfully by various combinations of erythromycin, newer macrolides, sulphonamides, trimethoprim, amikacin, gentamicin, imipenem, extended-spectrum cephalosporins and fluoroquinolones. Intensive treatment with multiple agents is often recommended when infections are first detected in patients with cystic fibrosis. In vitro susceptibility tests are not always a reliable guide of clinical response, and some infections, notably keratitis due to *M. chelonae*, frequently relapse and require surgical intervention, despite in vitro drug susceptibility.

Mycobacterium marinum disease is usually self-limiting, although chemotherapy with minocycline, co-trimoxazole or rifampicin with ethambutol hastens its resolution, and surgical debridement is required if the disease involves joints or tendons. More aggressive antimicrobial therapy, usually based on rifampicin, ethambutol and clarithromycin, is required for extensive and disseminated disease.

The early, preulcerative lesions of Buruli ulcer can be treated by excision and primary closure by suture, while excision and skin grafting has been used for ulcerated lesions. It now seems that extended antibiotic therapy with rifampicin plus clarithromycin or a fluoroquinolone may obviate or reduce the need for surgical intervention.

EPIDEMIOLOGY

Mycobacteria are widely distributed in the environment and are particularly abundant in wet soil, marshland, streams, rivers and estuaries. Some species, such as *M. terrae*, are found in soil, whereas others, including *M. marinum* and *M. gordonae*, prefer free water. Many species, including potential pathogens such as the *M. avium* complex, *M. kansasii* and *M. xenopi*, are able to colonise piped water supplies. Human beings are therefore regularly exposed to mycobacteria as a result of drinking, washing, showering and inhalation of natural aerosols. Such repeated subclinical infection may induce sensitisation to tuberculin and other mycobacterial skin-testing reagents.

Evidence is emerging that NTM may be transmitted between patients, particularly those with cystic fibrosis.

Both local and international spread of particular strains of *M. abscessus* have been described.

The number of cases of disease due to environmental mycobacteria relative to cases of tuberculosis increases in regions where the latter is uncommon and declining in incidence. In addition, the absolute incidence is increasing as a result of the growing number of immunocompromised individuals, notably patients with AIDS.

A few 'epidemics' of falsely diagnosed mycobacterial pulmonary disease and urinary tract infection have resulted from the collection of sputum and urine specimens in containers rinsed out with water from taps colonised by mycobacteria. Inadequate cleaning of endoscopes has also led to mycobacterial contamination of clinical specimens and diagnostic confusion. Likewise, false positive sputum smear examinations for acid-fast bacilli have occurred when staining reagents were prepared from contaminated water.

Conversely, contamination of clinical equipment has led to nosocomial infections with NTM. Notoriously, the recent emergence of *M. chimaera* endocarditis in patients undergoing procedures requiring cardiac bypass was tracked down to the presence of this organism in heater-cooler units and the aerosols they produce.

CONTROL

The incidence and type of disease in any region are determined by the species and numbers of mycobacteria in the environment and the opportunities for human transmission. The incidence of NTM disease is independent of that of tuberculosis and unaffected by public health measures designed to control the latter. Recent evidence of person-to-person spread of *M. abscessus* has led some institutions to implement respiratory control measures.

OTHER ACTINOMYCETALES

Gram-positive bacteria with branching filaments that sometimes develop into mycelia are included in the rather loosely defined order Actinomycetales. Although mostly soil saprophytes, five genera, *Actinomyces*, *Nocardia*, *Actinomadura*, *Propionibacterium* and *Bifidobacterium* (the latter two are considered briefly in Ch. 30), occasionally cause chronic granulomatous infections in animals and human beings. Members of the genera *Gordona*, *Oerskovia*, *Rothia* and *Tsukamurella* very rarely cause similar infections.

Tropheryma whippelii, first recognised in association with Whipple's disease, has been detected by PCR in a wider range of situations. Another genus, *Streptomyces*, is an extremely rare cause of disease, but is the source of

several antibiotics. Repeated inhalation of thermophilic actinomycetes, notably *Faenia rectivirgula* and *Thermoactinomyces* species, causes extrinsic allergic alveolitis (farmer's lung, mushroom worker's lung, bagassosis) in those who are occupationally exposed to mouldy vegetable matter.

ACTINOMYCES

Description

Actinomyces are branching Gram-positive bacilli. They are facultative anaerobes, but often fail to grow aerobically on primary culture. They grow best under anaerobic or microaerophilic conditions with the addition of 5%–10% carbon dioxide. Almost all species are commensals of the mouth and have a narrow temperature range of growth of around 35–37°C. They are responsible for the disease known as actinomycosis. Three-quarters of human cases are caused by *Actinomyces israelii*. Twenty-five species of the genus *Actinomyces* have now been described in association with human samples, and infections are considered endogenous in origin.

Multiple other bacteria are often found in association with actinomycotic lesions. These include the nonsporing anaerobes *Fusobacterium* and *Bacteroides* as well as the Proteobacteria *Aggregatibacter* and *Campylobacter*.

Pathogenesis

Actinomycosis is a chronic disease characterised by multiple abscesses and granulomata, tissue destruction, extensive fibrosis and the formation of sinuses. Within diseased tissues, the actinomycetes form large masses of mycelia embedded in an amorphous protein–polysaccharide matrix and surrounded by a zone of Gram-negative, weakly acid-fast, club-like structures. These clubs were once thought to consist, at least in part, of material derived from host tissue, but it now appears that they are formed entirely from the bacteria. The mycelial masses may be visible to the naked eye, and, as they are often light yellow in colour, they are called sulphur granules. In older lesions the sulphur granules may be dark brown and very hard because of the deposition of calcium phosphate in the matrix. Various species of actinomyces may colonise diseased tissue, such as lung cancer, but sulphur granules are not seen.

The principal forms of human actinomycosis are:

- Cervicofacial infection, which accounts for more than half of reported cases; the jaw is often involved. The disease is endogenous in origin; dental caries is a predisposing factor, and infection may follow tooth extractions or other dental procedures. Men are affected more frequently than women, and in some regions the disease is more common in rural agricultural workers than in town dwellers, probably owing to lower standards of dental care in the former.

- Thoracic actinomycosis commences in the lung, probably as a result of aspiration of actinomyces from the mouth. Sinuses often appear on the chest wall, and the ribs and spine may be eroded. Primary endobronchial actinomycosis is an uncommon complication of an inhaled foreign body.
- Abdominal cases commence in the appendix or, less frequently, in colonic diverticulae.
- Pelvic actinomycosis occurs occasionally in women fitted with plastic intrauterine contraceptive devices.
- Actinomyces have been isolated from cases of chronic granulomatous disease and should be vigorously sought in this rare condition.

The lymphatics are not usually involved, but haematogenous spread to the liver, brain and other internal organs occurs occasionally. Involvement of bone is uncommon in human actinomycosis and is usually the result of direct extension of adjacent soft tissue lesions.

Laboratory investigation

Specimens should be obtained directly from lesions by open biopsy, needle aspiration or, in the case of pulmonary lesions, fibreoptic bronchoscopy. Examination of sputum is of no value as it frequently contains oral actinomycetes. Material from suspected cases is shaken with sterile water in a tube. Sulphur granules settle to the bottom and may be removed with a Pasteur pipette. Granules crushed between two glass slides are stained by the Gram and Ziehl–Neelsen (modified by using 1% sulphuric acid for decolourisation) methods, which reveal the Gram-positive mycelia and the zone of radiating acid-fast clubs. Sulphur granules and mycelia in tissue sections are identifiable by use of fluorescein-conjugated specific antisera. In situ PCR has been used to detect *A. israelii* in tissue biopsies.

For culture, suitable media, such as blood or brain–heart infusion agar, glucose broth and enriched thioglycolate broth, are inoculated with washed and crushed granules. Contamination is reduced by the incorporation of metronidazole and nalidixic acid or cadmium sulphate in the media. Cultures are incubated aerobically and anaerobically for up to 14 days. After several days on agar medium, *A. israelii* may form so-called spider colonies that resemble molar teeth. Identity is generally confirmed by 16S rRNA gene sequencing although MALDI-based methods have been also established.

Treatment

Actinomyces are sensitive to many antibiotics, but the penetration of drugs into the densely fibrotic diseased tissue is poor. Thus, large doses are required for prolonged periods, and recurrence of disease is not uncommon. Surgical debridement reduces scarring and deformity, hastens healing and lowers the incidence of recurrences. Prolonged penicillin-based regimens are increasingly being replaced by shorter regimens based on amoxicillin with clavulanic acid (the clavulanic acid is required because lesions are often concomitantly infected with β-lactamase–producing bacteria) or cephalosporins, especially ceftriaxone. Alternative agents include tetracyclines, macrolides, fluoroquinolones and imipenem but in vitro sensitivity testing is unreliable. Additional drugs, including aminoglycosides and metronidazole, may be required when concomitant organisms are present.

NOCARDIA

Description

The nocardiae are branched, strictly aerobic, Gram-positive bacteria that are closely related to the rapidly growing mycobacteria. Like the latter, but unlike actinomyces, they are environmental saprophytes with a broad temperature range of growth. The properties of nocardiae and actinomycetes are compared in Table 28.2. Most isolates are acid-fast when decolourised with 1% sulphuric acid.

Many species of nocardia are found in the environment, notably in soil, and a range of species cause human opportunist disease, notably *Nocardia asteroides,* so named because of its star-shaped colonies, *N. abscessus, N. farcinica, N. brasiliensis, N. brevicatena, N. otitidiscaviarum, N. nova* and *N. transvalensis.* A wider range of species are encountered in profoundly immunosuppressed patients.

A related group of non–acid-fast species are assigned to the genus *Actinomadura,* which includes the species *Actinomadura madurae* and *A. pelletieri,* common causes of Madura foot (see later in the chapter).

Table 28.2 Differences between the genera Actinomyces and Nocardia

Actinomyces spp.	*Nocardia* spp.
Facultative anaerobes	Strict aerobes
Grow at 35–37°C	Wide temperature range of growth
Oral commensals	Environmental saprophytes
Non–acid-fast mycelia	Weakly acid-fast
Endogenous cause of disease	Exogenous cause of disease

Pathogenesis

Nocardiae, principally *N. asteroides,* are uncommon causes of opportunist pulmonary disease, which usually, but not always, occurs in immunocompromised individuals, including those receiving posttransplant immunosuppressive therapy or chemotherapy for cancer and those with AIDS. Corticosteroid therapy is a strong risk factor. As a result, the frequency and diversity of clinical manifestations of nocardial disease have increased over the past few decades. Preexisting lung disease, notably alveolar proteinosis, also predisposes to nocardial disease. The infection is exogenous, resulting from inhalation of the bacilli. The clinical and radiological features are very variable and nonspecific, and diagnosis is not easy. In most cases, there are multiple confluent abscesses with little or no surrounding fibrous reaction, and local spread may result in pleural effusions, empyema and invasion of bones. In some cases, the disease is chronic, whereas in others it spreads rapidly through the lungs. Secondary abscesses in the brain and, less frequently, in other organs occur in about one-third of patients with pulmonary nocardiasis. Acute dissemination with involvement of many organs occurs in profoundly immunosuppressed persons, notably those with AIDS. Recurrence is common in immunosuppressed patients, and mortality is high.

Nocardiae also cause primary posttraumatic, postoperative or postinoculation cutaneous infections (primary cutaneous nocardiasis). The most frequent cause is *N. brasiliensis* but some cases are caused by *N. asteroides* or other species. In the United States and the southern hemisphere, but rarely in Europe, cutaneous infections may result in fungating tumour-like masses termed *mycetomas.*

Madura foot is a chronic granulomatous infection of the bones and soft tissues of the foot resulting in mycetoma formation and gross deformity. It occurs in Sudan, North Africa and the west coast of India, principally among those who walk barefoot and are therefore prone to contamination of foot injuries by soil-derived organisms. A common causative organism is *Actinomadura madurae,* but Madura foot is also caused by other actinomycetes including *Streptomyces somaliensis* and by fungi (see Ch. 58).

LABORATORY INVESTIGATION

A presumptive diagnosis of pulmonary nocardiasis may be made by a microscopical examination of sputum. In many cases, the sputum contains numerous lymphocytes and macrophages, some of which contain pleomorphic Gram-positive and weakly acid-fast bacilli, and occasional extracellular branching filaments. Nocardiae are not so easily seen in tissue biopsies stained by the Gram or modified Ziehl–Neelsen methods, but may be seen in preparations stained by the Gram–Weigert or Gomori methenamine silver methods.

Nocardiae grow on blood agar, although growth is better on enriched media including Löwenstein–Jensen medium, brain–heart infusion agar and Sabouraud's dextrose agar containing chloramphenicol as a selective agent. Growth is visible after incubation for between 2 days and 1 month; selective growth is favoured by incubation at 45°C. Colonies are cream, orange or pink coloured; their surfaces may develop a dry, chalky appearance, and they adhere firmly to the medium.

Identification of species is usually undertaken in reference laboratories, with the most common technique being analysis of 16S rRNA gene sequences, a technique that has delineated over 30 species.

Treatment

A widely used regimen is sulfamethoxazole with trimethoprim (co-trimoxazole) for 3–6 months, although this prolonged course often causes adverse drug reactions. In addition, some strains, especially of *N. farcinica,* are resistant to sulphonamides. An alternative regimen, particularly in severe disease, is high-dose imipenem with amikacin for 4–6 weeks. Minocycline, third-generation cephalosporins, amoxicillin–clavulanate combinations, and linezolid, an oxazolidinone, are also effective. Drug susceptibility testing is subject to several variables, and no standardized methods have been proposed. Mycetomata due to nocardiae are much easier to treat than those due to fungi. Even long-standing cases with extensive mycetoma formation respond well to chemotherapy. Despite therapy, mortality of pulmonary and disseminated nocardiasis is high.

TROPHERYMA WHIPPELII

Whipple's disease is a rare multisystem disease with variable features including intermittent arthralgia, fever, weight loss, diarrhoea and malabsorption, lymphadenopathy and neurological symptoms. The intestine is principally affected but involvement of the lung, heart and skeletal muscle also occurs. PCR studies indicate that the central nervous system is often involved, even in the absence of neurological signs and symptoms. Most cases occur in middle-aged white males. The causative organism, *Tropheryma whippelii,* has a depleted genome and was originally cultivated in human embryonic lung cells, but sequencing of the genome has permitted the development of a medium for its cultivation in vitro. The organism is an environmental saprophyte and has been detected by PCR in stool samples from healthy individuals. Suspicion of

Whipple's disease should lead to PCR of faecal samples and at least one other site (e.g., saliva or blood). At least two positive results should trigger histological examination of periodic acid–Schiff stained biopsies of the duodenum or other affected organs. The ideal treatment, especially for relapses, has not yet been defined but penicillin, ceftriaxone, co-trimoxazole, tetracyclines and meropenem in various combinations for extended courses have all been considered effective. Most recently, doxycycline with hydroxychloroquine followed by lifelong doxycycline appears to provide prospects for a relapse-free response.

RECOMMENDED READING

Ambrosioni, J., Lew, D., & Garbino, J. (2010). Nocardiosis: updated clinical review and experience at a tertiary center. *Infection*, *38*(2), 89–97. doi:10.1007/s15010-009-9193-9.

Bryant, J. M., Grogono, D. M., & Rodriguez-Rincon, D. (2016). US Cystic Fibrosis Foundation and European Cystic Fibrosis Society consensus recommendations for the management of non-tuberculous mycobacteria in individuals with cystic fibrosis. *Thorax*, *71*, 1–22. doi:10.1136/thoraxjnl-2015-207360.

Bryant, J. M., Grogono, D. M., Rodriguez-Rincon, D., Everall, I., Brown, K. P., Moreno, P., ... Floto, R. A. (2016). Emergence and spread of a human-transmissible multidrug-resistant nontuberculous mycobacterium. *Science*, *354*(6313), 751–757. doi:10.1126/science.aaf8156.

Dolmans, R. A., Boel, C. H., Lacle, M. M., & Kusters, J. G. (2017). Clinical manifestations, treatment, and diagnosis of *Tropheryma whipplei* infections. *Clinical Microbiology Reviews*, *30*(2), 529–555. doi:10.1128/cmr.00033-16.

Friedman, N. D., Athan, E., Walton, A. L., & O'Brien, D. P. (2016). Increasing experience with primary oral medical therapy for Mycobacterium ulcerans disease in an Australian cohort. *Antimicrobial Agents and Chemotherapy*, *60*(5), 2692–2695. doi:10.1128/aac.02853-15.

Hay, R. J. (2010). Nocardiasis. In D. A. Warrel, J. D. Firth, & T. M. Cox (Eds.), *Oxford textbook of medicine* (5th ed.). Oxford: Oxford University Press.

Hoefsloot, W., van Ingen, J., Andrejak, C., Angeby, K., Bauriaud, R., Bemer, P., ... Nontuberculous Mycobacteria Network European Trials Group. (2013). The geographic diversity of nontuberculous mycobacteria isolated from pulmonary samples. An NTM-NET collaborative study. *Eur Respir J*, *42*(6), 1604–1613. doi:10.1183/09031936.00149212.

Kononen, E., & Wade, W. G. (2015). Actinomyces and related organisms in human infections. *Clinical Microbiology Reviews*, *28*(2), 419–442. doi:10.1128/cmr.00100-14.

Tortoli, E. (2014). Microbiological features and clinical relevance of new species of the genus *Mycobacterium*. *Clinical Microbiology Reviews*, *27*(4), 727–752. doi:10.1128/cmr.00035-14.

Walker, J., Moore, G., Collins, S., Parks, S., Garvey, M. I., Lamagni, T., ... Chand, M. (2017). Microbiological problems and biofilms associated with *Mycobacterium chimaera* in heater-cooler units used for cardiopulmonary bypass. *Journal of Hospital Infection*, *96*(3), 209–220. doi:10.1016/j.jhin.2017.04.014.

Wallace, J. R., Mangas, K. M., Porter, J. L., Marcsisin, R., Pidot, S. J., Howden, B., ... Stinear, T. P. (2017). *Mycobacterium ulcerans* low infectious dose and mechanical transmission support insect bites and puncturing injuries in the spread of Buruli ulcer. *PLoS Neglected Tropical Diseases*, *11*(4), 16. doi:10.1371/journal.pntd.0005553.

29 Clostridium

Gas gangrene; tetanus; food poisoning; pseudomembranous colitis

THOMAS V. RILEY

KEY POINTS

- All clostridial infections are characterized by toxin production by the infecting species.
- The major toxins produced by the species are neurotoxins affecting nervous tissue, histotoxins affecting soft tissue, and enterotoxins affecting the gut.
- *Clostridium perfringens* is the major cause of gas gangrene.
- Tetanus, particularly neonatal tetanus, is still a major public health issue in developing countries.
- Botulism occurs predominantly as a severe form of food poisoning.
- *C. difficile* is the most common cause of infectious diarrhoea in hospital patients in the developed world, and an increasing cause of community-acquired infection.

The clostridia are Gram-positive spore-bearing anaerobic bacilli. Most species are saprophytes that normally occur in soil, water and decomposing plant and animal matter; they play an important part in natural processes of putrefaction. Some, such as *Clostridium perfringens* and *C. sporogenes*, are commensals of the animal and human gut. On the death of the host, these organisms and other members of the intestinal flora rapidly invade the blood and tissues and initiate the decomposition of the corpse. The genus has undergone a major taxonomic revision. Initially this had little impact on clostridia of medical significance; however, *C. difficile* has been renamed very recently as *Clostridioides difficile*, and moved to within the Peptostreptococcaceae family. Whether the new name will be accepted by the *C. difficile* community around the world remains to be seen.

Pathogenic species include:

- *C. perfringens*, *C. septicum*, *C. novyi* and *C. sordellii*, the causes of gas gangrene and other infections. *C. perfringens* is also associated with a form of food poisoning.
- *C. tetani*, the cause of tetanus.
- *C. botulinum*, the cause of botulism.
- *C. difficile*, the cause of pseudomembranous colitis and antibiotic-associated diarrhoea.

Genome sequencing of the toxin-producing pathogens *C. perfringens*, *C. tetani*, *C. botulinum* and *C. difficile* has provided important data on pathogenic determinants and the regulatory events governing their expression as well as revealing the contribution of extrachromosomal elements to a pathogenic phenotype.

GENERAL DESCRIPTION

The clostridia are typically large, straight rods with slightly rounded ends. Pleomorphic forms, including filaments or elongated cells, club and spindle-shaped forms (*clostridium* is Latin for "little spindle") are commonly seen in stained smears from cultures or wounds. They are Gram-positive, but may appear to be Gram-negative. All produce spores, which enable the organisms to survive in adverse conditions (e.g., in soil and dust and on the skin).

Most species are obligate anaerobes: their spores do not germinate and growth does not normally proceed unless a suitably low redox potential (E_h) exists. A few species grow in the presence of trace amounts of air, and some actually grow slowly under normal atmospheric conditions.

Clostridia are biochemically active, frequently possessing both saccharolytic and proteolytic properties, although in varying degrees. Many species are highly toxigenic. The toxins produced by the organisms of tetanus and botulism attack nervous pathways and are referred to as neurotoxins. The organisms associated with gas gangrene attack soft tissues by producing toxins and aggressins and are referred to as histotoxic. *C. difficile* and some strains of *C. perfringens* produce enterotoxins.

CLOSTRIDIUM PERFRINGENS

DESCRIPTION

C. perfringens is a relatively large Gram-positive bacillus (about 4–6 × 1 μm) with blunt ends. It is capsulate and nonmotile. It grows quickly on laboratory media, particularly at high temperatures (approximately 42°C), when the doubling time can be as short as 8 minutes, and can be classified into one of five types (A to E). It can be identified by the *Nagler reaction,* which exploits the action of its phospholipase on egg yolk medium; colonies are surrounded by zones of turbidity, and the effect is specifically inhibited if *C. perfringens* antiserum containing α-antitoxin is present on the medium. Typical food-poisoning strains produce heat-resistant spores that can survive boiling for several hours, whereas the spores of the type A strains that cause gas gangrene are inactivated within a few minutes by boiling.

GAS GANGRENE

C. perfringens is the most common cause of gas gangrene, although various other species of clostridia, including *C. septicum, C. novyi* type A, *C. histolyticum* and *C. sordellii,* are occasionally implicated, either alone or in combination. Gas gangrene is almost always a polymicrobial infection involving anaerobes and facultative organisms.

The disease is characterized by rapidly spreading oedema, myositis, necrosis of tissues, gas production and profound toxaemia occurring as a complication of wound infection. The diagnosis is made primarily on clinical grounds with laboratory confirmation.

The main source of the organisms is animal and human excreta, and spores of the causative clostridia are distributed widely. Infection usually results from contamination of a wound with soil, particularly from manured and cultivated land. However, it may be derived indirectly from dirty clothing, street dust, and even the air of an operating theatre if the ventilating system is poorly designed or improperly maintained. The skin often bears spores of *C. perfringens,* especially in areas of the body that may be contaminated with intestinal organisms.

Pathogenesis of gas gangrene

Impairment of the normal blood supply of tissue with a consequent reduction in oxygen tension may allow an anaerobic focus to develop. The patient's condition may deteriorate rapidly with the development of severe shock (Fig. 29.1).

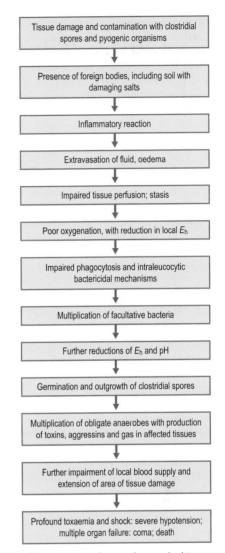

Fig. 29.1 Circumstances and events that may lead to gas gangrene.

Crushing of tissue and the severing of arteries in accidental injuries, rough handling of tissue and overzealous clamping during surgery, or shock waves from gunshot injuries may compromise the microcirculation in an extensive area of tissue and prejudice tissue perfusion. The presence of devitalized or dead tissue, blood clot, extravasated fluid, foreign bodies and coincident pyogenic infection are all factors that promote the occurrence of gas gangrene in a wound. The spores of the clostridia and their vegetative bacilli cannot readily initiate infection in healthy tissues, presumably because the E_h is too high, and the organisms are unable to avoid destruction and clearance by phagocytosis. Predisposing host factors include debility, old age, and diabetes.

When clostridial infection has been initiated in a focus of devitalized anaerobic tissue, the organisms multiply rapidly and produce a range of toxins and aggressins. These damage tissue by various necrotizing effects, and some have demonstrable lethal effects. They spread into adjacent viable tissue, particularly muscle, kill it, and render it anaerobic and vulnerable to further colonization, with the production of more toxins and aggressins.

- Hyaluronidase produced by *C. perfringens* breaks down intercellular cement substance and promotes the spread of the infection along tissue planes.
- Collagenase and other proteinases break down tissues and virtually liquefy muscles. The whole of a muscle group or segment of a limb may be affected.
- α-Toxin, a phospholipase C (lecithinase), is generally considered to be the main cause of the toxaemia associated with gas gangrene, although other clostridial species can produce similar manifestations.

In puerperal infections or in cases of septic abortion, the organisms may gain access from faeces-contaminated perineal skin or contaminated instruments to necrotic or devitalized tissues in the uterus or adnexa. Here they set up a dangerous and often fulminating pelvic infection, possibly with prompt invasion of the bloodstream. There may be intravascular haemolysis and anuria.

C. perfringens may also participate in peritoneal infections that occur as a result of extension of pathogens from the alimentary tract, as in cases of gangrenous appendicitis, intestinal obstruction, or mesenteric thrombosis.

If a preparation of adrenaline (epinephrine) used for injection is contaminated with clostridial spores, the combination of an infective inoculum with the local ischaemia that follows the injection may be catastrophic. Gas gangrene may complicate surgical operations on the lower limb or hip of patients whose blood supply is inadequate to maintain oxygenation in the postoperative period.

Clostridia may be associated with less severe forms of infection without the toxaemia and aggression of gas gangrene. Moreover, potentially pathogenic anaerobes may be cultivated from a wound that never shows any sign of gas gangrene, and sometimes the laboratory isolation may be attributed to the germination of a few contaminating spores when the specimen was being processed. Thus the onus is on the clinician to relate a laboratory report to the patient's circumstances.

Clinical clues include *crepitus*, the sponge-cake consistency caused by small bubbles of gas in adjacent tissues. In the early stages, the patient has an anxious, frightened appearance. Local pain is increased, and there is swelling of the affected tissues. Toxaemia and shock supervene, and the patient becomes drowsy and drifts into coma.

Prompt diagnosis and intensive surgical and antimicrobial treatment greatly influence the patient's chance of survival and may avoid the loss of the affected limb, but all devitalized tissue must be excised (see upcoming discussion).

LABORATORY INVESTIGATION

If there are sloughs of necrotic tissue in the wound, small pieces should be transferred aseptically into a sterile screw-capped bottle and examined immediately by microscopy and culture. Specimens of exudate should be taken from the deeper areas of the wound where the infection seems to be most pronounced. Gram smears are prepared. If gas gangrene exists, typical Gram-positive bacilli may predominate, often with other bacteria present in a mixed infection; however, there is usually a pronounced lack of inflammatory cells. Initiation of treatment should not await a full laboratory report, and early discussion with the bacteriologist is crucial. A direct smear of a wound exudate is often of great help in providing evidence of the relative numbers of different bacteria that may be participating in a mixed infection or may merely be present as contaminants, but the distinction is not invariably easy and joint discussions are important.

Treatment

Prompt and adequate surgical attention to the wound is of the utmost importance (Fig. 29.2).

- Sutures are removed, and necrotic and devitalized tissue is excised with careful debridement.
- Fascial compartments are incised to release tension.
- Any foreign body is found and removed.
- The wound is not resutured but is left open after thorough cleansing, and loosely packed.

Antibiotic therapy is started immediately in very high doses. This must take account of the likely coexistence of coliform organisms, Gram-positive cocci, and faecal anaerobes. Accordingly, penicillin, metronidazole, and an aminoglycoside have been given in combination for many years. Experimental studies in mice suggest that protein synthesis inhibitor antibiotics, such as clindamycin, have significantly greater activity than penicillin. Thus clindamycin plus an aminoglycoside or a broad-spectrum antibiotic, such as meropenem or imipenem, should be considered. In addition, clindamycin down modulates the production of cytokines involved in shock and organ failure. Much intensive supportive therapy is needed.

Enthusiastic claims have been made for the efficacy of hyperbaric oxygen therapy, but clinical trials have given conflicting results. Patients are placed in a special pressurized chamber where they breathe oxygen at 2- to 3-atm

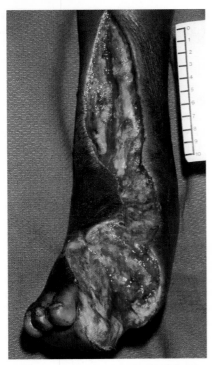

Fig. 29.2 Gas gangrene. Wound after debridement.

pressure for periods of 1 to 2 hours twice daily on several successive days. This may limit the amount of radical surgery needed; however, the necessity for surgical debridement should not be delayed.

A polyvalent antiserum containing *C. perfringens*, *C. septicum* and *C. novyi* antitoxins was used formerly, but has been replaced by intensive antimicrobial therapy.

Prophylaxis

Surgical wounds

C. perfringens is normally present in large numbers in human faeces, and its spores are found regularly on the skin, especially of the buttocks and thighs. As clostridial spores are very resistant to most disinfectants, they are likely to survive normal preoperative skin preparation and persist in the area of the planned incision. The numbers can be reduced by more prolonged skin preparation with the sustained action of an antiseptic such as povidone–iodine for a day or two; this procedure has a place in orthopaedic surgery.

When inevitable skin contamination is combined with circumstances that predispose to devitalization of tissue and reduced oxygen tension, a patient may be vulnerable to the development of postoperative gas gangrene. These circumstances arise when an elderly patient or a patient with vascular insufficiency undergoes major surgery to the hip or lower limb. Perioperative antimicrobial prophylaxis with penicillin is justified in such cases.

Accidental wounds

The prevention of gas gangrene in accidentally sustained wounds must take account of the endogenous factors already noted and the exogenous sources of clostridial spores and vegetative forms in soil, on contaminated clothing, and the like. In addition, there is an increased risk of anaerobic infection developing when foreign bodies such as soil, clothing, metal (nails, wire, bullets, shrapnel), and skin are driven into devitalized tissues. Prompt and adequate surgical attention is of paramount importance, but prophylactic administration of benzylpenicillin for patients presenting with serious contaminated wounds is also worthwhile. Prophylaxis may be omitted if the state of the wound and the patient's general condition are expertly and frequently monitored throughout the recovery period.

FOOD POISONING

Carrier rates for "typical food-poisoning strains" of *C. perfringens* range from about 2% to more than 30% in different surveys across the world. These bacteria also occur in animals; thus meat is often contaminated with heat-resistant spores. When meat is cooked in bulk, heat penetration and subsequent cooling is slow unless special precautions are taken. During the cooling period surviving spores may germinate and multiply in the anaerobic environment produced by the cooked meat. Anyone eating this will consume the equivalent of a cooked meat broth culture of the organism. The organisms are protected from the gastric acid by the protein in the meal and pass in large numbers into the intestine.

Ingestion of large numbers of viable organisms is necessary for the production of the typical disease syndrome, which is mediated by an enterotoxin that is released when sporulation occurs in the gut, *C. perfringens* enterotoxin (CPE). The gene for CPE (*cpe*) can be found on both the chromosome and plasmids. Typical symptoms are abdominal cramps beginning about 8 to 12 hours after ingestion, followed by diarrhoea. Fever and vomiting are not usually encountered and symptoms generally subside within a day or two. No specific treatment is indicated. The carrier state persists for several weeks, but this should not be regarded as an indication for exclusion from any duties, as carriers may be quite numerous in various communities.

The vehicle of infection is usually a precooked meat food that has been allowed to stand at a temperature conducive to the multiplication of *C. perfringens*. Although the heat resistance of spores of typical food-poisoning strains ensures their survival in cooked foods, and presumably accounts for the association of these strains with most of the reported outbreaks of *C. perfringens* food poisoning, similar trouble can be caused by classic heat-sensitive type A strains if they gain access to food during the cooling period under conditions suitable for their subsequent multiplication.

LABORATORY INVESTIGATION

This can be difficult as some people carry large numbers of *C. perfringens*. Diagnosis depends upon the isolation of similar strains of *C. perfringens* from the faeces of patients and from others at risk who have eaten the suspected food, and from the food itself. Numbers usually exceed 10^6 organisms/g faeces. The isolates can be sent to a reference laboratory for special typing to prove their relatedness. Detection of the *cpe* gene is becoming increasingly important for the diagnosis of *C. perfringens* food poisoning.

Prevention

The occurrence of this type of food poisoning is an indictment of the catering practices concerned, as food has to be mishandled to allow the chain of events to take place. Nevertheless, *C. perfringens* is among the most common causes of food poisoning.

COLITIS

A sporadic diarrhoeal syndrome, usually occurring in elderly patients during treatment with antibiotics, has been described. The circumstances differ substantially from those of *C. perfringens* food poisoning. A cytopathic enterotoxin can be detected in the patient's faeces.

ENTERITIS NECROTICANS (PIG–BEL)

A subgroup of *C. perfringens* type C that produces heat-resistant spores is the cause of a disease that affects New Guinea natives when they have pork feasts. The method of cooking the pork allows the clostridia to survive. When the contaminated meat is eaten along with a sweet potato vegetable that contains a proteinase inhibitor, a toxin (the β-toxin) is able to act on the small intestine to produce a necrotizing enteritis. A successful vaccination programme has reduced the incidence of pig-bel dramatically.

CLOSTRIDIUM SEPTICUM

DESCRIPTION

The bacilli are generally large and actively motile with numerous flagella. It is one of the less exacting anaerobes and grows well at 37°C on ordinary media. Spores are readily formed, and, as they develop, various pleomorphic forms arise ranging from swollen Gram-positive "citron bodies" to obviously sporing forms in which the oval spores may be central or subterminal and are clearly bulging.

PATHOGENESIS

C. septicum is one of the gas gangrene group of clostridia. It occurs harmlessly in the human intestine, but if the integrity of the gut epithelium is impaired, for instance by leukaemic infiltration, bacteraemia may occur. Cyclic or other forms of neutropenia are also associated with spontaneous, nontraumatic gas gangrene that begins with a bacteraemic phase. *Typhlitis*, a rapidly fatal terminal ileal infection and septicaemia in immunocompromised patients, is most commonly associated with *C. septicum*.

Intramuscular injection of cultures into laboratory animals produces a spreading inflammatory oedema, with slight gas formation in the tissues. Organisms invade the blood, and the animal dies within a day or two. Smears from the liver show long filamentous forms and citron bodies. *C. septicum* produces several toxins (α, β, δ and ε). The α-toxin, which has lethal, haemolytic, and necrotizing activity, appears to be the most important; it does not have phospholipase C activity and thus differs from the α-toxin of *C. perfringens*.

CLOSTRIDIUM NOVYI

C. novyi resembles *C. perfringens* in morphology, but is larger, more pleomorphic and more strictly anaerobic; it is readily killed when vegetative cells are exposed to air. The spores are oval, central or subterminal. The organism occurs widely in soil and is associated with disease in humans and animals. There are four types—A, B, C and D—distinguished on the basis of permutations of the toxins and other soluble antigens they produce. Only type A strains are of medical interest as they cause some cases of gas gangrene in humans. In 2000, an outbreak of *C. novyi* type A infections among injecting heroin users killed 13 people in the United Kingdom.

C. novyi gas gangrene is associated with profound toxaemia. Culture filtrates are highly toxic and possess at least four active substances (α, β, δ and ε toxins) that account for the various haemolytic, necrotizing, lethal, phospholipase and lipase activities of this organism.

CLOSTRIDIUM SORDELLII

C. sordellii belongs to the gas gangrene group of clostridia. It is part of the normal intestinal flora, and up to 10% of healthy women harbor *C. sordellii* in their vagina. *C. sordellii* is a cause of soft-tissue infections and sepsis in injecting drug users, but recently infections complicating childbirth, abortion and gynaecological procedures have received attention. *C. sordellii* infections are highly lethal and associated with a toxic shock syndrome–like presentation. The virulence of *C. sordellii* is related to the production of two exotoxins (lethal toxin and haemorrhagic toxin) that belong to the large clostridial toxin (LCT) family.

CLOSTRIDIUM TETANI

DESCRIPTION

The tetanus bacillus is a motile, straight, slender, Gram-positive rod. A fully developed terminal spore gives the organism the appearance of a drumstick with a large round end. Gram-negative forms are usually encountered in stained smears. It is an obligate anaerobe that grows well in cooked meat broth and produces a thin spreading film when grown on enriched blood agar. The spores may be highly resistant to adverse conditions, but the degree of resistance varies with the strain. Spores of some strains resist boiling in water for up to 3 hours. They may resist dry heat at 160°C for 1 hour, and 5% phenol for 2 weeks or more. Iodine (1%) in water is said to kill the spores within a few hours, but glutaraldehyde is one of the few chemical disinfectants that is assuredly sporicidal.

PATHOGENESIS

As in gas gangrene (see Ch. 29), germination of spores and their outgrowth depend upon reduced oxygen tension in devitalized tissue and nonviable material in a wound. When infection occurs, often assisted by the simultaneous growth of facultatively anaerobic organisms in a mixed inoculum, the tetanus bacillus remains strictly localized, but tetanus toxin is elaborated and diffuses, as described next.

Toxins

C. tetani produces an oxygen-labile haemolysin (tetanolysin), but the organism's neurotoxin (tetanospasmin) is the essential pathogenic product. Strains vary in their toxigenicity; some are highly toxic. Most strains produce demonstrable toxin after culture in broth for a few days.

The gene encoding the neurotoxin is located on a plasmid. The toxin is synthesized as a single polypeptide with a molecular weight of 150,000 Da, which undergoes posttranslational cleavage into a heavy chain and a light chain linked by a disulphide bond. The estimated lethal dose for a mouse of pure tetanospasmin is 0.0001 μg. It is toxic to humans and various animals when injected parenterally, but not by the oral route.

When tetanus occurs naturally, the tetanus bacilli stay at the site of the initial infection and are not generally invasive. Toxin diffuses to affect the relevant level of the spinal cord (local tetanus) and then to affect the entire system (generalized tetanus). These stages, including the intermediate one of "ascending tetanus," are demonstrable in experimental animals, but the stages tend to merge in their clinical presentation in humans.

The toxin is absorbed from the site of its production in an infective focus, but may be delivered via the blood to all nerves in the body. The heavy chain mediates attachment to gangliosides and the toxin is internalized. It is then moved from the peripheral to the central nervous system by retrograde axonal transport and transsynaptic spread. The tendency for the first signs of human tetanus to be in the head and neck is attributed to the shorter length of the cranial nerves. In fact, descending involvement of the nervous system is seen as the tetanus toxin takes longer to traverse the longer motor nerves and also diffuses in the spinal cord.

Once the entire toxin molecule has been internalized into presynaptic cells, the light chain is released and affects the membrane of synaptic vesicles. This prevents the release of the neurotransmitter γ-aminobutyric acid. Motor neurons are left under no inhibitory control and undergo sustained excitatory discharge, causing the characteristic motor spasms of tetanus. The toxin exerts its effects on the spinal cord, the brainstem, peripheral nerves, at neuromuscular junctions and directly on muscles.

Clinical features of tetanus

Cases of tetanus have been reported in which the infection was apparently associated with a superficial abrasion, a contaminated splinter, or a minor thorn prick. *Otogenic tetanus* may be attributable to overzealous cleansing of the external auditory meatus with a small stick. In other patients, the site of infection remains undiscovered *(cryptogenic tetanus).* Tetanus infection may also occur in or near the uterus in cases of septic abortion.

Tetanus neonatorum follows infection of the umbilical wound of newborn infants (see upcoming discussion). Cases of *postoperative tetanus* have been attributed to imperfectly sterilized catgut, dressings or glove powder, and sometimes to dustborne infection of the wound at operation.

The onset of signs and symptoms is gradual, usually starting with some stiffness and perhaps pain in or near a recent wound. In some cases the initial complaint may be of stiffness of the jaw *(lockjaw).* Pain and stiffness in the neck and back may follow. The stiffness spreads to involve all muscle groups; facial spasms produce the "sardonic grin," and in severe cases spasm of the back muscles produces extreme arching of the back *(opisthotonos).* The period between injury and the first signs is usually about 10 to 14 days, but there is a considerable range. A severe case with a relatively poor prognosis shows rapid progression from the first signs to the development of generalized spasms. Sweating, tachycardia and arrhythmia, and swings in blood pressure reflect sympathetic stimulation, which is not well understood but creates problems of management.

TREATMENT

The patient remains conscious and requires skilled sedation and constant nursing. If generalized spasms are worrying, the patient is paralysed and ventilated mechanically until the toxin that has been taken up has decayed; this may take some weeks.

The patient is given 10,000 units of human tetanus immunoglobulin (HTIG) in saline by slow intravenous infusion. Full wound exploration and debridement is arranged, and the wound is cleansed and left open with a loose pack. Penicillin or metronidazole is given for as long as considered necessary to ensure that bacterial growth and toxin production are stopped. The antitoxin and antibiotics are given immediately, and preferably before surgical excision, but delay must be avoided.

LABORATORY INVESTIGATION

Gram smears of the wound exudate and any necrotic material may show the typical "drumstick" bacilli, but this is not invariably so, and thus provides only presumptive evidence as other organisms that resemble *C. tetani* have terminal spores. Simple light microscopy is often unsuccessful; immunofluorescence microscopy with a specific stain is possible but not generally available.

Direct culture of unheated material on blood agar incubated anaerobically is often the best method of detecting *C. tetani*. There are various other tricks that exploit the organism's motility and fine spreading growth; sometimes these are vitiated by overgrowth with *Proteus* species. Material from the wound or from a mixed sporing subculture may be heated at various temperatures and for various times to exclude nonsporing bacteria; the heated specimens are then seeded onto solid media and incubated anaerobically. Tetanus may be produced in mice by subcutaneous injection of an anaerobic culture prepared from wound material; control mice are protected with tetanus antitoxin.

EPIDEMIOLOGY

Tetanus bacilli may be found in the human intestine, but infection seems to be derived primarily from animal faeces and soil. The organism is especially prevalent in manured soil, and for this reason a wound through skin contaminated with soil or manure deserves special attention. However, tetanus spores occur very widely and are commonly present in gardens, sports fields, and roads; in the dust, plaster and air of hospitals and houses; on clothing; and on articles of common use.

Spores of *C. tetani* and other anaerobes may be embedded in surgical catgut and other dressings. However, the sterility of surgical catgut (prepared from the gut of cattle and sheep) is now rigorously controlled.

Tetanus ranks among the major fatal infections. During the 1980s there were between 800,000 and 1 million deaths annually from tetanus, of which 400,000 were due to neonatal tetanus. The incidence varies enormously from country to country and is inversely related to socioeconomic development and standards of living, preventive medicine, and wound management. In developed countries, the reported incidence of adult and childhood tetanus is low. There is a direct relationship with fertile soil and a warm climate; thus people living in the agricultural areas of developing tropical and subtropical countries are exposed to severe challenges associated with poor hygiene, lack of shoes, neglect of wounds and inadequate immunization.

In addition, some local customs promote the occurrence of tetanus:

- Treatment of the umbilical cord stump with primitive applications that include animal dung
- Tying of the umbilical cord itself with primitive ligatures
- Ear piercing and other operations performed with unsterile instruments

Fatality rates may exceed 50%, and neonatal tetanus carries a very high mortality rate. Case fatality rates can be greatly reduced to less than 10% by modern methods of treatment in specialist centres. Unfortunately, such

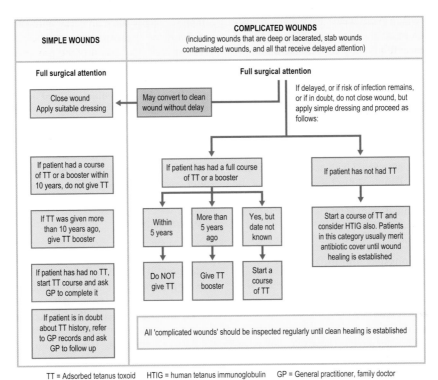

SIMPLE WOUNDS	COMPLICATED WOUNDS (including wounds that are deep or lacerated, stab wounds contaminated wounds, and all that receive delayed attention)	

Fig. 29.3 Wound management guidelines, with special reference to the prevention of tetanus.

TT = Adsorbed tetanus toxoid   HTIG = human tetanus immunoglobulin   GP = General practitioner, family doctor

expensive skilled help is available for only a small proportion of patients. Underprivileged people in countries with poorly developed or expensive medical services are at greatest risk and are least likely to receive sophisticated assistance; 80% of deaths occur in Africa and Southeast Asia. A maternal vaccination campaign mounted by the United Nations Children's Fund (UNICEF) during the past 20 years has reduced the incidence of neonatal tetanus by 50%.

PREVENTION AND CONTROL

Prompt and adequate wound toilet and proper surgical debridement of wounds are of paramount importance. There is an increased risk that tetanus spores may germinate in a wound if cleansing is delayed and if sepsis develops. Clean superficial wounds that receive prompt attention may not require specific protection against tetanus and it is unreasonable to insist that every small prick or abrasion requires protection with antitoxin or antibiotic.

Routine practice should take account of the local incidence of tetanus and the individual circumstances of the case. It is wise to recommend specific prophylaxis for a nonimmunized patient with a deep wound, puncture or stab wound, ragged laceration, a wound with much bruising and any devitalized tissue, a wound that is already septic or a bite wound or other type of wound that is likely to be heavily contaminated. Fig. 29.3 shows an approach that reflects current thinking in the United Kingdom.

The need for passive immunization is avoided if the patient is known to be properly immunized against tetanus (see Ch. 69). A patient may be regarded as immune for 6 months after the first two injections, or for 5 to 10 years after a planned course of three injections (or a subsequent booster injection) of adsorbed tetanus toxoid. Tetanus antitoxin should not be given to immune patients, but their active immunity may be enhanced when necessary by giving a dose of tetanus toxoid at the time of injury if the circumstances justify it.

A patient is considered nonimmune if there is no history of having had an injection of tetanus toxoid or if only one injection has been given. Take care: A patient may recall having had "a tetanus shot," but this may have been a previous dose of antitoxin for passive protection (which is transient and cannot be boosted by toxoid). If more than 6 months have elapsed after a course of two injections, or more than 10 years after a full primary course of three injections of adsorbed toxoid (or a booster injection), the patient should be regarded as nonimmune. A patient is nonimmune if more than 2 to 3 weeks have elapsed since a previous injection of equine antitoxin, or more than 6 to 8 weeks in the case of homologous (human) antitoxin. Nonimmunity should be assumed if there is any doubt about the immunization history.

Passive immunization with antitoxin

HTIG (homologous antitoxin) is available for passive protection and now supersedes equine antitoxin (heterologous antitoxin), which was associated with occasional adverse reactions. However, equine antiserum should not be prematurely discarded in countries that do not yet have HTIG. The prophylactic dose of HTIG is 250 to 500 units by intramuscular injection.

Combined active–passive immunization

A nonimmune patient receiving passive protection with HTIG after injury may be given the first dose of a course of active immunization with adsorbed toxoid at the same time, provided the injections are given from different syringes and into contralateral sites. The active immunization course must subsequently be completed.

Antibiotic protection

The prophylactic administration of antibiotics to all cases of open wounds is not recommended, although the use of penicillin or clindamycin is justified in some cases when there is a significant risk of infection. This precaution must not replace prompt and adequate surgical wound toilet.

CLOSTRIDIUM BOTULINUM

DESCRIPTION

C. botulinum is a strictly anaerobic, Gram-positive bacillus. It is motile and has spores that are oval and subterminal. It is a widely distributed saprophyte found in soil, vegetables, fruits, leaves, silage, manure, the mud of lakes, and sea mud. Its optimal growth temperature is about 35°C, but some strains can grow and produce toxin at temperatures as low as 1°C to 5°C.

The widespread occurrence of *C. botulinum* in nature, its ability to produce a potent neurotoxin in food, and the resistance of its spores to inactivation combine to make it a formidable pathogen. Spores of some strains withstand boiling in water (100°C) for several hours. They are usually destroyed by moist heat at 120°C within 5 minutes. Spores of type E strains (see upcoming discussion) are usually much less heat resistant. Insufficient heating in the process

of preserving foods is an important factor in the causation of botulism. The resistance of the spores to radiation is of special relevance to food processing.

Botulinum toxin is categorized as a biothreat level A biological warfare agent. Introduction of toxin into a target population by contaminating food or water is unlikely to succeed because of logistical problems, but botulinum toxin can also cause disease by inhalation.

Carefully controlled injections of toxin are used to treat involuntary muscle disorders, and as an "antiaging" remedy. Several cases of iatrogenic botulism have been diagnosed after cosmetic use of botulinum toxin.

PATHOGENESIS

Botulism is a severe, often fatal form of food poisoning characterized by pronounced neurotoxic effects. Botulinum toxins are among the most poisonous natural substances known. Seven main types of *C. botulinum*, designated A–G, produce antigenically distinct toxins with pharmacologically identical actions. All types can cause human disease, but types A, B and E are most common. The importance of this point is that, if antitoxin is given to a patient in an emergency, only the type-specific antitoxin will be effective.

The disease has been linked to a wide range of foods, usually preserved hams, large sausages of the salami type, home-preserved meats and vegetables, canned products such as fish and liver paste, and even hazelnut purée and honey. Traditional dishes such as fish or seal's flipper fermented in a barrel buried in the ground cannot be recommended by a bacteriologist! Type E strains are particularly but not invariably associated with a marine source, whereas type A and type B strains are usually associated with soil.

Foods responsible for botulism may not exhibit signs of spoilage. The preformed toxin in the food is absorbed from the intestinal tract. Although it is protein, intestinal proteolytic enzymes do not inactivate it. After absorption, toxin binds irreversibly to the presynaptic nerve endings of the peripheral nervous system and cranial nerves, where it inhibits acetylcholine release.

Clinical features

The period between ingestion of the toxin and the appearance of signs and symptoms is usually 1 to 2 days, but it may be much longer. There may be initial nausea and vomiting. The oculomotor muscles are affected, and the patient may have diplopia and drooping eyelids with a squint. There may be vertigo and blurred vision.

There is progressive descending motor loss with flaccid paralysis but with no loss of consciousness or sensation, although weakness and sleepiness are often described. The patient is thirsty, with a dry mouth and tongue. There are difficulties in speech and swallowing, with later problems of breathing and despair. There may be abdominal pain and restlessness. Death is due to respiratory or cardiac failure.

Wound botulism

Rare cases of wound infection with *C. botulinum* resulting in the characteristic signs and symptoms of botulism have been recorded.

Infant botulism

The "floppy child syndrome" describes a young child, usually less than 6 months old, with flaccid paralysis that is ascribed to the growth of *C. botulinum* in the intestine at a stage in development when the colonization resistance of the gut is poor. Some cases have been attributed to the presence of *C. botulinum* spores in honey; when the honey was given as an encouragement to feed, the ingested spores were able to germinate and produce toxin in the infant gut.

LABORATORY INVESTIGATION

The organism or its toxin may be detected in the suspected food, and toxin may be demonstrated in the patient's blood by toxin–antitoxin neutralization tests in mice. Samples of faeces or vomit may also yield such evidence. Take care: Bear in mind that botulinum toxin is very dangerous—specialist help should be summoned and the laboratory alerted.

TREATMENT

The priorities are:

- To remove unabsorbed toxin from the stomach and intestinal tract
- To neutralize unfixed toxin by giving polyvalent antitoxin (with due precautions to avoid hypersensitivity reactions to the heterologous antiserum)
- To give relevant intensive care and support

CONTROL

Great care must be taken in canning factories to ensure that adequate heating is achieved in all parts of the can contents. Home canning of foodstuffs should be avoided.

The amateur preservation of meat and vegetables, especially beans, peas and root vegetables, is dangerous in inexperienced hands. Acid fruits may be bottled safely in the home with heating at 100°C, as a low pH is inhibitory to the growth of *C. botulinum*.

A prophylactic dose of polyvalent antitoxin should be given intramuscularly to all persons who have eaten food suspected of causing botulism. Injecting three doses of mixed toxoid at intervals of 2 months can produce active immunity, but the very low incidence of the disease under normal conditions does not justify this as a routine. Active immunization should be considered for laboratory staff who might have to handle the organism or specimens containing the organism or its toxin.

CLOSTRIDIUM DIFFICILE

DESCRIPTION

C. difficile is a motile, Gram-positive rod with oval subterminal spores. It commonly occurs in the faeces of neonates and babies of all mammals until the age of weaning, but it is not generally found in adults.

The organism produces an enterotoxin (toxin A) and a cytotoxin (toxin B) both belonging to the LCT family; some strains produce a third (binary) toxin, the importance of which is still not yet understood. *C. difficile* causes antibiotic-associated diarrhoea, occasionally leading to a life-threatening condition, *pseudomembranous colitis* (PMC) (Fig. 29.4). There is almost always a history of previous antibiotic therapy although exposure to any agent that perturbs the gut flora, including cytotoxic drugs, may lead to clinical disease. Clindamycin and lincomycin are associated with a particularly high risk, but extended-spectrum cephalosporins are also commonly incriminated and are much more commonly used; virtually

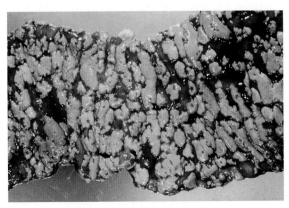

Fig. 29.4 Pseudomembranous colitis.

no antimicrobial drug has escaped blame. An epidemic of fluoroquinolone-resistant ribotype 027 *C. difficile* infection predominantly in North America is probably due to excessive use of these agents. The US Centers for Disease Control and Prevention consider *C. difficile* the number one antibiotic-resistant threat to public health in the United States.

LABORATORY INVESTIGATION

C. difficile can be isolated from the faeces by enrichment and selective culture procedures. Toxin B can be detected in the patient's faeces by testing extracts against monolayers of susceptible cells, or both toxins may be demonstrated by immunological methods such as enzyme-linked immunosorbent assay (ELISA). The sensitivity of many ELISA kits is only 50% to 70%, and results should be interpreted with caution. Moreover, toxin A negative strains, which still cause disease and are prevalent in certain regions of the world, are not detected by some kits. Because of these issues, highly sensitive polymerase chain reaction (PCR) detection of the toxin B gene is now the favoured approach. However, this approach is not without its difficulties as detection of *C. difficile* in the absence of faecal toxin does not correlate with disease and therefore *C. difficile* infection (CDI) is being overdiagnosed.

TREATMENT

It is essential to discontinue the antibiotic that is presumed to have precipitated the disease and to suppress the growth and toxin production of *C. difficile* by giving oral metronidazole or vancomycin. PMC may be fatal if it is not quickly recognized and treated. The current importance of *C. difficile* has led to a plethora of new treatment/prevention options such as antibiotics (fidaxomicin) and active or passive vaccination. Faecal microbiota transplantation has become a successful alternative therapy for recalcitrant cases of CDI but this procedure is not without its problems, both administrative and technical.

EPIDEMIOLOGY

The organism is usually acquired from an exogenous source by a patient whose intestinal colonization resistance has been compromised by antibiotic exposure. Patients developing infection have often spent lengthy periods in hospital. Reinfection occurs in 20% to 50% of cases as it may take the gut 2 to 3 months to normalize after perturbation.

Many production and companion animals are colonized by *C. difficile* before weaning; thus meat and meat products in North America can be contaminated by *C. difficile* spores. Although the suggestion that *C. difficile* is a foodborne pathogen has not been proven, animals may be an important reservoir of disease. Animal manure may be heavily contaminated with *C. difficile* spores that survive for many months in soil. An apparent increase in community-acquired infection, in the absence of risk factors such as antibiotic exposure, has led to suggestions that all patients with community-acquired diarrhoea should be tested for *C. difficile*.

PREVENTION

Clinical awareness is the keynote. *C. difficile* is the most common cause of hospital-acquired diarrhoea, and an important cause of community-acquired diarrhoea. If a patient develops diarrhoea after at least 48 hours in hospital, especially while taking antibiotics, the possibility of CDI must be considered. If several cases occur in a hospital unit, cross-infection should be considered as the hospital environment can become extensively contaminated with *C. difficile* spores. The existing antibiotic and infection control policies of the unit should be reviewed. Haematology and oncology patients who are increasingly treated in the community, and patients with inflammatory bowel diseases, are at great risk of community-acquired infection.

RECOMMENDED READING

Caya, J. G., Agni, R., & Miller, J. E. (2004). *Clostridium botulinum* and the clinical laboratorian. *Archives of Pathology & Laboratory Medicine*, *128*, 653–662.

Crobach, M. J., Planche, T., Eckert, C., et al. (2016). European Society of Clinical Microbiology and Infectious Diseases: update of the diagnostic guidance document for *Clostridium difficile* infection. *Clinical Microbiology and Infection, 4*, S63–S81.

Farrar, J. J., Yen, L. M., Cook, T., et al. (2000). Tetanus. *Journal of Neurology, Neurosurgery, and Psychiatry, 69*, 292–301.

Freeman, J., Bauer, M. P., Baines, S. D., et al. (2010). The changing epidemiology of *Clostridium difficile* infections. *Clinical Microbiology Reviews, 23*, 529–549.

McLauchlin, J., & Little, C. (2007). *Hobbs' food poisoning and food hygiene* (7th ed.). London: Hodder Arnold.

Popoff, M. R. (2014). Clostridial pore-forming toxins. *Anaerobe, 30*, 220–238.

Rood, J. I., McClane, B. A., Songer, J. G., et al. (1997). *The clostridia—molecular biology and pathogenesis*. San Diego: Academic Press.

Rossetto, O., Pirazzini, M., & Montecucco, C. (2014). Botulinum neurotoxins: genetic, structural and mechanistic insights. *Nature Reviews. Microbiology, 12*, 535–549.

Stevens, D. L., Aldape, M. J., & Bryant, A. E. (2012). Life-threatening clostridial infections. *Anaerobe, 18*, 254–259.

30 Nonsporing anaerobes

Wound infection; periodontal disease; abscess; normal microbiota

ROBERT P. ALLAKER

KEY POINTS

- Nonsporing anaerobes are found as part of normal microbiota in health.
- Most infections with anaerobes are of endogenous origin and are often polymicrobial. They act as opportunistic pathogens at damaged and necrotic tissue sites.
- Production of putrid odour is a common feature of infection.
- *Fusobacterium nucleatum* is often recovered from head and neck infections.
- Anaerobic Gram-negative rods, especially *Bacteroides fragilis* and anaerobic Gram-positive cocci, are the most common cause of nonclostridial anaerobic infections.
- Black-pigmented *Porphyromonas* and *Prevotella* species occur in abscesses and soft tissue infections in various parts of the body.
- Penicillins and nitroimidazoles, especially metronidazole, are the main agents used for treatment.

The significance of obligate anaerobes in general and of nonsporing anaerobes in particular is now well recognised. This heightened awareness of the important role that such organisms play, as part of the normal microbiota of the body and in a wide variety of infections, has come about largely through the application of greatly improved laboratory techniques for the isolation and cultivation of anaerobic bacteria, and the pioneering efforts of 'anaerobe enthusiasts' in various parts of the world.

A bewildering range of anaerobes is found in the mouth and oropharynx, gastrointestinal tract and female genital tract of healthy individuals as part of the commensal microbiota. These include Gram-positive and Gram-negative cocci, rods and filaments, as well as a number of spiral forms (Table 30.1). Most infections with these organisms are of endogenous origin, except in the case of animal and human bite wounds, where the infecting organisms, usually mixed, are derived from the mouth of the aggressor.

The microbiota of the lower intestinal tract, in particular, harbour vast numbers of anaerobes; quantitative studies on the microbiota of human faeces (Table 30.2) reveal a total content of over 10^{10} anaerobes per gram of faeces.

Many of the bacteria isolated from anaerobic infections are opportunist pathogens. Such organisms are particularly likely to set up infections in damaged and necrotic tissue, when they are translocated to sites other than their normal habitat, or in a host that is compromised or debilitated in a way that leads to impairment of immunological or other defence mechanisms. Anaerobic infections of the head, neck and respiratory tract are often associated with organisms found in the mouth, whereas infections in the abdominal and pelvic regions are more commonly associated with gut bacteria.

FEATURES OF ANAEROBIC INFECTIONS

CLINICAL SIGNS

A common but not invariable feature is the production of a foul or putrid odour. Foul-smelling pus or discharge should always alert the clinician to the likelihood that anaerobes are present, as no other organisms produce this effect, but the absence of this sign does not necessarily exclude the involvement of anaerobic bacteria. Other clues to the clinical diagnosis are listed in Box 30.1.

POLYMICROBIAL INFECTIONS

Infections involving nonclostridial anaerobes are often polymicrobial. The composition of these mixed infections varies according to the site affected. The complexity may vary from two or three species up to a dozen or more, and may include strict anaerobes, facultatively

Table 30.1 Anaerobic bacteria found as part of normal microbiota in humans[a]

	Skin	Mouth	Gastrointestinal tract	Genitourinary tract[b]
Gram-positive bacilli				
Actinomyces	–	+	+	+
Bifidobacterium	–	+	+	+
Clostridium	–	–	+	+
Eubacterium	–	+	+	+
Lactobacillus	–	+	+	+
Propionibacterium	+	+	+	+
Gram-positive cocci				
Coprococcus	–	–	+	–
Gemmiger	–	–	+	–
Peptococcus[c]	–	+	+	+
Peptostreptococcus[c]	+	+	+	+
Ruminococcus	–	–	+	–
Sarcina	–	–	+	–
Streptococcus	+	+	+	+
Gram-negative bacilli				
Anaerobiospirillum	–	+	+	(?)
Anaerorhabdus	–	–	+	(?)
Bacteroides	–	–	+	+
Bilophila	–	–	+	+
Butyrivibrio	–	–	+	–
Centipeda	–	+	+	(?)
Desulfomonas	–	–	+	–
Fusobacterium	–	+	+	+
Leptotrichia	–	+	+	–
Mitsuokella	–	+	+	(?)
Porphyromonas	–	+	+	+
Prevotella	–	+	+	+
Selenomonas	–	+	+	–
Succinimonas	–	–	+	–
Succinivibrio	–	–	+	–
Wolinella	–	+	+	–
Gram-negative cocci				
Acidaminococcus	–	–	+	+
Megasphaera	–	–	+	–
Veillonella	–	+	+	+
Spirochaetes				
Treponema	–	+	+	+
Other spiral forms	–	+	+	+

–, Not usually found; +, commonly present; (?), presence uncertain (further data required).
[a]Data from various sources.
[b]Female genitourinary tract.
[c]Includes recently reclassified species of 'anaerobic cocci'.

anaerobic and micro-aerophilic organisms. Such combinations frequently comprise mixtures of Gram-negative rods (such as *Bacteroides*, *Prevotella* and *Fusobacterium* species) and Gram-positive cocci (such as streptococci). In most cases, with the occasional exception of actinomycosis, it is not possible to accurately predict which organisms are present from the clinical presentation, although the detection of red fluorescing pus under ultraviolet light usually indicates the involvement of one of the black-pigmented *Porphyromonas* species.

LABORATORY INVESTIGATION

When anaerobic infection is suspected, it is important that adequate clinical specimens are collected and

Table 30.2 The bacterial microbiota of faeces of English subjects

Bacterial group	Mean bacterial count[a]
Gram-negative anaerobic rods	9.8
Bifidobacterium spp.	9.8
Clostridium spp.	5.0
Veillonella spp.	4.2
Lactobacillus spp.	6.5
Bacillus spp.	3.7
Enterobacteria	7.9
Streptococcus spp.	7.1
Enterococcus spp.	5.8
Total anaerobes	10.1
Total aerobes	8.0

[a]Log_{10} viable organisms per gram of faeces.
From Hill, M. J., Drasar, B. S., Hawksworth, G., Aries, V., Crowther, J. S., & Williams, R. E. (1971). Bacteria and aetiology of cancer of large bowel. *Lancet*, 1(7690), 95–100.

Box 30.1 Some clinical signs and indicators of nonclostridial anaerobic infections

- Presence of foul-smelling pus, discharge or lesion
- Production of a large amount of pus (abscess formation)
- Proximity of lesion to mucosal surface or portal of entry
- Failure to isolate organisms from pus ('sterile' pus)
- Infection associated with necrotic tissue
- Deep abscesses
- Gas formation in tissues (crepitus)
- Failure to respond to conventional antimicrobial therapy
- Pus that shows red fluorescence under ultraviolet light (*Porphyromonas* spp.)
- Detection of 'sulphur granules' in pus (actinomycosis)
- Infection of human or animal bite wound
- Gram-negative bacteraemia
- Septic thrombophlebitis

transported as soon as possible to the bacteriology laboratory, preferably under reducing conditions. After direct microscopical examination of the material, appropriate culture media should be inoculated for incubation in an anaerobic cabinet or in anaerobic jars. As many anaerobes are relatively slow growing, it is essential that cultures be incubated for several days before being discarded. In mixed infections, fast-growing aerobic or facultatively anaerobic organisms are often detected within 24 hours, whereas some anaerobes may require incubation for 7–10 days before their colonies can be recognised and identity confirmed using appropriate biochemical, mass spectrometry or nucleic acid amplification tests.

In some laboratories, gas–liquid chromatography is carried out directly on pus and other clinical specimens in order to detect metabolic products, such as butyric and propionic acids, that are characteristic of certain anaerobes. Molecular-based techniques are also used for the rapid identification of anaerobes. Rapid molecular methods include polymerase chain reaction-restriction fragment length polymorphism (PCR-RFLP), multi-locus sequence typing (MLST), *rpoB* and 16S gene sequencing and whole genome sequencing (WGS). All of these approaches should allow subtyping of strains, but differ in their accuracy, discriminatory power and reproducibility.

GRAM–NEGATIVE BACILLI

Fusobacterium spp.

Fusobacteria colonise the mucous membranes of human beings and animals and are generally regarded as commensals of the upper respiratory and gastrointestinal tracts. They tend to form long filamentous rods, often with pointed ends, sometimes described as fusiform or spindle shaped. Species such as *F. nucleatum*, *F. periodonticum* and *F. naviforme* are generally isolated from the oral cavity and are often associated with infections of this and related sites. *F. nucleatum*, the most studied species, is frequently recovered from mixed infections of the head and neck region, including dental abscesses and the central nervous system, and is quite commonly isolated from transtracheal aspirates and pleural fluid. Five subspecies are recognised: *animalis, fusiforme, nucleatum, polymorphum* and *vincentii*. *F. nucleatum* subspecies *nucleatum* is an important periodontal pathogen, particularly during the period when quiescent periodontitis becomes active.

F. necrophorum is an important animal pathogen. It is associated with human necrobacillosis and occasionally infections similar to those caused by *F. nucleatum*.

F. mortiferum, *F. necrogenes*, *F. gonidiaformans* and *F. varium* are generally isolated from the gastrointestinal and urogenital tracts of humans and animals. These species, together with *F. nucleatum*, are often associated with mixed intraabdominal infections, perirectal abscesses, osteomyelitis, decubitus and other ulcers and various soft tissue infections. *F. ulcerans* is associated with tropical ulcers but may be found in other sites.

Leptotrichia buccalis

This species shares a number of properties with the fusobacteria. It is normally considered to be an oral species but also occurs outside the oral cavity. It has been reported in acute necrotising ulcerative gingivitis (Vincent's disease), together with *Treponema, Porphyromonas* and *Fusobacterium* species. Some isolates described as *L. buccalis* probably represent separate species within the genus.

Table 30.3 Current taxonomic status of *Bacteroides*, *Porphyromonas* and *Prevotella* species

Group	Species
Saccharolytic (*B. fragilis* and related species)	*B. fragilis, B. caccae, B. eggerthii, B. ovatus, B. stercoris, B. thetaiotaomicron, B. uniformis, B. vulgatus, Parabacteroides distasonis, Para. merdae*
Moderately saccharolytic (*Prevotella* spp.)	*Prev. melaninogenica, Prev. bivia, Prev. buccae, Prev. buccalis, Prev. corporis, Prev. denticola, Prev. disiens, Prev. enoeca, Prev. heparinolytica, Prev. intermedia, Prev. loescheii, Prev. nigrescens, Prev. pollens, Prev. oralis, Prev. oris, Prev. oulorum, Prev. tannerae, Prev. veroralis, Prev. zoogleoformans, Prev. salivae, Prev. shahii, Prev. multiformis, Prev. marshii, Prev. baroniae*
Asaccharolytic (*Porphyromonas* spp.)	*P. asaccharolytica, P. catoniae, P. gingivalis, P. endodontalis, P. uenonis*

Bacteroides, Porphyromonas and *Prevotella* species

Bacteria once thought of as typical members of the genus *Bacteroides,* especially those isolated from human beings, form three broad groups according to whether they are asaccharolytic, moderately saccharolytic or strongly saccharolytic (Table 30.3):

1. The asaccharolytic, pigmented species are classified in the genus *Porphyromonas,* which includes the important periodontal pathogen *P. gingivalis.*
2. The moderately saccharolytic species that are inhibited by 20% bile and are largely indigenous to the oral cavity are assigned to the genus *Prevotella.*
3. The genus *Bacteroides* is now restricted to *B. fragilis* and related species that are saccharolytic and grow in the presence of 20% bile.

To add to the taxonomic complexity, many other former *Bacteroides* species that are usually isolated from nonhuman sources have undergone reclassification. *B. gracilis* and *B. ureolyticus* now belong to the genus *Campylobacter,* and the former *B. ochraceus* now belongs to the genus *Capnocytophaga.*

INFECTIONS WITH *BACTEROIDES, PORPHYROMONAS* AND *PREVOTELLA* SPECIES

Bacteroides species and related Gram-negative rods are, together with anaerobic cocci, the most common cause of nonclostridial anaerobic infections in humans. Organisms of the *B. fragilis* group are particularly significant, as they are the most commonly isolated and tend to be more resistant to antimicrobial agents than are most anaerobes.

B. fragilis itself is substantially outnumbered by other *Bacteroides* species in the normal bowel microbiota, but is often associated with intraabdominal and soft tissue infections below the waist. *B. fragilis* is also the most common anaerobe found in bacteraemia, and has even occasionally been reported from head and neck infections,

Box 30.2 Currently recognised species (human) of Gram-positive anaerobic cocci of possible clinical relevance

- *Peptococcus niger*
- *Peptostreptococcus anaerobius*
- *Peptoniphilus asaccharolyticus*
- *Peptoniphilus harei*
- *Peptoniphilus ivorii*
- *Peptoniphilus lacrimalis*
- *Finegoldia magna*
- *Parvimonas micra*
- *Anaerococcus hydrogenalis*
- *Anaerococcus lactolyticus*
- *Anaerococcus octavius*
- *Anaerococcus prevotii*
- *Anaerococcus tetradius*
- *Anaerococcus vaginalis*

despite its apparent absence from the normal flora of the mouth. Species of the *B. fragilis* group account for about a quarter of all anaerobes isolated from clinical specimens.

Black-pigmented species, including those from the genera *Porphyromonas* and *Prevotella,* occur in abscesses and soft tissue infections in various parts of the body. They are rarely isolated in pure culture. *P. gingivalis* is associated with chronic adult periodontitis and *P. endodontalis* with dental root canal (endodontic) infections.

GRAM–POSITIVE ANAEROBIC COCCI

Gram-positive anaerobic cocci comprise part of the normal microbiota of the mouth, gastrointestinal tract; genitourinary tract and skin (see Table 30.1). Most are found as part of the microbiota of the bowel and are not usually considered to be significant in infections.

However, several genera of clinically significant strictly anaerobic Gram-positive cocci, formerly regarded as belonging to the genus *Peptostreptococcus,* are now recognised (Box 30.2). They are not easy to identify precisely and are often described simply as anaerobic cocci.

- Blood cultures
- Central nervous system (including brain abscesses)
- Head and neck infections (including ear)
- Dental abscesses and infected root canals
- Periodontal diseases and infected oral implants
- Human and animal bites
- Pleural infections
- Abdominal infections
- Genitourinary tract infections
- Decubitus ulcers
- Foot ulcers
- Osteomyelitis

Table 30.4 Some characteristics of anaerobic nonsporing Gram-positive rods

Genus	Common sites	Acid end-products
Propionibacterium	Skin, mouth, gut, vagina	Propionic acid
Bifidobacterium	Gut, mouth, vagina	Acetic and lactic acids
Lactobacillus	Mouth, gut, vagina	Lactic acid (major end-product)
Actinomyces	Mouth, gut, vagina	Succinic, lactic and acetic acids
Eubacterium	Mouth, gut, vagina	Butyric and other acids

mouth, skin, gastrointestinal and female genitourinary tracts and are isolated from a variety of types of infection. The main genera and some of their characteristics are listed in Table 30.4.

INFECTIONS WITH ANAEROBIC COCCI

Anaerobic cocci are isolated from infections in various parts of the body, particularly from abscesses (Box 30.3). They are often found in association with other anaerobic, facultatively anaerobic or aerobic organisms. As with all mixed infections, it is difficult to assess the contribution of each individual organism to the pathogenic process. However, there is sufficient evidence from both clinical and experimental studies to confirm their pathogenic potential.

GRAM-NEGATIVE ANAEROBIC COCCI

Among genera recorded as part of the normal microbiota of the gastrointestinal tract (see Table 30.1), only *Veillonella* is found regularly at other sites. In the mouth, for example, this genus is a regular component of supragingival dental plaque and the tongue microbiota. Veillonellae are able to use some of the lactic acid produced by bacteria such as streptococci and lactobacilli that potentially induce dental caries.

The role of *Veillonella* species and other anaerobic Gram-negative cocci in disease, if any, has not been clearly established, although they may be isolated from a variety of clinical conditions. In general, they are regarded as a minor component of mixed anaerobic infections, and antimicrobial chemotherapy is not generally directed specifically against them.

NONSPORING GRAM-POSITIVE RODS

The spore-forming genus *Clostridium* is well known for its involvement in serious infections (see Ch. 29). The role of anaerobic nonsporing Gram-positive rods, on the other hand, is less well understood, although they are present in significant numbers in the normal flora of the

INFECTIONS WITH GRAM-POSITIVE RODS

Any of these bacteria can occur as components of mixed anaerobic infections, and *Actinomyces* species can undoubtedly adopt a pathogenic role. Most cases of actinomycosis are caused by *Actinomyces israelii* and are cervicofacial, although the disease can also occur in the thorax, abdomen and female genital tract. *Actinomyces* species are not themselves strict anaerobes, but *A. israelii* requires good anaerobic conditions for primary isolation, and agar plates should be incubated for 7–10 days.

Propionibacterium propionicum is morphologically and biochemically very similar to *A. israelii*. It is particularly associated with infection of the tear duct in the condition called lachrymal canaliculitis. The significance of other genera in infections is not clear. Some species are found in acne; they are also isolated occasionally in infective endocarditis and in infections associated with implanted prostheses. *Eubacterium* species are a large group (possibly mistaken for *Actinomyces* species in some reports), many of which have been reclassified into new genera, including *Slackia* and *Eggerthella*. These bacteria may play a role in infections around intrauterine devices; others, for example, *Slackia exigua,* may be involved in human periodontal disease. There is only limited evidence for the pathogenicity of *Bifidobacterium* species, although *Bif. dentium* has been isolated occasionally from pulmonary infections; bifidobacteria can also be isolated from dental caries lesions by use of appropriate cultural methods.

SPIRAL-SHAPED MOTILE ORGANISMS

Several *Treponema* species are found in the mouth and elsewhere in the body (see Table 30.1). They are thought to be an important component of the mixed anaerobic infection associated with acute necrotising ulcerative gingivitis along with fusobacteria and *Prev. intermedia*, and may also contribute to other forms of periodontal disease. The proportion of motile spiral organisms seen by dark-ground microscopy in samples from the gingival pocket increases markedly when there is evidence of periodontal destruction.

Motile, spiral-shaped, Gram-negative anaerobes of the genus *Anaerobiospirillum* have been isolated from patients with diarrhoea and from bacteraemia. Although comparatively rarely isolated from humans, they can cause serious infections. The distribution and normal habitat of this and other morphologically similar organisms are not well understood. In some cases, the source of infection may be domestic animals and pets.

TREATMENT

In many infections caused by anaerobes, the most important aspect of treatment is surgical. This often involves drainage of pus from abscesses, but may also include debridement, curettage and removal of necrotic tissue. For minor infections, surgical drainage alone may be sufficient, but in many cases, antimicrobial chemotherapy is also indicated. The main groups of agents used are the penicillins and the nitroimidazoles, particularly metronidazole. Other agents with good anti-anaerobe activity include chloramphenicol, clindamycin and cefoxitin, but resistant strains occur.

Metronidazole is effective against virtually all obligate anaerobes, including *Bacteroides, Porphyromonas, Prevotella* and *Fusobacterium* species, but not against facultatively anaerobic or microaerophilic bacteria such as actinomyces and streptococci. Resistance to metronidazole among anaerobic pathogens is still relatively low.

Most anaerobic species are sensitive to benzylpenicillin, but members of the *B. fragilis* group are usually resistant. Such resistance is associated with β-lactamase production, and these organisms are usually susceptible to combinations of penicillins with β-lactamase inhibitors (e.g., co-amoxiclav) and to carbapenems such as imipenem.

RECOMMENDED READING

Allaker, R. P., Young, K. A., Langlois, T., de Rosayro, R., & Hardie, J. M. (1997). Dental plaque flora of the dog with reference to fastidious and anaerobic bacteria associated with bites. *Journal of Veterinary Dentistry, 14*(4), 127–130.

Borriello, S. P., Murray, P. R., & Funke, G., (Eds.) (2007). *Topley and Wilson's microbiology and microbial infections, Vol. 1 Bacteriology.* Oxford: Wiley.

Brook, I. (2007). *Anaerobic infections diagnosis and management.* New York: Informa Healthcare USA, Inc.

Marsh, P., & Martin, M. V. (2009). *Oral microbiology.* Edinburgh: Churchill Livingstone.

Wilson, M. (2008). *Bacteriology of humans.* Oxford: Blackwell Publishing.

Website

List of Prokaryotic Names with Standing in Nomenclature. Available at http://www.bacterio.cict.fr/. (Accessed Jul 2006).

31 *Brucella, Bartonella* and *Streptobacillus*

Brucellosis; Oroya fever; trench fever; cat scratch disease; bacillary angiomatosis; rat bite fever

ADRIAN M. WHATMORE

KEY POINTS

- Brucellae are highly infectious coccobacilli that cause a septicaemic illness, undulant fever. Most human disease is caused by *Brucella melitensis*, *B. abortus* or *B. suis*.
- The disease is a typical zoonosis most commonly acquired from infected animals or from infected meat or dairy products.
- Brucellosis is diagnosed by isolation of the organism from blood; alternatively, serology or molecular tests can be used.
- Brucellosis is treated with a tetracycline, usually in combination with an aminoglycoside or rifampicin.
- *Bartonella bacilliformis* is a highly infectious agent causing the sandfly-disseminated diseases, Oroya fever (Carrion's disease) and verruga peruana in parts of South America.
- The organism infects blood cells and can be diagnosed in stained blood or tissue aspirates or by molecular methods.
- Other bartonellae cause trench fever and cat scratch disease. Endocarditis can complicate these infections.
- Chloramphenicol, macrolides, aminoglycosides, fluoroquinolones and tetracyclines are used in the treatment of *Bartonella* infections.
- *Streptobacillus moniliformis* is one of the causes of a septicaemic illness, rat bite fever. Treatment with penicillin or a tetracycline is usually effective.

BRUCELLA

The genus *Brucella* comprises a group of Gram-negative coccobacilli that can infect a wide range of mammals. They are of particular zoonotic and economic importance as a cause of highly transmissible disease in cattle, sheep, goats and pigs. Infection in pregnant animals often leads to abortion, and involvement of the mammary glands may cause excretion in milk for months or even years. Human infections arise through direct contact with infected animals, including handling of infected carcasses; indirectly from a contaminated environment; or through consumption of infected dairy produce or improperly cooked meat.

Brucellosis is a typical zoonosis, and person-to-person infection does not play a significant role in transmission. Infection may remain latent or subclinical, or it may give rise to symptoms of varying intensity and duration. Brucellosis can present as an acute or subacute pyrexial illness that may persist for months or develop into a focal infection that can involve almost any organ system. Acute febrile illness begins with nonspecific flulike symptoms such as fever, headache, malaise, myalgia and drenching sweats. While some patients recover spontaneously others develop persistent symptoms that wax and wane—these characteristic intermittent waves of increased temperature that gave the name undulant fever to human disease are now usually seen only in long-standing untreated cases. Complications include arthritis, spondylitis, chronic fatigue, neurological signs, internal abscesses and endocarditis. Estimated mortality rates in the absence of treatment are low, with fatalities usually reflecting endocarditis or meningitis.

DESCRIPTION

Classification

The *Brucella* genus comprises an expanding group of closely related bacteria that differ in their preferred animal host, genetic arrangement, phage sensitivity pattern, and oxidation of certain amino acids and carbohydrates. The main human pathogens are *Brucella abortus*, *B. melitensis*, *B. suis* and rarely *B. canis*. The first three may be further subdivided into biovars, which, in the case of *B. suis*, are associated with various animal hosts. *B. abortus* has a preference for cattle and other Bovidae, *B. melitensis* for

309

sheep and goats and *B. canis* for dogs. The first three biovars of *B. suis* preferentially infect pigs, whereas the fourth and fifth biovars have reindeer or caribou and rodents, respectively, as natural hosts. The biovars differ in their sensitivity to dyes, in production of hydrogen sulphide and in agglutination by sera specific for epitopes found in the *Brucella* surface lipopolysaccharide. Various molecular typing methods are also used to differentiate subtypes down to the level of individual strains. In recent years, many novel *Brucella* species have been described, but their pathogenicity for humans, if any, remains unclear: *B. ceti* (dolphins and porpoises), *B. pinnipedialis* (seals), *B. inopinata* (from a human wound infection), *B. papionis* (from abortions in nonhuman primates), *B. vulpis* (from foxes) and *B. microti* (from voles).

Morphology

Brucellae are Gram-negative coccobacilli or short bacilli, occurring singly, in groups or short chains. They are usually nonmotile, noncapsulate and nonsporing.

Culture characteristics

Brucella spp. are aerobic. However, *B. ovis* and many strains of *B. abortus*, when first cultured, are unable to grow without the addition of 5%–10% carbon dioxide. All strains grow best at 37°C in a medium enriched with animal serum and glucose.

On clear solid medium, smooth, transparent and glistening (honey droplet) colonies appear after several days. However, the organisms can mutate, especially in liquid media, forming rough colonies on subculture. There is a corresponding loss in virulence and an antigenic change, so that they are no longer readily agglutinated by homologous antisera prepared against normal smooth strains. Identification as *Brucella* and to the species/subspecies level can be made by various polymerase chain reaction (PCR)-based tests or by a combination of biochemical, cultural, phage typing and serological tests. Rapid gallery tests may misidentify *Brucella* spp., and this has historically resulted in laboratory-acquired infections; they are not recommended.

Sensitivity and survival

Brucellae may be killed at a temperature of 60°C for 10 minutes, but dense suspensions, such as laboratory cultures, can require more drastic heat treatment to ensure their inactivation. Infected milk is rendered safe by efficient pasteurisation. Brucellae are very sensitive to direct sunlight and moderately sensitive to acid, so that they tend to die out in sour milk and in cheese that has undergone lactic acid fermentation. The organisms can survive in soil, manure and dust for weeks or months and remain viable in dead fetal material for even longer. They have been isolated from butter, cheese and ice cream prepared from infected milk. They may survive in carcass meat for several weeks under refrigeration. Pickling and smoking reduce survival. They are susceptible to common disinfectants if used at appropriate concentration and temperature. They are sensitive in vitro to a wide range of antibiotics, only a few of which are effective therapeutically.

Antigenic structure

In all smooth strains, the dominant surface antigen is a lipopolysaccharide (LPS) O chain, which, depending on the three-dimensional structure of the polysaccharide portion, forms A, M or C epitopes. These are common to all smooth species, but the distribution of A and M depends on biovar. Rough strains do not produce the O chain but have a common R epitope. The LPS has endotoxin activity of relatively low pyrogenicity and elicits limited antibody-mediated protection. The organisms behave as stealth pathogens and evade innate immune responses; effective immunity is dependent on specific cell-mediated and cytotoxic responses elicited by a variety of protein antigens.

PATHOGENESIS

The incubation period is usually about 10–30 days, although infection may persist for several months before causing any symptoms. *B. melitensis* and *B. suis* tend to cause more severe human disease than *B. abortus* or *B. canis*. Infection by any species may give rise to a variety of non-specific symptoms, and, without the fluctuating temperature to act as a guide, diagnosis may be difficult. Pointers to diagnosis are a history of occupational exposure or recent travel to endemic areas with consumption of unpasteurised dairy products.

Brucellae can enter the body through skin abrasions, through mucosal surfaces of the alimentary or respiratory tracts, and sometimes through the conjunctivae, to reach the bloodstream by way of regional lymphatics. The organisms are facultative intracellular parasites and subsequently localise in various parts of the reticuloendothelial system with the formation of abscesses or granulomatous lesions, resulting in complications that may involve any part of the body. Brucellae surviving within cells may cause relapses of acute disease, or a chronic syndrome may develop that is associated with continued illness and vague symptoms of malaise, low-grade fever, lassitude, insomnia, irritability and joint pain. Such chronic brucellosis may follow an acute attack or develop insidiously over several years without previous acute manifestations.

LABORATORY INVESTIGATION

Brucellosis is confirmed in humans by isolating the organisms from blood or other tissue samples and by serological and other tests. In animals, culture may be attempted from abortion material, placenta, milk, semen or samples of lymphoid tissue, mammary gland, uterus or testis collected postmortem.

Brucellae are easily transmitted by aerosols, ingestion and percutaneous inoculation. Samples suspected to contain brucellae must be treated as high risk. Cultures must be handled under containment conditions appropriate to Hazard Group 3 pathogens.

Blood culture

When brucellosis is suspected, blood culture should be attempted repeatedly and not exclusively during the febrile phase. Because the organisms may be scanty, at least 10 mL of blood should be withdrawn on each occasion, 5 mL being added to each of two blood culture bottles containing glucose–serum broth. One of these bottles should be incubated in an atmosphere containing 10% carbon dioxide. Preliminary lysis and centrifugation of the blood improve the isolation rate. Other materials such as bone marrow, solid tissue samples or exudates are also suitable for culture.

Subculture should be made onto serum–dextrose agar every few days; alternatively, a two-phase Castaneda culture system, in which the broth is periodically allowed to flow over agar contained within the blood culture bottle, may be used. Blood cultures should be retained for 6–8 weeks before being discarded as negative. Automated blood culture systems may also be used.

Serological tests

In the absence of positive cultures, the diagnosis of brucellosis usually depends on serological tests, the results of which tend to vary with the stage of the infection (Table 31.1). In some rural communities the sera from a proportion of the normal population are reactive in low dilutions in serological tests because of previous subclinical infection.

Serum agglutination test

This test is considered the reference method for diagnosis of human brucellosis and usually becomes positive 7–10 days after onset of symptoms. During the acute stage of

Table 31.1 Results of serological tests used in the diagnosis of brucellosis

Type of brucellosis	Agglutination test	Complement fixation test	ELISA
Acute	+	+	+
Chronic	v	+	+
Past infection	(–)	–	(–)

(–), usually weak or negative; v, variable; ELISA, enzyme-linked immunosorbent assay.

the disease, levels of agglutinins associated with both immunoglobulin (Ig) M and IgG continue to rise. As high-titre sera may not cause agglutination in low dilution (the prozone effect), a range of serum dilutions from 1 in 10 to >1 in 1000 should be made.

As the disease progresses from the acute to the chronic phase and the organisms become localised intracellularly in various parts of the body, the IgM antibodies decrease; the agglutination titre falls and may become undetectable, even while the patient is still ill. The absence of agglutination therefore does not rule out the possibility of infection. Persisting antibodies that are no longer capable of agglutinating may be detected by complement fixation, antiglobulin or enzyme-linked immunosorbent assay (ELISA) tests. In latent or chronic infection, the complement fixation test is likely to be positive, whereas in cases of past infection it is negative.

Enzyme-linked immunosorbent assay

The ELISA for IgG and IgA antibodies shows a good correlation with active disease, especially in long-standing infection. It has largely replaced the antihuman globulin (Coombs') test, formerly used for detecting nonagglutinating (IgG) antibodies.

Because the O chain of smooth *Brucella* LPS is structurally related to the LPS antigens of various other Gram-negative bacteria, false-positive cross-reactions can occur in agglutination, complement fixation and ELISA tests by antibodies to *Yersinia enterocolitica* O9, certain *Salmonella* serotypes, *Escherichia coli* O157, *Francisella tularensis, Stenotrophomonas maltophilia* and *Vibrio cholerae*. Tests using protein antigens are more specific though less sensitive and may cross react with *Ochrobactrum* spp.—environmental bacteria closely related to *Brucella* that are occasionally implicated in opportunistic infections.

Rose bengal test

The rose bengal test, a rapid agglutination test with a buffered stained antigen, is widely used as a screening test in farm animals, but also gives good results in human brucellosis, and is often used for rapid screening in endemic countries. Positive results should be confirmed by a more specific quantitative method.

Other diagnostic tests

PCR methods can detect *Brucella* specifically and also give an indication of species and some biovars. Some promising results have been obtained, particularly with regard to human diagnostics, but no standard procedures are yet agreed.

TREATMENT

Brucella infections respond to a combination of streptomycin or gentamicin with tetracycline or to rifampicin and doxycycline. Tetracycline alone is often adequate in mild cases. Fluoroquinolones may be used in combination with rifampicin or tetracyclines but are not recommended for monotherapy. Treatment should be continued for at least 6 weeks. Co-trimoxazole and rifampicin can be used in children. In patients with endocarditis and neurobrucellosis, a combination of a tetracycline, aminoglycoside and rifampicin is recommended.

EPIDEMIOLOGY

B. abortus has been eradicated from cattle in most developed countries, although there have been occasional reemergences in some parts of Europe. It was formerly common in dairy farmers, veterinarians and abattoir workers but is now rare. All human brucellosis cases in the United Kingdom, other than the very occasional recrudescence of historical UK-acquired *B. abortus* infection, are now acquired abroad; most are caused by *B. melitensis,* which is still highly prevalent in some Mediterranean countries, the Middle East, central and southern Asia, and parts of Africa and South America.

Human brucellosis due to *B. suis* is largely an occupational disease arising from contact with infected pigs or pig meat. It was once common in the United States, chiefly among those who handled raw meat shortly after slaughter. It occurs in feral pigs in Australia and the United States and is a hazard to hunters. It is widespread in domesticated pigs in various African, Asian and South American countries; biovar 4 is found only in the Arctic regions of North America and Russia.

Brucellae have potential as agents of biological warfare or bioterrorism, and this possibility should be borne in mind in the event of unexplained outbreaks.

CONTROL

The live-attenuated *B. abortus* strain S19 vaccine has been used to protect cattle from abortion and so reduce spread of the disease. It can interfere with subsequent diagnostic serology and has been replaced in some areas by the rough strain *B. abortus* RB51, which may give comparable protection, is claimed to induce less interfering antibodies and is less hazardous to humans.

The live-attenuated smooth strain *B. melitensis* Rev I is used to protect sheep and goats from *B. melitensis* infection. Vaccination of pigs is not widely practised, although the attenuated *B. suis* strain 2 has been used in China.

Effective and safe vaccines are not currently available for humans. Pasteurisation eliminates the risk of brucellosis from the consumption of infected dairy products. However, there remains the possibility of infection due to contact with infected animals or their tissues. Veterinary surgeons, farmers and laboratory workers are particularly at risk.

Eradication ultimately depends on elimination of the infection from domestic animals by a policy of compulsory testing of the animals and slaughtering of positive reactors.

BARTONELLA

The genus *Bartonella*, which is distantly related to *Brucella*, comprises at least 20 species of very small Gram-negative bacilli, most of which have been implicated in various febrile and localising diseases in humans.

- *Bartonella bacilliformis* is the cause of Oroya fever or Carrion's disease and verruga peruana. It is spread by sandflies.
- *Bart. quintana* is the cause of louse-borne trench fever.
- *Bart. henselae* and *Bart. clarridgeiae* are the most common causes of cat scratch disease and can be transmitted by fleas and possibly ticks.

Other *Bartonella* species have been identified as pathogens of dogs and other mammals. Some, including *Bart. vinsonii* (and its various subspecies), *Bart. elizabethae, Bart. alsatica, Bart. koehlerae* and *Bart. rochalimae* occasionally cause a range of syndromes involving many organ systems in humans including bacteraemia and endocarditis. *Bart. grahamii* has been implicated in ocular disease.

BARTONELLA BACILLIFORMIS

Bart. bacilliformis is responsible for outbreaks of a severe and often fatal disease of humans classically associated with high-altitude valleys of the Andes, although the geographical range is reportedly expanding. The name Oroya fever was given after an epidemic of the disease in 1870 during the building of a railway between Lima and Oroya, when 7000 labourers died within a few weeks. The infection is spread by sandflies, usually *Lutzomyia verrucarum* and *L. peruensis*.

After recovery from Oroya fever the patient may develop a skin eruption known as verruga peruana. Individuals may remain bacteraemic and act as reservoirs of infection long after recovery from the illness, or after asymptomatic infection, which probably occurs in >50% of those exposed. *Bart. bacilliformis* is pathogenic only to humans.

Description

Bart. bacilliformis is a small, strictly aerobic, Gram-negative coccobacillus. The organisms occur singly, in pairs, chains or clumps. In older cultures, they tend to be extremely pleomorphic. They are motile through a cluster of about 10 flagella situated at one end of the cell. The organism grows best at 25–28°C and at pH 7.8.

Pathogenicity

After an incubation period of about 20 days, Oroya fever presents as a high fever followed by progressively severe anaemia due to blood cell destruction. There may be enlargement of the spleen and liver and haemorrhages into the lymph nodes.

Case fatality rates of around 10% are typical for Oroya fever. Verruga peruana is a form of bacillary angiomatosis; it may occur without the initial attack of Oroya fever or may develop several weeks after recovery. A pleomorphic skin eruption of reddish, round, elevated, hard nodules may become secondarily infected, producing ulcers and haemorrhagic lesions. The rash usually appears mainly on the legs, arms and face, although all parts of the body may be affected. The condition may persist for as long as a year but is rarely fatal.

Laboratory investigation

Diagnosis of *Bartonella* infections is based on a combination of analysis of risk factors, clinical history and laboratory testing including culture, direct staining, serology, histopathology and molecular techniques. None of the techniques is ideal—culture can take several weeks, many of the serological tests have low sensitivity and specificity and PCR approaches, while explored, are not widely available. *Bart. bacilliformis* antibodies can be detected by various serological tests, but they are common in inhabitants of endemic areas and not necessarily diagnostic of active disease.

In Oroya fever, bartonellosis is confirmed by demonstrating the organisms in smears of blood or stained by Giemsa or immunofluorescent stain often in conjunction with direct culture and serology. Growth can take 5–30 days on a semisolid nutrient agar supplemented with rabbit serum and haemoglobin. In the case of verruga peruana a skin biopsy should be taken for culture and staining to reveal the organism.

Treatment

Chloramphenicol can dramatically reduce the mortality rate in Oroya fever. Penicillin, streptomycin, tetracyclines, rifampicin, fluoroquinolones and clarithromycin may also be effective in uncomplicated cases. A combination of two antimicrobials is recommended in severe cases. Blood transfusion may be necessary in severe cases of anaemia.

Control

No vaccine is available. Insecticides are used to eliminate the sandfly vector in likely breeding sites inside and outside houses and surrounding areas. As the insects bite only at night, individuals may protect themselves by withdrawing from affected areas at nightfall.

BARTONELLA QUINTANA

This organism was formerly classified among the rickettsiae as *Rochalimaea quintana*. However, unlike the rickettsiae, these organisms can grow in cell-free media, and they tend to be epicellular rather than strictly intracellular parasites of humans. Unlike *Bart. bacilliformis* the organism does not possess flagella, although it may exhibit a twitching movement owing to fimbriae.

Bart. quintana was first identified as the cause of the febrile illness known as trench fever among the troops in the First World War. It is transmitted by the body louse, *Pediculus humanus,* under unhygienic living conditions and is not uncommon among homeless people in some countries. Trench fever is a bacteraemic condition typically associated with periodic febrile episodes lasting for about 5 days. *Bart. quintana* has also been implicated in cases of angiomatosis and endocarditis. Various serological tests are available, and the organism may be isolated from the blood of patients by culture on blood agar. *Bart. vinsoni* and its subspecies are similar and can cause an identical syndrome.

BARTONELLA HENSELAE

Bart. henselae has been isolated from the blood and lymph nodes of patients suffering from cat scratch disease, a severe condition of regional lymphadenopathy and fever resulting from the scratch or bite of an infected cat. Cat fleas and ticks may be responsible for transmission. *Bart. clarridgeiae,* which can be differentiated from *Bart. henselae* by its flagella, can cause an identical syndrome.

An organism known as *Afipia felis* has also been implicated in a small proportion of cases of cat scratch disease. It is morphologically similar to *Bart. henselae,* but differs biochemically, genetically and in being culturally less fastidious.

Bart. henselae and, less frequently, *Bart. quintana* and other species have been identified in the blood and tissues of individuals suffering from two severe clinical syndromes associated with human immunodeficiency virus (HIV) or other immunosuppressant conditions:

1. *Bacillary angiomatosis,* which produces proliferative vascular lesions in the skin, regional lymph nodes and various internal organs
2. *Bacillary peliosis,* which affects the liver and spleen

Diagnosis

Bart. henselae may be cultured from the pus or from lymph node samples of patients with cat scratch disease and from blood, lymphoid tissue, liver or spleen of patients with bacillary angiomatosis or peliosis. In tissue sections the organisms are best demonstrated by silver stain or an immunospecific stain. ELISA, with various protein antigens, is the most useful serological test.

Treatment

Tetracyclines, aminoglycosides, chloramphenicol, clarithromycin and fluoroquinolones are all effective against *Bartonella* infections. In cases of endocarditis, a combination of gentamicin and doxycycline is recommended. Treatment may need to be prolonged for at least 6 weeks.

STREPTOBACILLUS MONILIFORMIS

Streptobacillus moniliformis is one of the causes of rat bite fever in humans, the other being *Spirillum minus* (see Ch. 21). It is a common commensal of the nasopharynx of rodents and sometimes causes epizootic disease in mice and rats, resulting in otitis media, multiple arthritides and swelling of the feet and legs. Laboratory workers who handle rodents are most at risk. Rarely, outbreaks of infection occur as a result of the ingestion of milk or other food contaminated by rats.

DESCRIPTION

S. moniliformis is Gram-negative, nonmotile, noncapsulate and highly pleomorphic. The organisms appear as short bacilli, forming chains interspersed with long filaments that may show oval or spherical lateral swellings.

It is a highly fastidious facultative anaerobe that benefits from added carbon dioxide and a moist atmosphere. It grows best at 37°C and pH 7.6. Culture media must contain blood, serum or ascitic fluid. Media may be made selective by addition of colistin and nalidixic acid. After incubation for 2 days, discrete, granular, greyish yellow colonies 1–5 mm in diameter are visible on the surface, and minute fried egg colonies appear in the depth of the medium. The latter are cell wall deficient L-phase variants that develop spontaneously and have little or no virulence for laboratory animals.

S. moniliformis is killed in 30 minutes by a temperature of 55°C. In culture it survives for only a few days, although it may remain viable for up to a 1 week in serum broth at 37°C. With the exception of the L-forms, *S. moniliformis* is susceptible to penicillin, and both forms are sensitive to streptomycin and tetracycline.

PATHOGENICITY

In humans the organism usually enters the body through wounds caused by rodent bites. It multiplies and invades the lymphatics and bloodstream, causing a feverish illness with severe toxic symptoms and sometimes complications such as arthritis, endocarditis and pneumonia.

Infection acquired by ingestion of contaminated water, milk or food is known as Haverhill fever, a condition characterised by fever, sore throat, rash, polyarthritis and erythema. The duration of the illness varies from a few days to several weeks. Endocarditis, hepatitis and amnionitis may develop as complications. In the preantibiotic era a case fatality rate of about 10% was reported; the rate is much lower nowadays with effective treatment.

LABORATORY INVESTIGATION

An acute febrile illness associated with asymmetric arthropathy, a maculopapular rash involving the extremities and a history of contact with rodents may point to the diagnosis.

S. moniliformis can be isolated in culture from the patient's blood during the acute phase of the illness and from the synovial fluid of those who develop arthritis and identified by conventional biochemical and carbohydrate fermentation analysis. Growth occurs in serum broth as a characteristic granular sediment, appearing like cotton wool balls that do not disintegrate on shaking.

Inoculation into rodents was used for diagnosis in the past, but other techniques such as PCR are now preferred if culture is unsuccessful. Serological tests were used historically but were not considered reliable, and there remains no validated serological test for human diagnosis.

TREATMENT

Penicillin is the treatment of choice, but clarithromycin or oral tetracycline is also effective.

RECOMMENDED READING

Al Dahouk, S., Sprague, L. D., & Neubauer, H. (2013). New developments in the diagnostic procedures for zoonotic brucellosis in humans. *Revue Scientifique et Technique (International Office of Epizootics)*, *32*(1), 177–188.

Ariza, J., Bosilkovski, M., Cascio, A., et al. Institute of Continuing Medical Education of Ioannina. (2007). Perspectives for the treatment of brucellosis in the 21st century: the Ioannina recommendations. *PLoS Medicine*, *4*(12), e317.

Corbel, M. J., & Beeching, N. J. (2011). Brucellosis. In A. S. Fauci, E. Braunwald, & D. L. Kasper (Eds.), *Harrison's Principles of Internal Medicine* (18th ed., pp. 1296–1300). McGraw-Hill.

Elliott, S. P. (2007). Rat bite fever and *Streptobacillus moniliformis*. *Clinical Microbiology Reviews*, *20*(1), 13–22.

Gaastra, W., Boot, R., Ho, H. T., & Lipman, L. J. (2009). Rat bite fever. *Veterinary Microbiology*, *133*(3), 211–228. doi:10.1016/j.vetmic.2008.09.079.

Lopez-Goni, I., & O'Callaghan, D. (Eds.). (2012). *Brucella Molecular Microbiology and Genomics*. Norfolk: Caister Academic Press.

Minnick, M. F., & Anderson, B. E. (2014). *Bartonella*. In Y.-W. Tang, M. Sussman, D. Liu, I. Poxton, & J. Schwartzman (Eds.), *Molecular Medical Microbiology* (2nd ed., pp. 1911–1939). London: Academic Press.

Murray, P. R., & Corbel, M. J. (2010). *Brucella*. In *Topley and Wilson's Microbiology and Microbial Infections*. Online.doi:10.1002/9780470688618.taw0066.

Rolain, J. M., Brouqui, P., Koehler, J. E., Maguina, C., Dolan, M. J., & Raoult, D. (2004). Recommendations for the treatment of human infections caused by *Bartonella* species. *Antimicrobial Agents and Chemotherapy*, *48*(6), 1921–1933.

32 *Treponema* and *Borrelia*

Syphilis; yaws; relapsing fever; Lyme disease

MATTHEW DRYDEN

KEY POINTS

- The genus *Treponema* includes the agents of syphilis *(T. pallidum)*, yaws *(T. pertenue)*, bejel *(T. endemicum)* and pinta *(T. carateum)*. All are essentially morphologically and antigenically identical spirochaetes, which cannot be cultivated in vitro.
- These diseases, if untreated, characteristically progress to chronic disease through distinct early and late stages and pathologies whose appearance is separated by latent periods of variable length.
- Diagnosis of syphilis, which is primarily sexually transmitted, is made by clinical observation and confirmed serologically.
- All of these organisms are sensitive to benzylpenicillin, which can be used to treat the early stages of disease.
- The genus *Borrelia* includes agents of Lyme disease *(B. burgdorferi, B. afzelii, B. garinii* and possibly others) and relapsing fevers *(B. recurrentis* and others), all of which are transmitted to humans by ticks or lice.
- Lyme disease, if untreated, may progress through distinct clinical phases (stages 1–3), resulting in later pathology (e.g., arthritis, neurological damage) in some individuals.
- Relapsing fevers are characterised by recurring periods of fever and remission associated with antigenic variation of the borreliae. Infection may be fatal.
- Lyme disease is diagnosed clinically and confirmed serologically. Doxycycline may be used to treat the early stages.

Members of the genera *Treponema* and *Borrelia* are spirochaetes. Human diseases caused by these bacteria (Table 32.1) include syphilis, whose origin is debated but which was present in the Americas before European contact and became prevalent in Europe from the 15th century onwards, and infections such as Lyme disease, the true prevalence and geographical distribution of which are still being evaluated.

Treponemal infections may be spread from person to person by intimate physical contact, by contact with infectious body fluids or, in some instances, by fomites. The treponemes that infect humans are obligate human parasites, and no other natural hosts are known. In contrast, borreliae are transmitted to humans by infected ticks or lice. There are many species of borreliae throughout the animal kingdom, and the borreliae that cause Lyme disease and endemic relapsing fever also infect many other animal species, which act as reservoirs of infection; humans are an unfortunate incidental host in the natural history of these pathogens.

Characteristically, treponemal and borrelial infections occur in several distinct clinical stages. These may be separated by periods of remission, and each stage may have a particular associated pathology. Commonly, the causative organism is detectable in early lesions but is much more difficult to identify in later disease. The pathogen spreads from the initial site of infection to many organs via the bloodstream, and, despite a vigorous immune response, in some untreated cases these infections may be progressive, destructive and, in some instances (e.g., tertiary syphilis), fatal. In other cases, only the early symptoms are apparent, and the later pathology is not seen.

Antigenic variation contributes to bacterial virulence for the relapsing fever borreliae, but in general the pathogenic mechanisms employed by spirochaetes are poorly understood. No extracellular toxins have yet been identified, and the mechanisms that enable these organisms to persist in tissues despite vigorous immune responses remain unclear. *Borrelia burgdorferi* and other borreliae can vary their surface lipoproteins to avoid the immune system. The paucity of exposed antigenic proteins on the surface of *Treponema pallidum* may contribute to immune evasion. It is also likely that the later manifestations of the treponemal and some borrelial infections involve autoimmune phenomena.

Table 32.1   Principal human diseases caused by spirochaetes

Organism	Disease	Distribution	Primary mode of transmission	Animal reservoirs
T. pallidum	Syphilis	Worldwide	Sexual, congenital	None
T. pertenue	Yaws	Tropics and subtropics	Direct contact	None
T. endemicum	Bejel	Arid, subtropical or temperate areas	Mouth to mouth via utensils	None
T. carateum	Pinta	Arid, tropical Americas	Skin-to-skin contact	None
B. recurrentis	Epidemic relapsing fever	Central, East Africa; South American Andes	Louse bites	None
Borrelia spp.	Endemic relapsing fever	Worldwide[a]	Tick bites	Yes
B. burgdorferi sensu lato	Lyme disease	Northern hemisphere; temperate climates	Tick bites	Yes

[a]Distribution governed by presence of tick vectors.

In addition to the pathogenic species, many other spirochaetes form part of the normal bacterial flora of the mouth, gut and genital tract. Morphological and antigenic similarities between pathogenic and commensal spirochaetes may cause problems in the clinical and serological diagnosis.

DESCRIPTION

Spirochaetes are slender unicellular helical or spiral rods (Fig. 32.1) with a number of distinctive ultrastructural features used in the differentiation of the genera (Fig. 32.2). The cytoplasm is surrounded by a cytoplasmic membrane, and a peptidoglycan layer contributes to cell rigidity and shape. In *Treponema* species, fine cytoplasmic filaments are visible in the bacterial cytoplasm (Fig. 32.3), but these are absent in *Borrelia* species. Members of both genera are actively motile; several flagella are attached at each pole of the cell and wrap around the bacterial cell body. In contrast to other motile bacteria, these flagella do not protrude into the surrounding medium but are enclosed within the bacterial outer membrane. Treponemal flagella are complex, comprising a sheath and core (Fig. 32.4), whereas those of *Borrelia* species are simpler and similar to the flagella of other bacteria. The spirochaetal outer membrane is unusually lipid rich and, at least in some treponemes, appears to be protein deficient and to lack lipopolysaccharide. This may account for the susceptibility of these organisms to killing by detergents and desiccation.

Although the treponemes are distantly related to Gram-negative bacteria, they do not stain by Gram's method, and modified staining procedures are used. Moreover, the pathogenic treponemes cannot be cultivated in laboratory media and are maintained by subculture in susceptible animals. In contrast, borreliae stain Gram-negative, and many pathogenic species can be cultured in vitro in enriched, serum-containing, media.

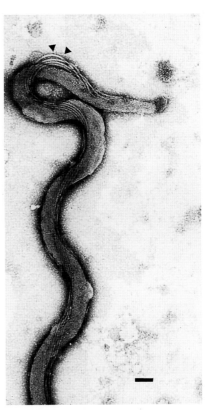

Fig. 32.1   Electron micrograph of *T. pallidum*. The flagella *(arrowheads)* are inserted at the tip and follow the helical contour of the bacterial cell enclosed within the outer membrane. Bar = 0.1 μm. (Photograph courtesy Professor C. W. Penn.)

TREPONEMA

Treponema species pathogenic for humans include the causative agents of venereal syphilis and the nonvenereal treponematoses, yaws, bejel and pinta.

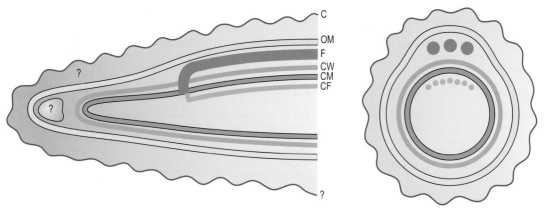

Fig. 32.2 Schematic representation of the structure of *T. pallidum* in longitudinal and cross section. *C*, Postulated capsular layer; *OM*, outer membrane; *F*, flagellum; *CW*, cell wall peptidoglycan; *CM*, cytoplasmic membrane; *CF*, cytoplasmic filaments (absent in borreliae). Areas of uncertainty (indicated by *question marks*) include the existence and form of the capsule, the continuity or otherwise of the outer membrane over the tip of the organism, the nature and form of the tip structure, and the exact juxtaposition of the ends of the cytoplasmic filaments with the bacterial flagellar basal bodies. (After Strugnell, R., Cockayne, A., & Penn, C. W. (1990). Molecular and antigenic analysis of treponemes. *Critical Reviews in Microbiology*, *17*(4), 231–250.)

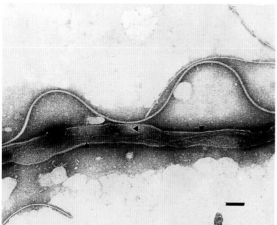

Fig. 32.3 Electron micrograph of a detergent- and protease-treated *T. pallidum* cell showing cytoplasmic filaments *(arrowheads)* in the bacterial cytoplasm. Bar = 0.1 μm.

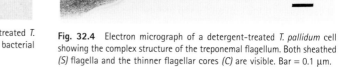

Fig. 32.4 Electron micrograph of a detergent-treated *T. pallidum* cell showing the complex structure of the treponemal flagellum. Both sheathed *(S)* flagella and the thinner flagellar cores *(C)* are visible. Bar = 0.1 μm.

The spirochaetes causing these different infections are microaerobic and morphologically identical: tightly coiled helical rods, 5–15 μm long and 0.1–0.5 μm diameter. They show only subtle antigenic differences and are characterised primarily by the clinical syndromes they cause and minor differences in the pathology induced in experimental animals.

TREPONEMA PALLIDUM SSP. PALLIDUM (T. PALLIDUM)

T. pallidum, the causative agent of syphilis, was first isolated from syphilitic lesions in 1905. Infection is usually acquired by sexual contact with infected individuals and is most common in the most sexually active age group of 15- to 30-year-olds. Congenital syphilis usually occurs following vertical transmission of *T. pallidum* from the infected mother to the foetus in utero, but neonates may also be infected during passage through the infected birth canal at delivery. Infection in utero may have serious consequences for the foetus. Rarely, syphilis has been acquired by transfusion of infected fresh human blood.

Pathogenesis

Untreated syphilis may be a progressive disease with primary, secondary, latent and tertiary stages. *T. pallidum* enters tissues by penetration of intact mucosae or through abraded skin.

The bacteria rapidly enter the lymphatics, are widely disseminated via the bloodstream and may lodge in any organ. The exact infectious dose for humans is not known, but in experimental animals, <10 organisms are sufficient to initiate infection. The bacteria multiply at the initial entry site forming a chancre, a lesion characteristic of primary syphilis, after an average incubation period of 3 weeks. The chancre is painless and most frequently on the external genitalia, but it may occur on the cervix, perianal area, in the mouth or anal canal. Chancres usually occur singly, but in immunocompromised individuals, such as those infected with the human immunodeficiency virus (HIV), multiple or persistent chancres may develop. The chancre usually heals spontaneously within 3–6 weeks, and 2–12 weeks later the symptoms of secondary syphilis develop. These are highly variable and widespread but most commonly involve the skin where macular or pustular lesions develop, particularly on the trunk and extremities. The lesions of secondary syphilis are highly infectious.

These lesions gradually resolve and a period of latent infection is entered, in which no clinical manifestations are evident, but serological evidence of infection persists. Relapse of the lesions of secondary syphilis is common, and latent syphilis is classified as early (high likelihood of relapse) or late (recurrence unlikely). Individuals with late latent syphilis are not generally considered infectious but may still transmit infection to the foetus during pregnancy, and their blood may remain infectious.

Late or tertiary syphilis may develop decades after the primary infection. It is a slowly progressive, destructive, inflammatory disease that may affect any organ. The three most common forms are neurosyphilis, cardiovascular syphilis and gummatous syphilis—a rare granulomatous lesion of the skeleton, skin or mucocutaneous tissues. Isolation of T. pallidum from patients with late syphilis is usually impossible, and much of the observed pathology may be due to autoimmune phenomena.

TREPONEMA PALLIDUM SSP. PERTENUE (T. PERTENUE)

T. pertenue is the causative agent of yaws, a disease that is endemic among rural populations in tropical and subtropical countries such as Africa, South America, Southeast Asia and Oceania. Eradication programmes sponsored by the World Health Organization reduced the number of cases to fewer than 2 million in the 1970s, but termination of the programmes led to a resurgence of pockets of disease, particularly in West Africa.

Nonvenereal infection with T. pertenue occurs following contact of traumatised skin with exudate from early yaws lesions. Infection is usually acquired before puberty. The incubation period is 3–5 weeks, and the initial lesions usually occur on the legs. The papular lesions enlarge, erode and usually heal spontaneously within 6 months. Eruption of similar lesions occurs weeks to months later, and relapse is common. Secondary lesions may involve bones, particularly the fingers, long bones and the jaw. Late yaws is characterised by cutaneous plaques and ulcers and thickening of the skin on the palms and soles of the feet. Gummatous lesions may also develop. This inflammation along with secondary bacterial infection can result in significant peripheral tissue destruction and disfigurement. In contrast to syphilis, neurological and cardiovascular damage does not occur. As affected individuals acquire infection early in life, they are essentially noninfectious at childbearing age, and congenital yaws is unknown.

TREPONEMA PALLIDUM SSP. ENDEMICUM (T. ENDEMICUM)

This organism causes a nonvenereal, syphilis-like disease called endemic syphilis or bejel. Bejel is endemic in Africa, western Asia and Australia and affects mainly children in rural populations where living conditions and personal hygiene are poor. Transmission is by direct person-to-person contact and by sharing of contaminated eating or drinking utensils.

The initial lesion is usually oral and may not be detected. Secondary lesions include oropharyngeal mucous patches, condyloma lata and periostitis. Late lesions involve gummata in the skin, nasopharynx and bones. As in yaws, the cardiovascular and central nervous systems are not involved, and congenital infection is rare because of the early age of infection.

TREPONEMA CARATEUM

Unlike the other treponematoses, the manifestations of pinta, caused by T. carateum, are confined to the skin. Although these lesions are nondestructive, they cause disfigurement with associated social problems for infected individuals. Pinta is probably the oldest human treponemal infection, with distribution now restricted to arid rural inland regions of Mexico, Central America and Colombia.

Spread of infection is by direct contact with infectious lesions. After a 7- to 21-day incubation period, small erythematous pruritic primary lesions develop, most commonly on the extremities, face, neck, chest or abdomen. The primary lesions enlarge and coalesce and once healed may leave areas of hypopigmentation. Disseminated secondary lesions appear 3–12 months later and may become dyschromic. Recurrence of lesions is common for up to 10 years after the initial infection. The depigmented lesions are characteristic of the later stages of pinta but do not cause any serious harm.

OTHER *TREPONEMA* SPECIES

Treponemes are implicated in several other human infections. The microbial flora associated with these conditions is complex, and the exact role of the spirochaetes in the aetiology of infection remains to be determined. Moreover, the taxonomic status of some of these organisms is uncertain.

Oral infections

T. denticola, T. socranskii and *T. pectinovorum* form part of the normal flora, and the numbers of these organisms increase in acute necrotising ulcerative gingivitis and chronic adult periodontal disease. *T. vincentii* (or Vincent's spirillum) is similarly associated with ulceromembranous gingivitis or pharyngitis, Vincent's angina. Several spirochaetes appear to be involved in the aetiology of a similar condition called trench mouth.

Gastrointestinal infections

Several as yet unidentified weakly haemolytic spirochaetes have been implicated in the aetiology of persistent diarrhoea and rectal bleeding in certain human populations. A morphologically similar but genetically distinct organism, *Brachyspira* (formerly *Serpulina*) *hyodysenteriae,* is the cause of swine dysentery.

Skin lesions

Tropical ulcer is a chronic skin condition in which spirochaetes of unknown identity have been implicated, usually in association with fusiform bacteria and other organisms.

LABORATORY INVESTIGATION

The inability to grow most pathogenic treponemes in vitro, coupled with the transitory nature of many of the lesions, makes diagnosis of treponemal infection impossible by routine bacteriological methods. Although spirochaetes are detectable by microscopy in primary and secondary lesions, diagnosis is based primarily on clinical observations and confirmed by serological tests. For practical purposes, the serological responses to all these pathogens are identical, and only their use in the serodiagnosis of syphilis is considered here.

Direct microscopy

Treponemes can be visualised directly in freshly collected exudate from primary or secondary lesions by dark-ground or phase-contrast microscopy. Although this method allows a rapid definitive diagnosis to be made, it is rather insensitive because primary lesions may contain relatively few bacteria. In addition, care must be taken to differentiate between pathogenic and commensal spirochaetes, which may occasionally contaminate such material. More sensitive and specific results may be obtained using fixed material in an immunofluorescence assay with an antitreponemal antibody.

Serological tests

Infection with *T. pallidum* results in the rapid production of two types of antibodies:

1. Specific antibodies directed primarily at polypeptide antigens of the bacterium
2. Nonspecific antibodies (reagin antibodies) that react with a nontreponemal antigen called cardiolipin

The mechanism of induction of nonspecific antibodies remains unclear. Cardiolipin is a phospholipid extracted from beef heart, and it is possible that a similar substance, present in the treponemal cell or released from host cells damaged by the bacterium, may stimulate antibody production.

Historically, assays for nonspecific antibody were used as routine screening tests for evidence of syphilis because of their low cost and technical simplicity. Enzyme immunosorbent assays that detect specific treponemal antibodies are increasingly replacing the older tests for screening purposes.

Nonspecific serological tests for syphilis

The rapid plasma reagin (RPR) test, which has now largely superseded the earlier Venereal Disease Research Laboratory (VDRL) test, is a nonspecific serological test for syphilis that uses cardiolipin as antigen. Immunoglobulin (Ig) M or IgG antibody present in positive sera causes a suspension of this lipoidal antigen to flocculate, and the result can be read rapidly by eye. Both of these assays may be used as screening tests and are positive in approximately 70% of primary and 99% of secondary syphilitics but are negative in individuals with late syphilis. These tests can be used quantitatively, and increases in antibody titres with time may be used to confirm a diagnosis of congenital syphilis. The RPR assay is not suitable for use with cerebrospinal fluid.

As a positive result in these tests usually indicates active infection, they can also be used to monitor the efficacy of antibacterial therapy.

Tests for specific antibody

Fluorescent treponemal antibody absorption (FTA-Abs) test   This is an indirect immunofluorescence assay in which *T. pallidum* is used as an antigen. Acetone-fixed treponemes are incubated with heat-treated sera, and bound antibody is detected with a fluorescein-labelled conjugate and ultraviolet microscopy. The serum is first absorbed with a suspension of a nonpathogenic treponeme, which removes nonspecific cross-reactive antibodies that may be directed against commensal spirochaetes. The FTA-Abs test is positive in approximately 80%, 100% and 95% of primary, secondary and late syphilitics, respectively, and, unlike the RPR and VDRL tests, remains positive following successful therapy.

T. pallidum haemagglutination assay (TPHA)   In this test, *T. pallidum* antigen is coated onto the surface of red blood cells, and specific antibody in test sera causes haemagglutination. As in the FTA-Abs assay, sera are preabsorbed with a nonpathogenic treponeme to remove antibody against commensal spirochaetes. The TPHA test is less sensitive than the FTA-Abs test in primary syphilis (positive in 65%), but both give similar results for secondary and late syphilis; the TPHA also remains positive for life following infection. This assay can be used to detect localised production of antitreponemal antibodies in cerebrospinal fluid, a marker of neurosyphilis. The *T. pallidum* particle agglutination (TPPA) test works on the same principle as the TPHA, but treponemal antigen is coated onto coloured gelatin particles rather than red blood cells.

Enzyme immunoassay   In these tests monoclonal anti–*T. pallidum* antibodies are used to detect antibody responses to individual treponemal antigens. This allows rapid screening of large numbers of samples with potentially enhanced specificity. Assays that detect either IgM or IgG are available. Positive results should be confirmed by a second specific test such as the TPHA.

Problems in the serological diagnosis of syphilis

Occasionally, both the nonspecific and specific tests produce false-positive results. The RPR and VDRL assays may give a transient positive result following any strong immunological stimulus such as acute bacterial or viral infection or after immunisation. More persistent false-positive results occur in individuals with autoimmune or connective tissue disease, in drug abusers and in individuals with hypergammaglobulinaemia. False-positive results

usually become apparent when negative results are found in specific serological tests, but in some cases FTA-Abs results may also be positive or borderline.

Rarely, the FTA-Abs test may be positive and the nonspecific VDRL test negative. Lyme disease (see later in the chapter) induces antibodies that react in the FTA-Abs but not in the VDRL assay. Other spirochaetal diseases such as relapsing fever, yaws, pinta and leptospirosis may give positive results in both specific and nonspecific tests. Of particular difficulty is the differential diagnosis of syphilis and yaws in immigrants from areas in which yaws is endemic.

Some of the newer enzyme immunoassays are less sensitive in cases of primary syphilis.

Direct detection of spirochaetal deoxyribonucleic acid (DNA) in clinical material by molecular methods, such as the polymerase chain reaction (PCR), may have a future role in confirming a diagnosis of syphilis in difficult or atypical cases.

TREATMENT

All the pathogenic treponemes are sensitive to benzylpenicillin, and prolonged high-dose therapy with procaine penicillin has been the traditional method of treatment for primary and secondary syphilis. So far there have been no reports of penicillin resistance. If penicillin allergy is a problem, erythromycin, tetracycline or chloramphenicol may be used. There are reports of treatment failure with erythromycin, and an erythromycin-resistant variant of *T. pallidum* has been isolated. In late syphilis, aqueous benzylpenicillin is used, as this penetrates better into the central nervous system. In neurosyphilis, successful eradication of the organism may not result in a clinical cure. More aggressive and prolonged antibiotic therapy may be required in HIV-positive patients with syphilis owing to impaired immune function.

Antibiotic therapy of syphilitics, particularly with penicillin, characteristically induces a systemic response called the Jarisch–Herxheimer reaction. This is characterised by the rapid onset (within 2 hours) of fever, chills, myalgia, tachycardia, hyperventilation, vasodilatation and hypotension. The response is thought to be due to release of an endogenous pyrogen from the spirochaetes.

EPIDEMIOLOGY AND CONTROL

Syphilis

The widespread introduction of antibiotic therapy shortly after the Second World War produced a dramatic decrease in the incidence of syphilis, but the disease remained endemic within the general population. Geographically localised outbreaks of syphilis, associated with specific recreational activities and lifestyles, now occur in countries such as the United Kingdom.

In the mid-1980s most cases of syphilis in developed countries occurred in male homosexuals. The advent of HIV and the acquired immune deficiency syndrome (AIDS) in the 1980s reduced the incidence among this group owing to changes in sexual practices. The early 1990s saw a resurgence of syphilis among the heterosexual population in the United States, resulting in an increased incidence among women and in the number of cases of congenital syphilis. Subsequent changes in sexual practices among homosexual men have reversed this trend: significantly more cases of primary and secondary syphilis now occur in men than women, and, among males, >60% of cases occur in men who have sex with men. The incidence of congenital syphilis has fallen from 2435 cases in 1994 to 427 in 2009. Total reported numbers of cases of syphilis in the United States were 46,291 in 2008 and 44,828 in 2009.

In the United Kingdom, ongoing outbreaks of syphilis in various regions have seen the number of cases rise consistently from 2000, peaking at around 3700 cases of infectious syphilis in 2007. Most cases of infectious syphilis (>70%) currently occur among men who have sex with men but significant numbers of cases are still detected in heterosexual men and women. Syphilis therefore continues to pose major public health issues. The potential for congenital infection and the acquisition of syphilis by blood transfusion means that screening programmes of all pregnant women and blood donations are still required.

Control of syphilis is achieved by treating index cases and any known contacts. Treatment of contacts is important as some may be incubating the infection even if they have no overt signs of disease.

Control of the disease may have additional benefits: primary syphilis increases the risk of HIV infection two- to five-fold, presumably by permitting easier access of the virus through damaged skin or mucosal membranes.

Other treponematoses

The incidence of the other treponematoses is influenced primarily by socioeconomic factors. Prevention and control involve treatment of individuals with active or latent disease and contacts and improvement of living conditions and personal hygiene.

BORRELIA

The two principal human diseases associated with borreliae are relapsing fever, caused by *Borrelia recurrentis* and

several other *Borrelia* species, and Lyme disease or Lyme borreliosis, a multisystem infection caused by *B. burgdorferi sensu lato*. The bacteria causing these infections are morphologically similar helical rods, 8–30 μm long and 0.2–0.5 μm in diameter, with three to ten loose spirals. Antigenic and genetic differences are used to differentiate the species.

RELAPSING FEVERS

Relapsing fevers are characterised clinically by recurrent periods of fever and spirochaetaemia.

Endemic or tick-borne relapsing fever is a zoonosis caused by several *Borrelia* species, including *B. duttoni, B. hermsii, B. parkeri* and *B. turicatae,* and is transmitted to humans by soft-bodied *Ornithodoros* ticks. The natural hosts for these organisms include rodents and other small mammals on which the ticks normally feed. The disease occurs worldwide, reflecting the distribution of the tick vector. A recently characterised strain, *B. miyamotoi,* has been placed within the relapsing fever group of borreliae. It has been associated with a febrile illness in patients bitten by ticks, but the full extent of its pathogenicity and geographical distribution has yet to be determined.

Epidemic or louse-borne relapsing fever is caused by *B. recurrentis,* an obligate human pathogen transmitted from person to person by the body louse, *Pediculus humanus.* The incidence is influenced by socioeconomic factors such as lack of personal hygiene, and, historically, increases during periods of war, famine and other social upheaval. The disease still occurs in central and eastern Africa and in the South American Andes.

The spirochaetes causing the two forms of relapsing fever differ in their mode of growth in the arthropod vector, and this influences the way in which human infection is initiated. *B. recurrentis* grows in the haemolymph of the louse but does not invade tissues. As a result the louse faeces are not infectious, and the bacterium is not transferred through eggs to the progeny. Human infection occurs when bacteria released from crushed lice gain entry to tissues through damaged or intact skin or mucous membranes. Spirochaetes causing tick-borne relapsing fever invade all the tissues of the tick, including the salivary glands, genitalia and excretory system. Infection occurs when saliva or excrement is released during feeding. Transovarial transmission to the tick progeny maintains the spirochaete in the tick population.

Pathogenesis

In both forms of relapsing fever, acute symptoms, including high fever, rigors, headache, myalgia, arthralgia, photophobia and cough, develop about 1 week after infection.

A skin rash may occur, and there is central nervous system involvement in up to 30% of cases. During the acute phase there may be up to 10^5 spirochaetes per cubic millimetre of blood. The primary illness resolves within 3–6 days, and terminates abruptly with hypotension and shock, which may be fatal. Relapse of fever occurs 7–10 days later, and several relapses may take place.

Each episode of spirochaetaemia is terminated by the development of specific antispirochaete antibody. Subsequent febrile episodes are caused by borreliae that differ antigenically, particularly in outer membrane protein composition, from those causing earlier attacks. As the cycle of fever and relapse continues, the borreliae tend to revert back to the antigenic types that caused the original spirochaetaemia, and ultimate clearance of the infection appears to be due to antibody-mediated killing.

In general, louse-borne relapsing fever has longer febrile and afebrile periods than tick-borne infection but fewer relapses. The case fatality rate varies from 4% to 40% for louse-borne infection and from 2% to 5% for tick-borne relapsing fever, with myocarditis, cerebral haemorrhage and liver failure the most common causes of death.

Laboratory investigation

Definitive diagnosis of relapsing fevers is made by detection of borreliae in peripheral blood samples. Thick or thin blood smears are stained with Giemsa or other stains such as acridine orange.

Although antibodies to the borreliae are produced during infection, serological tests are complicated by antigenic variation and the tendency to relapse. Serological tests for syphilis are positive in 5%–10% of cases.

Molecular diagnostics, PCR, for relapsing fever strains of borreliae on blood, is being developed for improved diagnosis.

Treatment

Tetracycline, chloramphenicol, penicillin and erythromycin have been used successfully. As in the treatment of syphilis, antibiotics may elicit a Jarisch–Herxheimer reaction.

Prevention of infection involves avoidance or eradication of the insect vector. Insecticides can be used to eradicate ticks from human dwellings, but elimination from the environment is not feasible. Prevention of louse-borne infection involves maintenance of good personal hygiene and delousing if necessary.

LYME DISEASE

Lyme disease, originally called Lyme arthritis, was recognised as an infectious condition in 1975 following an epidemiological investigation of a cluster of cases of suspected juvenile rheumatoid arthritis that occurred in Lyme, Connecticut, United States. A common factor in these cases was a previous history of an arthropod bite, and the infectious agent, *B. burgdorferi*, was subsequently isolated from an *Ixodes* tick. Retrospective serological data suggest that Lyme disease was endemic in the United States as early as 1962, and the clinical manifestations of this infection have been known in Europe, including the United Kingdom, since the early 1900s. Lyme disease has also been reported in Scandinavia, Eastern Europe, China and Japan. It is a disease of northern boreal forests.

The natural hosts for *B. burgdorferi* are wild animals, principally small rodents and birds. The larger animal hosts such as deer are probably more important in maintaining the size of tick populations and disseminating the pathogen rather than acting as a major source of *B. burgdorferi*. Infection in these animals may be inapparent, although clinical infection has been observed in domestic animals such as cattle, horses and dogs.

B. burgdorferi is transmitted to humans by ixodid ticks that become infected while feeding on infected animals. The principal vectors in the United States are *Ixodes dammini* and *I. pacificus* and in Europe *I. ricinus*. The life cycle of these ticks involves larval, nymph and adult stages, all of which are capable of transmitting infection, although the nymphal stage is most commonly implicated. In areas endemic for Lyme disease, 2%–50% of ticks may carry *B. burgdorferi*. Carriage rates vary geographically and by season. The bacterium grows primarily in the midgut of the tick, and transmission to humans occurs during regurgitation of the gut contents during the blood meal. Transmission efficiency appears to be relatively low but increases with the duration of feeding.

Although there is general similarity, clinical manifestations may differ in the United States and Europe. Host tissue tropism varies depending on the infecting strain. This variation is due in part to significant differences in the antigenic structure of bacterial strains causing infection in the two continents and has resulted in the division of *B. burgdorferi* into three distinct genospecies:

- *B. burgdorferi sensu stricto* is the sole cause of Lyme disease in the United States, where Lyme arthritis is a common complication of infection.
- *B. afzeli* and *B. garinii* are responsible for most Lyme disease in Europe and are associated with chronic skin and neurological manifestations, respectively.

Several other genetically distinct isolates of *B. burgdorferi* have been identified in ticks, but their importance in human infection has yet to be established.

Lyme disease may be a progressive illness and is divided into three stages:

- **Stage 1** is characterised by a spreading annular rash, *erythema chronicum migrans* (ECM), which occurs at the site of the tick bite 3–22 days after infection. Lesions may contain very small numbers of bacteria, and the disproportionate intensity of the pathology seen may be due to stimulation of cytokines such as tumour necrosis factor-α and secondary mediators. The bacterium also spreads to various other organs. In the United States, secondary lesions similar to those of ECM are common. Malaise, fatigue, headache, rigors and neck stiffness may also be apparent. The rash and secondary lesions fade within 3–4 weeks.
- **Stage 2** develops in some patients after several weeks or months. These patients exhibit cardiac or neurological abnormalities, musculoskeletal symptoms or intermittent arthritis. The neurological manifestations include cranial nerve palsies, radiculopathy, peripheral neuritis, myelitis and meningoencephalitis.
- **Stage 3** may ensue months to years later, when patients present with chronic skin *(acrodermatitis chronicum)*, nervous system or joint abnormalities.

Congenital infection has been rarely described with serious, potentially fatal, consequences for the foetus.

Borreliosis may also be entirely asymptomatic. Occupational exposure may occur, and groups such as forestry workers have been found to have a high rate of seropositivity along with a complete absence of reported symptoms. A small minority of patients with treated Lyme may experience persistent nonspecific symptoms of fatigue, myalgia and abnormal sensation. Clinical examination and routine investigations are generally normal. The concept of chronic Lyme is controversial, and there is much misleading information online regarding the diagnosis, investigation and management. It has become a fashionable label for patients with chronic non-specific symptoms, although it is difficult to demonstrate the presence of any active infection in such patients and also difficult to disprove that they have not had Lyme disease. Patient advocacy groups promoting and politicising this diagnosis have become prominent in many, mostly Anglo-Saxon countries, including Australia, where *B. burgdorferi* has never been identified and no cases of locally acquired Lyme have ever been confirmed. Such groups claim that serology has poor diagnostic sensitivity and that Lyme must be diagnosed clinically by 'Lyme literate' doctors.

Laboratory investigation

Once a clinical diagnosis has been made, serological tests are used routinely for the confirmation of Lyme disease, although antibodies are slow to rise and are not generally helpful in the first stage of infection, which should be treated empirically on clinical diagnosis. Serology is the mainstay of laboratory investigation. PCR can be performed on biopsies of skin lesions and other sterile sites such as CSF. Culture of the spirochaete from suitable biopsy material in specialist media is possible in research facilities.

The antibody response is very variable. Specific IgM and certain IgG antibodies develop within 3–8 weeks of infection. The earliest response appears to be against the bacterial flagellum and certain binding and outer surface proteins. Antibodies to different structural proteins develop during the course of the disease. Early treatment is said to abrogate the antibody response, presumably by successful eradication of the borreliae. High levels of IgG are generally produced in active infection. IgM may persist for many months and years but in some cases never be present at all. Antibody levels fall in time after successful treatment. Enzyme-linked immunosorbent assay (ELISA) is now widely used, and these tests for outer membrane and flagellar antibodies are very sensitive, except in the early weeks of infection. Immunoblotting with a panel of carefully selected recombinant antigens is used to confirm serological results. Immunoblotting was introduced to rule out false-positive ELISAs rather than as a back-up test. Serological diagnosis of early Lyme disease may still pose problems, as antibodies to the bacterium are slow to develop in some individuals and the formation of immune complexes may affect the test results. Antibodies that cross-react with *B. burgdorferi* may be produced after infection with other spirochaetes, and indeed some viral infections. Sera from patients with Lyme disease may give a positive FTA-Abs test, although the VDRL test is negative. Samples from patients who have received pooled human immunoglobulin often give false-positive results.

Serological evidence of infection may be detectable in the apparent absence of overt disease. The significance of these findings is unclear, but it is possible that such individuals may develop late complications of Lyme disease.

Indirect tests such as lymphocyte transformation tests and lymphocyte subset analysis have no place in the diagnosis of Lyme as yet. These tests have not been clinically validated.

Treatment

Early Lyme (ECM with or without a flulike illness following a tick bite) should be treated empirically with 14 days of doxycycline (amoxicillin for children or pregnant women). Penicillins, macrolides, cephalosporins and tetracyclines have all been used successfully. About 15%

of patients experience a Jarisch–Herxheimer reaction after antibiotic therapy. There have been relapses with macrolide treatment. Despite antibiotic treatment, a minority of patients suffer from nonspecific late complications of the disease, which may be mediated immunologically. Long-term antibiotic treatment has not been shown to improve symptoms.

Early-stage Lyme disease responds to 2 weeks of oral antibiotics. Longer courses of oral antibiotics (21–28 days) can effectively treat most early and uncomplicated neuroborreliosis, for example, facial palsy or radiculopathy. Severe neuroborreliosis such as meningoencephalitis, myelitis and widespread involvement usually requires initial intravenous treatment with a cephalosporin such as ceftriaxone.

Epidemiology and control

The geographical distribution of Lyme disease is governed by that of the tick vector and its associated animal hosts. Forestry workers and farmers are particularly at risk, but infection is also increasingly associated with recreational activities. In the United Kingdom, Lyme disease occurs in areas that support large populations of wild or domesticated animals on which ixodid ticks feed. In the United Kingdom the geographical distribution appears to be extending, although the incidence of infection remains much lower than in some central and Eastern European countries. Infection may also be acquired after travel to countries where Lyme disease is endemic. It is difficult to accurately assess the true incidence of Lyme disease because infection may be mild or asymptomatic and, consequently, not detected. In 2015 there were 720 laboratory-confirmed cases in the United Kingdom, but estimated case numbers range from 1000 to 3000 per year because some cases are treated empirically in primary care, and aetiology is never established. By comparison, approximately 30,000 confirmed cases were reported in the United States in 2009. Patient advocacy groups claim much higher numbers, but this is not supported by validated diagnostic methods.

Prevention of infection involves education of the public regarding avoiding tick bites and tick removal as well as the possible risks of infection. Eradication of the tick vectors or mammalian hosts from such areas is not feasible. A vaccine to protect residents and visitors in areas in which Lyme disease is endemic would be useful, but attempts to develop effective and safe recombinant vaccines against *B. burgdorferi* have so far been unsuccessful.

RECOMMENDED READING

Antal, G. M., Lukehart, S. A., & Meheus, A. Z. (2002). The endemic treponematoses. *Microbes and Infection, 4*(1), 83–94.
British Infection Association. (2011). The epidemiology, prevention, investigation and treatment of Lyme borreliosis in United Kingdom patients: a position statement by the British Infection Association. *The Journal of Infection, 62*(5), 329–338.
Cullen, P. A., Haake, D. A., & Adler, B. (2004). Outer membrane proteins of pathogenic spirochetes. *FEMS Microbiology Reviews, 28*(3), 291–318.
Dryden, M., Saeed, K., Ogborn, S., & Swales, P. (2014). Lyme borreliosis in southern United Kingdom and a case for a new syndrome, chronic arthropod-borne neuropathy. *Epidemiology and Infection, 9*, 1–12. doi:10.1017/S0950268814001071.
Edwards, A. M., Dymock, D., & Jenkinson, H. F. (2003). From tooth to hoof: treponemes in tissue-destructive diseases. *Journal of Applied Microbiology, 94*(5), 767–780.
Egglestone, S. I., & Turner, A. J. (2000). Serological diagnosis of syphilis: PHLS Syphilis Serology Working Group. *Communicable Disease and Public Health, 3*(3), 158–162.
Herremans, T., Kortbeek, L., & Notermans, D. W. (2010). A review of diagnostic tests for congenital syphilis in newborns. *European Journal of Clinical Microbiology & Infectious Diseases: Official Publication of the European Society of Clinical Microbiology, 29*(5), 495–501. doi:10.1007/s10096-010-0900-8.

Larsson, C., Andersson, L. C., & Bergstrom, S. (2009). Current issues in relapsing fever. *Current Opinion in Infectious Diseases, 22*(5), 443–449.
Lee, V., & Kinghorn, G. (2008). Syphilis: an update. *Clinical Medicine (London, England), 8*(3), 330–333.
Mygland, A., Ljøstad, U., Fingerle, V., Rupprecht, T., Schmutzhard, E., Steiner, I., & European Federation of Neurological Societies. (2010). EFNS guidelines on the diagnosis and management of European Lyme neuroborreliosis. *European Journal of Neurology, 17*(1), 8–16, e1–4. doi:10.1111/j.1468-1331.2009.02862.x.
O'Connell, S. (2010). Lyme borreliosis: current issues in diagnosis and management. *Current Opinion in Infectious Diseases, 23*(3), 231–235. doi:10.1097/QCO.0b013e32833890e2.
Stanek, G., Fingerle, V., Hunfeld, K. P., Jaulhac, B., Kaiser, R., Krause, A., ... Gray, J. (2011). Lyme borreliosis: clinical case definitions for diagnosis and management in Europe. *Clinical Microbiology and Infection, 17*(1), 69–79. doi:10.1111/j.1469-0691.2010.03175.x.

Websites

Centers for Disease Control and Prevention. Syphilis. Available at http://www.cdc.gov/std/syphilis/.
Public Health England. https://www.gov.uk/government/collections/lyme-disease-guidance-data-and-analysis.

33 *Leptospira*

Leptospirosis; Weil's disease; multi-system pathology

MATHIEU PICARDEAU

KEY POINTS

- The term *leptospirosis* is used to describe all infections in humans and animals, regardless of the clinical presentation or strain of *Leptospira* involved.
- The incidence rate is low in Europe (<1 case/100,000 inhabitants) and associated predominantly with occupational or recreational exposure.
- Leptospirosis is considered as an emerging or reemerging zoonotic disease.
- Antibiotics offer some benefit if started within 4 days of the onset of illness and preferably within 24–48 hours.
- Animals that acquire infection may not develop discernible disease but become long-term carriers, so-called maintenance hosts.
- More than 200 pathogenic serovars are known, and each is able to infect a range of animals that may become long-term carriers capable of infecting others. The organisms can also survive for long periods in the environment. Together, these features make control of leptospirosis a substantial challenge.

The recognition of human leptospirosis as a distinct clinical entity is usually attributed to Adolf Weil of the University of Heidelberg in 1886, although the disease had been described in animals since the mid-19th century. The term *Weil's disease* acknowledges Weil's observations in differentiating what was later proven to be a leptospiral infection from other forms of infective jaundice.

In 1914, Ryokichi Inada and his colleagues in Kyushu, Japan, observed spiral organisms in the livers of guinea pigs inoculated with blood taken from Japanese miners with infectious jaundice, presumed to be Weil's disease. They named the organisms *Spirochaeta icterohaemorrhagiae,* reflecting their spiral shape and the fact that human infections were associated with jaundice (icterus) and haemorrhage. In Europe, similar organisms were demonstrated in some cases of jaundice in German soldiers involved in the First World War. In 1917, another Japanese scientist, Hideyo Noguchi, recognised that the organisms associated with Weil's disease differed from other known spirochaetes and proposed the genus name *Leptospira,* meaning a slender coil. Today, >300 serovars have then been isolated from the environment, animals and humans.

Leptospirosis is a zoonosis and has one of the widest geographical distributions of any zoonotic disease. The highest incidence is found in tropical and subtropical parts of the world. Probably every mammal has the potential to become a carrier of some serovar of *Leptospira*. These carriers harbour leptospires in their kidneys and excrete the bacteria into the environment when they urinate. This enables spread among their own kind and to other species, including humans, who may directly or indirectly come into contact with their urine.

In humans, the disease varies in severity from a mild self-limiting illness to the fulminating and potentially fatal disease described by Weil. Fortunately, full recovery without long-term morbidity is the most frequent outcome.

DESCRIPTION

Classification

The family Leptospiraceae belongs to the order Spirochaetales and can be subdivided into three genera: *Leptospira, Leptonema* and *Turneriella*. Only *Leptospira* spp. are considered to be pathogenic for animals and humans.

The genus *Leptospira* contains 22 species that can be divided into three groups:

- ten pathogenic species *(L. interrogans, L. kirschneri, L. borgpetersenii, L. santarosai, L. noguchii, L. weilii, L. alexanderi, L. alstoni, L. kmetyi* and *L. mayottensis)*
- six saprophytic species *(L. biflexa, L. wolbachii, L. meyeri, L. vanthielii, L. terpstrae* and *L. yanagawae)*
- six 'intermediate' species *(L. inadai, L. broomii, L. fainei, L. wolffii, L. idonii* and *L. licerasiae),* which are of unclear pathogenicity

Pathogens and saprophytes differ in their nutritional requirements and other phenotypic properties. For example, the growth of pathogenic strains is inhibited by the purine analogue 8-azaguanine, whereas saprophytic strains grow normally in the presence of this compound. Similarly, unlike *L. interrogans*, *L. biflexa* can grow at low ambient temperature (11–13°C).

Leptospires are serologically classified in serovars, defined on the basis of structural heterogeneity in the carbohydrate component of the lipopolysaccharide (LPS). More than 200 different pathogenic serovars are currently recognised.

The genetic classification of *Leptospira* does not correlate with the phenotypic classification because serovars of the same serogroup may be distributed among different species. However, the serological classification is still widely used as it provides useful information for clinical or epidemiological investigations. The accepted nomenclature is generic name, followed by species name, followed by serovar, followed by strain (if appropriate). For example:

- *Leptospira* (generic name) *interrogans* (species name) serovar Icterohaemorrhagiae
- *Leptospira* (generic name) *interrogans* (species name) serovar Hardjo strain Hardjoprajitno.

The complete DNA sequence of hundreds of strains belonging to saprophytic and pathogenic strains has been determined, and comparative genomics should provide insight into the molecular mechanisms of the survival and persistence of *Leptospira* in host and environment.

The organism

Leptospires range between about 6 and 20 μm in length but are only about 0.1 μm in diameter, which allows them to pass through filters that retain most other bacteria. They are Gram-negative but take up conventional stains poorly. They can be visualised by Giemsa staining, silver deposition, fluorescent antibody methods or electron microscopy. These bacteria are so thin that they are best viewed by dark-field microscopy. They have a helical-cell shape with one or both ends appearing hooked, and they rotate rapidly around their long axis (Fig. 33.1).

Leptospira spp. possess a double-membrane structure composed of a cytoplasmic membrane, the periplasm and the outer membrane that contains the LPS and many membrane-associated lipoproteins, which are the main targets for the host immune response. Two endoflagella with their free ends towards the middle of the bacteria lie in the periplasmic space between the cell wall and the outer envelope and are wrapped around the cell wall. Each flagellum is attached to a basal body located at either end of the cell. The flagella are similar in structure to those

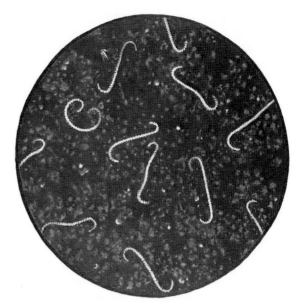

Fig. 33.1 Appearance of living leptospires as seen by dark-field microscopy. Note the very fine coils and characteristic hooked ends. (From an original painting by Dr Cranston Low. In Low, R. C., & Dodds, T. C. (1947). *Atlas of Bacteriology*. Edinburgh: Livingstone.)

of other bacteria and are responsible for motility, but the mechanism involved in their rapid movement is incompletely understood.

Leptospires are killed rapidly by desiccation, extremes of pH (e.g., gastric acid) and antibacterial substances that occur naturally in human and bovine milks. They are susceptible to low concentrations of chlorine and are killed by temperatures above 40°C (after about 10 minutes at 50°C and within 10 seconds at 60°C).

METABOLISM

Leptospires require aerobic or microaerophilic conditions for growth. Adequate sources of nitrogen, phosphate, calcium, magnesium and iron (as a haem compound or ferric ions) are essential. They can use fatty acids as their major energy source but are unable to synthesise long-chain fatty acids with 15 or more carbon atoms. Pathogenic species require the presence of unsaturated fatty acids to utilise saturated fatty acids. Vitamins B_1 (thiamin) and B_{12} (cyanocobalamin) are also essential, and the addition of biotin is needed for the growth of some strains. These components are provided in Ellinghausen–McCullough–Johnson–Harris (EMJH) medium.

Optimal growth of pathogenic species in culture takes place at 28–30°C, at pH 7.2–7.6. They are slow growing, with a generation time of about 20 hours: colonies are visible after 3–4 weeks on solid medium, whereas saprophytes grow more rapidly (colonies are visible after 1 week). Culture media do not generally contain selective agents as leptospires may be sensitive to them, so great care must be taken to avoid bacterial or fungal contamination at the time of inoculation and during the prolonged incubation period.

PATHOGENESIS

The molecular mechanisms of virulence of pathogenic strains remain poorly understood.

Infection is acquired by direct or indirect contact with infected urine, tissues or secretions. Ingestion or inhalation of leptospires is not thought to pose a risk, and human-to-human spread is very rare. Leptospires generally gain entry through small areas of damage on the skin or via mucous membranes. It is possible that they may also pass through waterlogged skin, although this is probably not a major route of infection.

The term *leptospirosis* is used to describe all infections in both humans and animals, regardless of the clinical presentation or strain of *Leptospira* involved. There are no serovar-specific disease patterns, although some serovars tend to cause more severe disease than others. In the past, many names (epidemic pulmonary haemorrhagic fever, cane cutter's disease, Fort Bragg fever, Weil's disease, autumnal fever etc.) were used to describe the particular clinical presentation or to reflect occupational, geographical, seasonal or other epidemiological features of leptospiral disease. Because of this, the full range of disease presentations was not appreciated and, even now, leptospiral infection may not be suspected unless the patient has the classically severe disease involving the liver and kidneys described originally by Weil. Some reports suggest that human infection with some serovars can, in rare cases, cause abortion.

CLINICAL FEATURES

Typically, acute symptoms develop 5–14 days after infection, although rarely the incubation period can be as short as 2–3 days or as long as 30 days. The infection presents with an influenza-like illness characterised by the sudden onset of headache, muscular pain, especially in the muscles of the lower back and calf, fever and occasionally rigors. Conjunctival suffusion and a skin rash may be seen in some cases.

During a bacteraemic phase lasting 7–8 days after the onset of symptoms, the leptospires spread via the blood to many tissues, including the brain. In severe

cases the illness often follows a biphasic course: the bacteraemic phase is followed by an immune phase, with the appearance of antibody and the disappearance of recoverable leptospires from the blood. In this phase patients may show signs of recovery for a couple of days before the fever, rigors, severe headaches and meningism return. Bleeding may occur, together with signs and symptoms of jaundice and renal impairment. Typically, bilirubin concentrations are markedly raised, but other liver function test results may be only moderately increased.

In some cases of leptospirosis, pulmonary manifestations of infection are predominant. Patients can present with cough, shortness of breath or haemoptysis. In severe cases, adult respiratory distress syndrome and pulmonary haemorrhage can supervene and lead to death.

In severe fulminating disease the patient may die within the first few days of illness, but with appropriate treatment the prognosis is usually good. Many deaths throughout the world are due to the failure to provide adequate supportive management, especially in relation to the maintenance of renal function. Generally, patients are well within 2–6 weeks, but some require up to 3 months to recover fully. In a few patients, symptoms persist for many months, but neither long-term carriage of leptospires nor chronic disease has been conclusively demonstrated in humans.

After infection, immunity develops against the infecting strain but may not fully protect against infection with unrelated strains.

LABORATORY INVESTIGATION

The initial diagnosis must rely on the medical history and clinical findings backed up with details of possible occupational or recreational exposure.

Serology

Antibodies can usually be demonstrated by the sixth day after symptoms have developed (Fig. 33.2), although their detection may be delayed if antibiotics were administered early in the course of the illness.

The microscopic agglutination test (MAT), which can indicate the likely infecting serogroup, is generally accepted as the gold standard. Doubling dilutions of patient's serum are titrated against pools of reference serovars representing the most common serogroups. After incubation, tests are read by dark-field microscopy; 50% agglutination of the leptospires by the patient's or control serum represents a positive result. Sera collected soon after the onset of symptoms often show cross-reactivity to different serogroups in the microscopic agglutination test. In contrast,

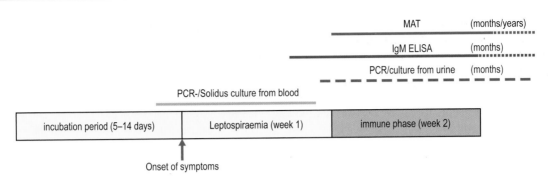

Fig. 33.2 Disease kinetics of leptospirosis. Infection produces leptospiraemia in the first few days after exposure. Leptospires are then cleared from the bloodstream as the titres of serum agglutinating antibodies increase (immune phase). Leptospires are also transiently shed in urine for long periods. *ELISA*, Enzyme-linked immunosorbent assay; *MAT*, microscopic agglutination test; *PCR*, polymerase chain reaction.

sera obtained during the convalescent phase of the illness generally show a significantly higher titre to the infecting serogroup.

Most other tests give no indication of the infecting serovar or serogroup. Several enzyme-linked immunosorbent assay (ELISA) kits offer ease of use together with relatively good sensitivity and specificity. Most detect IgM antibodies, which are detectable in the acute phase of the illness and may remain for several months after infection (Fig. 33.2).

Examination of blood and urine

The detection of leptospires in blood offers the earliest confirmation of infection. In theory, leptospirosis can be diagnosed by dark-field microscopy of blood taken during the first week of illness or, much less reliably, in urine during the second week. Dark-field microscopy of blood is technically demanding as Brownian movement of collagen fibrils, red blood cell membranes and other artefacts can resemble viable leptospires.

Culture of blood is useful for the identification of infecting serovars by specialised techniques that are available only in national reference laboratories. In recent years, PCR-based methods have been described, and these assays are now used in many diagnostic and reference laboratories for the detection of leptospires in biological fluids (blood, urine and cerebrospinal fluid) of patients. Molecular diagnostic techniques offer the potential for more rapid diagnosis of leptospirosis than the currently available serological methods. This is of particular value in the critically ill patient.

TREATMENT

Antibiotics offer some benefit if started within 4 days of the onset of illness and preferably within 24–48 hours.

In severe illness, intravenous benzylpenicillin is the drug of choice. For milder infections a 7- to 10-day course of oral amoxicillin is appropriate. Patients allergic to penicillins can be treated with erythromycin.

The value of antibiotic treatment is probably overestimated, and few trials have been conducted. However, supportive management to maintain tissue and organ function, such as the temporary maintenance of renal function by dialysis, may be lifesaving.

EPIDEMIOLOGY

Animals that acquire infection may not develop discernible disease but become long-term carriers—so-called maintenance hosts. Many rodents fall into this category. For example, rats acquiring inapparent infection with pathogenic strains may carry the bacteria in the convoluted tubules of the kidney (possibly life-long), resulting in chronic excretion of viable leptospires in their urine. Similarly, cattle may become a maintenance host for serovar Hardjo, dogs for serovar Canicola, and pigs for serovar Pomona or Bratislava. The reasons for this tolerance are unclear, as infection with other serovars may cause illness of varying severity followed by the transient shedding of the leptospires in the urine for only a few weeks.

Changes in industrial, agricultural and social practices may result in the rapid change of both the densities and types of animal populations in an area, with subsequent change in the predominant serovars of *Leptospira* causing disease in people and animals.

Viable leptospires are present in the semen of infected animals; in rodents a significant increase in the carriage of leptospires is seen once sexual maturity has been reached. Spread across the placenta occurs in several animal species, leading to infection and possibly death of the foetus.

Outside the animal host, leptospiral survival is favoured by warm, moist conditions at neutral or slightly alkaline pH. This no doubt contributes to the seasonal pattern of human infections, which peak in the summer months in both hemispheres. Even small reductions below pH 7.0 markedly reduce the survival of leptospires. The anaerobic conditions and low pH of raw sewage explain their short survival time compared with that in aerated sewage. Salt water is also relatively toxic to leptospires. They do not survive well in undiluted cow's milk, and therefore drinking unpasteurised milk poses minimal risk. However, they will survive in water at pH 7.0 or in damp soil for up to 1 month. If the soil is saturated with urine they may survive for up to 6 months, indicating the potential for long-term exposure to an infection risk even if the reservoir host has been removed for some time.

Leptospirosis in humans is an emerging disease with more than 1,000,000 severe cases occurring annually; case fatality rates may exceed 10%. The disease is expected to become more important because of predicted global climate changes and rapid urbanisation in developing countries where slum settlements have produced the conditions for epidemic rat-borne transmission of the disease.

Exposure to virulent leptospires may be direct, through contact with the urine or tissues of infected animals. Direct exposure is generally associated with particular occupations that bring human beings into contact with animals (e.g., butchers, veterinary surgeons, animal breeders, hunters or pet owners). Indirect exposure, through contact with freshwater or a humid environment contaminated with the urine of an infected animal, is more common. Such indirect exposure is associated with particular occupations (e.g., sewer workers, rice-field workers) or situations (e.g., triathlon participants, military manoeuvres). In slum communities in developing countries, indirect exposure from rats is thought to be the main source of infection.

Infections related to exposure to surface waters have shown a significant rise in industrialised countries. The increase is almost certainly due to the greater recreational use of surface waters for activities such as canoeing, rafting, fishing, and the use of rivers for the swimming section of triathlon competitions. There has also been an increase in cases of leptospirosis acquired abroad in endemic countries (Latin America and Southeast Asia), particularly among travellers on adventure holidays with water contact.

Morbidity and mortality from leptospirosis have declined markedly because of improved hygiene levels in industrialised countries. In countries with limited facilities for medical care death may occur in 25% or more cases.

CONTROL

With >200 known pathogenic serovars, each able to infect a wide range of animals that may become long-term carriers capable of infecting others, together with the organisms' ability to survive for long periods in the environment, the complete prevention or eradication of leptospirosis is impossible.

Mass immunisation of domestic livestock will prevent clinical disease in the animals and reduce the risk of human acquisition of infection.

To be fully effective, a vaccine should not only protect against disease in the animal but also prevent the establishment of the carrier state and the shedding of viable leptospires in the urine. It is also important that the vaccine contains antigens representing circulating serovars, as protection will be optimal only against the vaccine components. Current vaccines protect for only 1–2 years, and the economics of farming may influence a farmer's decision as to whether or not to immunise cattle. Cuba and China have used vaccines for mass prevention campaigns in human populations, and France has used a human vaccine containing only serovar Icterohaemorrhagiae since 1981.

Awareness of leptospirosis through the education of doctors, employers and the general public has helped to develop safer practices or procedures in the workplace and during recreational pursuits. This awareness should include consideration of leptospirosis in the differential diagnosis of fever in the returning tourist. Measures to reduce rodent populations in the vicinity of human activity, such as removing rubbish, especially waste food, and prevention of the access of rats into buildings is most important. Simple measures to reduce the risks of acquiring infection also include covering cuts and abrasions with waterproof plasters and wearing protective footwear before exposure to surface waters.

In parts of the world where the prevalence of human infection in certain groups is high, selective human immunisation schemes may be of benefit if a suitable vaccine is available. Antimicrobial prophylaxis with doxycycline may be of value in high-risk exposure situations in which prompt medical help is unavailable.

RECOMMENDED READING

Adler, B. (2015). *Leptospira and Leptospirosis, Current Topics in Microbiology and Immunology.* Springer-Varlag Berlin Heidelberg.

Costa, F., Hagan, J. E., Calcagno, J., Kane, M., Torgerson, P., Martinez-Silveira, M. S., ... Ko, A. I. (2015). Global morbidity and mortality of leptospirosis: a systematic review. *PLoS Neglected Tropical Diseases, 9*(9), e0003898. doi:10.1371/journal.pntd.0003898.

Kmety, E., & Dikken, H. (1993). *Classification of the Species Leptospira interrogans and History of Its Serovars.* Groningen: University Press.

Ko, A. I., Goarant, C., & Picardeau, M. (2009). Leptospira: the dawn of the molecular genetics era for an emerging zoonotic pathogen. *Nature Reviews. Microbiology, 7*(10), 736–747. doi:10.1038/nrmicro2208.

Levett, P. N. (2001). Leptospirosis. *Clinical Microbiology Reviews, 14*(2), 296–326.

Websites

International Leptospirosis Society (ILS). Available at http://www.leptosociety.org/.

World Health Organization. Leptospirosis. Available at http://www.who.int/topics/leptospirosis/en/.

34 *Chlamydia*

Genital and ocular infections; infertility; atypical pneumonia

DAVID MABEY AND ROSANNA W. PEELING

KEY POINTS

- Chlamydiae are obligate intracellular bacterial pathogens with a unique growth cycle.
- *C. trachomatis* is the most common bacterial sexually transmitted infection and the leading infectious cause of blindness.
- *C. pneumoniae* is an important cause of community-acquired pneumonia.
- Chlamydial infections are frequently asymptomatic.
- Serious sequelae of chlamydial infection (blindness, pelvic inflammatory disease, infertility) are caused by immune response–driven scarring and fibrosis.
- Diagnosis requires laboratory tests, preferably nucleic acid amplification tests.
- Treatment is with doxycycline, erythromycin or azithromycin.
- It is important to treat sexual partners of patients with chlamydial genital tract infection.
- Prevention depends on interrupting the transmission chain: there are no effective vaccines.

Chlamydiae are obligate intracellular bacterial pathogens of eukaryotic cells with a characteristic dimorphic growth cycle quite distinct from that of other bacteria, involving alternation between a metabolically inert, infectious, spore-like elementary body, which can survive in the extracellular environment, and a metabolically active, replicating reticulate body, which cannot. They are widely distributed in nature and are responsible for a variety of human infections affecting the eye, and the genitourinary and respiratory tracts.

Chlamydiae were first described in 1907 by Halberstaedter and von Prowazek, who observed cytoplasmic inclusions in conjunctival scrapings taken from children with trachoma and from monkeys inoculated with ocular material from these children. They named them *Chlamydozoa,* from the Greek words χλαμυς (cloak) and ζοον (animal) because of the way in which the inclusions were draped around the nucleus. Similar inclusions were soon observed in conjunctival scrapings taken from neonates with conjunctivitis, and from the cervix of their mothers. Most human infections are caused by *Chlamydia trachomatis,* which was first grown, in mouse brain and subsequently in eggs, from a patient with lymphogranuloma venereum (LGV) in the 1930s. The more fastidious trachoma biovar was not isolated until 1957. It was first grown in tissue culture in 1965, making it possible for the first time to study the epidemiology and clinical features of *C. trachomatis* infection on a large scale.

DESCRIPTION

CLASSIFICATION

The *Chlamydia* genus (order Chlamydiales; family Chlamydiaceae) comprises nine species of which two are primarily human pathogens: *C. trachomatis,* causing ocular and genital infections; and *C. pneumoniae,* causing mainly respiratory disease. The other species infect animals: *C. psittaci* (chiefly birds), *C. abortus* (sheep), *C. felis* (cats), *C. pecorum* (cattle), *C. suis* (pigs), *C. muridarum* (mice) and *C. caviae* (guinea pigs). *C. psittaci, C. abortus* and *C. felis* are occasionally transmitted to humans. A taxonomic reclassification, based on ribosomal DNA sequence data, assigned *C. pneumoniae, C. psittaci* and *C. abortus* to a new genus, *Chlamydophila.* However, this new taxonomy has not been universally accepted and is not used here.

The species *C. trachomatis* contains two biovars: the more invasive LGV biovar (serovars L1–L3) replicates in macrophages, invades lymph nodes and causes a systemic infection; the more common trachoma biovar is largely confined to squamo-columnar epithelial cells of the eye (serovars A–C) and genital tract (serovars D–K) (Table 34.1). Serovars are defined by the presence of specific epitopes on the major outer membrane protein. Serovars A–C differ from serovars D–K in that they are

Table 34.1 Human infections caused by chlamydiae

Site of infection	Disease	Sequelae	Organism (serovars)
Eye	Trachoma	Conjunctival scarring, trichiasis, blindness	C. trachomatis (A, B, Ba, C)
	Inclusion conjunctivitis		C. trachomatis (D–K)
	Ophthalmia neonatorum		C. trachomatis (D–K)
Genital tract			
Male	Nonspecific urethritis, proctitis, epididymitis	Urethral stricture	C. trachomatis (D–K)
Female	Cervicitis, urethritis, endometritis, salpingitis, PID, perihepatitis	Tubal infertility, ectopic pregnancy	C. trachomatis (D–K)
	Abortion, premature birth		C. trachomatis (D–K)
Male and female	Lymphogranuloma venereum	Scarring, lymphoedema, rectal stricture	C. trachomatis (L1–L3)
Respiratory tract	Neonatal pneumonia		C. trachomatis (D–K)
	Pharyngitis, bronchitis, pneumonia		C. pneumoniae
	Psittacosis, ornithosis		C. psittaci

PID, Pelvic inflammatory disease.

unable to synthesise tryptophan, owing to disruption of the *trpA* gene.

Chlamydiae have one of the smallest bacterial genomes, containing around 1 million base pairs. Virtually all strains of *C. trachomatis* also contain a 4.4-MDa plasmid of unknown function. Genomes of several *C. trachomatis* serovars have been sequenced and show a high level of conservation of gene order and content (>99%). A high degree of genetic conservation is also seen across *Chlamydia* species, with *C. trachomatis* and *C. muridarum,* for example, being >95% identical. The fact that chlamydiae replicate within an intracellular vacuole probably explains the high degree of conservation, as it does not allow them to exchange genetic material with other bacteria.

BIOLOGY

Chlamydiae probably evolved from host-independent, Gram-negative ancestors. They are 'energy parasites' relying on the host cell for synthesis of ATP. The chlamydial envelope possesses bacteria-like inner and outer membranes. The infectious elementary body is electron dense, DNA rich and approximately 300 nm in diameter. The cell wall does not contain peptidoglycan, and its rigidity is maintained by extensive disulphide linking of the major outer membrane protein, which makes up some 60% of the outer membrane. The elementary body binds to the host cell and enters by 'parasite-specified' endocytosis. Fusion of the chlamydia-containing endocytic vesicle with lysosomes is inhibited, and the elementary body begins its unique developmental cycle within the eukaryotic cell. The major outer membrane protein is reduced to a monomeric form and acts as a porin, allowing nutrients to enter the organism from the host cell. After about 8

hours the elementary body differentiates into the larger (800–1000 nm), noninfectious, metabolically active reticulate body, which divides by binary fission. By 20 hours postinfection, a proportion of reticulate bodies have begun to reorganise into a new generation of elementary bodies (Fig. 34.1). These reach maturity up to 30 hours after entry into the cell and rapidly accumulate within the endocytic vacuole, which may contain >1000 organisms. They are released by lysis of the host cell 30–48 hours after the start of the cycle.

PATHOGENESIS

After an incubation period of 5–10 days, *C. trachomatis* elicits an acute inflammatory response with a purulent exudate. A period of chronic inflammation ensues, with the development of sub-epithelial follicles, and this leads eventually, in some cases, to fibrosis and scarring. This scarring process is responsible for much of the morbidity associated with *C. trachomatis,* in both the genital tract and the eye. It is particularly likely to be seen after repeated infections.

Study of virulence determinants of *C. trachomatis* is difficult because it has not so far proved possible to manipulate chlamydiae genetically. However, the availability of the complete genome of several *C. trachomatis* strains has provided some insights. The serovar D genome contains genes homologous with those coding for virulence factors in other bacteria, including a cytotoxin gene, and genes encoding a type III secretion pathway (see Ch. 10). A conserved chlamydial protease, proteasome-like activity factor, is secreted into the host cell cytoplasm, where it interferes with the assembly and surface expression of HLA (human leucocyte antigen) molecules and inhibits apoptosis. In a nonhuman primate

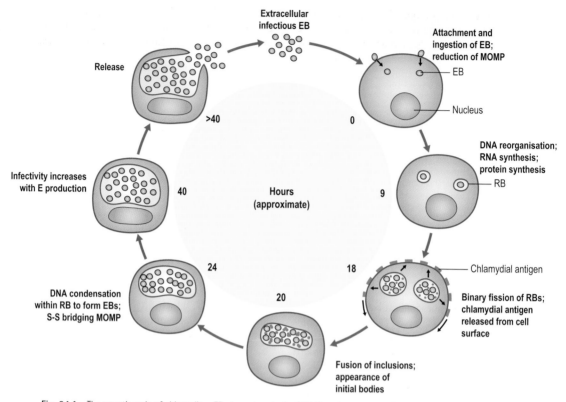

Fig. 34.1 The growth cycle of chlamydiae. *EB*, elementary body; *MOMP*, major outer membrane protein; *RB*, reticulate body.

model, genetic variations in six *C. trachomatis* genes that appear to be associated with increased virulence have been identified.

The epidemiology of *C. trachomatis* infection suggests that a degree of protective immunity follows natural infection. The prevalence and bacterial load of ocular infection are lower in adults than in children in trachoma endemic communities, and the duration of infection is shorter. Similarly, genital *C. trachomatis* infection is most prevalent in the youngest sexually active age groups, and the chlamydial isolation rate for men with non-gonococcal urethritis is lower in those who have had previous episodes. Killed whole organism vaccines provide some degree of protection against ocular *C. trachomatis* infection in human and nonhuman primates. Serovar-specific monoclonal antibodies to the major outer membrane protein neutralise *C. trachomatis* in vitro, but there are few data to suggest that either IgG or IgA antibody is protective. The intracellular development of *C. trachomatis* is inhibited by interferon-γ, and evidence from animal models and studies of human ocular infection suggest that cell-mediated immune responses, mediated by CD4+ lymphocytes are important for the clearance of infection.

Vaccine studies in primates suggest that vaccination could provoke more severe disease on subsequent challenge, implying that much of the damage caused by *C. trachomatis* infection may be immunopathological in origin. This would be in keeping with the histopathology of *C. trachomatis* infection, in which the lymphoid follicle is the hallmark. Follicles contain typical germinal centres, consisting predominantly of B lymphocytes, with T cells, mostly CD8+, in the parafollicular region. The inflammatory infiltrate between follicles comprises plasma cells, dendritic cells, macrophages, and polymorphonuclear leucocytes, with T and B lymphocytes. Fibrosis is seen at a late stage, typically in trachoma and pelvic inflammatory disease. T lymphocytes are also present and outnumber B cells and macrophages.

A chlamydial heat-shock protein (hsp 60), homologous with the GroEL protein of *Escherichia coli*, elicits antibody responses that are associated with the damaging sequelae of *C. trachomatis* infections in both the eye and genital tract. In vitro interferon-γ interferes with the chlamydial development cycle, leading to persistent infection with continuing release of hsp 60. It is not known whether the immune response to hsp 60 is itself the cause of immunopathological damage, or merely a marker of more severe or prolonged infection. Studies of gene expression at the site of ocular infection have shown the importance of innate immune pathways and natural killer (NK) cell activation and suggest that matrix metalloproteinases 7 and 9 play an important role in the scarring process. Polymorphisms in immune response genes encoding tumour necrosis factor-α, interferon-γ and interleukin-10 are associated with the development of severe scarring following ocular *C. trachomatis* infection.

CLINICAL FEATURES

CHLAMYDIA TRACHOMATIS

Genital infection

The clinical manifestations of genital *C. trachomatis* infection are similar to those of gonorrhoea, but are usually less severe, as *C. trachomatis* infection elicits a less intense acute inflammatory response than *Neisseria gonorrhoeae*. Many chlamydial infections are asymptomatic. Long-term sequelae such as infertility and ectopic pregnancy are generally caused by fibrosis and scarring of the fallopian tubes following prolonged or repeated infections and may develop even in those with few or no symptoms.

Infection in men

C. trachomatis is detectable in the urethra of up to 50% of men with symptomatic non-gonococcal urethritis. The incubation period is 7–21 days, compared to 2–5 days for gonorrhoea. Patients present with a history of dysuria, usually accompanied by a mild to moderate mucopurulent urethral discharge. *C. trachomatis* is responsible for a proportion of cases of chronic (persistent or recurrent) non-gonococcal urethritis. Since mixed infections are common, treatment of gonococcal urethritis with an antibiotic ineffective against *C. trachomatis* may result in post-gonococcal urethritis.

C. trachomatis is responsible for up to 70% of cases of acute epididymitis in young men (35 years of age or less) in developed countries. Patients present with unilateral scrotal pain, swelling and tenderness, often accompanied by fever. Most give a history of current or recent urethral discharge. In older patients, epididymitis and epididymoorchitis tend to be caused by urinary tract pathogens. There is no good evidence that chlamydial infection leads to male infertility or to acute or chronic prostatitis.

Both LGV and non-LGV strains of *C. trachomatis* can cause proctitis in those who practise receptive anal intercourse. Non-LGV strains cause a milder disease, which may be asymptomatic or give rise to rectal pain, bleeding and mucopurulent anal discharge.

Infection in women

C. trachomatis typically infects the columnar epithelial cells of the endocervix. It does not affect the squamous epithelium of the vagina. Infection is associated with a mucopurulent discharge from the cervix visible on speculum examination, and with hypertrophic cervical ectopy that tends to bleed on contact. Most infected women have no symptoms. The prevalence of cervical infection is no higher among women who complain of vaginal discharge than among those who do not, suggesting that it is not a cause of symptomatic vaginal discharge.

C. trachomatis has been implicated as a cause of the urethral syndrome, characterised by dysuria, frequency and sterile pyuria. Clinical signs of urethritis, such as urethral discharge or meatal redness, are not usually found.

Infection may spread from the endocervix to the endometrium and fallopian tubes, causing pelvic inflammatory disease. This is more likely to occur after trauma to the cervix due, for example, to termination of pregnancy, insertion of an intrauterine contraceptive device or delivery. Histological evidence of endometritis can be found in up to 50% of women with mucopurulent cervicitis due to *C. trachomatis* and is more common in those with a history of abnormal vaginal bleeding. Classic signs of pelvic inflammatory disease may be present (fever, lower abdominal pain and tenderness, and cervical motion tenderness), but chlamydial pelvic inflammatory disease may be subclinical. Spread to the peritoneum may result in perihepatitis (the Curtis–Fitz-Hugh syndrome), which may be confused with acute cholecystitis in young women. *C. trachomatis* infection has also been associated with postpartum endometritis.

C. trachomatis is the major cause of pelvic inflammatory disease in developed countries. Infertility may be the first indication of asymptomatic tubal disease. It occurs in about 10% of women following a single upper genital tract infection and in up to 50% after two or three episodes. Infertility may result from endometritis, from blocked or damaged fallopian tubes, or from abnormalities of ovum transportation caused by damage to the ciliated epithelial surface. Other consequences of salpingitis are chronic pelvic pain and ectopic pregnancy. Following chlamydial pelvic inflammatory disease, the risk of ectopic pregnancy increases 7–10-fold.

Some studies have shown *C. trachomatis* infection to be associated with low birth weight and pre-term delivery, but others have failed to confirm this. In general, infection was diagnosed and treated at a later stage of gestation in those studies that found a correlation between infection and adverse birth outcome than in those that did not.

Infection has been weakly associated with bartholinitis and should be considered in the absence of other known pathogens. A significant association between cervical chlamydial infection and cervical squamous cell carcinoma, but not adenocarcinoma, has been established, and it has been suggested that chlamydial infection may enhance the effect of oncogenic papillomaviruses.

Adult paratrachoma (inclusion conjunctivitis) and otitis media

Adult chlamydial ophthalmia commonly results from the accidental transfer of infected genital discharge to the eye. It usually presents as a unilateral follicular conjunctivitis, acute or subacute in onset. The features are swollen lids, mucopurulent discharge, papillary hyperplasia and, later, follicular hypertrophy, and occasionally punctate keratitis. About one-third of patients has otitis media and complains of blocked ears and hearing loss. The disease is generally benign and self-limiting. Patients and their sexual contacts should be investigated for genital chlamydial infection and managed appropriately.

REACTIVE ARTHRITIS

Arthritis occurring with or soon after non-gonococcal urethritis is termed *sexually acquired reactive arthritis*. Conjunctivitis and other features characteristic of Reiter's syndrome are seen in about one-third of patients. *C. trachomatis* has also been associated with 'seronegative' arthritis in women. Viable chlamydiae have not been detected in the joints of patients with this condition, which is probably the result of immunopathology. Despite this, early tetracycline therapy has been advocated by some investigators.

NEONATAL INFECTIONS

Conjunctivitis appears in 20%–50% of infants exposed to *C. trachomatis* infecting the cervix at birth. A mucopurulent discharge and occasionally pseudomembrane formation occur 1–3 weeks later. It usually resolves without visual impairment.

About half of the infants who have conjunctivitis also develop pneumonia, although a history of recent conjunctivitis and bulging eardrums are found in only half of the cases. Chlamydial pneumonia usually begins between the fourth and eleventh week of life, preceded by upper respiratory symptoms. There is tachypnoea, a prominent, staccato cough but usually no fever, and the illness is protracted.

Radiographs show hyperinflation of the lungs with bilateral diffuse, symmetrical, interstitial infiltration and scattered areas of atelectasis. Children infected during infancy are at increased risk of obstructive lung disease and asthma.

LYMPHOGRANULOMA VENEREUM

The clinical course of LGV can be divided into three stages: the primary stage at the site of inoculation; the secondary stage in the regional lymph nodes and/or the anorectum; and the tertiary stage of late sequelae affecting the genitalia and/or rectum.

Primary stage

After an incubation period of 3–30 days, a small, painless papule, which may ulcerate, occurs at the site of inoculation. The primary lesion is self-limiting and may pass unnoticed by the patient. Among patients with LGV presenting with buboes in Thailand, more than half had not been aware of an ulcer.

Secondary stage

This occurs some weeks after the primary lesion. It may involve the inguinal lymph nodes, or the anus and rectum. The inguinal form is more common in men than in women because the lymphatic drainage of the upper vagina and cervix is to the retroperitoneal rather than the inguinal lymph nodes. LGV proctitis occurs in those who practise receptive anal intercourse, probably due to direct inoculation.

The cardinal feature of the inguinal form of LGV is painful, usually unilateral, inguinal and/or femoral lymphadenopathy (bubo). Enlarged lymph nodes are usually firm and often accompanied by fever, chills, arthralgia and headache. Biopsy reveals small discrete areas of necrosis surrounded by proliferating epithelioid and endothelial cells, which may enlarge to form stellate abscesses that may coalesce and break down to form discharging sinuses. In women, signs include a hypertrophic suppurative cervicitis, backache and adnexal tenderness.

Clinical features of anorectal disease include a purulent anal discharge, pain and bleeding due to an acute haemorrhagic proctitis or proctocolitis, often with fever, chills and weight loss. Proctoscopy reveals a granular or ulcerative proctitis. Computed tomography or magnetic resonance imaging scans may show pronounced thickening of the rectal wall, with enlargement of iliac lymph nodes. Enlarged inguinal nodes may also be palpable.

Cervical adenopathy due to LGV has been reported after oral sex. A follicular conjunctivitis has also been described following direct inoculation of the eye, which may be accompanied by preauricular lymphadenopathy. Other rare manifestations of the secondary stage include acute meningoencephalitis, synovitis and cardiac involvement.

Tertiary stage

This appears after a latent period of several years, but is rare. Chronic untreated LGV leads to fibrosis, which may cause lymphatic obstruction and elephantiasis of the genitalia in either sex, or rectal strictures and fistulae. Rarely, it can give rise to the syndrome of esthiomene (Greek: 'eating away') with widespread destruction of the external genitalia.

TRACHOMA

The clinical signs of trachoma are best seen in the conjunctival surface of the everted upper eyelid. Active or inflammatory trachoma, which is usually seen in children in endemic communities, is a follicular keratoconjunctivitis. Subjects in whom five or more follicles of >0.5-mm diameter are seen in the central subtarsal conjunctiva are defined by the World Health Organization (WHO) as having follicular trachoma. In some cases, the inflammation is severe enough to obscure the conjunctival blood vessels. If more than half the blood vessels are obscured, this is defined as intense inflammatory trachoma. Blood vessels may be seen growing into the cornea, usually at its superior margin; this is known as pannus. *C. trachomatis* can be detected in a proportion of cases of follicular trachoma, but not in all cases, since the follicles can persist for weeks or months after the infection has resolved. Repeated episodes of inflammatory trachoma lead eventually to conjunctival scarring. As the scars contract they cause the lid margin to turn inwards (entropion) and the lashes to abrade the cornea (trichiasis). This causes extreme discomfort, damages the cornea, and leads eventually to blindness due to corneal opacity.

C. PNEUMONIAE

C. pneumoniae causes pneumonia, pharyngitis, bronchitis, otitis and sinusitis, with an incubation period of about 21 days. It may be a significant cause of acute exacerbations of asthma and is one of the most common causes of community-acquired pneumonia, but it is seldom identified as the causal agent because laboratory tests for its diagnosis are not widely used. It is a chronic, often insidious, respiratory pathogen to which there appears to be little immunity. Seroepidemiological studies indicate that some 60%–80% of people worldwide become infected with *C. pneumoniae* during their life.

C. PSITTACI

C. psittaci is an important cause of infections in a wide range of birds and is shed in nasal secretions and droppings. Nasal secretions contaminate the feathers, where they dry and produce a highly infectious dust in which the organism can survive for months. This may give rise to severe pneumonia in humans, called ornithosis or psittacosis depending on the bird species from which the infection was derived. The agricultural economy is also affected, as large outbreaks of ornithosis have been reported in turkeys, geese and ducks. There are import controls in many countries to restrict the movement of birds, which are rendered more infectious by travel-induced stress.

The incubation period is about 10 days, and the illness ranges from an influenza-like syndrome, with general malaise, fever, anorexia, rigors, sore throat, headache and photophobia, to a severe illness with delirium and pneumonia. The illness may resemble bronchopneumonia, but the bronchioles are involved as a secondary event and sputum is scanty. The organism disseminates through the body, and there may be meningoencephalitis, arthritis, pericarditis or myocarditis, or a predominantly typhoidal state with enlarged liver and spleen. Endocarditis has been described.

LABORATORY INVESTIGATION

The laboratory diagnosis of chlamydial infection depends on detection of the organisms or their antigens or nucleic acid and, to a much lesser extent, on serology (Table 34.2). In urogenital infection, the highest bacterial load of *C. trachomatis* is found in the endocervix in women and in the urethra in men. An endocervical swab is therefore needed for the diagnosis of infection by culture or antigen detection assay. However, the greater sensitivity of nucleic acid amplification tests for *C. trachomatis* means that self-administered vaginal swabs and first-catch urine specimens give equivalent results to endocervical swabs when using these assays. Samples to be tested can be transported to the laboratory at room temperature, making home-based screening for *C. trachomatis* possible.

CULTURE

Centrifugation of specimens onto cycloheximide-treated McCoy or HeLa cell monolayers, followed by incubation and then staining with a fluorescent monoclonal antibody or with a vital dye, to detect inclusions, has been widely used for the diagnosis of *C. trachomatis* infection. One

Table 34.2 Advantages and disadvantages of diagnostic tests for *C. trachomatis*

Factor considered	Culture	Direct fluorescent antibody	Enzyme immunoassay	Nucleic acid amplification
Sensitivity	<70%	70%–100%	<50%–70%	Up to 100%
Specificity	100%	Up to 98% (reader dependent)	95%–98%	Up to 99%
Appropriate specimens	Cervical/urethral/ocular swabs	Cervical/urethral/ocular swabs	Cervical/urethral/ocular swabs	Cervical/urethral/ocular swabs, urine (men), vaginal swabs
Speed/temperature for transport of specimen	Rapid or at low temperature	Room temperature	Room temperature if specimen in buffer	Room temperature if <48 h, 4°C if >48 h
Storage requirements	4°C if overnight, −70°C or liquid nitrogen if long term	4°C if short term	4°C if 3–5 days, freezing if longer	4°C if not processed in 7 days; −70°C if long term
Evaluation of adequacy of specimen	Not possible	Host cells seen under microscope	Not possible	Determine whether host DNA present
Special equipment or procedure	Centrifuge, biological safety cabinet, CO_2 incubator, microscope	Fluorescence microscope	ELISA reader	Dedicated equipment for nucleic acid amplification and detection
Processing of specimen	Laborious	Simple	Relatively simple, amenable to batching	Requires precautions against false positive results due to laboratory contamination
Reading of test	Subjective and moderately tedious	Subjective and tedious	Objective and simple	Objective and simple
Time to result	48–72 h	30 min	3 h	2–4 h
Cost	High	Moderate	Low	Very high

blind passage may increase sensitivity. However, cell-culture techniques are no more than 70% sensitive compared to nucleic acid amplification tests and are slow and labour intensive. Because culture is essentially 100% specific, it still has a role in medicolegal cases. *C. pneumoniae* is even more difficult to grow than C. *trachomatis*. *C. psittaci* is a hazard group 3 pathogen and few laboratories attempt to grow it.

DIRECT IMMUNOFLUORESCENCE

Microscopic detection of elementary bodies with species-specific fluorescent monoclonal antibodies is rapid and, for *C. trachomatis* oculogenital infections, highly sensitive and specific in the hands of skilled observers. However, the test is laborious and interpretation is subjective. It is best used in settings where few specimens are tested, or for confirming positive results obtained with other tests.

NUCLEIC ACID AMPLIFICATION TESTS

By enabling amplification of a nucleic acid sequence specific to the chlamydial species, the polymerase chain reaction assay, the strand displacement assay and the transcription-mediated amplification technique have overcome problems of poor sensitivity. Commercial assays for *C. trachomatis* based on each of these three amplification

methods are available and widely used. The first two assays amplify nucleotide sequences of the cryptic plasmid, which is present in multiple copies in each chlamydial elementary body. However, a rare variant of *C. trachomatis* has been described, which lacks the plasmid, giving rise to false negative results with these assays. The transcription-mediated amplification reaction is directed against rRNA, which is also present in multiple copies. These sensitive assays have replaced culture as the gold standard for the diagnosis of *C. trachomatis* infection. Nucleic acid amplification tests for *C. pneumoniae* and *C. psittaci* are not commercially available.

ENZYME IMMUNOASSAYS

Enzyme immunoassays that detect chlamydial antigens, usually the genus-specific lipopolysaccharide, have largely been replaced by the more sensitive nucleic acid amplification test.

POINT–OF–CARE TESTS

Over 20 rapid strip tests based on the immunochromatographic detection of chlamydial lipopolysaccharide are commercially available. They can give a result within 15–20 minutes of sample collection, but most lack sensitivity compared to nucleic acid amplification methods.

SEROLOGICAL TESTS

Serological tests are of no value in uncomplicated genital *C. trachomatis* infection. In pelvic inflammatory disease, in LGV and in the Curtis–Fitz-Hugh syndrome, serology may be useful if a rising titre can be demonstrated. *C. trachomatis* IgM antibody is the gold standard for the diagnosis of chlamydial pneumonia in babies. Pneumonia due to *C. pneumoniae* and *C. psittaci* is usually diagnosed serologically, but depends on the demonstration of IgM antibodies or an IgG titre >512 by microimmunofluorescence, or a rise in antibody titre in a convalescent sample. Immunofluorescence and enzyme immunoassays are commercially available, but have not been rigorously evaluated.

TREATMENT

Chlamydiae are intracellular and hence insensitive to aminoglycosides and other antibiotics that do not penetrate cells efficiently. Tetracyclines and macrolides are the mainstay of treatment. Treatment is often started before a microbiological diagnosis can be established, so additional broad-spectrum antibiotics are needed to cover gonococcal and, in the case of pelvic inflammatory disease, anaerobic infections. Treatment of sexual partners is essential to prevent reinfection.

Uncomplicated *C. trachomatis* infections are treated with a single dose of azithromycin 1 g, or with doxycycline 100 mg twice daily for 7 days. Chlamydial pelvic inflammatory disease is treated with a 14-day course of doxycycline 100 mg twice daily. Clinically significant resistance to these antibiotics has not been reported. Doxycycline is contraindicated in pregnancy. Azithromycin 1 g as a single dose, and amoxicillin 500 mg three times daily for 7 days, are safe and effective in pregnant women. Ofloxacin is active against *C. trachomatis* at a dose of 300 mg twice daily for 7 days, but is not widely used. Ophthalmia neonatorum and neonatal pneumonia due to *C. trachomatis* should be treated with erythromycin syrup by mouth, 50 mg/kg daily divided into four doses, for 14 days.

There has been no adequate study comparing antibiotic regimens for LGV, *C. pneumoniae* or *C. psittaci* infection. Recommended treatment for LGV is doxycycline 100 mg twice daily, or erythromycin 500 mg four times daily, for 21 days. Azithromycin has been used successfully in some cases, although a 1-g single dose is unlikely to be sufficient. Large collections of pus should be aspirated, using a lateral approach through normal skin. Macrolides or tetracyclines are recommended for the treatment of infection with *C. pneumoniae* and *C. psittaci*. Prolonged courses may be required in patients with pneumonia.

Ocular infection can be effectively treated with a single oral dose of azithromycin (20 mg/kg, maximum 1 g) but, in trachoma-endemic communities, reinfection rapidly occurs and mass treatment of entire communities is therefore recommended.

EPIDEMIOLOGY

C. trachomatis is the most common bacterial sexually transmitted infection and the most common infectious cause of blindness. Genital infection is common in all sexually active populations, and prevalence is usually highest in the young. In the United Kingdom, the number of reported chlamydial infections trebled between 1996 and 2005. Similar increases were seen in other Western countries over this period, including Sweden and Canada, despite active screening programmes. It is not clear to what extent this is due to an increased incidence, or to an increase in the number of people tested with the sensitive nucleic acid amplification tests that have been widely used since the late 1990s. The overall incidence of reported chlamydial infection in the United Kingdom in 2005 was 223 per 100,000 total population, with the highest rate (1300 per 100,000) in women aged 16–19. The WHO has estimated that, in 2005, there were 101 million new cases of genital chlamydial infection.

LGV is rare in industrialised countries, but is endemic in parts of Africa, Asia, South America and the Caribbean. Its epidemiology is poorly defined because LGV is often indistinguishable clinically from chancroid and other causes of genital ulceration with bubo formation, and it has been difficult to obtain laboratory confirmation. Among patients presenting with buboes to a sexually transmitted disease clinic in Bangkok, 10% were found to have LGV, and an epidemic of LGV has been reported among crack cocaine users in the Bahamas. In 2003, an outbreak of LGV proctitis due to the L2 serovar was reported among homosexual men in the Netherlands, and since then over 1000 cases have been reported in homosexual men in Europe and North America; most affected men were HIV positive.

Trachoma, caused by *C. trachomatis* transmitted from eye to eye, disappeared from Europe and North America in the 20th century as living standards improved, but remains endemic in poor rural populations in Africa and Asia. WHO estimates that at least 40 million people have trachoma and that 8 million are blind or visually impaired as a result.

MOLECULAR EPIDEMIOLOGY

Typing isolates of *C. trachomatis* is potentially of great value. It could help to map sexual networks, and to distinguish between treatment failure and reinfection in clinical trials. If associations could be found between particular strains and particular clinical findings, it could help to identify virulence determinants of *C. trachomatis* and increase understanding of the pathogenesis of infection.

The first typing method for *C. trachomatis,* the microimmunofluorescence test, was based on the ability of monoclonal antibodies to distinguish 13 (later increased to 17) serotypes of *C. trachomatis.* More recently, genital and ocular strains of *C. trachomatis* have been genotyped following amplification of the *ompA* gene, which encodes the major outer membrane protein, either by sequencing or by restriction fragment length polymorphism analysis of the amplified product; but *ompA* genotyping is not sufficiently discriminatory to distinguish between persistent infection and reinfection with a common genotype.

A multilocus sequence typing method, targeting six variable genes identified through genome sequencing projects, has been used to investigate a variant of *C. trachomatis* lacking the plasmid detected by commonly used nucleic acid amplification tests.

CONTROL AND PREVENTION

Health education and condom promotion, especially for the youngest sexually active age groups, may help to reduce the incidence of genital *C. trachomatis* infection. Syndromic management of symptomatic infections, and partner notification, may also play a role, but since a high proportion of chlamydial infections is asymptomatic in both sexes, these measures are unlikely to be successful on their own. A screening programme for *C. trachomatis* at primary health-care level in the United States has been shown to reduce the incidence of upper genital tract infection and its complications in women. Screening programmes have been introduced in some European countries, in which young people presenting to health services for any reason are offered a test for *C. trachomatis*; but the public health impact of such opportunistic screening programmes remains to be demonstrated. Where reinfection rates are high, retesting of positive cases 6 months after treatment has been recommended.

No vaccine is presently available. Recent research has focused on the development of a subunit vaccine against *C. trachomatis,* which provides protection without eliciting immunopathology. Purified preparations of major outer membrane protein were protective in murine models, provided the native trimeric structure of the protein was maintained. In nonhuman primates, a similar preparation of major outer membrane protein reduced peak shedding from the ocular surface, but had no effect on the duration of infection or on ocular disease.

The strategy for trachoma control recommended by WHO is based on the acronym SAFE: *S*urgery for trichiasis; mass treatment with *A*ntibiotics; *F*acial cleanliness; and *E*nvironmental improvement to reduce the transmission of *C. trachomatis* from eye to eye.

RECOMMENDED READING

Brunham, R. C., & Rey-Ladino, J. (2005). Immunology of chlamydia infection: implications for a *Chlamydia trachomatis* vaccine. *Nature Reviews. Immunology, 5*(2), 149–161.

Kuo, C. C., Jackson, L. A., Campbell, L. A., & Grayston, J. T. (1995). *Chlamydia pneumoniae* (TWAR). *Clinical Microbiology Reviews, 8*(4), 451–461.

Low, N., Bender, N., Nartey, L., Shang, A., & Stephenson, J. M. (2009). Effectiveness of chlamydia screening: systematic review. *International Journal of Epidemiology, 38*(2), 435–448. doi:10.1093/ije/dyn222.

Mabey, D., Solomon, A., & Foster, A. (2003). Trachoma. *Lancet, 362*(9379), 223–229.

Stephens, R. S., Kalman, S., Lammel, C., Fan, J., Marathe, R., Aravind, L., … Davis, R. W. (1998). Genome sequence of an obligate intracellular pathogen of humans: *Chlamydia trachomatis. Science, 282*(5389), 754–759.

Van der Bij, A. K., Spaargaren, J., Morré, S. A., Fennema, H. S., Mindel, A., Coutinho, R. A., & de Vries, H. J. (2006). Diagnostic and clinical implications of anorectal lymphogranuloma venereum in men who have sex with men: a retrospective case-control study. *Clinical Infectious Diseases, 42*(2), 186–194.

35 Mycoplasmas

Respiratory and genital tract infections

VICKI J. CHALKER AND REBECCA BROWN

KEY POINTS

- Mycoplasmas pathogenic for humans include the genera *Mycoplasma* and *Ureaplasma*. They are found in the respiratory and genital tracts of humans and many animal species. On occasion they may cause invasive infection, gaining access to joints and other organs.
- Mycoplasmas are small organisms that grow in cell-free enriched bacteriological media. They lack peptidoglycan; hence they are not susceptible to β-lactam or glycopeptide antibiotics. Infections are treated principally with macrolides, tetracyclines or fluoroquinolones. Increasing resistance to macrolides is documented.
- *Mycoplasma pneumoniae* is a pathogen for the human respiratory tract, sometimes resulting in pneumonia, especially in children.
- *Mycoplasma genitalium* and *Ureaplasma urealyticum* cause acute nongonococcal urethritis in men and are also implicated in chronic disease; *M. genitalium* also causes balanoposthitis.
- Mycoplasmas and ureaplasmas are associated with genital infections in women, including bacterial vaginosis, postpartum fever, cervicitis, endometritis, and salpingitis.
- Mycoplasmas have been associated with suppurative arthritis occurring in patients with hypogammaglobulinaemia (ureaplasma/*M. hominis*). *Mycoplasma fermentans* has been detected in the joints of patients with chronic arthritides.

DESCRIPTION

Mycoplasma (Greek: *mykes*, fungus; *plasma*, something moulded) refers to the filamentous (funguslike) nature of the organisms of some species and to the plasticity of the outer membrane resulting in pleomorphism. *Mycoplasma* species are taxonomically placed in the phylum Firmicutes, class Mollicutes ("soft skins"), order Mycoplasmatales, family Mycoplasmataceae and genus *Mycoplasma*. The taxonomic description of species within the Mollicutes class has been complicated and was first established in the 1960s. This class now contains four orders, five families, eight genera and more than 200 known species that have been detected in humans, vertebrate animals, arthropods, fish/shellfish and plants. In 1989, phylogenetic analysis based on 16S ribosomal ribonucleic acid (rRNA) sequences was reported for the Mollicutes where 47 species were included, revealing five distinct phylogenetic clades of descent, namely: anaeroplasmas, asteroleplasmas, hominis, pneumoniae and spiroplasmas. The term *mycoplasma(s)* is often used, as here, in a trivial fashion to refer to any member of the class Mollicutes. Mycoplasmas are of importance in human, animal and plant health and in agriculture.

Nineteen *Mycoplasma* species (Table 35.1) have been isolated from or detected in humans and at least six of these species are considered to be of pathological significance, including *M. genitalium, M. pneumoniae* and *M. hominis*. Zoonotic infection with other species has also been described, such as *M. phocerebale* and "seal finger" in cases post seal bite infection. The first report of a mycoplasma to be recovered directly from a human in association with a pathological condition occurred in 1937, when *M. hominis* was isolated from a Bartholin gland abscess. Shortly after this, *M. pneumoniae*, formally known as "Eaton agent," was isolated in the sputum from a patient with primary atypical pneumonia. Ureaplasmas were known originally as T strains or T mycoplasmas—T for "tiny," to indicate the small size of the colonies in comparison with those produced by other mycoplasmas. Many animals are infected by ureaplasmas. There are two species of *Ureaplasma* in humans that were previously classified as a single species: *U. urealyticum* and *U. parvum*.

The lack of a rigid peptidoglycan cell wall prevents mycoplasmas from staining by Gram stain, confers pleomorphism to their cells and makes them susceptible to osmotic stress. They have small genomes and limited

Table 35.1 Human *Mycoplasma* species, their colonisation site, and primary metabolite

Human species	Colonisation site	Primary metabolite
Mycoplasma salivarium	Oral cavity	Arginine
Mycoplasma orale	Oral cavity and oropharynx	Arginine
Mycoplasma pneumoniae	Respiratory tract	Glucose
Mycoplasma amphoriforme	Respiratory tract	Glucose
Mycoplasma fermentans	Urogenital tract	Glucose and arginine
Mycoplasma hominis	Urogenital tract	Arginine
Mycoplasma penetrans	Urogenital tract	Glucose and arginine
Ureaplasma urealyticum	Urogenital tract	Urea
Ureaplasma parvum	Urogenital tract	Urea
Mycoplasma genitalium	Urogenital tract	Glucose
Mycoplasma buccale	Oropharynx	Arginine
Mycoplasma faucium	Oropharynx	Arginine
Mycoplasma lipophilum	Oral cavity	Arginine
Mycoplasma pirum		Glucose and arginine
Mycoplasma primatum	Oral cavity and urogenital tract	Arginine
Mycoplasma spermatophilum	Genital tract	Arginine
Acholeplasma laidlawii	Oropharynx	
Hemoplasma	Systemic	
Candidatus Mycoplasma girerdii	Urogenital tract	

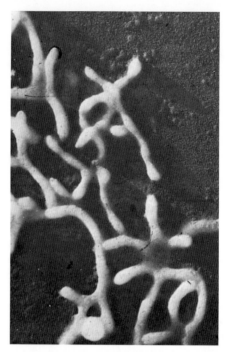

Fig. 35.1 Electron micrograph of *M. mycoides* ssp. *mycoides* (bovine origin), gold shadowed, to show branching filaments. Original magnification ×28,000. (From Rodwell, A. W., & Abbot, A. (1961). The function of glycerol, cholesterol and long-chain fatty acids in the nutrition of *Mycoplasma mycoides*. *J Gen Microbiol*, 25, 201–214.)

biosynthetic capabilities, restricting them to a parasitic existence in association with host cells. A majority of mycoplasmas exhibit strict host and tissue specificities.

Replication

Mycoplasmas multiply by binary fission; however, division is not always synchronous with genome replication, resulting in the formation of multinucleate filaments and other shapes. Subsequent division of the cytoplasm by constriction of the membrane at sites between the genomes leads to chains of beads that later fragment to give single cells. Budding occurs when the cytoplasm is not divided equally between the daughter cells. The minimal reproductive unit of mycoplasmas is a roughly spherical or bottle-shaped cell about 200 to 250 nm in diameter. Organisms of this order initiate growth in cell-free medium and make up, with larger forms (0.5–1 μm diameter), the substance of the characteristic agar-embedded colonies.

Morphology

Cell morphology varies with the *Mycoplasma* species, environmental conditions and the stage of the growth cycle.

Light microscopy reveals pleomorphic organisms, which may range from spherical through coccoid, coccobacillary, ring and dumb-bell forms, to short and long branching (Fig. 35.1), beaded or segmented filaments. Several species of human origin [including *amphoriphorme, genitalium* (Fig. 35.2), *penetrans* and *pneumoniae*] have specialised structures at one or both ends by which they attach to respiratory or genital tract mucosal surfaces. Transmission electron microscopy (TEM) of *M. pneumoniae* colonising bronchial epithelia reveal this "attachment organelle" directly associated with the host cell surface. The attachment organelle is thought to be multifunctional and is involved in gliding motility, cell division and adhesion.

Mycoplasmas lack many of the genes encoding peptidoglycan synthesis (unlike L-forms) and are susceptible to osmotic stress. The presence of cholesterol in the cytoplasmic membrane renders them susceptible to agents such as saponin, digitonin and some polyene antibiotics (e.g., amphotericin B) that complex with sterols (Fig. 35.3).

On agar, mycoplasmas often produce colonies that have a "fried egg" appearance, which results from the bacteria burrowing into the agar, and both bacteria and colonies are pleomorphic in size and shape (Fig. 35.4). However, some, such as *M. pneumoniae* on primary isolation, have

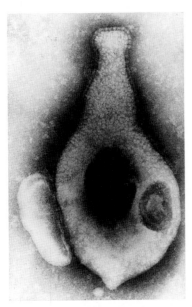

Fig. 35.2 Electron micrograph of *M. genitalium* (human origin), negatively stained, to show flask-shaped appearance and terminal specialized structure covered by extracellular "nap". Original magnification ×120,000. (From Tully, J. G., Taylor-Robinson, D., Rose, D. L., et al. (1983). *Mycoplasma genitalium*, a new species from the human urogenital tract. *Int J Sys Bacteriol*, 33, 387–396.)

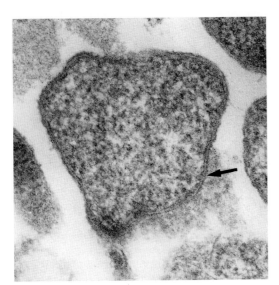

Fig. 35.3 Electron micrograph of *M. pulmonis* (of murine origin); thin section illustrating trilaminar membrane *(arrow)*. Original magnification ×75,000.

a mulberry appearance without the peripheral zone. The size of the colonies varies widely: colonies of some bovine mycoplasmas and most acholeplasmas may exceed 2 mm in diameter and are visible to the naked eye. Nevertheless, most require low-power microscopic magnification. Colonies

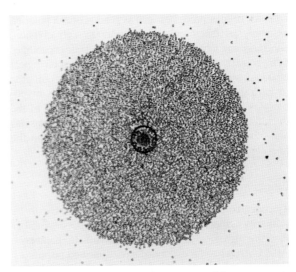

Fig. 35.4 Colonies of *M. hominis* (of human origin) (up to 110 µm in diameter) with typical "fried egg" appearance (oblique illumination). Original magnification ×150.

of ureaplasmas are characteristically small (15–60 µm in diameter), mainly because they usually lack the peripheral zone of growth. The size and appearance of all mycoplasmal colonies depend on the constituents and degree of hydration of the medium, the agar concentration, atmospheric condition, and age of the culture.

Genome

Mollicutes have small genomes compared to other bacteria, consisting of a single circular chromosome with low G+C (40%) content. This is believed to reflect a gradual reduction from a common ancestor by "degenerative evolution"; the selective pressure for this is unknown. Mycoplasmas are most closely related to the *Streptococci*, *Bacilli* and *Lactobacilli*.

The *M. pneumoniae* genome comprises 8.16 kb encoding 687 genes. Almost all of the genes in *M. genitalium* are present in *M. pneumoniae*, and the genome of the former is considered the smallest of any free-living organism (580,070 bp; 470 genes; G+C 32%); *M. hominis* is intermediate in size (665,445 bp; G+C 27.1%). The UGA codon, one of the universal translational stop codons (opal), encodes for tryptophan in mycoplasmas. The reduced genome size and streamlined metabolism of *M. pneumoniae* provide an ideal model for systemwide studies. The *M. pneumoniae* type strain M129 has been extensively characterised including full analysis of its transcriptome, metabolome and proteome. Since the small genome size results from loss of major anabolic pathways and a reduction in the complexity of gene expression regulation, *mycoplasmas* can still serve as models for other kinds of complex cellular processes such as genesis of cell polarity, assembly of macromolecular structures, cell division, adherence and motility. The limited biosynthetic capabilities of mycoplasmas are responsible for many of their biological characteristics, including the requirement for complex in vitro growth media. Genome reduction limits mycoplasmas to obligate parasitism. For example, loss of the thymidine kinase enzyme salvage pathway in mycoplasmas and other Mollicutes leads to complete reliance on the host for this function.

Biochemical reactions

The metabolic activities of mycoplasmas appear to be primarily associated with the generation of energy rather than the provision of substrates for synthetic pathways. All *Mollicutes* so far examined have truncated respiratory systems, lacking a complete tricarboxylic acid (TCA) cycle, quinones and cytochromes and consequently cannot generate adenosine triphosphate (ATP) by oxidative phosphorylation. Therefore it is assumed that mycoplasmas produce low ATP yields and relatively large quantities of metabolic end-products. *Mycoplasmas* can be divided into fermentative and nonfermentative organisms depending on their ability to metabolise carbohydrates (see Table 35.1) and some show both properties. *Ureaplasma* species generate ATP through the hydrolysis of urea, resulting in an accumulation of intracellular ammonia creating an electrochemical gradient from which ATP is generated.

Mycoplasma, Ureaplasma and certain other species require sterols in growth media, usually provided by serum. Sterols are critical components of the mycoplasma cell membrane that provide stability and structural support to the organisms in the absence of peptidoglycan. Thus they fail to grow in serum-free media and are inhibited by digitonin, distinguishing them from the species that do not require sterol. In addition, most mycoplasmas and ureaplasmas produce hydrogen peroxide, which produces α-type haemolysis in agar. *M. pneumoniae* produces clear zones of β-haemolysis, and about one-third of all *Mycoplasma* species display the phenomenon of haemadsorption (Fig. 35.5).

Cultivation

Mycoplasmas have limited biosynthetic abilities; therefore they need a rich growth medium containing natural animal protein (usually blood serum) and, in most cases, a sterol component. Serum supplies not only cholesterol but also saturated and unsaturated fatty acids for membrane synthesis, components that the organisms cannot synthesize. A medium that has been widely used for isolation contains bovine heart infusion (PPLO broth) with fresh yeast extract and horse serum. However, these components vary in

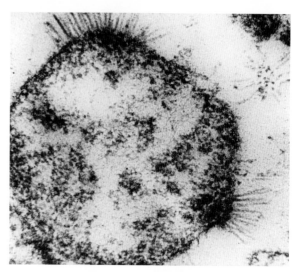

Fig. 35.5 Colony of *M. agalactiae* (of caprine origin) showing adherent guinea-pig erythrocytes (phenomenon of haemadsorption).

their ability to support growth, and success may depend on use of different batches of the components, sera from other animal species or the addition of various supplements. Cultivation of spiroplasmas is more difficult. A medium designated SP-4 has been helpful in their isolation and also in the isolation of fastidious mycoplasmas, such as *M. pneumoniae*, *M. fermentans* and *M. genitalium*, which is notoriously difficult to isolate. Most mycoplasmas are facultatively anaerobic but, because organisms from primary tissue specimens often grow only under anaerobic conditions, an atmosphere of 95% nitrogen and 5% carbon dioxide is preferred for primary isolation. The optimal temperature for growth of most mycoplasmas and ureaplasmas from humans or animals is 36°C to 38°C, but is lower for acholeplasmas and spiroplasmas and for some mycoplasma species from nonhuman sources. Commercial media are available, and various specific formulations have been described for the isolation of mycoplasmas and ureaplasmsas. Mycoplasmas are fastidious, and not all can be cultivated; some such as *M. amphoriforme* may require several weeks. Isolation of *M. genitalium* has been achieved using growth in cell cultures. Inoculated cell cultures are monitored for mycoplasmal growth by polymerase chain reaction (PCR) followed, when there are signs of growth, by subculture to mycoplasmal medium.

Viruses and plasmids

Viruses have been identified in *Acholeplasma*, *Mycoplasma* and *Spiroplasma* species. They are rod-shaped (Fig. 35.6) or enveloped spheres that bud from the mycoplasma membrane surface, or are polyhedral with a tail. They

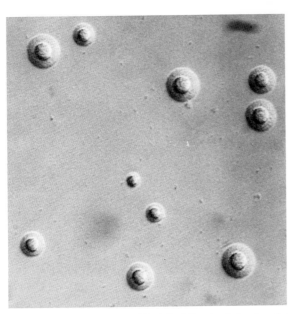

Fig. 35.6 Rod-shaped virus particles (75 × 7.5 nm) radiating from the surface of an *A. laidlawii* cell. Original magnification ×100,000.

have double-stranded DNA in circular or linear form. There is evidence for integration of the viral genome into the mycoplasmal chromosome, especially in spiroplasmas, and this may provide a mechanism for the promotion of genetic diversity. Viral release is continuous and is not accompanied by cell lysis. Plasmids have been detected in *Acholeplasma, Mycoplasma, Spiroplasma* and *Phytoplasma*.

PATHOGENESIS

Mycoplasmas are usually pathogens of the respiratory or urogenital tracts but can also be associated with a wide range of sequelae.

Respiratory infections

M. pneumoniae infections affect both the upper and lower respiratory tracts and occur both endemically and epidemically worldwide in children and adults. *M. pneumoniae* is a leading cause of community-acquired pneumonia (CAP) and is responsible for 15% to 20% of CAP cases in adults and up to 40% of cases in children. Though normally mild and frequently asymptomatic in adults, *M. pneumoniae* infections are often more serious in children and immunocompromised individuals. Radiographic evidence of pneumonia shows patchy opacities, usually of one of the lower or middle lobes. About 20% of patients suffer bilateral pneumonia, but pleurisy and

pleural effusions are unusual. The infection may show an indolent time course with cough, abnormal chest signs, and radiographic changes extending over several weeks; relapse is a prominent feature. A prolonged paroxysmal cough similar to whooping cough may occur in children. Despite these signs and symptoms, most patients are not seriously ill and few warrant admission to hospital. However, very severe infections have been reported in adults, usually in those with immunodeficiency or sickle cell anaemia, although death is rare. The clinical symptoms that manifest due to infection can be diverse with the most severe infections resulting in CAP and occasionally abscesses persisting for weeks to months. Apart from being involved in some exacerbations of chronic bronchitis, there is increasing evidence that *M. pneumoniae* might not only exacerbate asthma but sometimes be a primary cause of asthma in children due to the effects of the community-acquired respiratory distress syndrome (CARDS) toxin and modulation of the immune response to infection.

Disease caused by *M. pneumoniae* is usually limited to the respiratory tract; however, extrapulmonary manifestations include Stevens–Johnson syndrome and other rashes, arthralgia, meningitis or encephalitis (and other neurological sequelae including, rarely, Bell palsy), haemolytic anaemia (associated with cold agglutinins; anti-I antibodies), myocarditis, pericarditis and septic arthritis. *M. pneumoniae* has on rare occasions been isolated from and detected in cerebrospinal fluid.

M. pneumoniae infection occurs worldwide. Although endemic in most areas, seasonal variation can be observed with a preponderance of infection in late summer and early autumn in temperate climates. In some countries, such as the United Kingdom, epidemic peaks have been observed about every 4 years with seasonal peaks from December to February. Spread is fostered by close contact, for example, in a family, schools or military barracks. Overall, *M. pneumoniae* may cause only about one-sixth of all cases of pneumonia but has been quoted in up to 40% of cases. Infection is seen in all ages; however, it is detected more frequently in children and their parental age group.

Other agents associated with respiratory infection include *M. amphoriforme* (immunocompromised), *M. hominis* and ureaplasmas (both in neonates). *M. fermentans* has been associated with adult respiratory distress syndrome with or without systemic disease, and with pneumonia in a few children with community-acquired disease.

Urogenital and neonatal infections

As listed in Table 35.1, various mycoplasmas and ureaplasmas, most frequently *M. hominis* and *Ureaplasma*, have been isolated from the urogenital tract.

In men

Although *M. hominis* may be isolated from about 20% of men with acute nongonococcal urethritis (NGU), it has not been incriminated as a cause. There is increasing evidence to implicate *U. urealyticum*, but not *U. parvum*, in this acute condition; *U. urealyticum* is the most likely species involved in some chronic cases.

M. genitalium is now a well-established sexually transmitted infection and has been strongly implicated worldwide as a cause of about 10% to 35% of cases of nonchlamydial NGU (NCNGU), contributing significantly to the overall burden of disease. Failure to eradicate *M. genitalium* infection leads to persistent or recurrent signs and symptoms of urethritis in a significant proportion of men. In addition, there is preliminary evidence that *M. genitalium* causes balanoposthitis and it might be involved in some cases of acute epididymitis. There is evidence that ureaplasmas may occasionally cause acute epididymitis, but it is very doubtful that they have any role in male infertility.

In women

M. hominis and, to a lesser extent, ureaplasmas are found in the vagina of women who have bacterial vaginosis in much larger numbers, up to 10,000-fold in the case of *M. hominis*, than in healthy women. Thus it is possible that with various other bacteria they may contribute to the development of the condition; however, it seems very unlikely that *M. hominis* causes disease if present in small numbers.

M. genitalium has been associated strongly with cervicitis, despite the criteria used to define the condition being variable, and with pelvic inflammatory disease. *M. hominis* has been isolated from the endometrium and fallopian tubes of about 10% of women with laparoscopically confirmed pelvic inflammatory disease (PID), together with a specific antibody response. There is a strong association with endometritis, and antibody responses to mycoplasmas are present in some patients. The part that *M. hominis* is likely to play in infertility in women as a result of tubal damage is small. In contrast, serology has shown a strong association between *M. genitalium* and tubal factor infertility.

M. hominis has been isolated from the blood from women diagnosed with febrile abortion and postpartum fevers. These fevers are often transient and self-limiting, but dissemination has been seen associated with trauma or immunocompromise.

M. hominis and ureaplasmas have been isolated from the amniotic fluid and placentae of women with severe chorioamnionitis who have preterm labour. Similarly, ureaplasmas have been isolated from spontaneously aborted foetuses and stillborn or premature infants and they may have a role in abortion. However, bacterial vaginosis is strongly associated with preterm labour and late miscarriage. Thus it is not possible to differentiate the effects of these Mollicutes from those of the components of the vaginal microbiota.

In neonates

Ureaplasmas can be isolated from the respiratory tract of infants, including those born prematurely weighing less than 1 kg. Acquired peripartum is associated with a twofold risk of pneumonia, death or chronic lung disease compared to that in uninfected infants of similar or greater birthweight.

Meningitis may be associated with *M. hominis* or ureaplasmas gaining access to the cerebrospinal fluid within the first few days of life. These organisms have also been associated with postpartum fever after an abortion or even a normal delivery, possibly by causing endometritis.

Other clinical manifestations

Evidence that ureaplasmas are involved in the aetiology of sexually acquired reactive arthritis is based on synovial fluid mononuclear cell proliferation in response to specific ureaplasmal antigens. Ureaplasmas also have a role in suppurative arthritis in hypogammaglobulinaemic patients. *M. genitalium* has been reported in the joints of patients with Reiter disease or rheumatoid arthritis, but the significance of this remains unclear. Cases of *M. hominis* septic arthritis have been documented to occur in patients who were postpartum, had recently undergone urogenital surgery or manipulation or were immunocompromised, as well as in immunocompetent hosts following closed trauma.

M. pneumoniae pneumonia in immunodeficient patients may be severe, and the organisms may persist for many months in the respiratory tract of hypogammaglobulinaemic patients, despite apparently adequate antibiotic treatment. A few hypogammaglobulinaemic patients develop suppurative arthritis, and mycoplasmas are responsible for at least two-fifths of the cases. The mycoplasmas mainly involved are *M. pneumoniae*, *M. salivarium* (usually regarded as nonpathogenic), *M. hominis* and particularly ureaplasmas. Haematogenous spread of *M. hominis* leading to septic arthritis, surgical wound infections and peritonitis seems to occur more often after organ transplantation and in other patients on immunosuppressive therapy. The suggestion that *M. fermentans* infection of the peripheral blood monocytes of human immunodeficiency virus (HIV)–positive subjects may lead to a more rapid development of acquired immunodeficiency syndrome (AIDS) now seems highly unlikely. Similarly, nothing has emerged to support the notion that *M. penetrans* is associated with HIV positivity or with Kaposi sarcoma.

Pathogenic mechanisms

Not all mycoplasmas isolated from humans are known to be pathogenic. *M. pneumoniae, M. genitalium, M. hominis, M. fermentans* and *U. urealyticum* unequivocally cause disease or are strongly associated with disease. *M. amphoriforme* has been recovered from or detected in the respiratory tract of patients with antibody deficiency and chronic bronchitis and from children with respiratory disease, but its relation to this disease or, indeed, others is not clear.

Virulence is thought to be conferred by the following:

- The ability of some mycoplasmas to invade host cells
- The production of toxins by *M. pneumoniae* and some other mycoplasmas
- The stimulation of proinflammatory cytokines
- Antigenic variation that enables the mycoplasma to evade the protective immune systems of the host
- Immunological responses of the host including autoimmunity and exaggerated responses to repeat infection leading to greater pathology

M. pneumoniae is known to cause direct injury to the host through the generation of activated oxygen and the production of a pertussis toxinlike protein, the CARDS toxin. In addition to direct damage, *M. pneumoniae* can modulate the immune response of the host, generating inflammatory reactions causing the pulmonary and extrapulmonary symptoms associated with infection. *M. pneumoniae* expresses a variety of adhesion proteins and glycolipids that share structural homology to host cells; these may induce host immune responses that lead to cross-reactive antibodies and autoimmune damage. In *M. pneumoniae,* as well as other Mollicutes, pathogenicity is closely linked to carbon metabolism. The utilisation of glycerol and phospholipids plays an important role in the virulence of *Mycoplasma* species because the hydrogen peroxide generated is cytotoxic.

The CARDS toxin of *M. pneumoniae* is an adenosine diphosphate (ADP)–ribosylating and vacuolating cytotoxin that provides a mechanism to explain the observed epithelial damage that occurs with infection. This cytotoxin exhibits similarities to pertussis toxin. The CARDS toxin binds alveolar surfactant protein A and is likely to contribute to additional colonisation and pathogenic pathways. The CARDS toxin has an enzymatic action on both similar and distinct human cell proteins when compared with the S1 catalytic subunit of pertussis toxin. This leads to a cascade of events such as tissue disorganisation, inflammation, and airway dysfunction along with cell vacuolisation.

Following transmission to a new host, *Mycoplasmas* colonise epithelial linings localised to the base of the cilia where they interact directly with the host cell surface. *M. pneumoniae* and *M. genitalium* colonisation results from the interaction between adhesin proteins on the mycoplasma surface and sulphated glycolipid or sialoglycoprotein molecules on the host respiratory epithelium. There are many proteins associated with cytoadherence of *M. pneumoniae*, of which the membrane protein P1 is thought to have a major receptor-binding role. Antibodies to P1 inhibit *M. pneumoniae* adherence to tracheal epithelium. P1 is primarily localised to the attachment organelle but it is also found distributed over the entire surface of *M. pneumoniae*. The major adhesion of *M. genitalium* is the 140-kDa protein MgPa.

Some pathogenic *Mycoplasma* species have the capability to enter nonphagocytic host cells. The capability to enter a protecting niche provides these organisms with a unique opportunity for resisting host defenses and selective antibiotic therapies, establishing chronic infections and in some cases passing through cellular barriers to cause systemic infections. The mechanisms by which mycoplasmas enter host cells still, in the most part, need to be elucidated. Mycoplasmas such as *M. pneumoniae* and *M. genitalium* appear to enter the cells via their attachment organelle whereas other mycoplasmas, such as *M. fermentans* and *M. hominis,* do not have such a structure.

The ability of pathogenic microorganisms to adhere to and colonise host targets involves complex interactions and molecular cross-talk between microbial adhesins and host cell receptors. *M. pneumoniae* utilises glycolysis as the major pathway to produce ATP as it lacks the enzymes for the citric acid cycle. The surface localisation of glycolytic enzymes and their interaction with host factors has been described for several different *Mycoplasma* species including *M. gallisepticum, M. suis, M. bovis, M. fermentans* and *M. pneumoniae*. Many host targets are utilised by microbial pathogens and a broad spectrum of proteins of the human fibrinolysis system and ECM act as binding partners for glycolytic enzymes of microorganisms with fibronectin being among the most common. Elongation factor Tu, pyruvate dehydrogenase subunit B, and glyceraldehyde-3-phosphate dehydrogenase of *M. pneumoniae* have been reported as being surface-localised and function as binding proteins to human fibronectin. In comparison, elongation factor Tu of *M. genitalium*, which shares 96% homology with elongation factor Tu of *M. pneumoniae*, is unable to bind fibronectin due to a difference in 13 amino acids, 7 of which are located in a region of the protein implicated in fibronectin interaction of the *M. pneumoniae* protein.

Cytoadhesins of *M. hominis* have been shown to bind to sulphated structures on human cells and ECM molecules. Upregulation of laminin, thrombospondin and collagen as ligands and integrins as receptors for *M. hominis* cytoadherence and internalisation has been shown on the host cell membrane as a response to infection with *M. hominis*. The method by which *M. hominis* is internalised into host cells is unknown; however, the protein Vaa is thought to be one of the major adhesins.

Mycoplasmas are heterogeneous organisms, and many display antigenic variation and pronounced variation of surface proteins. This is thought to be an important way of evading the host immune response, particularly the humoral immune response, resulting in the chronic infection characteristic of many *Mycoplasma* infections.

LABORATORY INVESTIGATION

The clinical manifestations of *Mycoplasma*-induced disease are often insufficiently distinct for definitive diagnosis; therefore, laboratory-based detection is required. Laboratory-based detection of mycoplasmas in clinical specimens is gaining greater attention largely due to the availability of improved methods for detection.

Isolation of mycoplasmas is not often attempted because of insensitivity and the time required (several weeks for some species). Culture still has a place in the detection of some fast-growing mycoplasmas and ureaplasmas and is required for definitive diagnosis of active infection. Furthermore, isolation of mycoplasmas allows for further strain characterisation and antibiotic resistance testing. Mycoplasmas can be cultured using an enriched growth medium supplemented with nucleic acid precursors, fatty acids, amino acids, and, depending on the metabolic requirements of the *Mycoplasma*, glucose, arginine or urea. When mycoplasmas are cultured in liquid media, phenol red is used as an indicator of growth. Definitive identification of *Mycoplasma* species is required following culture, which is usually confirmed by PCR.

In the past, reliance was often placed on serology; however, this is now supplemented with molecular detection that is specific to the species under investigation. Methods such as qPCR are commercially available for the main pathogenic species in humans. Molecular detection enables testing within one day, the possibility of obtaining a positive result more quickly after the onset of illness than when using serology or culture, the need for one specimen containing organisms that do not have to be viable, and the ability to detect nucleic acid in preserved tissue. It can also be valuable in identifying mycoplasma aetiology in people with a variety of extrapulmonary syndromes due to the ability to detect the organism in blood and cerebrospinal fluid, which has rarely been successful by culture.

Serological testing was the first method developed for the detection of infection with *M. pneumoniae*. *M.*

pneumoniae has both lipid and protein antigens, which elicit an antibody response that can be detected after about 1 week of illness, with a peak at 3 to 6 weeks followed by a gradual decline. Initially IgM antibodies occur 6 to 10 days after infection; however, only about 80% of patients younger than 20 years develop IgM antibodies and this reduces to about 40% in patients that are older than 20 years. This means that a specific IgM response can be absent, especially in older patients. It has also been shown that IgM antibodies can still be detected at least 1 year after the onset of symptoms. Specific IgG antibodies appear 9 to 14 days after infection and may persist for up to 4 years. Specific IgA antibodies appear 1 week after the start of infection and decrease after about 5 weeks. Due to this antibody response, acute and convalescent patient sera, taken 2 to 3 weeks apart, are required for confirmation of infection. This is a significant limitation for prompt point-of-care diagnosis, particularly in adults over 40 years of age who may not mount an IgM response. It is difficult to obtain clear specificity ascertainment of serological assays in relation to cross-reactions with antibodies from other mycoplasma infections such as with *M. genitalium*. Comparative studies between commercially available EIAs show variability in diagnosis results, highlighting the need for standardisation and improved sensitivities and specificities among serological reagents used for detecting acute *M. pneumoniae* infection.

Comparison of PCR with culture and/or serology has yielded varied results that are not always in agreement. Positive PCR results in culture-negative persons, without evidence of respiratory disease, suggest inadequate assay specificity, persistence of the organism after infection, asymptomatic carriage of the organism or poor culture technique. Positive PCR results in serology-negative persons may be due to an inadequate immune response, early successful antibiotic treatment or the collection of specimens before the specific antibody response occurs. Serological and molecular test methods are not routinely available for all species, leaving reliance on identification to specialised reference laboratories and academia.

Molecular typing

There are two main clades of *M. pneumoniae* that can be distinguished by sequencing of the gene encoding the P1 cytoadhesin, multiple-locus variable-number tandem-repeat (VNTR) analysis (MLVA) and multiple-locus sequence typing (MLST) (see Ch. 3). MLVA has successfully been used for typing an increasing number of microbial species, including *M. pneumoniae* and, more recently, *M. hominis*. More than 26 differing types have been described for *M. pneumoniae*. However, in comparison to *M. pneumoniae*, *M. hominis* displays high genetic heterogeneity among isolates and 40 MLVA types have been described for 210 isolates tested. Other molecular typing methods have been developed for *M. hominis,* including methods based on sequence analysis of the *p75, p120'* and *vaa* genes, and MLST derived from whole genome. Several typing methods have been developed for *M. genitalium* including short tandem repeat (STR) analysis of the PLP gene MG309, single nucleotide polymorphisms (SNPs) of the rRNA operon and the MG191 *(mgpB)* gene, and restriction fragment length polymorphisms of the MG192 *(mgpC)* gene; however, combination of MG309-STRs and MG191-SNPs is considered sufficient for general epidemiological studies.

TREATMENT

Antimicrobial therapy is used to treat infections with *Mycoplasma;* however, because of resistance within these species, therapy is restricted to a small number of agents including the tetracyclines, macrolides and fluoroquinolones. The in vitro sensitivity of several mycoplasmas and ureaplasmas to various antibiotics used in treatment is shown in Table 35.2. These microorganisms are completely resistant to β-lactam or glycopeptide antibiotics due to their lack of peptidoglycan.

Macrolides are currently recommended as the first-line treatment for *M. pneumoniae* infection in the United Kingdom. The 2011 British Thoracic Society guidelines for the management of CAP in children and adults suggest empirical macrolide treatment at any age if there is no response to first-line β-lactam antibiotics or in the case of very severe disease. Tetracyclines and fluoroquinolones can be used to treat *M. pneumoniae* infections as an alternative to macrolides when clinically relevant. Evidence suggests that the first-line treatment for *M. genitalium* infections is with macrolides, and typically an extended course of azithromycin is recommended.

Since 2000, a significant worldwide increase in the prevalence of (multiclonal) macrolide-resistant *M. pneumoniae* strains has been observed. In Asia, resistance rates of over 90% have been reported, particularly in China, whereas in Europe and North America rates of up to 25% have been found. Macrolide-resistant *M. pneumoniae* can have serious consequences in children with prolonged clinical symptoms and more severe radiological findings. Additionally, an increase in extrapulmonary manifestations has been observed in patients infected with macrolide-resistant *M. pneumoniae.*

Similarly high levels of macrolide resistance are being reported with *M. genitalium* with more than 30% to 100% of cases showing resistance. In most cases, patients with macrolide-resistant *M. genitalium* can be treated with a fluoroquinolone but treatment failure can occur, particularly in the Asia-Pacific region, where preexisting fluoroquinolone resistance is common. Multidrug-resistant *M. genitalium* has been detected.

Resistance to tetracyclines conferred by the *tetM* gene has been documented in several species including *M. hominis* and *Ureaplasma* species.

In urogenital infections treatment must take into account the fact that several different microorganisms may be involved and that a precise microbiological diagnosis may not be attainable. Thus, patients with NGU should receive an antibiotic that is active against *C. trachomatis*, ureaplasmas and *M. genitalium.* Azithromycin, which is used increasingly for chlamydial infections, is also active against mycoplasmas, and its widespread short-term use for *Chlamydia* may be contributing to increasing resistance in mycoplasmas. A broad-spectrum antibiotic should also be included for the treatment of PID to cover *C. trachomatis, M. genitalium* and *M. hominis* as well as various anaerobic bacteria.

EPIDEMIOLOGY

M. pneumoniae

Infection is endemic with epidemic peaks occurring every 4 to 7 years. Typically, outbreaks of *M. pneumoniae* infection occur in areas of close personal contact—for example, in schools and military barracks. Individuals with an active *M. pneumoniae* infection carry the organism in their nose, throat, trachea and sputum; it is transmitted from person to person via aerosols. The spread of *M. pneumoniae* is greatly facilitated by the persistent cough that accompanies the infection. Current opinion suggests that asymptomatic carriage of *M. pneumoniae* occurs, facilitating the spread of infection. Epidemics of *M. pneumoniae* infections can be prolonged; this could be due to the long incubation period of 1 to 3 weeks of *M. pneumoniae* as well as the relatively low transmission rate of infection. Long-term morbidity due to *M. pneumoniae* infection is uncommon; however, the acute illness is often disruptive and can consume significant resources.

Epidemics of *M. pneumoniae* infections historically occur every 4 years in the United Kingdom with epidemic periods lasting on average 18 months. Sporadic infection occurs at low levels with seasonal peaks from December to February. From January 1989 to June 2015 seven epidemics of *M. pneumoniae* were noted in England and Wales of declining amplitude with a recent peak in 2015. For some epidemic periods, clear annual fluctuations can also be seen, apparent as a double peak over two winter seasons. The clarity of epidemic periods has, in recent years, declined with fewer reported cases overall. From 1975 to 2009, incidence was found to be similar by gender, both during epidemic and interepidemic periods. The annual notification rate in 2010 to 2014 was consistently highest in those aged 15 to 44 years.

Globally, epidemics of *M. pneumoniae* are considered to occur every 3 to 7 years; however, recent epidemiological studies have documented varying trends in epidemic patterns. In Jerusalem, historically, epidemics were observed every 3 to 5 years with seasonal peaks in October and early spring; however, since autumn 2014 a constant rate of infection has been observed, diverging from the historic pattern.

M. genitalium

Infection is sexually transmissible with a significantly higher prevalence in partners of patients positive for *M. genitalium* than for partners of patients negative for *M. genitalium* presenting with urethritis or cervicitis. Transmission seems to be at an equivalent rate, too, but independent of that of *Chlamydia trachomatis* when assessed by concordance; up to 63% of sexual partners of *M. genitalium*–positive patients are infected. Transmission is more frequently related to unprotected vaginal intercourse, but asymptomatic rectal carriage has been reported in men who have sex with men and no pharyngeal carriage has been reported. The risk factors associated with *M.*

genitalium infection in women are recent sexual intercourse, a greater number of sex partners, the shorter duration of a stable relationship, younger age of first intercourse, tobacco use, African ethnic origin and bacterial vaginosis. In men, risk factors associated with *M. genitalium* infection are young age and sexual intercourse in the month prior to consultation, with a sex partner with a recent history of STI diagnosis or treatment.

Studies of *M. genitalium* prevalence have demonstrated global infection rates of 1% to 4% in men and from 1% to 6.4% in women. Furthermore, carriage of *M. genitalium* may be asymptomatic. *M. genitalium* carriage is higher in populations at high risk of STI, that is, 4% to 38% in STI testing centres.

M. hominis and Ureaplasma species

Global infection rates of *M. hominis* and *Ureaplasma* species are not well documented and are mostly presented as case reports. However, the presence of *M. hominis* or *Ureaplasma* species on the mucosal surfaces of the cervix or vagina of sexually mature, asymptomatic women has been indicated at 21% to 53% and up to 80%, respectively; this is somewhat lower in the urethra of males.

RECOMMENDED READING

Blanchard, A., & Browning, G. (Eds.). (2005). *Mycoplasmas: molecular biology, pathogenicity and strategies for control.* Wymondham, UK: Horizon Scientific Press.

Furr, P. M., Taylor-Robinson, D., & Webster, A. D. B. (1994). Mycoplasmas and ureaplasmas in patients with hypogammaglobulinaemia and their role in arthritis: microbiological observations over 20 years. *Annals of the Rheumatic Diseases, 53,* 183–187.

Maniloff, J., McElhaney, R. N., Finch, L. R., *et al.* (Eds.). (1992). *Mycoplasmas: molecular biology and pathogenesis.* Washington, DC: American Society for Microbiology.

Taylor-Robinson, D. (1996). Mycoplasmas and their role in human respiratory tract disease. In S. Myint & D. Taylor-Robinson (Eds.), *Viral and other infections of the human respiratory tract* (pp. 319–339). London: Chapman and Hall.

Taylor-Robinson, D. (2002). *Mycoplasma genitalium*–an update. *International Journal of STD and AIDS, 13,* 145–151.

Taylor-Robinson, D., & Bebear, C. (1997). Antibiotic susceptibilities of mycoplasmas and treatment of mycoplasmal infections. *The Journal of Antimicrobial Chemotherapy, 40,* 622–630.

Taylor-Robinson, D., Gilroy, C. B., & Jensen, J. S. (2000). The biology of *Mycoplasma genitalium. Venereol, 13,* 119–127.

Taylor-Robinson, D., & Jensen, J. S. (2011). Genital mycoplasmas. In S. A. Morse, R. C. Ballard, K. K. Holmes, *et al.* (Eds.), *Atlas of sexually transmitted diseases and AIDS* (4th ed., pp. 64–75). London: Mosby.

Taylor-Robinson, D., & Jensen, J. S. (2011). *Mycoplasma genitalium*: from chrysalis to multicolored butterfly. *Clinical Microbiology Reviews, 24,* 498–514.

Totten, P. A., Taylor-Robinson, D., & Jensen, J. S. (2008). Genital mycoplasmas. In K. K. Holmes, P. F. Sparling, W. E. Stamm, *et al.* (Eds.), *Sexually transmitted diseases* (4th ed., pp. 709–736). New York: McGraw Hill.

Tully, J. G., & Razin, S. (Eds.). (1996). *Molecular and diagnostic procedures in mycoplasmology. Diagnostic procedures* (Vol. 2). London: Academic Press.

Waites, K. B., & Taylor-Robinson, D. (2011). *Mycoplasma* and *Ureaplasma.* In P. R. Murray, E. J. Baron, J. H. Jorgensen, *et al.* (Eds.), *Manual of clinical microbiology* (10th ed., Vol. 1, pp. 970–985). Washington, DC: American Society for Microbiology.

36 *Rickettsia, Orientia, Ehrlichia, Anaplasma* and *Coxiella*

Typhus; spotted fevers; scrub typhus; ehrlichioses; Q fever

DAVID H. WALKER AND XUE-JIE YU

KEY POINTS

- Rickettsiae are small obligate intracellular bacteria that are associated with insects or ticks during at least part of their transmission cycle.
- *Rickettsia* and *Orientia* cause spotted fevers, typhus fevers and scrub typhus by infecting and damaging endothelial cells, resulting in increased vascular permeability, oedema, adult respiratory distress syndrome, meningoencephalitis and rash.
- *Ehrlichia* and *Anaplasma* reside in persistently infected vertebrate hosts such as deer, dogs or rodents, and are transmitted by feeding ticks.
- *Ehrlichia* and *Anaplasma* target human monocytes or granulocytes, where they grow to microcolonies in cytoplasmic vacuoles.
- The frequent absence of antibodies to rickettsiae, orientiae and ehrlichiae early in the course of illness hinders laboratory diagnosis, making clinicoepidemiological suspicion of the diagnosis and empirical treatment, preferably with doxycycline, essential.
- *Coxiella burnetii* thrives in the acidic autophagolysosome of macrophages, has a stable extracellular form and infects human beings who inhale aerosols from birth fluids or the placenta of infected animals. Unlike the above mentioned obligate intracellular Rickettsiales, *Coxiella* has been cultivated in acellular medium.

Few diseases have had a greater impact on the course of human history than epidemic typhus. Hans Zinsser's classic book *Rats, Lice and History* provides a graphic account of how *Rickettsia prowazekii*, the aetiological agent of this louse-borne disease, has caused millions of deaths and much human suffering in conditions of famine, poverty and war. Epidemic typhus now occurs mainly in poor populations in developing countries, as world conditions have improved, but various other rickettsial diseases are still widely distributed.

The rickettsiae (*Rickettsia* and *Orientia* species) and anaplasmas (*Anaplasma, Ehrlichia, Neorickettsia,* and *Neoehrlichia* species) of medical importance are obligate intracellular bacteria mostly transmitted by arthropod vectors. Molecular studies reveal that *Rickettsia* species, *Orientia tsutsugamushi, Ehrlichia* species, *Anaplasma* species and *Neoehrlichia mikurensis* belong to the Alphaproteobacteria and have evolved from a common ancestor.

Coxiella burnetii, an intracellular bacterium found in ticks, is more closely related to *Legionella pneumophila* (Gammaproteobacteria), but is conveniently considered here alongside the rickettsia group.

RICKETTSIA AND ORIENTIA

DESCRIPTION

The genera *Rickettsia* and *Orientia* include organisms responsible for numerous diseases in many parts of the world (Table 36.1). The pioneering research of Ricketts and others in the early 20th century demonstrated the rickettsial aetiology of Rocky Mountain spotted fever and epidemic louse-borne typhus. Several other diseases, including murine typhus and Mediterranean spotted fever, were later shown to be rickettsial infections. Previously unrecognised spotted fevers caused by *R. japonica, R. africae* and *R. honei* were discovered in the 1980s and 1990s in Japan, Africa and Australia, indicating that much remains to be learned about these organisms. Other rickettsiae, poorly understood and presumed to be nonpathogenic, have been isolated, primarily from arthropods, including herbivorous insects. Some rickettsiae isolated from ticks and presumed to be nonpathogenic have been found to cause human diseases.

Rickettsiae are small (0.3–0.5 × 0.8–1.0 μm) Gram-negative bacilli. They reside in the cytosol of host cells

Table 36.1 Human diseases caused by *Rickettsia* and *Orientia* species

Species	Disease	Geographical distribution	Mode of transmission	Primary vectors	Main vertebrate hosts
Typhus group					
R. prowazekii	Epidemic typhus	Extant foci in Africa, North and South America	Louse faeces	*Pediculus humanus corporis*	Humans, flying squirrels
R. typhi	Murine typhus	Primarily tropics and subtropics	Flea faeces	*Xenopsylla cheopis* and other fleas	Rodents and other small mammals
Spotted fever group					
R. akari	Rickettsialpox	USA, Ukraine, Croatia, Korea, Turkey, Mexico	Bite of mouse mite	*Liponyssoides sanguineus*	House mice; possibly other rodents
R. australis	Queensland tick typhus	Australia	Bite of tick	*Ixodes holocyclus*	Unknown
R. conorii	Boutonneuse fever	Europe, Africa, Middle East, India	Bite of tick	*Rhipicephalus sanguineus*	Unknown
R. japonica	Japanese spotted fever	Japan and northeastern Asia	Bite of tick	*Dermacentor, Haemaphysalis, Ixodes* spp.	Unknown
R. rickettsii	Rocky Mountain spotted fever	North and South America	Bite of tick	*Dermacentor* spp., *Rh. sanguineus, Amblyomma cajennense, A. aureolatum*	Rodents, opossums, dogs and other small mammals
R. africae	African tick bite fever	Africa and West Indies	Bite of tick	*A. hebraeum, A. variegatum*	Unknown
R. parkeri	American tick bite fever	North and South America	Bite of tick	*A. maculatum, A. americanum, A. triste*	Unknown
R. sibirica	North Asian tick typhus	Northern Asia	Bite of tick	*Dermacentor, Haemaphysalis* spp., etc.	Rodents and other small mammals
R. honei	Flinders Island spotted fever	Australia and Asia	Bite of tick	*Bothriocroton hydrosauri*	Unknown
R. slovaca	Tick-borne lymphadenopathy	Eurasia	Bite of tick	*Dermacentor marginatum, D. reticularis*	Unknown
R. felis	Flea-borne spotted fever	Worldwide	Flea; transovarial transmission	*Ctenocephalides felis*	Opossums
Scrub typhus group					
Orientia tsutsugamushi	Scrub typhus	Asia, Australia, islands of south-west Pacific and Indian oceans	Bite of larval mite	*Leptotrombidium* spp.	Rodents (especially rats)

(Fig. 36.1). All pathogens are associated with a flea, louse, mite or tick vector. Species pathogenic for humans parasitise endothelial cells almost exclusively. Rickettsiae have a small genome (approximately 1 Mb) and lack genes encoding many essential enzymes. Thus they depend on the host for nutrition and building blocks and are yet to be cultivated outside eukaryotic cells. Like the chlamydiae (see Ch. 34), rickettsiae have a typical Gram-negative bacterial cell wall, including a bilayered outer membrane that contains lipopolysaccharide, and are energy parasites that transport adenosine triphosphate (ATP) with a unique translocase.

The genus *Rickettsia* is divided into two antigenically distinct groups based on their lipopolysaccharide: the typhus group and the spotted fever group. The immuno-dominant rickettsial outer membrane protein A (OmpA) exists only in the spotted fever group rickettsiae. Another

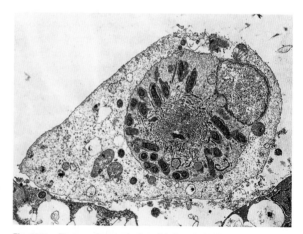

Fig. 36.1 Electron micrograph of a cell infected with *R. rickettsii*, showing the dilatation of the endoplasmic reticulum of host cells that occurs as a result of injury associated with infection by spotted fever group rickettsiae.

major outer membrane protein, OmpB, exists in all *Rickettsia* species. OmpA and OmpB both contain cross-reactive and species-specific epitopes.

The scrub typhus rickettsiae are antigenically distinct and appear to be fundamentally different. They have been classified into a related but distinct genus as *Orientia tsutsugamushi* (see Table 36.1). The cell wall lacks lipopolysaccharide, peptidoglycan and a slime layer and appears to derive its structural integrity from proteins linked by disulphide bonds. *O. tsutsugamushi* exhibits a major 56-kDa surface protein with both strain-specific and cross-reactive epitopes.

PATHOGENESIS

Invasion and destruction of target cells

Rickettsiae normally enter the body through the bite or faeces of an infected arthropod vector. They are disseminated through the bloodstream, attach to endothelial cells by OmpA, OmpB and other autotransporter surface proteins, enter endothelial cells by induced phagocytosis, escape from the phagosome, multiply intracellularly and eventually destroy their host cells. Cell culture studies suggest that spotted fever and typhus group rickettsiae destroy the host cell by different mechanisms. After infection with *R. prowazekii* or *R. typhi*, the rickettsiae continue to multiply until the cell is packed with organisms (Fig. 36.2) and then bursts, possibly as a result of membranolytic activity; before lysis, host cells appear ultrastructurally normal.

Spotted fever group rickettsiae seldom accumulate in large numbers and do not burst the host cells, but stimulate polymerisation of host-derived F-actin tails that propel them through the cytoplasm and into filopodia, from which they escape the cell or spread into an adjacent cell (Fig. 36.3). Two proteins, RickA and Sca2, act as critical regulators of actin-based movement in spotted fever group, but not in typhus, rickettsiae. Infected cells exhibit signs of membrane damage associated with an influx of water, which is sequestered within cisternae of dilated rough endoplasmic reticulum (see Fig. 36.1). Rickettsiae damage host cell membranes, at least in part, by stimulating production of free oxygen radicals by endothelial cells.

Scrub typhus rickettsiae also escape from the phagosome, reside free in the cytosol and are released from host cells soon after infecting them, but little is known about the mechanism(s) by which these organisms damage cells.

Pathological lesions

All members of the genera *Rickettsia* and *Orientia* cause widespread microvascular infection leading to the destruction and dysfunction of infected endothelial cells. The pathological manifestations appear to result more from direct rickettsial injury but also from immunopathological mechanisms mediated via cytokines, and cytotoxic T lymphocytes and inflammation play pathogenic as well as protective roles, but disseminated intravascular coagulation and endotoxin are not pathogenic factors. Interference with normal circulation and increased vascular permeability following damage of blood vessels can cause life-threatening encephalitis and noncardiogenic pulmonary oedema.

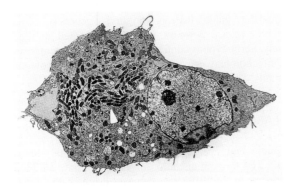

Fig. 36.2 Electron micrograph of a cell infected with *R. prowazekii*. The rickettsiae continue to multiply within the cell until it is completely packed with organisms and bursts. In contrast to cells infected with spotted fever group rickettsiae, the ultrastructural appearance of cells infected with typhus group rickettsiae remains normal until the cell lyses. The region of the cell containing rickettsiae is indicated by the *arrowhead*.

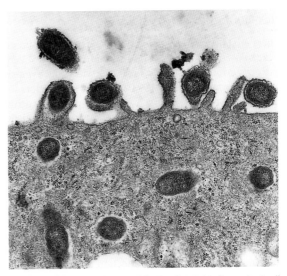

Fig. 36.3 Electron micrograph of *R. conorii* escaping from a host cell. Note the location of the rickettsiae within host cell filopodia.

CLINICAL ASPECTS OF RICKETTSIAL DISEASES

Epidemic typhus

Headache and fever develop 6–15 days after infection with *R. prowazekii*. A macular rash, often noted 4–7 days after the patient becomes ill, first appears on the trunk and axillary folds and then spreads to the extremities. In mild cases, the rash may begin to fade after 1–2 days, but, in more severe cases, it may last much longer and become haemorrhagic. Severe cases may also develop pronounced hypotension and renal dysfunction. The mental state of the patient may progress from dullness to stupor and even coma. Although the prognosis is grave for comatose patients, prompt appropriate treatment may be lifesaving.

Individuals who survive a primary infection of louse-borne typhus may develop a relatively milder reactivation of latent infection many years later. This is referred to as recrudescent typhus or Brill–Zinsser disease. Such individuals are nevertheless immune to a second louse-borne infection.

Flea-borne fevers

Patients infected with *R. typhi* develop symptoms similar to those of epidemic typhus. Fatal cases are uncommon but occasionally occur, particularly in the elderly. Although murine typhus is much milder than epidemic typhus, it is still severe enough to require several months of convalescence. *R. felis* is maintained transovarially in cat fleas and causes a less well-characterised illness.

Tick-borne spotted fever

There are many clinical similarities among the tick-borne rickettsioses of the spotted fever group. The most severe is Rocky Mountain spotted fever, for which the average case fatality rate for 1981–1998 was 3.3%. Risk factors for fatal infection include older age, glucose-6-phosphate dehydrogenase deficiency and delayed tetracycline treatment.

Patients become ill within 2 weeks of infection. Early symptoms include fever, severe headache and myalgia, often accompanied by anorexia, vomiting, abdominal pain, diarrhoea, photophobia and cough. An eschar *(tache noire)* frequently occurs at the site of the tick bite in all spotted fever group infections except Rocky Mountain spotted fever. A maculopapular rash usually develops within 3–5 days. The rash of spotted fever usually develops first on the extremities rather than on the trunk. Absence of a rash does not exclude rickettsial infection because a disproportionate number of fatal cases of Rocky Mountain spotted fever are of the 'spotless' variety. Spotted fever group

rickettsiae are found within the endothelial cells and less often macrophages of vertebrate hosts, but *R. rickettsii* can also invade vascular smooth muscle.

Vascular damage in severe cases may result in haemorrhagic rash, hypovolaemia, hypotensive shock, noncardiogenic pulmonary oedema and impairment of central nervous system function. A fulminant form of Rocky Mountain spotted fever sometimes kills the patient within 5 days of the onset of symptoms; this form of the disease is more common in black males who are deficient in glucose-6-phosphate dehydrogenase and may be related to haemolysis in these patients. Infection confers long-lasting immunity.

Rickettsialpox

The clinical course of rickettsialpox is similar to that of other spotted fever group infections and includes development of fever, headache and an eschar at the site where the infected mite fed. The rash is initially maculopapular but often becomes vesicular. Fever lasts for about a week, and patients usually recover uneventfully.

Scrub typhus

Scrub typhus may be mild or fatal, depending on host factors and presumably the virulence of the infecting strain. Symptoms develop 6–18 days after being fed upon by infected mite larvae (chiggers). The disease is characterised by sudden onset of fever, headache and myalgia. A maculopapular rash often develops 2–3 days after onset of the illness. An eschar is often apparent at the site of the chigger bite, with enlargement of local lymph nodes prior to the onset of febrile illness. Progression of the disease may be accompanied by interstitial pneumonitis, generalised lymphadenopathy and splenomegaly. Death may result from encephalitis, respiratory failure and circulatory failure. Patients who survive generally become afebrile after 2–3 weeks, or sooner if treated appropriately. Scrub typhus confers only transient immunity, and reinfection may occur with heterologous or homologous strains.

LABORATORY INVESTIGATION

Timely and accurate diagnosis of rickettsial disease followed by administration of an appropriate antibiotic may mean the difference between death of the patient and uneventful recovery. The lack of widely available, reliable diagnostic tests that can detect the disease in its early stages remains a problem, particularly as symptoms are often nonspecific. The rash may appear at a late stage in the infection or not at all and may resemble exanthemata of many other diseases. The presence or significance of an eschar, if present, is also commonly overlooked.

Serological methods

Rickettsial diseases are usually acute and short lasting. Antibodies appear in the second week of illness, when the patient is usually on the way to recovery. Death may occur before detectable levels of antibody are present. Serology is therefore not suitable for early diagnosis of rickettsial infections and is used mainly to confirm the diagnosis for epidemiologic investigations.

The traditional Weil–Felix test, which relies on agglutination of the somatic antigens of non-motile *Proteus* species, is no longer recommended because of unacceptably poor sensitivity and specificity. More reliable diagnostic tests, including immunofluorescence and enzyme immunoassay, are now commercially available.

Isolation of rickettsiae

Isolation of the organism provides conclusive proof of rickettsial infection. However, it is seldom attempted because of lack of facilities or expertise and because of the presumed danger to laboratory personnel. Such dangers have been overemphasised in this era of antibiotics, but use of containment facilities is appropriate.

Rickettsiae can be isolated in cell culture, in laboratory animals such as mice or guinea pigs, or in embryonated chicken eggs. Cell culture may yield timely results but is seldom used for isolation of rickettsiae from clinical samples. Rickettsiae can be detected in cell culture 48–72 hours after inoculation by the shell vial assay.

Detection of rickettsiae in tissue

Skin biopsies from the centre of petechial lesions or from eschars can be examined by immunohistochemistry. This approach is virtually 100% specific and has a sensitivity of 70%. Rickettsiae can be visualised for up to 48 hours after the administration of appropriate drugs, allowing diagnosis of infection postmortem. A method has been developed for capturing detached, circulating endothelial cells by antibody-coated magnetic beads and immunocytological detection of intracellular rickettsiae.

Polymerase chain reaction (PCR)

Detection of rickettsial DNA by PCR is more rapid than isolation and allows specific identification, but the test is not generally available. Detection in blood is insensitive, particularly early in the course of the infection when therapeutic decisions should be made. Peripheral blood mononuclear cells, biopsy of rash or eschar specimens may provide a more sensitive diagnostic yield.

PCR amplification of highly conserved rickettsial genes can also be used. A single primer pair that amplifies all or most rickettsiae can be designed from the genes encoding 16S ribosomal ribonucleic acid *(rrs)*, a 17-kDa protein *(htr)*, citrate synthase *(gltA)* or *sca5*. A suitable approach is to use a conserved genus-specific primer pair to amplify a rickettsial gene and then to identify the species by restriction fragment length polymorphism analysis or DNA sequencing. Scrub typhus can be diagnosed by PCR amplification of the 47-kDa or 56-kDa protein gene of *O. tsutsugamushi*.

TREATMENT

The drug of choice for treating rickettsial infections of all types and in all age groups is doxycycline. Chloramphenicol is an alternative, but is less effective and carries a higher risk of death. Both drugs are rickettsiostatic and allow the patient's immune system time to respond and control the infection. Sulphonamides should not be administered as they exacerbate rickettsial infections; β-lactam and aminoglycoside antibiotics are ineffective. Some new quinolones and macrolides have antirickettsial effects in vitro, but clinical experience in severe rickettsioses is lacking. Azithromycin is an effective drug for the treatment of scrub typhus. Short courses of doxycycline do not cause significant dental staining in young children.

Owing to the difficulties of accurate diagnosis and the risks involved in misdiagnosis, empirical doxycycline therapy is appropriate for patients who have had a fever for 3 days or more and a history consistent with the epidemiological and clinical features of rickettsial disease. The case fatality rate is increased significantly if treatment is delayed for >5 days.

Intensive nursing care, management of fluids and electrolytes, and administration of red blood cells to patients who develop anaemia may be needed. Surgery may also be necessary to remove digits and extremities that develop ischaemic necrosis.

EPIDEMIOLOGY

Typhus group infections

Epidemic typhus

R. prowazekii is transmitted from person to person by the body louse *Pediculus humanus corporis*; the organisms are present in the faeces of infected lice and enter through the bite wound or skin abrasions. *R. prowazekii* causes a fatal infection of the louse, which is therefore incapable of long-term maintenance of the rickettsiae, and human beings appear to be reservoirs of epidemic typhus. Patients who suffer a bout of recrudescent typhus (Brill–Zinsser disease) circulate sufficient rickettsiae in their blood to infect approximately 1%–5% of lice that feed on them—enough to initiate new epidemics of the disease. *R. prowazekii* is maintained in an enzootic cycle in North America involving flying squirrels and their fleas and lice and has been detected in ticks in Mexico.

Murine typhus

Murine typhus is distributed worldwide, particularly in tropical and subtropical coastal regions where the disease is an occupational hazard of working in rat-infested areas such as markets or ports. This disease is maintained in an enzootic cycle involving rats and their fleas, which remain infected for life. Even the inefficient rate of transovarial transmission in fleas may play an important role in maintaining the rickettsiae in nature. Humans are infected by the contamination of abraded skin, respiratory tract or conjunctiva with infective flea faeces, in which the rickettsiae can survive for as long as 100 days under optimal conditions of temperature and humidity. Murine typhus is also reemerging as a zoonosis involving cat fleas and opossums in the United States.

Spotted fever group infections

Tick-borne infections

Tick-borne rickettsiae of the spotted fever group are maintained in enzootic cycles involving ticks and their wild animal hosts. Ticks are the primary reservoirs of the rickettsiae and maintain the organisms by both transstadial transmission (during moulting of larva to nymph and thence to adult tick) and transovarial or vertical transmission. Some horizontal transmission (tick to vertebrate host to tick) is likely to be essential to the survival of virulent rickettsiae in nature because these rickettsiae are somewhat pathogenic to ticks.

Humans become infected following the bite of infected ticks or through contamination of abraded skin or mucous membranes. People place themselves at risk when they enter areas infested with infected ticks. Infection may also occur through bites of ticks of domestic dogs or if partially fed ticks rupture during manual de-ticking of dogs. Rocky Mountain spotted fever, *R. parkeri* infection, and other rickettsiae of unknown pathogenicity are endemic in the Americas, especially in the southeastern and south-central United States. A nonfatal illness, African tick bite fever, is often observed in travellers returning from safari in southern Africa.

Rickettsialpox

R. akari is maintained in an enzootic cycle that involves house mice *(Mus musculus)* and their mites. The arthropod vector is also the primary reservoir and can maintain the organism by transstadial and transovarial transmission. Rickettsialpox is primarily an urban disease associated with mice-infested buildings.

Scrub typhus

The nymphal and adult stages of the mites transmitting *O. tsutsugamushi* are free living and do not feed on animals. The parasitic larvae (chiggers) occur in habitats that have been disturbed by the loss or removal of the natural vegetation. The area becomes covered with scrub vegetation, which is the preferred habitat for chiggers and their mammalian hosts, and gives the disease its name. The disease is often localised because of the restricted habitat of the chiggers. Persons entering infected areas are at risk.

CONTROL

It is virtually impossible to eradicate rickettsial infections because of their enzootic nature. Measures aimed at reducing rodent or ectoparasite populations may help to reduce the risk of infection. In addition to delousing infested persons, their clothing and bedding should be decontaminated.

Persons entering areas endemic for spotted fever group infections should wear protective clothing treated with tick repellent. Individuals should also examine themselves carefully for ticks as soon as possible after returning from tick-infested areas. The probability of infection is decreased if the tick is removed soon after it attaches. Transmission may require up to 24 hours of feeding, perhaps because starved ticks require a partial blood meal if they are to reactivate the virulence of the rickettsiae as well as inject organisms into the feeding site in their saliva.

There is no safe, effective vaccine for any of the rickettsial diseases. The attenuated E strain of *R. prowazekii* induces protective immunity, but is unsuitable for general use because it causes a mild form of typhus in 10%–15% of those inoculated and reverts to a virulent state after animal passage. Inactivated Rocky Mountain spotted fever and epidemic typhus vaccines afford incomplete protection and are no longer available. A recombinant or attenuated vaccine that contains cross-protective antigens stimulating cellular immunity could protect against both typhus and spotted fever rickettsioses. Scrub typhus vaccines derived from killed rickettsiae do not prevent infection, and experimental recombinant subunit vaccines are insufficiently effective in animals.

Antimicrobial prophylaxis is not recommended for infections with *Rickettsia* species, as they are only rickettsiostatic and disease develops as soon as the antibiotic is discontinued. Prolonged prophylaxis with weekly doses of doxycycline is effective against scrub typhus, but is probably inappropriate except under exceptional circumstances, for instance during military operations.

EHRLICHIA AND *ANAPLASMA*

DESCRIPTION

Human ehrlichial disease was first recognised in 1954 when *Neorickettsia* (formerly *Ehrlichia*) *sennetsu* was identified as the cause of an illness resembling glandular fever in Japan. *Ehrlichia chaffeensis, Anaplasma phagocytophilum, E. ewingii* and *E. muris* later emerged as the causes of tick-borne diseases in the United States. *Ehrlichia* and *Anaplasma* species are transmitted through the bite of ticks. *N. sennetsu* is suspected to infect a fluke and to cause infection when ingested with parasitised raw fish (Table 36.2).

These organisms are small Gram-negative bacteria. They multiply within membrane-bound cytoplasmic vacuoles, usually in various phagocytes, and form characteristic microcolonies resembling mulberries, termed *morulae* (Latin: *morum*, mulberry) (Fig. 36.4). Electron microscopy reveals two distinct morphological forms, larger reticulate and smaller dense-core cells, which are the replicating and infectious forms, respectively, in a developmental cycle.

PATHOGENESIS

Anaplasma and *Ehrlichia* species can establish prolonged, even persistent, infections in vivo, and some species, including *E. chaffeensis,* kill heavily infected cells in vitro.

Cytokine-associated immunopathological mechanisms are probably important. *A. phagocytophilum* and *E. chaffeensis* evade the host immune system by antigenic variation and by modulating the host defences, respectively.

The tropism for phagocytes indicates that these organisms have evolved strategies for evading the microbicidal activities of the macrophage or granulocyte. Within phagocytes *A. phagocytophilum* and *E. chaffeensis* block the fusion of phagosome-containing bacteria with lysosomes to prevent killing by lysosomal enzymes. *A. phagocytophilum* prevents killing mediated by reactive oxygen species by lowering reduced nicotinamide adenine dinucleotide phosphate (NADPH) oxidase activity in neutrophils. To accommodate a slow generation time (about 8 hours), *Anaplasma* and *Ehrlichia* prolong their host cells' lifespan by inhibiting apoptosis.

Antibody to ehrlichiae confers passive protection, and cellular immunity is crucial to recovery. Suppression of neutrophil function by *A. phagocytophilum* may predispose to opportunistic infection.

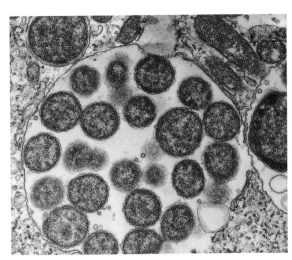

Fig. 36.4 Electron micrograph of *E. chaffeensis* within a cytoplasmic vacuole. (Micrograph courtesy Dr Vsevolod L Popov.)

Table 36.2 Human diseases caused by *Ehrlichia, Anaplasma* and *Neorickettsia* species

Species	Disease	Geographical distribution	Means of transmission	Primary vectors
E. chaffeensis	Monocytic ehrlichiosis	North and South America, Africa, Asia	Tick bite	*Amblyomma americanum*
A. phagocytophilum	Granulocytic anaplasmosis	USA, Eurasia	Tick bite	*Ixodes* spp.
E. ewingii	Ehrlichiosis ewingii	USA	Tick bite	*A. americanum*
N. sennetsu	Sennetsu ehrlichiosis	Japan, Southeast Asia	Fluke-infested fish	fluke
E. muris	Unnamed ehrlichiosis	USA	Tick bite	*Ixodes scapularis*
Neoehrlichia mikurensis	Unnamed	Eurasia	Tick bite	*Ixodes* spp.

Clinical aspects of infection

Human monocytic ehrlichiosis

The disease begins 1–2 weeks after a bite of an infected tick. Clinical features frequently include fever, headache, myalgias, nausea, arthralgias and malaise. Other manifestations include cough, pharyngitis, lymphadenopathy, diarrhoea, vomiting, abdominal pain and changes in mental status. A fleeting or transient rash involving the extremities, trunk, face or, rarely, the palms and soles appears in 30%–40% of patients about 5 days after onset. The rash may be petechial, macular, maculopapular or diffusely erythematous.

Cytopenia early in the course of the illness may provide presumptive clues to the diagnosis. Mild to moderate leucopenia is observed in approximately 60%–70% of patients during the first week of illness, with the largest decreases occurring in the total neutrophil count. Thrombocytopenia occurs in 70%–90% of patients. Mildly or moderately raised hepatic transaminase levels are noted in most patients at some point during their illness.

About 50% of patients need admission to hospital. Those with severe disease may develop acute renal failure, metabolic acidosis, respiratory failure, profound hypotension, disseminated intravascular coagulopathy, myocardial dysfunction and meningoencephalitis; about 2% die. Death is more common in elderly men and immunocompromised individuals, including those infected with human immunodeficiency virus (HIV).

Human granulocytic anaplasmosis

The incubation period is 7–10 days after a bite by an infected tick. Clinical signs and symptoms are similar to those of human monocytic ehrlichiosis, but the disease is less severe and the mortality rate is <1%. Rash and central nervous system involvement are rare.

Human ehrlichiosis caused by *E. ewingii* elicits similar signs and symptoms. The infection has often been observed in immunocompromised patients with no fatalities. Another ehrlichiosis with similar symptoms and no fatalities is caused by *E. muris*.

LABORATORY INVESTIGATION

Ehrlichia and *Anaplasma* species grow intracellularly, and isolation is difficult. Human infections are diagnosed mainly by demonstrating the development of specific antibodies during convalescence. Indirect immunofluorescence methods use cell culture–propagated organisms. *E. chaffeensis*, *A. phagocytophilum*, *E. ewingii* and *E. muris* are detected diagnostically by PCR with specific primers to amplify the ehrlichial DNA. Human granulocytic anaplasmosis can often be diagnosed by identification of characteristic morulae in Giemsa-stained peripheral blood neutrophils; *E. chaffeensis* is seldom detected in monocytes in blood smears.

TREATMENT

Doxycycline shortens the course of infection and reduces mortality. The use of chloramphenicol is not recommended.

EPIDEMIOLOGY

Deer and ticks are involved in the ecology of human monocytic and granulocytic ehrlichioses. Rodents and ticks comprise the ecology of granulocytic anaplasmosis and *E. muris*. Deer, canines, rodents and domestic ruminants are important reservoirs. Immature ticks obtain ehrlichiae from the blood of infected animals; the organisms are maintained transstadially but not transovarially and are transmitted during a subsequent blood meal. Human infections are strongly associated with the season of tick activity, history of tick bite and geographical distribution of the vectors. Most cases of human monocytic ehrlichiosis are reported between March and November and the geographic distribution is expanding from the south-central and southeastern United States, where *Amblyomma americanum* is prevalent. Human granulocytic anaplasmosis occurs from March to December in the northern states. Infections caused by *E. muris* have been acquired in Wisconsin and Minnesota but may have a greater global distribution.

COXIELLA

DESCRIPTION

Query, or Q fever, first identified as a distinct clinical entity in 1935 after an outbreak of typhoid-like illness among abattoir workers in Australia, is a widespread disease with an almost global distribution. The aetiological agent, *C. burnetii*, is a fastidious intracellular prokaryote that has been cultivated in cell-free medium and is genetically related to *Legionella* species.

C. burnetii is a pleomorphic coccobacillary bacterium with a Gram-negative type of cell wall. The organisms typically grow within the phagolysosome of macrophages of the vertebrate host (Fig. 36.5). Structurally distinct large and small cell variants have been described, suggesting that the organism has a developmental cycle. In acidic conditions, similar to those found within a phagolysosome, it actively metabolises a variety of substrates

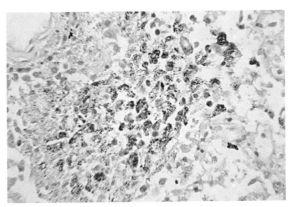

Fig. 36.5 Immunoperoxidase staining of *C. burnetii* in alveolar macrophages in a patient with Q fever. (Micrograph courtesy Dr J. Stephen Dumler.)

and can accomplish significant levels of macromolecular synthesis. Prolonged cultivation in vitro results in phase variation due to deletion of genes involved in the synthesis of lipopolysaccharides analogous to the smooth to rough transitions observed in other bacteria. Phase I organisms are representative of strains in nature, whereas phase II organisms appear in laboratory cultures and are avirulent for laboratory animals.

PATHOGENESIS

Human infection usually follows inhalation of aerosols containing *C. burnetii*. Entry into the lungs results in infection of the alveolar macrophages and a brief rickettsaemia. Most infections are subclinical, and only 2% of persons infected with *C. burnetii* are admitted to hospital. The incubation period for the acute form of the disease is usually about 2 weeks but can be longer.

Typical acute Q fever is a self-limiting flulike syndrome with high fever (40°C), fatigue, headache and myalgia. The patient may also suffer pneumonitis, hepatic and bone marrow granulomata, and meningoencephalitis. Chronic infections can develop, with the organism persisting in cardiac valves and possibly other foci. Endocarditis is rare, but potentially fatal, and may be accompanied by glomerulonephritis, osteomyelitis or central nervous system involvement.

Reactivation of latent infection may occur during pregnancy, and the organism is shed with the placenta or abortus.

LABORATORY INVESTIGATION

Diagnosis relies on the demonstration of specific antibodies in an indirect immunofluorescence assay or enzyme immunoassay. Immunofluorescence assay titres peak at 4–8 weeks. PCR amplification has been used to detect *C. burnetii* DNA in clinical samples from acute and chronic Q fever patients.

Isolation of *C. burnetii* from patient specimens is a specialised procedure and is not generally recommended because of the extremely infectious nature of the organism.

TREATMENT

Most infections resolve without antibiotic treatment, but administration of doxycycline reduces the duration of fever in the acute infection and is definitely recommended in cases of chronic infection. In Q fever endocarditis, long-term administration of a combination of two drugs among doxycycline, ciprofloxacin and rifampicin has been suggested.

C. burnetii may be recovered from some patients after months or even years of continuous treatment. In addition to antibiotic therapy, the haemodynamic status should be monitored. Valve replacement may be necessary in some cases of Q fever endocarditis.

EPIDEMIOLOGY

Q fever has been found on all continents except Antarctica, but most cases are reported from the United Kingdom and France. Elsewhere, the disease often goes unreported, is misdiagnosed, or causes such a mild infection that treatment is not sought. The main reservoirs of the disease are wild and domestic cattle, sheep and goats. Ticks can maintain *C. burnetii* by transstadial and transovarial transmission. Faeces of infected ticks contain very large numbers of *C. burnetii*, but arthropods are not an important source of infection.

C. burnetii may be the most infectious of all bacteria. Human infections generally follow inhalation of aerosols or direct contact with the organisms in the milk, urine, faeces or birth products of infected animals. The organism can survive on wool for 7–10 months, in skimmed milk for up to 40 months and in tick faeces for at least 1 year. Most individuals acquire the disease as an occupational hazard. Cases are common among abattoir workers and those associated with livestock rearing or dairy farming. Although Q fever normally occurs as isolated, sporadic cases, well-documented outbreaks have been reported.

CONTROL

Elimination of infected reservoir hosts is probably impossible because of chronic infections among the animals and the ability of the organism to survive for long periods in the external environment. Exposure can be reduced by construction of separate facilities for animal parturition, destruction of suspect placental membranes, heat treatment of milk (74°C for 15 seconds) and efforts to reduce the tick population. Abattoir workers should take care while handling carcasses, especially in the removal and dissection of mammary glands and inner organs. Animal hides should be kept wet until the salting procedure begins. Appropriate containment procedures should be observed in laboratories working with this highly infectious organism.

Inactivated whole-cell vaccines derived from phase I organisms have been developed and generate a protective response.

RECOMMENDED READING

Audy, J. R. (1968). *Red mites and typhus.* London: Athlone Press.

Blanton, L. S., & Walker, D. H. (2015). *Rickettsia prowazekii* (epidemic or louse-borne typhus). In J. E. Bennett, R. Dolin, & M. J. Blaser (Eds.), *Mandell, Douglas, and Bennett's principles and practice of infectious diseases* (8th ed., pp. 2217–2220). Canada: Elsevier Saunders.

Dalton, M. J., Clarke, M. J., Holman, R. C., Krebs, J. W., Fishbein, D. B., Olson, J. G., & Childs, J. E. (1995). National surveillance for Rocky Mountain spotted fever, 1981–1992: Epidemiologic summary and evaluation of risk factors for fatal outcome. *American Journal of Tropical Medicine and Hygiene, 52*(5), 405–413.

Dumler, J. S. (2010). Ehrlichioses and anaplasmosis. In R. L. Guerrant, D. H. Walker, & P. F. Weller (Eds.), *Tropical infectious diseases. Principles, pathogens, and practice* (3rd ed., pp. 339–341). Philadelphia: Elsevier Saunders.

Hechemy, K. E., Avsic-Zupanc, T., Childs, J. E., & Raoult, D. A. (Eds.). (2003). *Rickettsiology: Present and future directions.* New York: Academy of Sciences.

Kawamura, A., Tanaka, H., & Tamura, A. (1995). *Tsutsugamushi disease.* Tokyo: University of Tokyo Press.

Kim, I. S., & Walker, D. H. (2010). Scrub typhus. In R. L. Guerrant, D. H. Walker, & P. F. Weller (Eds.), *Tropical infectious diseases. Principles, pathogens, and practice* (3rd ed., pp. 334–338). Philadelphia: Elsevier Saunders.

Lina, T. T., Farris, T., Luo, T., Mitra, S., Zhu, B., & McBride, J. W. (2016). Hacker within! *Ehrlichia chaffeensis* effector driven phagocyte reprogramming strategy. *Frontiers in Cellular and Infection Microbiology, 6*(58), doi:10.3389/fcimb.2016.00058.

Maurin, M., & Raoult, D. (1999). Q fever. *Clinical Microbiology Reviews, 12*(4), 518–553.

Paddock, C. D., & Childs, J. E. (2003). *Ehrlichia chaffeensis*: A prototypical emerging pathogen. *Clinical Microbiology Reviews, 16*(1), 37–64.

Treadwell, T. A., Holman, R. C., Clarke, M. J., Krebs, J. W., Paddock, C. D., & Childs, J. E. (2000). Rocky Mountain spotted fever in the United States, 1993–1996. *American Journal of Tropical Medicine and Hygiene, 63*(1-2), 21–26.

Walker, D. H., & Blanton, L. S. (2015). *Rickettsia rickettsii* and other spotted fever group rickettsiae (Rocky Mountain spotted fever and other spotted fevers). In J. E. Bennett, R. Dolin, & M. J. Blaser (Eds.), *Mandell, Douglas, and Bennett's principles and practice of infectious diseases* (8th ed., pp. 2198–2205). Canada: Elsevier Saunders.

Zhang, J. Z., Sinha, M., Luxon, B. A., & Yu, X.-J. (2004). Survival strategy of obligately intracellular *Ehrlichia*: Novel modulation of immune response and host cell cycles. *Infection and Immunity, 72*(1), 498–507.

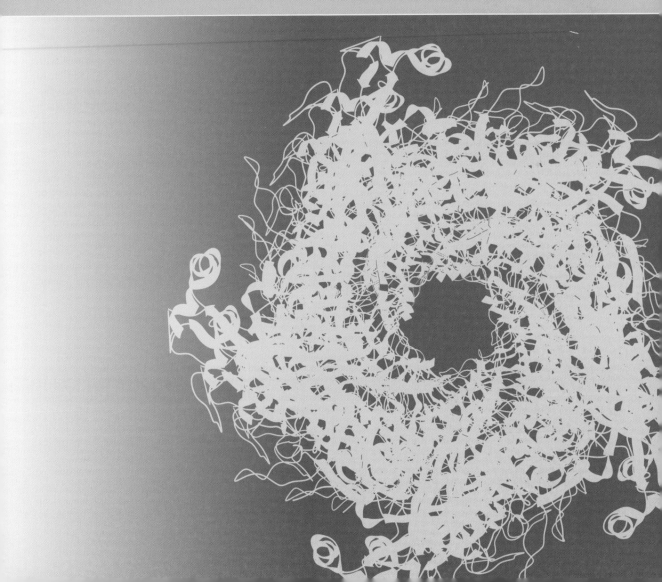

PART 4

VIRAL PATHOGENS AND ASSOCIATED DISEASES

37 Adenoviruses

Respiratory disease; conjunctivitis; gut infections

ALBERT HEIM

KEY POINTS

- Adenoviruses, comprising 75 types in seven species (A–G), commonly infect humans and can persist in lymphoid tissue.
- They cause (mostly) mild respiratory infections, especially in children, but can cause severe multiorgan disease in immunocompromised patients (disseminated disease).
- Types 1, 2, 5 and 6 of species C are mostly endemic; types 4 (species E), 3, 7, 14 and 21 (of species B) may be associated with epidemic lower respiratory tract infections.
- Types 31 (of species A), 40 and 41 (of species F) cause diarrhoea, but other types are also found in faeces without associated disease.
- Types 8, 37, 53, 54 and 64 (previously: 19a) of species D cause epidemic keratoconjunctivitis.
- Similar viruses infect a wide range of animals and birds but are not known to cross species boundaries (except occasional transmissions from nonhuman primates to humans).
- The use of adenoviruses as vectors for gene therapy is being explored but is not yet suitable for clinical use.

Adenoviruses were named from their original source, adenoid tissue, removed at operation and cultured as explants in vitro. Cellular outgrowth occurred readily, but this often deteriorated about 10 days later. The cause of the cytopathic effect was found to be adenovirus(es) present in the original tissue.

This discovery initiated much research, which established that there were a considerable number of types, mostly associated with mild upper respiratory tract infections. In addition, there were outbreaks of upper and lower respiratory tract infections in military recruits. Readily transmissible eye infections, pharyngoconjunctival fever and epidemic keratoconjunctivitis, were also found to be caused by adenoviruses. The focus of adenovirus research then shifted away from clinical virology with the discovery that some species could cause malignancies in laboratory rodents.

Clinical interest revived in the mid-1970s with the discovery of new types (40 and 41) linked (with several other hitherto unknown viruses) to that previously elusive entity viral gastroenteritis.

Starting with the description of type 53, new type numbers were given to genotypes (defined as adenoviruses with novel or at least recombinant genomes) in addition to serotypes (defined by unique neutralisation properties). Many of the new types (53–75) are genotypes but share neutralisation properties with an older serotype (see later in the chapter, under Classification). Consequently, this chapter uses the term *type* throughout, except when emphasising that a certain type is a serotype or genotype.

As many adenovirus infections are asymptomatic, their possible use as vectors for gene or vaccine delivery or tumour treatment has been developed. Human genes have been inserted into replication-crippled adenoviruses. Although these approaches show promise, formidable technical problems remain to be overcome. These include difficulties in making the transferred genes persist and in overcoming preexisting immunity to the adenovirus vector.

DESCRIPTION

Adenovirus virions provide a very good example of a nonenveloped icosahedron. Fig. 37.1A shows a group of typical adenovirus particles, whereas Figs. 37.1B–D compare a single virus particle, as seen by electron microscopy, with a model. The particles seen in Fig. 37.1A do not show the apical fibres (they are rarely seen in situ by the electron microscope), but otherwise the particles in Figs. 37.1A and B resemble the model closely.

The virion is 70–75 nm in size, and there are probably minor variations between preparations and, possibly, types. The surface has 252 visible capsomers. Twelve apical capsomers, each surrounded by five others, are known as

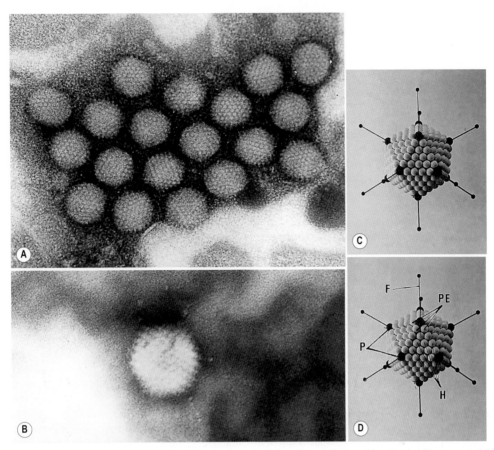

Fig. 37.1 (A) Group of adenovirus particles from a stool extract showing typical adenovirus morphology, although apical fibres are not visible. Individual capsomers can be seen as surface spots. These virus particles should be compared with the model seen in (C). Negative contrast, 3% potassium phosphotungstate, pH 7.0 (magnification ×160,000). (B) Single adenovirus particle showing some of the apical fibres. This is an unusual finding. Negative contrast, 3% potassium phosphotungstate, pH 7.0 (magnification ×280,000). (C and D) Photograph of a model with pentons *(P)*, peripentons *(PE)* and hexons *(H)* indicated. Note that the fibres *(F)* are attached to the penton.

pentons, consisting of a penton base and a fibre. All other 240 capsomers are surrounded by six others and are therefore called hexons (Fig. 37.1D).

From each penton base projects an apical fibre consisting of a shaft whose length is type specific (9–33 nm) and a terminal knob.

Adenoviruses contain a single piece of double-stranded DNA, about 35 kbp in size in human adenoviruses, which codes for a considerable number of structural and non-structural proteins with molecular weights of 7500–400,000 Da. There are three main structural proteins: one that forms the hexon (as a trimer), one that forms the penton base (as a pentamer) and a trimeric glycoprotein for the fibre.

There is a type-specific antigenic determinant (main neutralisation determinant ε) on the hexons, which also carry genus-specific antigens. The same genus-specific antigens are found on all mastadenoviruses (see later in the chapter), the genus to which the medically important human adenoviruses belong. These genus-specific antigens provide a basis for tests to detect adenoviruses and antibodies to them. The penton bases and fibres also bear antigenic determinants that are type specific, and antibodies binding to the fibre knob determinant γ can inhibit the haemagglutinating properties of adenoviruses. There are also studies showing that antibodies against pentons are more significant for neutralisation in human immune sera than antihexon antibodies, but this issue is controversial.

CLASSIFICATION

The family Adenoviridae comprises five genera: *Mastadenovirus* (including all human adenovirus species), *Aviadenovirus*, *Ichtadenovirus*, *Siadenovirus* and *Atadenovirus*.

According to the last International Committee on Taxonomy of Viruses (ICTV) report all human adenoviruses should be labelled as human mastadenoviruses; however, this is unusual in medical microbiology. Definition of the seven species of human adenoviruses (A–G) was based on hemagglutination and oncogenic properties, but nowadays, differences in DNA homology are more appropriate, with members of the same species having >50% homology. By contrast, numbering of types is based on the date of first isolation and does not indicate any phylogenetic relationship. Previously, all types were serotypes defined by neutralisation tests in cell culture using animal antisera. Preparation of type-specific antisera was a laborious task, and these antisera were then used to compare novel strains with previously known serotypes. In recent years, an alternative approach using complete genomic sequences offers a quicker and less laborious way to identify new types. This technique was used for the first time to identify type 53, an adenovirus strain with neutralisation properties of serotype 22 but isolated from an outbreak of epidemic keratoconjunctivitis, a disease usually not associated with serotype 22. The genome of the new strain was found to be a multiple recombinant with a hexon neutralisation epitope sequence of serotype 22, whereas most other parts of the genome were derived from types 8 and 37 (which are both associated with epidemic keratoconjunctivitis) or were novel sequence stretches. From then on, the new type definition (genotype with novel genome) has been used in addition to the serotype definition. Whilst most of the new types (53–75) are genotypes, a few are serotypes (e.g., type 54). The alternative definition of new types as genotypes is advantageous because the association of genotypes with clinical syndromes is more reliable than in the case of serotypes. Table 37.1 shows current classification into species and types.

REPLICATION

The virus attaches to susceptible cells by the apical fibres and is then taken into the cell, losing both fibres and pentons in the process. Inside the nucleus the DNA is released and the process of replication is initiated (see Ch. 7). About 20 early proteins are made, most of which are not incorporated into new particles. The late proteins are produced in quantity in the cytoplasm, are mostly structural and are later transported back to the nucleus where new virus particles are assembled, appearing as crystalline arrays. The shutting down of host cell metabolism and the accumulation of thousands of new virions results in rupture (lysis) of the infected cell with dissemination of the particles. In cell cultures, infected cells round up, swell and aggregate into clumps resembling bunches of grapes before they lyse.

Table 37.1 Properties and classification of adenoviruses of species A–G

Species[b]	Types	Tissues most commonly infected
A	12, 18, 31, 61	Gut
B	3, 7, 14, 16, 21, 55, 66, 68	Respiratory tract, conjunctiva[a]
	11, 34, 35, 50	Urogenital tract, conjunctiva[a]
C	1, 2, 5, 6, 57	Respiratory tract, lymphoid tissue (tonsils and adenoids)
D	8, 37, 53, 54, 64[c]	Conjunctiva
	9, 10, 13, 15, 17, 19, 20, 22–30, 32, 33, 36–39, 42–49, 51, 53, 54, 56, 58–60, 62, 63, 65, 67, 69–75	Gut, respiratory tract (probably low virulence)
E	4	Respiratory tract, conjunctiva
F	40, 41	Gut
G	52	Gut

[a]Only types 3, 7, 11 and 14.
[b]More than 50% DNA homology among members.
[c]Previously subtype 19a.

CLINICAL FEATURES

Table 37.2 lists the more common associations of types with disease. The great majority of infections with adenoviruses are not confirmed virologically, and the full extent of adenovirus disease burden is underreported. In addition, virus infection and replication are not invariably associated with disease.

Respiratory diseases

These are usually mild upper respiratory tract infections with fever, runny nose and cough. Most are due to types 1–7, although higher types may be involved sporadically. Types 1, 2, 5 and 6 of species C are more commonly associated with endemic infections of children, and associated clinical diagnoses include upper respiratory tract infection, tonsillitis, wheezing and failure to thrive. Adenovirus infections can mimic whooping cough in some patients. In older children and young adults, some of these infections will be labelled colds. Types 3 and 7 of species B and type 4 of species E are more epidemic. Occasionally and unpredictably, infections with these types may progress to lower respiratory tract infections and even to pneumonia that is frequently fatal. The majority of these pneumonias occur in young children but also in US military recruits, where strenuous exercise and close proximity combine

Table 37.2 Disease associated with adenovirus types

Disease	Those at risk	Frequently associated types
Acute febrile pharyngitis		
Endemic	Infants, young children	1, 2, 5, 6
Epidemic	Infants, young children	3, 4, 7
Pharyngoconjunctival fever	Older school-aged children	3, 4, 7
Acute respiratory disease	Military recruits	4, 7, 14p1, 21a
Pneumonia	Infants	1, 2, 3, 5, 7
Follicular conjunctivitis	Any age	3, 4, 11
Epidemic keratoconjunctivitis	Adults	8, 37, 53, 54, 64 (=19a)
Haemorrhagic cystitis	Infants, young children	11, 34, 35
Diarrhoea and vomiting	Infants, young children, older children	40, 41
		12, 18, 31
Intussusception	Infants	1, 2, 5
Disseminated infection	Immunocompromised (e.g., bone transplant recipients)	1, 2, 5, 11, 31, 34, 35

both to make the victims more vulnerable and to facilitate spread. Moreover, a variant adenovirus, type 14p1 (also labelled as 14a), has emerged to cause an epidemic threat in the United States, especially in military encampments but also in the general population. Eye involvement is a common feature (see later in the chapter), leading to such outbreaks being called pharyngoconjunctival fever. More recently, another variant adenovirus, type 21a (of species B, as is type 14p1), has been identified as a cause of severe pneumonia. Unlike other viral respiratory infections, adenoviruses may be associated with a raised white cell count and enhanced levels of C-reactive protein and therefore may be confused with a bacterial infection.

Eye infections

Adenoviruses have been associated with several outbreaks of keratoconjunctivitis in the United Kingdom, referred to as shipyard eye because originally (but erroneously) it was thought to be due to particles of steel swarf thrown up during welding and grinding. The real cause was an adenovirus transmitted through eyebaths and instruments used to treat eye injuries in the shipyard first aid clinic and which had become contaminated by virus from the index case. Use of properly sterilised instruments and single-dose preparations of eye ointment have made this uncommon, but occasional nosocomial outbreaks can be still observed. Keratoconjunctivitis is a severe eye infection starting as a red eye with foreign body sensation, tearing, ocular/periorbital pain and impaired vision due to corneal infiltrates, which may persist as numuli for several months. Subsequently, the disease becomes bilateral due to auto-inoculation in most cases. Swelling of regional lymph nodes is frequently observed, but there are no systemic symptoms such as fever. Most of the early outbreaks were due to adenovirus type 8, but later a

variant adenovirus, type 19a, as well as types 37, 53 and 54 (all of species D) have been found as etiologic agents. Recently, type 19a was relabelled as type 64 using the novel genotype definition (see earlier in the chapter). By contrast, type 19 (the prototype) is not associated with keratoconjunctivitis.

Conjunctivitis caused by other types (most frequently of species B and E) may occur in outbreaks of pharyngoconjunctival fever. This is a follicular conjunctivitis resembling that caused by *Chlamydia,* from which it should be differentiated, but the associated and usually marked adenovirus respiratory symptoms will provide a clue to the cause.

Gut infections

When faecal extracts from infants and toddlers with diarrhoea were examined by electron microscopy, typical adenoviruses were seen in some of the cases, often in very large numbers. These viruses were later shown to be two hitherto unknown types, 40 and 41 of species F. They cause a significant proportion of cases of endemic childhood diarrhoea (as opposed to outbreaks, often due to rotaviruses and noroviruses). Small epidemics of diarrhoea in older children (kindergarten and school age) can be caused by type 31 and occasionally by types 12 and 18, all of species A, but these infections can also be asymptomatic. Many new types of species D (e.g., 42–49, 51, 58, 59, 62, 67, 70–75) and the only type 52 of species G have been found in faeces samples, most of these from adults and many of these from immunocompromised patients (e.g., from patients with AIDS). Chronic diarrhoea is a feature of AIDS, although no causal role for these adenoviruses has been proven. These new types may be opportunistic pathogens with a low virulence or completely innocent bystanders, which also may circulate in immunocompetent adults but remain undetected.

The role of adenovirus(es) in mesenteric adenitis and intussusception is unproven. Finding a coincidental adenovirus in faeces is not proof of involvement because of prolonged shedding of species C adenoviruses after respiratory infections.

Other diseases of immunocompetent patients

There have been occasional reports of adenovirus (mostly types 11, 21, 34 and 35 of species B) recovered from the urine of patients with haemorrhagic cystitis. There are reports in the literature of recovery of adenoviruses (type 2 of species C and type 37 of species D) from both the male and the female genital tracts. They may be transmitted sexually but are not recognised as the cause of a sexually transmitted disease. In addition, rare cases of adenovirus hepatitis and encephalitis were reported. In the newborn, adenoviruses may cause disseminated disease with a septic shock form of presentation. There is no good evidence for adenoviruses being involved in initiating human tumours (e.g., glioma, leukaemias), but studies are ongoing.

Disease in immunosuppressed transplant recipients

Adenoviruses are significant pathogens in transplant recipients. Recipients of allogeneic haematopoietic stem cells are far more affected than solid organ recipients. Transplantation-related mortality due to adenovirus was found in many studies to be as high as 5% in paediatric (and about 1% in adult) stem cell recipients. Adenovirus types 1, 2 and 5 (of species C) account for about 80% of the cases in paediatric patients, and most of these infections reactivate from prolonged asymptomatic infections (latent adenovirus infections or adenovirus persistence) of gut-associated lymphoid tissue. As these are not lifelong infections in contrast to herpesvirus latency, incidence of adenovirus reactivations is lower in adults, but disease is as severe as in children. Reactivations start with shedding of high adenovirus loads in faeces, and subsequently adenovirus viremia with increasing virus loads can be observed. Many internal organs can be infected, but the liver seems to be the main replication site in many cases. With increasing virus loads in peripheral blood a sepsis-like disseminated adenovirus disease is observed, and virus loads $>10^9$ genome equivalents/mL blood are almost always fatal. In addition to the types of species C, type 31 of species A can be found frequently in children, whereas in adults, types of species B and D can be found. In solid organ transplantation, adenoviruses can cause severe disease of the transplanted organ, which has to be discerned from acute rejection, for example, hepatitis (in liver transplant patients), nephritis (in kidney transplant patients)

and pneumonitis (in lung transplant but also in other solid organ transplant recipients). Nephritis is caused by the same types of species B (e.g., types 11, 34 and 35) as haemorrhagic cystitis of immunocompetent patients.

PATHOGENESIS

Adenoviruses mostly infect mucosal surfaces (respiratory tract, gut and eye). Different types appear to prefer different regions of the body, probably due to the presence or absence of particular cellular receptors; for example, all types of species C and several types of species B (3, 7, 14 and 21) have a tropism for the respiratory epithelium, but several other types of species B (11, 34 and 35) have a tropism for the urogenital epithelium. All types of species F (40 and 41) and species A (12, 18, 31 and 61) are primary pathogens of the gut, infecting and damaging cells lining it. Death of the infected cells may lead to temporary malabsorption and diarrhoea in children, though not invariably. Respiratory strains of species C are frequently recovered from faeces, and it seems improbable that this results solely from overflow from the upper respiratory tract. It is much more likely that faecal excretion follows a secondary gut infection, albeit asymptomatic in most cases. In general, productive adenovirus infection of an individual cell will cause its death, but several studies have documented prolonged respiratory and gut excretion in healthy children, lasting for many months. Such respiratory carriage in lymphoid tissue (tonsils and adenoids), and gut carriage in gut-associated lymphoid tissues of the immune host is facilitated by the immune-modulating gene products of the E3 region and can result in productive infection of a few epithelial cells and intermittent adenovirus shedding, although this has not been documented in detail.

LABORATORY INVESTIGATION

Direct demonstration of virus

Detection of viral DNA

Conserved parts of the adenoviral genomic DNA can be detected by molecular detection methods (e.g., the very sensitive polymerase chain reaction, PCR) in a variety of clinical specimens. PCR protocols that detect all adenovirus types should be preferred. Real-time PCR has the advantage of semiquantitative results that help to discern low-level adenovirus shedding in case of prolonged asymptomatic carriage from high-level shedding in case of acute disease. With adequate calibration, real-time PCR gives adenovirus loads for blood (plasma or whole EDTA-blood) and stool suspensions. This is essential for early diagnosis of adenovirus dissemination in immunosuppressed patients.

DNA sequencing of antigenic epitopes can be used for typing purposes, and complete genomic sequencing can be used to identify new types and variants. However, these approaches are only available in reference laboratories.

Virus antigen

The presence of viral antigen in the nasopharynx may be identified by immunofluorescence with genus-specific antibodies (polyclonal or monoclonal) directly on aspirates and swabs, provided that they contain respiratory cells of sufficient number and quality. The presence of such infected cells usually indicates a significant infection, in contrast to asymptomatic carriage. Alternatively, viral antigen may be detected by commercially available enzyme immunoassays and rapid lateral flow assays. The drawback of these assays is that the quality of diagnostic specimen and the specificity of the reaction cannot be checked as with immunofluorescence.

Viral antigen can also be detected in faeces suspensions by a variety of enzyme immunoassays and lateral flow assays.

Electron microscopy

Virus particles may be seen directly in stool extracts by electron microscopy, although this cannot identify species and types. Nonetheless, where virus is seen in cases of acute diarrhoea, this is usually of type 40 or 41, particularly where large numbers are present (the level may reach $>10^{10}$ particles per gram of faeces).

CULTURE

Adenovirus can be grown in cell culture from respiratory specimens (nasopharyngeal aspirates, and nose and throat swabs), eye swabs, faeces and, occasionally, urine. The speed of isolation is usually an indication of viral load in the specimen and can provide a pointer to the clinical significance of the finding. If isolation takes longer than 12 days it is less likely to be clinically significant, particularly with types 1, 2, 5 and 6.

Isolation of an adenovirus in cell culture from the faeces of patients with diarrhoea is, by itself, of little significance. The diarrhoea-causing adenovirus types 40 and 41 of species F are fastidious, and cultivable adenoviruses in the stool are not usually those associated with diarrhoea. Nevertheless, species F adenoviruses replicate in 293 cells (an adenovirus-transformed human embryo kidney cell line that provides *E1* gene products in trans).

Serology

A rise in antibody levels indicates recent infection (although not its site or its nature), but absence does not exclude it, especially in babies. In general, serology has little significance in adenovirus diagnostics. Complement fixation is the test most frequently used routinely; it provides only a genus-specific diagnosis. Genus- and type-specific enzyme immunoassays have also been developed but are not used widely and their cut-offs are set rather arbitrarily. Neutralisation tests are both type-specific and more sensitive but are not available as routine tests; neither is haemagglutination inhibition widely available. However, both tests may be used by reference laboratories or in research.

TREATMENT

As most adenoviral infections of immunocompetent patients are self-limiting and not severe, there is little demand for specific treatment. Ribavirin, ganciclovir, vidarabine and cidofovir have all been shown to have antiviral activity in vitro. Cidofovir is frequently used in immunocompromised patients, but there are only anecdotal reports on its efficacy. Reduction of immunosuppressive therapy (if feasible) is essential, and early use of cidofovir (before high virus loads in peripheral blood are reached) may be advantageous.

EPIDEMIOLOGY

Adenoviruses are endemic. Types 1–7 spread readily between individuals, presumably by droplets and direct or indirect contact with infected secretions. Faecal–oral transmission (particularly of diarrhoea-associated types) can also occur, and probably does, in areas with poverty, poor hygiene and overcrowding.

Typing and subtyping of variants shows subtypes of different virulence (e.g., 14p1 and 21a) and indicates geographical variation in distribution. Such detailed analysis is not routine, however.

CONTROL

For the reasons discussed earlier in the chapter, under Treatment, there is little demand for a vaccine in the general population. Nevertheless, the problems with adenoviruses encountered by US armed forces in recruit camps led them to develop and use a live virus vaccine containing nonattenuated adenovirus types 4 and 7, administered orally in enteric capsules. Primary infection of the gut, instead of the respiratory tract, induces immunity and provides adequate protection from disease. However, this vaccine was licensed for use only in military personnel.

A careful and rigorous attention to aseptic technique and single-dose vials of materials for use in the eye is the best approach to preventing outbreaks of adenovirus eye infections.

ADENOVIRUS-ASSOCIATED VIRUSES

The adenovirus-associated viruses (adeno satellite viruses) are members of the Parvoviridae family (see Ch. 43). They are about 22 nm in diameter, appear to be more hexagonal than circular in outline and contain insufficient single-stranded DNA to replicate on their own. They form a genus, dependoparvoviruses, indicating their dependence on a coinfection with an adenovirus to provide the missing functions.

True adeno-associated virus infection has not been implicated in clinical disease. However, as with any other virus found in faeces, large numbers of parvovirus-like particles have been seen in extracts of diarrhoeal faeces, sometimes (but not invariably) combined with smaller numbers of adenoviruses. Neither virus grows in cell culture, leaving the significance of these observations obscure.

RECOMMENDED READING

Adhikary, A. K., & Banik, U. (2014). Human adenovirus type 8: the major agent of epidemic keratoconjunctivitis (EKC). *Journal of Clinical Virology*, *61*(4), 477–486. doi:10.1016/j.jcv.2014.10.015.

Echavarria, M. (2009). Adenoviruses. In A. J. Zuckerman, J. E. Banatvala, & P. D. Griffiths (Eds.), *Principles & practice of clinical virology* (6th ed., pp. 463–488). Chichester: Wiley-Blackwell.

Ganzenmueller, T., & Heim, A. (2012). Adenoviral load diagnostics by quantitative polymerase chain reaction: techniques and application. *Reviews in Medical Virology*, *22*(3), 194–208. doi:10.1002/rmv.724.

Gray, G. C., & Chorazy, M. L. (2009). Human adenovirus 14a: a new epidemic threat. *The Journal of Infectious Diseases*, *199*(10), 1413–1415. doi:10.1086/598522.

Kosulin, K., Geiger, E., Vécsei, A., Huber, W. D., Rauch, M., Brenner, E., ... Lion, T. (2016). Persistence and reactivation of human adenoviruses in the gastrointestinal tract. *Clinical Microbiology and Infection*, *22*(4), 381.e1–381.e8. doi:10.1016/j.cmi.2015.12.013.

Lion, T. (2014). Adenovirus infections in immunocompetent and immunocompromised patients. *Clinical Microbiology Reviews*, *27*(3), 441–462. doi:10.1128/CMR.00116-13.

Walsh, M. P., Chintakuntlawar, A., Robinson, C. M., Madisch, I., Harrach, B., Hudson, N., ... Jones, M. S. (2009). Evidence of molecular evolution driven by recombination events influencing tropism in a novel human adenovirus that causes epidemic keratoconjunctivitis. *PLoS ONE*, *4*(6), e5635. doi:10.1371/journal.pone.0005635.

Wold, W. S., & Toth, K. (2013). Adenovirus vectors for gene therapy, vaccination and cancer gene therapy. *Current Gene Therapy*, *13*(6), 421–433.

38 Herpesviruses

Herpes simplex; varicella and zoster; infectious mononucleosis; B cell lymphomas; cytomegalovirus disease; exanthem subitum; Kaposi's sarcoma; herpesvirus B

TANZINA HAQUE AND INGÓLFUR JOHANNESSEN

KEY POINTS

- All herpesviruses persist for the lifetime of the host and establish a latent (non-replicating) state from which they may be reactivated under certain conditions.
- Cell-mediated immunity, especially the action of cytotoxic T lymphocytes, is essential in the control of herpesvirus infections.
- Acute necrotizing sporadic viral encephalitis caused by HSV is a medical emergency requiring urgent treatment with high-dose intravenous aciclovir that must be instigated empirically without delay and prior to laboratory confirmation.
- Genital herpes simplex may be due to HSV 1 or 2, and the individuals are often unaware that they have this recurring infection.
- A live-attenuated VZV vaccine can protect against chickenpox (varicella); it may boost immunity in older age groups with a reduction in the symptoms of zoster (shingles), which arises as a result of VZV reactivation.
- Glandular fever is a clinical presentation of primary EBV infection, mainly in the 15–25 years age group; most individuals have an asymptomatic infection in childhood.
- EBV is a recognised human tumour-forming virus associated with certain epithelial and lymphoid tumours (e.g., posttransplant B cell lymphoproliferative disease, PTLD).
- CMV is commonly acquired without symptoms; however, in the immunocompromised host, CMV disease is serious and requires prophylaxis or preemptive therapy.
- Less well-known herpesviruses (HHV 6 and 7) cause a common childhood rash illness (exanthem subitum), whereas HHV 8 is associated with Kaposi's sarcoma (KS).

Species-specific herpesviruses have been described for most animals, and they share several features including their structure, mode of replication and the capacity to establish lifelong latent infections from which virus may be reactivated. Together, they form the Herpesviridae family.

Latent infection

Latency reflects persistence of the viral genome within a cell during which no infectious virus is produced, except during intermittent episodes of reactivation.

Reactivation

Reactivation from the latent state may be restricted to asymptomatic virus shedding or manifest as clinical disease.

Recurrence or recrudescence

These terms are used when reactivated virus produces clinically apparent disease.

The Herpesviridae family is subdivided into three subfamilies: alpha (α)-, beta (β)- and gamma (γ)- Herpesvirinae (see Table 38.1). The human α-Herpesvirinae contain the genera *Simplexvirus* (herpes simplex virus [HSV] 1 and 2) and *Varicellovirus* (varicella-zoster virus, VZV); the β-Herpesvirinae consist of *Cytomegalovirus* (cytomegalovirus, CMV) and *Roseolovirus* (human herpesviruses [HHV] 6 and 7) genera; and the γ-Herpesvirinae contain the *Lymphocryptovirus* (Epstein–Barr virus [EBV]) and *Rhadinovirus* (Kaposi's sarcoma–associated herpesvirus [KSHV]) genera. Individual viruses are denoted by the taxonomic unit (family/subfamily) followed by an Arabic number (e.g., human herpesvirus [HHV] 4). However, vernacular and approved names are often used interchangeably (e.g., HHV 4 and EBV). At present, eight human herpesviruses (HHV 1–8) are recognised, and infection with each of HHV 1–7 has been shown to be common in all populations; studies with HHV 8 suggest it is an uncommon infection in developed countries.

Table 38.1	Human herpesviruses (HHV)		
Approved name	Vernacular name (see text)	Subfamily (-herpesvirinae)	Genus (-virus)
HHV 1	HSV 1	α_1	Simplex
HHV 2	HSV 2	α_1	Simplex
HHV 3	VZV	α_2	Varicello
HHV 4	EBV	γ_1	Lymphocrypto
HHV 5	CMV	β_1	Cytomegalo
HHV 6	–	β_2	Roseolo
HHV 7	–	β_2	Roseolo
HHV 8	KSHV	γ_2	Rhadino

CMV, Cytomegalovirus; *EBV*, Epstein–Barr virus; *HHV*, human herpesvirus; *HSV*, herpes simplex virus; *KSHV*, Kaposi sarcoma-associated herpesvirus; *VZV*, varicella-zoster virus.

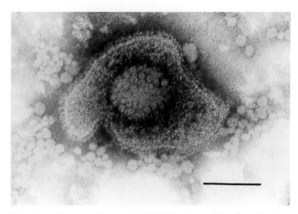

Fig. 38.1 Electron micrograph of HSV. Negative staining (2% phosphotungstic acid). Bar = 100 nm. (Prepared by Dr B. W. McBride.)

Herpesvirus B can transmit from (Old World) nonhuman primates to humans accidentally.

DESCRIPTION

Herpesviruses have a characteristic morphology (Fig. 38.1). The icosahedral protein capsid (average diameter 100 nm) consists of 162 hollow hexagonal and pentagonal capsomeres with an electron-dense core containing the DNA genome (together forming the nucleocapsid). Outside the capsid (in mature virus particles) is an amorphous proteinaceous layer, the tegument, surrounded by a lipid envelope derived from host cell membranes. Projecting from the trilaminar lipid host-derived envelope are spikes of viral glycoproteins. Cryo-electron micrographs indicate that the capsid is organised into at least three layers, with viral DNA inserted in the innermost layer. The average enveloped particle is approximately 200 nm in diameter.

The herpesvirus genome is linear double-stranded (ds) DNA that varies in length from 125–248 kbp with a base content ranging from 42–69 G+C mol% for the HHV. The presence of unique long and short (U_L, U_S) regions bounded by repeated and inverted short segments allows recombination and isomeric forms in some cases (Fig. 38.2). Genes coding for viral glycoproteins, major capsid proteins, enzymes involved in DNA replication and some transcripts associated with latency have been identified. Conserved sequences appear in certain regions, and some genes show homology with regions of human chromosomes. Restriction endonuclease and genome sequence analysis permit epidemiological comparison of strains (fingerprinting) within herpesvirus species.

Some herpesviruses are predominantly:

- Neurotropic (HSV and VZV)
- Lymphotropic (EBV, HHV 6 and 7).

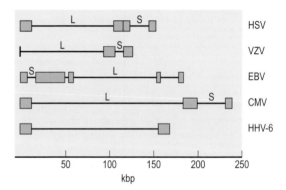

Fig. 38.2 Diagrammatic comparison of herpesvirus DNAs. Lines indicate long *(L)* and short *(S)* unique sequences; repeated regions are boxed.

BIOLOGICAL CLASSIFICATION

Broad characteristics of the three herpes subfamilies include:

- Alphaherpesvirinae (e.g., HSV, VZV and B virus): Rapid growth in cultured cells, latency in sensory ganglia
- Betaherpesvirinae (e.g., CMV): Slow growth in cultured cells, restricted host range
- Gammaherpesvirinae (e.g., EBV): Growth in lymphoid cells

The viruses are relatively thermolabile and readily inactivated by lipid solvents such as alcohols and detergents.

REPLICATION

After initial attachment of virus-encoded receptor-binding proteins to cell surface proteoglycans followed by specific binding to target cell receptors, the envelope of herpesviruses fuses with the cell membrane. The nucleocapsids cross the cytoplasm to the nuclear membrane; replication of viral DNA and assembly of capsids takes place within the nucleus. With HSV, it is known that the tegument proteins partake in transactivation of the first set of genes. Between 65 and 100 viral proteins are synthesised in an orderly sequence or cascade. Briefly, using HSV as an example, circularisation of the herpesvirus genome in the cell nucleus results in the orderly transcription (by host RNA polymerase II) of a cascade of immediate early (IE; α), early (E; β) and late (L; γ) genes. IE proteins activate expression of *E* genes that include virus-derived enzymes (including DNA polymerase and thymidine kinase [TK]) involved in replication, which is thought to proceed in a rolling circle manner yielding a concatomer that is cut to genome-length DNA units. Induction of *L* genes by *E* gene products results in production of viral structural proteins that package around progeny DNA to give rise to new nucleocapsids.

The viral capsid proteins migrate from the cytoplasm to the nucleus, where capsid assembly occurs and new viral DNA is inserted and located in the inner shell. Viral glycoproteins are processed in the Golgi complex and incorporated into host cell membranes from which the viral envelope is acquired—usually, from the inner layer of the nuclear membrane as the virus buds out from the nucleus. It then passes by way of membranous vacuoles to reach the cell surface. Generally, productively infected cells do not survive (lytic infection), and infectious virus (virions) are released during cytolysis.

HERPES SIMPLEX VIRUS

Herpes simplex virus (HSV) is ubiquitous, infecting the majority of the world's population early in life and persisting in a latent form from which reactivation with shedding of infectious virus occurs, thereby maintaining the transmission chain.

DESCRIPTION

In contrast to other members of the herpesvirus family, HSV can be grown relatively easily in cells from a wide variety of animals, so far more extensive studies have been undertaken with this virus than other members of the family.

There are two distinct types of HSV: type 1 (HSV 1) and type 2 (HSV 2). These two types are generally (but not exclusively) associated with different sites of infection in patients (see later in the chapter); type 1 HSV is associated primarily with the mouth and eyes (head), whereas type 2 HSV is most often found in the genital tract. Central nervous system (CNS) infections can be caused by both types.

HSV glycoproteins

The envelope of HSV contains at least 11 glycoproteins. Three of the glycoproteins (g) are essential for production of infectious virus: gB and gD, which (alongside gC) are involved in adsorption to (and entry into) cells, and gH, which (together with gL) is involved in fusion at entry and release of virus. Some of the glycoproteins have common antigenic determinants shared by HSV 1 and 2 (e.g., gB and gD), whereas others have specific determinants for one type only (gG).

PATHOGENESIS

Primary infection

The typical lesion produced by HSV is the vesicle, a ballooning degeneration of intraepithelial cells, which contains fluid with infectious virus. The basal epithelium is usually intact as vesicles penetrate the subepithelial layer only occasionally. The base of the vesicle contains multinucleate cells (Tzanck cells), and infected nuclei contain eosinophilic inclusion bodies. The roof of the vesicle breaks down and an ulcer forms. This happens rapidly on mucous membranes and non-keratinizing epithelia; on the skin, the ulcer crusts over, forming a scab that then heals. A mononuclear cell immune reaction is usual, with the vesicle fluid becoming cloudy with cellular infiltration in the subepithelial tissue. After resorption, or loss, of the vesicle fluid, the damaged epithelium is regenerated. Natural killer (NK) cells play a significant role in early defence by recognising and destroying HSV-infected cells. Herpesvirus glycoproteins synthesized during virus growth are inserted into host cell membranes, and some are secreted into extracellular fluid. The host's adaptive immune system responds to all these foreign antigens, producing both cytotoxic (CD4$^+$ and CD8$^+$) and helper (CD4$^+$) T lymphocytes, which activate primed B lymphocytes to produce specific antibodies; T cells are also involved in the induction of delayed hypersensitivity. The different glycoproteins have significant roles in generating these various cell responses; many induce neutralising antibodies.

During the replication phase at the site of entry in the epithelium, virus particles enter the sensory nerve endings that penetrate to the parabasal layer of the epithelium and are transported, probably as nucleocapsids, along the axon to the nerve body (neurone) in the sensory (dorsal root) ganglia by retrograde axonal flow. Virus replication in a neurone ends in lytic infection and neuronal cell death; however, in some ganglion cells, a latent infection is established in which surviving neurones harbour the viral genome; furthermore, neurones other than those in sensory ganglia can be the site of herpesvirus latency. It is not clear whether true latency occurs at epithelial sites; there is some evidence of persistence of virus at peripheral sites, but this may be due to a reactivation with a low level of virus replication.

Antibody reduces the severity of infections although it does not prevent recurrences. Thus, neonates receiving maternal antibody transplacentally are protected against the worst effects of neonatal herpes. HSV 2 infection seems to protect against HSV 1, but previous HSV 1 infection only partly modifies HSV 2 disease.

Latent infection

Latent infection of sensory neurones is a feature of the neurotropic herpesviruses, HSV and VZV; HSV 1 latency is the best understood. Only a small proportion (about 1%) of cells in the affected ganglion carry the viral genome as free circular episomes—estimated about 20 copies per infected cell. Very few viral genes are expressed in the latent state; in HSV, some viral RNA transcripts (latency-associated transcripts, LATs) are found in the nuclei, but no virus-encoded proteins have been demonstrated in the cells, so these infected neurons are not recognized as such by the immune system. Latent HSV genomes have been detected in postmortem studies on excised ganglia and other neuronal tissues. HSV 1 is regularly detected in the trigeminal ganglion, other sensory and autonomic ganglia (e.g., vagus) and adrenal tissue and the brain. HSV 2 latency in the sacral ganglia has been demonstrated. Either type may become latent in other ganglia.

Reactivation

Reactivation processes are still not clearly understood. It is suggested that HSV DNA passes along the nerve axon back to the nerve ending where infection of epithelial cells may occur. Not all reactivation will result in a visible lesion; there may be asymptomatic shedding of virus only detectable by culture or DNA detection by nucleic acid amplification tests (NAATs), which (in the United Kingdom) usually involves the use of polymerase chain reaction (PCR) assays.

The factors influencing the development of lesions due to reactivation are not clearly identified yet. An increase of CD8[+] T suppressor lymphocyte activity is common at the time of recurrences. Some mediators (e.g., prostaglandins), and a temporary decrease in immune effector cell function (particularly, delayed hypersensitivity), may enhance spread of HSV. Certainly, the known triggers for recurrences are accompanied by a local increase in prostaglandin levels, and depression of cell-mediated immunity predisposes to herpes recurrence. Thus, after bone marrow transplant or high-dose chemotherapy, HSV reactivation occurs in 80% of cases in the absence of prophylaxis.

Reactivation is a feature of HSV infection. It occurs naturally and can be induced by a variety of stimuli such as ultraviolet light (sunlight), fever, trauma and/or stress. The interval between the stimulus and the appearance of a clinically obvious lesion is 2–5 days; this has been demonstrated in patients undergoing surgical interference with their trigeminal ganglion, a common site of herpes latency.

CLINICAL FEATURES

Primary infection

Primary infection refers to the patient's initial acquisition of virus and, thus, occurs in those with no antibody against HSV (Table 38.2). It usually involves the mucous membranes of the mouth but may include the lips, skin of the face, nose or any other site, including the eye and genital tract.

Recurrent infection

Symptomatic recurrence is heralded by a prodrome in two-thirds of people who experience pain or paraesthesiae (tingling, warmth, itch) at the site, followed by erythema and a papule, usually within 24 hours. Progression to a vesicle and ulcer (with subsequent crusting) takes 8–12 days before natural healing occurs. Because of their

Table 38.2 Types of herpes simplex virus (HSV) infections	
Type of infection	Antibody status of patient
Primary: First HSV infection (any type at any site)	Seronegative
Latent: No symptoms	Seropositive
Recurrent: Recrudescence of the latent HSV type(s)	Seropositive
Initial (nonprimary): First episode of the heterologous HSV in a seropositive patient	Seronegative for infecting type; seropositive for latent type
Reinfection (exogenous): Infection with a strain that differs from the latent HSV type	Seropositive
HSV, Herpes simplex virus.	

association with febrile illness (e.g., the common cold), the lesions are popularly known as cold sores or fever blisters. The most common sites are at the mucocutaneous junction of the lip (seldom inside the mouth), on the chin, or inside the nose. However, recurrent lesions can manifest at any site innervated by the affected neuron, determined by the site of initial infection.

Severe pain, extensive mucosal ulceration and delayed healing are features of recurrent herpes in severely immunocompromised patients; the ulcers also provide entry for other (e.g., bacterial) infections. HSV viraemia after reactivation is uncommon, even in the immunocompromised individual but can lead to disseminated infection in internal organs. Some sufferers experience erythema multiforme following their recurrent herpes, associated with reaction to certain herpes antigens; this may take the form of the Stevens–Johnson syndrome.

Oral infection

Classically, primary HSV infection presents as an acute, febrile gingivo-stomatitis in preschool children. Vesicular lesions ulcerate rapidly and are present in the front of the mouth and on the tongue (stomatitis); gingivitis is usually present. Vesicles may also develop on the lips and skin around the mouth (herpetic dermatitis), and cervical lymphadenopathy can occur. The child is miserable for 7–10 days in an untreated case before the lesions heal. However, the majority of primary infections go unrecognized, the episode being attributed to teething or mistaken for thrush (candida infection). In primary infection in older children and adults, there may also be an associated mononucleosis; pharyngitis is also notable. Viraemia with dissemination of HSV to internal organs is rare, except in pregnancy (primary infection with hepatitis), the neonate (see later in the chapter) or the immunocompromised patient.

Skin infection
Herpetic whitlow

Hand infections with HSV are not uncommon, but other sites may be involved (e.g., as a result of sports, such as herpes gladiatorum in wrestlers or rugby players [as a result of direct skin-to-skin contact]). Three presentations of hand infections may be observed.

1. The classical primary lesion is on the fingers of the toddler with herpetic stomatitis as a result of autoinoculation.
2. Another classical and often primary infection is acquired by accidental inoculation in health-care workers (traumatic herpes). These infections may recur; the majority is caused by HSV 1.

3. The most common hand lesions are recurrent, associated with HSV 2 and genital herpes, and are seen in young adults. Pain and swelling occur, and the vesicles become pustular but, if in well-keratinized areas, do not always ulcerate. Associated lymphangitis is common. Primary and recurrent lesions take up to 21 and 10 days to heal, respectively. Fig. 38.3 shows recurrent lesions at an interval of 10 years.

Eczema herpeticum

A severe form of cutaneous herpes may occur in children with atopic eczema—eczema herpeticum or Kaposi's varicelliform eruption. Vesicles resembling those of chickenpox may appear, mainly on already eczematous areas. Extensive ulceration results in protein loss and dehydration, and viraemia can lead to disseminated disease with severe, even fatal, consequences. Occasionally, a similar picture is seen in adults with pemphigus when infected with HSV; patients with burns are also at risk. In each instance, early recognition and prompt antiviral therapy can be lifesaving.

Eye infection

HSV infection of the eye may be initiated during a childhood primary infection or occur from transfer of virus from a cold sore. There may be periorbital herpetic dermatitis together with conjunctivitis or keratoconjunctivitis associated with corneal ulceration. Typically, branching (dendritic) corneal ulcers are found. If these recur and are left untreated, the result is corneal scarring and visual impairment. More extensive ulceration occurs if steroids have been used, but deeper infiltrates are common in long-standing cases and benefit from combined steroid and antiviral therapy. The presence of typical herpes vesicles on eyelid margins is a useful clinical guide but is not always seen. The majority of eye infections are with HSV 1, and most patients with recurring eye disease are aged over 50 years. More than half of the corneal grafting performed in the United Kingdom is for HSV corneal scarring, although the disease may recur in the graft. Acute retinal necrosis associated with HSV 1 or 2 is also recognized and may affect the opposite eye in due course, leading to blindness.

Central nervous system (CNS) infection

HSV may reach the brain in several ways. Viraemia has been detected during primary herpetic stomatitis, and infection may be carried within cells into the brain and meninges. Direct infection from the nasal mucosa along the olfactory tract is another possibility, but the most likely route is central spread from the trigeminal ganglia.

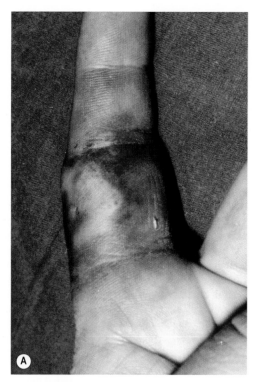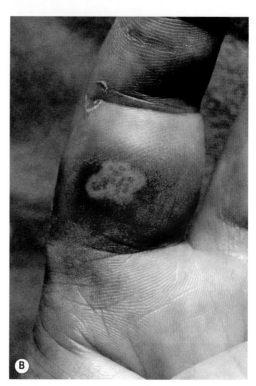

Fig. 38.3   Herpetic whitlow on the left index finger of the same individual photographed during recurrences in (A) 1984 and (B) 1994.

HSV encephalitis

Encephalitis caused by HSV is a rare condition but is the most common sporadic fatal encephalitis recognised in developed countries (1–2 cases per million population annually). The infection has a high mortality rate and significant morbidity in survivors of the acute necrotising form. It can present at any time of year and at any age—more frequently in those aged 50–70 years, but occasionally in the young.

Some 70% of cases are in people with serological evidence and often a clinical history of previous HSV infection. Recurrent lesions are seldom apparent at the same time as encephalitis. A prodrome of fever and malaise is followed by headache and behavioural change, sometimes associated with a sudden focal episode such as a seizure or paralysis; coma usually precedes death. The temporal lobe is most frequently affected, and virus replication in neurons, followed by the oedema associated with the inflammatory response, accounts for the haemorrhagic necrosis and space-occupying nature of this form of the disease. More diffuse, milder disease has been recorded. Brainstem (bulbar) encephalitis is another serious manifestation.

Examination of cerebrospinal fluid (CSF) often demonstrates the presence of red cells and a lymphocytic response, but these findings are nonspecific. Neuroimaging can often suggest the diagnosis, the typical feature being the presence of focal (e.g., temporal) lesions on computed tomography (CT) or magnetic resonance imaging (MRI; more sensitive) scans. Virus-specific diagnosis is described later in the chapter. Early clinical recognition, leading to prompt antiviral therapy, significantly reduces the 70% mortality rate and serious morbidity of untreated cases, but therapy must be started as soon as possible and before laboratory confirmation of the diagnosis. HSV 1 is responsible for most cases of encephalitis where virus has been identified (outside the neonatal period). HSV 2 encephalitis does occur in immunocompromised adults and may be seen more frequently in those infected with the human immunodeficiency virus (HIV).

HSV meningitis

Aseptic meningitis caused by HSV is much less serious than encephalitis. HSV 2 is the usual cause, and it reaches the CSF following radiculitis during genital herpes. A lymphocytic reaction is seen in the CSF, and there may be recurrent bouts of this meningitis without mucocutaneous manifestations (sometimes known as Mollaret's meningitis after Pierre Mollaret, a French neurologist who described it in 1944). HIV-infected patients may present with HSV meningitis.

Although meningitis and encephalitis are different clinical entities, they often have overlapping signs and symptoms, particularly in the case of meningoencephalitis and early in the disease course.

Genital tract infection

Both types of HSV can infect the genital tract. Although the more common association has been with type 2 virus, HSV 1 infection is not infrequent, particularly in young women, where it may account for more than half of genital infections. Genital infection may be acquired by auto-inoculation from lesions elsewhere on the body, but most often results from intimate sexual contact including orogenital contact. The lesions are vesicular at first but rapidly ulcerate.

- In the male, the glans and shaft of the penis are the most frequent sites of infection.
- In the female, the labia, vagina and/or cervix may be involved.
- In both sexes, lesions may spread to surrounding skin sites.

The incubation period is 2–20 days, with an average of 7 days. A primary infection is usually the most severe, especially in women. Fever and malaise are accompanied by regional lymphadenopathy and urethritis, and vaginal discharge may be present. The whole episode lasts for 3–4 weeks, and high titres of virus are shed. In some cases, a lymphocytic meningitis develops, and urinary retention can also be a problem; these are manifestations of sacral radiculopathy. Where the infection is an initial genital herpes (but not a primary HSV) infection (see Table 38.2), the attack is generally less severe but may still last for about 2 weeks.

Recurrent genital herpes

This can be as frequent as six or more episodes a year. Although the attacks are milder and shorter than first episodes (around 7–10 days), the results are socially and psychologically distressing. Some patients experience prodromal symptoms in the distribution of the sacral nerves, but the patient is already infectious by this stage. Virus shedding from the genital tract is often asymptomatic. The patient or general practitioner may not recognise recurrent lesions as herpetic in origin so that, in many instances, the risk of transmission to sexual partners is not appreciated. HSV 1 genital infection recurs less often than HSV 2 and thus carries a better prognosis. Either type is capable of transmission from mother to infant. Transplacental passage resulting in intrauterine damage

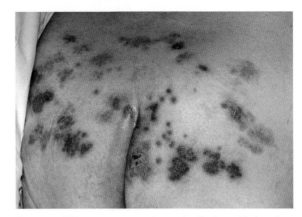

Fig. 38.4 HSV 2 recurrence over the sacral region in an elderly patient.

to the fetus has been recorded but is very rare and probably limited to cases with substantial maternal viraemia. Ascending infection from the cervix may be more significant, especially when the membranes are ruptured for some time before delivery.

Genital herpes can be a significant problem in immunosuppressed patients and may be seen as persistent, severe, perianal lesions (with or without proctitis) in many HIV-infected men who have sex with men (MSM). Genital herpetic ulcers are known to increase the risk of HIV transmission. Fig. 38.4 shows recurrent HSV 2 over the sacrum in an elderly person; the latent virus in the sacral ganglion travels to the skin dermatome served as well as the internal mucosal site; the patient had been nursed on a rubber ring.

Neonatal herpes

A rare (5 per 100,000 live births in the United Kingdom) but very serious infection, untreated neonatal herpes has a case fatality rate exceeding 60%, with half of the survivors severely damaged. Half are caused by each of HSV 1 and 2. Importantly, 85% of neonatal herpes is acquired perinatally by passage through an infected genital tract. The greatest risk, with around 50% transmission rate (because there is more virus present and no transplacental antibody transfer has occurred), is when the mother has a primary HSV infection within 6 weeks of delivery. In contrast, with recurrent herpes at term, the transmission rate is around 5%. The risk of transmission increases considerably after the membranes have been ruptured for >4 hours.

Neonatal infection may present in three different ways:

1. Skin, eye and mucous membrane (SEM) disease at about 10–12 days postpartum. Vesicular lesions on the skin may be absent, or few in number, and are

commonly located on the presenting part (e.g., the scalp; sites of trauma). Virus dissemination is the most serious complication, and, without prompt antiviral treatment, disseminated disease will occur in 75% of cases with signs of general sepsis including fever, poor feeding and irritability.

2. Disseminated disease presents during the first few days (often around day six) of life with pneumonitis and hepatitis (manifest as hepatomegaly and jaundice) with or without signs of aseptic meningitis and/or encephalitis. Progressive liver failure with coagulopathy leads to death in the most serious disseminated form.

3. CNS disease (with or without dissemination to internal organs) manifests itself at around 10–28 days of age and, in the absence of prompt antiviral treatment, causes severe neurological morbidity (70% risk) or death (6% mortality).

Prompt high-dose intravenous (IV) antiviral therapy for 2–3 weeks is the key to ensuring minimal morbidity and survival of the neonate, although local recurrent lesions can be expected, especially at skin sites, in the first year. Suppressive antiviral therapy given orally for 6 months after neonatal herpes may be considered to avoid recurrence of skin lesions and to improve neurological outcomes.

The prevention of neonatal herpes is difficult, the vast majority of infections occur in babies born to women with no past history of genital herpes and in whom the infection at term was either asymptomatic or unrecognised clinically. History of past and/or current genital herpes in pregnant women and/or their partners should be ascertained routinely and documented during antenatal appointments. With the availability of HSV type-specific antibody tests, susceptible women at risk of acquiring HSV from partners can be identified. The discovery of lesions compatible with primary HSV infection during pregnancy necessitates antiviral therapy for the mother. Lesion swabs (in virus transport medium, VTM) should be sent for HSV DNA tests by PCR alongside clotted blood samples for HSV type-specific antibody testing to determine whether the episode represents primary infection or reactivation. Suppressive antiviral therapy can be considered from 36 weeks of pregnancy until delivery. Caesarean section is recommended if primary genital herpes occurs in the third trimester or within 6 weeks of delivery. If clinically suspicious lesions are seen during labour, swabs should be tested for HSV DNA. Caesarean section may reduce the risk of infection if performed in the early stages of labour (before rupture of membranes or shortly thereafter). However, if the mother is known to have moderate levels of antibody, the baby is unlikely to develop HSV disease.

Some cases of neonatal herpes are acquired just after birth from contact with sources of HSV other than the mother's genital tract (e.g., oral or skin lesions of attendants or relatives). The clinical presentation is similar.

In a case of suspected neonatal herpes, swabs (in VTM) from the eyes, mouth, nasopharynx, rectum and skin at the site of the presentation in vaginal delivery (e.g., scalp) alongside CSF, urine and blood samples should be analysed by PCR assays and IV treatment started immediately using high-dose antivirals.

If vaginal delivery cannot be avoided in women with primary HSV infection during the third trimester or within 6 weeks of delivery, empirical treatment with high-dose IV antivirals should be started in asymptomatic neonates until active HSV infection is ruled out by PCR analyses of samples.

Laboratory investigation

Virus detection by PCR and serological studies both have their place in the diagnosis of HSV infection. In all instances of acute infection, be it primary or recurrent, virus detection by PCR (e.g., using direct vesicle swabs sent in VTM) is the method of choice as antibody responses are much less informative. Indeed, in recurrent episodes, the antibody titre may not vary. However, sensitive assays for immunoglobulin (Ig) G antibody, including type-specific antibody, have an important place in prospective testing.

Diagnosis of HSV

Direct diagnosis of HSV infection by detecting viral DNA by PCR is the most sensitive and specific method of diagnosis. The two HSV types can be differentiated by using either type-specific primers in the PCR or PCR using common primers followed by type-specific PCR analysis.

Isolation of HSV can be carried out in cultures of human diploid fibroblast cells. Growth is rapid, and within 24 hours a cytopathic effect (CPE) may be visible presenting as rounded, ballooned cells in foci that later expand and eventually involve the entire cell sheet. Virus is released from infected cells into the culture fluid; hence, the rapid spread of infection. Herpesvirus particles may be demonstrated by electron microscope (EM) analysis of vesicle fluid or tissue preparations. Detection of viral antigens in cells by immunostaining (the use of labelled monoclonal antibodies directed against viral antigens) provides a rapid diagnosis on cells scraped from the base of lesions. However, most clinical diagnostic laboratories in the United Kingdom have stopped using culture, EM and/or antigen detection assays for diagnosis of HSV infection in favour of PCR-based assessments.

Antibody tests for HSV

Commercially available enzyme immunoassays (EIAs) are sensitive and specific methods to detect total antibodies against HSV and type-specific antibodies against HSV 1 and HSV 2. However, treatment with antivirals can result in delayed appearance of these type-specific antibodies, and late convalescent samples (at 6 weeks) should be included.

Treatment

Over the past 30 years, specific antiviral therapy has revolutionised HSV management. Before the development of agents suitable for systemic use, topical application of the relatively non-selective idoxuridine was used successfully in the treatment of eye and skin infections. Aciclovir has a better therapeutic ratio and proven efficacy for the entire range of acute HSV infections. Aciclovir can be used prophylactically to prevent reactivation in the immunocompromised individual, and long-term suppressive therapy has been particularly successful in the management of frequently recurring genital herpes and HSV-related erythema multiforme. Patient-initiated early treatment can also abort or modify recurrences. Aciclovir inhibits viral DNA synthesis, and as such is effective only against replicative virus; it cannot eradicate latent virus.

Aciclovir is the most widely used agent for the treatment of HSV, and the drug has an excellent safety record, partly because of its dependence on virus TK for addition of the first phosphate group to the drug as a first step towards the triphosphate active form (subsequent phosphorylation is mediated by cellular kinases); it is available in preparations for topical, oral and intravenous use. It can be used in pregnancy as there is no evidence of adverse effects in infants of treated women, although such use is not specifically licensed in the United Kingdom and thus requires careful risk assessment. Topical cream or ointment is suitable only for mild epithelial lesions, such as recurrent cold sores. Oral or IV therapy with aciclovir should be given for:

- Any lesions that are not simply mild and superficial ones
- HSV-associated disease in the immunocompromised host
- CNS and systemic infections (IV therapy is required)
- Neonatal herpes (IV therapy must be used)
- Any of the serious manifestations of HSV disease

Dosage varies considerably, depending on the site of infection and whether the aim is suppression of recurrence or therapy of established disease. Because the level of aciclovir achieved in the CSF is only half that in plasma, the dosage for the treatment of CNS disease has to be higher than that for other systemic disease. Therapy must be maintained until clinical signs indicate a favourable response. In serious systemic disease or in the severely immunocompromised host, therapy is continued for 2–3 weeks or longer. In cases of neonatal HSV infection, a higher (IV) dose of aciclovir is given for at least 2 weeks for SEM disease and 3 weeks for CNS infection, followed by suppressive oral treatment for 6–12 months.

The poor bioavailability of oral aciclovir has led to the development of a prodrug, valaciclovir, which is rapidly converted into aciclovir, producing significantly higher plasma levels after oral dosing. Another effective antiherpes agent, penciclovir, is given in the form of an oral prodrug, famciclovir. Both of these agents are licensed for treatment of genital herpes and may be administered less frequently than aciclovir.

Resistance to aciclovir can develop. The most common forms are HSV strains with deficient or altered virus-encoded TK; hence, they cannot phosphorylate aciclovir to a monophosphate form, which is key to further phosphorylation by cellular kinases into the triphosphate active form that inhibits the HSV DNA polymerase. This has not been a significant clinical problem, but it must be remembered, particularly in the severely immunocompromised host (e.g., acquired immunodeficiency syndrome [AIDS] or following bone marrow transplant) that runs a greater risk of developing such resistance. A few resistant viruses with altered virus-encoded DNA polymerase have also been isolated and associated with clinical disease. With widespread use of aciclovir, more resistant strains may arise, and monitoring of the antiviral sensitivity of HSV isolates may be necessary. Usually, strains resistant to aciclovir are also resistant to famciclovir; in such instances, foscarnet is an alternative that may be used as it does not require activation by viral TK (but it does have serious side effects, such as nephrotoxicity).

Epidemiology

HSV is probably transmitted by direct contact with vesicular lesions and/or infectious fluid. Many children, especially in overcrowded conditions, acquire oral HSV 1 infections in the first few years of life. Spread may not occur so readily in better social conditions, with the result that primary infection is often delayed into young adulthood in developed countries. This is the usual time of exposure to genital herpes, and, as a result, primary infection may be HSV 1 or 2.

Sensitive EIAs, and type-specific assays, have shown that:

- 60%–90% of adults have had an HSV 1 infection
- Many more adults have had HSV 2 infection than give a history of genital herpes

Neonatal herpes is a rare complication in the United Kingdom. The rate of cases has increased in some populations as genital herpes has become more common.

Control

Transmission of herpes simplex can be reduced by:

- Simple hygiene measures (e.g., attention to adequate hand hygiene and use of alcohol-based gels)
- Education regarding the infectious stages
- Use of condoms

Reference has already been made to the prevention of neonatal infection as has the use of suppressive antiviral regimens to control predictable recurrence. Progress in understanding latency and reactivation will provide approaches to preventing reactivation. Protection from ultraviolet light and the use of inhibitors of prostaglandin synthesis may be useful in this context.

Experimental vaccines are under investigation, but none is licensed for use. Research into subunit vaccines based on the viral glycoproteins or other significant viral proteins may lead to an appropriate preparation to elicit the immune responses important in control of HSV. Recent trials have shown limited protection against genital tract disease. A vaccine that stimulates T cell immune responses may be required.

VARICELLA–ZOSTER VIRUS (VZV)

Infection with VZV presents in two forms:

1. Primary infection: Varicella (or chickenpox) is a generalised eruption.
2. Reactivated infection: Zoster (or shingles) is localised to one (or a few) dermatome.

DESCRIPTION

The viruses isolated from varicella and zoster are identical, and the virus has the morphology of all herpesviruses. Seventy genes code for 67 different proteins, including five families of glycoprotein genes. The glycoproteins gE, gB and gH are abundant in infected cells and are present in the viral envelope (Fig. 38.5).

Following attachment (mediated primarily by gB) to cell surface glycosaminoglycans and fusion, the nucleocapsid enters the cell and viral DNA is released into the nucleus where virus replication takes place. Histological examination of infected epidermis reveals typical nuclear inclusions and multinucleate giant cells identical to those of HSV. Human fibroblast cell cultures are most often

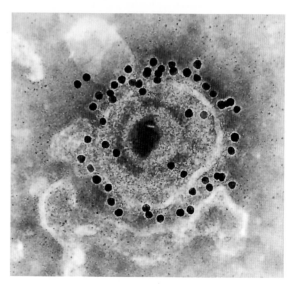

Fig. 38.5 VZV showing the virus envelope glycoprotein I (gE) labelled with monoclonal antibody and goat anti-mouse IgG conjugated with 15 nm colloidal gold (original magnification ×150,000). (Micrograph taken by C. Graham; supplied by Dr E. Dermott, Department of Microbiology and Immunobiology, Queen's University, Belfast, United Kingdom.)

used for isolation. Enveloped virus released from the nucleus remains closely attached to microvilli along the cell surface; studies of this cell-associated characteristic, with infection being passed from cell to cell, have been limited compared with studies of the lytic HSV. The typical CPE appears in cell cultures in 3 days to 2–3 weeks.

Recently, the presence of geographically distinct VZV genotypes has been described, but little is known about the clinical significance of these findings. Antibodies to the three main glycoproteins all neutralise virus infectivity. One of these glycoproteins, gB, shares 49% amino acid identity with the gB of HSV, and this may account for the cross-reactive, anamnestic, antibody response that may be detected during infections with either virus.

PATHOGENESIS

Varicella

This is a disease predominantly of children, characterised by a vesicular skin eruption (chickenpox; the origin of the term is unclear—from chickpea [the bean; refers to the look of the lesion] or the Old English term *gican* [to itch]). Virus enters through the upper respiratory tract or conjunctivae and may multiply in local lymph tissue for a few days before entering the blood and being distributed throughout the body. After replication in reticuloendothelial sites, a second viraemic stage precedes the appearance of the skin and mucosal lesions. An alternative model has been proposed, based on studies in a humanised severe combined immunodeficient (hu-SCID) mouse model (bearing human skin xenografts). The work showed that activated human tonsillar T lymphocytes could be infected and, if given to the mice intravenously, homed rapidly to the skin grafts where VZV could be detected by 7 days (although the typical epidermal vesicular lesion did not appear for 10–21 days).

The VZV vesicles lie in the middle of the epidermis, and the fluid contains numerous free virus particles. Within 3 days, the fluid becomes cloudy with the influx of leukocytes; fibrin and interferon are also present. The pustules then dry up, scabs form, and they desquamate. Lesions in all stages are present at any one time while new ones are appearing. The clearance of virus-infected cells is dependent on functional T lymphocyte-mediated immune mechanisms and antibody-dependent cell cytotoxicity (ADCC). Persons deficient in these responses, and in interferon production, have prolonged vesicular phases and great difficulty in controlling the infection.

Zoster

The pathogenesis of zoster (shingles) is not as well established as that of HSV recurrence. The latent virus is found in neurones and satellite cells in sensory ganglia, and more than one region of the genome is transcribed, although the state of the latent VZV is largely unknown. It seems likely that virus reaches the ganglion from the periphery by travelling up nerve axons, as HSV does, but there is also the possibility that, during viraemia, some virus enters ganglion cells. Another difference from HSV latency lies in the persistent VZV expression that has been detected in some mononuclear cells; this may have a role in VZV disease such as postherpetic neuralgia (see later in the chapter).

Reactivation of VZV as zoster can occur at any age in a person who has had a primary infection, which may or may not have been apparent clinically. The rate is greatest in persons aged ≥60 years and, as most primary infection takes place before the age of 20 years, there is usually a latent period of several decades. However, a much shorter latent period is seen in immunocompromised patients, and also in those who acquired primary infection in utero or in the first year of life. More than one episode of zoster is uncommon in any individual. The stimulus to reactivation is largely unknown, but virus travels from sensory ganglia to the peripheral site. Zoster is usually limited to one dermatome; in adults, this is most commonly in the thoracic or upper lumbar regions or in the area supplied by the ophthalmic division of the trigeminal nerve. It is thought that this distribution is related to the density of the original varicella rash. There are associations with preceding trauma to the dermatome—injury or injections—with an interval of 2–3 weeks before the zoster appears. There is an associated suppression of specific T cell–mediated responses in acute zoster, but rapid secondary antibody responses are usually found. Reactivation occurs more commonly in T cell immunodeficiency states.

Viraemia may occur in the course of zoster but is unusual, with preexisting immunity usually being boosted rapidly. In the immunocompromised host, however, viraemia may lead to dissemination of zoster, either to internal organs or in a generalized manner reminiscent of varicella (disseminated zoster).

CLINICAL FEATURES

Varicella

The incubation period averages 14–15 days but may range from 10–21 days. The patient is infectious for 2 days before and for some days after onset, while new vesicles are appearing and until all vesicles have crusted over.

The rash of varicella (chickenpox) is usually centripetal, being most dense on the trunk and head. Initially macular, the rash rapidly evolves through papules to the characteristic clear vesicles (dew drops).

Presentations vary widely, from the clinically inapparent through to a severe febrile illness with a widespread itchy rash, especially in secondary cases in older members of a household. Usually a relatively mild infection in the young child, the complications of varicella, which are much more likely in adults, may cause significant morbidity and even mortality.

In the past, the main differential diagnosis was smallpox (Table 38.3). Another possibility is monkeypox if the travel

Table 38.3 Key differences between rashes of varicella and smallpox		
Feature	Varicella	Smallpox
Characteristic lesions	Blisters: Domed small superficial single vesicles with clear fluid	Several layers of cells cover multifocal vesicles; early umbilication seen
Distribution	Centripetal: Most on trunk, neck, face, proximal parts of limbs	Centrifugal: Face, forearms and palms, soles of feet
Appearance at any one time	Pleomorphic: Papules, vesicles and crusts may all be seen in one area	Lesions all at same stage in one affected area

and/or occupational history (e.g., exotic pet handling) is suggestive of such exposure.

Secondary bacterial infection of skin lesions is the most common complication of varicella, mainly in the young child, and increases the amount of residual scarring. Thrombocytopaenic purpura occurs, especially in the immunocompromised host, and this may lead to haemorrhagic chickenpox, which is life threatening. A variety of organs may rarely be affected producing arthritis, myocarditis, hepatitis, glomerulonephritis and/or appendicitis. However, the two most frequent complications are related to the lungs and the CNS.

Pneumonitis

VZV pneumonitis is a serious complication, even in immunocompetent individuals. It is more likely to occur in adults, smokers, pregnant women, and immunocompromised hosts. Severity may vary from subclinical (evident only on radiography) to life threatening. Cough, dyspnoea, tachypnoea and chest pains begin a few days after the rash. Upon imaging, nodular infiltrates are seen in the lungs. Prompt antiviral therapy (see later in the chapter) must be used in sufficient dosage and started at the first sign of pneumonia. Early investigations (imaging and gas exchange) are indicated in all smokers and immunocompromised patients with chickenpox.

Central nervous system

Neurological complications include the common but benign cerebellar ataxia syndrome and aseptic meningitis. Acute encephalitis is rare but more serious and occurs mostly in the immunocompromised host. It may be confused with postinfectious encephalopathy, which, with other postinfectious manifestations such as transverse myelitis or Guillain–Barré syndrome (named after Guillain and Barré, who described the illness together with Strohl in 1916 following the initial description by Landry in 1859), is immunologically mediated and not related to viral cytopathogenicity.

Varicella in pregnancy

The infection may be more serious for the mother in pregnancy, with pneumonitis being the major problem. VZV can cross the placenta following maternal viraemia and infect the fetus. Two types of intrauterine infections are noted:

1. Congenital varicella syndrome (CVS) is a rare consequence of fetal infection in the first half of pregnancy (<1% of fetuses, if maternal infection occurs during first 12 weeks of gestation; 2%, if maternal infection occurs during 13–20 weeks of gestation). The characteristic features, usually unilateral, are scarring of the skin, damage to the musculoskeletal system (muscular atrophy, hypoplasia of the limbs, rudimentary or missing digits) as well as to the CNS (cortical atrophy, psychomotor retardation) and eyes (chorioretinitis, cataracts). Fetal infection is not inevitable. Silent intrauterine infection can also occur; no damage is seen, but the baby is born with latent VZV infection, which may manifest as zoster in the first year of life.

2. Neonatal varicella is defined as varicella developing within the first 4 weeks of life, usually acquired from maternal varicella in late pregnancy (although, rarely, the exposure may occur postnatally; e.g., to an older sibling with chickenpox). The interval between maternal viraemia and delivery is important. If the maternal rash begins 7 days or more before delivery, the woman's antibody response will have developed and protective IgG antibodies transferred across the placenta so that the baby does not develop disease. However, the infant is at serious risk if maternal varicella occurs 6 days or less before, or up to 2 days after, delivery; this allows viraemic spread across the placenta before maternal antibody is made and transferred to the baby. Because the usual respiratory entry route has been bypassed, the incubation period is reduced to (on average) 10 days. If infection arises, serious (even fatal) disseminated disease may develop, including pneumonitis and encephalitis. Such exposed neonates should be afforded passive immunity (see later in the chapter) and considered for prompt antiviral therapy as should neonates of seronegative mothers exposed to any source of VZV within the first 4 weeks of life.

Zoster

This is the manifestation of reactivated VZV infection; zoster takes the form of a localised eruption, which is unilateral and typically confined to one dermatome. Prodromal paraesthesiae and pain in the area supplied by the affected sensory nerve are common before the skin lesions develop; these are identical to those of varicella, except in their distribution. The evolution of the rash is similar with some new vesicles appearing, whilst the earliest ones are crusting; however, in the majority of cases, the entire episode is confined to the affected dermatome and heals in 1–3 weeks. Acute pain is not always a feature, but its presence should alert to the possibility of zoster and a search for early lesions (that may be internal but difficult to assess) is indicated. Occasionally there are no skin lesions—zoster sine herpete.

Disseminated zoster is indicated by lesions appearing in the skin at distant sites (resembling the clinical picture of chickenpox) or, more seriously, by involvement of internal organs such as the lung and CNS (meningitis, encephalitis and/or myelitis). In the immunocompromised host, this results in severe disease with occasional fatalities. Patients with internal organ zoster may or may not present with a typical skin rash.

Postherpetic neuralgia

This is the most common complication of zoster, a risk in 50% of patients aged >60 years, and results in significant morbidity in around 20% of cases. It is defined as intractable pain persisting for ≥1 month after healing of the skin rash. Constant pain at the site, or stabbing pains or paraesthesiae, may continue for 1 year, or much longer in a number of individuals. This is an exhausting and disabling condition for which no satisfactory cure has been found; adequate early antiviral therapy may reduce the incidence.

Ophthalmic zoster

Involvement of the ophthalmic division of the trigeminal nerve occurs in up to one-quarter of zoster episodes, with ocular complications in >50% of the patients. Corneal ulceration, stromal keratitis and anterior uveitis may result in permanent scarring, so this complication may threaten sight when the nasociliary branch is involved. Ocular complications are reduced in patients given oral aciclovir early in ophthalmic zoster. Occasionally, acute retinal necrosis is observed.

A contralateral hemiparesis due to granulomatous cerebral angiitis in the weeks following acute ophthalmic zoster is a recognised neurological complication. A more acute one, such as the Ramsay Hunt syndrome (named after the American neurologist James Ramsay Hunt; facial palsy with aural zoster vesicles; also known as herpes zoster oticus), suggests that motor neurones can also be involved. Sympathetic ganglia may also be the site of latency as indicated by cases in which the initial recrudescence has been in gastric mucosa with subsequent dissemination.

Recurrent and chronic VZV

Immunocompromised individuals, most particularly those with $CD4^+$ T cell lymphopenia due to HIV infection, may develop recurrent and chronic VZV infection. New lesions continue to appear, or reappear, after aciclovir therapy, often presenting an atypical hyperkeratotic appearance. Aciclovir-resistant VZV has been isolated in this situation.

LABORATORY INVESTIGATION

Typical presentations of varicella or zoster seldom need laboratory confirmation; however, atypical presentations merit investigation, especially in the immunocompromised host. Vesicular rashes due to enterovirus are sometimes confused with varicella and, in immunosuppressed individuals, various vesicular lesions may be mistaken for zoster. Localised vesicular lesions other than those on the face or genitalia are commonly misdiagnosed as being caused by zoster (see Fig. 38.4); many are due to recurrence of HSV, and this is readily shown by antigen detection and virus isolation or by PCR. Thus the approach to testing of vesicular lesions usually involves simultaneous HSV and VZV assessment of viral DNA by PCR.

Virus detection

Early vesicular lesions provide the best diagnostic material. Vesicle fluid is collected in a capillary tube, aspirated with a fine needle and syringe, or lesions are swabbed directly (and sent in VTM). Direct examination by EM will reveal herpesvirus particles; some of the fluid can be diluted in VTM and inoculated into tissue culture for virus isolation, which takes between 5 days and 3 weeks. More rapid detection is possible with centrifugation-enhanced cultures (shell vials). If cells swabbed from the base of lesions are available, or biopsy tissue, virus antigens may be sought by immunostaining assays. However, in the United Kingdom, VZV DNA amplification by PCR is now used for the detection of VZV in all types of samples including CSF and aqueous humour; equally, PCR is the approach now used for rapid diagnosis.

Serological diagnosis

Antibody testing with VZV antigens can confirm a diagnosis of varicella by demonstration of seroconversion or rising titres of antibody between acute and convalescent serum samples; IgM to VZV is detectable by IgM capture systems in both varicella and zoster, appearing early in zoster. It is common practice now to test for past infection (and, therefore, immunity) by measuring IgG antibody to VZV in those who are, or will become, immunocompromised, in women exposed antenatally to VZV or in health-care workers (or other adults) who are to be offered VZV immunization.

TREATMENT

VZV is not as sensitive to aciclovir as HSV, with 50% inhibitory dose (ID_{50}) values ranging from 4–17 μM aciclovir, compared with 0.1–1.6 µM for HSV. This means that frequent high-dose oral or IV therapy is required against the virus. High-dose aciclovir given intravenously is effective in the treatment of varicella and zoster in the immunocompromised host. Oral aciclovir can be used to accelerate healing and reduce new lesion formation during zoster in immunocompetent patients if given early enough and may lower the rate of postherpetic neuralgia. Alternative oral prodrug preparations such as valaciclovir and famciclovir require less frequent dosing. Trials have shown that high-dose oral aciclovir shortens the course of varicella in immunocompetent children by 1 day if commenced within 24 hours of the onset of rash. The practical difficulties of achieving such an early start of treatment rule out routine use of aciclovir for all cases of varicella in immunocompetent children, but consideration should be given to treating all adults as well as (where possible) adolescents and family contact cases who are known to develop more extensive disease. Treatment of VZV infection is given primarily to all 'high risk of complication' groups and should thus be considered for:

- Neonates (within the first 4 weeks of life)
- Immunocompromised patients
- Those with ophthalmic zoster
- Healthy individuals with varicella when there is an additional complicating factor such as pneumonia
- Infection involving motor nerves (e.g., facial palsy)

EPIDEMIOLOGY

Varicella is partly seasonal, being spread mainly by the respiratory route in winter and early spring. Some cases may result from contact with zoster (e.g., in the immunosuppressed) and occur sporadically in any season. Varicella is highly infectious (as a result of respiratory spread) to susceptible contacts upon direct exposure as in a household; however, a past history of varicella is a good indicator of existing immunity because the clinical picture is quite distinct and not easily confused with any other disease. The majority of children contract VZV between the ages of 4 and 10 years in Western countries, with around 8% of young adults remaining susceptible (Fig. 38.6). However, a much higher proportion of young adults remain susceptible in subtropical countries (for reasons that are not entirely clear). The rate of pneumonitis as a complication of varicella is surprisingly high in otherwise healthy adults (1 in 200; in children, the figure is 1 in 200,000), particularly in pregnant women and smokers who develop pneumonia in up to 10% of cases. Adult VZV pneumonitis may prove fatal without prompt

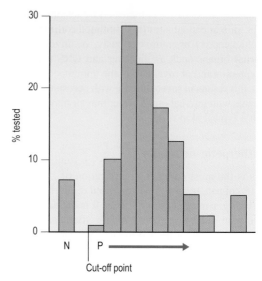

Fig. 38.6 Distribution of antibody (IgG) to VZV in a young adult population (southern England). The proportion confirmed as negative *(N)* was 7.8%. *P →*, increasingly positive result.

antiviral therapy. Zoster is associated with decreased T cell function and occurs with increased incidence in:

- Old age
- The pre-AIDS phase of HIV infection
- Organ transplant recipients
- Patients receiving chemotherapy and/or radiotherapy for lymphoid malignancies

In developed countries, the increasing survival of people beyond 65 years of age means that the incidence of zoster will increase. This may be exacerbated by less natural boosting of immune responses as VZV decreases in countries offering childhood immunization for varicella.

CONTROL

Passive immunization

Passive immunity is partly protective against varicella as seen in infants with maternal antibody or patients given varicella-zoster immunoglobulin (VZIG; ideally, within 72 hours of exposure). VZIG (in the United Kingdom), or another similar high-titre antibody preparation, is available for neonates, nonimmune pregnant contacts or immunocompromised contacts of VZV. As most pregnant contacts will be immune, testing for VZV IgG antibody after exposure may prevent unnecessary use of costly and scarce VZIG; conversely, VZIG may be considered for susceptible (VZV IgG antibody-negative) pregnant VZV contacts for up to 10 days post exposure (cf. for up to 7 days for susceptible immunosuppressed contacts). Current preparations seldom prevent infection but do ameliorate disease. Importantly, VZIG reduces the rate of VZV transmission to the fetus.

Varicella vaccine

A live-attenuated varicella vaccine has been in use for some years in Japan and some European countries and was approved in the United States for routine childhood immunization in 1995. The vaccine strain (Oka), which can be distinguished from wild-type VZV by molecular analysis, is given by intramuscular injection. The vaccine is immunogenic in children with leukaemia in remission and in healthy children and adults; vaccinees have resisted infection on close exposure to varicella. Some symptoms are noted around 10 days post vaccination, and vesicles appear at the site of injection in up to 5% of individuals. Immunization does not prevent latency developing; however, the incidence of zoster in vaccinees compared with that in the naturally infected is not increased. In the United States, surveillance has confirmed a significant reduction in the incidence of varicella, especially in the 1–4 years age group, and a substantial fall in mortality and complication rates. There have been reports of breakthrough epidemics locally, even in well-vaccinated cohorts, and a booster dose may be necessary. A large trial of vaccination in the elderly (>60 years old) showed a 60% reduction in the incidence of zoster and postherpetic neuralgia in those immunized with a high-titre preparation of Oka virus–based vaccine. Currently, in the United Kingdom, the VZV vaccine is not offered as part of the childhood immunization programme but, instead, to susceptible individuals who are in regular contact with those at risk of developing serious VZV illness. Thus, the vaccine is offered to nonimmune health-care workers and healthy contacts of immunocompromised patients. The primary course consists of two vaccine doses administered 4–8 weeks apart. Additionally, in the United Kingdom, a single dose of a higher titre (Oka-derived) vaccine is offered to adults aged 70 years (with a catch-up programme for those aged 70–79 years), with a view to lowering the incidence and severity of zoster in older populations.

EPSTEIN–BARR VIRUS

In 1964, Epstein, Barr and Achong described herpesvirus particles in cells from a lymphoma in African children studied by Burkitt, a British surgeon working in Africa, who suspected an infectious aetiology of the tumour (now known as Burkitt's lymphoma). The association of the then newly discovered herpesvirus, denoted Epstein–Barr virus (EBV), with a variety of epithelial and lymphoid tumours is now clear. Primary infection with EBV:

- Is most often acquired in childhood when it is generally asymptomatic
- Gives rise to infectious mononucleosis (also known as glandular fever) in up to a quarter of individuals when infection is delayed into adolescence

Humans are the only known natural host, but EBV infection can be transmitted experimentally to nonhuman (New World) primates (tamarin, marmoset; Old World primates are naturally immune as a result of infection with simian EBV homologues).

DESCRIPTION

The characteristic morphology of EBV seen on EM is that of a herpesvirus. EBV cannot be grown in human fibroblast or epithelial cell lines, and there is no completely productive or permissive system for its culture. This lymphotropic virus is classified in the Gammaherpesvirinae subfamily, genus *Lymphocryptovirus.*

REPLICATION

The full replication (productive, or lytic) cycle of EBV can take place in certain differentiated epithelial cells, although it is not clear whether this is an integral part of the natural life cycle of EBV infection in the human host. The B lymphocyte is the principal and essential cell infected through attachment of the major viral envelope glycoprotein gp350/220 to EBV receptors (primarily, the CD21 molecule) expressed on mature resting B lymphocytes. There are other receptors on cells of stratified squamous epithelium (e.g., in the oropharynx and ectocervix), and these epithelial cells can be infected through their basal aspect. Viral production is restricted to the differentiated cells of the granular layer and above, with virus shedding from the superficial cells. It is difficult to grow differentiating epithelia in culture, and most work on the lytic cycle of EBV has been done in B lymphoblastoid cell lines (BLCLs) in which a small proportion of the EBV-infected cells can be induced to produce virus.

The organization of the EBV genome differs from that of HSV, and some genes are present in one and not in the other. Approximately 80 proteins are encoded; many glycoproteins (gp) are known, including the major gp350/220, which mediates attachment to CD21, as well as gp25, gp42 and gp85 that bind a coreceptor (major histocompatibility [MHC] class 2 molecules) on the target cell and are involved in membrane fusion. The latent (nonproductive) state of EBV infection is established in a subset of resting memory B lymphocytes in which the EBV genome is maintained in the nucleus as multiple full-length covalently closed circular (CCC) episomes. Specific EBV-encoded small RNA species (EBERs) are found in abundance in all cells infected with the virus. A variable number of *EBV* genes are expressed in the different forms of the latent state. These are principally genes coding for one or more of six EBV nuclear antigens (EBNA leader protein [LP], 1, 2, 3a–c) and two latent membrane proteins (LMP 1, 2). EBNA 1 maintains the EBV episome as the B cells divide and is the only latent protein expressed in all types of EBV-associated tumours (see later in the chapter). EBNA 2 and LMP 1 are both viral oncogenes that promote B cell proliferation. Latency involves different expression patterns of these latent viral proteins—all are expressed by BLCLs in culture as well as at the outset of primary EBV infection (unrestricted latency), which is followed by downregulation of some, or all, of them (restricted latency) in the course of infection. Whilst all the lytic and latent proteins are involved in recognition by EBV-specific T cells that mediate immune control of the virus, such downregulation of latent genes is one mechanism that facilitates persistent infection and immune evasion. An unrestricted latent virus expression profile is observed during infectious mononucleosis and in EBV-associated posttransplant lymphoproliferative disease (PTLD), whilst more restricted patterns are seen in other malignancies associated with this virus. Interestingly, EBV encodes a homologue of interleukin (IL) 10 (viral IL 10, vIL10) that may play a role in immune modulation.

Although there are two types of EBV, types 1 and 2, their disease association is similar, and no unique clinical significance has been attributed to either type.

The full lytic cycle of EBV replication is accompanied by the production of a large number of lytic proteins that include virus structural antigens resulting in the assembly of progeny virus. Although EBV does encode a viral TK, aciclovir is phosphorylated by cellular kinases in cells producing EBV. The viral DNA polymerase is sensitive to the active aciclovir triphosphate, and treatment with aciclovir reduces EBV production in vitro but has no effect on latency or the B cell proliferation induced by the virus. However, aciclovir has very limited (if any) effectiveness in the clinical (patient) setting.

PATHOGENESIS

In primary infection, virus in saliva is thought to infect oropharyngeal B lymphocytes in tonsillar crypts; the exact role of epithelial cells in the process is still unclear. This leads to activation of the infected B cells, which progress to the local lymph nodes and on through the circulation with the potential to enter a productive (lytic) phase and release of progeny virus elsewhere in the body. Most shedding of virus takes place in the oral cavity (epithelial cells may have a role in this aspect of infection), and EBV can be detected regularly in the saliva of asymptomatic hosts, the amount increasing in immunosuppressed states.

Activated B lymphocytes secrete immunoglobulin, and EBV is a potent polyclonal activator of antibody production by B cells independent of any accessory cells.

Recovery from primary EBV infection is associated with humoral and, primarily, cellular immune responses involving T cells; any delay in cellular control, or overvigorous responses, will contribute to the severity of the infection. Thus, large initial infective doses may result in high numbers of circulating infected B lymphocytes followed by a marked T cell response. The polyclonal B cell activation results in the transient appearance of a variety of antibodies (predominantly IgM), both autophile and heterophile. The cellular response is detected as a mononucleosis with large numbers of atypical lymphocytes in blood and infiltrating tissues that are EBV-specific T cells.

Antibody responses after EBV infection follow a characteristic pattern, with the initial IgM response to virus capsid antigens (VCA) persisting for some months (being replaced by VCA IgG). The latent EBNA complex elicits antibodies in late convalescence only, perhaps after release from B cells lysed by EBV-specific T cells (Fig. 38.7). Failure to produce antibody to the EBNAs is a feature of immunodeficiency states that may also be associated with increased levels of antibodies to EBV lytic cycle antigens (early antigen [EA] and VCA), reflecting a high virus replication rate. High IgA levels to VCA are found in those at risk of developing EBV-associated nasopharyngeal carcinoma (NPC; see later in the chapter). Antibodies against the major viral envelope glycoprotein gp350/220 are neutralising and may protect against reinfection.

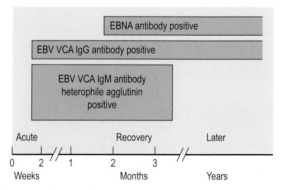

Fig. 38.7 Appearance and duration of diagnostic antibodies following primary EBV infection. *EBNA*, EBV, Nuclear antigen; *VCA*, viral/virus capsid antigen.

CLINICAL FEATURES

Primary infection with EBV is usually mild and unrecognised in the vast majority who acquire it in the first years of life.

Infectious mononucleosis/glandular fever

Infectious mononucleosis (IM; or glandular fever, GF) is seen predominantly in the 15–25 years age group when primary EBV infection is delayed into adulthood. The incubation period is 30–50 days, and the onset is abrupt, with a triad of sore throat, cervical lymphadenopathy and fever, often accompanied by malaise, headache, sweating (particularly at night) and gastrointestinal discomfort. A mononucleosis of atypical lymphocytes is observed in blood. Pharyngitis may be severe, accompanied by a greyish-white membrane and gross tonsillar enlargement. Lymphadenopathy becomes generalised, often with splenic enlargement and tenderness, mild hepatomegaly (and biochemical hepatitis) in some individuals and clinical jaundice in 5%–10% of cases. Intermittent fevers with drenching (at times, nocturnal) sweats may occur daily over 2 weeks. A faint transient morbilliform rash may be seen; a maculopapular rash may follow ampicillin administration due to immune complexes with antibody to ampicillin. The illness can last for several weeks; prolonged and debilitating fatigue and lack of concentration are common in the aftermath.

Complications of infectious mononucleosis/glandular fever

Complications are rare, but some can be serious:

- Acute airway obstruction may occur as a result of the lymphoid enlargement and oedema; this merits emergency tracheostomy in some cases but usually responds well to steroids.
- Splenic rupture (rare).
- Neurological complications include aseptic meningitis, encephalitis and the Guillain–Barré syndrome.

Other EBV–associated disease, tumours and immunosuppression

EBV is associated with an increasing number of diseases, including malignant tumours (Table 38.4). The role played by EBV in these conditions (whether cause, cofactor or otherwise) is not clear in all cases. Cellular immunodeficiency, associated with impaired T cell control of EBV-induced B cell proliferation, may result in EBV-driven B cell lymphoproliferations and lymphomas. This may be inherited (e.g., X-linked lymphoproliferative [or Duncan's] syndrome [X-LPS] due to a defective immunomodulatory *SAP* gene), acquired (e.g., in AIDS) or due to iatrogenic immunosuppression following transplantation surgery (PTLD). In African Burkitt's lymphoma (BL), characterized by translocation of the cellular proto-oncogene *c-myc* gene into chromosomal locations driven by the highly active immunoglobulin promoters, EBV infection at an early age combines with chronic immunosuppression due to holoendemic malaria to promote further the development of highly aggressive BL tumours (endemic BL, eBL). Sporadic BL (sBL), which arises outside equatorial Africa, is also associated with EBV in up to 50% of cases. Furthermore, Hodgkin's lymphoma (HL) is associated with EBV in approximately 50% of cases (particularly the mixed cellularity subset), and the anaplastic subset of nasopharyngeal carcinoma (NPC) is almost always associated with the virus. Haemophagocytic lymphohistiocytosis (HLH) is a rare but (if left untreated) potentially fatal primary (genetic) or secondary (e.g., infection-induced) condition characterised by defects in perforin and/or reduced NK cell function that may become apparent upon primary EBV infection, which the affected individuals cannot control adequately and results in overstimulation of T cells, a dysregulated cytokine storm and overactivation of macrophages/histiocytes leading to their phagocytosis of blood cell lineages (e.g., red and white blood cells as well as platelets) and clinical disease (including fever, splenomegaly, cytopenia, rash and haemophagocytosis).

LABORATORY INVESTIGATION

IM/GF is accompanied by the production of heterophile agglutinins that can be detected by a rapid slide agglutination test (the Paul–Bunnell test; related tests include the heterophile antibody test and the monospot test). Agglutination of horse or sheep red blood cells by serum absorbed to exclude a natural antibody is the basis of this test. Atypical lymphocytes, accounting for 20% of the lymphocytosis common in this condition, are seen in blood films. Definitive diagnosis requires the demonstration of IgM antibody to EBV VCA and/or seroconversion to VCA IgG antibody, followed by emergence (in due course; usually within 6 months) of EBNA IgG. These tests, using indirect immunostaining (immunofluorescence) or, more commonly nowadays, EIAs, are generally available; additional serological tests may be applicable to aid serological diagnosis in special situations (e.g., EA antibody tests).

Culture of EBV, from saliva or throat washings, is a research technique. Tissue sections can be immunostained

Table 38.4 Diseases associated with Epstein–Barr virus (EBV)

Disease	Cells infected	Link
Infectious mononucleosis (glandular fever)	Naive B lymphocytes	Causal; acute primary infection
Oral hairy leukoplakia (seen in AIDS)	Differentiated epithelium along edge of tongue	Causal; productive recurrence in immunocompromised host
Nasopharyngeal carcinoma (especially in Southeast Asia and China)	Anaplastic/undifferentiated nasopharyngeal epithelium (long latent period, >30 years)	All malignant cells contain EBV; cofactor(s) play a role and there is genetic risk
African (endemic) Burkitt's lymphoma	Monoclonal B cell tumour (short latent period, <5 years)	All malignant cells contain EBV; holoendemic malaria plays a role
Immunoblastic lymphoma (posttransplant/ AIDS; X-linked lymphoproliferative syndrome)	Activated B lymphocytes	Over 90% of malignant cells contain EBV; immunodeficiency states, genetic defect
Hodgkin's lymphoma	Hodgkin–Reed–Sternberg cells (germinal-centre B lymphocytes)	30%–90% of malignant cells contain EBV (particular disease subsets)
Anaplastic gastric carcinoma	Epithelial cells	Malignant cells contain EBV (particular disease subsets)
T/NK cell lymphoma	T/NK lymphocytes	30%–100% of malignant cells contain EBV (particular disease subsets)

AIDS, Acquired immunodeficiency syndrome; *EBV*, Epstein–Barr virus; *NK*, natural killer.

for LMP1, EBNA or other EBV proteins (Fig. 38.8) or may be probed for EBERs using in situ hybridisation (ISH) techniques; these approaches, as well as PCR assessment of EBV DNA in blood, are important in the diagnosis of disease in the immunocompromised host (including individuals suffering from HLH). The role of assessing levels of EBV DNA by PCR following transplantation to predict, diagnose or monitor treatment responses to PTLD is still being evaluated. Such measurements are not straightforward in the solid organ transplant (SOT) setting, although greater success has been achieved using EBV PCR to monitor high-risk haematopoietic stem cell transplant (HSCT) recipients. The availability of an international standard for such quantitative (real-time) EBV PCR assays facilitates meaningful comparison of results (viral load) among clinical laboratories when appropriate, thereby supporting continuity of care.

TREATMENT

Aciclovir is of little value against EBV disease, although it is sometimes included in regimes against PTLD. Whilst reducing immunosuppression in transplant recipients suffering PTLD is an option, this may put the grafted organ(s) at risk. Adoptive humoral immunotherapy using the agent rituximab, a humanised murine monoclonal antibody against the pan-B cell surface marker CD20, is effective against EBV-associated B cell tumours (including PTLD). Similarly, adoptive cellular immunotherapy employing autologous, or MHC-matched allogeneic, EBV-specific T lymphocytes has been shown to be effective in individuals who have not responded to any other treatment for PTLD. For HLH, treatment is specialized and

includes consideration of immunosuppressants as well as cytotoxic agents (e.g., etoposide).

EPIDEMIOLOGY

EBV is transmitted by saliva, and a potential role for sexual transmission has also been proposed. Rarely, transmission has been reported following transfusion of blood products to seronegative recipients. Infection is widespread, with most of the population infected in early life, even in developed countries. Increasing numbers of severely immunocompromised hosts are at risk of developing EBV-driven malignant lymphomas, including SOT and HSCT recipients. This can occur when donor virus is transmitted in grafted tissues or following reactivation of the recipient's own isolate. Primary EBV infection post transplantation is a high-risk situation for PTLD development, which explains why paediatric SOT recipients are at particular risk of the disease that can be fatal in up to 50% of cases despite therapy.

CONTROL

Subunit vaccines based on the major membrane glycoprotein gp350/220 have undergone trials and been shown to protect against tumour-inducing doses of EBV in a cottontop tamarin model and against IM/GF in seronegative healthy human populations (although not through sterile immunity as EBV infection is not prevented). However, such vaccines have not yet found their way into routine immunisation programmes. Screening for IgA antibodies to EBV VCA is used in populations

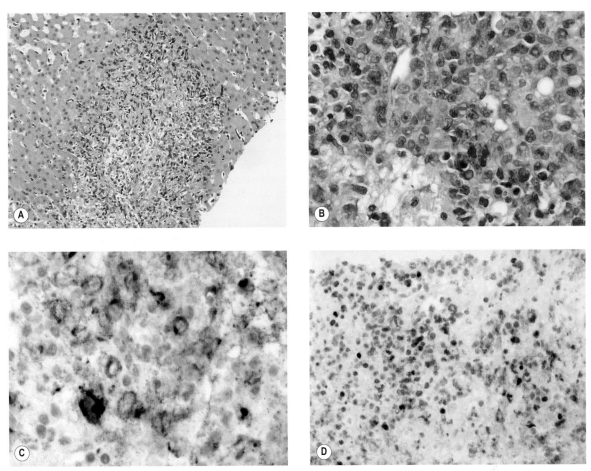

Fig. 38.8 Liver needle biopsy of posttransplant lymphoproliferative disease (PTLD) in a liver transplant recipient. (A) Portal area infiltrated with high-grade lymphoma showing slight spillover into adjacent and relatively normal-looking liver tissue. (B) High-power view of the neoplastic infiltrate showing large, atypical lymphoid blast cells. (C) Epstein–Barr virus (EBV) latent membrane protein (LMP) immunohistochemistry decorates many of the neoplastic lymphoid cells. (D) EBV nuclear antigen (EBNA) 2 immunohistochemistry also highlights many tumour cell nuclei (brown is positive). (Courtesy Dr C. O. C. Bellamy, Department of Laboratory Medicine, Royal Infirmary of Edinburgh, United Kingdom.)

at risk of NPC to detect preclinical cases, although EBV PCR analysis (primarily, of blood using viral load as marker of disease activity) is rapidly replacing such an approach.

CYTOMEGALOVIRUS

Human cytomegalovirus (CMV) infects humans, but there are other cytomegaloviruses that are specific for other animal species (e.g., murine CMV). The name derives from the cytopathic effects (CPE) of CMV infection that results in a swollen state of infected cells (cytomegaly) in culture and in tissues. Nuclei of productively infected cells contain a large inclusion body, giving rise to a typical 'owl's eye' appearance that can be seen by immunohistochemical staining under the light microscope. Whilst CMV is slowly proliferative in tissue culture, it replicates rapidly in the human body and can pose an immediate and serious threat to vulnerable individuals.

DESCRIPTION

CMV has the same general structure as other herpesviruses, but its target cell surface receptor is not yet known for certain. Human fibroblast cells are required for isolation of the virus in vitro. In contrast, CMV replicates in vivo in monocytes/macrophages and in epithelial/endothelial cells in salivary glands, kidneys, the respiratory tract and other epithelial/endothelial sites.

CMV remains highly cell associated and is sensitive to freezing and thawing. Virus shed in urine is stable at 4°C for many days.

REPLICATION

The temporal regulation of viral protein synthesis in the growth cycle is more obvious in laboratory culture of the slower growing CMV than with HSV. Nonstructural IE protein (p72) appears in nuclei within 16 hours of inoculation, whereas structural L proteins are produced after DNA synthesis; the typical CPE is often not recognisable for 5–21 days. Foci of swollen cells expand slowly as infection passes from cell to cell (Fig. 38.9). Passage and storage of virus are best achieved by trypsinisation and passage as infected cells.

Human CMV does not produce a virus-specified TK; instead, the protein kinase product of CMV gene *UL97* carries out initial phosphorylation of the antiviral drug ganciclovir in CMV-infected cells and cellular kinases then produce the active triphosphate form of the drug, which inhibits the CMV DNA polymerase.

There are several families of glycoproteins in CMV, and these are important antigenic targets. Most neutralising antibody is directed against gB.

PATHOGENESIS

Primary infection with CMV may be acquired at any time, possibly from conception onwards, and, similar to other herpesviruses, CMV persists in the host for life. Reactivation is common, and virus is shed in body secretions such as urine, saliva, semen, breast milk and cervical fluid. Mononuclear cells carry the latent virus genome, and viral RNA transcripts of *E* genes have been detected in such cells. Bone marrow progenitor cells of the myeloid line may be the prime site of latency. Once their descendants have been activated to differentiate into tissue macrophages, the virus can enter the replication cycle. Recurrent infections may follow reactivation of latent (endogenous) virus or reinfection with another (exogenous) strain. Isolates can be distinguished by restriction endonuclease analysis or (more often) PCR amplification followed by sequence analysis and by variations in envelope glycoproteins (gB and gH). Endothelial giant cells (multinucleate cells) have been found in the circulation during disseminated CMV infection. These cells are fully permissive for CMV replication.

Intrauterine infection

Maternal viraemia may result in fetal infection in approximately one in three cases of primary CMV infection during pregnancy, which may lead to disease in the fetus. Infection may also be acquired in utero when the mother suffers CMV reactivation or reinfection. Transplacental infection is probably carried by infected cells, and transmission is associated with a high viral load in blood. CMV causes damage to target cells once they have formed rather than acting as a teratogenic agent.

Perinatal infection

This is predominantly acquired from infected maternal genital tract secretions or from breast-feeding (3%–5% of pregnant women in Europe reactivate CMV). In the past, perinatal blood transfusion was also a recognised infection source, but, as leukodepletion (removal of white blood cells) is now the usual approach, this risk has been reduced.

Postnatal infection

This can be acquired in many ways. Saliva containing CMV is spread among young children and, at older ages, by kissing. Semen can contain high titres of virus and may be a source of sexual transmission or artificial insemination–associated infection. Whole blood transfusion used to be, and donated organs remain, an important source of CMV. It is not known which donors are most likely to transmit infection, so all CMV IgG antibody–positive (seropositive) cell and organ donors are considered as potentially infectious as the presence of antibody reflects the presence of persistent virus.

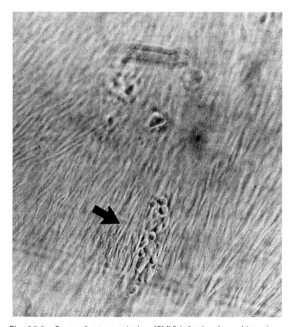

Fig. 38.9 Focus of cytomegalovirus (CMV) infection *(arrow)* in a tissue culture monolayer of human embryo fibroblasts.

Host responses

The host immune response to primary CMV includes humoral (IgM, IgG) and cellular (T lymphocyte) responses. Some of the T cell responses may contribute to immuno-pathology by cross-reacting to self molecules mimicked by CMV and presented in the appropriate self MHC context. CMV *E* genes transactivate other viral and cellular genes, and there may be an important interaction with HIV leading to the production of HIV from latently infected cells. Because CMV infects mononuclear cells, there is a degree of virus-induced immunosuppression associated with the acute infection. Cell-mediated responses are crucial to the control of CMV as evidenced by the serious consequences of disseminated infection in the immunocompromised host. The incubation period for primary infection is 4–6 weeks; reactivation, after transplantation, for instance, appears from 3 weeks onwards.

CLINICAL FEATURES

Congenital CMV infection

Congenital CMV infection is asymptomatic at birth in around 90% of infected babies, but around 10% of these may show sensorineural deafness and/or intellectual impairment in childhood as a result of progressive CMV infection. All congenitally infected infants excrete abundant virus in urine during the first year. Congenitally infected neonates who show symptoms of CMV infection at birth (around 10% of infected neonates) are said to have cytomegalic inclusion disease (CID). The classic presentations are:

- Intrauterine growth retardation
- Hepatosplenomegaly
- Jaundice (hepatitis)
- Thrombocytopenia and petechiae
- CNS involvement—a significant problem with CMV: Microcephaly, intracranial calcifications, chorioretinitis, encephalitis and sensorineural hearing loss are noted at birth (ultrasonography may detect such lesions in utero)
- Other organ involvement including myocarditis and/ or pneumonitis

Infection in children and adults

Postnatal infection with CMV is seldom recognised clinically. Respiratory tract infection is common in infancy, and a mononucleosis syndrome similar to symptomatic primary EBV infection is seen occasionally, especially in young adults or when CMV is acquired from blood transfusion. Fever, atypical lymphocytosis and abnormal liver function tests are noted, but pharyngitis and lymphadenopathy are unusual; heterophile agglutinins are not found. Importantly, adults can present mainly with features of acute hepatitis following primary CMV acquisition.

Infection in immunocompromised patients

Immunocompromised patients may develop symptoms as a result of primary, or reactivated, CMV infection. Dissemination of virus in the blood (viraemia), as indicated by a spiking fever and often leukopenia, is sometimes termed CMV syndrome. This can proceed to CMV end-organ diseases that include:

- Pneumonitis; a high mortality rate in recipients of bone marrow allografts
- Retinitis; may occur on its own (10%–40% of patients with AIDS)
- Oesophagitis/colitis; 5%–10% of transplant or AIDS patients
- Hepatitis
- Encephalitis; often fatal
- Pancreatitis and/or adrenalitis

CMV infection in transplant recipients is a significant cause of direct (caused by the virus) and indirect (caused by virus interactions with the immune system) morbidity that may culminate in loss of the grafted organ and even death. The mortality rate is high, particularly in allogeneic bone marrow recipients who develop an immunopathological pneumonitis associated with graft-versus-host disease. Transplant protocols include prophylaxis or preemptive therapy for the prevention of CMV disease. The former approach entails routine administration of the oral pro-drug valganciclovir for a period of time post transplantation; the latter involves regular measurements of CMV viral load in blood by PCR to detect virus so that early treatment (at preset viral load levels) can be started preemptively prior to the development of clinically overt CMV disease.

Retinitis due to CMV recurrence is a feature of late-stage AIDS. Early recognition, antiviral treatment and maintenance therapy are important in slowing the progression towards blindness.

LABORATORY INVESTIGATION

Detection of CMV at the site of disease is the aim (if possible). Samples should include urine, saliva, bronchoalveolar lavage fluid, vitreal fluid, biopsy tissue (if available), and peripheral blood collected in suitable (usually EDTA) anticoagulant.

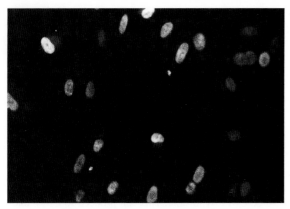

Fig. 38.10 Cytomegalovirus (CMV) early antigen demonstrated in nuclei of human embryo fibroblasts by immunofluorescence after incubation for 24 hours following centrifuge-assisted inoculation.

Virus detection

Viral DNA can be detected in samples using sensitive PCR assays. Diagnostic methods to detect CMV early antigen in cell cultures 24 hours post inoculation (Fig. 38.10) or conventional culture to isolate virus have been largely replaced by NAAT assays (primarily, PCR). CMV must be demonstrated in a sample (urine, saliva, blood or CSF) taken within the first 3 weeks of life to demonstrate congenital infection as later samples may reflect virus acquired in the postnatal period. Testing is usually performed in neonates who are symptomatic at birth. Conversely, those born without any symptoms of congenital CMV are unlikely to have tests done until later when they are investigated for hearing and/or intellectual impairment. In such cases, a stored dried blood spot (Guthrie card; named after the American microbiologist Robert Guthrie) taken in the first few days of life as part of neonatal screening programmes (if available) can be tested for CMV DNA by PCR; a positive PCR result is diagnostic of congenital CMV infection if the blood was taken within the first 3 weeks of life.

Confirmation that CMV is related to an end-organ disease process comes from showing the presence of virus (by immunohistochemical or nucleic acid detection methods) in the affected tissues. The demonstration of CMV viraemia (detection of CMV DNA in blood by PCR) is a significant prognostic finding; above certain levels, these approaches are predictive of clinical disease. The quantitative PCR assay is now the mainstay of detecting and monitoring CMV following transplantation; the availability of an international standard for such quantitative (real-time) CMV PCR assays ensures meaningful comparison of results (viral load) among clinical laboratories, thereby supporting continuity of care.

Serology for CMV

Commercially available EIAs are routinely used to screen for seropositive (CMV IgG antibody) status. These tests can be done urgently for organ donor–recipient assessments. CMV IgM can be detected by EIA following primary or secondary infection, but it may not be possible to detect IgM in the neonate or immunocompromised patient. Commercial assays are available to check the avidity of the CMV IgG antibody in pregnant women when investigating intrauterine growth retardation or other fetal anomalies; paired blood samples (current and antenatal booking/earlier samples) should be tested in parallel. A low avidity IgG result usually indicates that a primary infection has occurred within the past 3–4 months as the binding of recently acquired low-avidity IgG is easily disrupted by protein-denaturing agents; generally, IgG avidity increases over time as the antibody response matures.

TREATMENT

Ganciclovir, given intravenously or as its oral prodrug valganciclovir, is the antiviral agent most commonly used for active CMV infections. Valganciclovir provides systemic levels of ganciclovir equivalent to those achieved by IV therapy, provided gut absorption is not impaired. End-organ disease should be treated for at least 3 weeks, and treatment has been successful in CMV hepatitis, colitis and encephalitis; furthermore, progression of CMV retinitis in AIDS can be controlled with prolonged suppressive therapy. Ganciclovir can cause bone marrow toxicity resulting in neutropenia. Ganciclovir-resistant virus has been found; usually a mutation in the protein kinase gene *(UL97)* is responsible, but DNA polymerase (product of the *UL54* gene) mutations may also occur. Foscarnet is an alternative agent that does not require phosphorylation but has serious side effects (e.g., nephrotoxicity). Cidofovir is another alternative antiviral agent (but has similar serious nephrotoxic side effects). Conversely, aciclovir is not effective against CMV.

Symptomatic neonates diagnosed with congenital CMV infection within the first month of life should be considered for valganciclovir treatment for 6 months to improve long-term hearing and developmental outcomes.

In the transplant setting, valganciclovir is used routinely as a key component of either prophylaxis or preemptive treatment of CMV infection.

EPIDEMIOLOGY

CMV is acquired by 40%–60% of persons by mid-adult life and by more than 90% of those with multiple intimate exposures. Fewer than 5% of units of whole blood from seropositive donors result in transmission to seronegative recipients, whereas 80% of kidney donations transmit infection from seropositive donors. The full extent of congenital CMV disease is not known, but this infection occurs in approximately 3 of 1000 live births in the United Kingdom and is the most common viral cause of congenital infection. Primary CMV infection during pregnancy (i.e., in previously seronegative women) transmits to the foetus in 30%–40% of cases; conversely, it is estimated that 75% of babies with congenital CMV infection are born to mothers who were already CMV seropositive prior to pregnancy (i.e., born to mothers who experienced reactivation or reinfection during pregnancy).

CONTROL

Screening of organ donors (D) and recipients (R) is carried out prior to organ transplantation to prevent, where possible, a seronegative recipient (R−) receiving a solid organ from a seropositive donor (D+) in order to avoid the high-risk D+/R− SOT situation. In the bone marrow transplant setting, the equivalent high-risk situation involves D−/R+ HSCT procedures. Such tissue matching (when possible) reduces morbidity and mortality significantly for all forms of allogeneic transplant. Blood donor screening to select CMV-seronegative units for support of seronegative patients in transplant programmes, and for premature babies, is less important now with the use of leukodepletion. Antiviral prophylaxis (starting from time of transplant surgery), or preemptive treatment (starting from time of virus detection in blood), are routine procedures now in SOT and HSCT programmes for those at risk of CMV disease.

No CMV vaccine is licensed yet for routine use, but trials continue. Experimental live-attenuated vaccines have been tried, but hopes rest on subunit vaccines or a combined approach.

HUMAN HERPESVIRUSES 6 AND 7

DESCRIPTION

The existence of further herpesviruses infecting humans was not suspected until one was isolated in 1986 from the blood of patients with lymphoproliferative disorders, some of whom had AIDS. EM revealed a virus with characteristic herpesvirus features. DNA sequence studies showed this virus, now officially named HHV 6, to be distinct from the then five known human herpesviruses, but closer to human CMV, with which it has some homology. Two variants have been identified on sequence analysis: HHV 6A and 6B. Although first isolated from B cells, HHV 6 was shown to infect CD4$^+$ T lymphocytes preferentially. HHV 6B is the cause of a common disease of infancy called exanthem subitum or roseola infantum (sixth disease) and may cause febrile convulsions in childhood, whereas variant 6A has much less clear disease association. Both variants do seem to play a role in disease (bone marrow suppression, encephalitis) in immunocompromised patients following transplantation. The cell receptor for HHV 6 is CD46, a complement regulatory glycoprotein present on all nucleated cells. Bone marrow progenitor cells contain truly latent HHV 6; low-level persistent infection is found in salivary glands and brain cells.

In 1990 another new human herpesvirus was isolated in similar circumstances and has been shown to be sufficiently distinct from other HHV to be denoted HHV 7. Primary infection with HHV 7 has been identified in some cases of exanthem subitum and febrile convulsions in childhood, but its role following transplantation is unclear. A new genus, *Roseolovirus,* has been established for HHV 6 and 7, which are members of the subfamily Betaherpesvirinae, distantly related to human CMV but with much smaller genomes.

PATHOGENESIS AND CLINICAL FEATURES

Both HHV 6B and 7 are shed persistently in saliva, and both have been found in female genital secretions; only HHV 7 is found in breast milk. In most people, only low numbers of copies of HHV 6 or 7 are found in circulating cells. However, HHV 6 DNA may integrate into the human chromosome (1%–2% of individuals) and can thus be inherited from either parent. Such chromosomally integrated HHV 6 leads to a persistent very high level of viral DNA in all somatic cells in the body. As a result, the detection of high viral load in blood or other tissues may cause diagnostic confusion if these patients are ever investigated for HHV 6–related symptoms.

Exanthem subitum (roseola infantum)

Exanthem subitum (ES) was long considered to be an infection caused by a virus, and transmission by blood was confirmed experimentally years before HHV 6 was isolated. The infection is extremely common in the first few years of life, presenting between 6 months and 3 years of age, with a sudden onset of fever (up to 39°C). The acute febrile illness caused by these viruses accounts for 20% of all fevers in early childhood. The child is not usually ill, remaining alert and playful, with some throat congestion and cervical lymphadenopathy. Sometimes more pronounced respiratory symptoms occur with febrile convulsions. Fever usually persists for 3 days, when the temperature falls suddenly; a widespread maculopapular rash then appears in around 10% of cases. HHV 6B has been isolated from peripheral blood in patients during the acute febrile phase who subsequently either produced a rash or not. Seroconversion is noted in convalescence, confirming a primary infection with HHV 6B. Some cases are associated with HHV 7 infection, but no other firm disease association has been found for HHV 7 yet.

Neurological disease

A British survey has confirmed the importance of rose-oloviruses in neurological illness (febrile convulsions and encephalitis) in early childhood. Diagnosis is difficult as viral DNA is not always detected in CSF (and may then represent integrated HHV 6), but seroconversion to one of the viruses may confirm a primary infection. HHV 6 strains appear to remain thereafter in the brain, and these viruses are now considered to be commensal in CNS. No clear association with demyelinating diseases, particularly multiple sclerosis, has been shown.

Other associations

In the rare adult case, hepatitis and lymphadenopathy have been found and sometimes a heterophile agglutinin-negative mononucleosis. Reactivation in immunocompromised hosts may be diagnosed by viral load or on the basis of serology, but this is difficult to interpret. HHV 6 and 7 reactivate in the first weeks after transplant and appear to make CMV disease worse, but the full extent of disease in the transplant recipient has still to be established. HHV 6 may cause bone marrow suppression, encephalitis and pneumonitis following transplantation (HHV 6B is more often implicated than 6A).

Both HHV 6 and 7 infect T lymphocytes; indeed, HHV 7 uses the same receptor (CD4) as HIV. The potential significance of these interactions has still to be elucidated.

LABORATORY INVESTIGATION

Viral DNA detection (by PCR) is now the mainstay of routine diagnosis, with some laboratories providing a multiplex assay capable of distinguishing HHV 6A from 6B and 7. Isolation of HHV 6 or 7 involves cocultivation of peripheral blood lymphocytes with mitogen-activated cord blood lymphocytes. Very large, refractile multinucleate cells are produced in culture. These viruses may be isolated from saliva, particularly HHV 7.

A particular source of confusion is the ability of HHV 6 to integrate (on occasion) into target cell chromosomes. Also, antibody tests are not widely used as results can be confusing. Antibody avidity tests can help to establish whether a primary infection has occurred as the binding of low-avidity IgG is easily disrupted by protein-denaturing agents. Both this method and PCR can prove useful in establishing the diagnosis of HHV 6– and 7–associated exanthem subitum in a substantial proportion of suspected cases of infant measles.

TREATMENT

Usually, HHV 6 and 7 diseases are self-limiting, and treatment is seldom indicated clinically. HHV 6 and 7 are sensitive to ganciclovir, which can be used in serious cases (e.g., encephalitis or pneumonitis in immunocompromised patients). Foscarnet and cidofovir are alternative antivirals. Conversely, aciclovir is not effective against HHV 6 or 7. There is no vaccine available in routine clinical practice at this time.

EPIDEMIOLOGY

Antibody analysis to date has been based mainly on immunostaining studies with cells infected with either HHV 6 or 7 as antigens. High antibody titres to HHV 6 are found in young children in the first 4 years of life, reflecting recent primary infection in this age group. Primary infection, with viraemia and seroconversion, has also been detected in seronegative transplant recipients of liver or kidney grafts from seropositive donors. Possible transmission by blood transfusion has not been excluded. Infection with HHV 7 occurs, on average, slightly later in childhood. Older persons have lower levels of antibody, but more sensitive EIA tests reveal almost universal HHV 6B and 7 seropositivity. The full spectrum of disease associated with these viruses, and the extent of asymptomatic shedding, remains to be established.

HUMAN HERPESVIRUS 8 (KAPOSI'S SARCOMA–ASSOCIATED HERPESVIRUS)

Sequences of DNA representing a completely new human herpesvirus were identified in 1994 in tissues from the epidemic form of Kaposi's sarcoma in patients with AIDS. The DNA fragments unique to the tumour tissue were found to have some homology with the Gammaherpesvirus subfamily, including EBV. This virus, officially named HHV 8, but also referred to as Kaposi's sarcoma–associated herpesvirus (KSHV), is the latest human tumour-forming virus described.

HHV 8 is classified in the *Rhadinovirus* genus of the Gammaherpesvirinae along with known viruses of nonhuman primates. The genome is 165–170 kbp and encodes around 95 proteins, including a group that contains homologues of human proteins involved in cell growth regulation and cytokine production (e.g., IL6; viral IL6, vIL6). Like other herpesviruses, HHV 8 attaches to cells first via cell surface heparan sulphate and integrins through envelope glycoproteins gpK8.1 and gB. HHV 8 infects dividing B cells and then proceeds to either a lytic replication cycle, releasing infectious virus (virions), or enters latency, expressing only the latency-associated nuclear antigens (LANAs). Similar to EBV's EBNA 1, LANA 1 maintains the HHV 8 episome, whereas LANA 2 suppresses apoptosis via inhibition of p53-mediated transcription. Latency-associated membrane protein (LAMP) has functions reminiscent of EBV's LMP1 and 2 (see earlier in the chapter).

Kaposi's sarcoma

HHV 8 is strongly associated with all forms of Kaposi's sarcoma (KS) as being necessary for tumourigenesis. Classic KS was first described by the Austro-Hungarian dermatologist Moritz Kaposi in 1872 and affects elderly men of Mediterranean, Eastern European or Jewish backgrounds. The endemic form of KS was described in eastern Africa prior to the HIV epidemic, whereas AIDS-associated KS is an aggressive form of the disease that occurs in the context of HIV infection. Lastly, iatrogenic KS develops in immunosuppressed patients (e.g., organ transplant recipients) as a result of medical intervention. HHV 8 is not the sole driver of KS, and other factors (including immunosuppression) also play a role; however, KS only develops in individuals infected with HHV 8. The mucocutaneous neoplasm Kaposi described originally as 'a multifocal pigmented sarcoma' was the most common tumour in HIV-infected MSM before the advent of highly active antiretroviral therapy (HAART) and was one of the heralds of the AIDS pandemic in the early 1980s. A transmissible agent was long suspected in KS on epidemiological grounds, transmitted sexually, but rarely by blood. Endothelial cells of vascular or lymphatic origin are involved; they have a characteristic spindle shape and are arranged in bundles. Although occurring at multiple sites in skin, lymph glands and the gastrointestinal tract, the tumour itself does not lead to death. Local radiotherapy and systemic chemotherapy have been used in treatment. Lesions on exposed parts of the body are (sometimes raised) blue-reddish-purple-brown plaques that are a cause of considerable concern and distress for the affected individual.

Body cavity–associated B lymphoma/primary effusion lymphoma/multicentric Castleman's disease

HHV 8 genomes have been found in lymphoma cells from AIDS-related B cell lymphomas termed body cavity–associated B cell lymphomas (BCBL) or primary effusion lymphomas (PEL). This condition presents as a malignant effusion in pericardial, pleural and/or peritoneal spaces. Cell lines established from the tumours can be induced to produce viral proteins and particles; they have been used as a basis for diagnostic tests. A subset (plasma cell variant) of another condition, multicentric Castleman's disease (MCD; named after the American pathologist Benjamin Castleman), is also strongly associated with HHV 8. MCD is a lymphoproliferative disorder that is often localised in the mediastinum, mesenterium and/or peripheral lymph nodes.

LABORATORY INVESTIGATION

HHV 8 DNA amplification by PCR is used to detect and monitor HHV 8 (viral load in blood). Lytic growth of HHV 8 can be induced in latently infected B cell lymphoma cell lines (many are coinfected with EBV) and, as a result, reagents for antibody testing can be produced—both infected cell lysates for immunoblots and antigen-containing cells for immunostaining. Recombinant proteins have been synthesized and are useful for EIAs. Now that reagents free of EBV are available, the specific epidemiology of infection with this new herpesvirus is being studied.

EPIDEMIOLOGY

Molecular sequence data have revealed five clades of HHV 8, termed A–E. Clade B predominates in Africa, whereas in Europe and North America, clades A and C are more common. Serological surveys have shown that, unlike most of the human herpesviruses, HHV 8 infection is uncommon in developed countries (fewer than 5% of blood donors in North America and Northern Europe have anti-HHV 8 antibodies). Rates of seropositivity are higher in at-risk groups for KS, with up to 30% seropositivity rates in MSM. Confirmation of a high seropositivity rate (up to 60%) in adolescents and adults in most parts of Sub-Saharan African countries, and studies on transmission, have shown a link between mothers and their children and between siblings. Transmission from saliva is considered the most likely route, and the high rates in communities where overcrowding in childhood is seen support this. In Europe, there is increased seropositivity around the Mediterranean, and the presence of HHV 8 DNA in elderly Italians is highly predictive of the development of KS following organ transplantation or HIV infection.

TREATMENT AND CONTROL

Ganciclovir has activity against HHV 8, and its use in CMV prophylaxis after organ transplantation may contribute to reducing the risk of reactivation and disease due to HHV 8 in seropositive recipients or in seronegative recipients who have a seropositive donor. Foscarnet may be an alternative drug. Tumours associated with HHV 8 infection may regress if reduction of immunosuppression is possible (post transplant) or following improvements in immunity with combination anti-retroviral therapy (cART) (in patients with AIDS)—together with local radiotherapy and/or chemotherapy. The anti-CD20 agent rituximab may also have some effect in patients with BCBL/PEL. There is no vaccine available in routine clinical practice at this time.

CERCOPITHECINE HERPESVIRUS 1 (HERPESVIRUS B; B VIRUS; HERPESVIRUS SIMIAE)

DESCRIPTION

Herpesvirus B, antigenically related to HSV, commonly infects nonhuman Old World primates, in particular macaques (thought to be the natural host), causing a mild vesicular eruption on the tongue and buccal mucosa analogous to primary herpetic stomatitis in humans. The infection rate in these monkeys increases markedly if they are kept in crowded conditions, and, although relatively benign in the animals, this virus is potentially highly pathogenic for humans.

Human infection with herpesvirus B is rare. It is usually acquired from a monkey bite or from handling infected animals without appropriate personal protective equipment (PPE). In one instance, the wife of an infected monkey handler became infected through contact with her husband's vesicles; B virus has also been transmitted in the laboratory from infected monkey cell cultures. Within 5–20 days of exposure, local inflammation may appear at the site of entry, usually on the skin, accompanied by some itching, numbness and vesicular lesions. Ascending myelitis or acute encephalomyelitis may follow, occasionally as long as 5 weeks after exposure, and may not always be recognised. Delay in specific therapy leads to a high mortality rate and serious neurological sequelae in survivors.

DIAGNOSIS AND TREATMENT

Diagnosis by isolation of the virus from blood, vesicle fluid, conjunctival swabs and/or CSF is not always possible, and such approaches pose significant problems for the laboratory as a result of safety concerns (Advisory Committee on Dangerous Pathogens [ACDP] Category 4 organism; see Internet reference to ACDP). Herpesvirus particles may be detectable by EM of vesicle fluid. Definitive identification of the virus is available in specialist reference laboratories using immunostaining or herpesvirus B DNA analysis by PCR. Demonstration of specific antibodies is complicated by cross-reacting HSV antibody, but new specific antigens based on recombinant glycoproteins offer improved serology. B virus is not as sensitive to aciclovir as HSV, requiring concentrations equivalent to those used for VZV. Treatment needs to be given promptly to be effective, and very high-dose IV aciclovir for 2 weeks or longer is recommended in high-risk situations; alternative regimens in a lower risk context may include the oral prodrugs valaciclovir or valganciclovir. Ganciclovir should be used when there is evidence of CNS involvement. Because of the small number of cases, the best therapeutic regimen is not well established and remains somewhat empirical.

Prevention of B virus infection

Guidelines have been issued for the protection of those handling monkeys or monkey tissues. These include:

- Screening of macaque colonies when possible
- Recommendations for training to prevent exposure
- Safe handling and PPE procedures
- Immediate risk assessment, care of wounds and treatment (if appropriate)
- Information regarding the risks and nature of the infection

Prophylaxis in the event of possible exposure involves prompt, rigorous wound washing and cleansing with 10% iodine in alcohol. A course of high-dose oral aciclovir, or valaciclovir, is reserved for prophylaxis of high-risk exposures, namely, those on the head, neck and/or torso, deep wounds and where the source animal has lesions, suffered recent stress and/or illness or the material is of CNS or mucosal origin. After prophylaxis, a prolonged observation period is recommended as the onset of infection may be delayed.

RECOMMENDED READING

Awasthi, S., & Friedman, H. M. (2014). Status of prophylactic and therapeutic genital herpes vaccines. *Current Opinion in Virology, 6,* 6–12. doi:10.1016/j.coviro.2014.02.006.

De, S. K., Hart, J. C., & Breuer, J. (2015). Herpes simplex virus and varicella zoster virus: recent advances in therapy. *Current Opinion in Infectious Diseases, 28*(6), 589–595. doi:10.1097/QCO.0000000000000211.

De Vries, J. J., van Zwet, E. W., Dekker, F. W., Kroes, A. C., Verkerk, P. H., & Vossen, A. C. (2013). The apparent paradox of maternal seropositivity as a risk factor for congenital cytomegalovirus infection: a population-based prediction model. *Reviews in Medical Virology, 23*(4), 241–249. doi:10.1002/rmv.1744.

Gnann, J. W., Jr., & Whitley, R. J. (2016). Clinical practice: genital herpes. *The New England Journal of Medicine, 375*(7), 666–674. doi:10.1056/NEJMcp1603178.

Kimberlin, D. W., Jester, P. M., Sánchez, P. J., Ahmed, A., Arav-Boger, R., Michaels, M. G., ... National Institute of Allergy and Infectious Diseases Collaborative Antiviral Study Group. (2015). Valganciclovir for symptomatic congenital cytomegalovirus disease. *The New England Journal of Medicine, 372*(10), 933–943. doi:10.1056/NEJMoa1404599.

Kimberlin, D. W., Whitley, R. J., Wan, W., Powell, D. A., Storch, G., Ahmed, A., ... National Institute of Allergy and Infectious Diseases Collaborative Antiviral Study Group. (2011). Oral acyclovir suppression and neurodevelopment after neonatal herpes. *The New England Journal of Medicine, 365*(14), 1284–1292. doi:10.1056/NEJMoa1003509.

Knipe, D. M., & Howley, P. M. (Eds.). (2013). Herpesviridae. In *Fields virology* (6th ed., pp. 1802–2128). Philadelphia: Lippincott Williams & Wilkins.

Websites

Advisory Committee on Dangerous Pathogens. (2006). Biological agents. The principles, design and operation of Containment Level 4 facilities. Retrieved from http://www.dh.gov.uk/prod_consum_dh/groups/dh_digitalassets/@dh/@en/documents/digitalasset/dh_4135259.pdf. (Accessed Sep 2017).

British Transplantation Society: Active Standards and Guidelines. Retrieved from http://www.bts.org.uk/transplantation/standards-and-guidelines/. (Accessed Sep 2017).

UK Department of Health. (2015). Immunisation against infectious diseases. Retrieved from https://www.gov.uk/government/publications/varicella-the-green-book-chapter-34. (Accessed Sep 2017).

39 Poxviruses

Smallpox; molluscum contagiosum; parapoxvirus infections

T. HUGH PENNINGTON

KEY POINTS

- Poxviruses are large cytoplasmic DNA viruses that infect a wide range of species.
- Smallpox is a generalised disease with a vesicular rash and is associated with significant mortality.
- Live vaccine is used to eradicate disease but is not risk free.
- Eradication was successful because only human beings are infected, the disease is easily recognised, transmitted to only a few contacts, and there is no carrier state. Bioterrorism threatens the reintroduction of smallpox.
- Other human poxvirus infections are of minor significance and include molluscum contagiosum, monkeypox and orf.

The world's last naturally occurring case of smallpox was recorded in Merca, southern Somalia, in October 1977. This momentous event marked the end of a long campaign against smallpox, which in its 'modern' phase started with the introduction of vaccination by Edward Jenner at the end of the eighteenth century. With the eradication of smallpox, the importance of poxviruses in medical practice may appear to be much diminished, as the other naturally occurring viruses in this family that infect humans nearly always cause only self-limiting and trivial skin lesions. Smallpox caused a generalised infection with a high mortality rate and fell into that small group of viruses whose infections are commonly severe and frequently fatal. Notwithstanding their minor role today as human pathogens, poxviruses retain their importance, and their place in this book, for four reasons.

First, the successful smallpox eradication campaign is important in its own right as a major achievement. It is also important because it highlights the principles and problems associated with projects that aim to control infections by eradicating the pathogen. Smallpox was the first human disease to fall to this approach and remains the only successful example to date. [The announcement in June 2011 of the eradication of the cattle disease rinderpest marked the extinction of a second important pathogen; the end for polio (see Ch. 44) and guinea worm (see Ch. 60) is close.]

Second, work on the molecular biology of poxviruses has led to the identification of distinctive properties and to the development of techniques and approaches that have made it possible to move significantly towards constructing single-dose vaccines that protect simultaneously against a wide range of diseases. Genes coding for foreign nonpoxvirus antigens have been inserted into the poxvirus genome so that the antigens are expressed during virus infection and induce immunity.

Third, no account of virus diseases in general and poxvirus infections in particular is complete without consideration being given to the events that followed the introduction of myxomatosis into Australia—by far the best studied example to date of the evolution of a new virus disease.

Finally, new poxviruses continue to be discovered. In 2009 a novel deer parapox virus was identified as the cause of disease in two deer hunters in the United States.

DESCRIPTION

Classification

A large number of different viruses belonging to the family Poxviridae have been described. They infect a wide range of vertebrate and invertebrate hosts. The subfamily Chordopoxvirinae contains all of the viruses that infect vertebrates; it is divided into eight genera, each containing related viruses, which generally infect related hosts (Table 39.1). Members of the *Orthopox* and *Molluscipox* genera infect humans. By far the most intensively studied poxvirus is vaccinia virus, the Jennerian smallpox vaccine virus. This virus has been placed in the genus *Orthopoxvirus*, together with smallpox virus and some viruses that infect cattle and mice.

The virion

Poxviruses are the largest animal viruses. Their virions are big enough to be seen as dots by light microscopy after special staining procedures. They are much more complex than those of any other viruses (Figs. 39.1 and 39.2). They are also distinctive in that they do not show any discernible symmetry. The core contains the DNA genome and 15 or more enzymes that make up a transcriptional system whose role is to synthesise biologically active polyadenylated, capped and methylated virus messenger RNA (mRNA) molecules early in infection. The core has a 9-nm-thick membrane, with a regular subunit structure. Within the virion, the core assumes a dumbbell shape because of the large lateral bodies. The core and lateral bodies are enclosed in a protein shell about 12 nm thick (the outer membrane), the surface of which consists of irregularly arranged tubules, which in turn consist of a small globular subunit. Virions released naturally from the cell are enclosed within an envelope that contains host cell lipids and several virus-specified polypeptides, including haemagglutinin; they are infectious. Most virions remain cell associated and are released by cellular disruption. These particles lack an envelope, so the outer membrane constitutes their surface; they are also infectious. More than 100 different polypeptides have been identified in purified virions.

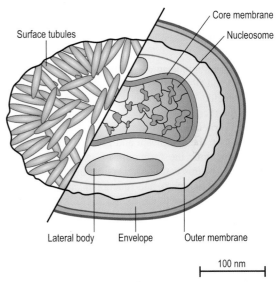

Fig. 39.1 Structure of the vaccinia virion. Right-hand side, section of enveloped virion; left-hand side, surface structure of nonenveloped particle. (Fenner, F., Henderson, D. A., Arita, I., Jezek, Z., Ladnyi, I. D., & World Health Organization. (1988). *Smallpox and Its Eradication.* Geneva: World Health Organization.)

Table 39.1   Family: Poxviridae

Subfamilies	Genera	Natural host
Chordopoxvirinae (contains all viruses that infect vertebrates)	*Leporipoxvirus*	Rabbits, squirrels
	Avipoxvirus	Birds
	Capripoxvirus	Goats, sheep
	Suipoxvirus	Swine
	Parapoxvirus	Cattle, sheep
	Yatapoxvirus	Monkeys, baboons
	Orthopoxvirus	Humans, cattle, mice
	Molluscipoxvirus	Humans
Entomopoxvirinae (viruses of insects)		Insects

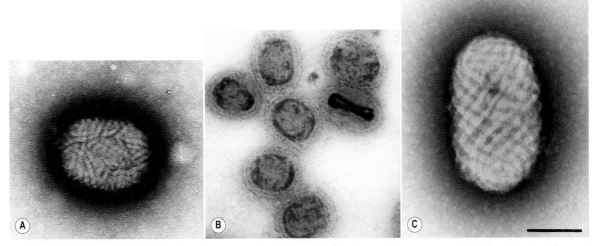

Fig. 39.2 Electron micrographs of poxviruses. (A) Molluscum contagiosum virus (MCV), ×15,000. (B) MCV showing internal structure, ×75,000 (prepared by Atack, N.). (C) Parapoxvirus: orf. Bar = 100 nm. (Courtesy of Gregory, D. W.)

The genome

Their DNA genomes range in mass from 85 MDa (parapoxviruses) to 185 MDa (avipoxviruses). The poxvirus genome is distinctive in that covalent links join the two DNA strands at both ends of the molecule, the genome thus being a single uninterrupted molecule that is folded to form a linear duplex structure. The occurrence of inverted terminal sequence repetitions is also a characteristic feature, identical sequences being present at each end of the genome.

REPLICATION

Poxviruses are unique among human DNA viruses in that virus RNA and DNA synthesis takes place in the cytoplasm of the infected cell and they code for all the proteins needed for their replication. They have early and late phases of protein synthesis (see Ch. 7). Virion assembly takes place in the cytoplasm and proceeds in a series of steps that include the formation of spherical immature particles. The virus causes irreversible inhibition of host protein synthesis due to the functional inactivation and degradation of host cytoplasmic RNA molecules, leading to the death of infected cells.

CLINICAL FEATURES

Smallpox virus had no animal reservoir and spread from person to person by the respiratory route. After infecting mucosal cells in the upper respiratory tract without producing symptoms, it spread to the regional lymph nodes and, after a transient viraemia, infected cells throughout the body. Multiplication of virus in these cells led to a second and more intense viraemia, which heralded the onset of clinical illness. During the first few days of fever, the virus multiplied in skin epithelial cells, leading to the development of focal lesions and the characteristic rash. Macules progressed to papules, vesicles and pustules, leaving permanent pockmarks, particularly on the face. Two kinds of smallpox were common in the first half of the twentieth century:

1. Variola major, or classical smallpox
2. Variola minor, or alastrim.

Variola major had case fatality rates varying from 10% to 50% in the unvaccinated. Variola minor caused a much milder disease and had case fatality rates of <1%. The viruses are very similar but can be distinguished in the laboratory by restriction enzyme fragment length polymorphisms of their genomes. Whilst diagnosis can be made on the basis of clinical features (although there may be some confusion with chickenpox), laboratory confirmation is essential. Historically this would have been by electron microscopic identification of virions in lesional material, but there are now genome amplification assays available in reference laboratories.

CONTROL OF SMALLPOX

Before vaccination

Before the introduction of vaccination, the control of smallpox relied on two approaches, variolation and isolation. Variolators aimed to induce immunity equivalent to that after natural infection. Susceptible individuals were deliberately infected with smallpox pus or scabs by scratching the skin or by nasal insufflation. Although the virus was not attenuated, infections had lower case fatality rates (estimated to be 0.5%–2%) and were less likely to cause permanent pockmarks than those acquired naturally. Variolation was first recorded in China nearly 1000 years ago and was practised in many parts of the world. In Afghanistan, Pakistan and Ethiopia the activities of variolators caused problems towards the end of the smallpox eradication programme in the 1970s because they spread virus in a way that evaded the measures erected to control natural virus transmission.

Vaccination

Edward Jenner vaccinated James Phipps with cowpox virus on 14 May 1796 and challenged him by variolation some months later. He repeated this 'trial', as he called it, in other children, and the description of these events in his 'Inquiry' in 1798 led to the rapid worldwide acceptance of vaccination. Introduction of the vaccine virus into the epidermis led to the development of a local lesion and the induction of a strong immunity to infection with smallpox virus that lasted for several years. Although the essentials of Jennerian vaccination remained unchanged for the rest of its history, early vaccinators developed their own vaccine viruses, which became known as vaccinia. The origin of these viruses is obscure, and modern vaccinia viruses form a distinct species of *Orthopoxvirus*, related to but very clearly distinct from the viruses of both cowpox and smallpox.

The eradication campaign

Smallpox was brought under control by:

- routine vaccination of children—compulsory in some countries
- outbreak control by isolation and selective vaccination

This was achieved gradually in Europe, the former USSR, North and Central America and Japan, and the virus had been eradicated from all these areas by the mid-1950s. In 1959 this achievement prompted the World Health Organization (WHO) to adopt the global eradication of smallpox as a major goal. At this time, 60% of the world's population lived in areas where smallpox was endemic. A slow reduction in disease was maintained for the next few years, but epidemics continued to be frequent. Consequently, the WHO initiated its Intensified Smallpox Eradication Programme. This started on 1 January 1967 when the disease was reported in 31 countries. It had the goal of eradication within 10 years. The goal was achieved in 10 years, 9 months and 26 days.

From a starting point of 10–15 million cases annually, and against a background of civil strife, famine and floods, success came because of a major international collaborative effort, aided by some virus-specific factors (Table 39.2). At the beginning of 1976 smallpox occurred only in Ethiopia. Transmission was interrupted there in August of that year, although an importation of virus into Somalia and adjacent countries had occurred by then. This was the last outbreak. The last case was recorded on 26 October 1977. There was a final, tragic death the following year after escape of the virus from a research laboratory; a reminder of the importance of biosecurity, reinforced by the laboratory infections caused by the SARS virus in 2004, and the escape of foot and mouth virus from a reference laboratory in 2007. In the final years of the programme, its emphasis moved from mass vaccination to a strategy of surveillance and containment. This strategy rapidly interrupted transmission because:

- cases were easy to detect owing to the characteristic rash
- patients usually transmitted disease to only a few people, and only to those in close face-to-face contact
- only persons with a rash transmitted infection

The WHO Global Commission for the Eradication of Smallpox formally certified that smallpox had been eradicated from the world on 9 December 1979.

Smallpox and bioterrorism

After eradication, virus strains were kept in government laboratories in Atlanta and Novosibirsk Region, Russia. The possibility that virus could fall into unauthorised hands is small, but vaccine stocks have been ordered and contingency plans prepared. The experience from outbreaks imported into Europe in the past suggests that outbreaks could be controlled rapidly. In some outbreaks, public pressure for protection led to unnecessary vaccinations, in turn leading to more deaths from vaccination (see later in the chapter) than from smallpox. Despite frequent misdiagnoses of early cases as chickenpox (see Ch. 38), the outbreaks were rapidly controlled. Fortunately smallpox spreads slowly. If a bioterrorist smallpox attack is suspected, brincidofir (used to treat cytomegalovirus infections) and the experimental drug tecovirimat might be used. They have antipoxvirus activity, but their effectiveness in treating smallpox is untested.

OTHER HUMAN POXVIRUS INFECTIONS

Molluscum contagiosum

The lesions of this mild disease are small, copper-coloured warty papules that occur on the trunk, buttocks, arms and face. It is spread by direct contact or by fomites. The lesion consists of a mass of hypertrophied epidermis that extends into the dermis and protrudes above the skin. In the epithelial cells, very large hyaline acidophilic granular masses can be observed. They crowd the host cell nucleus to one side, eventually filling the entire cell. When material

Table 39.2 Features of smallpox that facilitated its eradication	
Feature	Importance
Disease severe	Ensured strong public and governmental support for eradication programme
Detection of cases easy because of characteristic rash and subsequent development of facial pockmarks	Facilitated containment of outbreaks and audit of success of programme
Slow spread and poor transmissibility	Facilitated containment of outbreaks by vaccination and isolation
Transmission by subclinical cases not important	Meant that control of spread by isolation of cases was an effective procedure
No carrier state in humans	Meant that control of spread by isolation of cases was an effective procedure
No animal reservoir	Meant that control of spread by isolation of cases was an effective procedure
Vaccine technically simple to produce in large amounts, in high quality and at low cost (in skin of ungulates)	Meant that vaccine availability was not an important constraint in the eradication programme
Vaccine delivery simple and optimised by use of reusable, cheap, specially designed needles to deliver a standard amount of vaccine to scratches in skin	Meant that failure at the point of vaccination was not an important constraint in the eradication programme
Freeze-dried vaccine stocks were heat-stable with a very long shelf life in the tropics	Meant that vaccine viability under adverse environmental conditions was not an important constraint in the eradication programme

from the lesions is crushed, some of the inclusions burst open, liberating large numbers of virions. These have the size, internal structure and morphology of vaccinia virus. The infection has been transmitted experimentally to human subjects, but the virus has not been grown in cultured cells. The development of immunity is slow and uncertain. Lesions can persist for as long as 2 years, and reinfection is common.

Monkeypox

This has been implicated occasionally in a smallpox-like condition in equatorial Africa. Its natural hosts are rodents. It may be fatal in unvaccinated humans but is less transmissible from person to person than smallpox. Importation of infected Gambian pouched rats, which went on to infect captive prairie dogs, caused an outbreak of monkeypox in the United States in 2003.

Parapoxvirus infections

The virions of parapoxviruses are characterised by a crisscross pattern of tubes in the outer membrane (see Fig. 39.2C) and genomes that are considerably smaller (85 MDa) than those of other poxviruses. They infect ungulates and cause the human occupational diseases of orf and milker's nodes. The lesions of orf (which causes a disease in sheep known as contagious pustular dermatitis) are often large and granulomatous. Erythema multiforme is a relatively frequent complication. The lesions of milker's nodes are highly vascular, hemispherical papules and nodules. Both diseases are:

- self-limiting
- most common on the hands
- contracted by contact with infected sheep (orf) or cows (milker's nodes)
- occupational diseases, mainly seen in farm workers such as shepherds, slaughterhouse workers or butchers

VACCINIA

Vaccinia-like viruses infect cows and their milkers in Brazil. Whether they are remnants of the vaccination programme there, or naturally occurring viruses, is not clear.

Vaccinia virus as a vaccine vector

The vaccinia virus genome can accommodate sizeable losses of DNA in certain regions, to the extent that as many as 25,000 base pairs can be lost without lethal effect.

By replacing this nonessential DNA with foreign genes, it has been possible to construct novel recombinant virus strains, which express the foreign genes when they infect cells. Recombinant vaccinia strains containing as many as four foreign genes, coding for combinations of bacterial, viral and protozoal antigens, have been constructed.

The advantages of this ingenious way of developing new vaccines are:

- they are applicable to many different antigens
- the possibility of constructing multivalent vaccines that could give protection against several diseases after a single 'shot'
- stimulates cell-mediated immunity
- the ease of administration
- cheapness of vaccinia as a vaccine

A strain that expresses the rabies glycoprotein antigen is being used in Europe to protect foxes. Serious disadvantages remain for human diseases, however. These are primarily those associated with vaccinia virus itself, as its use was associated with a number of serious complications. The most important of these were:

- progressive vaccinia, a fatal infection that occurred in immunodeficient individuals
- eczema vaccinatum, a serious spreading infection that occurred in eczematous individuals
- postvaccinal encephalitis, which, although rare, was severe and occurred in normal healthy individuals
- myocarditis, a recently described complication identified following large-scale vaccination of the US military in 2003

These disadvantages preclude the use of vaccinia as a vector for foreign antigens in humans, and work is being done on the modification of its virulence to circumvent these problems. So far, studies on virulence genes have shown that poxviruses code for an impressive array of factors that interfere with host defences. These include proteins that bind complement components, act as receptors for interleukin-1β, interferon and tumour necrosis factor, and synthesise steroids. These factors are all exported from infected cells. Factors that act inside cells include proteins that block the action of interferon, inhibit the posttranslational modification of interleukin-1β and prevent the synthesis of a neutrophil chemotactic factor. It is possible that abrogation of virulence factors such as these may lead to safer vaccines.

MYXOMATOSIS: AN EVOLVING DISEASE

As a rule, virus infections are mild and self-limiting. Viruses are obligate parasites and it is not in their interests to cause the extinction or massive reductions in the size of host populations. It is reasonable to suppose that the type of disease caused by a virus reflects the outcome of a process in which host and virus have co-evolved to levels of resistance and virulence optimal for the maintenance of their respective population numbers. The high mortality rate of classical smallpox is considered by some to have been a major factor in the restriction of human population size, and this has been used to support the hypothesis that the association between smallpox and humans has been established, in evolutionary terms, only in recent times, co-evolution of the relationship being a long way from equilibrium. It is impossible to test this hypothesis directly for variola, but the relationship between another poxvirus, myxoma virus and the rabbit in Australia has provided a dramatic example. This is the only example of co-evolution where changes in an animal host and virus and the evolution of a disease have been studied in real time.

Myxoma virus is South American. It causes a benign local fibroma in its natural host, the rabbit *Sylvilagus brasiliensis*, but causes myxomatosis in the European rabbit, *Oryctolagus cuniculus*. This is a generalised infection with a very high mortality rate. Field trials to test its efficacy as a measure for controlling the European rabbit were carried out in Australia in 1950. The virus escaped and caused enormous epidemics in the years that followed. The original virus caused infections with a case mortality rate >99%, and rabbits survived for <13 days. Within 3 years, virus isolates from epidemics had become much less virulent, causing infections with mortality rates of 70%–95% and survival times of 17–28 days. Changes in the resistance of the rabbit also occurred, with mortality rates from infection falling (from 90% to 25% after challenge with strains of virus with modified virulence, for example), and symptomatology becoming less severe. In myxomatosis, natural selection favoured virus strains with intermediate virulence because such strains are transmitted more effectively than highly virulent strains, which kill their hosts too quickly, and nonvirulent strains, which are poorly transmitted.

RECOMMENDED READING

Baxby, D. (1981). *Jenner's smallpox vaccine*. London: Heinemann.
Damon, I. K. (2013). Poxviruses. In D. M. Knipe & P. M. Howley (Eds.), *Field's virology* (pp. 2160–2184). Philadelphia: Lippincott Williams and Wilkins.
Fenner, F., Henderson, D. A., Arita, I., Jezek, Z., Ladnyi, I. D., & World Health Organization. (1988). *Smallpox and its eradication*. Geneva: World Health Organization.
Jenner, E. (1798). *An inquiry into the causes and effects of the variolae vaccinae*. London: Sampson Low.

Kerr, P. J. (2012). Myxomatosis in Australia and Europe: a model for emerging infectious diseases. *Antiviral Research*, *93*(3), 387–415. doi:10.1016/j.antiviral.2012.01.009.
McCollum, A. M., & Damon, I. K. (2014). Human monkeypox. *Clinical Infectious Diseases*, *58*(2), 260–267. doi:10.1093/cid/cit703.

40 Papillomaviruses

KATE CUSCHIERI AND SHEILA GRAHAM

KEY POINTS

- HPV infections can cause skin cells to proliferate. Infection has subclinical, benign or malignant consequences according to viral and host factors.
- Some HPVs are associated with skin lesions, such as common hand warts and plantar verrucae.
- Persistent infection with high-risk or oncogenic HPV types can lead to the development of anogenital cancers, with HPV 16 being the most common high-risk type.
- *E6* and *E7* are the key transforming oncogenes of HPV.
- Current HPV prophylactic vaccines are highly efficacious against infection and associated disease but do not protect against all high-risk HPV types.

DESCRIPTION

Introduction including classification and major features

As ancient viruses that can infect an array of vertebrates, papillomaviruses (PVs) are extremely common, with the species name prefacing PV, e.g., bovine papillomavirus (BPV) and human papillomavirus (HPV); this chapter will focus on the latter. Papillomaviruses are epitheliotropic and can cause epithelia to proliferate; while this normally has subclinical or benign consequences, some infections can cause malignancy.

Papillomaviruses have:

- a diameter of 52–55 nm
- an icosahedral capsid composed of 72 capsomeres
- a supercoiled double-stranded DNA genome, with a single coding strand, a molecular weight of approximately 5×10^6 Da and consisting of about 7900 base pairs

- no envelope
- a strict tropism for epithelial cells

Classification

HPVs reside in the papillomaviridae and are formally classified by genome sequence analysis. Currently, HPVs are found in the *alpha, beta, gamma, mu* and *nu* genera, with most clinically relevant HPVs falling within the *alpha* genus (Fig. 40.1). An HPV type is defined by an HPV genome where the *L1* nucleotide sequence (the main structural gene of HPV) differs from that of any other genome by at least 10%. HPV types are distinguished by a number according to when they were discovered, and over 200 types of HPVs have been identified. HPV species then group related HPV types. Within types come several sub-lineages and variants, which have between 90% and 98% homology. While it has been long established that different HPV types have specific clinical associations (see Table 40.1), recent studies indicate that variants may confer different levels of clinical risk.

Beyond the systematic approach to classification, HPVs are frequently grouped according to the skin type or anatomical area they infect. Consequently, the descriptive terms *cutaneous HPVs, mucosal HPVs* and *genital HPVs*, while helpful, are not entirely robust (e.g., the genital types can be found in nongenital sites).

A further way of stratifying HPV is as low or high risk (LR or HR), according to the strength of oncogenic potential; currently, 12 HPV types are considered Group 1 carcinogens by the International Agency on Research: HPV 16, 18, 31, 33, 35, 39, 45, 51, 52, 56, 58, 59 (Fig. 40.1), with a further 1 (HPV 68) and 7 (26, 53, 66, 67, 70, 73, 82) types considered 'probable' or 'possible' carcinogens. HPV 16 is an order of magnitude riskier than the next most oncogenic type.

Genome organisation

The HPV genome contains an early region that encodes two large (*E1* and *E2*) and several smaller *(E4–E7)* genes

Alpha-papillomavirus
Mucosal and cutaneous

Group includes high-risk mucosal HPV types that are associated with cervical cancer, low-risk mucosal types that are associated with benign lesions, and low-risk cutaneous types that typically cause skin warts. Some types can be found in both mucosal and cutaneous lesions, although a preference is usually apparent. Low-risk HPV DNA is only rarely found in cancers. High-risk DNA is found in almost all cases of cervical cancer.

Mu-papillomavirus
Cutaneous

Benign cutaneous lesions usually at palmar and plantar epithelial sites. Not associated with cancer.

Nu-papillomavirus
Cutaneous

Benign cutaneous lesions. DNA occasionally detected in skin cancers.

Beta-papillomavirus
Cutaneous

Group includes high-risk and low-risk cutaneous types. Typically associated with unapparent infections in immunocompetent hosts, but can proliferate in immunosuppressed hosts and in EV patients. Persistent infection is thought to predispose to the development of skin cancer, especially in immunosuppressed individuals.

Gamma-papillomavirus
Cutaneous

Benign cutaneous lesions. Some types detected at oral sites. DNA only very rarely found in skin cancers.

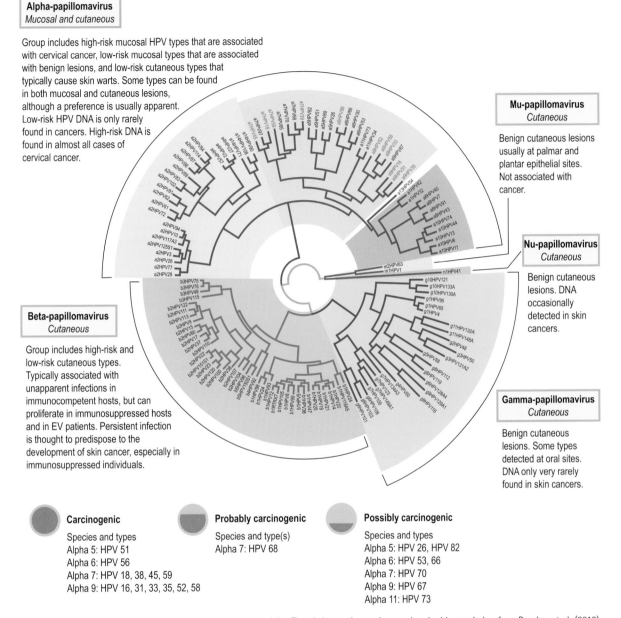

Carcinogenic

Species and types
Alpha 5: HPV 51
Alpha 6: HPV 56
Alpha 7: HPV 18, 38, 45, 59
Alpha 9: HPV 16, 31, 33, 35, 52, 58

Probably carcinogenic

Species and type(s)
Alpha 7: HPV 68

Possibly carcinogenic

Species and types
Alpha 5: HPV 26, HPV 82
Alpha 6: HPV 53, 66
Alpha 7: HPV 70
Alpha 9: HPV 67
Alpha 11: HPV 73

Fig. 40.1 HPV classification based on phylogeny and oncogenicity. The phylogenetic tree is reproduced with permission from Doorbar et al. (2012). The terminology *carcinogenic*, *probably carcinogenic* and *possibly carcinogenic* was conceived by the International Agency for Research on Cancer. EV, Epidermodysplasia verruciformis.

and a late region that encodes two large genes (*L1* and *L2*). Separating the two is a noncoding region, which contains various regulatory elements. The E region largely encodes the proteins responsible for pathogenicity, while the L region encodes the structural proteins. Cumulatively, HPV encodes nine main (plus a number of isoforms of these) proteins. The basic properties and functions of these proteins are outlined in Table 40.2.

EPIDEMIOLOGY

Major patterns including reservoir and transmission

HPV requires skin-to-skin contact for transmission, and it has been estimated that up to 80% of individuals will be

Table 40.1 Clinical manifestations of HPV types according to phylogeny and tropism

Genus	Tropism	Risk classification	Associated types	Clinical manifestations
Alpha-papillomavirus	Mucosal	High risk	16, 18, 31, 33, 35, 39, 45, 51, 52, 56, 58, 59, 68	Persistent infection can cause cancers of the cervix and anus and a component of cancers of the vulva, vagina, penis and oropharynx. Of the high-risk types, HPV 16 is the most common type associated with HPV-driven cancers.
	Mucosal	Low risk	6, 7, 11, 13, 26, 28, 29, 30, 32, 34, 40, 42, 43, 44, 53, 54, 61, 62, 67, 69, 70, 71, 72, 73, 74, 77, 81, 82, 83, 84, 85, 86, 87, 89, 90, 91, 94, 97, 102, 106, 114, 117A3, 125S1	Generally cause benign lesions including genital warts, oral lesions and papillomas of the conjunctiva and larynx. The Buschke–Lowenstein tumour is a rare complication of HPV 6 and 11 infection and is more common in males.
	Cutaneous	Low risk	2, 3, 10, 27, 57	Common warts (verruca vulgaris) and plantar, filiform and periungual warts. Occasionally these types can cause genital warts in children.
Beta-papillomavirus	Cutaneous		4, 5, 8, 9, 12, 14, 15, 17, 19, 20, 21, 22, 23, 24, 25, 36, 37, 38, 47, 49, 75, 76, 80, 92, 93, 96, 98, 99, 100, 104, 105, 107, 110, 111, 113, 115, 120, 122, 150, 151	Cutaneous lesions. General population can be infected, but immunocompromised individuals are more likely to be affected clinically, including those with the rare condition epidermodysplasia verruciformis (EV). Consequently, many of the types in the adjacent cell are referred to as EV types. Warts in EV patients can be extensive and have the capacity to transform into malignant lesions, particularly in those areas exposed to sunlight.
Gamma-papillomavirus	Cutaneous		4, 48, 50, 60, 65, 88, 95, 101, 103, 108, 109, 112, 116, 119, 121, 123	Cutaneous lesions, nearly always benign
Mu-papillomavirus	Cutaneous		1, 63	Cutaneous lesions, nearly always benign
Nu-papillomavirus	Cutaneous		41	Cutaneous lesions, nearly always benign

exposed to HPV infection. HPV is a stable virus and has been found in fomites including damp surfaces and towels. Wet skin is more vulnerable to surface breaks; hence verrucae are associated with swimming pools. Sexual intimacy is the main transmission route for HPV to the genitals, with female-to-male transmission more common. Transmission does not require penetration, and nonsexual transmission (including vertical transmission from parent to child) is possible. In women, the peak of genital infection occurs soon after onset of sexual activity and decreases sharply with age. Global prevalence of HPV infection in women with no disease is around 12%, with the highest prevalence observed in Sub-Saharan Africa (25%). In some settings, a second peak of HPV infection has been observed in women over 55, which may be attributable to waning immunity and/or lifestyle changes. Comparatively, prevalence of HR-HPV infection in males is relatively static, irrespective of age. In males, HPV has been detected on the penis, scrotum, rectum and buttocks. Similarly, in females, HPV can be found at all genital sites. Consequently, condoms, even if used consistently, are only partially protective.

Most HPV infections clear within 1–2 years, depending on both viral and host influences, including HPV type, viral load, smoking, age, persistent oral contraceptive use, coinfection with other STIs and immune capability. Persistent infection with HR-HPV carries a much greater risk of progression to cancer compared to transient infection.

REPLICATION

Life cycle

HPV can access basal epithelial cells via abrasions in the surface epithelial layers, sometimes referred to as micro wounds. However, for infections of the cervix, HPV can also directly infect the single-cell ectocervical layer prior to moving into the transformation zone, an area where columnar cells change into squamous cells and where most cervical abnormalities arise.

In most PVs, the L1 capsid protein binds to heparan sulphate proteoglycans on the basement membrane, which

Table 40.2 Papillomavirus gene functions

Gene	Function	Comments
E1	Viral DNA helicase that recruits the cellular DNA replication machinery	The only enzyme expressed by HPV. Frequently disrupted by integration.
E2	Regulation of transcription and replication and RNA processing. Episomal genome segregation. Nucleic acid–binding protein; very similar in BPV and HPV.	Regulates viral replication in association with E1. Frequently disrupted by integration.
E4	Virion maturation, disrupts keratinocyte fibre networks.	May facilitate release of virions from differentiated keratinocytes
E5	Alters signalling from growth factor receptors. Downregulates MHC.	Enhances transforming capabilities of E6 and E7. Facilitates immune evasion.
E6	Transforming function: binds to p53 and other proapoptotic proteins. Binds and degrades PDZ proteins.	Cooperates with E7 to stimulate cells into S phase, retard cell differentiation, inhibit apoptosis and increase efficiency of transformation
E7	Major transforming gene: binds to members of pocket protein family such as Rb	Induces proliferation. Works cooperatively with E6 but is capable of transforming cells independently of E6.
L1	Production of major capsid proteins, facilitates attachment and entry	Group- and type-specific determinants (for classification)
L2	Production of minor capsid proteins, facilitates attachment and entry	
URR (upstream regulatory region)	Regulation of gene function and initiator of viral replication	Noncoding region. Contains both positive and negative transcriptional and post-transcriptional control elements and the viral origin of replication.

facilitates a conformational change to the virus. This in turn exposes L2, which facilitates virus entry into the cell by micropinocytosis. The secondary cellular receptors for HPVs are not fully understood but may involve a number of proteins including growth factor receptors, laminins and the annexin-A2 heterotetramer. HPV travels in the cytoplasm from endosomes to the trans-Golgi network and reaches the nucleus approximately 24 hours after initial attachment, with the viral genome entering the nucleus following membrane breakdown during mitosis.

To produce daughter viruses, HPV invokes different processes at the different layers of the epithelium, and the program of epithelial differentiation actively supports completion of the virus replication cycle. The first stages involve uncoating and low-level genome amplification in the basal layer stem cells. Because these cells divide they can maintain viral genomes over a period of time, although there is limited viral gene expression. A full productive life cycle requires transit of these infected basal cells into the differentiating suprabasal layers to activate the full viral gene expression pattern. Normally, differentiating keratinocytes do not have active DNA replication, so HPV reactivates cell cycle entry in these cells in order to replicate its own genome. It does this through viral proteins E6 and E7, which stimulate cell cycle progression and inhibit cell death. High levels of genome amplification and particle assembly take place in the spinous and granular (suprabasal) layers, while particle release is confined to the uppermost layer. HPV completes these stages through a tightly regulated sequence of gene expression (Fig. 40.2)

and maintains a stable extrachromosomal state (referred to as an episome) throughout. A hallmark of the productively infected epithelium is that it retains an ability to differentiate despite activation of cell division. However, when the life cycle is aborted and the organised pattern of replication is lost, significant abnormal changes to the cell, called transformation, can occur.

Transformation

Transformation is an unlikely and unfortunate consequence of infection dependent on several interlinking factors including HPV type, location and duration of infection, immune capacity and environmental and constitutive risk factors. E6 and E7 are considered the primary oncoproteins, although E5 plays a supporting role.

Integration of the viral genome into the host chromosomes releases E6 and E7 from transcriptional control that keeps their levels low during a productive infection. This leads to high-level protein production necessary for cell transformation. Most HPV-associated tumours show integrated rather than episomal virus. However, at least 15% of tumours have episomal HPV genomes. The unifying factor in all HPV-driven tumours is a significant increase in E6 and E7 expression. E6 and E7 work cooperatively: E6 and particularly E7 induce proliferation of suprabasal cells, which avoid apoptosis through the actions of E6. These oncoproteins target and disable p53 and pRb, respectively, two key proteins involved in cell cycling that normally identify changes

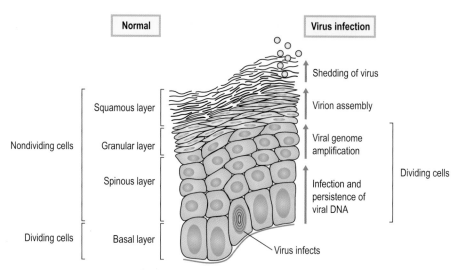

Fig. 40.2 The HPV replication cycle. HPV replication is tightly linked to the epithelial differentiation. HPV infects dividing basal epithelial cells and deposits its episomal genome in the nucleus. Upon cell division, daughter cells carrying virus genome copies can transit to the upper epithelial layers. This triggers HPV replication, including HPV genome amplification, virion assembly and release from the uppermost epithelial layer. Virions are depicted as blue circles. Epithelial cells are shown in beige with nuclei in pink.

in growth control signalling and prevent proliferation. *E7* can also act directly on centrosomes leading to genomic instability and abnormal mitoses, which would normally trigger p53-mediated apoptosis. E6 proteins also interact and degrade a set of so-called PDZ domain proteins that control cell shape and polarity, resulting in induction of proliferation and invasion. These viral–cellular interactions lead to unchecked growth of genetically unstable cells, vulnerable to secondary mutations and susceptible to malignant progression. The properties and affinities of E6 and E7 oncoproteins associated with high-risk HPV types are quite different from the properties of these proteins in low-risk HPV types.

CLINICAL FEATURES AND PATHOGENESIS

HPV infections

HPV can cause cells to proliferate where they otherwise would not. This can lead to the development of benign or malignant lesions. Table 40.1 summarises clinical manifestations of HPV infection.

Cutaneous warts

Cutaneous warts are relatively common, with an estimated prevalence of around 7%–12%. They are most common in childhood, decreasing in prevalence after age 20. Warts have varied clinical presentation; the common wart (verruca vulgaris), appears as a raised rough lesion, often on the

hands. Plantar warts manifest as painful thick hyperkeratotic plaques on the soles of the feet and have a mosaic-like appearance. Periungual warts, associated with nail biting, appear near nails. Planar, or flat, warts can occur singly or in groups, most commonly on the face. Filiform warts present as elongated protrusions and often manifest on eyelids or the lips (Fig. 40.3).

Histologically, warts are benign with hypertrophy of all layers of the dermis and hyperkeratosis of the horny layer (Fig. 40.4). They usually disappear spontaneously yet may be recalcitrant to treatment. Recurrence of lesions is probably due to persistence of the virus, either on the superficial skin or the basal cell layer.

Immunocompromised individuals are at increased risk of warts, which can be extensive. In those suffering from the rare genetic disorder epidermodysplasia verruciformis (EV) (characterised by a selective depletion of specific T cell clones), large warts associated with a variety of types including HPVs 4, 5, 8, 9 can persist for life, with UV-exposed warts harbouring the potential for malignant conversion. In addition, 40% of renal transplant recipients develop cutaneous warts within a year of receiving the graft.

Anogenital warts

Anogenital warts (Fig. 40.3C) are the most common clinical manifestation of anogenital infection, with HPV types 6 and 11 causing the majority. Four distinct subtypes have been described: condylomata acuminata (raised), flat warts, papular warts and keratotic lesions, the former two more

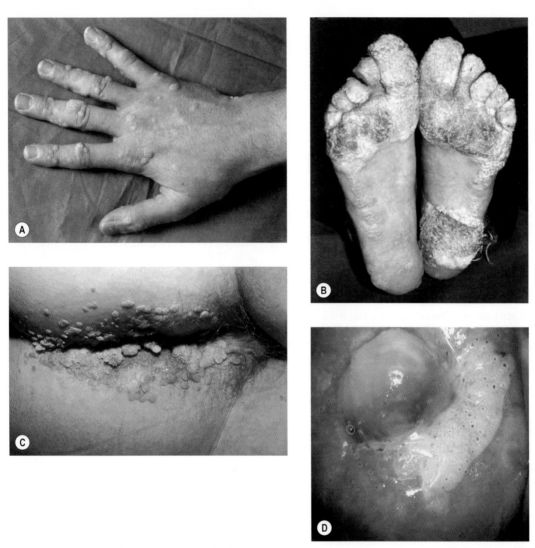

Fig. 40.3 Typical clinical presentations of HPV. A, Common hand warts on child. B, Extensive plantar warts in renal transplant patient. C, Genital warts (condylomata acuminata). D, Cervical flat wart after application of acetic acid. From Cubie, H.A. Diseases associated with human papillomavirus infection. (2013). *Virology*, 445(1-2). Copyright © 2013 Elsevier Inc. Figure supplied courtesy of Cubie and Benton.

likely to affect mucosa. Symptoms include burning itch, discharge and bleeding. Anogenital warts rarely follow a malignant course, although the Buschke–Lowenstein tumour is a rare example of this. The psychosexual morbidity and treatment costs associated with warts are nontrivial, particularly as recurrence within the first 3 months of treatment is not uncommon. Again, anogenital warts are more common in immunocompromised individuals and can become clinically apparent if the immune response is disturbed, as in pregnancy. In women, vulvar and vaginal warts are usually plainly visible. In men the most common sites for warts are the penile shaft, perianal skin and the anal canal.

Orolaryngeal warts
Recurrent respiratory papillomatosis (RRP)

This is a rare condition sometimes referred to as laryngeal papillomatosis, characterised by benign lesions affecting the mucosa of the airway. It has a bimodal distribution with peaks in children under 5 and adults over 15 years of age. Most cases are caused by HPV types 6 and 11. The disease is often more severe in children, who can acquire the infection in utero or intrapartum, whereas adults acquire the disease from orogenital contact with an infected partner, although the transmission rate is low. RRP may be indicative of an immunological incapacity, and signs and symptoms include hoarseness, chronic cough, dyspnea, recurrent upper respiratory infections, pneumonias and dysphagia. Lesions may cause life-threatening upper airway obstructions, which require surgery, and recurrence after treatment is common. Malignant conversion of laryngeal papillomas has been described.

Oral papillomatosis

A variety of benign lesions occur on the oral mucosa and tongue and are associated with a range of HPV types. The occurrence of multiple lesions on the buccal mucosa is known as oral florid papillomatosis. The virus types here are those found more commonly in the genital tract, and infection is acquired during orogenital contact.

HPV and cancer

Globally, 5%–8% of all human cancers are associated with HR-HPV. The most common HPV-driven cancer is cervical. An estimated 266,000 women died from cervical cancer worldwide in 2012, accounting for 7.5% of all female cancer deaths. The fact that HR-HPV is more likely to persist in cervical epithelia compared to other anogenital epithelia may explain its comparatively high incidence.

Other anogenital cancers that have an evidence-based HPV aetiology are vulvar, vaginal, anal and penile cancer. A component of squamous cell cancers of the head and neck, most notably the oropharynx, is also driven by HR-HPV. Figure 40.5 summarises HPV prevalence in cancers with a proven HPV aetiology. Anogenital cancers have a preinvasive phase defined as intraepithelial neoplasia grades 1, 2 and 3 according to histology, with 3 the most abnormal. Preinvasive lesions can take 4 decades to progress to cancer, providing an opportunity for screening, as is the case for cervix. The preinvasive phase of oropharyngeal cancer is not well defined.

Cervical cancer (CC)

Nearly all (~95%) CC are HR-HPV positive. The notion of an HPV-negative CC is often attributed to technical difficulties in detecting the virus as opposed to its absence. This said, certain rare cervical histological subtypes (such as clear cell adenocarcinoma) show a relatively low association with HPV (<30%). HPV 16 and 18 account for 70% of cervical cancers. The preinvasive phase of cervical cancer is referred to as cervical intraepithelial neoplasia (CIN) grades 1–3. CIN1 is termed low-grade disease, and CIN2 or CIN3 high grade, with the latter sometimes referred to as carcinoma in situ. The higher the grade, the greater the risk of progression to cancer. Clearance of CIN without intervention does occur, although 35% of CIN3 will progress to cervical cancer if left untreated. The most common type of cervical cancer is squamous cell cancer, which accounts for around 70%–80%; adenocarcinoma, which arises in glandular epithelium is rarer. Most cervical cancers arise in low- and middle-income countries because of the comparative absence of screening and vaccination programmes.

Anal and penile cancer (AC)

Around 90% of AC have an HPV aetiology. Preinvasive lesions are defined as anal intraepithelial neoplasia (AIN) grades 1–3 and can be detected by anoscopy. AC is 30- to 100-fold higher in renal transplant recipients, and HIV infection confers a 30-fold increased risk, independent of

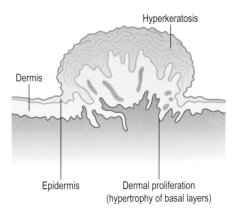

Fig. 40.4 Diagrammatic representation of the histological appearance of a wart.

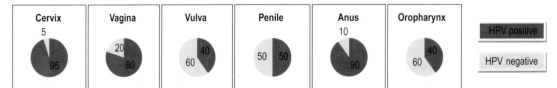

Fig. 40.5 HPV prevalence in cancers with a proven HPV aetiology. The darker and lighter red shows the HPV positive and negative component respectively. Numbers to percentages. Prevalence's are based on Plummer et al Lancet Glob Health 2016; 4: e609-16 and represent a global perspective.

sexual practices. Men who have sex with men have a greater risk of AC, which has informed recommendations for targeted vaccination of this group. Penile cancer is relatively rare, and ~50% are HPV positive, particularly the warty or basaloid tumours. Peak incidence is found in the seventh decade. Its precursor lesion takes the form of penile intraepithelial neoplasia (PeIN), which is classified as HPV related (undifferentiated PeIN) or non-HPV related (differentiated PeIN).

Vulvar and vaginal cancer

Around 40% of vulvar cancer is associated with HR-HPV, with HPV 16 dominating. The preinvasive vulval intraepithelial neoplasia (VIN) is defined as usual type (uVIN), which is HPV associated, affects younger women and is often multicentric disease, whereas differentiated type (dVIN) is not associated with HPV and generally occurs post-menopausally, often alongside chronic inflammatory dermatoses. Vaginal cancer is the rarest of all gynaecological cancers, and around 75% are associated with HPV, again largely HPV 16. It is found most frequently in postmenopausal women, and its precursor lesion is vaginal intraepithelial neoplasia (VaIN).

Squamous cancers of the head and neck

The most common HPV-associated cancer of the head and neck is oropharyngeal squamous cell carcinoma (OPSCC), incidence of which has risen in the past two decades, particularly in individuals <50 years old. The fraction of HPV-associated cancer ranges between 15% and 60%, depending on location, with HPV 16 the most prevalent type. HPV-negative cancers are more likely to be associated with the traditional risk factors of high alcohol consumption and smoking. OPSCC is also more common in males. Interestingly, HPV-associated OSCC has a better prognosis compared to HPV-negative OSCC; this is consistent with emerging evidence of a favourable prognosis in HPV-associated vulval and penile cancers (compared to negative counterparts).

DIAGNOSIS

Clinical and morphological identification

HPV infection may be readily diagnosed when there are typical, visible clinical lesions. Diagnosis of cutaneous anogenital warts is performed clinically, obviating the need for confirmatory laboratory testing. In cervical cytology preparations or smears, HPV infection can be recognised morphologically by the presence of vacuolated cells with enlarged hyperchromatic nuclei described as koilocytes. However, koilocytes are not always present and are not sufficiently specific for HPV. Histological examination of a biopsy taken from a lesion will show more specific features of HPV infection, including papillomatosis, hyperkeratinisation of the surface layer, hypertrophy of the basal layers and, crucially, disorganisation of the epithelial layers.

Serology

As HPV has no viraemic phase, is nonlytic and creates little inflammation, natural infection induces low-level antibody responses with a seroconversion rate of around 50%. Consequently, serology tests lack sensitivity for use in clinical management, although they are important for natural history studies and for monitoring vaccine-induced immunity.

Molecular detection

Nucleic acid (NA)-based HPV detection has been extensively applied for research, epidemiological and clinical use. With respect to disease management, HR-HPV testing is most frequently used in the context of cervical screening where assays involve the detection of NA for a group of HR-HPV types. Detection of low-risk HPV types is not helpful for cervical screening and management. Sensitivity of HR-HPV NA tests is high, but they cannot distinguish between clinically significant and transient infections. Consequently, biomarkers, which further delineate risk, are of value and include measuring transcription of *E6* and *E7*, detecting proteins that indicate abnormal cellular proliferation through immunohistochemistry and measuring host or viral methylation signatures.

In cervical screening, HR-HPV NA tests are sensitive for the detection of high-grade CIN (~95%). Also, women who test negative are very unlikely to have disease. Consequently, the method of primary cervical screening is changing from a morphology-based test (cervical cytology) to a molecular HR-HPV test, and algorithms based on HPV primary screening, followed by cytology of HPV-positive cases, are being introduced. HPV testing can also be used to risk stratify cytologically defined low-grade abnormalities, with HPV-negative women requiring less intense follow-up. Finally, in women treated for cervical lesions, HPV testing can help in posttreatment monitoring for residual disease (see Clinical Scenario).

TREATMENT AND CONTROL

Application of salicylic acid with regular paring is the preferred treatment for cutaneous warts, with cryotherapy in combination with salicylic acid recommended as a second-line treatment. Treatment of genital warts is more problematic and depends on the size and location of the warts and other comorbidities. Options include:

- antiproliferative agents such as podophyllin or 5-fluorouracil, although close monitoring is required
- destructive therapies such as trichloracetic acid, liquid nitrogen or surgical excision
- immunomodulators, such as imiquimod, which activate monocytes/macrophages and cause direct release of interferon-α (applied topically)

Interferon, photodynamic therapy and indole-3-carbinol have been used for treatment of recurrent laryngeal warts after the reduction of tumour load by cautery or excision.

All of these treatments will remove the lesions but do not always eradicate the virus from surrounding epithelium. Incomplete treatment is the most common cause of recurrence of warts; all of a patient's warts must have disappeared with restoration of normal skin texture before a cure is considered.

Treatment for intraepithelial lesions usually requires removal of the affected area through ablative techniques or surgical removal, with the latter approach permitting histological assessment. Low-grade lesions are often monitored closely rather than treated given their high natural clearance rate. Currently, no virus-specific antiviral agents exist for HPV infection.

VACCINES

Prophylactic HPV vaccines constitute a massive breakthrough in the management of HPV infection and associated disease. The vaccines are composed of adjuvant plus virus-like particles made from the L1 protein, which assemble into empty shells of the virus and which generate a neutralising antibody response yet cannot replicate given the absence of the other viral genes. Antibody responses to the vaccine are significantly higher than those associated with natural infection.

Three are currently licensed:

- Bivalent: protects against 16 and 18
- Quadrivalent: protects against 6, 11, 16 and 18
- Nonavalent: protects against 6, 11, 16, 18, 31, 33, 45, 52 and 58

The vaccines exist as prefilled syringes delivered via intramuscular injection into the arm. Initially a three-dose schedule over 6 months was recommended, although a two-dose approach at time 0 and ≥6 months has been implemented in certain settings more recently. The vaccines are safe and efficacious, providing almost complete protection from anogenital disease driven by the vaccine types with evidence of cross protection against closely related types. For maximum effectiveness, immunisation before sexual debut should be implemented, and vaccine programmes have led to a significant decrease in HPV infection and associated disease. Most programmes target females, although an increasing number are gender neutral. Another approach is to impose a female-only programme but perform targeted vaccination of MSM given their additional risk of HPV-associated disease.

As the key drivers of immune clearance of virus and disease are not fully characterised, the development and application of therapeutic vaccines has been slower than that of prophylactic vaccines. Therapeutic vaccines need to stimulate production of cytotoxic T cells, which recognise MHC molecules bound to viral antigens, and relevant antigens to achieve this have included E6 and E7 but also L1, L2 and E2. Candidates for therapeutic vaccines have included DNA vaccines and peptide vaccines, and both have been shown to induce T cell responses in clinical trials.

ACKNOWLEDGMENT

Cervical cytology slides reproduced with kind permission from Mrs Sue Mehew.

RECOMMENDED READING

Denny, L., Herrero, R., Levin, C., & Kim, J. J. (2015). Cervical cancer. Ch. 4. In H. Gelband, P. Jha, R. Sankaranarayanan, & S. Horton (Eds.), *Cancer: Disease control priorities* (3rd ed., Vol. 3). Washington, DC: The International Bank for Reconstruction and Development/The World Bank.

Doorbar, J., Quint, W., Banks, L., Bravo, I. G., Stoler, M., Broker, T. R., & Stanley, M. A. (2012). The biology and life-cycle of human papillomaviruses. *Vaccine, 30*(Suppl. 5), F55–F70. doi:10.1016/j.vaccine.

Drolet, M., Bénard, É., Boily, M. C., Ali, H., Baandrup, L., Bauer, H., ... Brisson, M. (2015). Population-level impact and herd effects following human papillomavirus vaccination programmes: a systematic review and meta-analysis. *The Lancet Infectious Diseases, 15*(5), 565–580. doi:10.1016/S1473-3099(14)71073-4.

Groves, I. J., & Coleman, N. (2015). Pathogenesis of human papillomavirus-associated mucosal disease. *The Journal of Pathology, 235*(4), 527–538. doi:10.1002/path.4496.

Lynch, M. D., Cliffe, J., & Morris-Jones, R. (2014). Management of cutaneous viral warts. *British Medical Journal, 348,* g3339. doi:10.1136/bmj.g3339.

Plummer, M., de Martel, C., Vignat, J., Ferlay, J., Bray, F., & Franceschi, S. (2016). Global burden of cancers attributable to infections in 2012: a synthetic analysis. *Lancet Glob Health, 4*(9), e609–e616. doi:10.1016/S2214-109X(16)30143-7.

41 Polyomaviruses

C. Y. WILLIAM TONG

KEY POINTS

- At least 13 polyomaviruses have been identified in humans, though only a minority has clear disease association.
- Merkel cell polyomavirus is the only human polyomavirus so far that is clearly associated with malignant tumours in humans.
- BKV and JCV are associated with diseases in immunosuppressed individuals.
- Polyomavirus-associated nephropathy (PVAN) caused by BKV is a significant cause of allograft dysfunction and graft loss after renal transplantation.
- Progressive multifocal leuco-encephalopathy (PML) caused by JCV is found in patients with advanced HIV disease and patients using immune-modulating therapeutic monoclonal antibodies.

INTRODUCTION

The term *polyomaviruses* literally stands for many (poly) tumour (oma) viruses, so called because of their ability to induce various tumours in experimental animals. More than 13 human polyomaviruses have been identified so far, but only a minority is recognised to have disease association (Table 41.1). Initially, only murine and hamster polyomaviruses appeared to be oncogenic in their natural hosts. However, the more recently discovered Merkel cell polyomavirus has a clear association with Merkel cell carcinoma, a rare human neuroendocrine cutaneous tumour found in the immunosuppressed or those exposed to sunlight. The older members BK virus and JC virus have no clear association with malignancy, and both were named after the initials of the patients from whom they were first isolated.

The virions are 42–45 nm in size, with a 72-capsomere icosahedral capsid. The genome consists of a double-stranded super-coiled loop of DNA, approximately 5100 bp in length, with both strands coding for virus proteins. Capsids contain three structural proteins, VP1, VP2 and VP3. Current taxonomy divides the Polyomaviridae family into four genera. Human polyomaviruses can be found in the *alpha*, *beta* and *delta* genera, whereas the *gamma* genus only contains avian polyomaviruses.

REPLICATION AND TRANSFORMATION

There are three noncapsid regulatory proteins: large T antigen ($T\,Ag$), small $T\,Ag$ and agnoprotein. Some polyomaviruses have an additional middle $T\,Ag$. These are the first antigens to appear after infection; they accumulate in the nucleus, stimulate cellular growth and are important for replication. This is followed by a switch to transcription of the late region of the genome and production of the three structural capsid proteins. The growth cycle in culture is 36–44 hours, and the release of mature virus particles follows lysis of the cell. The structural proteins determine host range and infectivity. BKV can be grown with difficulty in human embryonic kidney cells, whereas JCV, which is not only species but also tissue specific, replicates only in human embryo glial cell cultures. Recently, the 5-hydroxytryptamine 2A ($5HT2_A$) receptor for serotonin on the surface of glial cells was identified as the receptor protein for entry of JCV.

The early proteins are associated with immortalisation and transformation of host cells. Large T antigen binds to both retinoblastoma protein (Rb) and p53 and prevents the induction of cell death. Polyomaviruses do not have a viral DNA polymerase. Instead, they utilise the host DNA polymerase α/primase complex to which $T\,Ag$ binds. $T\,Ag$ also binds to double-stranded (ds) DNA and has helicase activity to help to unwind the viral dsDNA for DNA replication.

CLINICAL FEATURES AND PATHOGENESIS

Primary infections with polyomaviruses are mostly asymptomatic. Rarely, upper respiratory tract symptoms,

411

Table 41.1 Polyomaviruses that have been linked with human diseases

Designation	Common name	Year of discovery	Disease association
Genus: *Alphapolyomavirus*			
Human polyomavirus 5	Merkel cell polyomavirus (MCPyV)	2009	Merkel cell carcinoma, a rare primary neuroendocrine malignant tumour of the skin
Human polyomavirus 8	Trichodysplasia spinulosa–associated polyomavirus (TSPyV)	2010	Trichodysplasia spinulosa, a rare dermatological condition found only in immunosuppressed patients
Genus: *Betapolyomavirus*			
Macaca mulatta polyomavirus 1	Simian vacuolating agent (SV40)	1960	Contamination of polio vaccines; association with human cancer controversial
Human polyomavirus 1	BK polyomavirus (BKV, BKPyV)	1971	Ureteric stenosis, haemorrhagic cystitis, polyomavirus-associated nephropathy in transplant recipients
Human polyomavirus 2	JC polyomavirus (JCV, JCPyV)	1971	Progressive multifocal leuco-encephalopathy in immunosuppressed patients
Human polyomavirus 3	KI polyomavirus (KIPyV)	2007	Respiratory tract infection in young children, clinical significance unclear
Human polyomavirus 4	WU polyomavirus (WUPyV)	2007	Respiratory tract infection in young children, clinical significance unclear
Genus: *Deltapolyomavirus*			
Human polyomavirus 7	Human polyomavirus 7	2010	HPyV7-associated keratosis in immunosuppressed patients

cystitis and encephalitis have been described. SV40 is primarily a simian virus. Its association with human infection is related to the inadvertent use of SV40-contaminated poliovirus vaccines in the 1950s and 1960s. The role, if any, of SV40 in human diseases is controversial. WUPyV and KIPyV are found in respiratory samples. Their role in human respiratory tract infection is at present unclear.

Reactivation of BKV and JCV is common, particularly in organ transplant patients, with up to 40% of renal allograft recipients and haematopoietic stem cell transplant (HSCT) patients excreting a polyomavirus in urine in the early months after transplantation. BKV reactivation is associated with haemorrhagic cystitis (HC) in HSCT patients and PVAN in renal transplant patients. JCV is associated with PML, seen in immunosuppressed patients, most commonly patients with advanced HIV infection.

Haemorrhagic cystitis (HC)

This is a common complication after HSCT. Early-onset HC (<2 weeks) is probably not related to viral infection. However, late-onset HC (>2 weeks) is often related to BK reactivation. BK virus excretors are four times more likely to develop HC than non-excretors, and there is a strong temporal relationship between BK excretion and onset of HC. Pathogenesis may be related to immune reconstitution as its onset often coincides with engraftment.

Polyomavirus-associated nephropathy (PVAN)

The association of BKV reactivation in the renal allografts of transplant recipients with graft dysfunction was made only in the past 10 years. Its discovery coincided with the introduction of newer, more potent immunosuppressive agents such as tacrolimus and mycophenolate mofetil. So far no specific immunosuppressive agents have been clearly associated with PVAN.

PVAN is mostly reported in patients receiving renal allografts and only rarely after other transplantations. Onset of PVAN occurs at a median time of about 6 months after transplantation, and up to 1%–5% of renal allografts are affected. Men are more likely to develop PVAN than females in most case series. The only presenting clinical feature is that of deterioration in graft function. Hence, the major differential diagnosis is allograft rejection. Since the management of graft rejection is to increase immunosuppression, whereas that of PVAN is to decrease it, an accurate diagnosis is necessary to inform management.

Progressive multifocal leuco-encephalopathy (PML)

This condition, associated with the reactivation of JCV in the brain, was first described in 1958 in patients with Hodgkin's lymphoma and chronic lymphocytic leukaemia. Over the past 10 years, PML has been found almost exclusively in patients with acquired immune deficiency syndrome (AIDS). More recently, PML has also been described in patients receiving monoclonal antibody therapy such as natalizumab (used in the treatment of multiple sclerosis) and rituximab.

Patients with PML have multiple foci of demyelination, usually affecting white matter in the cerebral hemispheres, but occasionally elsewhere in the central nervous system. Affected oligodendrocytes become swollen, with hyperchromatic nuclei and occasional basophilic inclusions pathognomonic of PML. Replication of the virus occurs in the nucleus, causing cell destruction and breakdown of the myelin sheath.

The clinical features depend on the areas affected. Symptoms include visual, mental and speech impairment, hemiplegia, loss of memory, personality change and dementia. Death usually occurs within 6 months of the first signs of the disease. Other causes of similar symptoms such as cerebral lymphoma, toxoplasmosis and tuberculosis need to be excluded.

LABORATORY INVESTIGATION

In HC, polyomaviruses can be detected in large quantity in urine. The presence of BKV in the urine can be confirmed by BKV-specific PCR. Patients with uncomplicated HC do not normally have significant BK viraemia (i.e., virus detectable in peripheral blood).

The gold standard of PVAN diagnosis is histological examination of renal biopsy and identification of viral inclusion bodies in the renal tubular cells. The presence of polyomavirus can be confirmed by immunohistological staining using monoclonal antibodies against polyomavirus *T Ag*. Histology can also exclude or detect concomitant presence of graft rejection. Noninvasive methods such as urine cytology looking for polyomavirus-infected uroepithelial cells (decoy cells) or detection of polyomavirus in urine by electron microscopy, though sensitive, are nonspecific and have poor positive predictive values. The best noninvasive diagnostic method, with the highest positive predictive value, is quantitative plasma BK viral load. Surveillance of renal transplant recipients using serial plasma viral load is being advocated, which can also be used to monitor the progress of the disease.

The gold standard for diagnosis of PML depends on a combination of neuroimaging and biopsy. JCV DNA may not be detectable in the cerebrospinal fluid (CSF) even with the use of highly sensitive nested PCR. Intrathecal antibody detection may be useful if JCV DNA is negative in CSF.

Antibodies to polyomaviruses can be measured using haemagglutination inhibition (HAI) and enzyme-linked immunosorbent assay (ELISA). HAI uses whole virions and gives a species-specific result, whereas in ELISA, disrupted virions or purified VP1 can be used to give a more sensitive and type-specific result. Rising titres and the presence of immunoglobulin M are diagnostic of recent infection. Serum JCV antibody index is a semi-quantitative immunoassay used to guide the management of multiple sclerosis patients treated with natalizumab. Patients with an index of >1.5 have a high risk of development of PML and would require intensive imaging follow-up or consideration of stopping therapy.

TRANSMISSION AND EPIDEMIOLOGY

Very little is known about the transmission of polyomaviruses. Both BKV and JCV are frequently detected in urine. Respiratory, sexual and fecal–oral routes of transmission are all possible. In human tissues, BKV DNA may be found in tonsils, lung, lymph nodes and spleen and JCV DNA in lung, liver, spleen, lymph nodes and leucocytes.

Serological studies show that BKV infection is a common event in early childhood. By 3 years of age, 50%–60% of children have antibody, rising to almost 100% by the age of 10 years. JCV circulates independently of BKV in the community, and acquisition of antibodies is slower and increases steadily with age to about 60%–70% in adulthood.

TREATMENT

Cidofovir is active against polyomaviruses in vitro. As polyomaviruses do not carry viral DNA polymerase, the action of cidofovir is likely to be targeted against other proteins such as host polymerase or viral *T Ag*. Its clinical use in HC or PVAN has not been particularly successful. In addition, cidofovir is nephrotoxic and can only be used in very small doses in renal patients. Leflunomide is a mild immunosuppressive agent licensed for the treatment of rheumatoid arthritis. It also has antiviral properties and has been used as a treatment for PVAN. It has significant haematological toxicity. which can be restrictive and dose limiting. The main management of PVAN is preemptive reduction of immunosuppression. In order to achieve this, noninvasive surveillance methods for PVAN such as quantitative plasma viral load measurement need to be available.

There is no established treatment for PML. In multiple sclerosis patients, the treatment, which acts as the trigger for PML, needs to be stopped to prevent further progression. Plasma exchange could be used to rapidly remove natalizumab. In HIV patients, the use of combination antiretroviral therapy (cART) may prolong survival, but this could paradoxically also increase the damage through immune reconstitution inflammatory syndrome (IRIS). Several chemotherapeutic agents, including cytosine arabinoside (ARA-C, cytarabine), cidofovir and mefloquine, have been tried. With the recent discovery of JCV utilising the serotonin receptor to enter into glial cells, there has been interest in investigating the use of 5HT2a antagonists.

RECOMMENDED READING

DeCaprio, J. A., Imperiale, M. J., & Major, E. O. (2013). Polyomaviruses. In D. M. Knipe & P. M. Howley (Eds.), *Fields virology* (6th ed.). Philadelphia: Lippincott Williams & Wilkins.

Khalili, K., & Stoner, G. L. (Eds.). (2001). *Human polyomaviruses. Molecular and clinical perspectives.* New York: Wiley-Liss.

Pinto, M., & Dobson, S. (2014). BK and JC virus: a review. *The Journal of Infection, 68*(Suppl. 1), S2–S8. doi:10.1016/j.jinf.2013.09.009.

Tavazzi, E., White, M. K., & Khalili, K. (2012). Progressive multifocal leukoencephalopathy: clinical and molecular aspects. *Reviews in Medical Virology, 22*(1), 18–32. doi:10.1002/rmv.710.

42 Hepadnaviruses

Hepatitis B virus infection; hepatitis delta virus infection

C. Y. WILLIAM TONG

KEY POINTS

- Hepatitis B virus (HBV) causes acute hepatitis and chronic infection leading to chronic liver disease, cirrhosis and hepatocellular carcinoma.
- HBV is a partially double-stranded DNA virus, carrying a reverse transcriptase-like enzyme to replicate viral DNA from an RNA intermediate.
- HBV is transmitted in blood, e.g., through intravenous drug use, by sexual intercourse and from mother to child during childbirth.
- There is considerable geographical variation in infection rates; the highest rates are in the Far East, Sub-Saharan Africa, Oceania and South America.
- An effective vaccine is available, given in three doses over 6 months. Universal vaccination of young children will reduce the chronic infection rate and long-term sequelae, including hepatocellular carcinoma.
- Treatment of chronic HBV infection includes a course of pegylated interferon or the use of long-term suppressive therapy with nucleos(t)ide analogues.

The Hepadnaviridae are a family of hepatotropic DNA viruses with a unique life cycle involving an RNA intermediate and the use of a viral polymerase enzyme with reverse transcriptase activity. There are two recognised genera whose members are species-specific and cause acute and chronic infection of the liver. The genus *Orthohepadnavirus* infects vertebral hosts including humans, great apes, woodchucks and ground squirrels, while the genus *Avihepadnavirus* infects birds such as ducks, herons and storks. Hepatitis B virus (HBV) is the type species of *Orthohepadnavirus* and a major cause of chronic liver disease and hepatocellular carcinoma (HCC) in humans. HBV infection also occurs in the wild in a number of nonhuman primate species, such as chimpanzees, orangutans and gibbons. Each of these species harbours variants of HBV distinct from those found in humans.

HEPATITIS B VIRUS

STRUCTURE

The virion of HBV is a 42-nm double-shelled particle known as the Dane particle. The outer envelope of the virion is formed by hepatitis B surface antigen (HBsAg). The inner core, 27 nm in diameter, consists of hepatitis B core antigen (HBcAg), which encloses the viral genomic DNA and polymerase.

The outer envelope protein, HBsAg, is overproduced by HBV, and the excess HBsAg is found in abundance in the blood of chronically infected individuals as subviral particles. Two different forms of subviral HBsAg can be seen in the blood (Figs. 42.1 and 42.2). The predominant form is a small, spherical particle with a diameter of 22 nm. A filamentous form is also present. Both types of particles are composed of lipid, protein and carbohydrate; they are not infectious and consist solely of surplus virion envelope.

The viral DNA is about 3200 nucleotides long and is circular in configuration (Fig. 42.3). The long negative sense strand is complete, but there is a gap of variable length of about 1000 nucleotides in the complementary positive sense strand. This incomplete strand is closed by the viral polymerase when virus replication starts. There are four overlapping open reading frames on the circular viral DNA coding for the core, surface, polymerase and an X protein, which is possibly an activator of transcription. An additional viral protein, the hepatitis B e antigen (HBeAg), is translated from the precore/core open reading frame that encodes the HBcAg protein using an upstream initiating codon. HBeAg is not found in the virion but is secreted from infected cells into the bloodstream, particularly during active viral replication. It is therefore frequently used as a marker indicating significant viral activity. The surface antigen gene is transcribed to produce three messenger RNAs (mRNAs): L, M and S. The S mRNA is the shortest but most abundantly produced. The product of

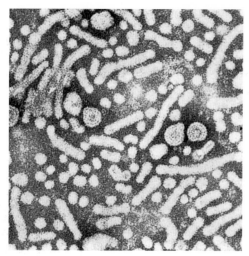

Fig. 42.1 Electron micrograph of the particles in the blood of a patient infected with HBV (original magnification ×130,000). (Courtesy Dr A. Keen, University of Cape Town.)

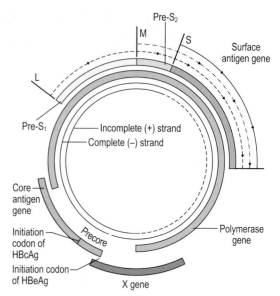

Fig. 42.3 Gene organisation of HBV DNA showing the four overlapping reading frames of core, polymerase, surface and X.

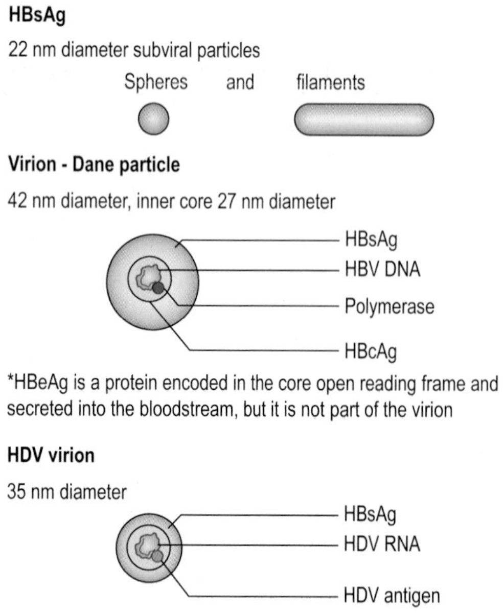

HBsAg

22 nm diameter subviral particles

Spheres   and   filaments

Virion - Dane particle

42 nm diameter, inner core 27 nm diameter

— HBsAg
— HBV DNA
— Polymerase
— HBcAg

*HBeAg is a protein encoded in the core open reading frame and secreted into the bloodstream, but it is not part of the virion

HDV virion

35 nm diameter

— HBsAg
— HDV RNA
— HDV antigen

Fig. 42.2 Schematic diagram of particles and antigens of HBV and HDV.

the M mRNA is medium in length and consists of an additional portion of the S reading frame known as pre-S_2. The protein from the L mRNA is the longest and comprises an additional pre-S_1 segment in addition to pre-S_2 and S. The L product is present only in the virions, whereas the M and S proteins are found in the virions as well as the subviral particles.

GENETIC VARIATION

HBV can be classified into ten genotypes, A–J, by comparison of their nucleotide sequences. Some genotypes have a restricted geographical distribution; for example, genotype E is found predominantly in Sub-Saharan Africa, genotypes B and C in the Far East, and genotypes F and H in Central and South America. The HBsAg of all HBV genotypes contains a common 'a' determinant, which is the main target of the protective antibody response. Immunity induced by infection or immunisation with one HBV genotype cross-protects against infection with others.

STABILITY

There is only limited success culturing HBV using primary hepatocyte cell culture, and viral expression is often studied using cell lines with transfected HBV. It is therefore difficult to assess the stability of HBV. Indirect evidence has been obtained from the study of recipients of blood products treated in various ways and from chimpanzee inoculation experiments. Infectivity is lost after autoclaving at 121°C for 20 minutes or dry heat at 160°C for 1 hour. HBV remains active after storage at 30–32°C for at least 6 months and when frozen at −15°C for 15 years. HBV in blood can withstand drying for at least 1 week. Effective chemical disinfectants include treatment with hypochlorite (10,000 ppm available chlorine) for 10 minutes and 2% glutaraldehyde for 5 minutes. In clinical practice, chlorine-based disinfectants are the most commonly used to disinfect environments contaminated with HBV. Glutaraldehyde was previously used to decontaminate endoscopes but was withdrawn because of toxicity. Effective substitutes include 0.2%–0.35% peracetic acid, hypochlorous acid (superoxidised water) and chlorine dioxide.

REPLICATION

The pre-s1 domain of the large HBsAg molecule is believed to bind to a transmembrane transporter protein, sodium taurocholate cotransporting polypeptide, to gain entry into hepatocytes. Once in the cytoplasm, the nucleocapsid is transported to the nucleus where replication of viral nucleic acid starts. The viral polymerase completes the positive sense strand to form a covalently closed circular (ccc) DNA. This cccDNA forms a minichromosome in association with host histone proteins and establishes the basis of the persistent infection. From the cccDNA, mRNAs are transcribed, which are then translated to form the various viral proteins including HBsAg and HBcAg. A 3.5-kb mRNA that spans the entire length of the genome (known as the pregenome) is packaged with the viral polymerase and a protein kinase into the core particles. The multifunctional viral polymerase then reverse transcribes the pregenomic RNA into the negative strand genomic DNA. The same viral enzyme then creates the complementary positive strand DNA using the negative strand as a template, but this process is left incomplete as the process stops when the nucleocapsid matures. The mature nucleocapsid is then transported to the cytoplasm to be associated with the envelope protein HBsAg in the endoplasmic reticulum to form progeny virions. Some nucleocapsids remain in the nucleus and contribute to the intranuclear pool of cccDNA, thus leading to amplification of infection. Integration of viral DNA genome into a host chromosome can occur during the replication cycle, preferentially at sites of transcriptional activity, which may be important in the mechanism of carcinogenesis. However, unlike other viruses such as HIV, integration is not essential for the replication of HBV.

ACUTE INFECTION

The incubation period of HBV infection ranges from 6 to 24 weeks but is often about 2–3 months. Acute infection can be asymptomatic, particularly in children. Symptoms in the prodromal phase may include malaise, anorexia, weakness, myalgia, nausea and vomiting. Presence of hepatitis is signalled by the appearance of jaundice and right upper quadrant abdominal pain, accompanied by pale stool and dark coloured urine. Paradoxically, the patient often feels physically better when the jaundice appears. Hepatocellular damage is detectable biochemically with elevated alanine transaminase (ALT) levels before the onset of clinical jaundice and persists after it has resolved. In some cases, immunological reactions due to circulating immune complexes may manifest as arthralgia, urticarial or maculopapular skin rash, polyarteritis nodosa or glomerulonephritis. Up to 1% of acute hepatitis B infections become fulminant, resulting in acute liver failure.

PATHOLOGY OF ACUTE INFECTION

All types of viral hepatitis produce similar changes at the histological level. In the acute stage there are signs of inflammation in the portal tracts; the infiltrate is mainly lymphocytic. In the liver parenchyma, infected hepatocytes show ballooning and form acidophilic (Councilman) bodies as they die.

HBV replicates in the hepatocytes, reflected in the detection of viral DNA and HBcAg in the nucleus and HBsAg in the cytoplasm and at the hepatocyte membrane. During the incubation period, high levels of virus are present before the host immune response develops to control the virus. During replication, HBcAg and HBeAg are also present at the cytoplasmic membrane. These antigens induce both B and T cell responses; damage to the hepatocyte can result from antibody-dependent, natural killer (NK) and cytotoxic T cell action. Expression of major histocompatibility complex (MHC) class I antigens is poor in hepatocytes but can be enhanced as interferons are produced in response to the infection. This in turn leads to increased antigen recognition and lysis of the infected hepatocytes. Thus, liver damage in HBV infection is mediated by an immunopathological mechanism.

CHRONIC INFECTION

Most adults with acute HBV infection recover completely. Chronic infection occurs in 5%–10% of adults, 20%–50% of children under the age of 6, and over 90% of newborns who acquire the infection (Fig. 42.4). Five stages of chronic infection are recognised (Table 42.1):

1. High replicative/low inflammatory (immune tolerance) phase
2. Immune clearance phase
3. Low (non)replicative phase (previously known as chronic inactive carriage)
4. HBeAg negative chronic hepatitis B; through emergence of hepatitis B variants
5. HBsAg loss, occult hepatitis B phase

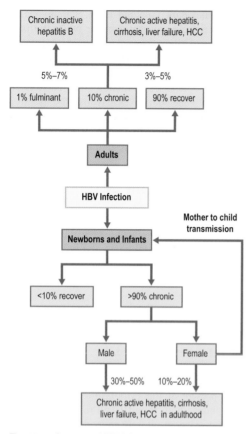

Fig. 42.4 Outcome of HBV infection in adults and children.

The high replicative/low inflammatory phase occurs mostly in children who acquired the infection at a young age but is also seen in immunocompromised individuals. During this phase, the infected individual is immunologically tolerant to the presence of the virus, allowing the virus to replicate to very high levels without showing any symptoms. Serum HBV DNA levels are typically very high (>1 million IU/mL), and HBeAg is present with normal ALT levels. There is little evidence of necroinflammation or fibrosis on liver biopsy. Because of the high level of viraemia, these patients are highly infectious.

The immune clearance phase occurs when immune tolerance is lost. This typically occurs in early adulthood for those who were infected at a young age. This phase is characterised by HBeAg positivity, slightly lower level of HBV DNA (>200,000 IU/mL) compared to the immune tolerance phase, fluctuating levels of ALT and evidence of moderate to severe liver necroinflammation and rapid progression of fibrosis. This phase may be confused with acute hepatitis because of similarity in symptoms and presence of low level of IgM anti-HBc. The longer the duration of immune clearance, the more is the resultant liver damage.

For individuals who successfully control active HBV replication, the low (non)replicative phase follows. Seroconversion from HBeAg to anti-HBe occurs, and HBV DNA levels become very low (<2000 IU/mL) or undetectable, while ALT levels normalise. These individuals are asymptomatic, but most remain HBsAg positive. As a

Table 42.1 Laboratory markers in different clinical phases of chronic hepatitis B

	ALT	HBsAg	Anti-HBc	Anti-HBc IgM	Anti-HBs*	HBeAg	Anti-HBe	HBV DNA
Uninfected, susceptible	N	−	−	−	−	−	−	−
Uninfected, immune through vaccination	N	−	−	−	+	−	−	−
Acute hepatitis B	+++	+++	+	+++	−	+/−	−/+	+++++
Chronic high replicative/low inflammatory phase	N	++++	+	−	−	++	−	+++++++
Immune clearance phase	++/+++	+++	+	+/−	−	+/−	−/+	++++
Chronic low (non) replicative phase	N	+	+	−	−	−	+	++
HBeAg negative chronic hepatitis B	++/N	++	+	−	−	−	+	++/+++
Past hepatitis B, resolved with immunity	N	−	+	−	+	−	+	−
HBsAg loss – occult hepatitis B	N	−	+	−	−	−	+	+

N: normal
−: negative
+: positive, number of + indicate level of positivity
Anti-HBs*: − <10 mIU/mL; + >10 mIU/mL

result of successful immunological control of HBV, these patients tend to have a more favourable long-term outcome. Traditionally, these patients are often referred to as healthy hepatitis B carriers. However, the use of such a term may result in a false sense of security, as between 10% and 20% may revert to active infection (reactivation) or change to the phase of HBeAg negative chronic hepatitis B through the emergence of viral variants. It is therefore necessary to have lifelong follow-up of patients with chronic inactive HBV infection.

In some patients, viral activity remains after seroconversion from HBeAg to anti-HBe. It is characterised by periodic fluctuating levels of HBV DNA and ALT. In these patients, a viral variant emerges (see later in the chapter), which is HBeAg negative but remains virologically active. The HBV DNA levels of these patients tend to be at a moderate level between 2000 and 200,000 IU/mL. Because of the fluctuating course, it is sometimes difficult to distinguish between patients in this phase with patients in the inactive phase. Nevertheless, a distinction is important as these patients have active disease and may progress to develop cirrhosis and HCC.

Approximately 0.5% per year of patients with inactive chronic hepatitis B will clear HBsAg. These individuals have resolved HBV infection, and the presence of a past HBV infection is indicated by the presence of anti-HBc, with or without anti-HBs. However, in most cases, HBV is not completely cleared, and reactivation can occur in the presence of immunosuppression such as after organ transplantation or treatment with immunosuppressive drugs. The risk of development of HCC is significantly reduced in these patients with resolved infection but not completely eliminated, particularly in older patients or those who have already developed cirrhosis. In some individuals, HBV DNA is persistently detectable in the absence of HBsAg. These patients are said to have occult HBV infection.

PATHOLOGY AND PATHOGENESIS OF CHRONIC INFECTION

In chronic hepatitis, damage extends out from the portal tracts, giving a piecemeal necrosis appearance. Some lobular inflammation is also seen. As the disease progresses, fibrosis and, eventually, cirrhosis develops. Chronic liver damage results from continuing, immune-mediated destruction of hepatocytes expressing viral antigens. In addition, autoimmune reactions may contribute to the damage as immune responses are induced to various liver-specific antigens.

Persistence of HBV is indicated by the continued presence of HBsAg and HBV DNA in the blood for more than 6 months. It is not yet clear what determines whether an individual will progress to the chronic state. There may be host genetic factors, but the absence, or relative inefficiency, of the immune response is important, as shown by the increased likelihood of chronic infection in the very young and the immunocompromised. In the neonate, infection occurs in the presence of maternal anti-HBc and HBeAg, which can cross the placenta. It is speculated that this results in tolerance through masking of HBcAg on hepatocyte membranes, and thus prevention of its recognition by cytotoxic T cells and other immune mechanisms that could lead to clearance of the virus.

Other factors associated with increased risk of cirrhosis include older age or longer duration of infection, infection with HBV genotype C, high level of HBV DNA, heavy alcohol consumption and concurrent infection with hepatitis C virus (HCV), hepatitis D virus (HDV) or human immunodeficiency virus (HIV).

Hepatocellular carcinoma (HCC)

There is considerable evidence that up to 80% of HCC worldwide is caused by chronic infection with HBV. Thus, the highest rates are found in areas where HBV is endemic and where infection occurs at a very early age. Risk factors for HCC include male gender, a family history of HCC, older age, cirrhosis, infection with HBV genotype C, presence of core promoter variants (see section on variants later in the chapter) and coinfection with HCV.

While only 5% of patients with cirrhosis develop HCC, between 60% and 90% of patients with HCC have underlying cirrhosis. Thus, a proportion of HCC occurs in the absence of cirrhosis. The prolonged presence (>40 years) of HBeAg and high levels of HBV DNA are independent risk factors for HCC. Integration of viral DNA is a possible mechanism of carcinogenesis as HBV DNA is often integrated in tumour cells, but the site differs in different tumours. HCC could be prevented by vaccination. Experience from Taiwan, which has a high prevalence of both HBV infection and HCC, demonstrated that the introduction of universal childhood vaccination against HBV is effective in reducing the incidence of HCC in young adults.

HBV VARIANTS

The frequency with which mutations appear in HBV is related to the high rate of replication of the virus and its dependence on replicating DNA via RNA and an RNA-dependent DNA polymerase. In highly viraemic individuals, as many as 10^{10} mutant genomes may arise each day. Most mutants are defective, but some may explain treatment failure or breakthrough infection.

HBsAg variants

HBsAg variants arise as an escape mechanism during infection in the presence of anti-HBs. In babies exposed to maternal virus during birth given hyperimmune hepatitis B globulin (HBIG) and active immunisation to reduce the risk of infection, the immune selection pressure from the HBIG and vaccine may result in the selection of HBsAg escape mutants. This is seen particularly in countries where universal childhood HBV vaccination has been practised for many years, leading to breakthrough infection despite vaccination. Another scenario where immune selection pressure is intense is following liver transplantation for chronic hepatitis B. Immune selection pressure is exerted through the posttransplantation use of HBIG to protect the new liver from being reinfected with HBV.

HBsAg escape mutants mainly affect the 'a' determinant of HBsAg, the principal target of anti-HBs. The most common mutation observed is in position 145 of the *HBsAg* gene with an amino acid change from glycine to arginine (G145R). HBsAg escape mutants are transmissible, and the widespread occurrence of HBsAg mutants would create considerable problems for the hepatitis B vaccination programme. In addition, many existing diagnostic assays for HBsAg use specific monoclonal antibodies that detect epitopes associated with the 'a' determinant. The presence of such mutations could lead to false negative diagnostic results when the monoclonal antibodies fail to bind to the mutated epitopes. Some cases of so-called occult HBV infection are in fact due to false negative HBsAg, with detectable HBV DNA and no detectable antigenaemia.

HBcAg variants

Mutations in the core promoter or pre-core coding regions of the core antigen open reading frame suppress the production of HBeAg, without affecting the synthesis of HBcAg and the assembly of complete virions. In the pre-core mutation variant, a stop codon is introduced between the initiation codons of HBeAg and HBcAg so that full-length HBeAg is no longer produced, but the production of HBcAg is unaffected. Individuals with these mutations are HBeAg negative but positive for HBV DNA. The absence of expression of HBeAg in such mutants is also believed to be an escape phenomenon enabling the virus to survive the cell-mediated immune selection pressure from the host during the immune clearance phase. Core promoter mutations have been associated with the development of HCC in some studies.

Polymerase variants

These are detected during therapy with nucleoside analogues and confer drug resistance. Their presence can affect the choice of drugs. The most well-recognised mutation affecting the drug lamivudine is a change from methionine to valine or isoleucine at position 204 (M204V/I). This is often accompanied by another change at position 180 (L180M), which helps to maintain viral fitness and continuing replication. In HBV-infected patients who receive a liver transplantation, antiviral prophylaxis is often given together with HBIG. Because the polymerase gene and the surface gene in HBV share the same region of the genome, although read in a different reading frame, mutations in the polymerase gene could force a mutation in the surface gene and vice versa. This could lead to complicated selections of mutants affecting both HBsAg and HBV polymerase.

LABORATORY INVESTIGATION

The laboratory can test for a wide range of HBV antigens and antibodies, using immunoassays based on enzyme reactivity (EIA) or chemiluminescence (CLIA). HBV DNA can be quantified in serum or plasma using real-time polymerase chain reaction (PCR) assays. The standard screening test is for HBsAg, which, if present in the serum, indicates that the patient is currently infected with HBV. The source of chronic infection is intrahepatocytic cccDNA, which is difficult to measure. Recently, the quantitative serum HBsAg level has been used as a surrogate marker of the level of cccDNA, with a high level correlating with the high replicative/low inflammatory phase and a low level associated with the low replicative phase.

ACUTE INFECTION

HBV DNA is the first detectable HBV marker in an acute infection, followed shortly by HBsAg (Fig. 42.5), and both are present for some weeks before the onset of symptoms. In patients who have rapid viral clearance, antigenaemia is of short duration and may no longer be detectable at the onset of symptoms. If successive serum samples are examined, the development of anti-HBs will confirm recent primary infection, although there is considerable variation in the appearance of this antibody. HBV DNA may remain positive after disappearance of HBsAg. This creates the so-called window period when an individual is HBsAg negative but remains infectious. In such cases, detection of IgM anti-HBc indicates that a primary infection has occurred recently.

HBeAg is produced when virus is replicating and thus is usually found soon after HBsAg. IgM anti-HBc is a transient response and, if present in high titre, indicates a recent acute infection. Early disappearance of HBeAg and replacement with anti-HBe is a good prognostic sign

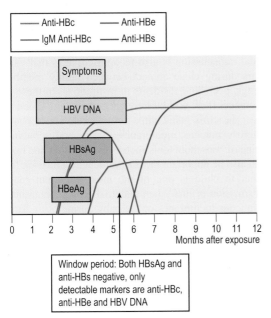

Anti-HBc   Anti-HBe
IgM Anti-HBc   Anti-HBs

Symptoms

HBV DNA

HBsAg

HBeAg

0   1   2   3   4   5   6   7   8   9   10   11   12
Months after exposure

Window period: Both HBsAg and
anti-HBs negative, only
detectable markers are anti-HBc,
anti-HBe and HBV DNA

Fig. 42.5 HBV antigens, antibodies and DNA in a patient recovering from acute infection.

for recovery. The presence of anti-HBs, occurring in about 90% of individuals after HBsAg clearance, indicates the development of immunity to further infection with HBV.

CHRONIC INFECTION

Chronic infection with HBV is defined by the presence of HBsAg for more than 6 months. During this time, IgM anti-HBc is replaced with IgG anti-HBc, although in some individuals with chronic active infection, IgM anti-HBc may persist at a low level. HBeAg remains detectable during the high replicative/low inflammatory and immune clearance phases. It is replaced by anti-HBe either following successful immune clearance into the low replicative phase or the development of HBeAg negative mutants during chronic HBeAg negative hepatitis B. These two possible outcomes can be recognised by testing for HBV DNA levels. Chronic inactive HBV infection has a persistent low HBV DNA viral load, whereas chronic HBeAg negative HBV infection often has fluctuating levels of HBV DNA at moderate to high levels.

TREATMENT

The management of acute hepatitis B is usually supportive. Those with fulminant liver failure following acute infection or end-stage liver failure following chronic infection may be candidates for liver transplantation.

The goal of treatment for chronic hepatitis B is to suppress HBV replication, prevent the progression of liver disease and thereby the development of cirrhosis, liver failure and HCC. Patients in the high replicative/low inflammatory phase with high HBV DNA levels but normal ALT are not candidates for antiviral therapy. Instead, they should be monitored closely at 3–6-monthly intervals. Patients who have low replicative infection do not need antiviral treatment. For those who need treatment, the choice is between a course of interferon or long-term suppression with nucleoside or nucleotide analogues.

Interferon alpha (α-IFN) is the first-line treatment option for patients without cirrhosis. Interferon has antiviral, antiproliferative and immunomodulatory effects. However, its efficacy is limited and only benefits a small proportion of patients. The current strategy is to use long-acting pegylated interferon α for a finite duration of 24–48 weeks. In HBeAg positive individuals, a high pretreatment ALT level, high histological activity score on liver biopsy, low HBV DNA levels and infection with genotype A or B, rather than C or D, are favourable prognostic indicators of treatment response. Seroconversion from HBeAg to anti-HBe occurs in approximately 30%, but <10% eventually clear HBsAg. Response in HBeAg negative disease is much less predictable and often requires a longer duration of therapy. Side effects are common and include influenza-like symptoms, neutropenia, thrombocytopenia, autoimmune thyroid disorders and psychiatric symptoms such as depression. An exacerbation of hepatitis is common, which is often a favourable indication of a subsequent response. However, in some patients, particularly those with existing cirrhosis, this can lead to hepatic decompensation. Increasingly, quantitative HBsAg level is used to guide interferon therapy. Those who show a significant decline in HBsAg level within 12 weeks of therapy are advised to continue, whereas those showing no decline in level are advised to stop.

Nucleoside or nucleotide analogues act as a false substrate after phosphorylation in infected hepatocytes and are incorporated into the growing DNA chains resulting in premature chain termination of HBV DNA synthesis. Lamivudine is a first-generation nucleoside analogue in widespread use for some years. At a dose of 100 mg daily, lamivudine leads to a marked reduction or elimination of detectable HBV DNA in plasma in about 40% of HBeAg-positive and 60%–70% of HBeAg-negative patients. Between 40% and 60% of patients have ALT normalisation. Although toxicity is low, and in the long term the drug is generally tolerated well, prolonged administration is complicated by the emergence of antiviral resistance, manifested by the reappearance of HBV DNA in plasma and raised ALT levels after initial normalisation. Development of resistance-associated mutations in the polymerase enzyme, particularly that of M204V/I, is common and can be detected in 14%–32% after 1 year and increases to 60%–70% after 5 years of treatment. Resistance is more frequent in those who are immunosuppressed. Because of the rapid development of high-level resistance, lamivudine is now rarely used as a first-line therapeutic agent. Instead, it is increasingly being used as a short-term prophylactic agent to prevent HBV reactivation in the immunosuppressed.

Telbuvidine is an L-nucleoside analogue with potent anti-HBV activity. It is similar to lamivudine in mechanism of action and resistance profile but is more potent. However, its use is limited because of a high rate of resistance and cross-resistance with lamivudine. Emtricitabine is another L-nucleoside analogue with similar activity to that of lamivudine.

Adefovir is a nucleotide analogue of deoxyadenosine monophosphate that has demonstrated efficacy in suppressing HBV DNA (20%–50%) and normalising liver function (50%–70%). Resistance to adefovir emerges less frequently than lamivudine, and adefovir is effective against lamivudine-resistant mutants. However, adefovir is not a very potent agent, and its use is now mostly superseded by newer antiviral agents such as entecavir and tenofovir.

Entecavir is a carbocyclic analogue of 2′ deoxyguanosine. It is a potent suppressor of HBV replication, resulting in loss of serum HBV DNA in 70%–90% and ALT normalisation in 70%–80% of patients. However, it is partially susceptible to the resistance-associated mutations selected by lamivudine. Hence, a higher dose (1 mg instead of 0.5 mg) is required in the presence of lamivudine resistance. Development of full resistance to entecavir requires a two-hit mechanism with initial selection of M204V/I followed by several entecavir-specific mutations. As a result, treatment failure due to entecavir resistance is rare and is observed only in 3.6% of patients after 96 weeks of treatment. Entecavir-resistant HBV is susceptible to adefovir or tenofovir.

Tenofovir is a nucleotide analogue initially approved for the treatment of HIV. It is often used in a coformulation with emtricitabine. Though structurally similar to adefovir, it is less nephrotoxic. After 48 weeks of therapy with tenofovir, HBV DNA loss is achieved in 80%–90% and ALT normalisation in 70%–80% of patients. So far, very little resistance against tenofovir has been described. It is necessary to monitor renal function, and tenofovir is contraindicated in patients with renal insufficiency. The combination of tenofovir with lamivudine or emtricitabine is often used in HIV/HBV coinfection in order to treat both viruses.

EPIDEMIOLOGY

HBV is present in the blood as well as in body fluids such as semen, vaginal secretions and saliva. The presence of HBV in blood underlines the original association of infection with blood transfusion or the use of blood products and infections associated with needlestick injuries. Sexual transmission is also recognised, as is that which occurs during close contact between family members, siblings, peers and residents in institutions. In these circumstances there will be frequent contact with blood and saliva; the virus gains entry through cuts and abrasions or across mucous membranes. Biting and scratching, sharing of household tools such as toothbrushes and razors could also be important factors. Vertical transmission from mother to child is one of the most important routes. Transmission occurs when maternal blood contaminates the mucous membranes of the baby during birth. Transplacental infection is thought to be quite rare unless maternal viral load is very high.

The World Health Organization (WHO) has categorised three levels of HBV endemicity, high ($\geq$8%), intermediate (2%–7%) and low (<2%), based on the local prevalence of HBsAg. High-prevalence regions include Sub-Saharan Africa, most of Asia and the Pacific Islands. Intermediate-prevalence regions include the Amazon, southern parts of Eastern and Central Europe, the Middle East and the Indian sub-continent. Low-prevalence regions include most of Western Europe and North America. Overall, it is estimated that one-third of the world's population has been infected with HBV and that 248 million individuals worldwide are chronically infected. Of these, between 15% and 40% will develop serious sequelae in their lifetime. In areas of low endemicity, the risk of infection varies widely in different groups according to behaviour. Most cases occur in parenteral drug injectors sharing needles and syringes and by sexual transmission both homosexual and heterosexual. Screening of all blood donations using HBsAg and HBV DNA has virtually eliminated transmission by transfusion and blood products.

Health-care personnel and laboratory workers are at risk of HBV infection through exposure to blood and body fluids of infected patients, although the degree of risk varies with the place and nature of their work, the care with which it is performed and their immune status. High-risk occupations include surgery, dental surgery, obstetrics and gynaecology, which involve working with sharp instruments, often in restricted spaces. Operators may injure themselves and inoculate patients' blood. The spilling of a patient's blood will pose a threat only if there is contamination of unprotected abraded skin (intact skin is resistant to HBV penetration) or mucous membranes.

Patients are also at risk from staff, and episodes have been identified in which health-care workers have transmitted HBV to their patients during invasive procedures, especially in difficult operations where the operator's hands are hidden and needles and instruments are guided by touch (exposure-prone procedures).

CONTROL

Broadly, there are two approaches to the prevention of infection with HBV—modification of risk behaviour and immunisation. Measures for the former include avoiding unprotected sexual contact by the use of condoms and reducing needle sharing among injecting drug users through needle exchange schemes. Implementation of sensible infection control policies can reduce the risks considerably to health-care workers and patients. It is essential that blood for transfusion and organ donors for transplantation are screened.

Passive immunization

HBIG is prepared from donors with high titres of anti-HBs. Doses of 200–500 IU in 2–4 mL are given intramuscularly. The use of HBIG is indicated in the following situations:

- After accidental exposure if the victim is not vaccinated, or did not respond to the vaccine.
- Babies born to infected mothers (in conjunction with active immunisation).
- To prevent infection of a new liver transplanted into a recipient with chronic HBV infection.

HBIG must be given as soon as possible after exposure and preferably within 48 hours; a second dose is given 4 weeks later to those who do not respond to current vaccines. Such a regimen does not give absolute protection, but an efficacy of 76% has been reported. In cases of needlestick injuries, if the victim has not been vaccinated, HBIG should be used and a course of active immunisation started, injecting the two materials into different body sites. To prevent mother-to-child transmission of HBV, where the mother is highly infectious—for example, the mother is HBeAg positive or HBV DNA viral load >1 million IU/mL—a combination of HBIG with active immunisation given to the baby within 24 hours of birth is effective in as much as 90% of cases.

Active immunisation

Currently available vaccines are produced by cloning the surface antigen gene in yeast cells. The product is particulate and resembles the small particles seen in patients, although it is not glycosylated. The vaccine is administered with alum as adjuvant and injected intramuscularly; care should be taken to avoid injection into fat as this can reduce seroconversion rates. For this reason, injection into the deltoid muscle of the upper arm is recommended. The vaccine is free from major side effects; local swelling and reddening may occur in up to one in five recipients, with a slight fever in only a few cases.

Three doses of vaccine are given at 0, 1 and 6 months. Shorter schedules may be appropriate in some circumstances. The seroconversion rate is influenced by a number of factors, the most important of which are the age and sex of the vaccinee. Rates in excess of 95% are seen in young women, whereas the rate may drop to 80% in older men. Immunosuppressed patients show even lower rates—for example, only 50%–60% in patients on maintenance dialysis.

The duration of the response to vaccine is variable and dependent on the titre of anti-HBs after completion of the course. A postvaccination anti-HBs level >10 mIU/mL is considered as protective. However, to ensure a higher level of protection, a booster dose is often recommended if the anti-HBs level taken within 2–3 months after the third dose is <100 mIU/mL. If no response is detected (i.e., <10 mIU/mL), a vaccine course of three further doses should be given. A vaccine nonresponder is defined as an individual who fails to develop immunity after two vaccine courses. Such individuals are not protected and must seek prophylaxis by passive immunisation if they suffer accidental exposure. Those who are known to have responded can be given a booster if they are exposed to the virus. Some individuals show a drop in antibody level with time, but memory B cells will become activated on exposure to the virus and will provide sufficient protection against infection or at least to prevent the development of chronic infection.

Who should be immunised?

Transmission from mother to child is an important route and requires intervention at birth (within 24 hours) to protect the child. As most babies infected at birth will become chronically infected, it is essential to target this group. Dependent on the infectiousness of the mother, combined passive and active immunisation or active immunisation alone can be used. WHO has recommended universal childhood vaccination against HBV. Many countries have now incorporated this into their childhood vaccination programmes.

In the absence of a universal vaccination programme, the following groups should be targeted for HBV vaccination:

- Occupational risk groups: All health-care workers who may have direct contact with patients' blood or body fluids, including doctors, nurses, cleaners, laboratory workers and paramedics. Other occupational risk groups such as police, fire and prison service staff, military personnel, morticians and embalmers.
- Babies of chronically infected mothers

- Injecting drug users
- Individuals who change sexual partners frequently
- Close family contacts and sexual partners of a case
- Families adopting children from endemic countries and foster carers
- Individuals with learning difficulties living in long-stay homes
- Patients needing frequent transfusions and/or blood products
- Patients with chronic renal failure
- Patients with chronic liver disease (not related to HBV infection)
- Inmates of custodial institutions
- Long-stay travellers to endemic countries

THE DELTA AGENT (HEPATITIS D VIRUS, HDV)

The delta (δ) antigen was first identified in the late 1970s. Initially, it was thought to be an antigen of HBV, but it is part of another virus that cannot replicate without assistance from HBV. The specific helper function provided by HBV is its surface antigen, HBsAg, which also serves as the outer envelope of hepatitis D virus (HDV). HDV is a small (35–37 nm), enveloped particle containing a single, small, circular molecule of RNA of 1.7 kilobase pairs with an internal δ antigen enveloped by HBsAg (Fig. 42.2). The origin of the virus is unknown, and it has no homology with HBV. It has some resemblance with the satellite viruses of plants. However, it is also possible that the circular RNA of HDV is derived from an aberrant splicing event in human cells.

CLINICAL FEATURES AND PATHOGENESIS

HDV can only infect simultaneously with HBV (coinfection) or as a superinfection of an individual chronically infected with HBV. Coinfection has a better prognosis than superinfection, which often results in increase in severity of the chronic hepatitis with increased risk of developing cirrhosis, liver failure and HCC.

DIAGNOSIS

Tests are available for HDV antigen, antibody and RNA. The sequence of appearance of the various markers in a patient coinfected with HBV and HDV is shown in Fig. 42.6. The initial antibody to HDV is IgM. In cases of superinfection, the test results are as illustrated in Fig. 42.7. During the episode there may be a drop in the HBsAg

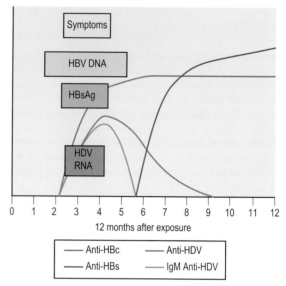

Fig. 42.6 Typical serological profile of simultaneous HBV and HDV coinfection.

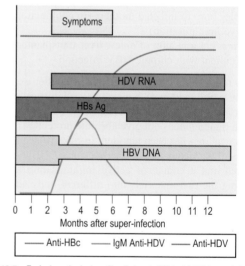

Fig. 42.7 Typical serological profile of chronic HBV with HDV superinfection.

titre, which, although usually still detectable, may disappear temporarily in a few cases. This can cause some diagnostic confusion. There may also be a reduction in HBV DNA levels, which may result in a false assurance that the HBV infection is not active if HDV superinfection is not recognised.

EPIDEMIOLOGY

There are an estimated 25 million HDV-infected individuals in the world, but there is considerable geographical variation. Analysis of the RNA from different isolates has shown that there are at least eight different genotypes. Genotype 1 is of worldwide distribution; genotype 3 is found in the Amazon region; genotypes 2 and 4 in the Far East; and genotypes 5–8 in Sub-Saharan Africa.

In the 1980s, it was thought that HDV was mainly associated with drug users and that controlling HBV through HBV vaccination or needle exchange schemes would be effective in eliminating HDV infection. There was an initial decrease in the prevalence of HDV in Europe, but more recently, it is increasingly recognised that HDV is not disappearing. Intravenous drug use is still an important factor, but it is no longer the sole driver of HDV spread. Immigrants from regions endemic for both HBV and HDV, such as Eastern Europe and Sub-Saharan Africa, now constitute a higher proportion of infected cases in many cities. Despite having the highest prevalence of chronic HBV infection, the prevalence of HDV in Southeast Asia and China is very low.

TREATMENT AND CONTROL

The only proven treatment of HDV infection is a prolonged course of pegylated interferon. However, this is not particularly successful as the sustained response rate after 48 weeks of treatment is <30%. There is no benefit in adding ribavirin or nucleos(t)ide analogues against HBV. The same general control measures as for HBV are also relevant for the control of HDV. HBV vaccine will prevent HDV coinfection, but there is no means of protecting against HDV superinfection.

RECOMMENDED READING

European Association for the Study of the Liver. (2017). EASL 2017 Clinical practice guidelines on the management of hepatitis B infection. *Journal of Hepatology, 67*(2), 370–398. doi:10.1016/j.jhep.2017.03.021.

Schweitzer, A., Horn, J., Mikolajczyk, R. T., Krause, G., & Ott, J. J. (2015). Estimations of worldwide prevalence of chronic hepatitis B virus infection: a systematic review of data published between 1965 and 2013. *Lancet, 386*(10003), 1546–1555. doi:10.1016/S0140-6736(15)61412-X.

Seeger, C., Zoulim, F., & Mason, W. S. (2013). Hepadnaviruses. In D. M. Knipe & P. M. Howley (Eds.), *Field's virology* (Ch. 68). Philadelphia: Lippincott–Raven.

Taylor, J. M., Purcell, R. H., & Farci, P. (2013). Hepatitis D. In D. M. Knipe & P. M. Howley (Eds.), *Field's virology* (Ch. 69). Philadelphia: Lippincott–Raven.

Trépo, C., Chan, H. L., & Lok, A. (2014). Hepatitis B virus infection. *Lancet, 384*(9959), 2053–2063. doi:10.1016/S0140-6736(14)60220-8.

Websites

Department of Health. Immunisation against infectious disease: *The Green Book.* Ch. 18. Hepatitis B. Retrieved from https://www.gov.uk/government/uploads/system/uploads/attachment_data/file/503768/2905115_Green_Book_Chapter_18_v3_0W.PDF. (Accessed Jul 2017).

NICE guidelines CG165: Hepatitis B (chronic): diagnosis and management. Retrieved from https://www.nice.org.uk/Guidance/cg165. (Accessed Jul 2017).

Parvoviruses

B19 infection; erythema infectiosum

KEVIN E. BROWN

DESCRIPTION

Parvoviruses (parvum means small) have been isolated from a wide range of organisms, from arthropods to human beings. The family Parvoviridae is divided into two subfamilies: the Parvovirinae and the Densovirinae. The latter group infects only invertebrates. The Parvovirinae contain eight genera: *Amdoparvovirus, Aveparvovirus, Bocaparvovirus, Copiparvovirus, Dependoparvovirus, Erythroparvovirus, Protoparvovirus* and *Tetraparvovirus* (Table 43.1). They are differentiated by the sense of the single-stranded DNA, genomic organisation and replication strategy.

- Autonomous *(Protoparvovirus)*
- Requirement for a helper virus *(Dependoparvovirus)*
- Preferential replication in erythroid progenitor cells *(Erythroparvovirus)*

Parvovirus B19 (B19V) within the genus *Erythroparvovirus* was the first member of the Parvovirinae shown to be a human pathogen. Human bocaviruses *(Bocaparvovirus)* are a probable cause of some cases of lower respiratory tract infections in children. Although adeno-associated viruses (within the genus *Dependoparvovirus*), human parvovirus 4 *(Tetraparvovirus)*, Bufavirus and Tusavirus (both members of *Protoparvovirus*) can be detected in human beings at various sites, they have not been linked definitely with human disease. The rest of this chapter will confine itself to human parvovirus B19.

The B19 virion (Fig. 43.1) is 20–25 nm in diameter, nonenveloped and contains a single strand of DNA (5.6 kilobases). There are two capsid proteins, VP1 and VP2. B19 is genetically and antigenically stable with only one serotype and is extremely resistant to lipid solvents, acid, alkali and high salt concentrations. It is relatively heat resistant, as infectivity from clotting factor concentrates with high B19 viral loads can persist even after treatment at 80°C for 72 hours. The name *B19* was given because it was first found in the blood of an asymptomatic blood donor (coded 19 in panel B) where it caused a false positive result in an early test for hepatitis B surface antigen.

EPIDEMIOLOGY

B19 infection is common and worldwide in distribution. Serological studies indicate that infection is most commonly acquired between 4 and 10 years of age, and by 15 years approximately 50% of children have antibody. Infection occurs throughout adulthood and up to 90% of elderly people are seropositive.

B19 virus infections are endemic throughout the year in temperate climates, with a seasonal increase in frequency in late winter, spring and early summer months. There are also longer term cycles of infection, with a periodicity of about 4–5 years. Most infections are transmitted by close contact by the respiratory route, with a seroconversion rate of 20%–30% for day-care personnel in close contact with infected children. Asymptomatic blood donors with

Table 43.1 Taxonomic organisation of Parvoviridae, their natural hosts and the diseases they cause

Subfamily	Genus	Virus	Host	Disease
Densovirinae	Four genera	Densonucleosis viruses	Arthropods	Many fatal diseases
Parvovirinae	*Amdoparvovirus*	Aleutian disease virus	Mink	Pneumonitis
	Aveparvovirus	Chicken parvovirus	Chickens	
	Bocaparvovirus	Bovine parvovirus 1	Cattle	Mild gastroenteritis
		Human bocaviruses 1-4	Humans	Respiratory illness
	Copiparvovirus	Bovine parvovirus 2	Cattle	Not known
	Dependoparvovirus	Adeno-associated viruses	Humans and others	Unknown
	Erythroparvovirus	Human parvovirus B19	Humans	Transient aplastic crisis, erythema infectiosum/fifth disease, foetal hydrops
		Simian parvovirus	Monkey	Anaemia
	Protoparvovirus	Minute virus of mice	Mice	Subclinical
		Feline panleucopenia virus	Cats	Enteritis, leucopenia, cerebellar ataxia
		Canine parvovirus I	Dog, fox	Enteritis, myocarditis
		Porcine parvovirus	Pigs	Reproductive failure
		Bufavirus	Humans	Not known
		Tusavirus	Humans	Not known
	Tetraparvovirus	Human parvovirus 4	Humans	Not known

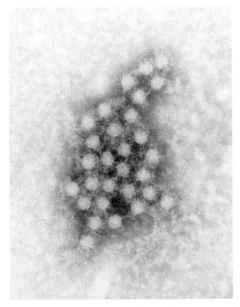

Fig. 43.1 B19 particles in an immune electron microscopy preparation of serum from a child with a petechial rash and arthritis (original magnification ×200,000). (Courtesy Dr Hazel Appleton, Public Health England, London.)

high viral loads enable transmission by blood or blood products, and the stability and heat resistance of B19 enable transmission by heat-treated factor VIII and IX to haemophiliacs. Although individual blood samples are not routinely tested, directives in Europe and the United States require screening of pooled blood products to reduce the risk of transmission through pooled products.

REPLICATION

The parvovirus B19 genome is a single strand of DNA of either sense (i.e., positive or negative), with long (365 nucleotide) repeats at each end. Parvoviruses encode no DNA polymerase, and so replication requires either host or helper virus polymerase activity. B19V is highly erythrotropic and thus requires actively dividing erythroid progenitor cells in S-phase of cell division for efficient replication. Replication is initiated at the terminal hairpins through a process known as rolling hairpin replication. Transcription of mRNA, DNA replication and assembly all occur in the cell nucleus, and infected cells typically have intranuclear inclusions and marginated chromatin (Fig. 43.2). Expression of the non-structural protein, essential for transcription of the capsid proteins, also induces cellular apoptosis, cytolysis and viral release.

PATHOGENESIS

The clinical manifestations of B19V infection are due to either the direct effect of viral replication, which causes cell death, or the subsequent immune response. B19V attaches to cells through the blood group P antigen (globoside), and rare individuals who lack P antigen (p phenotype) are not susceptible to B19V infection. P antigen is present on mature erythrocytes, erythroid progenitors, megakaryocytes, vascular endothelium, placental cells and foetal myocardial and liver cells. Because of the requirement for actively dividing cells, the cells most affected by B19V are the rapidly dividing erythroid precursors in the bone marrow (or in the foetal liver). The outcomes

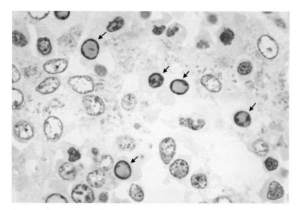

Fig. 43.2 Foetal liver (haematoxylin and eosin stain) from foetal hydrops showing characteristic B19-infected erythroblasts *(arrows)* with intranuclear inclusions and marginated chromatin. (Courtesy Dr Elizabeth Gray, Pathology, Aberdeen Royal Infirmary.)

of infection depend on the immune competence and any red cell–related haematological dysfunction in the infected person. Development of antibody is needed to control B19V replication; capsid protein VP1 is the target for neutralising antibody. After recovery, immunity is lifelong in normal individuals. Persistent and sometimes relapsing infection occurs in the immunocompromised as the little antibody they may produce in response to infection is not capable of neutralising the virus and controlling the infection. Persistent infection can also develop in the foetus, the maternal viraemia giving ample opportunity for infection of the placenta and foetus. Reinfection may occur but is associated with illness only in the immunosuppressed.

Experimental infection of healthy volunteers has revealed the steps in the pathogenesis of B19V infection (Fig. 43.3). The virus is infectious when given in nasal drops. One week later there is an intense viraemia with infectious

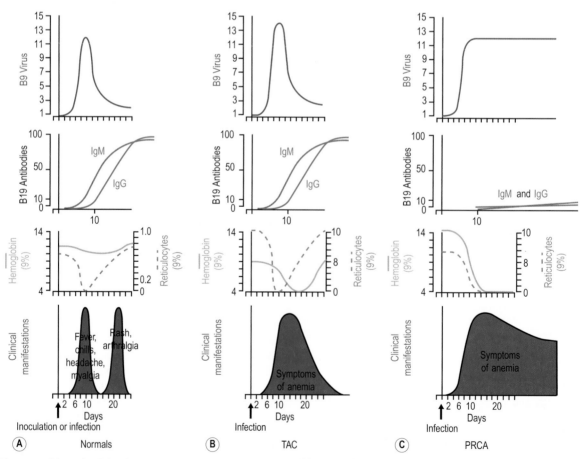

Fig. 43.3 Schematic of the time course of parvovirus B19V infection in (A) normals (erythema infectiosum), (B) transient aplastic crisis (TAC), and (C) chronic anemia/pure red cell aplasia (PRCA). (Reprinted with permission from Young and Brown, 2004. © 2004 Massachusetts Medical Society. All rights reserved.)

virus also present in respiratory secretions but not in faeces or urine. At this time, a febrile influenza-like illness may occur, thought to be cytokine induced. The intense viraemia (up to 10^{14} IU [or genome equivalents] per mL) lasts for only a few days before there is a brisk antibody response, initially of the immunoglobulin (Ig) M class, but followed rapidly by the appearance of IgG antibody, and a drop in the viral load. B19V viral loads of $>10^4$ IU/mL generally persist for 3–6 months, but lower levels of viraemia may be detectable for years following acute infection.

Haematological changes take place in the second week after inoculation. At 10 days after inoculation erythroid precursors are absent from the bone marrow, and reticulocytes disappear from the peripheral blood; there is a small subclinical fall in the haemoglobin level. Lymphocyte, neutrophil and platelet counts sometimes fall transiently, but this is not due to lack of precursors in the bone marrow. Haematological changes are the direct result of virus-induced cell death of erythroid progenitor cells in bone marrow with interruption of erythrocyte production. No effect on the precursor cells of the myeloid series is observed.

The rash and arthralgia associated with B19V infection occur in infected volunteers during the third week after inoculation and occur as the immune response becomes detectable. Similar symptoms are seen in immunosuppressed patients treated with immunoglobulin and are assumed to be immune mediated.

CLINICAL FEATURES

There is a wide spectrum of clinical consequences of B19V infection, depending on the haematological and immune competency of the individual (Table 43.2).

Minor illness or subclinical infection

Asymptomatic or mild infection can occur at any age. In children this accounts for about half of all infections. A nonspecific febrile respiratory tract illness is common at the viraemic phase; it is usually mild but may mimic influenza.

Rash illness

In healthy individuals, B19V can cause erythematous, macular or maculopapular or, less commonly, purpuric rashes. In its most distinct form the erythematous rash is called erythema infectiosum or slapped cheek syndrome, so called because of the intense erythema of the cheeks (Fig. 43.4). Rash illness is most common in children aged 4–11 years and is sometimes called fifth disease, as it was the fifth of six erythematous rash illnesses of childhood in an old classification. Classically, it starts with facial erythema, followed by a maculopapular rash of the trunk and limbs. It lasts only a day or two, although transient recurrences may occur over 1–3 weeks. It may be exacerbated when the individual is hot—for example, after exercise or a hot bath—and may be itchy. As it spreads out, there may be central clearing of the erythema, which can give a lacy or reticular appearance (Fig. 43.5). There may be associated lymphadenopathy and joint symptoms.

Even during a community outbreak of slapped cheek syndrome, clinical diagnosis is unreliable as the illness can be very similar to rubella (where arthropathy and lymphadenopathy may also occur), HHV 6 or enterovirus infection. Cheek erythema is not always prominent, the rash may not appear lacy and it may be on the palms and soles; rarely, there are vesicles. A purpuric rash limited to the hands and feet in a gloves-and-socks distribution with pain, pruritus and oedema can also occur. In the absence of virology tests the most frequent clinical diagnoses made are rubella, allergy and viral illness. Where the rash is purpuric, the platelet count is usually normal, but a transient thrombocytopenia may occur.

Joint disease

Symptoms and signs of joint involvement may occur with or without rash illness, and B19V infection should be considered in the differential diagnosis of acute arthritis. This is more common in adults, especially women, of whom 80% have joint symptoms, compared with about 10% in childhood. Like the rash, the arthropathy is very similar to that seen with rubella, being a symmetrical arthralgia or

Table 43.2 Spectrum of disease due to B19 related to host factors			
Disease	Host	Diagnosis	Treatment
Rash illness (erythema infectiosum, fifth disease, slapped cheek syndrome)	Normal children and adults	IgM	None
Arthralgia	Normal adults	IgM/IgG	Nonsteroidals
Transient aplastic crisis	Patients with increased erythropoiesis	Quantitative PCR	Blood transfusion
Persistent anaemia	Immunocompromised patients	Quantitative PCR	Intravenous immunoglobulin
Congenital anaemia or hydrops	Foetus <20 weeks	Paired serum/ Quantitative PCR	Consider intrauterine blood transfusion

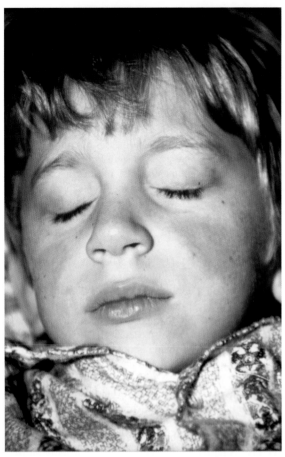

Fig. 43.4 Slapped cheek syndrome. Note the intense cheek erythema and circumoral pallor. (Courtesy Dr Ken Mutton, Medical Microbiology, Manchester Royal Infirmary.)

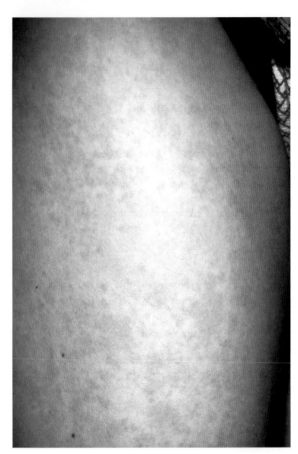

Fig. 43.5 Late stage of B19 rash with central clearing showing lacy appearance.

arthritis involving mainly the small joints of the hands, although feet, wrists, knees, ankles and other joints may be affected. In children, the arthropathy may be less symmetrical. Arthropathy usually resolves within 2–3 weeks but may occasionally persist or recur for months and, very rarely, for years. Some of these patients may be classified clinically as having early benign rheumatoid arthritis. However, B19V arthropathy is not destructive; if rheumatoid factor is detected it does not persist, and B19V virus infection is not causally linked to rheumatoid arthritis.

Transient aplastic crisis (TAC)

This is an acute transient event seen in those with various underlying haematological problems who have a competent immune system:

- decreased red cell survival (e.g., haemolytic disorders)

- where the bone marrow is stressed, for example, because of haemorrhage or iron deficiency anaemia

There is a virtual absence of red blood cell precursors in the bone marrow at the beginning of the crisis, followed by disappearance of reticulocytes from the peripheral blood and a subsequent fall in haemoglobin concentration. The cessation of erythropoiesis lasts for 5–7 days, and patients present with symptoms of acute anaemia, which can be life threatening. Blood transfusion is required, but after a week or so specific antibody production controls viral replication, the bone marrow recovers rapidly, there is a reticulocytosis and the haemoglobin concentration returns to steady-state values.

Throughout the world, B19V infection is responsible for 90% of cases of transient aplastic crisis in those with underlying haemolytic disorders, most commonly in children with, for example, sickle cell anaemia, hereditary spherocytosis or thalassaemia.

Persistent infection in the immunocompromised

The inability to mount an effective neutralising antibody response to B19V results in persistent infection. This has been described in patients with:

- congenital immunodeficiency
- leukaemia
- acquired immune deficiency syndrome (AIDS)
- transplant recipients

The bone marrow picture is typical of that seen in transient aplastic crisis with absent red cell precursors but here results in pure red cell aplasia, ongoing viraemia and a nonspecific febrile illness presenting with symptoms of chronic anaemia or a remitting and relapsing anaemia, without rash or joint disease. Rarely, other lineages in addition to the erythroid lineage may be affected, but B19V is not a cause of aplastic anaemia.

B19V in pregnancy

Although B19V infection can cause foetal loss, most pregnancies result in the birth of a normal baby. Congenital B19V infection is not associated with birth defects, although in very rare cases it has been associated with developmental abnormalities.

Transplacental infection can occur during acute maternal infection, whether or not symptoms of B19V infection occur in the mother, before maternal antibody has developed and crossed the placenta to protect the foetus. Infection in the first 20 weeks can lead to intrauterine death (increased risk 9%) and nonimmunological foetal hydrops (risk 3%), of which about half die and are included in the 9%. This is in contrast to hydrops, which occurs following Rhesus incompatibility and is immune mediated. The greatest risk of foetal loss is during the second trimester.

These effects are due to the immaturity of the foetal immune response and the shorter survival of foetal red cells. The large increase in red cell mass (in both the bone marrow and extramedullary sites of erythropoiesis) during the second trimester leads to the increased risk of developing anaemia at this time. The anaemia persists and becomes chronic because of ongoing viral replication. Infection of foetal myocardial cells can also occur, causing myocarditis. Both the anaemia and the myocarditis contribute to the development of cardiac failure, leading to the development of ascites and foetal hydrops (Fig. 43.6). Foetal loss is usually 4–6 weeks after maternal infection but can be as long as 12 weeks later. Overall, B19V probably accounts for 10% of cases of foetal hydrops. A more effective foetal immune response reduces the risk of foetal loss in the third trimester; very rarely, chronic anaemia in the newborn has followed intrauterine infection.

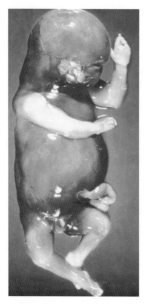

Fig. 43.6 Foetal hydrops due to B19. Note pallor of limbs. In utero autolysis of foetus disguises pallor of body.

Other

In healthy people, case reports suggest that the manifestations of B19V may on occasion be very wide (e.g., meningitis, hepatitis, haemophagocytic syndrome or myocarditis). However, as both IgM and DNA may persist for months, some associations may be casual rather than causal.

DIAGNOSIS (Table 43.2)

Clinical

Although the rash can be characteristic, a diagnosis based on clinical features alone is unreliable. Because of the possible consequences to the foetus, all possible B19V infections in pregnant woman should be confirmed or refuted by laboratory testing.

Cultivation

B19V does not grow in standard tissue culture but only in selected erythro- or megakaryocytic cell lines or primary bone marrow culture. Cell culture does not have a role in clinical diagnosis of B19V infection.

Molecular

During pure red cell aplasia, and the acute illness of transient aplastic crisis, B19V viral loads are high and coincide with haematological changes, so detection of the viral genome in serum by quantitative PCR (calibrated against the WHO standard, and results in IU/mL) is the method of choice. While awaiting B19V quantitation in those with anaemia, the reticulocyte count is a quick test that can be helpful as a low or absent count is consistent with current active B19V infection. A positive qualitative PCR result is unhelpful, as it only indicates a previous B19V infection at some time as B19V DNA can remain detectable for life. B19V viral loads $>10^9$ IU/mL indicate a current infection; viral loads $>10^4$ IU/mL indicate recent infection.

Immunological

In most cases, B19V-specific IgM and IgG is detectable within a day or two of onset of the rash. Once B19V-specific IgM has appeared in the serum, it rapidly reaches peak concentrations and is usually detectable for 2–3 months. B19V IgG antibody usually remains detectable for life. Diagnosis of recent infection can be made by detection of B19V IgM, demonstrating seroconversion or increasing amounts of IgG antibody. As false-positive IgM infections can occur with other rash illness, a good practice is to confirm all B19V IgM-positive results in pregnant women by quantitative PCR as above.

Investigations during pregnancy and infection in the foetus

At booking, all pregnant women should be advised to inform their general practitioner, midwife or obstetrician as soon as they develop a rash, unexplained arthropathy or are in contact with someone with a possible viral rash. Recommendations for investigating a pregnant woman who has had significant contact with possible B19V are summarised in Fig. 43.7. Testing of a current sample for IgG and IgM should be initiated. Comparison to results in a stored blood (e.g., booking sample) taken prior to the contact may also be helpful. Where maternal infection is proven, whether or not symptoms have occurred, obstetric referral for investigations (e.g., foetal ultrasonography) should be arranged without delay as deterioration from early hydrops to intrauterine death can be rapid. Although foetal loss has been documented only with infection up to 20 weeks' gestation, investigation of rash or contact is recommended at any gestation and is also indicated for nonimmune foetal hydrops.

The diagnosis of B19V infection in a foetus is complex. When foetal hydrops is found in an asymptomatic pregnant woman, maternal infection is likely to have occurred some weeks previously, and B19V IgM may not be detectable in the mother. Samples from mother and foetus, if available, should be tested by quantitative

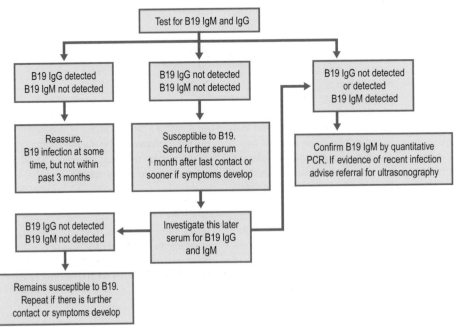

Fig. 43.7 Investigation for B19 in a pregnant woman with significant exposure to rash illness. (Reproduced with modifications with permission of Public Health England, London.)

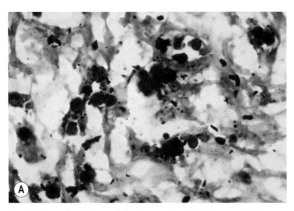
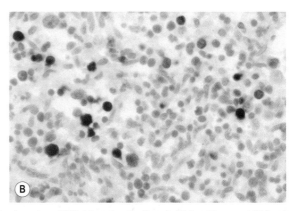

Fig. 43.8   In situ hybridisation using a pool of B19 oligonucleotide probes showing enlarged B19-infected erythroblasts in (A) foetal heart and (B) foetal liver from a fatal case of foetal hydrops. (Courtesy of Professor Heather Cubie, Specialist Virology Centre, Royal Infirmary, Edinburgh.)

PCR. If available, a previously stored blood sample (i.e., booking blood) should be tested in parallel for evidence of seroconversion. Testing of amniotic fluid for B19V DNA can also be informative. Confirmation of infection by testing placental or foetal tissues taken at autopsy can be made by quantitative PCR, in situ hybridisation for B19V DNA on formalin-fixed, paraffin-embedded tissue sections (Fig. 43.8) or immunohistochemistry/immunofluorescence for B19V antigens or by demonstrating characteristic intranuclear inclusions in erythroid precursors (Fig. 43.8).

TREATMENT (Table 43.2)

Most cases of B19V infection are mild and self-limiting, and specific treatment is not required other than symptomatic relief for joint disease. No antiviral drugs are available. However, there are three situations (see Table 43.2) in which severe anaemia occurs as a consequence of B19V infection, and in each of these blood transfusion or intravenous immunoglobulin is indicated. In transient aplastic crisis, blood transfusion tides patients over the relatively short period of erythroid aplasia before the immune response rapidly clears the virus infection. In the immunocompromised there is a failure to produce neutralising antibody, so management consists of a course of intravenous immunoglobulin, with blood transfusion support if needed. This leads to reduction of the viraemia, sometimes accompanied by the development of rash illness. If high-level viraemia recurs ($>10^9$ IU/mL), further immunoglobulin is usually necessary. With infection during pregnancy, termination of pregnancy is not indicated as a foetus that survives B19V infection has a good prognosis. Although spontaneous resolution of hydrops due to B19V with the birth of a healthy baby has been documented, the overall foetal mortality rate is decreased with intrauterine transfusion.

CONTROL

Prevention of disease by isolating susceptible individuals is generally impractical as infections may be subclinical, and symptomatic individuals are infectious before distinctive symptoms appear. In addition, as the rash and arthralgia of B19V infection are caused by immune reactions, not viraemia, those with rash or arthropathy are not infectious. However, susceptible pregnant health-care workers should not care for those with transient aplastic crisis or pure red cell aplasia; those with these manifestations are likely to be infectious. Theoretically, susceptible individuals at risk of significant anaemia (e.g., immunocompromised children) could be protected temporarily by the administration of human immunoglobulin, but this has not been tried. Good hand hygiene should be encouraged.

There is as yet no licensed vaccine against B19V, but recombinant B19V virus–like particles can be produced that induce neutralising antibodies and so are potentially suitable candidates for a human vaccine. At present, screening of at-risk groups is not recommended as vaccine and prophylaxis are not available.

ACKNOWLEDGMENT

The author would like to thank Dr Pam Molyneux who wrote the previous version of this chapter and who provided the information for the case history.

RECOMMENDED READING

Cotmore, S. F., Agbandje-McKenna, M., Chiorini, J., Mukha, D. V., Pintel, D. J., Qiu, J., ... Davison, A. J. (2014). The family Parvoviridae. *Archives of Virology, 159*(5), 1239–1247. doi:10.1007/s00705-013-1914-1.

Crabol, Y., Terrier, B., Rozenberg, F., Pestre, V., Legendre, C., Hermine, O., ... Groupe d'experts de l'Assistance Publique-Hôpitaux de Paris. (2013). Intravenous immunoglobulin therapy for pure red cell aplasia related to human parvovirus b19 infection: a retrospective study of 10 patients and review of the literature. *Clinical Infectious Diseases, 56*(7), 968–977. doi:10.1093/cid/cis1046.

Kerr, J. R., Cotmore, S. F., Bloom, M. E., Linden, R. M., & Parrish, C. R. (Eds.). (2006). *Parvoviruses* (1st ed.). London: Hodder Arnold.

Maple, P. A., Hedman, L., Dhanilall, P., Kantola, K., Nurmi, V., Söderlund-Venermo, M., ... Hedman, K. (2014). Identification of past and recent parvovirus B19 infection in immunocompetent individuals by quantitative PCR and enzyme immunoassays: a dual-laboratory study. *Journal of Clinical Microbiology, 52*(3), 947–956. doi:10.1128/JCM.02613-13.

Schildgen, O. (2013). Human bocavirus: lessons learned to date. *Pathogens, 2*(1), 1–12. doi:10.3390/pathogens2010001.

Söderlund-Venermo, M., Brown, K. E., & Erdman, D. D. (2017). Human parvoviruses. In D. D. Richman, R. J. Whitely, & F. G. Hayden (Eds.), *Clinical virology.* (4th ed.). Washington: American Society for Microbiology Press.

Young, N. S., & Brown, K. E. (2004). Parvovirus B19. *The New England Journal of Medicine, 350*(6), 586–597. doi:10.1056/NEJMra030840.

Website

CDC: Parvovirus B19 and fifth disease. About Parvovirus B19. Retrieved from http://www.cdc.gov/parvovirusb19/about-parvovirus.html. (Accessed Jul 2017).

NHS choices: Slapped cheek syndrome. Retrieved from http://www.nhs.uk/conditions/Slapped-cheek-syndrome/Pages/Introduction.aspx. (Accessed Jul 2017).

Public Health England: Viral rashes in pregnancy. Retrieved from https://www.gov.uk/government/uploads/system/uploads/attachment_data/file/322688/Viral_rash_in_pregnancy_guidance.pdf. (Accessed Jul 2017).

44 Picornaviruses

Meningitis; paralysis; rashes; intercostal myositis; myocarditis; infectious hepatitis; common cold

HELI HARVALA AND INGÓLFUR JOHANNESSEN

KEY POINTS

- Picornaviruses pathogenic for humans belong to the *Enterovirus* (includes the former *Rhinovirus* genus), *Parechovirus* and *Hepatovirus* genera.
- Enteroviruses cause a wide range of diseases including aseptic meningitis, poliomyelitis, encephalitis, maculopapular skin rashes, ulcerative exanthems and myocarditis.
- Rhinoviruses are responsible for the most frequent of all human infections—the common cold.
- There are effective vaccines against polioviruses and hepatitis A virus.
- Enteroviruses are among the most environmentally stable viruses.
- Diagnosis of enterovirus infection now relies on nucleic acid detection.
- New strains of enteroviruses regularly emerge and can cause major epidemics of disease.

The family *Picornaviridae* comprises small (pico) RNA viruses with a diameter of 27–30 nm. It currently consists of 31 genera of which members of the *Enterovirus* (incorporating the former *Rhinovirus* genus), *Parechovirus* and *Hepatovirus* genera are of considerable human importance, resulting in a variety of clinical manifestations including aseptic meningitis, encephalitis, myocarditis, respiratory tract infections, rashes, ulcerative exanthemas, hepatitis and the common cold. The *Enterovirus* genus is divided according to genetic phylogeny into 10 species, from which 7 species *(Enterovirus A–D* and *Rhinovirus A–C)* contain (sero)types known to infect humans (Table 44.1). In the following text, the *Enterovirus A–D* species will be discussed under the heading Enteroviruses and the *Rhinovirus A–C* species under the heading Rhinoviruses.

ENTEROVIRUSES

DESCRIPTION AND CLASSIFICATION

Enteroviruses are known to infect humans primarily via the gut and include polioviruses, coxsackie A and B viruses, echoviruses and chronologically numbered enteroviruses discovered since the 1970s. This traditional subgrouping of enteroviruses was mainly based on human disease manifestation and the pathogenicity of virus isolates in laboratory animals (Table 44.2). The viral etiology of poliomyelitis was discovered in 1909 by Landsteiner and Popper; they induced paralysis in monkeys by inoculation of specimens from two cases of paralytic polio. Forty years later, Dallford and Sickles discovered a second group of enteroviruses when searching for appropriate animal models for polio and isolated a new virus from faecal extracts of two children with paralysis in the town of Coxsackie, New York. These coxsackieviruses were divided into subgroups A and B based on their different pathogenicity in newborn mice. Following the development of cell culture systems, a third group of enteroviruses was isolated from human stool samples. These viruses replicated only in cell cultures and at the time it was uncertain whether they could cause disease in humans. Thus, they were named echoviruses based on the descriptive acronym: *e*nteric (isolated mainly from stool samples), *c*ytopathogenic (in cell culture), *h*uman (no disease in monkeys or newborn mice), *o*rphan (disease association uncertain). Furthermore, it became obvious that all three groups of viruses were antigenically distinct based on laboratory neutralisation assays and that each group consisted of several different serotypes. A total of 3 poliovirus, 23 coxsackie A virus (CAV), 6 coxsackie B virus (CBV) and 28 echovirus serotypes are currently known (Table 44.2).

A new classification system based on the genetic clustering of viruses was proposed in the late 1990s as the traditional enterovirus serotypic differentiation based on

435

neutralisation was shown to correlate with genetic data obtained from the virus protein 1 (VP1) coding region. Based on the phylogenetic analysis of these capsid coding region sequences, enteroviruses are divided into four species, A–D (Table 44.1). The representative species letter is now also included in the virus type name; for example, enterovirus 71 belongs to species A and is called enterovirus A71 (EV-A71). Furthermore, enteroviruses showing >75% nucleotide similarity in the VP1 region belong to the same enterovirus type, whereas those with <70% nucleotide similarity are distinct types.

Composition

The RNA genome is approximately 7500 nucleotides long, single stranded and of positive sense (ss+ve RNA)

Table 44.1 Phylogenetic classification of enteroviruses (n = 116) and rhinoviruses (n = 167) within the genus *Enterovirus* that are known to infect humans

Enterovirus species	(Sero)types known to infect humans
Enterovirus A	Coxsackievirus A2–8, 10, 12, 14, 16 Enterovirus A71, A76, A89–A91, A114, A119–A121
Enterovirus B	Coxsackievirus A9 Coxsackievirus B1–6 Echovirus 1–7, 9, 11–21, 24–27, 29–33 Enterovirus B69, B73–B75, B77–B88, B93, B97–B98, B100–B101, B106–B107, B110–B113
Enterovirus C	Coxsackievirus A1, 11, 13, 17, 19–22, 24 Poliovirus 1–3 Enterovirus C95–C96, C99, C102, C104–C105, C109, C113, C116, C117–C118
Enterovirus D	Enterovirus D68, D70, D94, D111
Rhinovirus A	Rhinovirus A1–A2, A7–A13, A15–A16, A18–A25, A28–A34, A36, A38–A41, A43–A47, A49–A51, A53–A68, A71, A73–A78, A80–A82, A85, A88–A90, A94–A96, A98, A100–A101
Rhinovirus B	Rhinovirus B3–B6, B14, B17, B26–B27, B35, B37, B42, B48, B52, B69–B70, B72, B79, B83–B84, B86, B91–B93, B97, B99
Rhinovirus C	Rhinovirus C1–C55

and, therefore, can be translated directly by host ribosomes to generate viral proteins. It is surrounded by a virus-encoded capsid consisting of a protein shell arranged in icosahedral symmetry around the genomic RNA (together forming the nucleocapsid), the complete sequence of which is now known for most classified types. Four major peptides are recognised in the shell: viral protein (VP) 1, VP2, VP3 and VP4. Specific neutralising antibodies are considered to be the major mechanism of protection against infection. For example, four major antigenic sites on exposed surface loops of the VP1–3 proteins of polio type 3 have been identified. The virus is nonenveloped.

In addition to the properties listed in Table 44.2, all enteroviruses:

- attach to cells of the intestinal tract at specific receptor sites and replicate in the cytoplasm of the intestinal cells
- commonly cause asymptomatic immunising infections, which protect against future infection with the same virus
- occasionally spread to, and infect, the central nervous system (CNS) and other target organs
- cause infections more commonly in children than in adults
- usually cause infections in late summer and early autumn (in temperate climates)

PROPERTIES OF ENTEROVIRUSES

In the presence of moist organic material, enteroviruses:

- survive at room temperature for weeks
- survive at 4°C for months
- are killed at 50–55°C

They are stable in acid pH but rapidly inactivated by 0.3% formaldehyde and solutions giving a free residual chlorine concentration of 0.3–0.5 parts per million (ppm). However, chemical inactivation is ineffective if organic matter is present (e.g., in swimming pools).

Table 44.2 Specific features of polioviruses, coxsackieviruses and echoviruses

Group	No. of serotypes	Growth in MK[a] cells	Pathology in monkeys	Pathology in newborn mice
Poliovirus	3	+	Paralysis	None
Coxsackie A viruses	23	− or −/+	None	Infect striated muscle and cause flaccid paralysis
Coxsackie B viruses	6	+	None	Destroy the pyramidal tracts and cause spastic paralysis
Echoviruses	28	+	None	None

[a]Monkey kidney.

REPLICATION

Knowledge of enterovirus replication is based on studies of poliovirus. Briefly, the ss+RNA genome acts as mRNA for translation of a single precursor polyprotein that is digested at specific sites by internal protease activity giving rise to viral proteins including a viral polymerase and individual proteases. As a pool of viral proteins accumulates, cytoplasmic RNA replication is favoured using the ss+RNA as a template for production of an ss-RNA copy giving rise to a double-stranded RNA (dsRNA) replicative intermediate that acts as a template for the production of further ss+RNA progeny genomes. The capsid coat is assembled as 12 pentamers of the structural VP1–4 proteins around the ss+RNA giving rise to infectious virus (virion). The end of replication is signalled by lysis of the host cell with the release of new progeny virus particles.

CLINICAL FEATURES

The enteroviruses are associated with a wide variety of clinical presentations although the majority of infections are asymptomatic. Many enterovirus types can cause similar clinical disease. The main sites affected are:

- CNS (paralytic poliomyelitis, meningitis, encephalitis), particularly in children; persistent encephalitis may develop in immunocompromised patients
- skin and mucosa (maculopapular rashes, ulcerative exanthem)
- striated muscle (intercostal myositis, myocarditis accompanied by pericarditis)
- respiratory tract (rhinitis, pharyngitis, bronchiolitis, pneumonia)
- eyes (conjunctivitis)

- disseminated neonatal infections can be severe, extensive and occasionally fatal

Maternal infection in pregnancy is not known to be associated with congenital defects. There are additional controversial links between enterovirus infections and chronic fatigue syndrome (unlikely) and the onset of insulin-dependent (type 1) diabetes mellitus (possible); ongoing research aims to clarify the latter association.

Paralytic poliomyelitis

Most poliovirus infections are asymptomatic; up to 10% of infections result in recognisable clinical illness. The virus is excreted in faeces, and an immunological response develops that protects against reinfection with the same strain. Most symptomatic cases present with mild influenza-like or gastrointestinal symptoms (4%–8%). Evidence of CNS involvement with headache, photophobia, neck stiffness and back pain is observed in 1%–2% of infected individuals (10% of those with symptoms); rapid and complete recovery in <10 days is usual.

The most severe outcome of poliovirus infections is acute flaccid paralysis (AFP). All three poliovirus types can cause paralysis (Table 44.3). This occurs in approximately 1 in 1000 poliovirus-infected children (0.1%) and 1 in 75 adults (1.3%). The paralysis is usually flaccid due to destruction of lower motor neurones, but virus invasion of the brainstem can lead to incoordination of muscle groups and painful spasms. Paralysis occurs early in the illness, but the extent is variable; often the paralysis is most severe initially, and some function may return over the next 6 months as inflammation and oedema subside. Damage to nerve cells in the brainstem (bulbar paralysis) can cause dysfunction of vital autonomic centres with the inability to breathe and swallow. The time between infection and the development of paralytic symptoms is usually 14 days but ranges from 3 to 21 days. During this

Table 44.3 Types of polioviruses		
	Wild polioviruses (WPV)	Circulating vaccine-derived poliovirus (cVDPV)
Definition	Infectious virus, which can invade the CNS and cause paralysis, occasionally leading to death	A rare circulating infectious virus, which has mutated from the weakened poliovirus strains used in oral polio vaccine. The longer the virus circulates, the more genetic changes it undergoes. In rare instances, the vaccine virus can genetically change into a form that can paralyse; this is known as a circulating vaccine-derived poliovirus (cVDPV).
Strains	Type 1: Caused all cases in 2015 Type 2: Eradicated in 1999 Type 3: Last case in 2012	Type 1: 20 cases in 2015 Type 2: 12 cases in 2015 Type 3: Rare
Cases in 2015	70	32

period, several factors have an adverse effect on the outcome of infection:

- Increased muscular activity can lead to paralysis of the limbs used, possibly due to enhanced vascularity, either in the limb or the affected area of the spinal cord, allowing increased access of virus to nerve endings.
- Women in the third trimester of pregnancy can suffer severe disease, but there is no known evidence of congenital defects in infants born to mothers with poliomyelitis; maternal infection acquired late in pregnancy may lead to perinatal infection and disease of the newborn.
- Injection of adjuvant-containing vaccines, and irritant substances such as heavy metals, can result in paralysis in the limb(s) that received the inoculation; paralysis develops (incidence 1 in 37,000 injections) when poliovirus is contracted within 1 month of receiving such inoculations.
- Patients who have had their tonsils removed have a higher chance of developing bulbar poliomyelitis, which has been attributed to the reduction of secretory immunoglobulin (Ig) A in the pharynx and, thus, reduced virus neutralisation.

Vaccine-associated paralytic poliomyelitis (VAPP) is caused by a rare complication of oral live-attenuated polio vaccine. During initial replication, the Sabin strains used in the oral poliovirus vaccine (OPV) can revert back to neurovirulent variants, and these can then enter the CNS system and cause paralysis (Table 44.3). VAPP is indistinguishable clinically from polio caused by wild-type polioviruses, occurring in recently vaccinated individuals or in susceptible individuals exposed to vaccine virus indirectly.

Viral meningitis

Viral meningitis occurs most commonly in young children and adults under the age of 40 years. Generally, enteroviruses are the most common cause of meningitis in countries where mumps and bacterial causes have been controlled by vaccination. The incubation period varies from 3 to 5 days. The onset is abrupt, with severe headache and vomiting, and is sometimes associated with a non-specific or maculopapular rash. Symptoms are self-limiting, and after a variable convalescent period, a full recovery is made, although rare cases of paralysis do occur. Patients with enterovirus meningitis have clear cerebrospinal fluid (CSF) and normal or slightly increased pressure; a pleocytosis with increased lymphocyte count is often, but not always, present.

Viral meningitis can be caused by many different enterovirus types, but most commonly by species B

enteroviruses including CBV1-6, CAV9 and echoviruses (notably types 6, 9, 11 and 30). In addition, polioviruses and some species A enteroviruses including EV-A71 have been associated with meningitis. A number of enterovirus types have considerable epidemic potential, but most of the meningitis outbreaks have been associated with echovirus 30. Although these outbreaks are often local, the virus strains associated with new recombinant forms show spread through large geographical areas, often within 1–2 years of their first emergence.

Encephalitis

Enterovirus encephalitis can be associated with viral meningitis or may present without, or with only minimal, meningeal involvement. Typical presentation includes fever, headache, lethargy, drowsiness, acute onset of flaccid muscle weakness, and, in some cases, signs of brainstem dysfunction. Several enterovirus types have been associated with encephalitis, mostly including enteroviruses from species A (EV-A71, EV-A76 and EV-A89) and B (CAV9, CBV5, EV-B75, echovirus 11 and 30).

Neonatal infections

All coxsackie B viruses as well as echoviruses 6, 9 and 11 can cause severe neonatal infections. The virus is probably transmitted during birth, or postnatally, from the (often asymptomatic) mother or nursery attendants. Circulatory collapse, myocarditis, hepatitis and meningoencephalitis may develop, and infection can spread rapidly to other infants in the nursery or special care baby unit. The type of virus circulating in the community at the time is usually implicated.

Epidemic pleurodynia

Epidemic pleurodynia, or Bornholm disease (first described on the Danish island of Bornholm), is characterised by fever and the sudden onset of agonising stitch-like pains in the muscles of the chest, epigastrium or hypochondrium. Although the disease is most frequently recognised in its epidemic form, many sporadic cases occur. Pleurisy and pericarditis may complicate epidemic myalgia, although most cases recover within a week. This disease has been associated mainly with all coxsackie B viruses but also occasionally with CAV9 and echoviruses (notably types 1, 6, 9, 16 and 19).

Myocarditis, pericarditis and dilated cardiomyopathy

In newborn infants, severe and often fatal myocarditis has been reported, and the virus can be found in high concentrations in the myocardium at autopsy. Epidemics have occurred in nurseries when there is evidence of coxsackie B virus activity in a community. Myocarditis and pericarditis can occur in children and adults, and virus has been isolated occasionally from pericardial fluid.

Coxsackie B viruses (CBV1–6) are major causes of human myopericarditis, but this is a difficult diagnosis to confirm. Although severe in the neonate, it tends to follow a more benign course in the adult. The initial symptoms are often of an upper respiratory or influenza-like illness, followed 7–10 days later by clinical heart disease. Chest pain is a feature, and electrocardiographic abnormalities such as tachycardia and arrhythmias have been found. On clinical examination, murmurs, rubs and, occasionally, pericardial effusions are detected.

The myocardial inflammation can persist, leading to chronic myocarditis, which may progress to dilated cardiomyopathy. In dilated cardiomyopathy (also linked to coxsackie B viruses), the function of the enlarged heart is severely impaired, with up to 50% of these patients requiring heart transplantation.

Herpangina

Herpangina is an acute feverish disease with sore throat and pain on swallowing, usually in young children, characterised by (usually small numbers of) lesions in the mouth consisting of papules on the anterior pillars of the fauces, soft palate, uvula, pharynx and tonsils; these papules become vesicles and finally shallow ulcers with a greyish base and punched-out edge. Many species A enteroviruses (notably CAV6, CAV10 and CAV16) are associated with herpangina.

Maculopapular rash

Enterovirus infections, especially those caused by CAV9 and echovirus 9, are often accompanied by a fine maculopapular, rubella-like, rash. Outbreaks may be seen in nurseries and schools.

Hand, foot and mouth disease

Hand, foot and mouth disease (HFMD) presents as a mildly febrile ulcerative exanthem with painful stomatitis and a painful vesicular rash on the hands and/or feet (less frequently on the buttocks and external genitalia). Typically, it lasts about a week; most cases are seen in summer in children aged 1–10 years, but cases can occur in clusters and in families. HFMD has been associated with several enterovirus types, but most commonly with CAV16 and EV-A71, and more recently with CAV6 and CAV10 (all from species A).

Large outbreaks of HFMD caused by EV-A71 have been described in Asia and the Pacific region since the late 1990s. An unexpectedly large outbreak with high mortality was seen in Malaysia in 1997 that was followed by a related outbreak in Taiwan in 1998; since that time, regular epidemics have occurred in the Asia–Pacific region. Although most affected children will develop self-limiting HFMD, a small proportion develop neurological and systemic complications. In the most severe cases, EV-A71 causes a brainstem encephalitis, which is often accompanied by severe cardiorespiratory symptoms. Sporadic cases of severe meningoencephalitis are also seen in Europe, but outbreaks there are rare.

An atypical form of HFMD has been associated with infections caused by CAV6 and CAV10. The first outbreak was described in Finland in 2008; a link between atypical forms of HFMD (also termed eczema coxsackium) and CAV6 was established and these infections have been observed worldwide since that time. These infections are associated with high fever, vesiculobullous eruptions and/or an eczema-form rash affecting the back of the hands and legs, trunk and buttocks (often followed by onychomadesis [nail loss]). Infections often mimic chickenpox and/or disseminated eczema; infected children with pre-existing eczema appear to be predisposed to more severe disease.

Respiratory infections

Respiratory infections caused by enteroviruses vary from mild rhinitis and pharyngitis to more severe bronchiolitis, pneumonia and respiratory failure. Traditionally, species C enteroviruses (CAV21) have been associated with epidemics of rhinitis and pharyngitis in camps of military recruits. In 2014 a large outbreak of EV-D68 causing a severe respiratory infection mainly in children was first noted in the United States and Canada and subsequently in Asia, Europe and South America. EV-D68 (classified as human rhinovirus 87 until 2002) shares physiochemical properties with human rhinoviruses including acid lability, optimal growth at 33°C and isolation primarily from respiratory samples. Most common symptoms include coughing, wheezing and fever that are very similar to those caused by rhinoviruses. Severe respiratory infections caused by EV-D68 are usually seen in children but also in adults with underlying respiratory diseases and/or immunosuppression. Patients suffering severe EV-D68 infection often require hospital admission, and some need even further care, including ventilatory support in an intensive care unit. EV-D68 infections have also been associated with neurological complications, including paralysis. However, EV-D68 is rarely detectable in CSF and stool samples; hence, a respiratory specimen is needed to confirm the diagnosis.

Conjunctivitis

Acute haemorrhagic conjunctivitis (AHC), a highly infectious enterovirus disease, is characterised by sudden onset, periorbital swelling, severe eye pain and subconjunctival haemorrhages. It has a short incubation period of 1–2 days. Although subconjunctival haemorrhage is a complication, most patients recover within 7 days. Neurological complications can occur, including polio-like paralysis. In 1969, outbreaks of AHC caused by EV-D70 spread throughout Africa and Asia; 10 years later, the disease also occurred in the Americas. Species C enterovirus, CAV24, is another identified cause of AHC, first identified in Singapore in 1970. Since that time, it caused a major outbreak affecting more than a million people in South Korea in 2002 and has spread worldwide subsequently.

PATHOGENESIS

Most enterovirus infections follow a similar pattern, as illustrated in Fig. 44.1 for poliovirus, with differences in the target organs (e.g., CNS, skin, heart or muscle). Although the pathogenesis of CBV3 and EV-A71 infections have now been well studied with the support of transgenic animal models, what follows pertains to poliomyelitis.

Virus is ingested and, after multiplication in the lymphoid tissue of the tonsils or Peyer's patches (gut-associated lymphoid tissue, GALT) and the local lymph nodes, it enters the blood and then the CNS. The paralytic effect of poliovirus is due to destruction of motor neuron cells in the anterior horns of the spinal cord or bulbar regions. Once within the brain or spinal cord, virus can spread directly (or indirectly via the CSF) to neighbouring cells.

The viraemic phase marks the end of the incubation period and is manifest in the patient by fever and generalised symptoms; it is followed by a period of about 48 hours of relative well-being (the disease is biphasic) whilst the virus is invading nerve tissue followed by the signs of paralysis. If antibody is present in blood, virus can be prevented from reaching the CNS.

Enteroviruses are lytic, destroying the infected cell within a few hours to days. Cell damage will trigger an inflammatory response; the resultant oedema may affect neurones other than those infected with the virus. As the oedema resolves, function will recover in these uninfected cells, thereby explaining the apparent improvement in the degree of paralysis in the weeks to months following the acute stage.

EPIDEMIOLOGY AND TRANSMISSION

Humans are the only known natural source of poliovirus. The virus is spread from person to person, and no intermediate host is known. Other enteroviruses have a similar epidemiology, but homologues of human enteroviruses have also been identified in Old World primates. Enteroviruses are excreted in large numbers from the gut and cause infection upon ingestion. Although faecal contamination is the usual source of enterovirus infection, acid labile enteroviruses such as EV-D70 have been found almost exclusively in conjunctival and throat specimens, and EV-D68 is spread typically by respiratory routes.

Enterovirus infection can be achieved in the following ways:

- by direct transfer on fingers (faecal–oral transfer)
- on eating utensils
- through contaminated food or drink
- by inhalation of droplets expelled by infected individuals (mostly EV-D68)
- through contaminated surfaces (mostly EV-D68)
- by entry through the conjunctiva (mostly EV-D70)

Outbreaks often occur in closed communities (e.g., military establishments) and schools. In the acute phase of infection, virus is present in the throat and, although droplet spread can occur, the faecal–oral route is the usual means of transmission. After the acute phase, it is the only possible route. Cases are most infectious late in the incubation period, but infection can be transmitted at any time during virus excretion in faeces.

Infection rates can reach 100% in closed communities and households, particularly where children are present. Social factors, such as standards of hygiene and overcrowding, are also important. Sewage can contain polioviruses, particularly when there is infection in a community. Enteroviruses can survive for several months in river water but are unlikely to survive in chlorine-treated water or swimming pools where the recommended level of chlorination (without protein contamination) is achieved.

PREVENTION AND CONTROL

After natural infection, immunity is long lasting. Virus-neutralising antibodies are formed early during the disease (often before day 7) and persist for several decades. Secretory IgA is produced in the gut. In the clinical setting, standard infection prevention and control (SIPC) precautions (including adequate hand hygiene) are critical in preventing spread.

Immunisation

Polio is a vaccine-preventable disease; there are two types of vaccines: inactivated polio vaccine (IPV) and live-attenuated oral polio vaccine (OPV) (Table 44.4).

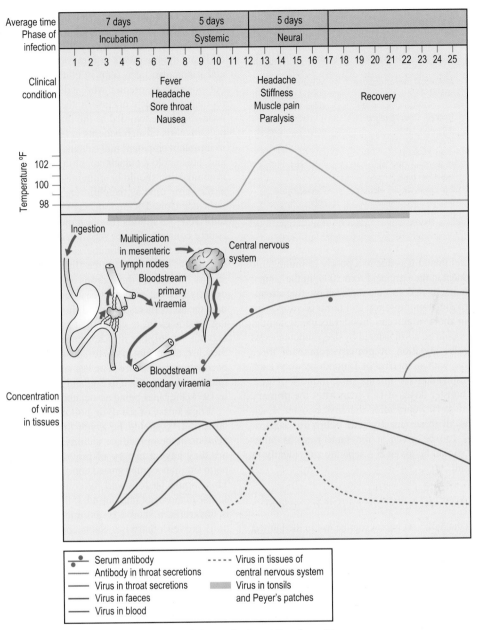

Fig. 44.1 Pathogenesis of paralytic poliomyelitis.

Inactivated polio vaccine (Salk vaccine)

Developed by Jonas Salk (United States) and introduced in 1956 for routine immunisation, IPV contains strains of the three types of viruses grown in monkey kidney cell culture and inactivated by exposure to formaldehyde. The batches of vaccine are tested for the presence of residual live poliovirus and must be free of contaminants. IPV is used widely, and with many countries achieving acceptance

rates in excess of 90% (e.g., the Nordic countries), such regions have eliminated poliovirus infection despite the fact that inactivated vaccine does not induce much secretory IgA in the alimentary tract or afford protection to individuals who are not vaccinated. A high rate of immunisation is necessary, and antibody levels need to be maintained as the outcome of exposure to virus is directly related to the level of antibody at the time of exposure. For example,

Table 44.4 Types of polio vaccines

	Oral polio vaccine (OPV)	Inactivated polio vaccine (IPV)
Nature	Mixture of live-attenuated strains	Mixture of inactivated, killed strains
Contains	Trivalent OPV: All three poliovirus types Bivalent OPV: Poliovirus types 1 and 3 Monovalent OPV: Any individual type	All three poliovirus types
Risk of polio	Can cause vaccine-derived polio in underimmunised population	Cannot cause polio

an outbreak in Finland was due to a poorly immunogenic type 3 component in the vaccine. From 2004, in the United Kingdom, the inactivated vaccine replaced the live attenuated one for routine immunisation and forms a component of the current multivalent childhood vaccine schedule. The vaccine should be administered by deep subcutaneous or intramuscular injection. A primary course of three injections given with an interval of 1 month between each dose is recommended for infants of 2 months of age, followed by booster doses at 1–3 years after the primary course and at 5–10 years after the first booster. Each dose contains all three (inactivated) poliovirus strains. The vaccines can be given at the same time as other vaccines but should be given at a separate site, ideally in a different limb.

Live-attenuated oral polio vaccine (Sabin vaccine)

This replaced the Salk vaccine for routine use in the United Kingdom in 1962 and is used extensively in many other countries. Developed by Albert Sabin (United States) in 1959, OPV contains live but attenuated strains of the three types of viruses grown in cultures of either monkey kidney cells or human diploid cells. The strains were obtained by growing less virulent polioviruses and, after passage, selecting strains that had lost their neurovirulence.

The vaccine is administered orally and thus mimics natural infection with stimulation of circulating IgG and local secretory IgA in the pharynx and alimentary tract, thereby producing local resistance to subsequent infection with wild-type polioviruses. Herd immunity is important in preventing the circulation of the wild-type virus and high levels of immunisation uptake are necessary. The wide circulation of vaccine virus, which helps to maintain immunity in the community, aids this. However, vaccine strains are not completely stable, and studies of sequential isolates of virus from vaccine recipients show very rapid

reversion to neurovirulence with multiple rounds of replication in the vaccinee and after transmission to contacts. Vaccine-associated poliomyelitis has been reported in oral vaccine recipients at a rate of 1 in 2 million doses, and it has also been seen in contacts of recipients. It is not possible to predict who will be affected; extended replication, which occurs in the immunocompromised host, should be avoided as the rate of vaccine-associated poliomyelitis in such patients is 10,000 times greater than in immunocompetent individuals. Nonimmunised parents and household contacts of children receiving primary immunisation should be immunised against poliomyelitis at the same time as the children.

In the United Kingdom, OPV was recommended up until 2004 for infants from 2 months of age. The primary course consists of three separate doses given at the same time as the then used diphtheria/tetanus/pertussis vaccine. Each dose contains all three (live-attenuated) poliovirus strains. In infants, three drops are dropped from a spoon directly into the mouth. Breast-feeding does not interfere with the antibody response and should continue. A reinforcing dose is given to children at school entry and prior to leaving school, but it is not necessary for adults unless they are at special risk, for instance, through travel or occupational exposure. The last cases of indigenous polio infection were notified in England in 1984, and in Scotland in 1994, the latter being associated with the vaccine itself.

When a case of paralytic poliomyelitis is diagnosed, a dose of IPV should be given to all immunocompetent persons in the immediate vicinity of the case, whether or not they have a history of previous vaccination against polio (immunocompromised contacts should receive IPV). This should be followed by completion of the primary course in those not immunised. If the source of the outbreak is uncertain, it should be assumed to be wild-type virus until proven otherwise. Such circumstances necessitate coordinated efforts of the relevant health-care and public health bodies to ensure a prompt and appropriate response.

Global eradication

The World Health Organization (WHO), through an expanded programme on immunisation, has increased the rate of polio immunisation, chiefly with the use of live-attenuated OPV. The Global Polio Eradication Initiative (GPEI) was formed by the World Health Assembly (WHA; the governing body of the WHO) in 1988. At that time, polio paralysed >350,000 people a year. The programme has been extremely successful; although the virus is still circulating, the number of clinical polio cases has decreased by >99%.

The GPEI strategy relies on using the live-attenuated OPV on national immunisation days (NIDs), with the aim of immunising all young children (<5 years of age) in a particular region in a short period of time followed by repeat session(s) to break polio transmission. Using this strategy, the Americas were declared free of indigenous poliovirus in 1994, the western Pacific region in 2000, Europe in 2002 and Southeast Asia in 2014. Type 2 wild polio was eradicated in 1999. Currently, endogenous poliovirus is circulating only in three countries: Pakistan, Afghanistan and Nigeria; much recent progress has been achieved in Nigeria. Other countries have notified reimportation of the virus, and outbreaks that threaten national and international spread do occur. Difficulties associated with the vaccination campaign, some of which are specific to the use of live-attenuated OPV, include interference from other enteroviruses leading to poor responses, malnutrition, inhibitory factors in the gut, social/cultural resistance to polio vaccination, problems in maintenance of the cold chain, delivery of vaccine in war zones and programme funding. No decision will be made to discontinue immunisation against polio until all countries are free of wild-type poliovirus infections. In countries where no such virus is reported, surveillance systems must be introduced that are effective at detecting wild-type poliovirus infections, and all cases of paralytic illness must be investigated. Only then is a country certified poliovirus free. Currently, the main obstacle to achieving the WHO's goal of global polio eradication is funding, but recent data show that completing this task within the next 5 years may translate into a net benefit of £25–35 billion for the world community.

Prospects for the future

Routine and mass administration of live-attenuated OPV since 1961 has prevented many millions of cases of paralytic poliomyelitis; however, when the incidence of poliomyelitis falls dramatically, as in the United States, for example, the proportion of paralytic cases attributable to vaccine (VAPP), although very low, becomes increasingly significant. Furthermore, recombination of live-attenuated vaccine and wild-type virus in areas of poor vaccine coverage as well as long-term excretion of vaccine virus in immunocompromised individuals pose additional OPV-related problems. There is thus a considerable rationale for shifting to use of the inactivated vaccine (IPV). In the long term, whilst eradication of poliovirus may be achievable, some problems will remain. Reemergence of wild-type polio from stored stocks (e.g., laboratory virus, stored clinical samples) is a possibility that needs to be addressed, and a decision made whether the oral vaccine should still be manufactured to deal with such an occurrence or, alternatively, emphasis placed on the inactivated vaccine (that requires inoculation).

RHINOVIRUSES

Although many other viruses cause similar illness, rhinoviruses within the *Enterovirus* genus are responsible for the most frequent of all human infections, the common cold. Most people suffer two to four colds every year, and although the primary infection is not often a severe one, secondary bacterial infection can follow and symptoms may be more severe. Sinusitis and otitis media are quite common. Rhinoviruses have also been associated with acute exacerbations of asthma and may even contribute to its development. These viruses are of major economic significance because they cause the loss of many million man-hours of work each year, accounting for up to half of upper respiratory tract infections. The recently discovered human rhinoviruses within species C seem to be more likely to cause wheezing illness and asthma exacerbations than rhinovirus within species A and B.

PROPERTIES

As the name *rhinovirus* implies, the viruses are associated with the nose. Rhinoviruses can be distinguished from most other enteroviruses by their acid lability. Although rhinoviruses are detectable in human faeces, they are not thought to infect the intestinal tract. There are over 100 serotypes of rhinoviruses; all are fastidious in cell culture. Electron microscopy (EM) cannot differentiate them from other family members (Fig. 44.2). The capsid of

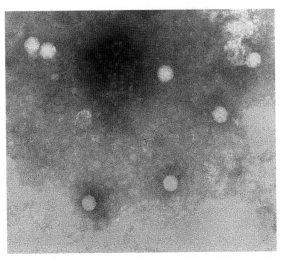

Fig. 44.2 Human rhinovirus. This virus is indistinguishable in appearance from other picornaviruses. Approximate size 25–30 nm. (From Madeley C. R., & Field, A. M. (1988) *Virus morphology* (2nd ed.). Edinburgh: Churchill Livingstone.)

rhinoviruses appears to be less rigid than that of other enteroviruses. This loose packaging is consistent with its greater buoyant density and sensitivity to acid.

Classification

The first rhinovirus was identified in 1953, and, by 1987, over 100 rhinovirus serotypes were classified based on their antigenic properties. These viruses were divided into major (90% of viruses) and minor (10%) groups based on their cellular receptor specificity; major group viruses attach to the intercellular adhesion molecule 1 (ICAM-1) and the minor group viruses to members of the low-density lipoprotein receptor (LDLR) family. The first systematic genetic characterisation of all designated 102 rhinovirus serotypes was performed in 2002; based on that, all viruses were divided into two groups (A [76 rhinovirus types] and B [25 rhinovirus types]). These groups were subsequently named as *Rhinovirus* A and B species within the *Enterovirus* genus. The advanced use of molecular detection methods led to the discovery of a third rhinovirus species in 2006, *Rhinovirus* C species, and, to date, a total of 55 rhinovirus types within species C have been classified (Table 44.1). Furthermore, human cadherin-related family member 3 (CDHR3) has been identified as the first receptor for rhinoviruses within species C. Interestingly, a coding single nucleotide polymorphism (SNP) is linked to the greater cell-surface expression of CDHR3 protein and an increased risk of wheezing and hospitalisation of children with asthma.

Stability

Inactivation of rhinoviruses occurs below pH 6.0 and is more rapid the lower the pH. Complete inactivation occurs at pH 3.0. Some rhinoviruses may survive heating at 50°C for 1 hour. They are relatively stable in the range of 20–37°C and can survive on environmental surfaces such as door handles for several days. They can be preserved at −70°C. Rhinoviruses are resistant to 20% ether and 5% chloroform but are sensitive to aldehyde and hypochlorite.

REPLICATION

The viruses replicate in the cytoplasm of infected cells to give a cytopathic effect (CPE) that coincides with release of the virus. If the infected cultures are incubated at 37°C, the yield is reduced to 30%–50% of that at 33°C.

CLINICAL FEATURES AND PATHOGENESIS

The typical illness is generally referred to as the common cold. The onset, after contact with infection, is usually within 2–3 days, sometimes as long as 7 days. The symptoms are:

- clear watery nasal discharge, which often becomes mucoid or purulent due to secondary bacterial infection
- sneezing and coughing
- sore throat
- headache and malaise

The symptoms are most severe for 2–3 days when nasal virus titres are maximal, and, although recovery is usually complete within a week, symptoms can persist for 2 weeks or longer. The ratio of symptomatic to asymptomatic infection is about 3 : 1, and the illness is generally worse in cigarette smokers. Rhinoviruses have frequently been isolated from patients during acute exacerbation of chronic obstructive pulmonary disease (COPD) and are the most common viruses to be associated with wheeze in preschool children. Rhinoviruses are responsible for most first wheezing episodes in young children; rhinovirus detection rates of up to 76% have been described. Rhinovirus-induced early wheezing is seen as an important risk factor for recurrent wheezing and childhood asthma.

All respiratory viruses may cause symptoms of the common cold, and dual infections with rhinovirus and another respiratory agent are not uncommon. In the immunocompetent individual, colds are mostly trivial and an inconvenience. Conversely, rhinovirus infection of an immunocompromised host can cause serious respiratory disease.

In organ cultures, the virus settles on the ciliated nasal epithelial cells, enters, infects and spreads from cell to cell in the epithelium. The cilia become immobilised, and both cilia and cell degenerate as the virus replicates. Bacterial invasion of the damaged epithelium can then occur. Interferon is usually detectable shortly after the peak of virus shedding and probably plays a part in recovery. Virus shedding ceases when antibody is detected in nasal secretions, suggesting that this may be the main factor leading to recovery. Little is known of the importance of cell-mediated immunity. The symptoms probably relate to the local inflammatory response and interferon release. Rhinoviruses have been recovered in pure culture from sinus fluids collected from patients with acute sinusitis, but secondary bacterial infection is thought to be the usual cause. Acute otitis media is the most common complication in children suffering upper respiratory tract infection, and rhinoviruses can be detected (by nucleic acid amplification tests, NAATs) in the middle ear in up to 40% of such cases.

Lower respiratory tract infection may occur on some occasions since:

- patients with colds may also have lower respiratory tract symptoms with abnormal lung function

- children who develop colds may develop wheeze
- adults with colds may suffer exacerbation of COPD (e.g., asthma)

Immunity

After the acute illness, neutralising antibody can be detected in both serum and nasal secretions. It can continue to rise in titre for 4–5 weeks after infection and may persist for up to 4 years, although some infections may provoke only a poor response, leaving the patient susceptible to the same serotype after a few weeks or months.

EPIDEMIOLOGY AND TRANSMISSION

Rhinoviruses can be isolated from patients with respiratory illnesses throughout the year, but in temperate climates, the incidence of colds due to rhinoviruses increases in autumn and spring and is lowest in the summer months. In the tropics, the peak incidence occurs in the rainy season. Although deliberate exposure of volunteers to wet and chilling conditions does not per se cause colds, the association is notable. Rhinoviruses may be transmitted by inhalation of droplets expelled from the nose of a patient and also by hand-to-surface contact (environmental contamination). During the acute phase of the illness, high concentrations of virus are present in nasal secretions and may contaminate the fingers, and thereafter the contaminated fingers may touch the eye or nasal mucosa. The incidence of rhinovirus infections is highest in preschool children, who often introduce colds to their homes, and, therefore, people who are in contact with young children are at increased risk of infection.

PARECHOVIRUSES

Parechoviruses are widespread pathogens, infecting mainly young children. Generally, parechoviruses cause a similar range of clinical disease as members of the closely related *Enterovirus* genus. The first parechoviruses were discovered in 1961 during a diarrhoea outbreak in the United States. They were first described as echovirus 22 and 23 in the *Enterovirus* genus but later reclassified into their own genus and renamed human parechoviruses (HPeV1 and HPeV2) because of differences in genomic organisation and biological properties. New HPeV types were not recognised until the late 1990s: HPeV3 was isolated in 1999 in Japan from a 1-year-old child with transient paralysis, fever and diarrhoea and (almost contemporaneously) three Canadian HPeV3 isolates were isolated from the nasopharyngeal aspirates of neonates with sepsis-like

Table 44.5 Identification of human parechovirus (HPeV) types 1 to 16

HPeV type	Year of isolation	Country of origin	Associated symptoms
1	1956	United States	Diarrhoea
2	1956	United States	Diarrhoea
3	2004	Japan	Transient paralysis
4	2002	Netherlands	Isolated fever
5	1986	United States	Isolated fever
6	2007	Japan	Reye syndrome
7	2009	Pakistan	No symptoms[a]
8	2007	Brazil	Diarrhoea
9	Unknown	Unknown	Unknown
10	2006	Sri Lanka	Diarrhoea
11	2005	Sri Lanka	Diarrhoea
12	2008	Pakistan	Acute flaccid paralysis
13	2008	Pakistan	Diarrhoea
14	2008	Netherlands	Isolated fever
15	2008	Pakistan	Diarrhoea
16	Unknown	Unknown	Unknown

[a]Child had been in contact with a case of acute flaccid paralysis.

illness. Since that time, 13 further HPeV types have been identified (Table 44.5).

PROPERTIES

The genomic organisation of parechoviruses resembles that of enteroviruses, with the exception that the structural protein VP0, which is a precursor for VP4 and VP2 in most picornaviruses, is not cleaved. As a result, parechoviruses have only three structural proteins (VP0, VP1 and VP3).

CLINICAL FEATURES

Parechovirus infections vary from asymptomatic or mild infections to more severe diseases including sepsis and encephalitis, which are mostly seen in young children. A total of 14 out of 16 parechovirus types have been associated with human infections so far; parechovirus type 3 (HPeV3) is the most significant cause of sepsis-like and CNS infections in young children. In general, neonates with HPeV infections present similarly to enterovirus infections with clinical signs including fever, seizures, irritability, rash and feeding problems.

A number of studies have documented specific association between HPeV3 and sepsis-like illness in children under the age of 3 months. A first outbreak of sepsis-like disease due to HPeV3 was also recently reported from

Australia; the outbreak involved 118 infants of whom 25% required intensive care admission, demonstrating the severity of these infections. In addition, HPeV type 4 has occasionally been linked to severe sepsis-like infection in young children.

HPeV3 has been identified as an important cause of encephalitis with a typical white matter involvement characterised by restricted diffusion upon magnetic resonance imaging (MRI) of young infants. The initial presentations typically include seizures, fever and rash. Pleocytosis or biochemical alterations in CSF are absent in most cases of parechovirus encephalitis. Although parechovirus encephalitis can be fatal, it is generally a rare disease.

EPIDEMIOLOGY

Based on seroprevalence studies, parechovirus type 1 infections are very common, and seropositivity approaches 100% in adult populations. In contrast, lower seropositivity has been observed for parechovirus type 3. A study from Japan reported a seroprevalence of 40% among women of childbearing age, whereas European studies have obtained lower seropositivity rates (<10%).

LABORATORY INVESTIGATION OF ENTEROVIRUS, RHINOVIRUS AND PARECHOVIRUS INFECTIONS

CULTURE

Virus isolation is usually made from faeces (or rectal swabs) and/or throat swabs. As virus excretion can be intermittent, two specimens should be collected on successive days, as early as possible in the illness, ideally within 5 days of onset.

In paralytic poliomyelitis, the virus can be found in faeces for a few days preceding the onset of acute symptoms and is present in >80% of cases in faeces during the first 4 days of symptoms. Only a few patients continue to excrete the virus after the 12th week although prolonged excretion may occur in the immunocompromised host. The virus can be isolated from the oropharynx of many patients for a few days before and after the onset of illness. Conversely, isolation from the CSF is seldom successful in cases of paralytic poliomyelitis. Echoviruses, coxsackie B viruses and coxsackie A9 virus are readily isolated from nose and throat swabs, stools or CSF; they are present in 80% of cases in faeces for at least 2 weeks after onset of disease. However, the clinical relevance of virus isolation from faeces is not always clear as enteroviruses can be

excreted for some time after asymptomatic infection and may thus only be an incidental finding. Very few data are available for isolation of newly identified enterovirus types (i.e., enteroviruses identified in and after the 1980s). Parechoviruses have mostly been isolated from stool samples and rhinoviruses (as well as EV-D68) from respiratory specimens.

Enteroviruses, rhinoviruses and parechoviruses were traditionally identified by isolation in cell culture, followed by neutralisation using an antiserum pool. Acid lability is a further aid to identification of an isolate as a rhinovirus. However, successful virus isolation is largely dependent on the cell lines used and also on availability of antisera in pools applied. For example, species C rhinoviruses do not grow in traditional cell lines, and only parechovirus type 1 and 2 antisera are included in antiserum pools. Furthermore, virus isolation is laborious, time consuming, costly and requires considerable expertise; thus, it has largely been superseded by NAATs for RNA detection in clinical samples in diagnostic laboratories—primarily using reverse transcriptase polymerase chain reaction (RT-PCR).

Molecular methods

Enterovirus, parechovirus and rhinovirus infections are most often diagnosed in clinical samples by RT-PCR targeting the 5′ noncoding region (NCR) of the viral genome. Identification of conserved sequences within that region has resulted in the development of PCR primers that allow either the detection of enteroviruses only or the detection of both enteroviruses and rhinoviruses. A separate RT-PCR is required for the detection of parechoviruses. Many studies have confirmed that RT-PCR is faster and more sensitive than culture for the detection of enteroviruses, rhinoviruses and parechoviruses.

The current gold standard of diagnosis for meningitis is to detect the enterovirus or parechovirus genome in CSF by RT-PCR. Virus genomes can also be detected in stool, respiratory and vesicle fluid samples as well as blood depending on the diagnosis (Table 44.6). However, it should be noted that in cases of severe enterovirus and parechovirus encephalitis, virus may not be detectable in CSF and, in cases of EV-D68 infections, virus is usually only present in respiratory specimens.

Because the 5′ NCR of enteroviruses, rhinoviruses and parechoviruses is the most conserved among the viruses, it is used as a target for screening RT-PCR only. In contrast, the VP1 (and other parts of the capsid region) is highly variable and thus allows the previously assigned enterovirus, rhinovirus and parechovirus types to be identified reliably. This is often of most interest for the national public health laboratories performing nonpolio enterovirus surveillance.

Table 44.6 Preferred specimens for identification of picornavirus infections by RT-PCR

Clinical presentation	Stool[a]	CSF	Respiratory sample	Vesicle swab	Eye swab	Blood
Paralysis	Yes	Yes	Yes	No	No	No
Meningitis	Yes	Yes	Yes	No	No	No
Encephalitis	Yes	Yes	Yes	No	No	Maybe
Neonatal sepsis	Yes	Yes	Yes	Maybe	No	Yes
Epidemic pleurodynia	Yes	No	Yes	No	No	No
Myocarditis	Yes	No	Yes	No	No	Maybe
Herpangina	Yes	No	Yes	Maybe	No	No
HFMD or other rash	Yes	No	Yes	Yes	No	Maybe
Respiratory infection	No	No	Yes[b]	No	No	No
Conjunctivitis	No	No	No	No	Yes	No
Acute hepatitis A	Yes	No	No	No	No	Yes[c]

[a]Detection of enterovirus in stool does not always indicate causality; enteroviruses are excreted in stool for several weeks after the onset of symptoms and may not be the cause of current illness. However, in cases of suspected polio, such a finding is always of importance.
[b]In case of respiratory infection, consider testing for both rhinoviruses and enteroviruses.
[c]IgM serology is the key method for diagnosing acute hepatitis A virus infection.
CSF, Cerebrospinal fluid; *HFMD*, hand, foot and mouth disease; *RT-PCR*, reverse transcriptase polymerase chain reaction.

Serological tests

Although specific IgM and IgG enzyme immunosorbent assays (EIAs) for enteroviruses are available, their use is limited by the heterotypic and anamnestic responses associated with such infections. Serological methods cannot be used in the routine diagnosis of rhinovirus and parechovirus infections because of the multiplicity of serotypes and the lack of a common antigen.

TREATMENT AND CONTROL OF ENTEROVIRUS, RHINOVIRUS AND PARECHOVIRUS INFECTIONS

Although inactivated enterovirus vaccines can be produced, there remains the considerable problem of deciding on their antigenic composition. The only vaccines currently available are against polioviruses (IPV/OPV; discussed earlier in the chapter) and a whole virus vaccine against EV-A71 that has previously undergone Phase III clinical trials and is currently awaiting approval from the Chinese Food and Drug Administration.

Much effort has been devoted to the development of suitable antiviral therapy against enterovirus and rhinovirus infections. Three compounds are currently under clinical evaluation: pleconaril (Viropharma, United States), BTA798 (Biota Pharmaceuticals, United States) and pocapavir (ViroDefence, United States). All these compounds are capsid binders; they inhibit viral attachment to cell receptors and uncoating of virus. Pleconaril has shown some beneficial effect in clinical trials but was rejected by the US Food and Drug Administration in 2002 for treatment of the common cold because of safety fears. The other main issues with capsid binders are that enteroviruses readily develop resistance against them, and they do not inhibit all enterovirus and rhinovirus types or even strains. Other compounds including polymerase, protease and assembly inhibitors are currently under investigation.

Because of the lack of approved antiviral drugs for the treatment of picornavirus infections, treatment is limited to supportive care. Intravenous immunoglobulin (pooled immunoglobulin from multiple blood donors) is sometimes used, but success of this treatment is dependent on the presence of specific neutralising antibodies in the preparation used. In addition, isolation of the infected person, although perhaps desirable, is not always a practical method of preventing the spread of infection. Standard infection prevention and control (SIPC) measures, including adequate hand hygiene, reduce spread of infection in the hospital (and community) setting.

HEPATOVIRUSES

HEPATITIS A VIRUS

Hepatitis A has a worldwide distribution and occurs in epidemics as well as sporadically. The virus was first detected by EM examination of faeces. The genus *Hepatovirus* consists of hepatitis A virus (HAV) as its only species.

HAV is the causative agent of infectious hepatitis. It has similar polypeptides to the four major polypeptides of the enteroviruses and shares the same properties of resistance to physical and chemical agents. Recently, it has been adapted to cell culture; it will grow only in cells of primate origin.

Clinical features

Although the incidence has fallen in the past decade, HAV is still responsible for almost 60% of acute viral hepatitis in the United States. The illness is usually mild and occurs after an incubation period of 3–6 weeks. There is a prodrome of malaise, muscle pain and headache, and there may be a low-grade fever. The symptoms improve and disappear as jaundice develops. Serological tests show that many patients have a subclinical illness, and fulminant hepatitis and liver failure are rare. HAV does not cause chronic infection although the immunocompromised state may support longer term excretion. Infection is mild in young children, often asymptomatic or accompanied by nausea and malaise only. Of children aged under 3 years, only 5% develop jaundice, but this rises progressively to >50% in adults. The fatality rate also rises with age, to 2% in adults. Some patients develop diarrhoea, and some appear to have a relapse a few weeks after initial onset. Arthritis and aplastic anemia are rare complications. Treatment is supportive (e.g,, fluid replacement). There are no specific antiviral drugs. Severe cases of fulminant liver failure can be considered for receipt of a liver transplant.

Pathogenesis

Like the enteroviruses, HAV probably infects cells in the gut initially and then spreads to the liver through the blood-stream. The histopathological appearance of an affected liver shows periportal necrosis and infiltration of mononuclear cells. Viral antigens are seen in the cytoplasm of the hepatocytes. Virus is excreted in bile into the gut 1–2 weeks before the onset of jaundice, and excretion then declines rapidly over the ensuing 5–7 days. Virus is also present in urine during that same period.

Laboratory investigation

Although the virus has been grown in cell culture, it is not possible to do this routinely from the faeces of patients. Diagnosis relies on the demonstration of specific IgM antibody, which develops very early in the course of infection and is generally present by the time the patient is investigated (in the presence/absence of IgG). It is detectable in the serum for 2–6 months after the onset of symptoms (Fig. 44.3). IgG antibody usually persists for many years and is a useful indicator of immunity. Virus can be detected in stool (and, very early in the illness, in blood) samples by RT-PCR.

Epidemiology

Only one type of HAV has been recognised. Molecular typing is now available to investigate outbreaks and link

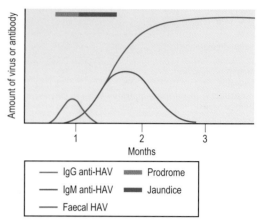

Fig. 44.3 Events during hepatitis A virus infection.

sporadic cases with common source outbreaks. Serological studies confirm that virus is prevalent in countries where sanitation is poor (consistent with the faecal–oral route of spread), and children are infected early in childhood. Even in developed countries, more than half of the population has been infected with the virus. However, with increasing use of vaccine, lower rates are seen. This can result in increased numbers of acute cases in young adults and older patients who may have a history of recent travel to an endemic area.

Outbreaks of HAV infection have been associated with food. Shellfish have often been incriminated, particularly when they are harvested from coastlines adjacent to sewage outlets. When shellfish is eaten raw, or only partially cooked, the virus retains its ability to infect. Contaminated raspberries were incriminated in a notorious outbreak in which uncooked frozen raspberries were eaten many months after picking. Infection is assumed to have come from an infected raspberry picker. The infectious dose is low—<100 virus particles. Because there is only a transient viraemic phase, only a few infections have been recognised after blood transfusion.

Prevention and control

A highly effective and immunogenic vaccine was licensed for use in the United Kingdom in 1991. It is a formaldehyde-inactivated vaccine prepared from virus grown in human diploid cells. A primary course of two doses (or, more recently, a single dose) of vaccine given intramuscularly produces good levels of neutralising antibody that are known to persist for at least 10 years. The vaccine is now preferred to human normal immunoglobulin (HNIG) for frequent travellers, for those with potential occupational exposure, and to protect contacts of cases. Recent vaccine formulations may combine hepatitis A and B antigens in the same vaccine.

RECOMMENDED READING

Harvala, H., Wolthers, K. C., & Simmonds, P. (2010). Parechoviruses in children: understanding a new infection. *Current Opinion in Infectious Diseases, 23*(3), 224–230.

Holm-Hansen, C. C., Midgley, S. E., & Fischer, T. K. (2016). Global emergence of enterovirus D68: a systematic review. *The Lancet Infectious Diseases, 16*(5), e64–e75. doi:10.1016/S1473 -3099(15)00543-5.

Knipe, D. M., & Howley, P. M. (Eds.), (2013). Picornaviridae. In *Fields virology* (6th ed., pp. 453–581). Philadelphia: Lippincott Williams & Wilkins.

Nathanson, N., & Kew, O. M. (2010). From emergence to eradication: the epidemiology of poliomyelitis deconstructed. *American Journal of Epidemiology, 172*(1), 1213–1229. doi:10.1093/aje/kwq320.

Ooi, M. H., Wong, S. C., Lewthwaite, P., Cardosa, M. J., & Solomon, T. (2010). Clinical features, diagnosis, and management of enterovirus 71. *The Lancet Infectious Diseases, 9*(11), 1097–1105.

Rhoades, R. E., Tabor-Godwin, J. M., Tsueng, G., & Feuer, R. (2011). Enterovirus infections of the central nervous system. *Virology, 411*(2), 288–305.

Zuckerman, A. J., Banatvala, J. E., Schoub, B. D., & Mortimer, P. (Eds.), (2009). *Principles and practice of clinical virology* (6th ed., pp. 273–279, 489-510, 601-642). Chichester: Wiley-Blackwell.

Websites

Global Polio Eradication Initiative. Available at http://www .polioeradication.org/. (Accessed Sep 2017).

UK Department of Health. UK hepatitis A immunisation policy. Available at http://www.dh.gov.uk/prod_consum_dh/groups/dh_ digitalassets/@dh/@en/documents/digitalasset/dh_124297.pdf. (Accessed Sep 2017).

UK Department of Health. UK polio immunisation policy. Available at http://www.dh.gov.uk/prod_consum_dh/groups/dh_digital assets/@dh/@en/documents/digitalasset/dh_108823.pdf. (Accessed Sep 2017).

45 Orthomyxoviruses

Influenza

MARIA ZAMBON

KEY POINTS

- Influenza viruses cause respiratory infections worldwide; there are three types: A, B and C.
- Influenza A is found in aquatic birds, poultry and pigs, and these play important roles in the epidemiology of human infections.
- Influenza viruses are segmented RNA viruses that regularly undergo genetic change.
- The surface proteins, the haemagglutinin and the neuraminidase, can show gradual change (antigenic drift) and sudden major change (antigenic shift).
- In humans, influenza A results in high morbidity and mortality rates in the winter months in temperate zones but throughout the year in more tropical climates.
- The spread pattern may be pandemic, epidemic or sporadic/zoonotic.
- Pandemic influenza typically arises when a new virus from an animal host emerges into a susceptible human population. The impact of pandemics may be mild, moderate or severe, depending on the virulence properties of the virus.
- Zoonotic influenza A infections in humans may have a high case fatality and different clinical manifestations compared with seasonal influenza A.
- Since 1997, H5 avian influenza has been a major problem in the Far East, with strains from domestic poultry occasionally infecting humans directly, resulting in high mortality rates; this virus could become adapted to humans.
- Vaccines have been available for many years, recommended for annual boosting of high-risk groups in interpandemic periods to reduce mortality, morbidity and hospital admission rates.
- Antiviral drugs act to inhibit viral replication and are clinically useful in treatment and prophylaxis.

The Orthomyxoviridae family comprises four genera: *influenza A, B* and *C* and *thogotoviruses*, within the negative-sense RNA virus order Mononegavirales. All of these are small enveloped viruses with a segmented genome. The thogotoviruses are the most recently discovered genus and are found in mosquitoes, ticks and the banded mongoose but are not so far associated with human disease and are not discussed further.

INFLUENZA A, B AND C HOST RANGE

Influenza B and C have limited genetic diversity and occur almost exclusively in humans, which are the natural animal reservoir. Occasional transmission of influenza B to mammalian species such as seals and influenza C to pigs has been described. In contrast, there are many different subtypes of influenza A viruses, all of which naturally infect water-based wild birds, usually with very little disease. Influenza A viruses have a broad host range with the potential to infect a wide range of animal species. Viral subtypes are distinguished according to their surface proteins, the haemagglutinin (HA) and neuraminidase (NA). Sixteen HA subtypes and nine NA subtypes are found in varying combinations circulating in wild birds. Only a limited number of influenza A subtypes have adapted to circulation in mammalian species, including humans, horses and pigs (Fig. 45.1). Very recent work has also identified new influenza viruses in New World bats.

Avian influenza A subtypes are transmitted through a faecal–oral route, and virus can be shed in high quantity in the environment following replication in the gastrointestinal tract. There is frequent spillover of avian influenza A subtypes into domestic poultry reservoirs, as a result of their shared habitat with wild birds. Replication in poultry may be associated with disease of varying severity or may be asymptomatic, depending on the viral subtype and the poultry species.

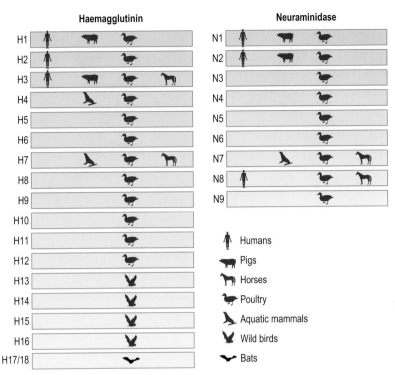

Fig. 45.1 Natural hosts for different influenza subtypes.

Nomenclature

The World Health Organization (WHO) system of nomenclature for influenza A includes the host of origin, geographical origin, strain number and year of isolation; then, in parentheses, the antigenic description of the haemagglutinin and neuraminidase is given—for example, A/swine/Iowa/3/70 (H1N1). If isolated from a human host the origin is not given—for example, A/Scotland/42/89 (H3N2).

Physical characteristics

In common with many enveloped viruses, influenza A, B and C are relatively labile and easily destroyed by common household cleaning agents and detergents. In the environment, influenza A virus can survive in cold seawater for several days and is detectable in dust beyond 1 week, although the infectivity of such material is not well understood.

THE VIRUSES

Influenza virions are spherical, 80–120 nm in diameter, but may be filamentous and up to 100-fold longer (Fig. 45.2A). They have a helical nucleocapsid comprising, in A and B, eight segments of single-stranded RNA and, in C, seven segments. Also present within the virion particle is the viral RNA-dependent RNA polymerase enzyme; this is essential for infectivity as the viral RNA is of negative sense and therefore has to be transcribed to produce viral messenger RNA. The nucleocapsid is surrounded by the M1 protein shell, immediately exterior to which is a lipid envelope derived from the host cell. The viral M2 protein projects through the envelope to form ion channels, which assist virus entry through an endosomal route, which involves pH changes. Two types of spikes project from the lipid envelope, the haemagglutinin (HA) and the neuraminidase (NA) enzyme (Fig. 45.2B). The HA, so-called because the virus agglutinates certain species of erythrocyte, is about 10 nm in length and consists of trimers of identical glycoprotein subunits, each consisting of two polypeptide chains, HA_1 and HA_2 joined by a linkage site that may be a single basic amino acid, usually arginine, or a string of basic amino acids (Fig. 45.3).

Influenza viruses bind to cells by the HA interacting with cell membrane receptors containing *N*-acetylneuraminic acid (sialic acid). The amino acid residues involved in receptor binding show variability according to host of origin. Differences in viral receptor binding characteristics have important biological significance for the transmission

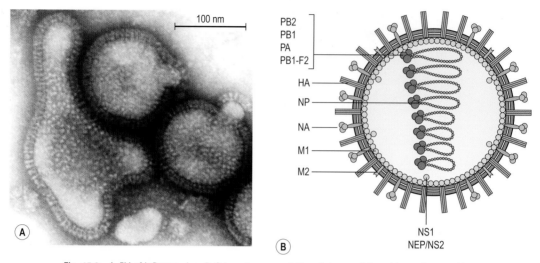

Fig. 45.2 A, EM of influenza virus. B, Schematic representation of virus particle and internal composition.

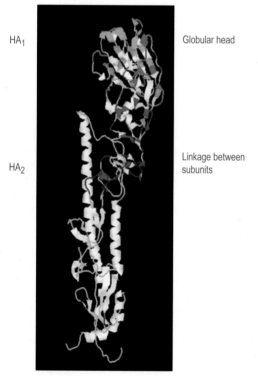

Fig. 45.3 Schematic of HA1 and HA2 monomer.

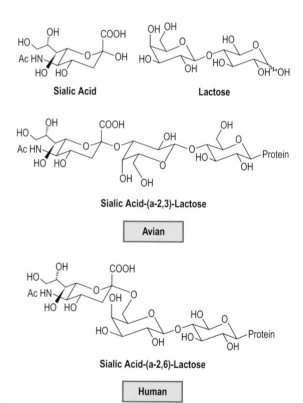

Fig. 45.4 Host virus receptor configuration in avian and human viruses, leading to differences in receptor binding preferences.

properties of the virus. Human influenza viruses recognise receptors that contain sialic acid attached to the penultimate sugar (usually lactose) via an $\alpha(2,6)$-linkage, whereas avian strains prefer receptors with an $\alpha(2,3)$-linkage (Fig. 45.4).

Between the HA spikes on the virus surface are the mushroom-shaped NA spikes. The NA protein is assembled from four subunits attached by a stalk containing a hydrophobic region, which is anchored in the viral lipid envelope. The NA enzyme catalyses the cleavage of sialic acid and an adjacent sugar residue from glycoproteins found in mucus. This action allows the virus to permeate through the mucin overlying host epithelial surfaces. Neuraminidase activity is also important in the release of new virus particles from infected cells. Sialic acid is always present in newly synthesised virions, and its removal by NA prevents the new virus particles clumping through the binding to viral HA, thus assisting the spread of the virus from the original site of infection.

Virus variability

All influenza viruses replicate via virally encoded RNA-dependent RNA polymerase enzymes. Such enzymes lack a proofreading (error correction) function, leading to high rates of mutation during replication. Viruses carrying mutations that do not provide a severe replication disadvantage therefore evolve rapidly, a feature described as genetic drift. Genetic recombination among diverse influenza A viral subtypes occurs when more than one subtype infects a single host, creating new combinations of viral gene segments (reassortment) and altering the replication and virulence properties of the progeny virus. Together, the combination of genetic drift and segment reassortment provides the mechanism for generation of genetic diversity amongst influenza A viruses. These genetic mechanisms generate adaptive flexibility, which is reflected in the wide variety of animal species (host range) that can be infected. Different genetic lineages of influenza B and C also show some evidence of segment reassortment, but this is very much more limited than for influenza A and is not associated with significant biological diversity.

EPIDEMIC AND PANDEMIC INFLUENZA

Major epidemics that may have been caused by influenza viruses have been described for >2000 years. Historically, it was rationalised that such unexpected events occurred under the influence of the stars, hence the term *influenza* (Italian for influence). It is well recognised that epidemics vary in severity. Occasionally, infection arising from a new strain spreads throughout the world and causes very significant marked waves of illness; such pandemics have been recognised at irregular intervals.

Pandemics occurred in 1918, 1957 and 1968, with the emergence of H1N1 Spanish influenza, H2N2 and H3N2 respectively, and most recently in 2009, with the emergence of H1N1 from swine (H1N1 2009 pdm) into the human population. The great pandemic of 1918–1919 was particularly severe, killing 20–40 million people as it spread over a few years. In 1957, the emergence of H2N2 as a pandemic virus displaced circulating H1N1, which

disappeared until 1977, when it re-emerged after 20 years (Fig. 45.5). The emergence of new influenza A viruses in humans that are able to transmit person to person and cause a global pandemic, is likely to have arisen from an initial rare event involving a novel influenza A virus with the capacity of replicating in humans and transmitting. Virus isolation studies from 1933 onwards, and analysis of isolates, have given an understanding of how the epidemic and pandemic behaviour relates to changes in the virus.

Major pandemics are associated with antigenic shifts—when the viral HA or NA (or both) is changed. Antigenic shift results from the acquisition of a complete new RNA segment 4 and/or 6, either as a result of reassortment or infection of humans with an animal virus. Until 1977, when H1N1 reappeared, it was considered that when a new pandemic virus appeared the old one disappeared, but since that time, two influenza A subtypes have been circulating concurrently, namely H3N2 and H1N1 (Fig. 45.5). H1N1 viruses in 1977 were antigenically very similar to H1N1 viruses from before the 1957 pandemic, and may have been reintroduced from frozen laboratory sources, as there is no evidence of latent or persistent infection of humans. The most recent pandemic of 2009 exemplifies the emergence of an influenza strain from an animal reservoir (H1N1 from swine reservoir), to cause widespread disease in humans of all age groups. Although H1N1 has been circulating since 1918, H1N1 swine viruses were sufficiently different to H1N1 viruses circulating in humans, so that preexisting immunity in the population was insufficient to prevent widespread transmission, especially in younger age groups. The impact of H1N1 in the population was mild to moderate overall, partly due to the lower intrinsic virulence of the strain and partly due to the preexisting immunity in the adult and elderly population, although susceptible groups such as pregnant women had an increased risk of serious outcome. Since 2010/11, H1N1 2009 pdm has completely displaced the previously circulating H1N1 strain, which is an example of replacement of one epidemic strain by a new pandemic strain.

Epidemics occurring regularly in winter months between pandemics are associated with genetic drift in the HA antigen. Amino acid changes arising as a result of genetic mutation provide a selection advantage for the virus if they occur on the globular head of the HA protein, where host antibody binds (Fig. 45.3). Mutation at these sites allows the virus to infect despite the presence of antibody to previous strains, a phenomenon known as antigenic drift.

The wild bird reservoir for influenza A is globally dispersed and mobile, creating a natural milieu for relentless evolution of genetic diversity. Consequently, there is a continuous threat to humans of the emergence of a new influenza A virus, capable of adapting to human

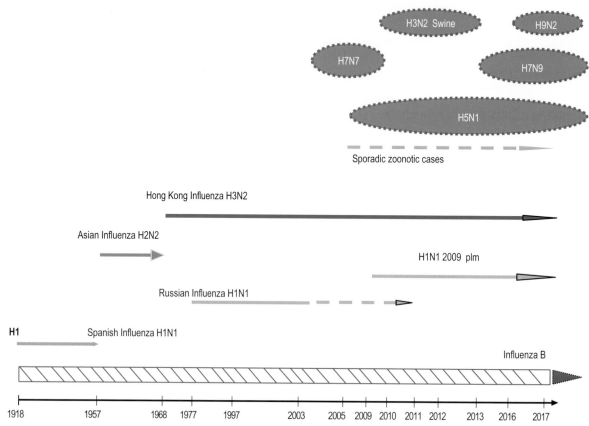

Fig. 45.5 Influenza viruses first isolated in 1933. Cocirculation of different viruses during the 20th and 21st centuries. Oval symbol denotes sporadic incidents and outbreaks with avian influenza viruses.

transmission, causing a pandemic of disease in a globally susceptible population. The criteria for the establishment of a new pandemic of influenza in humans include:

- a novel virus, with a new haemagglutinin (HA) subtype (antigenic shift)
- association with disease
- susceptible population
- ability of virus to transmit person to person

Sporadic zoonotic infections of influenza A are therefore closely monitored, in view of the potential they have to create a new pandemic influenza strain. All of the HA and NA subtypes are found in aquatic birds (both seabirds and ducks), but evolutionary pressures leading to the generation of viral diversity is not well understood in these animal reservoirs. Viral factors govern the ability to transmit and replicate in humans. These include receptor characteristics, replication competence and ability of virus to be shed directly into bodily secretions, which can be transmitted. In the laboratory it is easy to show that, if a cell is infected with two different strains, viruses arise

with RNA segments derived from each parent through reassortment of segments.

Pigs have receptors for both human and avian strains, and this mammalian host has long been considered a key mixing vessel for reassortment following simultaneous infection with human and avian viruses. The conditions in Southeast Asia, where there are high densities of people, poultry and pigs, favour reassortment (Fig. 45.6). The importance of the pig host in the generation of diversity is emphasized by the 2009 pandemic.

CROSS-SPECIES INFLUENZA A INFECTION

In recent years, influenza A viruses have been detected in a variety of mammalian species including dogs, mink, tigers, whales, cats and civets, usually arising from occasional transmission events from avians, which may cause a range of disease symptoms in the new host, depending on the infecting virus subtype. Influenza A infection in mammalian species is usually associated with

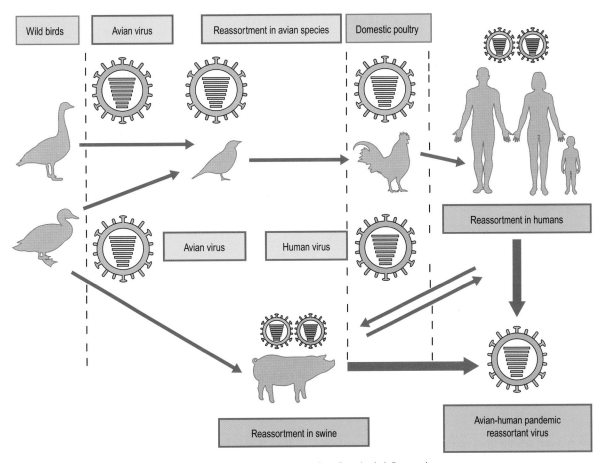

Fig. 45.6 Possible pathways for generation of pandemic influenza viruses.

viral replication in the respiratory tract leading to respiratory illnesses with some systemic features, and occasionally extra respiratory replication. Sporadic infection events have usually involved only limited transmission in the new host. Diseased poultry and domestic ducks usually serve as the source of infection for avian influenza in mammalian hosts (Fig. 45.6). Infection arises through a variety of routes including contact with contaminated water, avian faecal material or contact with carcasses of infected birds. However, adaptation to dogs in North America has occurred, as a result of transmission of H7 from horses, creating a new animal reservoir of endemic influenza A (Fig. 45.7).

Zoonotic transmission to humans

Sporadic zoonotic infection of humans with influenza A viruses should be distinguished from epidemic human influenza A seasonal infection, which occurs during the winter months and is attributable to subtypes of influenza

A (H3N2 and H1N1), which normally transmit between humans causing seasonal respiratory illness along with influenza B or C.

Human cases of infection with avian influenza viruses involving H5, H7, H10 or H9 subtypes have usually been acquired as a result of exposure to domestic poultry, material containing avian influenza virus or other mammalian species infected as an intermediate host with an avian influenza virus. The outcome of sporadic human infection ranges from severe disease of the respiratory system, which may also lead to multiorgan failure and death, to milder respiratory infection or simple conjunctivitis. The spectrum of disease is dependent on the nature of the infecting avian influenza A virus; for example, H5 infections are associated with severe respiratory infections with a high case fatality rate; H7N7 infections are associated with conjunctivitis and milder respiratory infections. Since 2013, H7N9 transmissions from poultry to humans have increased significantly, showing a clear seasonality in the sporadic human cases with several hundred cases

Expanding Host Range Influenza A

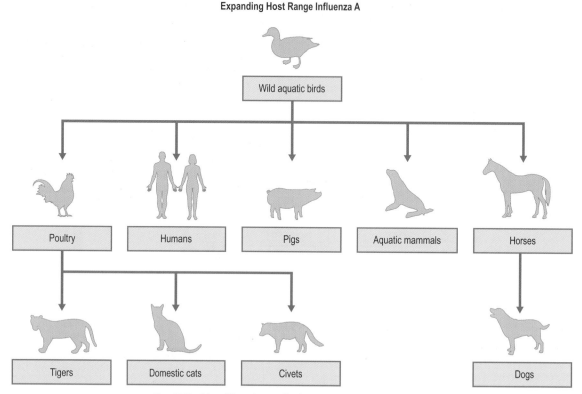

Fig. 45.7 Adaptable and expanding host range of influenza A viruses.

every year, arising from an expanding locus of endemic poultry infection in China. These infections have been associated with high case fatality between 30% and 40%. There have also been sporadic cases of human H5N6 and H9N2 associated with severe illness as a result of transmission from poultry sources in the Far East.

In contrast, in North America, there have been several hundred cases of swine-to-human transmissions of swine H3N2 or H1N1 viruses to children as a result of direct exposure to pigs, with illness in general being very mild and essentially undistinguishable from seasonal influenza.

The outcome of zoonotic infections of influenza viruses is therefore dependent on both the virus and the host, where the genetic makeup of the virus and the host immune responses both play a role in determining severity.

Risk factors for the acquisition of zoonotic avian or nonhuman influenza A include:

- close or direct contact with diseased poultry or other domestic fowl
- close or direct contact with other mammalian species infected with unusual influenza A viruses (swine, seals)
- inhalation, ingestion or mucosal contact with infectious material

Risk factors for severe human disease outcome following zoonotic infection of influenza A include:

- H5 or H7 subtype (30%–50% case fatality rate)
- young age
- preexisting lung disease
- pathogenicity of infecting virus in poultry reservoir

Human seasonal influenza A, B and C infections

As can be seen from the foregoing discussion, influenza A virus subtypes circulating in humans (H1N1 and H3N2) were ultimately derived from an animal reservoir. Several influenza A subtypes cocirculate globally in humans in varying proportion, causing respiratory disease during the winter months in temperate climates, and during months of highest humidity in dry climates. In tropical climates, distinct seasonality is less evident, with patterns of influenza transmission throughout the year. Influenza B viruses cocirculate globally with influenza A viruses and contribute to the burden of seasonal influenza (Fig. 45.5) but are not usually associated with such severe morbidity and mortality. Influenza B viruses do not undergo antigenic shift as there is no animal reservoir and, although epidemics do occur at 3- to 6-year intervals, they never reach pandemic proportions. The antigenic changes in influenza B result from genetic drift, as seen in influenza A after the appearance of new virus strains. Influenza C viruses are associated with much milder illness, with limited generation of genetic diversity and sporadic pattern of circulation.

Clinical features in human seasonal influenza A infection

Influenza is an acute infection of the human respiratory tract. Disease is characterised by the sudden onset of fever, chills, headache, muscle pain and extreme fatigue. Other common symptoms include a dry cough, sore throat and stuffy nose. For otherwise healthy individuals, influenza is an unpleasant but usually self-limiting disease with recovery usually within 2–7 days. The illness may be complicated by (and may present as) bronchitis, secondary bacterial pneumonia or with otitis media (ear infection) in children.

Serious illness and mortality are highest among the newborn, older people and those with underlying disease, particularly chronic respiratory or cardiac disease, or those who are immunosuppressed.

In classical seasonal influenza A infection:

- the incubation period is short, 2 days, but may vary from 1 to 4 days
- the illness is characterised by a sudden onset of systemic symptoms such as chills, fever, headache, myalgia and anorexia
- respiratory symptoms are also common but take second place to the systemic effects, especially early in the illness

Many patients have both upper and lower respiratory tract infection, often with a troublesome, dry cough. The main physical finding is pyrexia, which rises rapidly to a peak of 38–41°C within 12 hours of onset. Fever usually lasts for 3 days but may be present for 1–5 days. During the second and third days of the illness the systemic effects diminish, and by the fourth day, the respiratory symptoms and signs are predominant. In adults, systemic illness without respiratory symptoms is common. Some symptoms are age specific, for example febrile convulsions and otitis media in children and dyspnoea in the elderly. About one-third of patients suffer only a common cold-like illness, and as many as 20%–30% of cases are subclinical (asymptomatic). A long convalescence is common, and cough, lassitude and malaise may last for 1–2 weeks after the disappearance of other manifestations. Many other respiratory viruses can cause typical influenza-like illnesses, although the severity of the systemic symptoms is usually greatest with influenza virus.

Complications of human seasonal influenza

- Primary influenza pneumonia is an unusual complication that may occur at any age and carries a case fatality rate of 1%–5%, depending on age and underlying conditions. This can be fatal, especially in young adults during an outbreak, after a very short illness of sometimes <1 day. A similar rapid illness can occur in the elderly.
- More commonly, a bacterial pneumonia caused by *Staphylococcus aureus*, *Streptococcus pneumoniae* or *Haemophilus influenzae* occurs late in the course of the illness, often after a period of improvement, resulting in a classical biphasic fever pattern.
- Very rare complications include myocarditis, encephalitis or meningoencephalitis.

The incidence of chest complications is related to the age of the patient, increasing progressively after the age of 60 years. Severe infections and sudden death can occur, especially if there is some underlying disease, such as cerebrovascular, cardiovascular or chronic respiratory disease.

In the immunocompromised, symptoms may last longer and viral excretion may go on for weeks to months. Excess mortality was reported in pregnant women during the 1918 and 1957 pandemics, and even in nonpandemic outbreaks, an increase in hospital admission due to cardiorespiratory disease is seen in the second and third trimesters. Susceptibility of pregnant women to severe influenza was also evident in the 2009 pandemic.

Clinical features in zoonotic influenza A infections

There is a spectrum of illness associated with the presentation of zoonotic avian influenza A virus infection, which is associated with the infecting subtype. Conjunctivitis was a feature of H7N7 outbreak cases in the Netherlands but has not featured in several hundred H7N9 cases in China in the last few years. H5N1 infections are associated with illness onset up to 7 days post exposure, in contrast to the shorter incubation time of seasonal influenza, with associated delayed viral shedding. The early stages of infection may be difficult to distinguish from seasonal influenza or other respiratory infections that share many common presenting symptoms. The predominant clinical features include high temperature, cough and shortness of breath. Although the majority of cases have been respiratory in presentation, a handful of cases present atypically with fever, gastrointestinal disturbance and diarrhoea. Early clinical signs include alteration in liver function tests, particularly elevated aminotransferase enzymes, lymphopenia and evidence of interstitial pneumonia on chest X-ray. Progression of disease predominantly involves the respiratory tract and can lead to acute respiratory distress syndrome, with death most frequently being due to respiratory failure, often associated with multiorgan failure. Limited autopsy evidence from fatal H5 cases is consistent with respiratory failure and primary viral interstitial pneumonia but with little evidence of extra respiratory spread of virus to account for the multisystem dysfunction. The latter may be attributable to immune dysregulation leading to a cytokine storm (uncontrolled release of tissue damaging immune response molecules); there is some autopsy evidence for haemophagocytic syndrome, but the overall understanding of pathogenesis is limited. Recovery from H5 infection occurs from about 7 to 10 days post illness onset and is associated with a rise in neutralising antibody titres.

Clinical features in human seasonal influenza B infection

Symptoms closely resemble those associated with seasonal influenza A infections, consisting of a 3-day febrile illness with predominantly systemic symptoms. Overall, the infection is somewhat milder.

INFLUENZA C

Clinically, influenza C causes an afebrile upper respiratory tract infection usually confined to young children; outbreaks are not recognised.

SEASONAL INFLUENZA A EPIDEMICS

An individual throughout life can expect to experience multiple influenza infections. Viruses bearing mutations accumulated during error-prone replication (genetic drift) may have a replication advantage because they can evade the existing human immune response, giving a selection advantage due to antigenic drift in circulating strains. Over a period of several years, antigenic variants gradually predominate, displacing older strains, and cause epidemic disease.

Influenza virus is transmitted is by aerosol, droplets or direct contact with respiratory secretions of someone with the infection, for example, sneezing and coughing. Influenza spreads rapidly, especially in closed communities. Most influenza cases in temperate countries tend to occur during a 12- to 16-week period during the winter. The timing, extent and severity of seasonal influenza can all vary according to country. Winter activity is therefore unpredictable. Influenza A viruses cause outbreaks most years in most countries, and it is these viruses that are the usual cause of seasonal epidemics. More severe

epidemics occur intermittently, often associated with the emergence of an antigenic drift variant. Influenza B tends to cause less severe disease and smaller outbreaks, although in children the severity of illness may be similar to that associated with influenza A.

High rates of infection are generally found in preschool children; thereafter the rates are lower, even in the elderly. However, elderly patients in residential homes, if not protected, are at particular risk from acute illness and sudden death. Thus, even if the attack rate is low, the case fatality rate is high. Staff, visitors or other patients may introduce the virus, and this is an important consideration when planning intervention measures.

PATHOGENESIS

Inhaled virus is deposited on the mucous membrane lining the respiratory tract or directly into the alveoli, the anatomical location depending on the size of the droplets inhaled. The virus is exposed to mucoproteins containing sialic acid that can bind to the virus, thus blocking virus attachment to respiratory tract epithelial cells. However, the action of viral neuraminidase allows the virus to break any bonds formed. Specific local secretory immunoglobulin (Ig) A antibodies, if present from a previous infection, may neutralize the virus before attachment occurs, provided the antibody corresponds to the infecting virus type. If not prevented by one of these immune defence mechanisms, the virus attaches to the surface of a respiratory epithelial cell and the intracellular replication cycle is initiated.

The major site of infection for seasonal influenza in humans is the ciliated columnar epithelial cell. New viruses bud from the apical membrane, the cilia are lost and viruses spread to other areas of the respiratory tract. The cell damage initiates an acute inflammatory response with oedema and the attraction of phagocytic cells. The earliest response is the synthesis and release of interferons from the infected cells: these can diffuse to and protect both adjacent and more distant cells before the virus arrives. It appears that interferons released in this way cause many of the systemic features of the flulike syndrome. Although viral components are absorbed and trigger the immune system, the virus itself is confined to the epithelium of the respiratory tract. Specific antibody helps to limit the extracellular spread of the virus, whereas T cell responses are directed against the viral glycoproteins on the surface of infected cells, leading to their destruction by cytotoxic T cells and also by antibody-dependent cell cytotoxicity. The pathogenesis of severe sporadic influenza A zoonotic infections in humans can involve multisystem failure, but evidence of extra respiratory virus replication is rare. It is considered likely that aberrant innate immune responses, such as a cytokine storm arising from massive unregulated production of cytokines and chemokines contribute to poor outcome in severe cases, possibly arising from different respiratory cell tropism of viruses bearing different receptors.

The pathogenicity of influenza viruses is multifactorial and may involve viral, host and environmental factors. Pathogenicity is best understood with influenza A in birds. Host cell receptors are determinants of tropism in birds. Virus infectivity is dependent on host protease activity, cleaving HA into HA_1 and HA_2. There is a clear molecular correlate of pathogenicity associated with the presence of a string of polybasic amino acids at the HA_1–HA_2 cleavage site in certain H5 or H7 avian strains, as the HA protein containing such an insert can now be cleaved by a much wider range of host protease enzymes. In turn, virus dissemination within the avian host is enhanced, and replication occurs in a much wider range of tissues outside the gastrointestinal tract.

Understanding of pathogenesis in mammals is much less complete but is recognised to be multifactorial, involving several genes, including viral HA, NA, polymerase proteins and NS1. Receptor binding preference is an important determinant of tissue and cell tropism, which may influence innate immune responses. Polymerase replication proteins may influence the ability of virus to replicate efficiently, and the NS1 nonstructural protein may also influence pathogenicity by its role in antagonism of innate immune responses. Human H7N9 cases have many similar features to human H5N1 cases, but H7N9 viruses are much less pathogenic in birds than H5N1 viruses, emphasising the difference in mammalian and avian virulence factors.

IMMUNITY

After an attack of influenza, immunity to the particular strain of infecting virus is of long duration. It is related to the amount of local antibody (IgA) in the mucous secretions of the respiratory tract together with specific IgG serum antibody concentration. Immunity to infection, especially with influenza A, is subtype specific, giving little or no protection against subtypes possessing immunologically distinct H or N proteins. Once recovered from an initial influenza infection, exposure to more recent related strains will boost IgG levels to the earlier strains, the so-called original antigenic sin phenomenon.

LABORATORY INVESTIGATION

Prior to the 21st century, laboratory diagnosis of influenza depended on virus isolation through culture methods or

through detection of viral proteins in respiratory epithelial cells by immunofluorescence (IF) or enzyme-linked immunosorbent assays (ELISA). The application of reverse transcription–PCR to respiratory clinical material to detect viral genomic material has transformed the time taken to provide accurate and reliable diagnosis from days to within a matter of hours. Rapid diagnosis of respiratory infections has increased in importance, particularly in hospital or care facilities, such as homes for the elderly. Antiviral drugs given early in infection can be used to control disease and limit transmission. The best specimens for rapid diagnosis are nasal aspirates or nasal washes, but nasal or throat swabs containing epithelial cells are satisfactory if taken in the first few days of illness (Fig. 45.8). Detection of infected airway epithelial cells using direct IF is an insensitive technique and, if undertaken, should be recognised as a suboptimal diagnostic test.

In zoonotic influenza A infection (H5 or H7), virus shedding peaks several days after illness onset, and slightly later than in seasonal influenza, but may continue for up to 10 days, and declines in the recovery phase. In fatal cases, viral shedding may continue at very high levels. H5 virus replication occurs predominantly in the lower respiratory tract. Detection of virus genomic material by RT-PCR is optimal if secretions from the lower respiratory tract are obtained.

Whilst it is now possible to make a diagnosis of influenza without a virus isolate, it is important in the early stages of an outbreak or in sporadic cases that viruses should be isolated and analysed antigenically to provide the best possible information for vaccine production. For primary isolation the most suitable cells are Madin–Darby canine kidney (MDCK) cells.

SEROLOGY

Serological confirmation of a clinical diagnosis is by demonstration of a four-fold or greater rise in functional strain specific antibody titre. Strain differences can be demonstrated by means of haemagglutination inhibition (HI) and neutralisation antibody assays. Specific neutralising antibody can be detected from about 10 to 14 days post infection and reaches a plateau at around 28 days (Fig. 45.8). Complement fixation tests are still occasionally used. This test uses nucleocapsid antigens that are type-specific and can distinguish A from B and C infections, but cannot distinguish between different influenza A infections.

TREATMENT

Oral amantadine hydrochloride was introduced in the early 1980s, followed by a derivative, rimantadine. These drugs

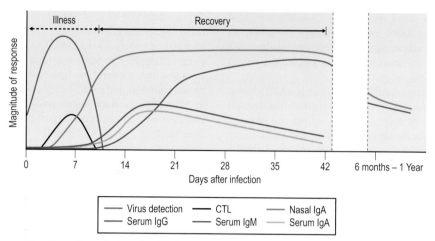

Fig. 45.8 Diagnostic detection of influenza infections in humans. *CTL*, Cytotoxic T cell response.

work by blocking the M2 ion channels in the envelope, thus preventing the pH changes that precede the membrane fusion step essential for nucleocapsid release. Unfortunately, these compounds have activity only against influenza virus type A. Amantadine is effective when given prophylactically and also therapeutically in patients treated within 24 hours of onset of illness. Viruses resistant to amantadine and rimantadine may appear within a few days of drug administration; however, resistant strains show no increased pathogenicity or transmissibility. In recent years, most circulating H3N2 and H1N1 viruses have been naturally resistant to amantadine. Therefore, amantadine is not a useful drug for seasonal influenza, though some clades of H5N1 retain sensitivity.

More recently, two neuraminidase inhibitors (NIs), zanamivir and oseltamivir, have been licensed for therapeutic use in both influenza A and B infections, and other drugs with a similar mode of action are in development (e.g., peramivir). They act to prevent the release of viral particles through the action of viral neuraminidase enzymes, which are conserved across all viral NA subtypes. They can reduce the duration of symptoms by 1–3 days if given within 36 hours of the onset of illness. Zanamivir has poor bioavailability and is administered by inhalation of a dry powder twice daily for 5 days. Oseltamivir is given by mouth as a prodrug and has excellent bioavailability, although nausea and vomiting may occur in some patients. Twice-daily dosage for 5–7 days has been used in those with normal renal function; once-daily dosage is recommended when renal function is impaired.

Both drugs have been licensed since 1999–2000, and a decade of global use indicates that mutations in viral NA are the major source of drug-resistant variants. Resistant viruses have usually had a fitness deficit that compromises their transmissibility. Oseltamivir has been used much

more extensively in this time, and as a consequence, most available data on the emergence of antiviral resistance are related to oseltamivir use. Some key principles have become evident about the emergence of NI drug resistance.

Influenza A virus NAs are classified into group I and group II NAs, which differ in configuration of the enzyme active site. Group I NAs, for example N1, have an active site cleft for substrate binding that is broader, so that the most common oseltamivir resistance mutation in N1 NA at position 275 is readily tolerated and inhibits drug action. Such mutations in H1N1 viruses arise during treatment, most commonly in younger or immunocompromised individuals, where viral shedding is higher, and in H5N1 viruses, where viral replication is not controlled by human immune responses. The spontaneous emergence and transmission of resistant H1N1 virus due to H275Y mutation during the northern hemisphere winter of 2007–2008 was a demonstration of the genetic evolution of influenza viruses. Compensatory mutations in the viral NA or other parts of the viral genome, arising from genetic drift have overcome the fitness deficit normally associated with mutation at position 275, enabling an otherwise disadvantaged virus to outcompete sensitive strains and predominate globally. Over a period of approximately 12 months, virtually all seasonal H1N1 viruses have become naturally oseltamivir resistant.

The patterns of mutations conferring drug resistance are subtype and drug specific. Although H275Y resistance is most common in N1 subtype containing viruses, such viruses remain susceptible to zanamivir (but not peramivir). N2 NAs fall into group 2 NA, for which the active site is narrower, and mutation at position 275 does not have the same effect. In H3N2, the most common mutation conferring NI resistance is at position 119 or position

272. As a consequence of the emergence of significant antiviral resistance, it is now important to ensure global surveillance of drug resistance and a rapid analysis of circulating subtypes so as to direct appropriate antiviral therapy.

During a pandemic there is a major role for the prophylactic use of antiinfluenza drugs such as oseltamivir and zanamivir in those at high risk, in health-care staff and in staff in long-term care facilities who have not been protected by an appropriate vaccine. Early studies have identified protection rates of over 80% with such chemoprophylaxis.

CONTROL MEASURES

The presence of a large global mobile animal reservoir of influenza A virus suggests that eradication of avian influenza A as a zoonotic infection of humans will be impossible. Control strategies focus on limiting the opportunities for cross-species transmission of novel subtypes. For example:

- housing domestic poultry in shelters to avoid contact with over-flying migrating birds
- eliminating wild-bird markets
- segregating different species of birds in markets
- housing aquatic birds and domestic poultry separately
- slaughtering domestic flocks infected with highly pathogenic influenza A viruses

These measures may achieve some success in preventing zoonotic transmission of influenza A to humans and have certainly reduced the circulation of H5 in domestic poultry in Hong Kong since 1997. However, they have little impact on the annual cycle of avian influenza in the wild bird population. Transmission of avian influenza by migrating birds is responsible for extending the geographical range of evolving avian influenza strains, as has been seen in 2005 and 2006, with the detection of H5N1 in birds and poultry in parts of Europe and Africa and the Middle East, whereas hitherto it was confined to Southeast Asia.

Infection control

Exposure to heat for 30 minutes at 56°C is sufficient to inactivate most strains. The viruses are inactivated by a variety of substances, detergents, soaps and other household compounds as well as 20% ethanol, halogens and phenolic compounds. These biological properties are the basis of most infection control advice and practices surrounding the management of nosocomial influenza infection and exposure of individuals to influenza viruses.

Immunisation

A key control strategy for reduction of morbidity and mortality due to influenza is immunisation. The aim is to produce haemagglutination inhibiting or neutralising antibody in all vaccinees. This protects against infection but only with strains closely related to those in the vaccine, and limits transmission. Whole virus, split and subunit inactivated influenza vaccines for intramuscular injection have been widely available for many years (Fig. 45.9), and live-attenuated vaccines have been available more recently for use in children in the United States. Inactivated vaccines are usually trivalent and contain the H and N

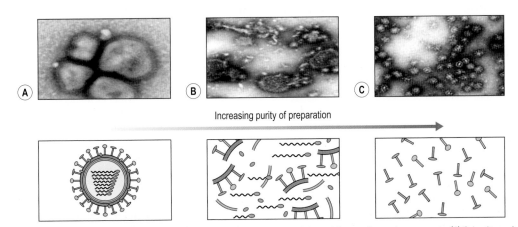

Increasing purity of preparation

Fig. 45.9 Inactivated vaccine preparations. (A) Whole virus. (B) Split vaccine preparation, with some internal components. (C) Subunit vaccine, highly purified surface proteins.

subunits from two type A strains and one type B strain. More recently, quadrivalent inactivated vaccines have also been introduced, with an additional influenza B component to improve the protection against diverse influenza B subgroups. The strains are updated annually on the recommendation of the WHO and, in the United Kingdom, are recommended for use in people aged over 65 years, and in those of any age in clinical risk groups who suffer from chronic cardiorespiratory problems, diabetes, renal or liver failure or an immunosuppressive illness. In interpandemic years, with the elderly given annual boosting, the mortality rate can be reduced by 75% and the rate of hospital admission with complications by about 50%. In recent years, recognition of the impact of seasonal influenza in pregnancy has led to global recommendations for vaccination in pregnancy, and the inclusion of pregnancy as an indication for vaccination in the United Kingdom.

Intervention during a pandemic is more difficult, often for logistic and vaccine supply reasons. Vaccine delivery may be delayed, and the risk groups for vaccination may differ from those normally vaccinated during seasonal influenza as was noted during the pandemic of 2009, where the key risk groups were children and pregnant women. The interval from isolation of a potential pandemic strain to release of an inactivated vaccine made by current methods using eggs is 4–6 months. Such vaccines rely on adequate quantities of virus with the appropriate H and N antigens being produced in cells or eggs inoculated with seed virus. Reassortment of two strains, one a high-yielding laboratory-adapted strain and the other containing the required H and N antigens, may be designed for growth in eggs so that vaccine is prepared as quickly as possible. More recently, using the newer process of reverse genetics, vaccine seed strains can be generated without using traditional reassortment methods. Appropriate vaccine strains are developed by cloning of relevant genes, and this is a successful innovation to speed up vaccine production, which is gradually being introduced in the vaccine industry.

Vaccine seed strains need to be grown in cell or egg substrates to make inactivated vaccines. Separated whole virus particles are inactivated by either formalin or β-propiolactone and may be used at this stage as whole virus vaccines. Whole virus vaccine should not be given to those who are allergic to egg protein. The H and N antigens may be separated from the whole virus by treatment with detergent, and such subunit or split-virus vaccines are better tolerated, especially by young children. Other types of vaccines have been tried, such as cold-adapted live-attenuated vaccines given intranasally. These have been generally effective in provoking a good local (IgA) antibody response and are particularly good at developing protective efficacy in children, though less so

in adults, and several countries, including the United States, USSR and the United Kingdom, are gradually implementing influenza childhood vaccination programmes with live-attenuated influenza vaccines (LAIV).

Clinical trials as part of pandemic vaccine development programmes have demonstrated an important role for vaccine adjuvants such as MF59 and ASO3 in antigen sparing, enabling reduced quantities of vaccine to go further and providing excellent immune responses, particularly in young children. Such vaccines were used for the first time as part of the response to the 2009 pandemic. Consideration of potential unexpected side effects such as narcolepsy may limit mass vaccination programmes using powerful adjuvants until there is a better understanding of mechanisms of action and potential adverse effects. Future vaccine development will concentrate on ensuring better understanding of human immune responses, improving immunogenicity of existing vaccines and developing processes and substrates for a more rapid response.

Global surveillance

The WHO Global Influenza Programme, with its network of reference laboratories, plays a very important role in monitoring the evolution of influenza viruses, selecting and developing prototype pandemic vaccine strains, and developing and updating WHO diagnostic reagents. Recent changes in International Health Regulations have increased the obligation in countries worldwide to have the capacity for preventive measures and to be able to detect and respond to infections of international concern. The emergence of the 2009 pandemic demonstrated the unpredictability of influenza virus evolution and the continuing threat to human health posed by this viral infection. Responses to the pandemic were the most sophisticated ever known following the emergence of a new virus, which despite its mildness still presented formidable challenges to healthcare systems in developed and developing countries. As a result of the global experiences during the first waves of the pandemic, incremental improvements in surveillance and vaccine production may be expected. Incremental improvements in vaccine virus strain selection, based on extensive genetic sequence analysis combined with advanced modelling and computational biology have been achieved in recent years and will improve the choice of strains for vaccine viruses to formulate annual seasonal vaccines. This, together with a renewed interest in developing vaccines that induce longer lasting and more durable immune responses and an enhanced search for antiviral combination therapies and new antiviral targets, will provide better countermeasures for future epidemic and pandemic influenza A strains, which will inevitably emerge.

RECOMMENDED READING

Bedford, T., Riley, S., Barr, I. G., Broor, S., Chadha, M., Cox, N. J., ... Russell, C. A. (2015). Global circulation patterns of seasonal influenza viruses vary with antigenic drift. *Nature, 523*(7559), 217–220. doi:10.1038/nature14460.

Cox, N. J., Hickling, J., Jones, R., Rimmelzwaan, G. F., Lambert, L. C., Boslego, J., ... Ortiz, J. R. (2014). Report on the second WHO integrated meeting on development and clinical trials of influenza vaccines that induce broadly protective and long-lasting immune responses: Geneva, Switzerland, 5-7 May 2014. *Vaccine, 33*(48), 6503–6510. doi:10.1016/j.vaccine.2015.10.014.

Hayward, A. C., Fragaszy, E. B., Bermingham, A., Wang, L., Copas, A., Edmunds, W. J., ... Zambon, M. (2014). Comparative community burden and severity of seasonal and pandemic influenza: results of the Flu Watch cohort study. *The Lancet. Respiratory Medicine, 2*(6), 445–454. doi: http://dx.doi.org/10.1016/S2213-2600(14)70034-7.

Hurt, A. C. (2014). The epidemiology and spread of drug resistant human influenza viruses. *Current Opinion in Virology, 8*, 22–29. doi:10.1016/j.coviro.2014.04.009.

Lafond, K. E., Nair, H., Rasooly, M. H., Valente, F., Booy, R., Rahman, M., ... Global Respiratory Hospitalizations—Influenza Proportion Positive (GRIPP) Working Group. (2016). Global role and burden of influenza in pediatric respiratory hospitalizations, 1982-2012: a systematic analysis. *PLoS Medicine, 13*(3), e1001977. doi:10.1371/journal.pmed.1001977.

Treanor, J. J. (2016). Clinical practice. Influenza vaccination. *The New England Journal of Medicine, 375*(13), 1261–1268. doi:10.1056/NEJMcp1512870.

Trock, S. C., Burke, S. A., & Cox, N. J. (2015). Development of framework for assessing influenza virus pandemic risk. *Emerging Infectious Diseases, 21*(8), 1372–1378. doi:10.3201/eid2108.141086.

Webster, R. G., Monto, A. S., Braciale, T. J., & Lamb, R. A. (Eds.). (2013). *Textbook of influenza* (2nd ed.). Wiley Blackwell, Oxford.

Zambon, M. (2014). Developments in the treatment of severe influenza: lessons from the pandemic of 2009 and new prospects for therapy. *Current Opinion in Infectious Diseases, 27*(6), 560–565. doi:10.1097/QCO.0000000000000113.

Websites

Centers for Disease Control and Prevention (CDC). Influenza (Flu). Available at https://www.cdc.gov/flu/. (Accessed Nov 2017).

European Centre for Disease Prevention and control (ECDC). Influenza. Available at http://ecdc.europa.eu/en/healthtopics/influenza. (Accessed Nov 2017).

International Society for Influenza and Respiratory Viruses. Available at http://www.isirv.org/. (Accessed Nov 2017).

Public Health England. Seasonal influenza: guidance, data and analysis. Available at https://www.gov.uk/government/collections/seasonal-influenza-guidance-data-and-analysis. (Accessed Nov 2017).

World Health Organization. Influenza. Available at http://www.who.int/csr/disease/influenza/en/. (Accessed Nov 2017).

46 Paramyxoviruses and Pneumoviruses

Respiratory infections; mumps; measles and Hendra/Nipah disease

J. S. MALIK PEIRIS, MARILDA M. SEQUEIRA AND DAVID W. BROWN

KEY POINTS

- Respiratory syncytial virus, parainfluenza viruses and human metapneumovirus are important and frequent causes of respiratory tract infections, especially in children.
- Seasonality of respiratory viruses is variable depending on the geographical region.
- Measles remains a serious disease, especially in malnourished young children in less developed countries where it contributes to significant morbidity and mortality and in patients with severely compromised cellular immunity in whom it is often fatal.
- Vaccines are available for measles and mumps viruses. Effective RSV vaccines have been developed and are likely to be licensed within the next few years.
- The global measles vaccination programme has made great progress. Measles has been eliminated from the Americas and is well controlled in many other regions. Maintaining high levels of vaccine coverage is critical, since it reappears quickly when the levels of herd immunity drop.
- There are no reliable antiviral drugs for any of the paramyxo/pneumoviruses other than for RSV.

The Paramyxoviridae and the Pneumoviridae are families of enveloped viruses containing negative sense single-stranded RNA genomes. They resemble the Orthomyxoviruses in morphology, but they are larger and more fragile (Fig. 46.1A–C).

Within the family Paramyxoviridae there are seven genera, four of which contain several members that cause disease in humans or animals (Table 46.1). The Pneumoviridae, a recently established virus family, contains human respiratory syncytial virus (HRSV) and Human metapneumovirus (HMPV), formerly classified as Paramyxoviridae (Table 46.2, Fig. 46.2). The renaming of HRSV to human orthopneumovirus has recently be proposed by

ITCV, but is not yet in general usage. The two families share a common morphology, biological activities and genome organisation, but there are distinct phylogenetic relationships (Fig. 46.3), differences in the RNP structure (Fig. 46.1B) and the *M2* gene.

In addition to these established human pathogens, zoonotic paramyxovirus infections are increasingly recognised. In the 1990s, two new paramyxoviruses, Hendra and Nipah, which cause encephalitis in humans, were discovered in Australia and Malaysia, respectively. In 2014, Sosuga virus, a rubula-like virus similar to bat viruses, was identified in a case of acute febrile disease acquired in Southern Sudan.

STRUCTURE AND REPLICATION

Structure

Parainfluenza, mumps, measles, Newcastle disease virus (NDV) and simian virus 5 are indistinguishable when seen in the electron microscope (and as described later in the chapter), whereas the pneumoviridae (HRSV and HMPV) have slightly longer surface spikes and are more difficult to visualise. The helical nucleocapsids have a herringbone or zipper-like appearance (Fig. 46.1B), which is more easily recognised than the complete particle when viewed using electron microscopy.

Functionally there are other differences. Parainfluenza viruses (1–4a, b), NDV and mumps virus have a surface haemagglutinin and neuraminidase located on the same spike; measles virus spikes have haemagglutinin but no neuraminidase activity while pneumoviruses have neither. In addition, measles virus has a haemolysin not possessed by the others. HRSV has a large surface glycoprotein, G, which has a cell-attaching function similar to that of a haemagglutinin; other surface spikes carry fusion (F) proteins, and all envelopes have matrix (M) proteins. In all members, the RNA is complexed with protein to form the nucleocapsid.

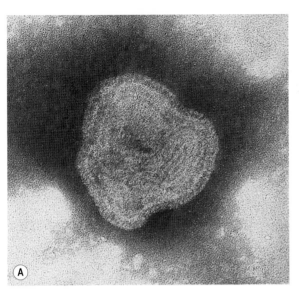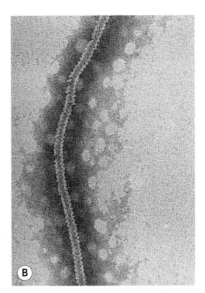

Fig. 46.1   A, Electron micrograph of a typical paramyxovirus. B, Separate internal helical nucleocapsid. Negative contrast, 3% potassium phosphotungstate, pH 7.0, magnification ×200,000.

Table 46.1   Classification and important pathogens of the Paramyxoviridae

Genus	Human viruses	Animal viruses
Respirovirus	Parainfluenza viruses types 1, 3 (HPIV1,3)	Newcastle disease virus (NDV) (poultry), simian virus 5
Rubulavirus	Mumps virus Parainfluenza viruses types 2, 4a, 4b (HPIV)	
Morbillivirus	Measles virus	Canine distemper virus, rinderpest virus, equine morbillivirus, morbilliviruses of seals, dolphins and porpoises
Henipavirus	Hendra virus[a] Nipah virus[a]	Hendra virus Nipah virus

[a]These viruses primarily infect animals but can cause serious zoonotic human disease (see text).

Table 46.2   Classification and important pathogens of the Pneumoviridae

Genus	Human viruses	Animal viruses
Orthopneumovirus	Human respiratory syncytial virus (HRSV)	
Metapneumovirus	Human metapneumovirus (HMPV)	

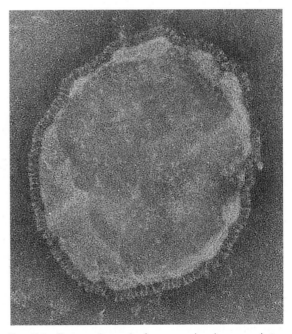

Fig. 46.2   Electron micrograph of a pneumovirus, human respiratory syncytial virus. Human metapneumovirus is indistinguishable in appearance. Negative contrast, 3% potassium phosphotungstate, pH 7.0, magnification ×200,000.

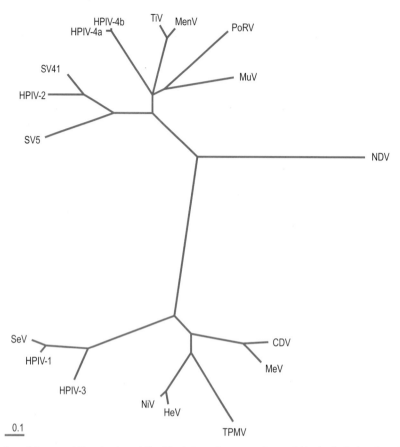

Fig. 46.3 Phylogenetic tree of Paramyxoviridae showing relationships between important viruses within the family based on the deduced amino acid sequences of the matrix protein. Branch lengths represent relative evolutionary distances. *NDV*, Newcastle disease; *CDV*, canine distemper virus; *MeV*, measles virus; *TPMV*, tupaia paramyxovirus; *HeV*, Hendra virus; *NiV*, Nipah virus; *HPIV3*, human parainfluenza virus 3; *HPIV1*, human parainfluenza virus 1; *SeV*, Sendai virus; *SV5*, simian virus 5; *HPIV2*, human parainfluenza virus 2; *SV41*, simian virus 41; *HPIV4a*, human parainfluenza virus 4a; *HPIV4b*, human parainfluenza virus 4b; *TiV*, Tioman virus; *MenV*, Menangle virus; *PoRV*, porcine rubulavirus; *MuV*, mumps virus. From Breed, A. C., Field, H. E., Epstein, J. H., & Daszak, P. (2006). Emerging henipaviruses and flying foxes – Conservation and management perspectives. *Biological Conservation*, 131(2), 211–220. doi: 10.1016/j.biocon.2006.04.007

REPLICATION

The replication of paramyxoviruses follows a common theme. After attachment, the F protein fuses the viral envelope to the cell membrane, becoming part of it and releasing the nucleocapsid into the cell. The negative-sense genome cannot act as messenger RNA (mRNA), making it necessary for the virus to carry its own RNA-dependent RNA polymerase. This polymerase produces subgenomic-sized mRNA transcripts, which are translated to produce some of the early virus-specific polypeptides. These include a second RNA polymerase, which copies the genome into full-length positive complementary strands that are, in turn, copied back into negative strands both for transcription into later mRNA (coding for structural proteins) and for incorporation into new virions. The virus haemagglutinin is

incorporated into the cell membrane, allowing the virus to bud off from the cell surface. Red blood cells will adsorb to the cell surface expressing the viral haemagglutinin (called haemadsorption), and this is used in the laboratory to identify virus-infected cells.

THE PARAMYXOVIRIDAE

PARAINFLUENZA VIRUSES

Classification

The parainfluenza viruses are distributed within two genera, *Respiroviruses* and *Rubulaviruses* (see Table 46.1). There are four parainfluenza viruses (HPIV1–4), which are antigenically distinct, but this is not clinically relevant. Across the wider group there are conserved antigenic epitopes on the paramyxovirus envelope proteins, which cause the serological cross-reactions that are found between the parainfluenza viruses, mumps virus and simian virus 5. HPIV4 has two subtypes, 4a and 4b, which can be distinguished only by neutralisation or haemadsorption inhibition tests.

NDV is a typical paramyxovirus. It infects chickens and other domestic birds. The severity of infection varies considerably from inapparent to fatal, depending on the strain of virus. Because some strains can cause major outbreaks with high mortality, an effective live chicken vaccine based on a virulent strain has been developed. Simian virus 5 (SV5) is often present in normal uninfected monkey kidney cell cultures but does not appear to reduce their sensitivity to other viruses and does not cause human illness. Additional paramyxoviruses are natural pathogens of cattle and other domestic species; they are not known to infect humans.

Clinical features and pathogenesis

The parainfluenza viruses are mostly associated with:

- croup, a harsh brassy cough in children familiar to many parents as a middle-of-the-night irritant caused by a combination of tracheitis and laryngitis
- minor upper respiratory tract illness
- bronchiolitis and pneumonia (particularly HPIV3)

They are responsible for 6%–9% of respiratory infections for which a viral cause can be identified. The incubation period is 3–6 days, during which the virus spreads locally within the respiratory tract. Infections occur in infants in the presence of circulating maternal antibody, but the latter appears to provide some protection in the first 4 months of life.

NDV may cause a mild conjunctivitis in humans, usually as a result of a laboratory accident.

Laboratory investigation

Molecular methods, particularly the reverse transcription–polymerase chain reaction (RT-PCR), are now the most widely used methods for diagnosis for the detection of parainfluenza virus RNA; HPIV PCR assays have been incorporated into multiplex nucleic acid amplification tests that detect a wide range of respiratory infections.

A rapid diagnosis may be made by immunofluorescent staining of exfoliated respiratory cells separated from well-taken nasopharyngeal secretions. There are monoclonal antibody reagents for immunofluorescent detection of parainfluenza virus types 1, 2 and 3, but reagents for type 4 are less widely available.

Similar antiviral antibodies may also be used in enzyme immunoassays to identify viral antigen in specimens from the patient. They have the advantage of requiring only antigen to be present in the specimen, whereas other assays require intact infected cells (for immunofluorescence) or infective virus (for culture).

Virus may be isolated in monkey kidney cell cultures, when available. Visible cytopathic effects in the cell sheets are minimal, and it is usually necessary to show infection of the cells by the haemadsorption of 1% guinea pig or human group O red blood cells. The infecting virus can be typed (or subtyped) by coating the cell cultures with type-specific antisera before adding the red cells. The typing can be confirmed by a neutralisation test or by immunofluorescence.

Serology is not used routinely in diagnosis. Type-specific antibodies may be detected by neutralisation or haemadsorption inhibition, but these tests are too complex for routine use.

Epidemiology and transmission

In temperate regions, HPIV1 infections exhibit a winter peak, whereas HPIV3 is a spring/summer infection, with small epidemics appearing reliably each year. HPIV2 and 4a and 4b infections peak in the winter and are less frequently associated with clinical disease. HPIV4 infections were underdiagnosed in the past because of a lack of suitable reagents, and reported figures are too low for epidemiological patterns to be clear. The reasons for these differing individual epidemiological patterns are unknown.

Numerically, parainfluenza infections cause far fewer clinical episodes than HRSV, and most diagnosed infections are in preschool and primary school children. Eighty percent of children aged 4 years have acquired HPIV3 antibody. Symptomatic reinfections occur in childhood. Fatalities are rare.

The viruses are present in respiratory secretions and are expelled during coughing and sneezing. Infection is acquired by inhalation of infected droplets and by person-to-person contact.

No specific antiviral treatment is available. A number of candidate vaccines including live-attenuated strains have been developed, but no vaccine is yet available for routine use.

MUMPS VIRUS

Description

Mumps virus is a typical paramyxovirus, indistinguishable in the electron microscope (EM) from parainfluenza viruses, measles virus and NDV, with a similar ribonucleocapsid, which may be the only virus-like material seen by electron microscopy. There is only one serotype, although monoclonal antibodies have shown antigenic differences in the surface proteins of different strains, and sequencing studies have revealed multiple genotypes.

Clinical features and pathogenesis

Mumps is an 'iceberg' disease, which, although common as a childhood infection, is often subclinical. Although the salivary glands are often involved, inapparent or minor infections are more common. Infections in adults may be more severe and more likely to lead to complications. The introduction of MMR (mumps, measles, rubella) vaccine as a universal vaccine of childhood has resulted in a significant age shift, with many clinical cases in countries using MMR occurring in older children and university-age adults.

Infection is acquired by inhalation of droplets and by direct and indirect contact with infected secretions. The incubation period is 14–18 days and is followed by a generalised illness with later localisation in the salivary glands, usually the parotids. The generalised phase presents as a flulike illness with fever and malaise, followed by pain in the parotid glands, which then swell rapidly. Much of the swelling is due to blockage of the efferent duct of the parotid gland, and sucking a lemon in front of a sufferer is a refined form of torture, although likely to be diagnostic!

Neurological involvement is common in mumps (in more than 50% of infections), although the majority of cases are not clinically apparent. However, clinical meningitis remains the most common serious complication, occurring in 1%–10% of patients with mumps parotitis. Meningitis (like any other complication) can occur before, during, after or even in the absence of salivary gland involvement. Before the widespread use of the MMR vaccine, mumps virus and the enteroviruses (see Ch. 44) accounted for most of the cases of aseptic meningitis in the United Kingdom. Mumps meningitis is rarely fatal, and complete recovery is usual. Meningoencephalitis has been described, but is much rarer, and carries a poorer prognosis and may result in long-term neurological sequelae or death. Deafness and tinnitus have also been described as complications but are very rare.

In prepubertal children the acute illness usually subsides in 4–5 days, with complete recovery. The best known complication, in postpubertal males, is orchitis. This, although painful and causing softening and atrophy of the affected testicle, is usually unilateral and rarely causes sterility. Oophoritis occurs in girls and should be distinguished from a ruptured ovarian cyst or acute appendicitis. Both orchitis and oophoritis commonly develop as the parotitis resolves, and a history of previous parotid pain and swelling usually provides the clue.

The role of mumps in pancreatitis is difficult to establish. There may be abdominal pain in acute mumps, but the levels of serum amylase do not correlate with the clinical picture. High levels may provide supportive evidence but are not diagnostic. Although uncomfortable, it resolves.

Laboratory investigation
Detection and isolation

Laboratory confirmation of suspected mumps cases is important in countries with MMR programmes. The detection of mumps virus RNA by genome amplification (RT-PCR) is the most sensitive and widely used diagnostic test using throat swab, saliva or urine samples collected in the acute phase of illness. Virus is detectable in the cerebrospinal fluid (CSF) of patients with mumps meningitis.

Isolation of the virus in cell culture (usually in monkey kidney or HEp2 cells) from throat swabs, saliva, urine or the CSF is possible, and the virus may take up to a week to grow to detectable levels. Virus presence can be reliably confirmed by indirect immunofluorescent staining of cultured cells. Alternatively, neutralisation or haemadsorption, which can be inhibited by specific antiserum, may be used to confirm the presence and identity of the virus.

Serology

Serological confirmation of mumps in a child is based on the detection of mumps-specific IgM by EIA using serum samples. In older adolescents and adults, especially those with a history of MMR vaccination, the IgM response may not be detectable, but high titres of IgG are detected and virus is detectable by PCR. This pattern suggests a mumps reinfection, and these cases are sometimes seen with a classical clinical presentation. Complement fixation tests, neutralisation and haemagglutination inhibition tests have been used in the past, but they are more complex and do not offer any advantages in routine diagnosis.

Epidemiology

Mumps is a worldwide disease, with humans the only known reservoir. Mumps is less infectious than measles or chickenpox. In the absence of vaccination, most infections are in children of school age, but, where MMR has been introduced, infection can be well controlled with the age of infection increased. It was thought that mumps infection conferred lifelong immunity, but recently mumps outbreaks have been described in well-vaccinated populations in the United States and Europe. A high proportion of cases have occurred in recipients of one and sometimes two doses of a mumps-containing vaccine, which suggest a waning of immunity following vaccination.

Control

Some, but not very reliable, protection may be given by passive immunisation, but this treatment is not used clinically.

Mumps-containing vaccines generally use one of Jeryl Lynn or Urabe-like strains, almost universally given as the triple MMR vaccine. All three vaccine components are live-attenuated viruses. The mumps component induces a good antibody response. Immunogenicity is lower with vaccines containing the Jeryl Lynn strain, and antibody levels wane in populations with good mumps control leading to mumps cases in vaccinees. Cases of mild postvaccine meningitis have also been described in vaccinees receiving mumps vaccine containing Urabe and related strains. This has led to their withdrawal in many vaccine programmes.

MEASLES VIRUS

Description

Measles virus (MeV) is a morbillivirus. The virus particles are enveloped, 100–200 nm in diameter and morphologically indistinguishable in the EM from other members of the group. The ribonucleoprotein helix is readily released from the virion and may be the only identifiable virus structure seen by electron microscopy. It has a single-stranded, nonsegmented negative-sense RNA genome that is 15,894 nucleotides in length. The genome contains six genes encoding nucleoprotein (N), phosphoprotein (P), matrix (M), fusion (F), haemagglutinin (H) and polymerase (L). The two viral membrane glycoprotein spikes (haemagglutinin tetramers and fusion protein trimers) play key roles in viral entry and are the main targets of virus-neutralising antibodies. The haemagglutinin binds to the cellular receptor (SLAM-CDw150), and the F protein causes the fusion of virus and host cell membranes, viral penetration, and haemolysis. Measles does not have a neuraminidase function.

There is only one serotype of measles virus, although monoclonal antibodies show that there may be minor antigenic differences between wild and cultivated strains. Sequencing of measles strains has enabled MeVs to be grouped into eight clades A–H, subdivided into 24 genotypes based on the highly variable 450 nucleotides coding for the *N* gene.

Measles is related to a number of animal morbilliviruses. Canine distemper and rinderpest in cattle are well-known relatives, although a global campaign to eradicate rinderpest was successful. In the past few years other related viruses have been isolated from seals (of several species), dolphins and porpoises. All are distinct and can cause serious illness in their natural species, although survivors develop solid immunity. There is partial cross-protection experimentally in ferrets between measles and canine distemper viruses.

Clinical features and pathogenesis

Measles is an acute febrile illness that usually occurs in childhood. After an incubation period of 10–12 days, the onset is flulike, with high fever, cough and conjunctivitis. Koplik's spots (red spots with a bluish-white centre on the buccal mucosa) may be present at this stage. After 1–2 days the acute symptoms decline, with the appearance of a widespread maculopapular rash. Rash is not seen in measles infection in severely immunocompromised individuals. Infection is usually rapidly fatal, and this is thought to point to the importance of T cell–mediated immunity in clearing the infection.

Over the next 10–14 days recovery is usually complete as the rash fades, with considerable desquamation. Complications include:

- giant cell pneumonia, more common in adults
- otitis media
- post-measles encephalitis

The pneumonia is due to direct invasion by virus, but the role of virus in the other two complications is uncertain. Measles encephalitis can cause severe and permanent mental impairment in those it does not kill. It is estimated to occur in 1 : 1000 cases, and so it is uncommon but disastrous.

The mortality rate associated with uncomplicated measles in immunocompetent, well-nourished children is low but rises rapidly with malnourishment, in the immunocompromised and, to a much lesser extent, with age. The virus has also been devastating in isolated populations (such as the Inuit in Greenland some years ago) into which it was introduced as a new disease. Measles infection causes immunosuppression, which has been linked to all-cause mortality in children in Africa.

One further rare complication of measles is subacute sclerosing panencephalitis (SSPE), estimated to occur in 1 : 25,000 cases. It occurs in children or early adolescents who have had measles early in life, usually when under 2 years of age. It is a progressive and inevitably fatal neurodegenerative disease. Within infected cells is a defective form of measles virus, which, because it is unable to induce the production of a functional M protein, is not released from the cells as complete virus. Patients deteriorate over several years, losing intellectual capacity before motor activities. Oligoclonal antibodies to measles virus proteins appear in the CSF, which are diagnostic, but the virus cannot be cultivated unless it is 'rescued' by cocultivating neuronal cells with a susceptible cell type.

There are reports linking measles with multiple sclerosis, Paget's disease of bone and Crohn's disease. In each disease, tubular structures resembling measles nucleocapsids were seen by thin-section electron microscopy. Immunofluorescence has been used to demonstrate measles antigens in biopsy material. The evidence linking measles virus to the aetiology of these diseases is not compelling.

Laboratory investigation

The widespread use of vaccine has made the disease rarer in the community, and, consequently, fewer clinicians are familiar with it. There are also a number of other diseases, which present with a similar picture of rash and fever, including HHV6, Dengue and Zika infections. Rubella and parvovirus B19 are part of the differential diagnosis. The clinical diagnosis of measles is therefore unreliable, and so all cases are investigated as part of surveillance programmes. Laboratory confirmation is most commonly by the detection of measles-specific IgM in a venous blood or oral fluid (avoiding the need for venesection). Increasingly, RT-PCR amplification of viral RNA from a throat swab, oral fluid or urine sample collected during acute infection is used for rapid diagnosis. In hospital, and particularly in immunocompromised patients in whom the disease is often without rash (and where the diagnosis may not be suspected at first), the diagnosis is best made by PCR detection of viral RNA. Recently, cases of IgM-negative, PCR-positive measles have been reported in vaccinees, which are compatible with a reinfection.

The virus may be isolated, though not readily, from blood or nasopharyngeal aspirates during the prodrome and until day 2 of rash, in human fibroblasts, primary monkey kidney cells and Vero cells. The virus can then be identified by neutralisation or immunofluorescence.

Epidemiology

Measles is highly infectious. Transmission is from person to person by aerosol of small respiratory droplets and by direct and indirect contact with infected respiratory and nasal secretions. The key features of measles were first described in an outbreak on the Faroe Islands in the 1840s. Three-quarters of the population were infected, although the mortality rate was low. Most of those who were not infected were aged over 65 years, the interval since the last time the disease had been present in the islands. These observations confirmed the high infectivity and that infection leads to lifelong immunity. Measles epidemics occurred every 2 years in the absence of vaccination.

This periodicity was absent in isolated populations too small to maintain transmission (<400,000), in poverty and overcrowding, and following the widespread use of vaccine.

In 1980, before measles vaccine was used globally, an estimated 2.6 million deaths due to measles occurred worldwide. The success of the global measles programme has led to a reduction in mortality to <150,000 by 2015. The feasibility of measles eradication has been discussed for more than 30 years. Measles meets all of the biological criteria for disease eradication: (1) humans are the sole pathogen reservoir; (2) accurate diagnostic tests exist and (3) an effective, practical intervention (vaccine) is available at reasonable cost. Interruption of transmission in large geographical areas, such as the Americas for prolonged periods, further supports the feasibility of eradication. Elimination of measles was achieved in the Americas in 2016, good progress has been achieved in most regions, although in Southeast Asia and Africa measles still circulates widely.

Control

The first measles vaccine was a formalin-inactivated one. Although inducing circulating antibody, it was found that vaccinees subsequently exposed to natural measles were likely to develop severe atypical disease. It was later recognised that the vaccine had failed to induce adequate levels of antibody to the haemolytic F protein, and the immune response it induced did not inhibit cell-to-cell spread of the virus. Consequently it was withdrawn.

All modern vaccines are now live-attenuated vaccines, containing the Edmonston B, Moreton or Schwarz strains, which give a seroconversion rate of over 90%. Antibody persists, although antibody titers in the community drop in the absence of circulating measles. A few cases of reinfection have been described in vaccinees.

Measles vaccine is now generally combined with rubella (MR) and mumps (MMR) and administered in either form as part of global control programmes. This combination of attenuated viruses was introduced initially in the United States and has been shown to induce good immune responses to all three infections. Two doses of MMR are given either as part of routine programmes (given between 9 and 18 months of age) or in targeted campaigns to ensure adequate population immunity, which needs to reach 95% to eliminate measles transmission.

The attenuated measles vaccine, alone or in combination with mumps and rubella, is both effective and safe. In the United Kingdom, vaccine uptake fell in the early years of this century because of fears over its safety, particularly as a possible cause of autism. These fears were shown to be unsubstantiated. The measles vaccine has an excellent safety profile.

NIPAH AND HENDRA VIRUSES

Nipah virus was first identified during an outbreak of respiratory disease in pigs, which was associated with encephalitis cases in humans in Malaysia in 1998. There were more than 200 human cases, with 105 deaths. The causative agent was a paramyxovirus. Nipah virus is closely related to Hendra virus, which was discovered in Australia in 1994 causing a fatal respiratory disease in horses. Zoonotic transmission to humans has occurred, resulting in a fatal encephalitis.

The natural host of these viruses are fruit bats of the Pteropodidae family, with transmission to other mammals including humans an unusual event. Rare human cases continue to occur within the geographical range of the host species. Subsequently, outbreaks of Nipah virus have been reported in India and Bangladesh, without obvious involvement of pigs as an intermediate host. Human infection has been linked to the consumption of date palm sap contaminated with the virus by fruit bats. There is also evidence of limited human-to-human transmission and nosocomial infection.

The incubation period for Nipah and Hendra infections is estimated as 10–21 days. Most Nipah cases present with an acute encephalitis characterised by fever and headache with a reduced level of consciousness. Myalgia, drowsiness, dizziness and vomiting are also common. The clinical picture is consistent with involvement of the brainstem and upper cervical spinal cord. A few patients present as an atypical pneumonia with cough and fever. The few Hendra cases presented with fever, myalgia and headaches, and one case developed a fatal encephalitis a year after first diagnosis. Both infections have a high mortality rate, and many survivors have residual neurological damage.

These viruses are members of the *Henipavirus* genus. Diagnostic tests based on virus detection by RT-PCR and the detection of specific IgM antibodies are available. Because of the high fatality rate, work with these viruses is under BSL4 containment. No vaccines are currently available.

THE PNEUMOVIRIDAE

HUMAN RESPIRATORY SYNCYTIAL VIRUS

Description

Human respiratory syncytial virus (HRSV) has a global distribution and is the most important cause of viral lower respiratory tract illness in infants and children. Virtually all infections occur before 2 years of age.

HRSV is a member of the *Orthopneumovirus* genus, Pneumoviridae family. The viral genome consists of 10 genes encoding 11 proteins. The virus envelope contains three encoded transmembrane surface glycoproteins, the fusion (F), the major attachment (G) and the small hydrophobic SH protein. There is also a nonglycosylated matrix (M) protein. The F and G glycoproteins induce most of the neutralising antibody response to infection. The virus lacks a haemagglutinin and a neuraminidase. The glycoprotein G is a receptor for cell attachment (but not for red blood cells). The F protein induces the syncytia in cell cultures from which the virus derived its name, and it is probably responsible for both virus/cell fusion and spread within the host.

HRSV has a single serotype with two antigenic subgroups A and B. HRSV antigenic differences were demonstrated using MABs, which defined extensive antigenic differences in the G protein. Less are seen in F and other viral proteins. The two subgroups exhibit a three- to four-fold reciprocal difference in neutralisation with convalescent polyclonal serum. Virus sequencing studies have shown distinct lineages or clades within each subgroup, which have a broad geographic distribution.

HRSV infects chimpanzees readily; indeed, early isolates were termed chimpanzee coryza agent. Cattle, goats and sheep may be infected naturally with human strains, and there is evidence that other domestic and rodent species are susceptible. Closely related viruses are seen in other species such as bovines (BRSV).

Clinical features

HRSV infections result in clinical syndromes that include upper respiratory tract infection, otitis media, bronchiolitis, lower respiratory tract infections including pneumonia and exacerbations of asthma- or viral-induced wheeze. In general, 25%–40% of healthy term infants exposed to HRSV at age 6 weeks to 9 months present with upper respiratory tract symptoms and/or bronchiolitis and pneumonia. The most serious illness caused by HRSV is bronchiolitis in young babies, in whom the bronchiolar inflammation can act as a one-way valve leading to hyperinflation of the lungs (very characteristic on radiography). Clinical signs and symptoms include wheezing, crepitations and increased transparency on a chest X-ray. Risk factors for severe disease include the degree of prematurity, chronic lung disease, some forms of congenital heart disease and immunodeficiency.

In normal babies, illness is rarely fatal where access to experienced medical staff and facilities for appropriate management is available.

While the main clinical feature is bronchiolitis, the upper respiratory tract is also infected, which makes virological diagnosis possible using nasopharyngeal aspirates or nasopharyngeal swabs. If HRSV is present in the nasopharynx and there is clinical evidence of lower respiratory tract involvement, HRSV is likely to be responsible.

HRSV is also common in healthy adults, especially in medical personnel or individuals caring for small children. These episodes generally present with rhinorrhea, pharyngitis, cough, bronchitis, headache and fever. A more severe illness and some fatalities can occurs in older persons, especially the elderly and high-risk groups such as the immunocompromised. Nosocomial hospital outbreaks are frequent and occur in multiple age groups and settings including neonatal intensive care, haematology, transplant and oncology units.

Laboratory investigation

Detection and isolation

During the acute phase of illness virus may be readily demonstrated in nasopharyngeal secretions (which are usually copious) by RT-PCR, immunofluorescence, enzyme immunoassays or cell culture.

Rapid diagnosis in <1 hour with commercially available immunofluorescence or enzyme immunoassay kits is sensitive, provided an adequate number of desquamated respiratory cells be collected in the secretions. Such assays may be less sensitive compared with culture, but the virus grows slowly, and positive results will come too late to influence management. As with other respiratory viruses, molecular methods such as real-time RT-PCR, either for a single virus or multiplexed to detect a panel of respiratory viruses, are more sensitive and specific and have become the diagnostic method of choice in many settings. RT-PCR testing is the optimum method in adults and the elderly because the virus titres in secretions may be lower.

Serology

Serological methods are rarely used for diagnosis. Since the infection occurs mainly in infants, many of the patients are too young to respond reliably, and even adults do not always produce a detectable rise in serum antibody levels. However, improved immunoassays for antibodies to the G and F proteins have become more widely available recently.

Treatment

National clinical guidelines for the management of infants and children with RSV infection are available. The only licensed antiviral drug available for the treatment of RSV infection is ribavirin. Despite many studies, its clinical efficacy remains controversial, and because of the drug toxicity and minimal clinical benefit measured, it is not recommended for routine clinical use. Currently, ribavirin is only recommended for use in children with substantial comorbidities (i.e., those with lung or cardiac disease or immunosuppressive disease and therapy) or those with very severe RSV disease.

Palavizumab is a humanised mouse monoclonal antibody directed against the fusion (F) glycoprotein of HRSV. As palavizumab is very expensive and monthly injections are required to maintain protective titres during RSV season, the American Academy of Pediatrics (AAP) and Public Health England (PHE) advise its use only for the most vulnerable infants. A biosimilar, less expensive version of palavizumab may become available commercially within a few years because of expiry of the patent, which may make it more widely available.

Another monoclonal antibody, motavizumab is showing promise in reducing hospitalisation due to HRSV. Trials of new antivirals (GS-5806, ALS-008176) are in progress.

Various treatment strategies have proven ineffective when examined in rigorous clinical trials. So bronchodilators, epinephrine, corticosteroids and antibiotics should be used with strict criteria.

Epidemiology

HRSV is a ubiquitous pathogen, found in all human populations, and is an important cause of child morbidity. Globally, an estimated 33.8 million new episodes occur in children under 5 years of age annually, and 3.4 million HRSV episodes required hospitalisation in 2005. Reinfections are common as initial HRSV infections do not generate substantial immunity. The severity of HRSV disease generally decreases in subsequent reinfections, and their frequency decreases with age.

HRSV is transmitted through close contact with an infected case. Routes of infection include through large droplets, by direct contact with infectious secretions on environmental surfaces and through contact with contaminated hands to nasal or conjunctival mucosa.

In the temperate zones of both the northern and southern hemispheres, HRSV circulates seasonally, causing a substantial epidemic every year usually between late autumn and early spring. In general, virus circulation lasts 3–5 months in the community. The exact timing varies. In tropical and subtropical regions, the seasonal relationship is less defined, with virus detectable all year round and epidemics usually peaking during the rainy season. Many developing countries do not have accurate data for virus seasonality.

The two HRSV subgroups can cocirculate during an epidemic, and frequently there is a predominant subgroup in each epidemic year. This pattern usually alternates but in a somewhat irregular pattern. Shifts in the predominant strains within each subgroup also occur.

Control

HRSV vaccines have been in development for many years. A formalin-inactivated, crude, whole-virus vaccine was first trialled in the 1960s. It induced good levels of circulating antibody but failed to protect the recipients, who became more ill than controls when subsequently exposed to HRSV. A wide range of HRSV vaccine candidates have been developed using different technologies and targeting diverse populations (the newborn, pediatric, pregnant women and elderly) and are being evaluated in preclinical and clinical trials. These include live attenuated, F protein–based candidates, other technologies such as pre- and post-F subunit protein, nucleic acid and gene-based vectors. Several have given encouraging results in clinical trials.

A major challenge to using these vaccines is that the peak of disease occurs within the first year of life. It has proved difficult to identify the right age to give the vaccine; early enough to prevent disease but late enough to be safe and immunogenic. Vaccines for the elderly are developed and may be the first to be used.

HRSV is a major nosocomial hazard. Hand washing (soap and water or alcohol based) is the single most important infection control measure, and its use should be stimulated in all health settings.

HUMAN METAPNEUMOVIRUS

Description

Human metapneumovirus (HMPV) was discovered in the Netherlands in 2001 as a cause of respiratory infections, which closely mimicked HRSV both in spectrum of disease caused and age group affected.

HMPV has a negative-sense single-stranded RNA genome that contains eight genes that code for nine proteins. These generally correspond to those of HRSV, except that HMPV lacks the genes for NS1 and NS2. The virus envelope contains the three surface glycoproteins (F, G and SH) in the form of spikes. Like HRSV, HMPV surface glycoproteins have no haemagglutinin, haemolysin or neuraminidase function.

Genetic analysis indicates that at least two separate lineages (A and B) circulate worldwide; subsequent phylogenetic analysis of additional sequences obtained for the *F* and *G* genes revealed that each lineage can be further divided into sub-lineages.

Clinical features

HMPV infection is associated with a range of symptoms, and it has been identified as one of the most frequent causes of upper (U-) and lower respiratory tract infections (LRTI) in childhood.

Children with HPMV infection most commonly present with URTI symptoms such as rhinorrhea, cough or fever. However, the most common causes of hospitalisation are bronchiolitis and pneumonia. There is some evidence that the virus may precipitate exacerbations of asthma in small children and adults. Wheezing is a common clinical symptom observed in multiple studies of children with HMPV-associated LRTI. Clinically, HMPV causes a very similar spectrum of disease to HRSV infection, although there are reports that fever is more frequent in HMPV and rhinorrhea in HRSV-infected patients. Risk factors for severe HMPV infection associated with acute respiratory failure are younger age and prematurity, the presence of severe chronic underlying diseases and the nosocomial acquisition of infection. Reinfections occur and young adults present with mild cold and flulike symptoms. However, in elderly patients, reinfection can lead to severe infection (such as pneumonitis) and even fatal cases.

Laboratory investigation

Routine diagnosis is becoming more widely available. Molecular detection using real-time RT-PCR is the method most often used as a single or multiplexed methodology in-house or in various commercial kits. Immunofluorescence and ELISA-based assays to detect viral protein are commercially available but are less sensitive. Cell culture using several cell lines are used for research purposes. ELISAs for detecting HMPV antibodies are available.

Epidemiology

HMPV has a worldwide distribution, and generally has a seasonal peak in the winter. Outbreaks occur mainly in January to March in the northern hemisphere and June to July in the southern hemisphere. Some studies suggest that the HMPV season follows the HRSV and influenza seasons, although it often overlaps the HRSV season.

HMPV spreads through infectious airborne droplets and by direct contact with infected secretions. The incubation period is usually 3–5 days. HMPV principally affects young children, infection is common, seropositivity approaches 100% in the population by 5–10 years of age. Infection is observed in all age groups, and reinfection can occur throughout life. The duration of symptoms is often less than a week, and some studies suggest that children shed virus for 1–2 weeks. The two HMPV lineages cocirculate. Predominant HMPV lineages vary from year to year. Studies on the severity of the two HMPV lineages have not shown any difference.

Treatment and control

Currently, there is no specific drug treatment, although animal models are being developed to evaluate potential treatments and vaccines. Current management of HMPV infection is primarily supportive. There are studies of monoclonal antibody and ribavirin treatment without clear evidence of efficacy against HMPV infection in humans.

Several vaccine candidates against HMPV, including those prepared from chimeric viruses, plasmid-based reverse genetics systems, live-attenuated viruses and subunits of the virus (mainly F protein), have been tested in rodent and nonhuman primate models but are not yet ready for study in humans.

ACKNOWLEDGMENT

Professor Dick Madeley, who wrote this chapter in earlier editions of the book.

RECOMMENDED READING

Bennett, J. E., Dolin, R., & Blaser, M. (2014). *Mandell, Douglas, and Bennett's principles and practice of infectious diseases* (8th ed.). Elsevier. Paramyxoviridae sects 157–162, pp. 1937–1981.

Higgins, D., Trujillo, C., & Keech, C. (2016). Advances in RSV vaccine research and development–a global agenda. *Vaccine, 34*(26), 2870–2875. doi:10.1016/j.vaccine.2016.03.109.

Knipe, D. M., & Howley, P. M. (Eds.). (2013). *Fields virology* (6th ed.). Philadelphia: Lippincott, Williams & Wilkins.

Schildgen, V., van den Hoogen, B., Fouchier, R., Tripp, R. A., Alvarez, R., Manoha, R., ... Schildgen, O. (2011). Human Metapneumovirus: lessons learned over the first decade. *Clinical Microbiology Reviews, 24*(4), 734–754. doi:10.1128/CMR.00015-11.

Wild, T. F. (2009). Henipaviruses: a new family of emerging Paramyxoviruses. *Pathologie Biologie (Paris), 57*(2), 188–196. doi:10.1016/j.patbio.2008.04.006.

Zuckerman, A. J., Banatvala, J. E., Griffiths, P. D., Schoub, B., & Mortimer, P. (Eds.). (2009). Chs. 17, 18, 22 and 24. *Principles & practice of clinical virology* (6th ed.). pp. 409–440, 441–462, 533–560). Chichester: Wiley-Blackwell.

47 Arboviruses: alphaviruses, flaviviruses and bunyaviruses

Encephalitis; yellow fever; dengue; haemorrhagic fever; miscellaneous tropical fevers; undifferentiated fever

ALAN D. T. BARRETT AND ANN M. POWERS

KEY POINTS

- Arboviruses are transmitted biologically by arthropod vectors (mosquitoes, ticks and biting flies).
- There are three major types of clinical diseases caused by these viruses: central nervous system, visceral organs/haemorrhagic fever and febrile infections, with many progressing from the latter to the former syndromes. Many arboviruses are highly pathogenic and require a high level of biocontainment.
- There are more than 500 recognised arbovirus species classified in six virus families: Togaviridae, Flaviviridae, Bunyaviridae, Rhabdoviridae, Reoviridae and Orthomyxoviridae.
- In the United Kingdom arboviruses are overwhelmingly of concern to travellers. Dengue, West Nile, yellow fever and Zika viruses are four widely distributed flaviviruses of global concern, but numerous other agents must be considered in specific locations.
- The *Alphavirus* chikungunya virus, which historically had a geographical range encompassing Sub-Saharan Africa, India and Southeast Asia, has spread throughout the world in the past decade and now maintains a global distribution matching that of dengue.
- The *Hantavirus* genus of the Bunyaviridae contains many pathogens associated with haemorrhagic fever with renal syndrome or hantavirus pulmonary syndrome. Hantaviruses are transmitted by rodents, not arthropods.
- Commercial vaccines are available only for yellow fever, dengue, Japanese encephalitis and tick-borne encephalitis, but a number of experimental vaccines show promise.
- The only effective antiviral treatment is ribavirin, which has efficacy only against selected bunyaviruses and alphaviruses.

The name arbo (arthropod-borne) virus denotes viruses transmitted biologically by arthropod (mainly insect and tick) vectors. Arboviruses are found in many different taxa, and over 550 individual arbovirus species are now officially classified in six virus families. Many arboviruses are highly pathogenic and are classified at biosafety level 3 or 4. As there are many similarities in their transmission cycles and in the diseases that they cause, they are considered together in this chapter.

Arboviruses were defined by a World Health Organization Scientific Group as 'viruses that are maintained in nature principally, or to an important extent, through biological transmission between susceptible vertebrate hosts by haemotophagous arthropods or through transovarian and possible venereal transmission in arthropods; the viruses multiply and produce viraemia in the vertebrates, multiply in the tissues of arthropods, and are passed on to new vertebrates by the bites of arthropods after a period of extrinsic incubation'.

Certain viruses within the six families containing arboviruses are not transmitted by arthropods but are maintained in nature within rodent reservoirs that may transmit infection directly to humans. These include the *Hantavirus* genus of the family Bunyaviridae.

DESCRIPTION

Classification

Most arboviruses are members of the families Togaviridae, Flaviviridae and Bunyaviridae; some are assigned to the families Reoviridae (genera *Coltivirus* [e.g., Colorado tick fever virus] and *Orbivirus* [e.g., Bluetongue viruses]), Orthomyxoviridae (e.g., Thogoto virus) and Rhabdoviridae (members of the genera *Vesiculovirus* [e.g., vesicular stomatitis virus] and *Lyssavirus*) (Table 47.1). Within the Togaviridae, only one *(Alphavirus)* of the two genera contains arthropod-borne viruses; the other genus, *Rubivirus*, contains rubella virus, which is

Table 47.1 Characteristic properties of arboviruses

Property	Arbovirus family (principal genus)					
	Togaviridae *(Alphavirus)*	Flaviviridae *(Flavivirus)*	Bunyaviridae *(Orthobunyavirus)*[a]	Rhabdoviridae *(Rhabdovirus)*[b]	Reoviridae *(Reovirus)*[c]	Orthomyxoviridae
Symmetry[d]	Icosahedral	Icosahedral	Helical	Bullet-shaped	Icosahedral	Icosahedral
Total diameter (nm)	60–70	50	80–120	180 × 85	60–80	15–120
Nucleic acid	(+)ssRNA	(+)ssRNA	(−)ssRNA and ambisense	(−)ssRNA	dsRNA	(−)ssRNA
Molecular weight (×10⁶) (Da)	4.2–4.4	4.2–4.4	0.3–3.1	3.5–4.6	0.2–3.0	
No. of nucleic acid molecules	1	1	3	1	10–12	6–7
No. of viruses in family	31	60	100	75	89	8
Inactivation by diethyl ether or sodium deoxycholate	+	+	+	+	−	+

ssRNA, Single-stranded RNA; *dsRNA*, double-stranded RNA.
[a]Other important genera: *Nairovirus*, *Phlebovirus* (arthropod-borne), *Hantavirus* (not arthropod-borne).
[b]See Ch. 55.
[c]See Ch. 51.
[d]All have enveloped virions (except Reoviridae).

not arthropod-borne, as its sole member (see Ch. 56). The Flaviviridae contain four genera *(Flavivirus, Pestivirus, Pegivirus,* and *Hepacivirus)*, but only the *Flavivirus* genus contains arthropod-borne viruses. Pestiviruses infect only vertebrate animals (e.g., bovine viral diarrhoea virus), pegiviruses cause persistent infection in a number of animal species (including humans) and hepatitis C virus is described in Ch. 48. The Bunyaviridae consist of five genera *(Orthobunyavirus, Hantavirus, Nairovirus, Phlebovirus* and *Tospovirus)*, containing over 300 species, and is the largest virus family. The *Tospovirus* genus contains plant viruses that are transmitted by vectors (thrips), whereas the *Hantavirus* genus contains viruses that are transmitted by rodents rather than arthropods.

The classification of arboviruses into individual species is now made on the basis of polythetic criteria including genetic as well as antigenic and other phenotypic characteristics. Clusters of viruses that show antigenic overlap are termed serogroups or antigenic complexes. Table 47.2 lists some of the important members.

Properties

Arboviruses share common biological attributes (see Table 47.1):

1. Most induce fatal encephalitis 1–10 days after intracerebral inoculation of mice aged less than 48 hours; some also induce fatal encephalitis after intracerebral inoculation of weaned mice aged 3–4 weeks.

2. Haemagglutination. Most arboviruses can agglutinate erythrocytes, an ability that is inhibited by antiserum against viruses within the same serogroup. Seroreactivity against viruses from dissimilar serogroups is generally weak.

3. Many arboviruses multiply in continuous polyploid tissue cultures of mammalian cells incubated at 37°C, such as grivet monkey kidney (Vero) and baby hamster kidney (BHK).

4. Many arboviruses, such as dengue and Ross River viruses, multiply in continuous cultures of mosquito cells when incubated at 34°C or lower temperatures; *Aedes albopictus* C6/36 mosquito cells are often used. In general, mosquito-borne viruses do not replicate in tick-cell cultures and *vice versa*.

5. Mosquito-borne arboviruses multiply after oral feeding or intrathoracic injection of virus into numerous mosquito species (after incubation at 4–28°C, depending on the mosquito species). Intrathoracic susceptibility of mosquitoes to dengue and California serogroup viruses is 10–100 times higher than that of mammalian tissue cultures or suckling mice. Some arboviruses, including members of the *Orthobunyavirus* and *Phlebovirus* genera of the Bunyaviridae, *Flavivirus* genus of the Flaviviridae, *Alphavirus* genus of the family Togaviridae and some members of the *Vesiculovirus* genus of the family Rhabdoviridae, are also transmitted transovarially by vectors. Ticks do not normally transmit mosquito-borne arboviruses and *vice versa*. Sandfly-borne viruses are transmitted only by sandflies *(Phlebotomus* spp. and *Lutzomyia* spp.).

Table 47.2 Some important arboviruses

Family and genus	No. of members	Some important members	Comments
Togaviridae *Alphavirus*	31	Western equine encephalitis virus Eastern equine encephalitis virus Venezuelan equine encephalitis virus Chikungunya virus Ross River virus	Mosquito-borne
Flaviviridae *Flavivirus*	60	St. Louis encephalitis virus Japanese encephalitis virus Murray Valley encephalitis virus Yellow fever virus Dengue virus West Nile virus Zika virus Louping ill virus Powassan virus Tick-borne encephalitis virus Kyasanur Forest virus Omsk haemorrhagic fever virus	Mosquito-borne Tick-borne
Bunyaviridae	100		
Orthobunyavirus	48	La Crosse virus Snowshoe hare virus Oropouche virus	California (CAL) serogroup
Phlebovirus	10	Rift Valley fever virus Punta Toro virus Sandfly fever virus Toscana virus	
Nairovirus	7	Crimean–Congo haemorrhagic fever virus	
Hantavirus	24	Sin Nombre virus (not arthropod-borne)	

6. Tick-borne arboviruses multiply after oral feeding to larval or nymphal ixodid ticks (hard ticks of the genera *Dermacentor* and *Ixodes*). The virus is transferred transstadially to the next developmental stage (nymph or adult, respectively), which then transmits virus by biting susceptible vertebrates.

REPLICATION

The replication of the various arboviruses differs significantly and is one of the major criteria used in their classification (see Ch. 7 for a general account).

Alphaviruses

Alphaviruses are 60–70 nm in diameter and enter cells by receptor-mediated endocytosis, but co-receptors or other factors probably also contribute to entry and cell specificity. The virion fuses with an endosomal membrane via a fusion peptide in the E1 envelope glycoprotein. The nucleocapsid is released and binds to ribosomes, and the nonstructural

proteins (nsP1–4) are translated directly from the genomic RNA. RNA replication occurs in complexes comprised of the nonstructural proteins and cellular proteins in association with cytoplasmic membranes. Genomic RNA is messenger sense (positive strand) and serves as a template for full-length negative-sense RNA synthesis; these negative-sense RNAs are templates for the production of positive-sense genomic RNA, as well as a subgenomic mRNA that encodes the structural proteins. Both of these RNAs are capped at the 5′ end and polyadenylated at the 3′ end. Regulation of positive- versus negative-strand synthesis occurs via changes in the nonstructural protease activity mediated by different cleavage patterns of the nonstructural polyprotein. The subgenomic message is translated to yield a polyprotein comprised of the capsid (C) and envelope glycoproteins (E1, E2) as well as two peptides (6K, E3) that may be present in the mature virion to varying degrees depending on the virus. The capsid is cleaved cotranslationally in the cytoplasm via its own protease activity, and the remaining polyprotein enters the endoplasmic reticulum, where it is processed through the secretory pathway to yield glycosylated E2 and E1 protein heterodimers in the plasma membrane. Genomic RNA combines in the cytoplasm with 240 copies of the capsid protein to form a nucleocapsid, and nucleocapsids interact with the cytoplasmic tail of the E2 envelope protein to mediate budding, whereby 240 E2/E1 protein heterodimers and a portion of the plasma membrane are incorporated into the mature virion.

Flaviviruses

Flavivirus virions are 50 nm in diameter and have three structural proteins; the genome is encapsidated by a small core protein and there are two proteins, the membrane (M) and envelope (E), on the outside of the virus particle. The E protein is the major protein of the virus. It is normally glycosylated, has haemagglutination activity, and is the target of neutralising antibodies. The NS3 protein contains the majority of T cell epitopes. The virus genome is one single-stranded, positive-sense RNA molecule. Flavivirus RNA is not polyadenylated. The 5′ one-third of the genome encodes the three structural proteins, and the remaining two-thirds encodes seven nonstructural (NS) proteins (NS1, NS2A, NS2B, NS3, NS4A, NS4B and NS5) involved in virus replication and form the replication complex in virus-infected cells, including an RNA-dependent RNA polymerase (NS5). NS2A, NS4B and NS5 are involved in interferon antagonism and counteract the host innate immune response. Flaviviruses replicate in the cytoplasm of cells. The input virion RNA is translated as a single open reading frame to generate a polyprotein precursor that is rapidly co- and posttranslationally processed by viral and cellular proteases to yield the structural and NS proteins. Flavivirus particles assemble by budding through Golgi vesicles and contain prM, a precursor to M protein, as a chaperone for the E protein. Mature virions are produced at the cell surface where the pr portion of prM is cleaved by the cell enzyme furin to yield the mature M protein found in virions.

Bunyaviruses

The Bunyaviridae are icosahedral enveloped viruses, with diameters of 80–120 nm. They have tripartite RNA genomes of negative sense, termed the large (L), medium (M) and small (S) segments. The L RNA encodes the RNA-dependent RNA polymerase carried in the virion. The L protein of Crimean–Congo haemorrhagic fever virus encodes an ovarian tumour-like cysteine protease motif, suggesting that the L polyprotein is cleaved autoproteolytically. The M RNA encodes two glycoproteins, Gc and Gn, found on the surface of virions. The S RNA encodes a nucleocapsid (N) protein.

The *Orthobunyavirus* genus also contains a nonstructural protein, NSs, which is an interferon antagonist that also inhibits host cell protein synthesis. The tripartite genome enables bunyaviruses to undergo genetic reassortment that occurs naturally between closely related bunyaviruses and contributes to genetic variation and evolution. The *NSm* gene of the *Tospovirus* genus and the *NSs* gene of the *Phlebovirus* and *Tospovirus* genera are encoded as genes in the positive-sense orientation. Thus, the S- and M-RNA segments of tospoviruses and the S-RNA of phleboviruses are termed ambisense RNAs. The *NSs* is a key virulence determinant of bunyaviruses and has a critical role in viral evasion from the host innate immune response via blocking host transcription.

Bunyaviruses replicate in the cytoplasm of cells and assemble by budding through Golgi vesicles.

PATHOGENESIS

Natural vertebrate infection by arboviruses is initiated when mosquitoes or other arthropods deposit saliva in extravascular tissues and blood vessels while blood-feeding. For some alphaviruses, murine model systems using needle inoculations indicate that the initial site of replication is the Langerhans cell. *Alphavirus* replication appears to stimulate both the migratory response of these cells to, and the accumulation of leucocytes in, the draining lymph nodes, where local replication produces viraemia. Arboviruses induce high titres of viraemia in many susceptible vertebrates 1–7 days after parenteral inoculation or following bites by infected arthropods, resulting in the potential for infection of additional vectors. Invasion of the central nervous system (CNS) via the olfactory nervous tract may ensue in some infections, whereas other viruses cross the blood–brain barrier. In alphavirus infections accompanied by rash and arthritis, virus replication and necrosis occur in the epidermis and possibly the muscles, tendons and connective tissue. Infection of macrophages may mediate musculoskeletal pathology via the release of inflammatory mediators. Wild bird and mammal reservoir hosts regularly exhibit viraemia without clinical symptoms.

Antibodies are first detected when the fever subsides, usually within 5–10 days after infection, and may persist for many years. Antibodies are of the immunoglobulin (Ig) M class, which are generated first and persist for 1–3 months after infection; subsequently, they are of the IgG class, which appear 2–3 weeks after infection and may last for years. In some cases, such as with West Nile virus, IgM can persist for months after the initial infection. The reason is unknown.

Arboviruses cause a spectrum of disease ranging from inapparent infection (often the most likely outcome) to acute encephalitis. Within the CNS, arboviruses multiply in and induce necrosis of neurones, which in turn become surrounded by microglia, forming glial knots. There is also evidence of apoptosis for some virus infections. An age dependence of CNS disease has been observed for many arboviruses, and animal model systems indicate that age-dependent apoptosis of neurones may explain this phenomenon. Perivascular cuffing with mononuclear cells affects many cerebral blood vessels. Usually there is concomitant meningitis with accumulation of mononuclear cells in the subarachnoid space and hyperaemia of adjacent capillaries. Invasion of the CNS appears to be a critical determinant in the pathogenesis and is due in some cases to the level of viraemia. The role of the immune system is not clear, although it may be involved in the pathogenesis of dengue haemorrhagic fever and dengue shock syndrome. Antigen–antibody complex formation may underlie the syndrome, which is associated with increased capillary permeability and shock, often with haemorrhage. It is known that the uptake of virus into macrophages is enhanced in the presence of nonneutralising antibody, as the virus–antibody complexes bind to Fc receptors, so there is likely to be a great increase in the uptake and release of virus from macrophages. The innate immune system may also be involved in the development of chronic arthralgia in chikungunya virus infections as the macrophages infiltrating the joint tissue during infection can result in a persistent inflammatory state.

Some arboviruses including alphaviruses (e.g., Ross River virus), flaviviruses (e.g., West Nile virus) and bunyaviruses (e.g., Bunyamwera virus) can disrupt the activation of specific innate immunity antiviral pathways, including interferon induction, to enhance their replication.

CLINICAL FEATURES

The tissue tropism of arboviruses can be divided into four categories:

1. the CNS (e.g., encephalitis, aseptic meningitis)
2. visceral organs (e.g., hepatitis and haemorrhagic fevers)
3. febrile infections
4. infection of reproductive tissues

Human arbovirus infections become clinically manifest according to the target organ principally infected (Table 47.3). These include the following syndromes.

Encephalitis

For many arboviruses, encephalitis is most common in children and/or the elderly. Illness typically has an abrupt onset within 1 week of infection, with headache, fever, myalgia and dysthesias, and sometimes lethargy, chills, dizziness, nausea, vomiting and prostration. Inflammation of the throat, cervical lymphadenitis and abdominal tenderness are also common. Signs and symptoms usually subside after several days but may recrudesce. Progression to encephalitis may occur rapidly, or a prodromal illness may last for 1 week or more. Severe CNS disease is accompanied by neck stiffness, motor weakness and paralysis, meningismus, cranial nerve palsy, confusion, convulsions and somnolence, leading to coma. Rigidity or weakness of the limbs may occur with reduction in reflexes. White blood cells, predominantly lymphocytes, and raised glucose levels may occur in the cerebrospinal fluid, which can exhibit increased pressure. Peripheral blood cell counts may be raised, with a left shift. During most outbreaks of arboviral encephalitis, a proportion of patients develop aseptic meningitis alone, without significant neuronal involvement, whereas up to 50% of patients recover from acute encephalitis to suffer from neuropsychiatric sequelae varying from physiological impairment to mental disorder, which may last from months to years.

Yellow fever

Yellow fever is caused by a mosquito-borne flavivirus that is found in tropical South America and Africa. The disease has an incubation period of 3–6 days, characterised by the sudden onset of headache and fever (temperatures may exceed 39°C), with generalised myalgia, nausea and vomiting. Jaundice may appear by the third day of illness, but frequently is mild or absent. Haematemesis, melaena, epistaxis and bleeding gums may also be noted. Albuminuria and oliguria may also begin suddenly during the first week of illness. In severe cases, death may occur 3–6 days after the onset of illness, and midzonal necrosis is observed in the liver. The case fatality rate is estimated as 20%–50%.

Dengue

Dengue is caused by four genetically and serologically related flaviviruses called dengue-1, -2, -3 and -4 and is considered the most important mosquito-borne virus in the world, with 390 million infections, including 90 million clinical cases, per year. Dengue presents as an acute febrile illness with chills, headache, retroocular pain, body aches and arthralgia in more than 90% of apparent cases, with nausea or vomiting and a maculopapular rash resembling measles lasting for 2–7 days in about 60% of cases. Illness persists for 7 days, fever remitting after 3–5 days, followed by relapse (saddleback fever) and pains in the bones, muscles and joints sufficiently severe to earn the epithet breakbone fever. Rash occurs more commonly in patients aged <14 years. Complete recovery is the rule. The incubation period is 5–11 days.

Table 47.3 Clinical syndromes associated with selected arboviruses and their geographical distribution

Syndrome	Genus	Serogroup (vector)	Causative	Arbovirus serotype	Geographical distribution
Encephalitis or aseptic meningitis	*Alphavirus*	(mosquito)	EEEV	Eastern equine encephalitis	Eastern Canada, USA, Caribbean
			VEEV	Venezuelan equine encephalitis	North, Central and South America
			WEEV	Western equine encephalitis	North, Central and South America, Caribbean
	Flavivirus	(mosquito)	JEV	Japanese encephalitis	Orient (Japan to Australia)
			MVEV	Murray Valley encephalitis	Australia
			SLEV	St. Louis encephalitis	Canada, USA, Central America
		(tick)	LIV	Louping ill	Scotland, Northern Ireland
			POWV	Powassan	Canada, Northern USA
			TBEV	Tick-borne encephalitis complex	Central and northern Europe, Siberia, Asia
	Orthobunyavirus	CAL (mosquito)	LACV	La Crosse	USA
			SSHV	Snowshoe hare	Canada
Yellow fever	*Flavivirus*	(mosquito)	YFV	Yellow fever	Tropical Africa, Caribbean, tropical South America
Dengue	*Flavivirus*	(mosquito)	DENV	Dengue (four types)	Entire tropical zone India, Philippines, Southeast Asia, Oceania
		(tick)	KFDV	Kyasanur Forest disease	India
			OMSKV	Omsk haemorrhagic fever	Siberia
	Nairovirus	CCHF (tick)	CCHFV	Crimean–Congo haemorrhagic fever	Central and southern Africa, Asia, Europe
Miscellaneous tropical fevers	*Alphavirus*	(mosquito)	CHIKV	Chikungunya	Africa, India, Southeast Asia, Oceania, Americas, Caribbean
			RRV	Ross River[a]	Australia, Oceania
	Flavivirus	(mosquito)	ILHV	Ilheus	Caribbean, South America
			WNV	West Nile	Central and northern Africa, Europe, North, Central and South America, Caribbean
	Orthobunyavirus	SIM (mosquito)	OROV	Oropouche	Caribbean, South America
	Phlebovirus	PHL (mosquito)	RVFV	Rift Valley fever	Northern, eastern and southern Africa
		PHL (sandfly)	PTV	Punta Toro	Central America
		PHL (sandfly)	SFNV	Sandfly fever – Naples	Mediterranean
	Vesiculovirus	VS (sandfly)	VSIV	Vesicular stomatitis – Indiana	USA, Central America
Undifferentiated fever	*Coltivirus*	CTF (tick)	CTFV	Colorado tick fever	Western USA
Reproductive tissues	*Flavivirus*		ZIKV	Zika	Africa, Asia, North, Central and South America

[a]Ross River virus infections frequently exhibit polyarthralgia.

Dengue haemorrhagic fever

This is a less common manifestation of dengue, with about 500,000 cases per year and a case fatality rate of 5%, mainly affecting children. It is occasionally accompanied by a shock syndrome, known as dengue shock syndrome, with a case fatality rate of up to 50%. These two severe forms of dengue are observed in patients who undergo successive infection with two different dengue viruses (e.g., a primary dengue-1 infection followed by a secondary infection with dengue-2 virus). After an acute onset, fever of 40°C, accompanied by vomiting and anorexia, enlarged liver and petechiae, persists for 5–10 days. This is followed by a complete recovery unless shock supervenes as occurs in 7%–10% of patients 2–7 days after onset, usually accompanied by haematemesis and melaena.

Miscellaneous tropical fevers

These manifest as generalised illness with increased temperature to above 39°C with any combination of headache, myalgia, malaise, nausea or vomiting and sometimes accompanied by maculopapular rash or polyarthralgia, that is, a dengue-like syndrome but without haemorrhagic manifestations or the shock syndrome. Tropical fevers arise from infection with a wide variety of arboviruses (see Table 47.3), and clinical diagnosis is impossible without access to serological tests for diagnosis. Many of the Old World alphaviruses such as Ross River, chikungunya, o'nyong-nyong and Sindbis viruses cause an arthritic syndrome accompanied by rash, which can persist for months or even years in the case of chikungunya and Ross River virus infections. Chronic or relapsing arthritic symptoms may be caused by inflammation associated with periodic increase in replication within persistently infected synovial macrophages, which persist despite neutralising antibodies and antiviral cytokine responses. Inhibition of cytokine responses by virus–antibody complexes binding to Fc receptors, and interleukin-10 induction, may facilitate persistence.

Undifferentiated fever

A US example is Colorado tick fever (genus *Coltivirus*) in which symptoms of chilliness, headaches, retroorbital pain and generalised aches, especially in the back and limbs, appear 3–6 days after bites by infected *Dermacentor andersoni* ticks in wooded areas of the Rocky Mountain region. Fever of 39–40°C often shows a biphasic course, with eventual defervescence within 1 week, followed by complete recovery.

Hantavirus pulmonary syndrome

This syndrome, due to the hantavirus Sin Nombre, was first recognised in southwestern United States during 1993. Sudden onset of fever, myalgia, headache, cough and nausea or vomiting is accompanied by rapid respirations exceeding 20 per minute, temperature above 38°C and hypotension. Extensive interstitial and alveolar infiltrates are observed in the lungs, accompanied by reduced oxygen saturation. Fatal cases develop progressive pulmonary oedema with hypoxia and severe hypotension and die 2–16 days after onset of symptoms; the case fatality rate may exceed 50%. Patients with nonfatal infection usually recover within 1–3 weeks.

Congenital Zika Syndrome

Although Zika virus causes a febrile illness, the virus readily infects cells in reproductive tissues with long-term infection of semen and vaginal tissues. The virus can infect the foetus leading to a variety of physical and mental clinical complications, including microcephaly (a condition where the circumference of the head of a newborn child is less than that of the normal circumference for gestational age, sex and race), that are collectively termed Congenital Zika Syndrome. In addition, Zika virus appears to cause up to a 20-fold increase in the incidence of Guillain–Barré syndrome (GBS), a condition where the immune system attacks the peripheral nervous system.

LABORATORY INVESTIGATION

Diagnosis of arbovirus infections depends on:

- the isolation of virus from blood, cerebrospinal fluid or tissues
- detection of arbovirus-specific RNA in blood, cerebrospinal fluid or tissues and sometimes urine or semen
- antigen detection (mostly viral surface envelope proteins) by indirect immunofluorescence, commonly used as a rapid diagnostic method, and for flavivirus NS1 protein, which is a nonstructural protein that is secreted from cells and found in serum during acute infection
- Serology, haemagglutination inhibition and enzyme-linked immunosorbent assays (ELISAs) for IgM and/or IgG and neutralisation tests can be used to detect serum antibodies from patients. However, these assays are dependent on availability of virus and/or antigens.

Virus isolation

Virus isolation was historically an important diagnostic tool but is a slow process and unlikely to generate results until after an acute disease. With the extensive development of molecular tests, virus isolation is now rarely used for diagnostic purposes but remains important for downstream research. The causative virus can often be isolated from blood collected during the initial 3–4-day febrile illness when viraemia titres peak. Some arboviruses can also be isolated from cerebrospinal fluid or brain biopsy or from brain at autopsy of fatal encephalitis cases. Liver may yield virus isolation from fatal cases of yellow fever.

Arbovirus–specific RNA detection

Detection of virus-specific RNA, by reverse transcriptase–polymerase chain reaction (RT-PCR) and the more sensitive realtime RT-PCR, are rapid approaches to diagnosis, but depend on the availability of specific oligonucleotide primers. Given the large number of arboviruses, there must be significant differential diagnosis before selection of appropriate primers. Genus-reactive primers have been described for alphaviruses, flaviviruses and bunyaviruses.

After amplification of extracted RNA, the product is analysed by restriction enzyme digestion, melt curve analysis, fluorescent probe detection and/or determination of the nucleotide sequence of the PCR product and comparison with sequences in Genbank or other nucleotide sequence databases.

Serology

Serological testing is often the only available means of laboratory diagnosis of encephalitis. The detection of a four-fold or greater rise of antibody titre by haemagglutination inhibition tests or ELISAs on paired sera collected during the acute and convalescent phases of illness may provide good, but not definitive, evidence of concurrent infection. Antibodies detected by complement fixation testing first appear 2 weeks or more after onset and become undetectable by 3 years. Haemagglutination inhibition and complement fixation test results are usually not as specific as those obtained by neutralisation. Virus-specific IgM antibody may be detected within 1 day of onset of clinical symptoms using an IgM capture ELISA. IgM antibody generally wanes 1–3 months after onset and is replaced by IgG antibodies beginning 2–3 weeks after infection. IgM antibodies are indicative of a recent infection.

TREATMENT

Currently, no specific antiarboviral therapeutic agent is available. Patients with encephalitis are managed supportively, using anticonvulsants as required, and ice packs are applied when indicated to reduce hyperthermia. Raised intracranial pressure can also be treated, and airway protection may be needed in unconscious patients, with hyperventilation accompanied by anaesthesia and sedation. Brain swelling can be minimised by regulating serum sodium levels and osmolarity. Nosocomial infections, especially pneumonia, should be prevented and treated aggressively when they occur. Similarly, in dengue and haemorrhagic fevers, supportive measures may include careful maintenance of fluid and electrolyte balance. Ribavirin shows activity against some bunyaviruses (and in combination with interferon-α) but has not been evaluated for most arboviruses and is not therapeutic in many arbovirus infections.

EPIDEMIOLOGY

Natural cycles

Arboviruses are maintained in natural transmission cycles involving reservoir hosts and arthropod vectors, typically:

- ticks
- mosquitoes
- other biting flies or bugs

Except for dengue virus and chikungunya virus in some locations, arboviruses are zoonotic pathogens that utilise wild animals as reservoir hosts. Many arboviruses also use nonhuman animals as amplification hosts during epidemics, and human beings are often tangentially infected, dead-end hosts during these outbreaks. Mosquitoes or other arthropods become infected by engorging on a viraemic vertebrate. In mosquitoes, infection begins in the midgut epithelium and spreads to the haemocele or open body cavity, where it may disseminate to other tissues and organs including the salivary glands. This extrinsic incubation period is completed when replication in salivary gland acinar cells leads to virus release into the apical cavities and salivary ducts. Transmission may then occur upon a subsequent blood meal, when mosquitoes deposit saliva in extravascular tissues while probing to locate a venule, or intravascularly. Infection of the vertebrate then leads to viraemia and the opportunity for infection of additional vectors. Nonviraemic transmission, whereby an infected vector transmits to an uninfected vector feeding at the same time on the same host before replicative viraemia can occur, has been described for tick-borne viruses and West Nile virus (WNV).

Examples of major natural cycles are:

- human–mosquito cycle, as in DENV, CHIKV, ZIKV and urban YFV (Fig. 47.1)
- mosquito–bird cycle, as in SLEV and WNV (Fig. 47.2)
- mosquito–mammal cycle, as in Venezuelan equine encephalitis virus (VEEV; Fig. 47.3).

Epidemiological aspects of arbovirus infections with major impact on human health are described according to syndrome and infecting serotype (see also Table 47.2).

Alphaviruses
Western equine encephalitis virus

Western equine encephalitis virus (WEEV) has caused periodic outbreaks of equine and human encephalitis in the western half of North America, as well as in Brazil and Argentina. Although massive outbreaks occurred during the mid-20th century in western North America, only one

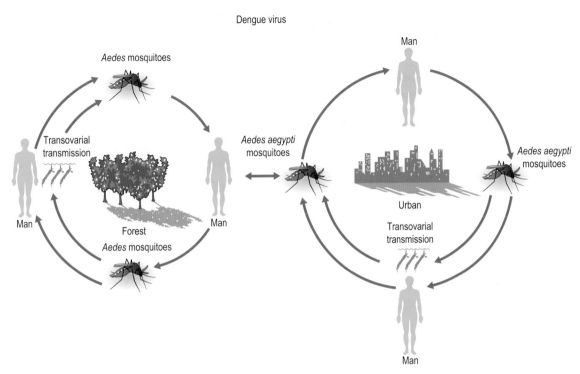

Fig. 47.1 Natural cycle of arbovirus infection: human–mosquito cycle (e.g., dengue and urban yellow fever).

human case has been documented since 1998. In North America, cases occurred only during June to September, when mosquitoes are abundant. Outbreaks of infection occurred at intervals of a few years and were preceded by epizootic peaks of encephalitis among horses. The principal mosquito vector species in Canada and the western United States is *Culex tarsalis*. Passerine birds constitute the principal reservoirs. Human beings and equids are considered dead-end hosts because they produce little viraemia. Although all age groups may be involved, encephalitis due to WEEV has most commonly affected children, in whom the disease is often severe.

Eastern equine encephalitis virus

Eastern equine encephalitis virus (EEEV) causes human and horse cases in Atlantic coastal areas extending from New Hampshire and Vermont to Florida and Texas and northeastern Mexico, and in a few inland locations such as Missouri, Michigan and Wisconsin. Occasionally, disease extends northwards into Canada. In the United States, an average of eight human cases of EEEV are reported annually. While encephalitis is the most severe disease manifestation, only 4%–5% of EEEV infections result in encephalitis. Severe illness affects mainly those aged <14 years and >55 years, with overall case fatality rates as high as 69%.

Surviving patients usually have severe neurological sequelae. Most human cases occur during late August and September, about 3 weeks after the peak of horse cases. EEEV was previously reported to occur throughout South and Central America, but the virus associated with these infections is now known as Madariaga virus. Madariaga virus is only rarely associated with human disease. In North America, EEEV is maintained enzootically in hardwood swamp habitats, where the mosquito *Culiseta melanura* transmits the virus among passerine birds. During years of hyper-enzootic transmission, horses and human beings residing near the swamp habitats become infected via bridge vectors such as *Aedes* spp. (*Cs. melanura* feeds primarily on birds). Equids and humans are considered dead-end hosts because they develop little viraemia, and outbreaks are therefore confined to regions of enzootic activity.

Venezuelan equine encephalitis virus

Venezuelan equine encephalitis virus (VEEV) causes outbreaks involving up to hundreds of thousands of human beings and equids, primarily in northern South America, with one outbreak extending as far north as Texas in the United States in 1971. During outbreaks, VEEV is transmitted among equids by a variety of mosquitoes such as *Aedes* and *Psorophora* spp. Equids are extremely effective

St. Louis encephalitis

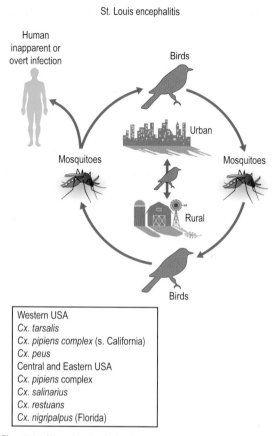

Fig. 47.2 Natural cycle of arbovirus infection: bird–mosquito cycle (e.g., St. Louis encephalitis).

Venezuelan equine encephalitis

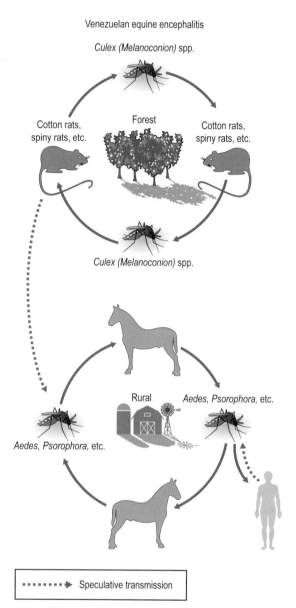

Fig. 47.3 Natural cycle of infection: mammal–mosquito cycle (e.g., Venezuelan equine encephalitis).

amplifying hosts because they develop high-titred viraemia and are attractive to mosquitoes. An equine vaccine is commercially available that has been effective in halting the spread of epidemics. Antigenically related viruses occur in sylvatic and swamp habitats through much of the neotropics and subtropics, as far north as Florida, in the United States, and as far south as northern Argentina. These viruses can cause febrile illness and sometimes fatal encephalitis in human beings that enter these foci, and one antigenic subtype (designated ID) can mutate to become capable of initiating widespread outbreaks. Rates of encephalitis (generally <5% of cases) and mortality (around 0.5%) are generally lower than for EEEV, with most fatal cases occurring in young children. Neurological sequelae are uncommon.

Ross River virus

Ross River virus (RRV) infection, known in Australia as epidemic polyarthritis, has also occurred in the South Pacific. In Australia, disease occurs primarily during the summer

and autumn as sporadic cases and small outbreaks. An average of 5000 cases is reported each year, with most of the cases historically occurring in rural areas. However, recent outbreaks have skirted major urban areas in coastal regions where urbanisation has brought people in closer proximity to vector and reservoir habitat. RRV is maintained in a zoonotic vertebrate–mosquito cycle, with *Culex annulirostris* and *Aedes vigilax* serving as the principal vectors, and flying foxes and marsupials implicated as reservoir hosts. Human infections have also been documented in New

Guinea, the Solomon Islands, New Caledonia, Fiji, American Samoa and the Cook Islands. During 1979–1980 a large, explosive epidemic of Ross River polyarthritis swept across the South Pacific, with 40%–60% of the population affected on some islands. *Aedes polynesiensis* was implicated as the vector, and epidemiological studies suggested a human–mosquito–human transmission cycle.

Chikungunya virus

Chikungunya virus (CHIKV) is named after a Makonde word meaning that which bends up, referring to the posture of patients with severe joint pains. It has its enzootic ancestry in Sub-Saharan Africa, where a sylvatic transmission cycle occurs between wild primates and possibly other vertebrates, and arboreal *Aedes* mosquitoes. Urban CHIKV epidemics causing hundreds of thousands of cases involve *Ae. aegypti* and/or *Ae. albopictus* transmission in a human–mosquito–human cycle. Unlike dengue, which is endemic in many of these Asian cities, CHIKV may disappear and reappear at irregular intervals. However, CHIKV infection is often overlooked because it is clinically indistinguishable from dengue fever. Since March 2005, epidemics have taken place in the Indian Ocean, Asia and Africa involving millions of people with a very small number of fatalities. The virus spread to the western hemisphere in 2013, where over 1.1 million cases were estimated to have occurred in the first year alone. Transmission in many locations has been enhanced by the adaptation of newly emerged strains to *Ae. albopictus* mosquitoes via a mutation in the *E1* envelope glycoprotein gene. The ability of this vector to mediate epidemic transmission in a temperate region of an industrialised nation (Italy) underscores the direct risk of CHIKV to many parts of the world including Europe and the Americas. Like dengue, CHIK intervention using vector control has been ineffective yet remains one of the limited control options in the absence of a vaccine.

O'nyong-nyong virus

O'nyong-nyong virus (ONNV), derived from the description by the Acholi tribe, meaning joint breaker, was first isolated during a 1959–1962 epidemic affecting 2 million people in Uganda, Kenya, Tanzania, Mozambique, Malawi and Senegal. Another major outbreak involving an estimated 1 million cases occurred in 1996 in Uganda and northern Tanzania. Attack rates are generally high and all age groups are affected during ONNV epidemics. Serological evidence in Kenya suggests active transmission to humans is occurring even in the absence of reported cases or epidemic activity. The transmission cycle involves *Anopheles funestus* and *Anopheles gambiae* mosquitoes; ONNV is the only known alphavirus with *Anopheles*

vectors. The reservoir and amplification hosts are unknown, but antibodies against ONNV have been found in a range of vertebrates including rodents, duikers, African forest buffalo and mandrills.

Flaviviruses: mosquito-borne

St. Louis encephalitis virus

St. Louis encephalitis virus (SLEV) was first isolated from the brain of a person dying from acute encephalitis in St. Louis, Missouri. The largest outbreak in recent times occurred in 1975, when 1815 (86%) of 2113 confirmed cases of arbovirus encephalitis were due to SLEV. Mosquito vectors in California, the Rocky Mountains and plains states comprise mainly *Cx. tarsalis*, but *Cx. pipiens* and *Cx. quinquefasciatus* are important along the Mississippi Valley and eastwards. The introduction of West Nile virus into North America has displaced SLEV in *Culex* mosquitoes, and SLEV infections are now rare.

Japanese encephalitis virus

Japanese encephalitis virus (JEV) was first isolated from the brain of a patient with fatal encephalitis in Tokyo in 1935. It continues to cause epidemics of encephalitis, affecting children, particularly in India, Korea, China, Southeast Asia and Indonesia, with case fatality rates often exceeding 20%. JEV is occasionally found in the Torres Straits and the tip of northern Australia. Approximately 68,000 cases occur each year, of which 15,000 are fatal. The ratio of apparent to inapparent infection is 1 : 50–400, depending on the geographical area. *Cx. tritaeniorhynchus* mosquitoes are the principal vectors, and maximal virus isolation rates from mosquitoes occur during late July, simultaneously with human and equine epidemics. Important vertebrate reservoirs are black-crowned night herons and other water birds, and pigs are considered to be an amplifying host.

West Nile virus

West Nile virus (WNV) was first isolated from a febrile patient in the West Nile district of Uganda in 1937. The virus has a wide geographical distribution, including southern Europe, Africa, central and south Asia, Oceania and most recently North America. In the late summer of 1999, the first outbreak of WNV infection was reported in the western hemisphere, in New York, and the virus subsequently spread into many parts of North America. Genetic studies have shown that the related Kunjin virus, found in Australasia, is a subtype of West Nile virus. Although the virus infects a wide variety of animals, including horses, cattle and humans, the major vertebrate hosts are wild birds, and migratory birds are important in the spread of the disease owing to long-term high-titre viraemia. The principal vectors are considered to be mosquitoes of the *Culex* genus. Both sylvatic and urban transmission cycles have been reported, with *Cx. pipiens* implicated as the major urban vector. WNV usually causes a febrile illness, but encephalitis is seen in patients over 50 years of age. Epidemics vary in size, with the largest reported in the United States in 2002, 2003 and 2012, each with 2500 cases of West Nile neurological disease (WNND). These are the largest recorded epidemics of arboviral meningo-encephalitis in the United States. Overall, in the United States there had been more than 43,000 human cases, including over 19,000 cases of WNND and over 1900 deaths by the end of 2016. During 2006 the virus spread as far south as Argentina, causing disease in equines. WNV has infected at least 326 species of birds, 30 other vertebrate species and 62 species of mosquitoes. In addition, outbreaks of WNV infection have been reported in southern European countries since 1999.

Usutu virus

Usutu virus, isolated in Africa, is a member of the Japanese encephalitis serogroup of the *Flavivirus* genus and was not known to cause disease. In 2001 the virus emerged in Austria, in Vienna and surrounding districts, and was responsible for a large epizootic with high mortality in birds, especially Eurasian blackbirds *(Turdus merula)* and owls. The virus has continued to spread in Europe and cause epizootics in birds plus sporadic human cases.

Murray Valley encephalitis virus

Murray Valley encephalitis virus (MVEV) was first isolated from the brain of a patient with fatal encephalitis at Mooroopna, Victoria, Australia. MVEV caused epidemics of encephalitis in irrigated farming regions of the Murray–Darling River basin during the summer months (January to March) of 1951 and 1974, with case fatality rates approaching 40%. The last outbreak was in 2011, with 17 cases, including three deaths. MVE virus was isolated from *Cx. annulirostris* mosquitoes only during 1974 but not during intervening years, which suggests epidemic introduction of virus into this dry temperate region. Although the virus causes clinically severe disease, the incidence is low. Natural cycles of transmission of MVEV involve *Cx. annulirostris* as the principal mosquito vector and water birds as reservoirs.

Yellow fever virus

Yellow fever virus (YFV) was first isolated in Ghana from the blood of a male patient with fever, headache, backache and prostration. YFV is found mostly in tropical Africa and tropical South America; 90% of cases are in Africa. There are two epidemiological patterns. In the sylvatic cycle, virus is transmitted among monkeys by mosquitoes (*Haemagogus* and *Sabethes* species in South America and *Aedes* species in Africa). Humans are infected incidentally when entering the area, for example, to work as foresters. In the urban cycle, person-to-person transmission is via *Ae. aegypti*, which uses larval habitats close to human habitation in water, pits and scrap containers such as oil drums.

In the Americas, the majority of YFV cases are reported in Brazil, Peru and Bolivia and involve males aged 15–45 years who are agricultural and forest workers. YFV usually occurs from December to May and peaks during March and April, when populations of *Haemagogus* mosquitoes are highest during the rainy season.

YFV is endemic in many parts of West, Central and East Africa, principally between latitudes 15°N and 15°S, extending northwards into Ethiopia and Sudan. Continuing activity has been encountered in parts of West Africa. There are relatively few outbreaks in East Africa, with the last major outbreaks in Sudan in 2003 and 2005. In 2016 a large outbreak took place in Angola and Congo with 6500 cases and over 400 deaths. *Ae. africanus* is the principal vector in Africa.

Dengue viruses

Dengue virus (DENV) infection is endemic in all tropical regions between latitudes 23.5°N and 23.5°S. Four genetically and serologically related viruses termed dengue-1, -2, -3 and -4 cause the disease dengue. The febrile clinical symptoms associated with dengue are similar to those of other arboviruses from other families; this has resulted in confusion in the diagnosis of dengue. In particular, the high incidence of dengue has resulted in the misdiagnosis of some arbovirus outbreaks as discussed earlier in the chapter. Serological studies are needed to differentiate these.

DENV is thought to have originated in Asia in a sylvatic cycle involving arboreal mosquitoes and monkeys. However, endemic viruses have evolved and are now maintained in nature by a cycle involving humans as both reservoir and amplification host, and domestic mosquitoes, principally *Ae. aegypti*, as vectors. DENV has caused numerous outbreaks throughout the South West Pacific region since it was first recognised among servicemen during the Second World War. Subsequently, in the South West Pacific, multiple dengue viruses have affected Tahiti, with haemorrhagic dengue first encountered in 1971. In addition to *Ae. Aegypti*, other species have been implicated as vectors, including *Ae. scutellaris hebrideus* in New Guinea, *Ae. polynesiensis* in Tahiti and *Ae. cooki* in Niue. Hawaii was dengue-free from 1944 to 2001 until, in 2001–2002, there was a DENV-1 outbreak involving at least 122 cases and *Ae. albopictus* as the vector. DENV activity continues in many tropical countries of the Pacific rim, including northern Australia. Most Southeast Asian countries, including Indonesia, Malaysia, Thailand, Vietnam, China, Philippines and India, experience repeated epidemics of dengue caused by all four viruses, with most cases occurring between June and November. Mostly children are affected; in some outbreaks up to 25% may develop haemorrhagic fever. Most epidemics occur in urban areas and villages where *Ae. aegypti* is abundant but not in rural environments. Up to 100 million clinical cases may occur each year, mostly in children; this is a major public health problem.

Dengue is endemic throughout tropical Africa, including Nigeria in the west and Mozambique in the east and also in Middle Eastern countries such as Saudi Arabia. Dengue disease is seldom severe in Africa, and dengue haemorrhagic fever is rare.

Caribbean countries have been involved in epidemic waves of dengue since 1827, with little evidence of clinical dengue during interepidemic periods. All four DENV have been implicated in outbreaks affecting residents of Caribbean islands and adjacent areas of Central and South America. Each year cases of dengue are imported into continental United States and Europe following visits to dengue-endemic countries. Although most infections in the United States occur among travellers returning from the Caribbean, small numbers of cases (<30 per year) of indigenous dengue occur regularly among residents of southern Texas who live near the border with Mexico. The semitropical climate in this area allows *Ae. aegypti* to flourish during the nine warmer months of each year. Recently, a small epidemic was detected in the Florida Keys, another subtropical area inhabited by *Ae. aegypti*. In 1985, *Ae. albopictus* was introduced from Asia into the Americas via used motor tyre casings that had been imported for retreading into Texas, from Japan, South Korea and several Southeast Asian countries. The mosquito rapidly established itself in Texas and spread into midwestern, northeastern and northwestern states of the United States and also into Mexico and other countries. A peridomestic mosquito, *Ae. albopictus*, was first identified as a dengue vector in Malaysia during the 1960s, and it transmits dengue both in the human–mosquito cycle and by transovarial transfer. However, to date, there have been few reports of dengue virus transmission in the Americas by *Ae. albopictus*.

Zika virus

Until recently, Zika virus (ZIKV) was considered endemic to Africa and Southeast Asia, with rare human cases. In 2007 ZIKV caused an outbreak of 49 confirmed, and 59 probable cases, of a relatively mild disease characterised by rash, arthralgia and conjunctivitis on Yap Island, Federated States of Micronesia, in the southwestern Pacific Ocean. Serological studies suggest that 73% of Yap Island residents aged three or older had been recently infected with ZIKV. This was the first time that ZIKV was detected outside of Africa and Asia. The virus was found in French Polynesia in 2013–2014, with subsequent spread across the South Pacific. During 2015 the virus expanded its geographical range from Asia into the Americas, with confirmed reports from Brazil in May 2015 onwards. Overall, during 2015–2016, 46 countries and territories in the Americas have reported 120,000 confirmed cases of Zika fever, with many times this number of suspected cases. In addition to Zika fever, multiple countries in the Americas have reported increased microcephaly and Guillain–Barré syndrome case numbers with respect to the current epidemic. Consequently, Zika fever is now considered an important emerging disease, and the World Health Organization declared the epidemic to be a Public Health Emergency of International Concern on 1 February 2016. As much of the Americas are in the southern hemisphere, the tropical season is November to May, and the number of cases greatly decreased in the second half of 2016. At the time of writing, it is unknown if the virus will cause an outbreak in the 2016–2017 season. In jungles, the virus is thought to exist in an *Aedes* mosquito–monkey cycle; however, it can also exist in a human–*Aedes aegypti* cycle, which is thought to be the major transmission cycle in the Americas.

Flaviviruses: tick-borne
Powassan virus

Powassan virus, the sole North American tick-borne flavivirus, was first isolated from the brain of a fatal human case of encephalitis in Powassan, Ontario, Canada. To date, it has caused approximately 40 cases of encephalitis and four deaths among residents of forested areas of Ontario, Quebec and Nova Scotia in Canada, as well as Massachusetts, New York State and Pennsylvania in the United States. All of these cases occurred between May and October. Principal tick vector species in Ontario are *Ixodes cookei*, which feeds on groundhogs, and *I. marxi*, which feeds on tree squirrels; both of these mammals serve as reservoirs.

Tick-borne encephalitis viruses

Tick-borne encephalitis virus (TBEV) is used to describe a serocomplex of related viruses that are transmitted by ticks and cause similar diseases. These include central European (also known as the western subtype) TBEV that causes central European encephalitis and Russian spring-summer encephalitis (also known as the far eastern subtype of TBEV). In addition, a third subtype, Siberian TBEV, has been described mainly on the basis of genetic studies. Russian spring-summer encephalitis occurs in eastern Europe and parts of Asia, including northern Japan, and causes a more severe disease than the central European encephalitis found in western Europe and Scandinavia. The case fatality rate of central European encephalitis is usually below 10%, whereas it can reach 30% for Russian spring–summer encephalitis. In Britain and Ireland and some parts of France and Scandinavia, a mild form of tick-borne encephalitis is caused by a related virus called louping ill. The latter virus also infects sheep and grouse and gets its name from the leaping gait in infected sheep; the virus rarely infects humans.

Human infections with TBEV may range in severity from mild biphasic meningoencephalitis, which is characteristic of the central European TBEV and louping ill virus, to a severe form of polioencephalomyelitis that is characteristic of Russian spring-summer encephalitis virus.

Natural cycles involve *I. ricinus* ticks as vectors, and mice, shrews and other small rodents as reservoirs, with infection transferred tangentially to sheep or other farm animals, and also to human beings. In Siberia, *I. persulcatus* ticks serve as vectors. Recently, additional viruses have been described from Spain, Turkey and other European countries that are related to louping ill virus and are members of the TBEV complex and cause TBEV-like disease symptoms in sheep and other animals.

The TBEV complex contains three viruses associated with haemorrhagic fever: Omsk haemorrhagic fever (OHF), Kyasanur Forest disease (KFD) and Alkhumra viruses. OHF was identified during the Second World War in Omsk, and the virus causes occasional outbreaks in Russia, whereas KFD is found only in India and causes regular outbreaks of haemorrhagic fever. Alkhumra virus was isolated in 1995, with subsequent sporadic outbreaks in Saudi Arabia; it caused haemorrhagic fever with a fatal outcome in 25% of patients. Genetic studies suggest that Alkhumra virus is a subtype of KFD virus.

Bunyaviruses: *Bunyavirus* genus
California (CAL) serogroup

There are at least 14 viruses related antigenically to the prototype California encephalitis virus. In the United States, encephalitis and aseptic meningitis arise commonly from infections with La Crosse virus, first isolated from the brain of a patient with fatal encephalitis in La Crosse, Wisconsin. Other viruses occasionally associated with aseptic meningitis are snowshoe hare virus, isolated from the blood of a snowshoe hare in Montana, and Jamestown Canyon virus (JCV), isolated from *Culiseta inornata* mosquitoes collected at Jamestown Canyon, Colorado. In

central Europe, febrile illness, sometimes with aseptic meningitis, arises from infection with Tahyna virus, isolated from *Ae. caspius* mosquitoes collected near Tahyna, in the former Czechoslovakia.

Currently, CAL serogroup viruses are the most common arboviruses associated with encephalitis in the United States. The highest attack rates occur in states adjoining the Great Lakes, affecting mainly children aged <15 years. Abundant tree holes in wooded areas provide optimal breeding sites for the principal mosquito vector *Ae. triseriatus*, but rainwater collected in disused motor tyres is a suitable breeding ground for *Ae. triseriatus* in suburban locations. As adult mosquitoes die in winter, CAL serogroup viruses survive through transovarial transmission. Principal vertebrate reservoirs are tree squirrels and chipmunks.

Oropouche (ORO)

This virus is the only human pathogen in the Simbu serogroup; it was isolated in Trinidad in 1955. Outbreaks of Oropouche fever, a febrile illness, have occurred in Brazil since 1961, involving urban transmission by the midge *Culicoides paraensis*. An outbreak was reported in Panama in 1989, and cases of Oropouche fever have been reported in Peru since 1992.

Garissa virus

In 1997–1998, Garissa virus was described as a reassortant bunyavirus. It was isolated from patients with acute haemorrhagic fever during an epidemic of Rift Valley fever in Kenya and southern Somalia. Acute sera from patients with haemorrhagic fever yielded either virus isolation or PCR evidence of infection. Initial studies indicated that the sequences of the L and S RNA segments were nearly identical to those of Bunyamwera virus, whereas the sequence of the M segment was very different (33% nucleotide and 28% amino acid differences). Very recent studies have shown that Garissa and Ngari virus M segments are nearly identical in sequence, whereas the L and S segments of Bunyamwera virus are similar to those of both Ngari and Garissa virus. These data indicate that Garissa virus is not a reassortant but an isolate of Ngari virus, which is a reassortant of Bunyamwera virus. Previously, Ngari virus had not been considered a cause of haemorrhagic fever; further studies are required to investigate the pathogenesis and epidemiology of Ngari virus.

Bunyaviruses: *Phlebovirus* genus
Rift Valley fever virus

Rift Valley fever virus (RVFV) was first isolated in 1930 from sheep during an epizootic causing abortion and death in the Rift Valley near Lake Niavasha, Kenya, but is present from South Africa to Egypt. The virus infects many large domestic animals and a wide variety of mosquito species, with sheep, cattle, buffaloes and rodents as reservoirs. RVFV is epizootic with long interepizootic periods. Outbreaks of Rift Valley fever occurred in Egypt during 1977 involving an estimated 200,000 human cases and 600 deaths. Subsequently, Rift Valley fever has been reported during 1998–1999 in Mauritania and Senegal, and in Yemen and south-west Saudi Arabia in 2000–2001, involving over 2000 clinical cases and a mortality rate of 14%. Genetic studies of the virus are consistent with the theory that infection came from East Africa.

Severe fever with thrombocytopenia syndrome virus

Severe fever with thrombocytopenia syndrome virus (SFTSV) was first isolated in China in 2009 from patients who had a haemorrhagic fever illness. Clinical symptoms include fever, thrombocytopenia, leukocytopenia and elevated serum enzyme levels, with multiorgan failure in severe cases. The case fatality rate for SFTSV is 6%–30%, and evidence of person-to-person transmission has also been described. Subsequently, haemorrhagic fever cases were recognised in other countries in Asia, including Japan and Korea. SFTSV is a phlebovirus that uses *Haemaphysalis longicornis* as the tick host. The vertebrate host has not been substantiated, although a number of animal species show evidence of infection by the virus. Humans appear to be accidental hosts.

A virus closely related to SFTSV has been identified in the United States and has been called Heartland virus. To date, eight cases of Heartland virus disease have been described among residents of Missouri and Tennessee with transmission through the bite of *Amblyomma americanum*, also known as the lone star tick.

Sandfly fever group

These viruses are distributed throughout the European and North African countries surrounding the Mediterranean Sea, extending eastward through Israel and Iran to West Pakistan and central India. Sandfly fever (Naples and Sicilian) viruses were first isolated from the sera of US servicemen during an outbreak in the Second World War.

Epidemics of dengue-like fever occur during the sandfly season (June to September) and affect mainly visitors rather than residents. Natural vectors are *Phlebotomus papatasi* and other phlebotomine sandflies. Isolation of virus from male sandflies collected during July suggests transovarial transfer of virus. The natural cycle of sandfly fever appears to involve solely human beings, as definitive host and reservoir, with sandflies as vectors.

Toscana virus

Toscana virus was first isolated from sandflies collected in Tuscany, Italy; it is transmitted by *Phlebotomus perniciosus* sandflies and can be transferred transovarially. Natural reservoirs of Toscana virus appear to be small rodents (*Apodemus sylvaticus*).

Bunyaviruses: *Nairovirus* genus
Crimean–Congo haemorrhagic fever virus

Crimean–Congo haemorrhagic fever virus (CCHFV) was originally described as two separate viruses: Crimean haemorrhagic fever virus, isolated from the serum of a human with fatal haemorrhagic fever near Samarkand, Uzbekistan, and Congo virus isolated from the serum of a child with fever and arthralgia in Zaire. Antigenic and genetic studies show that the two viruses are identical. CCHFV is distributed widely throughout tropical Africa, from Mauritania to Uganda and Kenya, the Middle East and West Pakistan, and southwards to South Africa. It is also found in Asia, including parts of China, and in Southern Europe. The geographical distribution of CCHFV corresponds to that of *Hyalomma* spp. ticks, from which the virus can be isolated. Human infection is rare, but mortality rates of up to 50% have been reported.

Bunyaviruses: *Hantavirus* genus

Unlike the other genera in the Bunyaviridae, members of the *Hantavirus* genus are rodent-associated viruses. They are zoonotic viruses of rodents (mainly mice or voles) that excrete virus in urine for prolonged periods. Virus is transmitted to humans by contact with aerosols of rodent urine.

Hantaan and Puumala viruses

These viruses induce either (1) a severe illness, termed haemorrhagic fever with renal syndrome, due to Hantaan virus in Japan, Korea, China and Siberia, and Puumala virus in Scandinavia, or (2) a mild illness, termed nephropathia epidemica, due to Puumala virus in Scotland, France, Belgium and Germany, the Balkans and Greece. Hantaan virus was first identified in soldiers serving in Korea in 1951 and named after the area where it was detected. Principal vertebrate reservoirs comprise *Apodemus agrarius* rodents in Asia and *Clethrionomys glareolus* (bank vole) in Europe.

Sin Nombre virus

Sin Nombre virus induces hantavirus pulmonary syndrome, a severe acute respiratory illness with a case fatality rate exceeding 50%. Initially encountered in May 1993 in the Four Corners region of the United States (Arizona, Colorado, New Mexico and Utah), cases have since occurred elsewhere in the United States, Canada and many countries in South America. The principal rodent reservoir is considered to be *Peromyscus maniculatus* (deer mouse), but each hantavirus pulmonary syndrome-causing virus occupies a geographical region defined by the rodent species that carries it. Thus, Black Creek Canal virus found in cotton rats *(Sigmodon hispidus)* in Florida is related to viruses found in South America, with a distinct rodent host.

This was the first occasion on which molecular methods identified an unknown arbovirus before the virus was isolated. Hantavirus group antibodies were detected in sera from human cases and rodents. RNA from lung and liver of fatal human cases and seropositive rodents was amplified by RT-PCR; positive bands were detected using primers for Prospect Hill (North American) and Puumala virus-like hantaviruses but not Hantaan and Seoul-like (Asian) hantaviruses. This was achieved within 3 weeks after death of the initial human cases. Several months later, Sin Nombre virus, genomically distinct from Prospect Hill and other hantaviruses, was isolated from tissue suspensions, initially from *P. maniculatus* and subsequently from humans.

CONTROL

Strategies for the prevention of arbovirus infections depend on either vector control or active immunisation with vaccine.

Vector control

Suppression of populations of vector mosquito species can halt virus transmission in urban and suburban localities as follows:

1. Use of insecticides to kill adult mosquitoes (adulticiding); however, nontarget insects may also be affected. The use of persistent insecticides on the interiors of houses has decreased because of environmental concerns; however, this approach may remain effective against certain vectors and in certain ecologies.
2. Removal of domestic larval development sites for *Ae. aegypti* such as tin cans and tyres that could contain rainwater, both near human habitations and in public parks and drainage systems; this has prevented the occurrence of dengue in Singapore and urban yellow fever in metropolitan areas in Caribbean countries.
3. Chemical control of larvae by applying insecticides or oil to small larval sites; this has reduced mosquito vector populations substantially in irrigated localities.
4. Biological control of larvae by microbiological agents such as *Bacillus thuringiensis israeliensis*, larvivorous fish, flatworms or mermethid nematodes, or insect growth regulators such as the juvenile hormone that mimics methoprene.
5. Personal protection against bites by mosquitoes involving a combination of protective clothing, preferably impregnated with permethrin, screening of dwellings to prevent entry of vectors and frequent application of repellents such as *N,N*-diethyl-*m*-toluamide (DEET) or picaridin to exposed skin. For tick-borne viruses, protective clothing should be worn outdoors, followed by rigorous inspection to remove attached ticks from the skin.

Vaccines

To date, relatively few vaccines have been developed to control arbovirus diseases.

Alphaviruses

There are no licensed vaccines for use in humans. However, formalin-inactivated vaccines for WEEV, EEEV and VEEV are used to immunise horses, researchers who work with the viruses and military personnel. A live VEE vaccine, known as TC-83, is also administered to horses and researchers. TC-83 is associated with adverse reactions and lack of seroconversion in many human vaccinees and is not suitable for use in the general population. Additional vaccines against VEEV and CHIKV are under development and in both preclinical and clinical trials.

Flaviviruses

Vaccines have been licensed against yellow fever, Japanese encephalitis and TBE viruses, plus a live dengue vaccine has been licensed recently. A live yellow fever vaccine, 17D, was developed in the 1930s by 176 passages of wild-type strain Asibi through chicken tissue. One dose of vaccine administered subcutaneously and containing 5000–200,000 plaque-forming units of virus gives protective immunity 10 days after immunisation. Until recently, the World Health Organization recommended booster immunisations every 10 years to maintain immunity; however, in 2016 booster doses were no longer recommended. The vaccine can be given to children over 9 months of age. Immunisation is contraindicated in immunocompromised individuals and pregnant women. More than 650 million doses of vaccine have been administered, leading to only a few cases of yellow fever–associated neurotropic disease (YEL-AND) and yellow fever–associated viscerotropic disease (YEL-AVD).

Both live and killed vaccines have been developed to control Japanese encephalitis. Formalin-inactivated vaccines were developed in the 1940s based on virus grown in mouse brain, but were recently discontinued because of the risk of allergic reaction following immunisation. Killed vaccines based on virus grown in Vero cell culture are now being used. Two doses of killed vaccine given 7–28 days apart are required for protective immunity. A booster is given at 1 year and subsequently every 3–4 years to maintain immunity. Two live vaccines have been developed: SA14-14-2 was generated in the People's Republic of China by 126 passages of wild-type strain SA14 in primary hamster kidney cell culture. It is given as two doses and has been administered to more than 300 million people in China without any reports of adverse reactions. To date, the vaccine has been used in nine other Asian countries. The second live human vaccine is a recombinant chimeric vaccine based on ChimeriVax technology. Here, recombinant DNA technology was used to take the live-attenuated yellow fever 17D vaccine virus and replace the membrane and envelope (M/E) structural proteins with those of live Japanese encephalitis vaccine strain SA14-14-2. In addition, a live vaccine is used to immunise pigs.

A formalin-inactivated TBE vaccine using virus grown in chicken eggs was developed in the 1970s to control central European tick-borne encephalitis virus. The vaccine was improved by transferring manufacture to primary chick embryo fibroblast cell culture. Two doses are given, 2 weeks to 3 months apart, followed by a booster given 9 months to 1 year later. Boosters are recommended every 3 years. The vaccine has proved to be very effective, with few adverse reactions, and has resulted in the near elimination of tick-borne encephalitis in Austria. The effectiveness of the vaccine against Russian spring-summer encephalitis (RSSE) is uncertain, but animal studies suggest the vaccine will protect against RSSE.

In 2015 the first dengue vaccine was licensed in five countries. This is a tetravalent recombinant chimeric live-attenuated dengue vaccine using the ChimeriVax technology. Four 17D viruses were generated containing the M/E protein genes of the respective DENV-1, -2, -3 or -4 virus and these were formulated into a tetravalent vaccine to protect against all four dengue viruses.

Bunyaviruses

Although there are no commercially available vaccines against diseases caused by bunyaviruses, a number of experimental live and killed vaccines have been developed against Rift Valley fever. In addition, experimental deoxyribonucleic acid (DNA)-based vaccines have been developed against several hantaviruses and show promise in preclinical studies.

RECOMMENDED READING

Elliott, R. M., & Brennan, B. (2014). Emerging phleboviruses. *Current Opinion in Virology*, 5, 50–57. doi:10.1016/j.coviro.2014.01.011.

Karabatsos, N. (1985). *International Catalogue of Arboviruses Including Certain Other Viruses of Vertebrates* (3rd ed.). San Antonio: American Society for Tropical Medicine and Hygiene.

Ksiazek, T. G., Peters, C. J., Rollin, P. E., Zaki, S., Nichol, S., Spiropoulou, C., ... Khan, A. S. (1995). Identification of a new North American hantavirus that causes acute pulmonary insufficiency. *American Journal of Tropical Medicine and Hygiene*, 52(2), 117–123.

Monath, T. P. (1988). *The Arboviruses: Ecology and Epidemiology* (Vol. 1–5). Boca Raton: CRC Press.

Petersen, L. R., Jamieson, D. J., Powers, A. M., & Honein, M. A. (2016). Zika virus. *The New England Journal of Medicine*, 374(16), 1552–1563. doi:10.1056/NEJMra1602113.

US Department of Health and Human Services. (2007). *Biosafety in Microbiological and Biomedical Laboratories* (5th ed.). Washington, DC: US Government Printing Office.

Weaver, S. C., & Barrett, A. D. (2004). Transmission cycles, host range, evolution and emergence of arboviral disease. *Nature Reviews. Microbiology*, 2(10), 789–801.

Weaver, S. C., Ferro, C., Barrera, R., Boshell, J., & Navarro, J. C. (2001). Venezuelan equine encephalitis. *Annual Reviews of Entomology*, 49, 141–174.

Weaver, S. C., & Reisen, W. K. (2010). Present and future arboviral threats. *Antiviral Research*, 85(2), 328–345. doi:10.1016/j.antiviral.2009.10.008.

Weaver, S. C., & Lecuit, M. (2015). Chikungunya virus and the global spread of a mosquito-borne disease. *The New England Journal of Medicine*, 372(13), 1231–1239. doi:10.1056/NEJMra1406035.

48 Hepatitis C virus

Hepatitis C; non-A; non-B hepatitis; hepacivirus

PETER SIMMONDS AND ELEANOR BARNES

KEY POINTS

- Hepatitis C virus (HCV) is principally transmitted by blood-borne routes. The development of antibody and PCR-based methods for the diagnosis of HCV infection is of major value in blood donor screening and investigation of clinical hepatitis.
- HCV infection is persistent in a large proportion of those exposed. Significant liver disease develops slowly (20–30 years) and can lead to cirrhosis, end-stage liver failure and hepatocellular carcinoma.
- Chronic HCV infection has been treated with pegylated interferon-α and ribavirin with variable response rates. More effective treatment is now based on directly acting antiviral agents that target virus replication (e.g., protease, NS5A and polymerase inhibitors).

Hepatitis C virus (HCV), discovered in 1989, was the long sought-after and highly elusive causative agent of posttransfusion non-A, non-B hepatitis. This hugely important discovery allowed rapid development of serological screening assays for HCV infection and their adoption for blood donor screening. This consequently virtually eliminated transmission of HCV by blood transfusion, and indeed the occurrence of transfusion-associated hepatitis.

Infection with HCV is widespread throughout the world and is particularly associated with risk groups for parenteral (blood-borne) exposure. Amongst these, drug users sharing needles and syringes are numerically the most significant in Western countries. HCV infection is frequently persistent, and leads to the development of significant liver disease, such as cirrhosis and hepatocellular carcinoma (HCC), but only after a long, usually asymptomatic carrier phase. HCV is currently the subject of intensive efforts to develop effective antiviral treatment for chronic infection, and protective vaccines.

PROPERTIES

STRUCTURE

HCV is a small, enveloped virus with a single-stranded RNA genome of positive (coding) polarity (Fig. 48.1). HCV has been visualised in the plasma of HCV-infected individuals as small (50 nm), round particles. The surface of the virus particle contains a number of small surface projections thought to be formed from complexes of the virally encoded envelope glycoproteins, E1 and E2. The RNA genome is approximately 9400 bases in length, of which over 98% contains protein-coding sequence. In common with many other small RNA viruses, the gene sequences of HCV are translated in a single block to produce a large (>3000 amino acid) polyprotein. During and after translation, proteases cleave this precursor into a total of nine mature proteins, which are involved in virus replication and virion assembly (p7, NS2–NS5B) or form structural components of virus particles (core, E1 and E2).

REPLICATION

The genome positions and functions of individual proteins encoded by HCV are summarised in Fig. 48.1. For example, NS5B is the RNA polymerase required by HCV for replication of its genetic material through a negative-stranded intermediate. NS3 contains protease and helicase activities; the former is required for the majority of cleavage reactions in the processing of the polyprotein after translation. The three proteins at the left-hand end of the genome are structural proteins. Multiple copies of the core protein assemble to form a nucleocapsid that packages the viral RNA, while E1 and E2 are synthesised on internal membranes within the infected cell, become heavily glycosylated and form the HCV envelope as the nucleocapsid buds out of the cell.

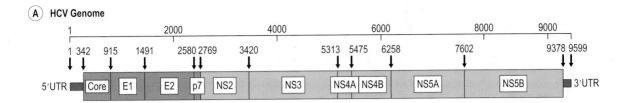

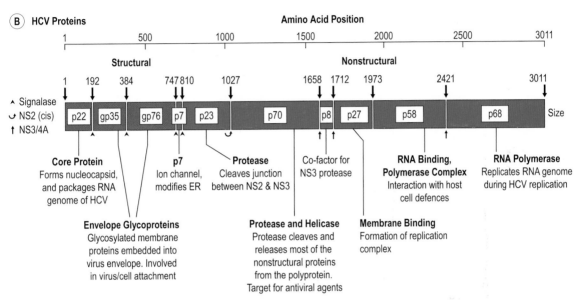

Fig. 48.1 Organisation of HCV genome, showing (A) the structural *(core, E1 and E2)* and nonstructural genes *(p7, NS2–NS5B)*, and (B) the proteins produced from them by proteolytic cleavage of the translated polyprotein. Properties and functions where known of the HCV proteins are summarised in the text.

The extreme ends of the HCV genome are noncoding and play a number of roles in the transcription and translation of the virus genome. Details of the factors that initiate and regulate HCV transcription still remain unclear, although the noncoding ends are likely to be involved in protein complexes with NS5B, NS3 and other HCV and cellular proteins to mediate binding and initiation of RNA copying. The 5′ untranslated region (5′UTR) plays an important role in directing the translation of the HCV polyprotein from an internal (methionine) codon. RNA secondary structure formation allows direct binding of the host cell ribosome to internal sequences in the 5′UTR, bypassing the conventional attachment to the (capped) end of the RNA molecule, as is found in the translation of cellular mRNAs. The 5′UTR additionally possesses two sites to which the cellular micro RNA, miR-122, may bind. This miRNA is preferentially expressed in the liver, and its interaction with HCV is required for virus replication.

The principal targets of HCV replication in vivo are hepatocytes in the liver. The entry mechanism of HCV into hepatocytes (and other cell types) is complex and incompletely understood. A variety of cellular proteins are involved in the initial attachment of HCV to the cell (the LDL receptor, heparan sulfate), binding and internalisation (CD81, DC-SIGN, L-SIGN, claudin-1 [CLDN1] and occludin [OCLN]), the latter process after endocytosis of the bound virion in a clathrin-coated endosome. In vivo, this likely occurs on the basolateral membrane surface of hepatocytes to allow concentration of the virion. Subsequently, interaction with other host factors such as scavenger receptor BI, CD81, CLDN1 and OCLN leads to viral internalisation via clathrin-mediated endosomes and fusion of viral and endosomal membranes. On entering the cytoplasm, the RNA genome is released from the viral capsid and translated. The newly synthesised RNA replicating and unwinding enzymes such as NS5B, NS5A and NS3 subsequently initiate transcription of the genomic RNA into a full-length negative-polarity copy, which in turn acts as the template for the production of multiple positive-stranded RNA copies. These can be used for further rounds of transcription or used for the production of further viral proteins.

Replication of HCV takes place in membrane compartments associated with the cellular endoplasmic reticulum (ER). Although the core protein remains within the cytoplasm after cleavage from E1, E1 and E2 are embedded in the ER membrane, and their extracellular domains are glycosylated. Details of the subsequent stages of capsid assembly and maturation, the insertion of HCV RNA, and the budding of HCV through the ER into extracytoplasmic space and release from the cell await further studies.

CLASSIFICATION

HCV shows the greatest similarity in structure, size and genome organisation with flaviviruses. Together, these viruses are classified as members of the *Flaviviridae* (Table 48.1), currently divided into four named genera. The *Hepacivirus* genus contains HCV, a recently discovered equine homologue of HCV (nonprimate hepacivirus) and GB virus B, originally isolated from a captive tamarind, in which it causes acute hepatitis and liver disease similar to that of HCV in humans. Recently, several more equally divergent hepaciviruses have been described in various species of bats, mice and in the common brown rat *(Rattus norvegicus)*. Hepaciviruses have been additionally characterised in Old World primates and cows and are

likely widespread throughout mammals. Both GBV-B and rodent hepaciviruses are currently under evaluation as possible experimental models for HCV vaccines.

Human pegivirus (HPgV, originally described as GB virus C or hepatitis G virus) is classified as a member of the recently described *Pegivirus* genus. This virus is widely distributed in humans and was originally thought to be a further agent involved in post-transfusion and chronic hepatitis of unexplained aetiology. This association has subsequently been disproved, and infection appears to be entirely asymptomatic, despite being persistent in a significant proportion of those it infects. Its genome shows a number of similarities to that of HCV, including a 5′UTR that has similar ribosomal binding and internal initiation to that of HCV (although a different RNA secondary structure and no miR-122 binding sites), while the coding region contains homologues to its structural and nonstructural proteins. However, it lacks a protein corresponding to the core protein of HCV that forms the nucleocapsid. Viruses similar to HPgV are widely distributed in a range of nonhuman primate species (simian pegiviruses including GBV-A), rodents, bats (originally described as GBV-D), and there are two different species in horses and pigs. The *Pestivirus* genus contains viruses that are structurally similar to HCV and infect a number of domestic and wild species of ruminants such as pigs, sheep and cows. Viruses in the Flavivirus genus are discussed in Ch. 47.

VIRUS STABILITY

HCV is inactivated by exposure to chloroform, ether and other organic solvents and by detergents. The effectiveness of a number of virus-inactivating procedures has been demonstrated by studies of the infectivity of products manufactured from plasma such as the factor VIII and IX concentrates used to treat haemophiliacs. For example, dry-heat treatment at 80°C or wet-heat treatment at 60°C, organic solvents (n-heptane) and detergents have been shown to efficiently remove infectivity for HCV in recipients.

DIAGNOSIS

SEROLOGICAL DIAGNOSIS

Chronic infection with HCV is associated with the presence of both plasma viraemia and virus-specific antibody. Methods to detect both antibody and HCV directly have been used for diagnosis of HCV infection.

The technical simplicity of antibody testing has favoured its use for general screening and diagnostic testing. Antibody tests for HCV are based on cloned HCV RNA

Table 48.1	Members of the *Flaviviridae* family
Genus	Examples
Hepacivirus	Hepatitis C virus Nonprimate hepacivirus (infects horses) GB virus B Numerous additional species infecting rodents, bats, cows, primates
Pegivirus	Human Pegivirus (formerly GB virus C, hepatitis G virus) Simian Pegivirus (formerly GBV-A) and other homologues in nonhuman primates Bat Pegivirus (described as GBV-D) Numerous additional species infecting rodents, bats, horses and pigs
Pestivirus	Bovine viral diarrhoea virus Types I and II swine vesicular disease virus (formerly hog cholera virus) Border disease virus Less well characterised variants in other ruminant species
Flavivirus 68 members (some examples)	Tick-borne encephalitis virus Louping ill virus Japanese encephalitis virus Dengue virus, serotypes 1–4 Yellow fever virus

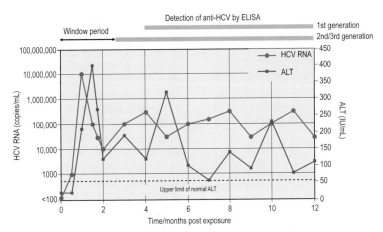

Fig. 48.2 Virological and biochemical markers of acute HCV infection. HCV RNA *(red line)* and abnormal ALT levels *(blue line)* appear approximately 30 days after exposure to HCV in a typical individual. The subsequent development of chronic hepatitis is indicated by persistent viraemia and by fluctuating abnormal ALT levels. Antibody to HCV first appears after the onset of acute hepatitis, in this example leading to 'window periods' of around 100–150 days for the first-generation serological assay (containing only NS3 and NS4 proteins) and approximately 60–80 days for second- and third-generation assays (containing additional NS3, [NS5], and core proteins).

sequences of HCV genotype 1a originally derived from an experimentally infected chimpanzee. Recombinant proteins expressed from these clones have formed and remain the basis for almost all assays for antibody to HCV since then. Current assays incorporate antigens from the core, NS3 and NS5 regions to produce assays of high sensitivity and specificity for antibody to HCV of all genotypes.

Testing for HCV antibody is normally carried out as a two-stage procedure. An enzyme-linked immunosorbent assay (ELISA) format is used for initial testing of serum or plasma from patients or blood donors. Repeatedly reactive samples are then retested by a second ELISA in a different format or by a supplementary assay such as the Ortho recombinant immunoblot assay (RIBA) that contains a number of separate HCV antigens. Currently used serological tests for anti-HCV are now highly sensitive and specific in most patient groups, although individuals who are immunosuppressed, such as those coinfected with HIV, renal dialysis or transplant patients, and those with congenital immunodeficiencies can produce false-negative serological test results. In these cases, direct detection methods for HCV, such as the polymerase chain reaction (PCR) to detect viral RNA, are required.

DIRECT DETECTION METHODS

Assays to detect HCV directly, such as viral RNA by PCR, are required to demonstrate active infection with HCV. Primary infection is characterised by a prolonged window period between exposure to HCV and development

of antibody detectable by the best current ELISAs (Fig. 48.2). For this reason, further direct methods for the detection of the virus itself are required for the effective diagnosis of HCV infection in acute hepatitis, or for diagnosis of HCV in immunosuppressed individuals who do not mount a detectable antibody response. Genome detection methods have also been widely adopted in addition to serological tests for the routine screening of blood donors for HCV in most Western countries.

Direct detection methods are based on either the detection of HCV RNA sequences by PCR or other nucleic acid amplification methods or of viral antigens by ELISA. Diagnostic PCR methods are commercially available and are capable of high sensitivity and specificity for the detection of HCV RNA sequences in plasma (or liver biopsy) specimens. Alternative, non–PCR-based methods, such as transcript-mediated amplification, have also been developed and provide comparable sensitivity to PCR. An alternative to nucleic acid detection is the use of ELISA-based methods for the detection of HCV core protein in plasma, and more recently combined antibody/antigen detection methods.

Direct virus detection is the only reliable method of following the effect of treatment with antiviral drugs on patients with chronic infection because normalisation of biochemical liver function tests is not always associated with virus clearance. Similarly, chronic HCV infection with associated disease is known in patients with normal liver functions tests. Quantitation of the virus genome titre is now increasingly possible with commercial tests based on PCR, other amplification methods or hybridisation and is used as a predictor for response to antiviral therapy (see TREATMENT).

GENETIC VARIATION

Nucleotide sequences of HCV frequently show substantial differences from each other. This has led to the current genotypic classification of HCV, in which variants from a variety of geographical locations can be classified into six main genotypes and a rarer genotype seven, and a number of subtypes (Fig. 48.3).

Genotypes show approximately 30% sequence divergence from each other, differences that greatly modify their antigenic properties and their biology (see TREATMENT).

Some genotypes of HCV (types 1a, 2a, 2b) show a broad worldwide distribution, while others such as type 5a and 6a are only found in specific geographical regions (South Africa and Southeast Asia, respectively). Blood donors and patients with chronic hepatitis from countries in Western Europe and the United States are most frequently infected with genotypes 1a, 1b, 2a, 2b and 3a. The relative frequencies of each may vary geographically, such as the trend for more frequent infection with type 1b in southern and Eastern Europe, and the association of genotype 1a and 3a infection with infection through drug use. HCV genotypes can be identified by analysis of sequences from the 5'UTR or from coding regions. Methods for rapid genotyping of HCV have been developed and play a role in the pre-treatment assessment of patients receiving antiviral treatment.

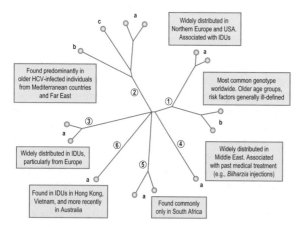

Fig. 48.3 Comparison of complete genome sequences of the common genotypes of HCV plotted as a phylogenetic tree, showing the six main genetic groups (genotypes 1–6) and a number of the more common subtypes (a, b, c). The distribution of the different genotypes in the principal risk groups for HCV infection is indicated (IDU, injecting drug user). A full listing of currently classified HCV genotypes and subtypes is provided at: https://talk.ictvonline.org/ictv_wikis/flaviviridae/w/sg_flavi/56/hcv-classification

EPIDEMIOLOGY

In Western Europe, Australia and North America, most HCV-infected patients have a history of parenteral exposure to the virus, and the majority are (or have been) people who inject drugs. The seroconversion rate in this risk group has been estimated at 20% per year, and so long-term drug users are almost invariably HCV-infected. Drug use was uncommon before the 1960s, and so infected drug users tend to be younger than patients infected by blood transfusion or other routes. Most drug users have asymptomatic infection with no history of jaundice but have chronic hepatitis; few have overt clinical signs or symptoms of liver disease or liver failure.

Other blood-borne routes of HCV transmission include blood transfusion before 1991 (when universal donor screening was initiated), recipients of pooled plasma products such as factor VIII, and immunoglobulin manufactured before 1986 (when virus-inactivation procedures for plasma-derived blood products became widely used). Other at-risk groups include transplant recipients, haemodialysis patients, and health-care workers from needlestick injuries. Tattooing and acupuncture may also be responsible for some percutaneous exposure, and in countries of high prevalence, the use of unsterilised needles for cultural rituals, medical treatment or vaccination programmes may result in HCV infection.

The lowest frequencies of HCV infection are found in Scandinavian and other Northern European countries such as the United Kingdom (0.3%–0.4%), with slightly higher prevalence in North America (1%) and Australia. Prevalence is intermediate in southern and Eastern European countries, even higher in Japan, and most prevalent in the Middle East; frequencies of HCV infection of up to 30% have been recorded in areas of Egypt. In this latter case, bilharzia treatment using reusable and unsterile needles in the 1960s has been identified as the main source of infection.

There is little evidence for nonparenteral transmission of HCV. For example, there is little convincing evidence for transmission by sexual contact where confounding factors have been removed. Mother-to-child transmission of HCV occurs at frequencies between 1% and 3% in the majority of studies. Transmission occurs generally at birth, presumably through contact with blood.

CLINICAL FEATURES

Chronic hepatitis C infection causes an indolent and slowly progressive liver disease that is asymptomatic until the development of decompensated liver disease and often liver cancer (Fig. 48.4).

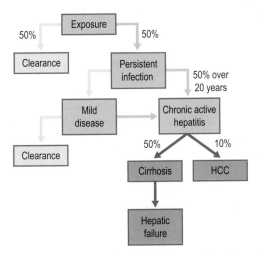

Fig. 48.4 Natural course of HCV infection showing approximate frequencies and time course of persistence and of progression to clinically significant disease. HCC, hepatocellular carcioma.

ACUTE HEPATITIS

Exposure to HCV usually results in an asymptomatic infection without jaundice, with approximately half to three-quarters becoming chronic carriers of the virus. Most studies have reported an interval of around 8 weeks to the development of abnormal liver function tests (such as alanine aminotransferase [ALT] levels) (Fig. 48.2). Clinically, hepatitis caused by HCV is indistinguishable from that caused by other hepatitis viruses; jaundice may develop, but, more usually, symptoms are nonspecific such as fatigue, anorexia and nausea. Viraemia can be detected in the early stages of acute hepatitis, appearing at the same time or slightly earlier than abnormal ALT levels, while seroconversion for antibody may be delayed for several weeks or months after the onset of hepatitis. Histologic features of acute HCV are similar to those associated with acute HAV and HBV infection; liver biopsy is rarely indicated to make a diagnosis of acute HCV infection.

CHRONIC HEPATITIS

The frequency of chronic infection following exposure to HCV is approximately 50% (Fig. 48.4). Persistent infection with HCV is generally associated with persistent and progressive hepatitis, with fluctuating or continuously abnormal ALT levels. Although viraemia is invariably detected in patients with chronic hepatitis, there is no correlation between level of viraemia and the severity of

liver disease, ALT levels or other biochemical abnormalities associated with hepatitis.

HCV infection causes a range of characteristic histological changes in the liver, although few allow a specific diagnosis of HCV infection to be made. These include lymphoid follicles within the portal tracts, a dense periportal inflammatory process, bile duct damage, and lobular hepatitis, with lymphocyte infiltration within sinusoids surrounding the hepatocytes. Liver histology in HCV infection is now commonly classified using scoring systems such as the Ishak or Metavir scores.

The percentage of chronically infected individuals who progress to cirrhosis and liver failure is not known. When chronic hepatitis does progress to clinically significant liver damage, then progression is almost invariably very slow (e.g., 20 years or more), although factors associated with faster progression include age at infection, male gender, patients who are immunosuppressed, or the presence of other risk factors such as heavy alcohol intake. Particularly aggressive HCV-associated liver disease has been observed in immunosuppressed organ transplant recipients and in patients with inherited immunodeficiency states. Cirrhosis is rarely observed within 10 years of infection, and as few as 20% of infected patients have cirrhosis after 20 years' follow-up. Cirrhosis may be complicated by liver failure (decompensated cirrhosis), manifested as jaundice, portal hypertension and variceal bleeding; these manifestations of liver failure are shared with other forms of cirrhosis. Hepatocellular carcinoma (HCC) frequently complicates chronic hepatitis C, although HCC is rare within 15 years of initial infection. In many Western countries such as Spain and Italy, and in Japan, HCV infection is found in 60%–90% of cases of HCC.

EXTRAHEPATIC MANIFESTATIONS

In a minority of infected patients, HCV may be responsible for extrahepatic clinical manifestations and disease. These include certain types of vasculitis and glomerulonephritis caused by immune complex deposition. Associations between HCV infection and Sjogren's syndrome, essential mixed cryoglobulinaemia and membranoproliferative glomerulonephritis type 1 have been suggested.

TREATMENT AND CONTROL

TREATMENT

Until recently, pegylated interferon-α (IFN-α) combined with ribavirin (RBV) was the standard treatment for chronic hepatitis associated with HCV infection. Typically, 6 mega units of IFN-α, three times a week given by injection, and RBV were used for 6–12 months. Cure was typically achieved in 45%–70% of patients. IFN-α therapy is associated with prolonged treatment courses and severe side effects, and treatment failure is common. Increasingly, directly acting antiviral therapies (DAAs) are replacing IFN-α as the mainstay of therapy (see Ch. 5 and Table 48.2). The success rate of therapy with DAAs is >95% in most patient populations with minimal side effects and represents an enormous advance in the field. Similar to treatment for HIV, DAA therapy is given as combination therapy with multiple drugs that have distinct viral targets. Combination therapy limits the ability of the virus to develop resistance-associated genetic substitutions (RAS) during therapy. Viral targets for DAA include the HCV

NS3 protease, NS5A protein and NS5B polymerase. Inhibitors of NS5B are either nucleoside analogues that cause chain termination of RNA transcripts, or nonnucleoside protein binding inhibitors of RNA polymerase. The genetic barrier for the development of RAS is generally lower for drugs that target the HCV NS3 protease or the NS5A protein, and RAS to the NS5A protein may persist long term. In contrast, RAS to drugs that target the NS5B polymerase are less commonly observed. Ribavirin is frequently combined with DAA therapy.

Quantitative PCR is widely used in preference to monitoring of serum transaminases for determining response to treatment. Three patterns are observed (Fig. 48.5). Uncommonly, patients may remain RNA positive despite treatment (nonresponders), whilst most respond with clearance of viraemia and normalisation of ALT. A proportion of this latter group relapse during therapy (breakthrough) or when therapy is withdrawn (relapse). The treatment objective is a sustained virological response defined as HCV RNA negativity, 3–6 months after therapy ends. This equates to long-term RNA clearance (and normal ALT) (i.e., cure). In an attempt to improve response rates, particularly with IFN-α–based therapies, and to avoid the unnecessary treatment of potential nonresponders, clinical and virological features associated with sustained response have been defined. The most important factors are:

HCV genotype. The infecting genotype has a major influence on frequency of response to treatment. For

Table 48.2 Directly acting antiviral agents for the treatment of chronic HCV infection

NS3/4A protease inhibitors	NS5A multifunctional protein inhibitors	NS5B RNA polymerase inhibitors
Simeprevir	Ledipasvir	Sofosbuvir
Paritaprevir	Daclatasvir	Dasabuvir
Grazoprevir	Ombitasvir	
Glecaprevir	Elbasvir	
	Velpatasvir	
	Pibrentasvir	

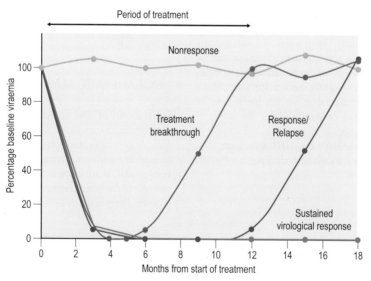

Fig. 48.5 Outcomes of therapy in chronic hepatitis C. Nonresponders are those where RNA levels remain close to baseline levels during or after cessation of treatment. Among those initially responding and showing virus clearance, a proportion will relapse during therapy *(treatment breakthrough)* and some will relapse at conclusion of therapy *(responder-relapser)*. The desired outcome is a sustained virological response, where individuals remain nonviraemic for 12 (SVR12) or 24 (SVR24) weeks from the cessation of treatment. HCV RNA levels parallel replication of HCV in the liver and the resulting inflammatory damage. Normalisation of the liver enzyme ALT and other transaminases normalise along with virus clearance.

IFN-α–based therapies, the rates of long-term response are higher among patients infected with genotypes 2a, 2b and 3a compared with those with types 1 or 4. Limited data indicate an intermediate response rate of genotypes 5 and 6. With peg-IFN-α and ribavirin therapy, sustained clearance of viraemia is typically observed in 50% of patients infected with type 1, and 80%–85% of those with type 2 and 3 infections. Prolonging combination treatment to 12 months significantly improved the frequency of response in those infected with type 1, but not nontype 1 genotypes. Interestingly, with DAA-based therapies, HCV genotype 3 infection has proven the more difficult genotype to treat. This is partly explained by the fact that the protease inhibitors were particularly designed to target the genotype 1 protease, but DAA combinations that include NS5A and NS5B inhibitors are also less effective in HCV genotype 3 infection.

The mechanism by which different genotypes might differ in their susceptibility to interferon-based treatments remains unknown, particularly as it remains unclear whether a directly antiviral action or enhancement of immune responses to HCV infecting cells in the liver contributes most to viral clearance. It is unlikely that the different response rates achieved with type 3 is simply secondary to differences in disease severity. Pretreatment assessment of genotype allows for more appropriate patient selection for treatment and is widely used to calculate the necessary dose and duration to obtain a sustained clearance of viraemia. Pretreatment genotyping is also recommended in those receiving DAAs that vary in efficacy between genotypes (such as the first-generation protease inhibitors, telaprevir and boceprevir)

IL-28B genotype. Recent genome-wide association studies of response to IFN-α–based therapies have identified a single nucleotide polymorphism close to IL-28B (or interferon lambda), a recently characterised antiviral cytokine distantly related to type I IFNs and IL-10, that is associated with treatment response. Individuals infected with genotype 1 treated with IFN-α/RBV show two-fold differences in frequencies of sustained response to therapy according to their IL-28B genotype, a finding that accounts at least in part for observed treatment response rates in different racial groups. This polymorphism is also associated with differences in spontaneous clearance of HCV infection after exposure. It likely represents, or is closely genetically linked to, a key factor governing infection outcome of HCV. IL-28B genotype also has a predictive value for treatment outcomes with DAA therapies, but the effect is much weaker than that observed with IFN-α–based therapies.

Immunosuppression. Subjects infected with HIV-1 (even when controlled with antiretroviral therapy) and immunosuppressed individuals (genetic immunodeficiencies, iatrogenic, those with systemic disease such as leukaemia) all show reduced response rates to IFN-α–based therapy, emphasising the necessary role of the adaptive immune system in virus clearance. However, with DAA-based therapies HIV-1 coinfection has no impact on HCV treatment outcomes.

Disease progression. Patients with advanced HCV-related disease such as cirrhosis or decompensated liver disease respond poorly to IFN-α–based therapy and such therapy may precipitate hepatic decompensation in patients with advanced fibrosis. However, DAA therapies have revolutionised the ability to treat patients with cirrhosis and may be given before, peri- or posttransplantation. Achieving viral eradication in these patients is particularly valuable, as this may ensure the long-term survival of the liver graft. Patients with liver cirrhosis and HCV genotype 3 infection remain the most challenging patient population to treat with DAA therapies, though it is expected that truly pangenotypic drugs for these patients will become available soon.

Baseline viral load and early treatment response. For genotype 1–infected individuals, high viral loads are associated with a reduced likelihood of achieving a sustained response to treatment. Monitoring of viral loads early in treatment is also predictive of outcome; slow reduction or unchanged RNA levels in the first 4 weeks of therapy are associated with a poor outcome and may be used to tailor dose and duration of therapy.

Liver transplantation. Liver transplantation is indicated for patients with decompensated HCV cirrhosis, and for some patients with hepatocellular carcinoma complicating HCV infection. Liver transplantation does not cure HCV infection, and without treatment, reinfection of the graft is inevitable. The recent development of DAA therapies means that for the first time, patients may be transplanted and HCV eradicated in the peri- or posttransplant period.

PREVENTION

Screening of blood donors has proved to be effective at preventing transmission of HCV infection through blood transfusion. A combination of blood donor screening and virus inactivation has virtually eliminated HCV transmission by blood products such as clotting factor concentrates and immunoglobulins.

The main continuing risks for HCV transmission are injecting drug abuse and the use of unsterile needles for medical and dental procedures, tattooing and other percutaneous exposures. Much of this could be prevented by education, greater availability of disposable needles, and for injecting drug users (IDUs), by needle exchange programmes. Many of the public health measures adopted to prevent transmission of HIV by parenteral routes will assist efforts at controlling HCV.

IMMUNISATION

The development of a vaccine for HCV faces a series of formidable obstacles, amongst which viral heterogeneity and the difficulty in evaluating candidate vaccines in suitable animal models are the most acute. Recombinant envelope proteins (E1 and E2) have been shown to generate specific anti-E1 and E2 humoral responses in immunised chimpanzees and phase-I human studies, and in chimpanzees shown to induce transient protection from challenge with the same virus strain. More recently, HCV vaccines that target the more conserved nonstructural proteins of HCV have been developed. A promising approach is the use of viral vectors to induce HCV specific T cell immune responses at high magnitude. These are further enhanced by the use of heterologous prime/boost viral vectored strategies. At the time of writing (2017) these vaccines have progressed through a series of phase I studies in healthy volunteers and are being assessed for efficacy in a large group of IDUs that are commonly exposed to HCV.

Infection with HCV is a growing medical problem worldwide. A combination of public health preventative measures, improved diagnosis, screening, antiviral treatment and immunisation will undoubtedly all be required to combat its spread in the future.

RECOMMENDED READING

Alter, M. J. (2007). Epidemiology of hepatitis C virus infection. *World Journal of Gastroenterology, 13*(17), 2436–2441.

Götte, M., & Feld, J. J. (2016). Direct-acting antiviral agents for hepatitis C: structural and mechanistic insights. *Nature Reviews. Gastroenterology & Hepatology, 13*(6), 338–351. doi:10.1038/nrgastro.2016.60.

Houghton, M. (2011). Prospects for prophylactic and therapeutic vaccines against the hepatitis C viruses. *Immunological Reviews, 239*(1), 99–108. doi:10.1111/j.1600-065X.2010.00977.x.

Lindenbach, B. D., & Rice, C. M. (2005). Unravelling hepatitis C virus replication from genome to function. *Nature, 436*(7053), 933–938 (and other articles in that issue).

Scheel, T. K., & Rice, C. M. (2013). Understanding the hepatitis C virus life cycle paves the way for highly effective therapies. *Nature Medicine, 19*(7), 837–849. doi:10.1038/nm.3248.

Swadling, L., Klenerman, P., & Barnes, E. (2013). Ever closer to a prophylactic vaccine for HCV. *Expert Opinion on Biological Therapy, 13*(8), 1109–1124. doi:10.1517/14712598.2013.791277.

Webster, D. P., Klenerman, P., & Dusheiko, G. M. (2015). Hepatitis C. *Lancet, 385*(9973), 1124–1135. doi:10.1016/S0140-6736(14)62401-6.

49 Hepeviruses

SAMREEN IJAZ AND RICHARD S. TEDDER

KEY POINTS

- There are four major hepatitis E virus (HEV) genotypes that infect humans, and they are remarkable in their associated divergences in relation to epidemiology, clinical features, transmission routes and reservoirs.
- The HEV genome is a single-stranded, 7.2 kb RNA of positive sense and has three open reading frames. Diagnosis for the virus can be made using tools for the detection of antibody, antigen and RNA.
- HEV is prevalent through the Indian subcontinent, parts of Southeast Asia, North and Central Africa and Central America and is transmitted mainly by the consumption of faecally contaminated food and water. In other regions, such as Europe and North America, the virus transmits via a zoonosis, with animals acting as a reservoir for infection in humans.
- The clinical features of HEV infection range from asymptomatic infection to mild hepatitis to fulminant liver failure. Genotype 1 infection has been associated with a high mortality rate in pregnant women, particularly in the third trimester of pregnancy. Persistent infections leading to chronic hepatitis have been reported in immunosuppressed populations and have been linked to genotype 3 viruses. A number of extrahepatic manifestations linked to acute and chronic hepatitis E have been described.
- Pegylated interferon and/or ribavirin have been used successfully to treat individuals with persistent HEV infections. An HEV vaccine has been developed and shown to be safe and immunogenic and to confer protection against HEV infection.

DESCRIPTION

Hepatitis E virus (HEV) belongs to the genus *Hepevirus* in the Hepeviridae family and infects humans and a range of animal hosts. The Hepeviridae family has been divided into the two genera: *Orthohepevirus* (all mammalian and avian HEV isolates) and *Piscihepevirus* (cutthroat trout virus). *Orthohepevirus* contains four species, A–D. *Orthohepevirus* A includes isolates from humans, pigs, wild boar, deer, mongoose, rabbit and camel (Fig. 49.1), *Orthohepevirus* B include isolates from chicken, *Orthohepevirus* C includes isolates from rat, ferret and mink, and *Orthohepevirus* D includes isolates from bats.

Studies of the evolutionary history indicate that HEV has evolved through a series of events, in which ancestral HEV may have adapted to a succession of animal hosts leading to human beings. Four major HEV genotypes infect humans (G1–G4) and are remarkable in their associated divergences, leading HEV to be aptly described as having two faces. The epidemiological picture, clinical features, transmission routes and reservoirs as well as outcome differ significantly depending on the region of the world and, accordingly, the HEV genotype (Table 49.1).

G1 and G2 are restricted to the human host. G1 occurs in Asia and Africa, with G2 reported from Mexico and also Africa. G3 has a worldwide distribution and is associated with infections in humans, pigs and other mammalian species; in contrast, G4 only infects humans and pigs, principally in Southeast Asia. G4 in pigs also occurs in India and occasionally in Europe.

EPIDEMIOLOGY

Developing world

HEV genotype 1 and 2 viruses remain major public health concerns in resource-poor settings where HEV is thought to be responsible for >50% of viral hepatitis cases. The virus is transmitted via the faecal-oral route through the consumption of contaminated food and water. Person-to-person spread is uncommon. There is a striking age-related clinical picture with disease mainly reported from young adults between the age of 15 and 39 years, with a slight male preponderance. Recent studies undertaken in

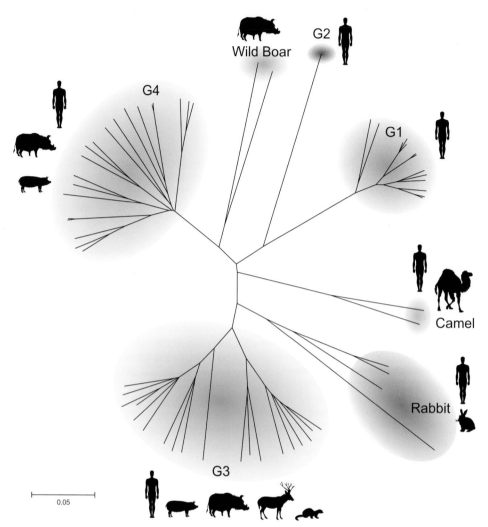

Fig. 49.1 Phylogenetic analysis across complete genome sequences showing relationship across the *Orthohepevirus* A members. G1–G4 denote genotypes 1–4. G1 and G2 are restricted to humans; G3 and G4 are found in humans and a range of animals including pigs, wild boar, mongoose and deer. The *Orthohepevirus* A species also comprises isolates from rabbits and camels. (Figure adapted from Debing Y, Moradpour D, Neyts J, Gouttenoire J. Update on hepatitis E virology: implications for clinical practice. J Hepatol 2016; 65(1): 200–212.)

Table 49.1 Epidemiology, clinical features and outcome in the four human HEV genotypes

	Genotype 1	Genotype 2	Genotype 3	Genotype 4
Distribution	Asia, Africa	Mexico, Africa	Worldwide	China, SE Asia and Central Europe
Reservoir	Human	Human	Pigs, boar, deer	Pigs
Transmission	Waterborne, faecal-oral	Waterborne, faecal-oral	Zoonotic, foodborne, vocational	
Disease pattern	Large waterborne outbreaks, sporadic		Sporadic, occasional small clusters related to food	
HEV as % hepatitis	Common		Infrequent	
Relation of attack rate with age	Most common in young adults (15–44 years)		Mostly middle/older age (>50 years)	Limited data
Gender (M:F)	2 : 1	2 : 1	>3 : 1	
Clinical outcome	Self-limiting	Self-limiting	Self-limiting	
Deaths in pregnancy	High	Not reported	Not reported	Not reported
Chronic infection	Not reported	Not reported	Yes	Yes, but limited number

populations from Nepal and Bangladesh indicate antibody prevalence rates of 47% and 50%, respectively, with no differences noted by gender. Seroprevalence increased with age and demonstrated low prevalence in children <10 years. As well as sporadic infections, the virus is linked to large waterborne outbreaks, which can affect many thousands of individuals. More recent outbreaks have been reported from camps for displaced persons and refugees in Africa where significant mortality is observed in pregnant women and in children under the age of 2 years.

Developed world

In the developed world, HEV G3 and G4 are known to transmit via a zoonosis, with animals acting as a reservoir for infection in humans. Case control questionnaires have indicated the consumption of mussels, game meat and in particular pork products to be associated with HEV infection. The pig remains the best-studied vector, and the concept of a zoonosis is supported by the close sequence homology shared between human and swine HEV sequences. Human infections are essentially dead-end infections, with person-to-person transmission being uncommon. Usually sporadic, a few clusters related to the consumption of undercooked meat have been observed. Surveillance shows a remarkably consistent demographic picture with the majority of clinical cases reported in males over the age of 50 years. Seroprevalence rates vary widely from 1% to 50%, a variation traditionally attributed

to the performance of the different assays used. However, it is now accepted that significant variances in seroprevalence exist between and within countries, indicating local differences in risk and exposure. Data from England collected over 10 years indicate that the infection is dynamic in the population, suggesting fluctuations in risk over time. What influences these fluctuations is unclear. Similar to data from the developing world, there is an observed cohort effect with an increase in seroprevalence with age and low rates in children.

REPLICATION

Hepatitis E virion is a 27 to 32 nm spherical particle that is icosahedral in symmetry and has spikes on the capsid surface. The genome is a single-stranded, 7.2 kb RNA of positive sense with a 7-methylguanylate (m7G-cap) cap at its 5′ end and a poly-A tail at its 3′ end. The genome has short 5′ and 3′ untranslated regions (UTRs) and three open reading frames (ORF) (Fig. 49.2). ORF1 encodes for a polyprotein with several putative functional motifs and domains including methyltransferase, papain-like cysteine protease (PCP), RNA helicase and RNA-dependent RNA polymerase (RdRp), which are involved in the replication and processing of viral proteins. The functions of the other predicted domains X, Y and variable domains remain uncertain. ORF2 encodes the major viral capsid protein that encapsidates the viral RNA genome. This protein carries an N-terminal signal sequence that translocates the

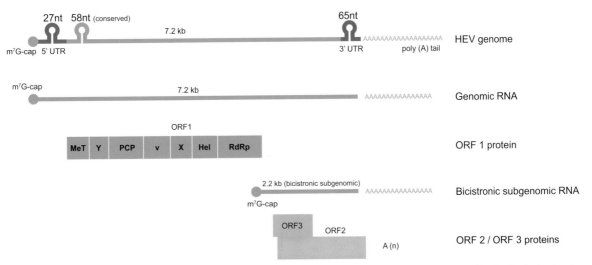

Fig. 49.2 Genome organisation and proteins of HEV. The 7.2 kb–positive-strand RNA genome of HEV is capped at the 5′ end and polyadenylated at the 3′ end. The genome has short 5′ and 3′ untranslated regions (UTRs) and three open reading frames (ORFs). ORF1 is translated from the genomic mRNA and encodes a nonstructural polyprotein with several putative functional motifs and domains involved in the replication and processing of viral proteins. ORF2 and 3 are translated from a 2.2 kb bicistronic subgenomic mRNA. ORF2 encodes the major viral capsid protein which encapsidates the viral RNA genome. The ORF3 encodes a small regulatory phosphoprotein.

protein into the endoplasmic reticulum where it acquires N-linked glycosylation. The viral capsid protein has three defined domains: the shell, middle and protruding domains. A number of studies investigating neutralising epitopes have mapped these to be in the protruding domain of the ORF2 protein with residues 452–617 identified to be important. The viral capsid is also thought to be involved with cellular proteins for the purpose of cell entry, capsid assembly and virus egress. The ORF3 encodes a small phosphoprotein that associates with the cytoskeleton and more specifically with microtubules, and is thought to be essential for the release of virus from infected cells.

The life cycle of HEV remains poorly understood mainly because of the lack of efficient in vitro culture methods. The viral particles are concentrated on the surface of hepatocytes, bind to an undefined receptor and are internalised. Following uncoating, the genomic RNA is released and translated in the cytoplasm into the nonstructural proteins. The viral polymerase RdRP then replicates the positive-sense genomic RNA into negative strand transcripts. These serve as templates for the synthesis of a 2.2 kb subgenomic RNA as well as full-length positive-sense transcripts. The positive-sense subgenomic RNA is translated into ORF2 and ORF3 proteins. The capsid proteins package the viral genome to assemble progeny virions. Viral egress is thought to require the cellular secretory machinery together with the ORF3 protein. More recent data have shown that virus secreted into the bloodstream is associated with the ORF3 protein and wrapped by a lipid cellular membrane whilst virus secreted into the bile is nonenveloped.

CLINICAL FEATURES

Acute HEV infection

The clinical features of HEV infection range from asymptomatic infection to mild hepatitis to fulminant liver failure. Symptoms, if they occur, include general malaise, abdominal pain, anorexia, nausea and fever and are followed by the onset of jaundice accompanied by dark urine, pale stools and itching. Most infections are self-limiting. Data reported mainly from the G1 virus in the developing world suggest a mortality rate of between 0.5% and 4% overall. This increases markedly to approximately 25% among pregnant women, particularly in the third trimester. Spontaneous abortions, stillbirths and neonatal deaths are also increased. This poor outcome of infection during pregnancy appears only to be associated with genotype 1 infection. Acute HEV infection in patients with underlying liver disease may lead to decompensation and a poor outcome, again in association with genotype 1 virus.

Chronic HEV infection

Persistent infections leading to chronic hepatitis have been reported in immunosuppressed populations including solid organ transplant recipients, patients with haematological disorders receiving chemotherapy and HIV-infected individuals. With the exception of one genotype 4 and one genotype 7 (camelid) virus, all chronic HEV infections have been genotype 3. Persistent infections with genotype 1 and 2 viruses have not been reported. The clinical features of persistent HEV infections are often unremarkable. Liver transaminases are usually very modestly raised, and few patients present with any symptoms. Once infected, 60% of solid organ transplant recipients fail to clear the virus and develop chronic hepatitis. Liver biopsy shows rapid progression of liver fibrosis, with 10% of patients progressing to cirrhosis over a few years. Factors such as low leucocyte, total-lymphocyte and T-cell counts were associated with failure to clear HEV. In the HIV setting, patients who develop chronic infection have low CD4 counts. Viral clearance following treatment in HIV-infected individuals is associated with the recovery of CD4 levels and can present as an immune reconstitution hepatitis.

Extrahepatic manifestations

A number of extrahepatic manifestations linked to acute and chronic hepatitis E have been reported. These include thrombocytopenia, glomerulonephritis, acute pancreatitis and acute thyroiditis. A range of neuropathologies have also been described including brachial neuritis, Guillain–Barré syndrome, peripheral neuropathy, neuromyopathy and vestibular neuritis.

DIAGNOSIS

Acute hepatitis E cannot be clinically distinguished from other causes of acute hepatitis. Diagnosis of the virus can be undertaken using methods for detecting antibody, antigen and RNA.

After an incubation period of 2–6 weeks, the immune response to HEV follows a typical pattern—an initial short-lived IgM response followed by more durable IgG antibodies. Although there are four human HEV genotypes, they elicit very similar antibody responses and appear to represent a single serotype. Enzyme immunoassays or rapid immunochromatographic kits use a range of recombinant viral antigens for the detection of specific IgM antibodies. The anti-HEV IgM titres increase rapidly and then wane over the weeks following infection. Anti-HEV IgG antibodies are detected shortly after the IgM and will continue to rise into the convalescence period, remaining detectable for months to years (Fig. 49.3).

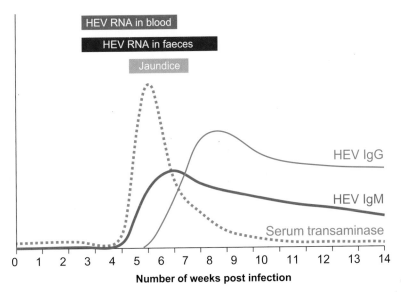

HEV RNA in blood

HEV RNA in faeces

Jaundice

HEV IgG

HEV IgM

Serum transaminase

Number of weeks post infection

Fig. 49.3 Virological and biochemical profile of acute HEV infection.

Antigen detection has been used for the diagnosis of HEV infections. Antigen ELISAs are less sensitive than molecular methods; however, they provide a more rapid and accessible method for identifying current HEV infections. Whilst some studies have shown a good correlation between HEV RNA and antigen, others have reported a weaker association. It remains unclear whether this reflects the populations tested or indeed differences in genotype reactivity.

Detection of HEV RNA is important in the diagnosis, confirmation and monitoring of HEV infections. In patients with an acute HEV infection, peak viraemia occurs during the incubation and early phase of the disease. Viral RNA can be detected just before the onset of clinical symptoms in both blood and stool samples. HEV RNA does not persist in the immunocompetent host becoming undetectable in blood approximately 3 weeks after the onset of symptoms. Viral shedding in stool continues for a short period after plasma viral clearance.

Clinical diagnosis of chronic hepatitis E is impossible as these infections are largely asymptomatic. Testing strategies for identifying individuals with persistent infections are not clear, and an underlying lack of awareness in physicians can mean that infections remain undiagnosed for years. As chronic infections occur in immunosuppressed individuals, the majority of whom will have complex underlying conditions and management strategies, chronic HEV infections can also be misdiagnosed as drug-induced liver injury or graft-versus-host disease. Laboratory diagnosis of chronic HEV must be through HEV RNA testing as antibody detection in the immunosuppressed population is not reliable.

Cell culture systems remain largely inefficient and are not used for routine HEV diagnostics.

TREATMENT

The prognosis for individuals with chronic hepatitis E has been poor. Reduction in levels of immunosuppression, in particular those that target T cells, has resulted in viral clearance but only in 30% of patients. Antiviral treatment is now an option for patients for whom this strategy is not possible or is not successful. Early reports on treatment described the efficacy of pegylated interferon alpha or ribavirin monotherapy or in combination to treat chronic HEV. Ribavirin is now established as the drug of choice demonstrating a potent response with plasma viral clearance usually achieved within a few weeks. Ribavirin has also been shown to be an effective treatment for severe acute hepatitis E. However, a number of side effects, in particular anaemia, have been linked to ribavirin treatment requiring dose reduction, blood transfusions or supportive erythropoietin. Treatment failures have also been reported that are often linked to suboptimal dosage. The selection of a G1634R mutation in the RdRp domain of ORF1 has been observed in three patients experiencing treatment failure. A subsequent report has described additional amino acid changes in the viral polymerase and also insertions in the hypervariable region linked to treatment failure and viral fitness. The clinical significance of these changes remains uncertain.

CONTROL

Immunisation

Two vaccines for HEV have been investigated in clinical trials, of which only one, Hecolin, has been progressed and is currently available. Hecolin was developed and is manufactured by Xiamen Innovax Biotech, Xiamen, and is to date licensed only in China for use in individuals aged 16 years and older. Hecolin is based on a 239 amino acid recombinant HEV G1 peptide of the capsid protein expressed in *E. coli*, which forms a homodimer and assembles into approximately 23 nm particles. The vaccine was shown in a phase II study to be safe and immunogenic and conferred protection against HEV infection with an efficacy of 83%. A randomised, double-blind, placebo controlled phase III trial included over 100,000 healthy adults and demonstrated the vaccine to be well tolerated and protected against hepatitis E with an efficacy of 100%. Data on this protection are primarily applicable to G4 disease; data on disease caused by other genotypes are either too limited (G1) or not available (G2 and G3). An extended assessment of the vaccine showed that, whilst HEV antibodies declined over time, the efficacy did not significantly decrease 4.5 years after the first dose. Evaluations throughout the prelicensing clinical trials showed serious adverse events following hepatitis E immunisation to be rare.

Reducing exposure

Reducing exposure to the virus clearly has a role in control. Sanitation, through the treatment and disposal of human waste, and availability of clean drinking water are the main prevention strategies in the developing world. Boiling and chlorination of water will inactivate HEV. Through the developed countries, focus remains on ensuring meat products are thoroughly cooked. Demonstration of HEV infections in blood donors has led to investigations into appropriate measures for reducing the acquisition of the virus through blood components.

TRANSFUSION–TRANSMITTED HEV

The high prevalence of asymptomatic infections in blood donors has raised the concern of infection via blood components. Studies in blood donors report a wide range of seroprevalence rates from 6% to 46%. With the exception of Scotland, data from Europe demonstrate a high HEV RNA prevalence rate in blood donations. In 2016, HEV RNA prevalence rates were approximately 1:1600 in English blood donors. In contrast, no HEV RNA–positive donations were reported from Canadian and Australian studies, with lower RNA prevalence rates seen in Japan and the United States. Unsurprisingly, data from India, where the virus is endemic, indicated a very high HEV RNA incidence.

An investigation undertaken in recipients of HEV-containing blood components, showed 18 (42%) of 43 to develop HEV infection. Follow-up of the HEV-infected recipients showed that outcome of infection was complex but that patients treated with medium or high doses of immunosuppressive drugs developed prolonged or persistent HEV with a delayed or absent immune response.

Mitigating the risk of HEV transmission through pathogen inactivation/reduction has shown limited efficacy. The HEV capsid is not sensitive to solvent/detergent treatment, and pathogen reduction protocols that block DNA and RNA replication have been shown to be ineffective. Some countries have implemented universal or selective screening protocols for the provision of HEV RNA–negative blood components.

RECOMMENDED READING

Hewitt, P. E., Ijaz, S., Brailsford, S. R., Brett, R., Dicks, S., Haywood, B., … Tedder, R. S. (2014). Hepatitis E virus in blood components: a prevalence and transmission study in southeast England. *Lancet, 384*(9956), 1766–1773.

Izopet, J., Labrique, A. B., Basnyat, B., Dalton, H. R., Kmush, B., Heaney, C. D., … Adhikary, D. (2015). Hepatitis E virus seroprevalence in three hyperendemic areas: Nepal, Bangladesh and southwest France. *Journal of Clinical Virology, 70*, 39–42. doi:10.1016/j.jcv.2015.06.103.

Kamar, N., Bendall, R., Legrand-Abravanel, F., Xia, N. S., Ijaz, S., Izopet, J., & Dalton, H. R. (2012). Hepatitis E. *The Lancet, 379*(9835), 2477–2488. doi:10.1016/S0140-6736(11)61849-7.

Khuroo, M. S., & Khuroo, M. S. (2016). Hepatitis E: an emerging global disease–from discovery towards control and cure. *Journal of Viral Hepatitis, 23*(2), 68–79. doi:10.1111/jvh.12445.

Park, W. J., Park, B. J., Ahn, H. S., Lee, J. B., Park, S. Y., Song, C. S., … Choi, I. S. (2016). Hepatitis E virus as an emerging zoonotic pathogen. *Journal of Veterinary Science, 17*(1), 1–11. doi:10.4142/jvs.2016.17.1.1.

Peters van Ton, A. M., Gevers, T. J., & Drenth, J. P. (2015). Antiviral therapy in chronic hepatitis E: a systematic review. *Journal of Viral Hepatitis, 22*(12), 965–973. doi:10.1111/jvh.12403.

Zhu, F. C., Zhang, J., Zhang, X. F., Zhou, C., Wang, Z. Z., Huang, S. J., … Xia, N. S. (2010). Efficacy and safety of a recombinant hepatitis E vaccine in healthy adults: a large-scale, randomised, double-blind placebo-controlled, phase 3 trial. *The Lancet, 376*(9744), 895–902. doi:10.1016/S0140-6736(10)61030-6.

50 Arenaviruses and filoviruses

Lassa; Junin; Machupo; Guanarito; Sabia; Marburg and Ebola viruses

DAVID SAFRONETZ, HEINZ FELDMANN AND DARRYL FALZARANO

KEY POINTS

- Infection with members of the arenavirus (e.g., Lassa, Junin, Machupo and Lujo viruses) and filovirus (Marburg and Ebola [EBOV] viruses) families can cause a spectrum of clinical symptoms, with the most severe form being a viral haemorrhagic fever.
- Viral haemorrhagic fever initially presents with nonspecific symptoms such as fever, headache and muscle and joint pain; pharyngitis; and, later, nausea, vomiting and diarrhoea. There follows increasing fever, abdominal pain, oedema and enlarged lymph nodes with bleeding from gums, nose, vagina and into the gut; however, overt bleeding is typically not the cause of death.
- The reservoirs for arenaviruses are specific rodent species, while the reservoirs for filoviruses may be multiple species of fruit bats.
- Person-to-person transmission typically requires close contact and/or exposure to contaminated body fluids or tissues. This transmission route is notorious for hospital-acquired infections.
- Experimental data and recent clinical trials (for EBOV only) suggest that vaccines against members of both the arenaviruses and filoviruses are possible; however, the only approved vaccine is for Junin and is only available for use in Argentina.
- Convalescent plasma and ribavirin appear to be possible treatments for certain arenavirus infections. Cocktails of monoclonal antibodies and possibly novel small molecules may be effective against filoviruses.

ARENAVIRUSES

INTRODUCTION

Until recently, the family Arenaviridae consisted of a single genus *(Arenavirus)*, which comprised 23 unique viral species, most of which utilised rodent reservoirs in nature. However, the discovery of unique arenaviruses in snakes in 2014 resulted in a reorganisation of the Arenaviridae into two unique genera; *Mammarenavirus* for those utilising mammalian reservoir hosts and *Reptarenavirus* for snake-borne members of the family. Currently the International Committee for Taxonomy of Viruses recognises 34 unique viral species within the Arenaviridae; 31 in the *Mammarenavirus* genus and three in the *Reptarenavirus* genus. At least 10 arenaviruses are known to be associated with human disease, all of which belong within the *Mammarenavirus* genus. Much remains to be elucidated about reptarenaviruses, including the pathogenic potential to humans; therefore, the focus of this chapter will be on mammarenaviruses.

Mammarenaviruses are categorised into two complexes based largely on antigenic properties and, more recently, genetic analysis. These groups correspond in general to the geographic distribution of the viruses and rodent reservoirs and are therefore classified as either Old or New World arenaviruses (Fig. 50.1; Table 50.1). The prototype arenavirus, lymphocytic choriomeningitis virus (LCMV), was initially discovered in 1933, and although classified as an Old World virus, has a worldwide distribution due to the global movement of its rodent reservoir, the common house mouse *(Mus musculus)*. In addition to LCMV, the Old World lineage contains several African arenaviruses, the most prevalent of which is Lassa virus. The New World arenaviruses are divided into three clades (A, B and C). The most prominent lineage is clade B, which contains the highly pathogenic arenaviruses responsible for South American haemorrhagic fevers. By comparison, clades A and C are much smaller and are mainly comprised of viruses currently believed to be nonpathogenic to humans. Recently, genetic analysis of arenaviruses isolated from North America has suggested the presence of a fourth clade (A/recombinant), which is comprised of viruses with genetic characteristics of both clade A and B viruses. Recent advances in genetic sequencing techniques coupled with increased surveillance is accelerating new arenavirus discoveries as evidenced by

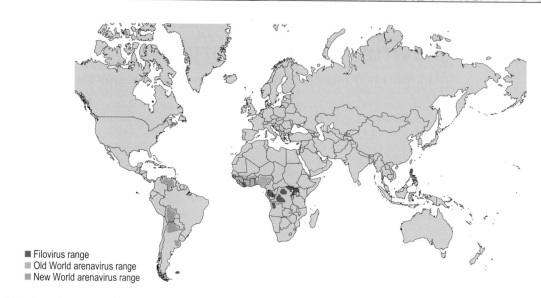

■ Filovirus range
■ Old World arenavirus range
■ New World arenavirus range

Fig. 50.1 Approximate geographical distributions of arenaviruses and filoviruses. The potential geographical ranges of the Old world and New world arenaviruses and the filoviruses are indicated based on known human cases and host reservoir sampling. LCMV has a predicted worldwide distribution and is not indicated.

the recent identification of Lujo virus, the first pathogenic arenavirus discovered in Africa in nearly 4 decades.

PROPERTIES

Members of the family Arenaviridae contain a genome of two segments of single-stranded, negative sense RNA (Fig. 50.2A). Each segment contains two nonoverlapping open reading frames of opposite polarity separated by a short hairpin configuration (ambisense coding strategy). The large (L) segment (approximately 7200 nucleotides) encodes in the genomic sense the viral polymerase and in the antigenomic sense the zinc-binding matrix protein (Z). The small (S) segment (approximately 3400 nucleotides) encodes in the genomic sense the nucleoprotein (NP), and in the antigenomic sense the glycoprotein precursor (GPC), which is post-translationally cleaved by cellular proteases into two envelope proteins, GP1 and GP2. The 5′ and 3′ terminal ends of both segments contain conserved complementary nucleotides, allowing for panhandle formation resulting in the appearance of circular genomic segments (Fig. 50.2B). The virions are pleomorphic, enveloped particles with diameters ranging from 50 to 300 nm (typically between 110 and 130 nm) on electron microscopy and enclose a helical nucleocapsid (Fig. 50.2C). Virions contain not only virus genome but also host ribosomes (both 28S and 18S ribosomal RNA), which give the virus its characteristic grainy morphology and the family name (arena is derived from the Latin word

for sand). The lipid envelope is derived from the host plasma membrane and T-shaped GP spikes extend 7–10 nm from its surface. Virions are relatively unstable, and infectivity is abolished by ultraviolet or gamma irradiation, heating to 56°C, exposure to detergents or other lipid solvents and pH outside the range 5.5–8.5.

REPLICATION

Arenaviruses can replicate in a number of mammalian hosts and in many tissues. Most Old World and clade C New World arenaviruses use α-dystroglycan as a cellular receptor, whereas the haemorrhagic New World arenaviruses (Junin, Machupo, Guanarito and Sabia) have been shown to use human transferrin receptor 1. Attachment is mediated by GP1, after which viral particles are taken up by endocytosis. Acidification of the endocytotic vesicle results in conformational changes in GP1/GP2 and allows the viral envelope to fuse with the vesicle membrane, releasing the nucleocapsid. Viral transcription and replication are restricted to the cytoplasm of infected cells and utilise a cap-snatching mechanism. The NP and viral polymerase mRNAs are transcribed from genomic RNA, whereas GP and Z mRNAs are transcribed only from antisense transcripts of the genome. The intergenic stem-loop hairpins on both L and S segments serve as transcription terminators. The RNA polymerase (molecular weight 250 kDa) catalyses the production of both RNA transcripts and new genomic RNA. The Z protein (11 kDa) is involved

Table 50.1 Members of the arenaviridae and filoviridae

	Year first isolated	Human disease	Natural host	Distribution
Old world				
Lymphocytic choriomeningitis	1933	Mild to severe meningitis	*Mus musculus, Mus domesticus*	Worldwide
Lassa	1975	Asymptomatic to severe LF	*Mastomys natalensis*	West Africa
Ippy	1970	Not known	*Arvicanthus* spp.	Central African Republic
Mopeia	1977	Not known	*Mastomys natalensis*	Eastern Africa
Mobala	1983	Not known	*Praomys jacksoni*	Central African Republic
Kodoko	2007[a]	Not known	*Mus minutoides*	Guinea
Lujo	2008	VHF	Not known	Southern Africa
Morogoro	2009	Not known	*Mastomys* spp.	Tanzania
Merino Walk	2010	Not known	*Myotomys unisulcatus*	South Africa
New world (clade)				
Junín (B)	1958	Argentinian HF	*Callomys musculinus*	Argentina
Machupo (B)	1965	Bolivian HF	*Callomys callosus*	Bolivia
Tacaribe (B)	1963	Not known	*Artibeus* bat	West Indies
Amapari (B)	1966	Not known	*Oryzomys goeldi, Neacomys guianae*	Brazil
Paraná (A)	1970	Not known	*Oryzomys buccinatus*	Paraguay
Tamiami (A/rec)[b]	1970	Not known	*Sigmodon hispidus*	USA
Cupixi (B)	1970	Not known	*Oryzomys capito*	Brazil
Pichinde (A)	1971	Not known	*Oryzomys albigularis*	Colombia
Latino (C)	1973	Not known	*Callomys callosus*	Bolivia
Flexal (A)	1977	VHF[c]	*Oryzomys* spp.	Brazil
Guanarito (B)	1989	Venezuelan HF	*Sigmodon alstoni, Zygodontomys brevicauda*	Venezuela
Sabiá (B)	1994	Brazilian HF	Not known	Brazil
Oliveros (C)	1996	Not known	*Necromys benefactus*	Argentina
Pirital (A)	1997	Not known	*Sigmodon alstoni*	Venezuela
Allpahuayo (A)	1997	Not known	*Oecomys bicolor, Oecomys paricola*	Peru
Whitewater Arroyo (A/rec)	2000	VHF, suspected[d]	*Neotoma albigula, Neotoma mexicana*	USA
Bear Canyon (A/rec)	2002	Not known	*Netotoma macrotis, Peromyscus californicus*	USA
Chapare (B)	2004	VHF	Not known	Bolivia
Catarina (A/rec)	2007	Not known	*Neotoma micropus*	USA
Pinhal (C)	2007[a]	Not known	*Calomys tener*	Brazil
Skinner Tank (A/rec)	2008	Not known	*Neotoma mexicana*	USA
Filoviruses				
Marburg (MARV)	1967	MVD	*Rousettus aegyptiacus, Hypsignathus monstrosus*	Angola, DRC, Kenya, Uganda, Zimbabwe
Ravn (RAVV)	1987	RVD	Not known	Kenya, DRC, Uganda
Ebola (EBOV)	1976	EVD	*Epomops franqueti, Hypsignathus monstrosus, Myonycteris torquata, Micropteropus pusillus, Mops condylurus, Rousettus aegyptiacus*	DRC, RC, Gabon, Guinea, Sierra Leone, Liberia
Sudan (SUDV)	1976	EVD	Not known	Sudan, Uganda
Reston (RESTV)	1989	Not known	Not known	Philippines
Taï Forrest (TAFV)	1994	EVD	Not known	Côte d'Ivoire
Bundibugyo (BDBV)	2007	EVD	Not known	Uganda, DRC
Lloviu (LLOV)	2010[a]	Not known	*Miniopterus schreibersii*	Spain

VHF, Viral haemorrhagic fever; *LF,* Lassa fever; *DRC,* Democratic Republic of the Congo; *RC,* Republic of the Congo.
[a]Identification based on nucleotide sequence only, virus has yet to be isolated.
[b]Recently identified arenaviruses in North America appear to have genetic characteristics of both lineage A and B, and therefore represent a fourth recombinant lineage (A/rec).
[c]Moderate laboratory-associated infection described.
[d]A causal relationship between Whitewater Arroyo and three fatal cases has yet to be proven.

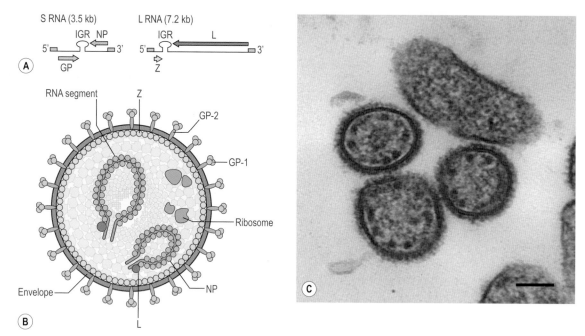

Fig. 50.2 Particle structure and genome organisation of arenaviruses. A, Schematic diagram of the arenavirus genome. B, An arenavirus particle. C, Electron micrograph of Lassa virus particles. *IGR*, Inter-genic region.

in viral transcription and as a structural protein, perhaps links the glycoproteins to the nucleocapsid. The NP (63 kDa) is the most abundant protein, with 1500–2000 copies per virion. The surface glycoproteins GP1 and GP2 are produced as a glycoprotein precursor on the rough endoplasmic reticulum. The precursor protein is glycosylated and cleaved by signal peptidase and SKI-1/S1P protease (or a closely related protease) to GP1 (43 kDa) and GP2 (35 kDa) in the Golgi apparatus and delivered to the cell surface. Together they form the T-shaped spikes, with an estimated 650 copies of each per virion. The assembled virus, together with host ribosomes, is released by budding.

CLINICAL FEATURES AND PATHOGENESIS

Lymphocytic choriomeningitis virus

LCMV is focally distributed throughout the world, though infection in humans is rare and is typically asymptomatic or mild, except in immunocompromised individuals. Most infections are acquired by contact with laboratory mice or hamsters, though fatal infections have occurred after transplantation of infected tissues from LCMV-positive donors. During pregnancy, LCMV infection can be severe and is associated with developmental defects in the foetus.

LCMV infection, although rare, may present as:

- an undifferentiated febrile illness
- aseptic meningitis
- encephalitis

The incubation period is 1–2 weeks, and the illness is of short duration. It can vary from a mild disease with headache and fever to neck stiffness, myalgia and photophobia. Long-term effects including persistent headache, paralysis and psychological changes have been described. Persistent infection and T-cell reactivity to epitopes on GP2 associated with disease manifestation have been described in mice. Whether persistent infection of human organ donors is responsible for rare transplant-acquired LCMV is not known.

Lassa fever

Lassa fever was first documented in 1969 and is now known to be endemic in West Africa, especially Nigeria, Liberia, Sierra Leone and Guinea. Lassa virus has also been described in Mali, Ivory Coast, Benin, Togo and surrounding countries, suggesting a larger range than previously thought. Throughout West Africa as many as 500,000 people are infected annually, with approximately 3000–5000 deaths. In addition, several imported cases of Lassa fever have been diagnosed in Europe and North America over the last few decades, making Lassa virus a prominent etiological agent of viral haemorrhagic fever with a high impact on public health systems worldwide. Similar to other arenaviruses, contact with infected rodent hosts *(Mastomys natalensis)*, or ingestion/inhalation of virus-laden particles is a common source of human infection; however, person-to-person transmission is also well documented and can result in outbreaks, especially in hospital settings.

The majority of Lassa virus infections are asymptomatic or mild in nature; however, approximately 20% of infections demonstrate moderate to severe disease and can be associated with haemorrhagic manifestations and multi-organ failure. The incubation period is 1–3 weeks, with a gradual onset of fever, headache and muscle and joint pain. Pharyngitis with a non-productive cough is a common feature. In severe cases there is vomiting, diarrhoea, increased levels of liver enzymes (ALT and AST) and a raised haematocrit. Abdominal and retrosternal pain, oedema of the face and neck, enlarged lymph nodes and/or haemorrhage in the conjunctiva or mucosal surfaces are particularly indicative of a poor prognosis. Recovery takes 1–3 weeks and can be associated with hearing loss.

In fatal cases the fever is maintained and rapid deterioration occurs over the first 2 weeks, associated with:

- hypovolaemia, hypotension, pleural effusion, ascites and anuria
- bleeding from the gums, nose, intestine or vagina, linked to platelet dysfunction
- acute neurological changes varying from unilateral or bilateral deafness (in one-third of patients), to signs of encephalopathy, including generalised seizures, dystonia and neuropsychiatric changes

Infection during pregnancy, especially the third trimester, is particularly severe, with maternal mortality rates of approximately 20%, and foetal mortality rates near 100%. In children, infection is associated with a swollen baby syndrome, consisting of widespread oedema, abdominal distension and bleeding. In clinically relevant infections, platelet and lymphocyte counts fall early in the illness. Endothelial cell damage leads to extravascular fluid loss, and thus oedema and, together with platelet loss and dysfunction, to the haemorrhagic manifestations. Viraemia can persist for weeks and reaches high levels in severe and fatal cases.

Until recently, Lassa virus was the only arenavirus associated with haemorrhagic fever in Africa. However, in 2008 a small outbreak of unexplained haemorrhagic fever occurred in South Africa after a severely ill patient was medically evacuated from Zambia. A novel arenavirus was isolated and named Lujo virus. In total, Lujo infected five people, four of whom contracted the virus through secondary or tertiary transmission, and resulted in four deaths.

South American haemorrhagic fever

Argentinian, Bolivian, Venezuelan and Brazilian haemorrhagic fevers are caused by Junin, Machupo, Guanarito and Sabia viruses, respectively. Of these, Argentinian haemorrhagic fever (AHF) represents the most significant public health concern, with cases occurring annually in a constantly expanding endemic region. AHF is seasonal (from April to June), and cases or epidemics occur every year, with several hundred cases being reported annually. In untreated individuals the mortality rate ranges from 15% to 30%. Approximately 80% of Junin infections demonstrate mild to moderate symptoms. Following a 1–2 week incubation period, AHF begins with a gradual onset of nondescript symptoms (e.g., fever, muscle ache, dizziness, lymph node swelling, flushing of the face, neck and upper chest). After 6–10 days, 20%–30% of patients progress to more serious, multisystem disease with neurological and haemorrhagic manifestations. Cardiovascular and renal involvements are uncommon but can occur. In severe disease, petechiae develop, and there can be bleeding from the gastrointestinal tract. Leakage of fluid through damaged vascular endothelium leads to hypotension, oliguria and hypovolaemic shock; encephalopathy occurs in many patients. Raised levels of tumour necrosis factor (TNF)-α and thrombopoietin are proportional to disease severity.

Severe AHF is associated with:

- neurological symptoms including confusion, ataxia and tremors, which can progress to convulsions and coma
- haemorrhagic manifestations, resulting from thrombocytopenia and possibly clotting factor consumption, which can include haematomas, blood in vomit, sputum and urine as well as bleeding from gums, nose, vagina and gastrointestinal tract
- secondary bacterial infections, especially pneumonia and septicemia, are common and complicate recovery

In contrast to Junin infections, Machupo and Guanarito viruses are typically associated with sporadic outbreaks with similar clinical manifestations and mortality rates as AHF. To date, Sabia virus has been associated with one confirmed naturally occurring infection (initially thought to be yellow fever), and two laboratory-acquired infections.

In 2004 a novel arenavirus, subsequently named Chapare virus, was isolated from a fatal case associated with a small outbreak of haemorrhagic fever in Bolivia. Because of the remote location, the scope of the original outbreak remains unknown as does the incidence and detailed manifestations of disease. Flexal and Tacaribe viruses have caused laboratory-acquired haemorrhagic fever, and in 2000 a variant (approximately 89% similar) of Whitewater

Arroyo virus is suspected to have caused three fatal cases of viral haemorrhagic fever in California, USA.

Despite the initial isolation of LCMV over 80 years ago, arenaviruses remain emerging viruses that are often considered among the most neglected pathogens worldwide. Over the last several years the Arenaviridae has continued to expand with discoveries of several novel viral species, a few through outbreak investigations and many more from ecological studies, as was the case with the discovery of snake-borne arenaviruses. The pathogenic potential of many of the new arenaviruses remains to be determined, and therefore they cannot be ruled out as human pathogens.

DIAGNOSIS

Diagnosis depends upon an initial clinical suspicion of infection and involves obtaining a history of potential contact associated with travel or with confirmed cases. Specific diagnosis depends on detection of the virus, its antigens and/or genome. A specific immune response may provide retrospective diagnosis or information on seroprevalence rates in given populations. With the exception of LCMV, diagnosis of arenaviral infections should involve a national or international reference laboratory to provide recommendations for specimen collection, storage and transport as well as appropriate diagnostics tests.

Genome detection

Genome detection by reverse transcriptase–polymerase chain reaction (RT-PCR) amplification either by conventional or real-time methods is commonly utilised for diagnosis of RNA viruses. RT-PCR is highly sensitive and specific and is particularly valuable for early diagnosis; however, appropriate assays must be carefully selected. For example, the genetic diversity associated with Lassa virus is detrimental to the development of a specific realtime RT-PCR assay. Rather, conventional multiplex RT-PCR assays, targeting conserved regions of Old and/or New World arenaviruses have been developed to detect, and in some cases differentiate, these viruses.

Antigen detection

Antigen detection from blood by antigen capture enzyme-linked immunosorbent assay (ELISA) or immunofluorescence assay (IFA) is useful for early diagnosis and for providing information on prognosis. Immunohistochemistry can be useful for laboratory confirmation of arenaviruses in tissue samples collected from fatal cases; however, this is rarely done because of the highly infectious nature of

these agents and the risks associated with performing postmortems.

Serology

Antibody detection by ELISA is the most useful serological test and can be adapted to detect specific immunoglobulin (Ig) M responses in acute sera as well as IgG in convalescent serum samples. Care should be taken, however, when interpreting apparently negative results in acute samples because with some arenaviruses, most particularly Lassa virus, the development of specific IgM and IgG antibody responses can be delayed.

Virus isolation

Arenaviruses that cause viral haemorrhagic fever are all considered category A, biosafety level 4 agents, and culture from confirmed cases should not be attempted except in designated high-containment facilities. Arenaviruses can be isolated from:

- blood or serum in acutely infected patients
- throat swabs, breast milk, cerebrospinal fluid, urine or a variety of tissues taken by biopsy/autopsy

Cell culture (BHK-21, Vero E6 or Vero 76 cells) is the most convenient and efficient mode of isolation. Animals (suckling mice, guinea pigs, hamsters) have also been used with limited success.

TREATMENT

For AHF (Junin virus), infusion of high-titre convalescent plasma is beneficial, especially if given within the first week of illness, and can reduce mortality rates to as low as 1%. However, approximately 10% of those receiving immunotherapy develop a reversible neurological syndrome 4–6 weeks later. Intravenous ribavirin, a broad-spectrum nucleoside analogue antiviral, is effective against Lassa virus infections and has been shown to reduce mortality rates in cases of severe disease from 55% to 5% if administered early in the infection (within 6 days). There is also anecdotal evidence of ribavirin being beneficial in the treatment of Junin, Sabia and Lujo virus infections; therefore, ribavirin therapy should be considered early after symptom onset of any suspected arenavirus infection. Recent laboratory investigations in animal models also suggest favipiravir, another broad-spectrum antiviral currently in licensing processes for treatment of influenza virus infections, may also be effective for treatment of arenaviral hemorrhagic fevers, though human trials have not been conducted to date. Short of specific treatments, supportive care, including maintaining fluid and electrolyte balance is critical for increasing survival rates.

EPIDEMIOLOGY AND TRANSMISSION

All arenavirus infections are zoonotic and the animal reservoir hosts, mammalian or reptilian, are thought to be largely unaffected following infection. For mammarenaviruses, rodent-to-rodent transmission likely occurs via both horizontal (i.e., between two animals not in a parent/offspring relationship) and vertical (i.e., mother to child) routes and results in persistent infections with excretion of the virus in excreta and secreta. Human infection usually occurs mainly by inhalation/ingestion of particles contaminated with urine or saliva from infected rodents and rarely by direct methods including bites or consumption of infected animals. Introduction of virus through open wounds also seems possible. In addition, laboratory-acquired infections have been documented for several pathogenic arenaviruses, and nosocomial transmission can be common when proper containment and infection control practices are not followed.

In general, mammarenaviruses persistently infect two of the rodent families:

1. The *Muridae* (house mice, *Mastomys* and *Praomys*) inhabit the same ecosystem as humans.
2. The *Cricetidae* (voles, deer-mice, gerbils) inhabit open grasslands, and it is only when they invade human territory, or vice versa, that human infections occur.

Tacaribe virus is the only *Mammarenavirus* isolated from outside these two rodent families, being excreted by the fruit-bat *Artibeus*.

CONTROL

As with all rodent-borne diseases, controlling reservoirs/vectors of disease is extremely difficult for arenaviruses. Therefore, medical interventions are paramount to controlling and preventing human illness; however, few approved vaccines or therapeutics currently exist. An effective Junin virus vaccine (Candid #1) is in use in Argentina. Experimental Lassa fever vaccines, including a chimeric of Mopeia and Lassa viruses (ML-29), recombinant vaccinia and vesicular-stomatitis viruses expressing structural proteins of Lassa virus have been shown to be highly effective in nonhuman primate models. Prophylaxis with oral ribavirin in contacts has also shown some benefit. In the absence of specific therapeutics and treatments, educational campaigns targeting rodent avoidance have become essential in infection control of arenaviruses. Suspected and confirmed cases must be cared for in strict isolation in designated hospitals to prevent exposure of the attendant staff to the high levels of virus present in acutely ill patients. Contact tracing is often carried out to assess the possibility of secondary transmission.

FILOVIRUSES

INTRODUCTION

Ebola and Marburg viruses belong to the family Filoviridae (filamentous or thread-like viruses) in the order Mononegavirales. The genus *Ebolavirus* contains viruses from five defined species based on serological cross-reactivity and genetic differences: Ebola virus (EBOV), Sudan virus (SUDV), Taï Forest virus (TAFV), Reston virus (RESTV) and Bundibugyo virus (BDBV) (Table 50.1). The *Marburgvirus* genus contains two virus groups: Marburg virus (MARV) and Ravn virus (RAVV). The newest recognised genus, *Cuevavirus*, contains a single virus, Lloviu virus (LLOV) that is based on sequences derived from bats in Spain; however, the actual virus has yet to be isolated. The most widely investigated isolates are EBOV strains Mayinga and Kikwit '95, and MARV strain Musoke. Infection with either Ebola or Marburg viruses can result in severe disease in humans and nonhuman primates, with case-fatality rates in human outbreaks as high as 90%.

PROPERTIES

The nonsegmented negative-sense RNA genome of filoviruses is approximately 19 kb in length, with the following gene order: 3′ leader, nucleoprotein (NP), virion protein (VP) 35, VP40, glycoprotein (GP), VP30, VP24, polymerase protein (L) and the 5′ trailer (Fig. 50.3B). Virus particles are filamentous and appear as U-shaped, 6-shaped, circular or branched (Fig. 50.3C). While they are uniformly 80 nm in diameter, they can vary in length from 800 to 14,000 nm, with peak infectivity ranging between 970 nm and 1200 nm. Virus particles possess a helical central core, known as the ribonucleoprotein complex (RNP), composed of NP, VP35, VP30, L and the viral RNA (Fig. 50.3A). RNP formation is aided by the membrane-associated protein VP24. The surface consists of a cell-derived lipid envelope containing the membrane-anchored glycoprotein ($GP_{1,2}$), which projects approximately 10 nm from the surface. The matrix protein VP40 underlies the membrane and is the driving force behind virus particle formation.

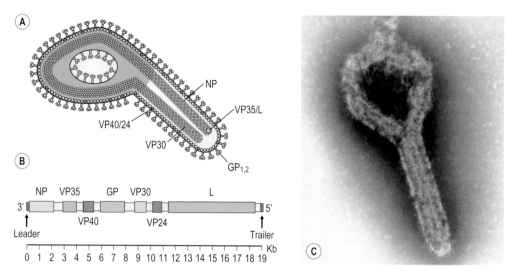

Fig. 50.3 Particle structure and genome organisation of filoviruses. A, Schematic diagram of a filovirus particle. B, A filovirus genome. C, Electron micrograph of a filovirus particle.

REPLICATION

In vitro and in vivo studies have indicated that most cell types, with the exception of lymphoid cells, can be infected by filoviruses. The spike glycoprotein, $GP_{1,2}$, is the sole protein on the surface of the virion and mediates binding and entry into target cells. GP_1 is thought to interact with attachment factors on the cell surface to initiate entry. A number of different molecules have been shown to enhance infection; however, a definitive surface receptor has not been identified. Following attachment, the current paradigm is that EBOV is taken up by macropinocytosis. For EBOV, it has been demonstrated that during endosomal maturation, decreasing pH and digestion of GP_1 by endosomal proteases leads to a structural rearrangement of $GP_{1,2}$ that allows the receptor-binding domain to become accessible for interactions with the host proteins Niemann-Pick C1 (NPC1) and two-pore calcium channel (TPC). This triggers the hydrophobic fusion peptide of GP_2 to drive fusion of the viral and endosomal membranes, allowing the release of the ribonucleoprotein (RNP) complex into the cytoplasm. While not extensively studied, it is assumed that similar mechanisms are responsible for the entry of MARV.

Following the release of the RNP into the cytoplasm, transcription is the first event to occur. Because of the similar genome organisation among all members of the Mononegavirales, transcription and replication are assumed to follow common mechanisms. The viral polymerase complex, consisting of at least L and VP35, produces polyadenylated, monocistronic mRNAs that are capped at the 5′ end for each viral gene in a 3′–5′ direction.

Similar to other members of the order, there seems to be a gradual decrease in mRNA levels from 3′ to 5′ end of the genome. Transcription requires NP, VP35, L and VP30 for EBOV but can proceed in the absence of VP30 for MARV. The genome ends are predicted to form stem-loop structures at the 3′ and 5′ ends of genomic and antigenomic RNAs that are important for replication, similar to other negative-sense RNA viruses. Replication proceeds from the *cis*-acting promoter at the 3′ end of the genomic RNA, resulting in the synthesis and encapsidation of antigenomic RNA molecules. These in turn serve as templates for the genomic RNA, which is also encapsidated. The balance between transcription and replication is thought to be regulated by the quantity of NP. The glycoprotein gene of EBOV undergoes transcriptional editing, which allows for the production of at least three different glycoprotein products: the primary, unedited product soluble glycoprotein (sGP) and its cleavage product (Δ-peptide), in addition to the full-length glycoprotein ($GP_{1,2}$) and the small secreted glycoprotein (ssGP). The full-length glycoprotein is only produced following the insertion of an additional adenosine residue into the editing site. The insertion results in a frame shift during translation that yields a protein that is distinct in sequence from sGP. This is the only example of an edited viral glycoprotein and is not known to occur for MARV.

Virus assembly and budding requires the major matrix protein VP40. When expressed alone, it is capable of forming virus-like particles (VLPs) that resemble authentic particles. During the production of viral proteins, NP induces the formation of inclusion bodies, which accumulate the other viral proteins of the RNP complex. RNPs are likely assembled in these inclusions when sufficient levels of viral proteins and negative-sense genomes are reached. Interactions between RNPs and VP40 direct the transport of RNPs to the plasma membrane via host cell proteins, where VP40 most likely initiates the assembly process. VP24 also associates with the plasma membrane and may play a role in particle formation. Once all the virus structural components are together in one location, VP40 octamers (which encompass the RNP via interactions with viral RNA) are tightly associated with $GP_{1,2}$ lipid rafts, allowing the entire complex to be enveloped and extruded from the host cell as infectious virions.

CLINICAL FEATURES AND PATHOGENESIS

Following an incubation period of 2–21 days, there is sudden onset of relatively nonspecific symptoms including:

- fever (>38.3°C)/chills
- fatigue
- anorexia
- myalgia
- headache
- nausea
- vomiting
- sore throat
- diarrhoea
- abdominal and/or chest pain.

A maculopapular rash associated with varying degrees of erythema may develop, primarily on the trunk. Disease progression may include evidence of coagulation abnormalities, which may manifest as:

- conjunctival injections/haemorrhage
- bruising
- bleeding from mucosal membranes and/or venipuncture sites
- melaena and haematuria.

Increased D-dimers, which are highly suggestive of coagulation abnormalities, were observed in nearly all patient plasma analysed during an outbreak of SUDV in Uganda in 2000; however, during an EBOV outbreak, clinical manifestations of coagulation disorders were noted in <45% of patients. In the 2013–2016 West African outbreak, clinical presentation of coagulation abnormalities was not frequently reported. Profuse bleeding is rare and when present is primarily restricted to the gastrointestinal tract. The later stages of the disease are characterised by severe nausea, obtundation, tachypnea, vomiting, prostration, increased respiratory rate, anuria and decreased body temperature indicative of the onset of shock. The specific cause of death is unclear; however, impairment of

cardiovascular regulation leading to a lack of control of blood pressure, coagulation/anticoagulation and fluid distribution coupled with the inability to mount an appropriate immune response together contribute to multiorgan failure leading to coma and death. An elevation of liver enzymes has also been noted. Individuals who survive frequently have prolonged myelitis, arthralgia, headache, lethargy, psychosis, recurrent hepatitis and ocular disorders (most commonly, uveitis) in addition to psychosocial difficulties integrating back into their community. Viral meningitis caused by EBOV, months after the initial recovery, has been reported.

The case-fatality rate and severity of symptoms appear to be viral species dependent: EBOV (40%–90%), MARV (25%–90%), SUDV (50%–60%), BDBV (25%), TAFV (0%) and RESTV (0%). In fatal cases, viraemia can reach 10^9 genome copies/mL, while survivors generally have lower levels of viraemia (<10^7 genomes/mL). Viral antigen can be found systemically but is most abundant in the spleen and liver.

The initial targets for filovirus replication are monocytes/macrophages and dendritic cells. Infection results in the activation of monocytes/macrophages with the systemic release of cytokines, chemokines and other mediators such as tissue factor. Infection of dendritic cells leads to impaired functioning, including a decreased ability to secrete proinflammatory cytokines, a lack of upregulation of costimulatory molecules, a decreased ability to stimulate T cells and a decreased ability to produce type I interferon (IFN). An effective IFN response may be the most useful mechanism to control filovirus replication, and early IFN-α production has been associated with survival. Unfortunately for the host, the IFN response is usually suppressed, resulting in the inability to control infection. For EBOV, VP35 and VP24 have been characterised as interferon antagonists, while for MARV, VP35 and VP40 appear to function as interferon antagonists.

Trafficking of the initial infected target cells to regional lymph nodes, liver and spleen, where resident macrophages and dendritic cells are subsequently infected, is thought to aid in the dissemination of the virus. Following replication in the initial target sites, the liver and adrenal cortex are important secondary sites of virus replication, with both showing evidence of extensive virus replication and necrosis. While liver impairment itself is not considered to be significant enough to be the sole cause of death, it likely contributes to overall pathogenesis by exacerbating coagulation and fluid distribution abnormalities through the decreased synthesis of coagulation factors and plasma proteins, including albumin, as a result of liver damage. Impairment of the adrenal cortex likely contributes to hypotension and sodium loss with hypovolemia.

Late in infection, extensive necrosis is observed in parenchymal cells of many organs, including the liver, spleen, kidney and gonads, with little infiltration of immune cells into infected tissues. Tissue damage correlates with the presence of viral antigens and nucleic acid. Though not directly infected, lymphocytes are depleted as a result of infection. The mechanism remains unknown, but several reports have suggested that lymphocytes undergo apoptosis; however, this has not been observed in all studies.

Poorly maintained fluid distribution and uncontrolled coagulation are hallmarks of filovirus infection. This is manifested as systemic oedema and disseminated intravascular coagulation (DIC). Additional fluid loss as a result of severe diarrhoea and vomiting was a more profound hallmark of the outbreak in West Africa than in previous outbreaks. Disruption of the endothelium seems to occur indirectly as a result of mediator-induced inflammatory responses from primary target cells (i.e., monocytes/macrophages). Coagulation and fibrinolysis are also severely disrupted during filovirus infection and can be observed as thrombocytopenia, consumption of clotting factors and increased levels of fibrin degradation products. This pro-coagulant state enhances inflammation, which subsequently induces further coagulation. Fibrin deposition results in the development of microvascular thrombi in various organs leading to ischemia and impaired organ perfusion, which contributes to multiorgan failure.

DIAGNOSIS

As filovirus outbreaks occur sporadically, typically in isolated regions of Africa, initial diagnosis is usually based on clinical symptoms. It is quite likely that single cases (or even small clusters) of filovirus infection are misdiagnosed, as the symptoms can be similar to other diseases, such as malaria, haemorrhagic measles, typhus, rickettsiosis and leptospirosis. This is especially true when cases occur outside of expected regions, and the delay in identifying cases was cited as a significant factor that led to the unprecedented outbreak in West Africa in 2013–2016. When possible, international reference laboratories should be involved in sample collection, storage and transport, especially when potential cases occur in nonendemic countries. During the 2013–2016 outbreak in West Africa, numerous mobile labs were established throughout Sierra Leone, Guinea and Liberia to provide diagnostic services.

Genome detection

Currently, the most common method to identify filovirus infections is RT-PCR on blood samples. Nucleic acid can be detected in blood as early as 3 days post-onset of symptoms. Most laboratories favour RT-PCR because of its sensitivity, specificity and rapidity. It has been successfully implemented in the mobile laboratory setting and has proven accurate and effective in both Ebola and Marburg virus disease outbreaks. More rapid tests, requiring little to no specialised equipment or training are currently being assessed. In future outbreaks, point-of-care testing may become more prominent. Because of the seriousness of a positive test for filoviruses, the diagnosis of index cases or of single imported cases should not be solely based on a single assay. Confirmation by an independent assay and/or laboratory should always be attempted.

Antigen detection

Classically, antigen detection was performed on blood samples by immunofluorescence assay (IFA). More recently, viral antigen detection is performed using ELISA-based methods. Rapid dip-stick tests are under development. Typically, this is performed to confirm results from RT-PCR.

Serology

Antibody detection can be performed by ELISA-based methods on both acute (IgM) and convalescent (IgG) serum. These assays are typically used to confirm diagnosis and for surveillance efforts.

Virus isolation

Filoviruses can be isolated from blood and tissue samples by cell culture, typically on Vero or Vero E6 cells. These viruses are considered category A agents and require biosafety level 4 for virus isolation.

TREATMENT

Currently there are no approved treatments for either Ebola or Marburg virus disease other than supportive care, which is directed towards the maintenance of effective blood volume and electrolytes. Oral rehydration therapy and in some settings intravenous fluid therapy are offered and may improve survival. In settings where advanced care is possible, treatment has included dialysis and mechanical ventilation. Survival where access to advanced care was possible has been substantially higher.

The size and duration of the 2013–2016 West African outbreak led to clinical trials to assess numerous therapeutics and vaccines. A cocktail of three monoclonal antibodies directed against the EBOV glycoproteins, called ZMapp (or ZMab), appeared to be effective at preventing death in the limited number of individuals who received this therapy. It has been shown to be highly effective in nonhuman primate studies. In nonhuman primate studies, two small molecule antivirals BCX4430 and GS5734 have recently been shown to provide promising protection postexposure.

EPIDEMIOLOGY AND TRANSMISSION

With the exception of RESTV and LLOV, all human filovirus infections have an origin linked to tropical Africa (Fig. 50.1; Table 50.2). The initial MARV outbreaks occurred in Germany and the former Yugoslavia (now Serbia) in 1967 following contact with infected monkey tissues imported from Uganda. Imported cases have also occurred in South Africa (MARV, 1975, and EBOV, 1996) where persons became infected while travelling in other African countries and subsequently infected health-care providers. In 2008 there were two imported cases of MARV, one in the United States and the other in the Netherlands, in individuals who had travelled to Uganda. While imported cases of filoviruses are uncommon (with the exception of cases crossing borders during the outbreak in West Africa), this nevertheless demonstrates that filoviruses have the potential to cause disease outside of Africa and that they need to be considered in travellers returning from regions where exposure is possible. Between 2013 and 2016 the largest outbreak of EBOV occurred in West Africa, primarily in Guinea, Sierra Leone and Liberia, resulting in 28,616 infections and 11,310 deaths (more than all other outbreaks combined). This was the first time a filovirus outbreak occurred primarily in large urban settings and completely overwhelmed the local health infrastructure.

When known, transmission has occurred as a result of direct contact with blood, secretions or tissues from infected patients or animals, such as gorillas and chimpanzees. EBOV has been found in saliva, stool, semen, breast milk, tears and blood as well as nasal and skin swabs from infected individuals. The persistence of EBOV in semen (observed up to 18 months postrecovery) has been a particular problem in the West African outbreak and has resulted in multiple cases of sexually transmitted EBOV from survivors, which have started new transmission chains following the declarations of being EBOV free. While aerosol exposure has only been conclusively demonstrated in experimentally infected animals, an airborne route has been suggested in a limited number of human cases as the mode of transmission.

The filovirus reservoir has not been definitively identified, but there is a strong association with multiple African fruit-bat species. Comparisons with other viruses that cause haemorrhagic fever, such as members of the Old World arenaviruses, suggest that chronic infection of an animal reservoir might be responsible for maintenance of filoviruses in nature. Both viral RNA and antibodies (IgG)

against EBOV and MARV have been detected in several species of fruit bats, suggesting these species may be a natural reservoir. Despite many attempts, only MARV has actually been isolated (from five bats of the species *Rousettus aegyptiacus*). Two of these species (*Hypsignathus monstrosus* and *Epomops franqueti*) were strongly associated with the start of an outbreak of EBOV in the Democratic Republic of the Congo (DRC) in 2007. While contact with monkeys, typically as food, has likely served as the source of infection in a number of outbreaks, they are not considered the reservoir. Contact with a bat was proposed in the retrospective index case in the West African outbreak.

The only filovirus species that has not appeared in tropical Africa is RESTV, which was identified in imported cynomolgus macaques in 1989 at a quarantine facility in Virginia, USA. Importation of RESTV-infected monkeys from one holding facility in the Philippines has subsequently occurred multiple times. In 2008, during an investigation regarding high swine mortality at multiple farms in the Philippines, a number of pigs that had died tested positive for RESTV; however, it is unclear if RESTV infection was the cause of death. While virulent in monkeys, to date there has been no apparent pathogenicity in humans despite at least 25 laboratory-confirmed infections.

CONTROL

In the early outbreaks, nosocomial spread was a major route of infection. In certain locations this was also a problem during the West African outbreak. The use of barrier nursing techniques, isolation of potentially infected patients, contact tracing and a rapid response from international agencies remain the primary mechanisms of control for filoviruses. The potential reservoir(s) (i.e., bats) are not well defined; regardless, population control of bats is not a feasible option. Multiple methods are available for disinfection including UV light, gamma irradiation, heat (>60°C for 30 minutes) and chemical inactivation; however, virus infectivity is quite stable at room temperature, particularly in clinical specimens.

While there are no approved vaccines against filoviruses, as a result of the West African outbreak multiple vaccines have been assessed in human clinical trials and shown to be immunogenic, with an acceptable safety profile. The filovirus glycoprotein appears to be the only antigen required in a vaccine, which has been expressed in both nonreplicating vaccines (DNA, recombinant adenoviruses and virus-like particles) and replication competent vaccines (recombinant human parainfluenza virus 3 and recombinant vesicular stomatitis virus). Recently, blended vaccines (i.e., containing antigens from more than one species)

Table 50.2 Occurrences of filovirus infections

Virus	Country	Year	No. of cases (CFR[a])	Epidemiology
MARV	Germany/Serbia (former Yugoslavia)	1967	32 (22%)	Contact with imported vervet monkeys and their tissues
	Zimbabwe/ South Africa	1975	3 (33%)	Index infected in Zimbabwe, two secondary cases in companion and nurse
	Kenya	1980	2 (50%)	Traveller to the area that was the source of vervet monkeys in 1967; secondary infection in doctor who survived
	Kenya	1987	1 (100%)	Traveller to Mount Elgon Cave (bat infested)
	DRC	1998–2000	154 (83%)	Community outbreak lasting more than 2 years
	Angola	2005	252 (90%)	Outbreak in an urban setting
	Uganda	2007	4 (25%)	Contact with workers or worked in mine (containing bats)
	Netherlands	2008	1 (100%)	Imported from Uganda (visited cave containing bats)
	USA	2008	1 (0%)	Imported from Uganda (visited same cave as above)
EBOV	DRC (former Zaire)	1976	318 (88%)	Unknown origin, nosocomial spread by needlestick
	DRC (former Zaire)	1977	1 (100%)	Sporadic case
	Gabon	1994	52 (60%)	Workers in gold-mining camps, identified retrospectively
	DRC	1995	315 (81%)	Index worked in forest, close contact, nosocomial transmission
	Gabon	1996	37 (57%)	Butchering dead chimpanzee, close contact transmission
	Gabon	1996	60 (75%)	Index case a hunter, close contact transmission
	South Africa	1996	2 (50%)	Index treated patients in Gabon, attending nurse in South Afric, nurse died
	Gabon/RC	2001–2004	302 (84%)	Multiple outbreaks, contact with dead monkeys
	RC	2005	12 (83%)	Eating a chimpanzee
	DRC	2007	264 (71%)	Unknown origin
	DRC	2008–2009	32 (47%)	Unknown origin
	Guinea Sierra Leone Liberia	2013–2016	28,616 (40%)	Presumed single introduction from bat. Other countries with cases included Mali, Senegal, Nigeria, United States, United Kingdom & Italy
	DRC	2014	66 (74%)	Occurred in multiple villages. Not linked to West African outbreak
SUDV	Sudan	1976	284 (53%)	Linked to bat-infested cotton factory, nosocomial transmission
	Sudan	1979	34 (65%)	Index linked to same cotton factory as 1976, nosocomial transmission
	Uganda	2000–2001	425 (53%)	Unknown source, nosocomial and community transmission
	Sudan	2004	17 (41%)	Index butchered monkeys, nosocomial and close contact transmission
	Uganda	2011	1 (100%)	Unknown source
	Uganda	2012	11 (4%)	
	Uganda	2012–2013	6 (50%)	
RESTV	USA	1989	Epizootic, 4 (0%)	Imported monkeys (Philippines), asymptomatic human infections
	USA	1990	Epizootic	Imported monkeys (Philippines), no human infections
	Italy	1992	Epizootic	Imported monkeys (Philippines), no human infections
	USA	1996	Epizootic	Imported monkeys (Philippines)
	Philippines	1996	Epizootic	Quarantine facility for all previous occurrences of REBOV
	Philippines	2008	Epizootic, 6 (0%)	Large outbreak in pigs, asymptomatic human infections
TAFV	Côte d'Ivoire	1994	1 (0%)	Performed autopsy on dead chimpanzee infected with CIEBOV
	Liberia	1995	1 (0%)	Serological diagnosis only
BDBV	Uganda	2007	149 (25%)	Unknown origin, community transmission
	DRC	2012	36 (36%)	

DRC, Democratic Republic of the Congo; *RC*, Republic of the Congo.
[a]All known incidents of naturally-acquired filovirus infections are listed including date and country of infections, in addition to the number of cases, the case-fatality rate and the available epidemiological data.

have been demonstrated to provide protection against multiple filovirus species. A vesicular stomatitis virus–based vaccine platform that had been demonstrated to protect nonhuman primates from either EBOV or MARV when given up to 48 hours post infection was shown to provide complete protection in a phase IIb clinical trial, within 10 days of vaccination. Unfortunately, clinical trials were not started until near the end of the outbreak, and in many cases it is unclear whether numerous treatments had any effect.

RECOMMENDED READING

Anthony, S. M., & Bradfute, S. B. (2015). Filoviruses: one of these things is (not) like the other. *Viruses, 7*(10), 5172–5190. doi:10.3390/v7102867.

Buchmeier, M. J., de la Torre, J.-C., & Peters, C. J. (2013). Arenaviridae. In D. M. Knipe & P. M. Howley (Eds.), *Field's virology* (6th ed.), 1283–1303. Philadelphia: Wolters Kluwer Health/Lippincott Williams & Wilkins.

Feldmann, H., & Geisbert, T. W. (2011). Ebola haemorrhagic fever. *Lancet, 377*(9768), 849–862. doi:10.1016/S0140-6736(10)60667-8.

Feldmann, H., Sanchez, A., & Geisbert, T. W. (2013). Filoviridae: Marburg and Ebola Viruses. In D. M. Knipe & P. M. Howley (Eds.), *Field's virology* (6th ed., p. 1), 923–956. Philadelphia: Wolters Kluwer Health/Lippincott Williams & Wilkins.

Messaoudi, I., Amarasinghe, G. K., & Basler, C. F. (2015). Filovirus pathogenesis and immune evasion: insights from Ebola and Marburg virus. *Nature Reviews. Microbiology, 13*(11), 663–676. doi:10.1038/nrmicro3524.

Mendoza, E. J., Qiu, X., & Kobinger, G. P. (2016). Progression of Ebola therapeutics during the 2014–2015 outbreak. *Trends in Molecular Medicine, 22*(2), 164–173. doi:10.1016/j.molmed.

Moraz, M. L., & Kunz, S. (2011). Pathogenesis of arenavirus hemorrhagic fevers. *Expert Review of Anti-infective Therapy, 9*(1), 49–59. doi:10.1586/eri.10.142.

Salvato, M. S., Clegg, J. C. S., Buchmeier, M. J., Charrel, R. N., Gonzalez, J. P., & Lukashevich, I. S. (2005). Family Arenaviridae. In M. H. V. Van Regenmortel, C. M. Fauquet, M. A. Mayo, J. Maniloff, U. Desselberger, & L. A. Ball (Eds.), *Virus taxonomy, eighth report of the International Committee on taxonomy of viruses* (pp. 725–733). San Diego: Elsevier.

51 Reoviruses

Gastroenteritis

NIGEL CUNLIFFE AND OSAMU NAKAGOMI

KEY POINTS

- The *Reoviridae* comprises five genera that infect humans; they are characterised by the possession of 9–12 segments of double-stranded RNA encased within a non-enveloped capsid of icosahedral symmetry.
- When viewed under the electron microscope, the characteristic wheel-shaped virus particles measure 70–75 nm in diameter.
- Rotavirus A is the major cause of acute gastroenteritis in infants and young children worldwide.
- A unique feature of rotavirus replication is the transient acquisition of an envelope during the process of budding into the endoplasmic reticulum.
- Rotaviruses produce the nonstructural protein NSP4, the first described viral enterotoxin.
- Diagnosis of rotavirus gastroenteritis is usually made by the detection of viral antigen (VP6) using enzyme-linked immunosorbent and immunochromatographic assays.
- A distinct winter seasonality of rotavirus infection is evident in temperate countries; infection is year-round in tropical countries.
- Rehydration and restoration of electrolyte balance are the primary aims of treatment of acute rotavirus gastroenteritis.
- A live, oral rotavirus vaccine has been included in the childhood immunisation schedule of numerous countries worldwide, with consequent reduction in the global rotavirus disease burden.

Viruses in the family *Reoviridae* contain 9–12 segments of linear double-stranded RNA as the genome. When viewed under negative-stain electron microscopy, the virion measures 65–85 nm in diameter and possesses icosahedral symmetry. Reoviruses are recovered from a wide range of host species including humans, mammals, birds, reptiles,

fish, crustaceans, marine protists, insects, ticks, arachnids, plants and fungi.

The family *Reoviridae* contains 15 genera of which five contain viruses that infect humans.

Orthoreovirus – reoviruses were originally recovered from both respiratory secretions and faeces but could not be associated with disease, hence the name *reo*virus (*r*espiratory *e*nteric *o*rphan).

The *Coltivirus* (e.g., Colorado tick fever virus), *Orbivirus* (e.g., Kemerovo virus, found in Russia and Eastern Europe) and *Seadoranvirus* (e.g., Banna virus, found in Southeast Asia and China) are transmitted by insects and are therefore classified as arboviruses (see Ch. 47). Infection gives rise to a febrile illness, occasionally with rash, leukopenia and meningitis/encephalitis.

Rotavirus – this genus contains eight species, Rotavirus A–H, which cause gastroenteritis in both human and animal species.

ROTAVIRUSES

Rotavirus was discovered by Bishop and colleagues in 1973, by electron microscopic examination of duodenal biopsies taken from infants with severe diarrhoea. Rotavirus A (also called group A rotavirus) was subsequently identified as the most important cause of severe childhood gastroenteritis throughout the world. Rotaviruses also infect and often cause diarrhoea in the young of a wide variety of avian and mammalian species including cattle, sheep, goat, horses, pigs, dogs, cats, mice, rabbits, monkeys and many others. Because the clinical significance of Rotavirus A far exceeds that of other species, the term rotavirus hereafter refers to Rotavirus A unless specified otherwise.

EPIDEMIOLOGY

Rotavirus infections occur worldwide, but the vast majority of deaths occur in children in developing countries, particularly in Sub-Saharan Africa and in the Indian subcontinent. Thus, rotavirus accounted for about 40% of an estimated 2 million diarrhoea deaths each year (equating to an estimated 527,000 rotavirus-associated deaths in 2004, the last year before the introduction of rotavirus vaccine). In industrialised countries, while deaths due to rotavirus are rare, the incidence of rotavirus hospitalisations ranged from 4–12 per 1000 child-years, and rotavirus accounted for 40%–50% of hospital admissions due to diarrhoeal disease in the prerotavirus vaccine era. Most symptomatic rotavirus infections are seen in children between 6 months and 2 years of age in industrialised countries, whereas in many developing countries >70% of rotavirus diarrhoea cases occur in infants younger than 1 year of age (Fig. 51.1). By the age of 5 years, virtually all children have been infected with rotavirus regardless of setting. In temperate countries, rotavirus infections display marked seasonality, with distinct peaks during the winter months and few infections identified outside this period, whereas rotavirus infections occur year-round in most tropical countries (Fig. 51.2).

Transmission of rotavirus occurs via the faecal-oral route, and its transmission within families to siblings and parents is well recognised. The shedding of enormous numbers of virions (up to 10^{11} per gram of faeces) during the acute phase, and a very small minimal infectious dose (100 infectious viral particles are sufficient for infection), contributes to the efficient human-to-human transmission of the virus.

Morphology

Viral particles (virions) have icosahedral symmetry and measure 75 nm in diameter with three concentric layers of capsid proteins but appear as characteristic sharp-edged, double-shelled particles under negative-stain electron microscopy. The virions look like spokes grouped around the hub of a wheel; hence *rota* meaning wheel in Latin. This appearance is diagnostic (Fig. 51.3). Under cryoelectron microscopy, the triple-layered particle is penetrated by 132 large channels and the virion has 60 spikes (VP4 trimers)

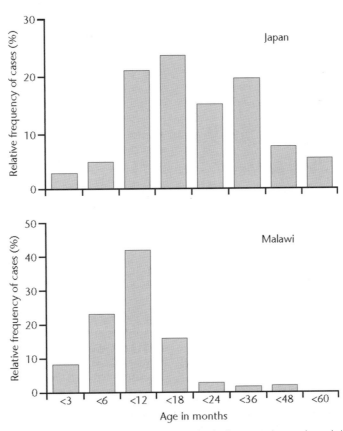

Fig. 51.1 Contrasting patterns of age distribution of rotavirus diarrhoea occurring in the prerotavirus vaccine period in Malawi (as an example of a developing country) and in Japan (developed country). (Reproduced from Cunliffe, N. A., Glass, R. I., & Nakagomi, O. (2014). Rotavirus and other viral diarrhoea. In J. Farrar, P. Hotez, T. Junghanss, G. Kang, D. Lalloo, & N. J. White (Eds.). *Manson's Tropical Diseases* (23rd ed.) (Ch. 18, pp. 207–214). Elsevier Saunders, Philadelphia.)

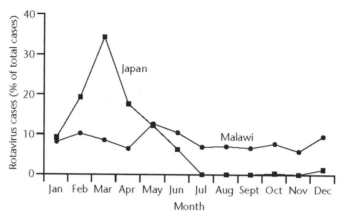

Fig. 51.2 Contrasting seasonality of rotavirus diarrhoea occurring in the prerotavirus vaccine period in Malawi (as an example of a tropical climate) and in Japan (temperate climate). (Reproduced from Hart, C. A., Cunliffe, N. A., & Nakagomi, O. (2009). Diarrhoea caused by viruses. In G. C. Cook & A. Zumla (Eds.) *Manson's Tropical Diseases* (22nd ed.) (Ch. 45, pp 815–824). Elsevier Saunders, Philadelphia.)

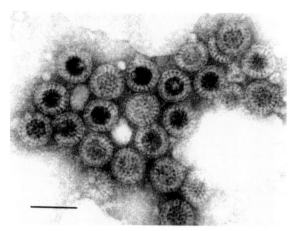

Fig. 51.3 Negatively stained electron micrograph of rotavirus particles in a faecal specimen. Potassium phosphotungstic acid stain. Bar = 100 nm.

protruding on its surface. Including the spikes, the virion measures approximately 100 nm in diameter (Fig. 51.3).

Genome and gene-coding assignments

The 11 segments of double-stranded RNA, encased in the virion, are extracted and separated by polyacrylamide gel electrophoresis to produce strain-specific electrophoretic migration patterns called electropherotypes (Fig. 51.4). As well as long and short electropherotypes (differing in the rates of relative migration of RNA segments 10 and 11), various minor differences in the migration of corresponding segments have been recognised and utilised extensively in epidemiological studies.

Each genome segment codes for one viral structural protein (VP) or nonstructural protein (NSP) except genome

segment 11, which encodes two out-of-frame nonstructural proteins: NSP5 and NSP6. The gene-coding assignments have been established (Fig. 51.4). RNA segments 1, 2 and 3 code respectively for the inner core proteins VP1 (which functions as the viral RNA polymerase), VP2 (the main scaffolding protein) and VP3 (the capping enzyme). RNA segment 6 codes for the middle layer protein, VP6, which is the single most abundant rotavirus protein and which interacts with the core protein VP2 and the outer capsid proteins VP7 and VP4. VP6 carries epitopes specifying group (rotavirus species specific antigen), whereas VP7 and VP4 independently carry neutralisation epitopes that define the virus G and P serotypes, respectively (see later in the chapter). VP4 is cleaved post-translationally into VP5* and VP8* (an asterisk is to denote posttranslational product); this proteolytic cleavage is essential for infectivity.

- Rotavirus A is responsible for the vast majority of cases of rotavirus diarrhoea in infants and young children. It also causes diarrhoeal disease in adults, including the elderly.
- Rotavirus B was initially discovered as the cause of outbreaks of acute diarrhoea among all age groups in China and is now endemic in several Asian countries including China, India, Bangladesh, Myanmar and Nepal.
- Rotavirus C causes occasional episodes of gastroenteritis in older children.
- Rotavirus H is a rare cause of diarrhoea in humans and to date has been detected only in Asia.

Six nonstructural proteins are coded for by genome segments 5 (NSP1), 7, 8 or 9 (NSP2 and NSP3, depending on the strain), and 10 or 11 (NSP4, and NSP5/NSP6, depending on the strain). NSP2 is proposed to act as a

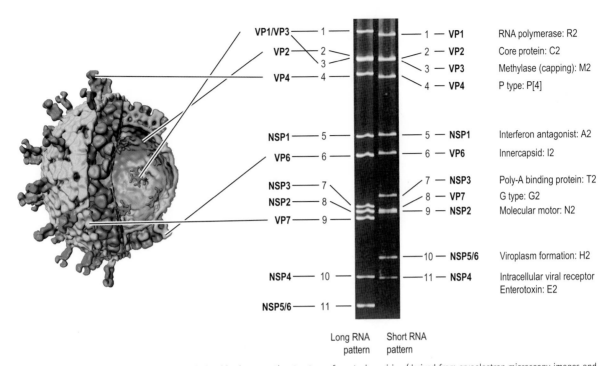

VP1/VP3 — 1 —
VP2 — 2 — 3
VP4 — 4 —

NSP1 — 5 —
VP6 — 6 —

NSP3 — 7
NSP2 — 8
VP7 — 9

NSP4 — 10 —

NSP5/6 — 11 —

1 — VP1   RNA polymerase: R2
2 — VP2   Core protein: C2
3 — VP3   Methylase (capping): M2
4 — VP4   P type: P[4]

5 — NSP1   Interferon antagonist: A2
6 — VP6   Innercapsid: I2

7 — NSP3   Poly-A binding protein: T2
8 — VP7   G type: G2
9 — NSP2   Molecular motor: N2

10 — NSP5/6   Viroplasm formation: H2
11 — NSP4   Intracellular viral receptor
               Enterotoxin: E2

Long RNA   Short RNA
pattern   pattern

Fig. 51.4 Schematic diagram showing the relationships between the structure of a rotavirus virion (derived from cryoelectron microscopy images and computer image processing) and the genomic double-stranded RNA segments separated by polyacrylamide gel electrophoresis. Two RNA patterns, long and short, are shown. The cut-away representation of the reconstructed virion shows the triple-layered icosahedral architecture and the locations of the various structural proteins. Note that coding assignment is slightly different between long and short RNA pattern strains. RNA segment 10 of the short RNA strain is the result of rearrangement of RNA segment 11 of the long RNA pattern. The outer (VP7 and VP4), middle (VP6) and inner (VP2) layers are shown in orange, blue and green, respectively. The flower-like structures inside the VP2 layer represent VP1–VP3 complexes, which function as RNA polymerase and capping enzymes. The genotype of each RNA segment of the short RNA strain (strain DS-1) is shown. The corresponding genotypes of the long RNA strain (strain Wa) are G1-P[8]-I1-R1-C1-M1-A1-N1-T1-E1-H1. The three-dimensional image structure of reconstructed rotavirus virion was generated by B. V. V. Prasad, Baylor College of Medicine, Houston, Texas, USA.

molecular motor to drive replicating mRNA into the nascent viral particles and so maintain nucleotide pools in viroplasms during replication. Both NSP2 and NSP5 are involved in viroplasm formation. NSP3 functions as polyadenylic acid (poly A)-binding protein (rotavirus mRNA is not polyadenylated) and binds to the 3′ end of viral mRNA and to cellular eIF4G, thus enhancing the translation of viral mRNA. While NSP4 is an intracellular viral receptor playing an important role in viral morphogenesis (see earlier in the chapter), it also functions as a viral enterotoxin (see later in the chapter).

Antigenic and genetic diversity

Rotavirus A is genetically diverse in each of the 11 genome segments (called genotypes), and a nucleotide sequence-based, complete genome classification system is used; the genome of individual rotavirus strains is given the complete descriptor of Gx-P[x]-Ix-Rx-Cx-Mx-Ax-Nx-Tx-Ex-Hx where x denotes the genotype number (Fig. 51.4). Of these 11 genotypes, the G and P genotypes have been extensively investigated because of their presumed importance in protective immunity. Reverse transcriptase–polymerase chain reaction (RT-PCR) with gene- and type-specific primers has been widely applied as a reliable typing procedure. There are thus far 35 G genotypes and 50 P genotypes reported among human and animal rotaviruses. Among rotavirus A strains, five genotype combinations comprise more than 85% of rotaviruses detected in humans, including G1P[8], G2P[4], G3P[8], G4P[8] and G9P[8] (Fig. 51.5). However, genotype G12 emerged globally over the last decade, and G8 has been commonly reported in many African countries.

At the molecular level, several factors have been identified that can explain the genomic and antigenic variability of cocirculating rotavirus strains.

- Like other viruses that depend on virion-associated, RNA-dependent RNA polymerases for their replication, rotavirus genomes undergo frequent point mutations that accumulate over time and give rise to multiple lineages and sub-lineages (when this

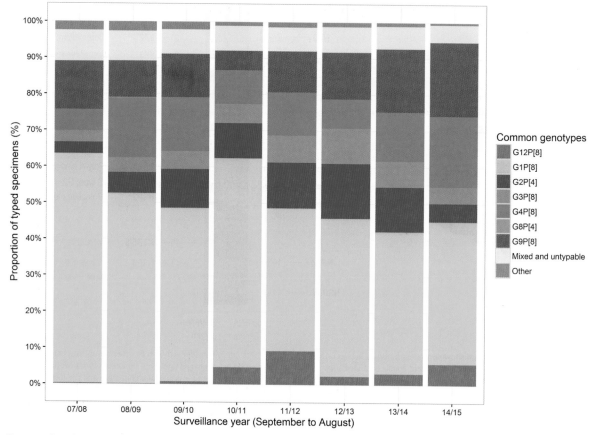

Fig. 51.5 Rotavirus genotype distribution for typed specimens from 11 European Union countries without routine rotavirus vaccination by surveillance year, September 2007 to August 2015. Includes data for Bulgaria, Denmark, France, Greece, Hungary, Lithuania, The Netherlands, Italy, Slovenia, Spain and Sweden. (Courtesy M. Iturriza-Gomara, EuroRotaNet.)

occurs in the neutralisation proteins, antigenic drift will result).

- Rotaviruses, like other segmented RNA viruses, undergo extensive reassortment in doubly infected cells. This has been shown to occur both in vitro and in vivo. If RNA segments coding for serotype-specific proteins are involved, major antigenic changes can result (antigenic shift).
- Genome segments of animal rotaviruses may be transferred to human rotaviruses either as a whole genome or in part (by reassortment), resulting in occasional detection of human Rotavirus A isolates that have genome segments highly similar to those of animal rotaviruses (e.g., cat, cow, pig), either as a whole or in part (interspecies transmission).
- Rotaviruses that establish chronic infections in immunocompromised hosts may undergo various forms of genome rearrangement, resulting in highly atypical RNA profiles.

REPLICATION

Rotavirus replicates exclusively in the cytoplasm of infected cells. Attachment is via VP4 to receptors on the cell surface: sialic acid and $\alpha 2\beta 1$ integrin for initial binding, and $\alpha 2\beta 1$ and other integrins, heat-shock protein 70 and histo-blood group antigens as postbinding receptors. The multistep attachment and entry process for rotaviruses is complex and involves a remarkable conformational change in the structure of VP4 induced by proteolytic cleavage, exposing additional attachment sites. When crossing the cell membrane, the outer capsid is removed (loss of the VP4 and VP7 proteins), but the viral particle is never completely uncoated, leaving the viral genomic RNA in the core of the double-layered particle. Soon after entry, the loss of the outer capsid activates the virion-associated, RNA-dependent RNA polymerase, which transcribes the minus-strand of each genomic RNA segment to produce messenger RNA (mRNA) molecules. The mRNA molecules are capped at the 5′ end (m7GpppG) by the action of VP3 (guanylyltransferase) but not polyadenylated and extrude to the cytoplasm through channels on the double-layered particle. The mRNA molecules are then translated to generate the viral proteins after the 5′ cap structure is recognised by the cap binding protein, eIF4E, which is complexed with the scaffolding protein, eIF4G, which also interacts with NSP3 that plays a role of poly-A binding protein (by recognising the consensus sequence and tightly binding at the 3′ untranslated region of the mRNA). As the binding affinity of eIF4G to NSP3 is stronger than that of eIF4G to the host poly-A binding protein, NSP3 evicts the host poly-A binding protein from its binding site in eIF4G, thereby the viral mRNA molecules being preferentially translated.

Following translation of viral proteins, the mRNA molecules act as templates for the minus-strand synthesis to yield double-stranded RNA (replication). Replication of the genome occurs within the nascent subviral particles in the viroplasms, which are localised adjacent to the nucleus and the endoplasmic reticulum (ER). The viroplasm is an electron-dense structure in the cytoplasm for which NSP2 and NSP5 provide a scaffold. Nascent double-layered particles, after binding to an intracellular viral receptor (NSP4), bud from viroplasms into the ER in a unique process during which double-layered particles transiently acquire an envelope (ER membrane). At the same time, the outer capsid proteins, VP7 and VP4, are incorporated into newly synthesised particles, which become mature, triple-layered particles by losing their envelope. These are then released from the apical surface of enterocytes after vesicular transport from the ER by a pathway bypassing the Golgi apparatus.

PATHOGENESIS AND IMMUNITY

Rotaviruses replicate exclusively in the differentiated epithelial cells at the tips of the small intestinal villi; the crypts, which contain undifferentiated enterocyte stem cells, are spared. Progeny virus is produced after 10–12 hours, and released in large numbers into the intestinal lumen ready to infect other cells. Biopsies show atrophy of the villi and mononuclear cell infiltrates in the lamina propria. The pathogenesis of rotavirus diarrhoea includes both malabsorption and increased secretion. Malabsorption of nutrients, electrolytes and water may be the consequence of the damage to mature absorptive enterocytes. Malabsorption may also be caused by virus-induced down-regulation of the expression of absorptive enzymes and functional changes in tight junctions between enterocytes leading to paracellular leakage. Secretory mechanisms include those mediated by activation of the enteric nervous system and the effect of NSP4, the latter being via activation of cellular

Cl⁻ channels (different from the cystic fibrosis transmembrane regulator), leading to increased Cl⁻ and, consequently, water secretion.

Rotavirus infection was previously thought to be limited to the intestine, but rotavirus causes viraemia for at least a short period in the acute phase of infection in immunocompetent infants as well as in experimentally infected animals. The clinical significance of this systemic spread of rotavirus is unclear, however.

Studies of the natural history of rotavirus infection show that immunity acquired following primary infection results predominantly in protection against the development of subsequent severe disease, but that protection against asymptomatic infection or mild disease is much less. Such postinfection immunity is believed to be mediated by both humoral and cell-mediated immune responses. Rotavirus-specific immunoglobulin (Ig) A antibodies on the enteric mucosal surface are thought to be the primary mediator of protective immunity.

As the role of the innate immune system in rotavirus infection is studied, the countermeasures taken by rotavirus against antiviral mechanisms have captured much attention. NSP1 functions as a viral ubiquitin ligase, interacting with and promoting the degradation of IFN regulatory factor (IRF) 3 and IRF7 through a ubiquitination-proteasome mechanism. NSP1 also inhibits activation of nuclear factor-κB. Thus, rotavirus counteracts the production of INFβ by host cells. In addition to its role as poly-A binding protein (see earlier in the chapter), NSP3 is proposed to cause nuclear retention of poly-A containing mRNA molecules of the host cell, severely inhibiting translation from host cell mRNA and weakening the host antiviral and stress responses.

CLINICAL FEATURES

Infection with rotavirus can result in a wide spectrum of clinical outcomes, ranging from asymptomatic infection to severe, life-threatening gastroenteritis. The onset of symptoms is abrupt after a short incubation period of 1–2 days. Fever, vomiting and watery diarrhoea are seen in the majority of infected children, lasting for 2–6 days. If body fluids are not replaced, dehydration ensues that may range in severity from mild to severe. There is little evidence that illness severity is related to virus serotype. Rotavirus infection can cause gastroenteritis in older children and adults, although severe disease is less common. Outbreaks of gastroenteritis due to rotavirus infection have been observed in the elderly, in whom severe dehydration can result. In the immunodeficient host, a persistent infection may occur, with severe chronic diarrhoea associated with rotavirus excretion that can last for many months.

LABORATORY INVESTIGATION

At the peak of infection, as many as 10^{11} virus particles per gram of faeces are present and can be detected by a variety of methods. Electron microscopy will detect the characteristic virus particles (Fig. 51.3). In the majority of cases there are sufficient numbers of virions in faeces to allow identification of RNA profiles (Fig. 51.4). However, most laboratories employ antigen detection tests, targeted on the middle-layer protein VP6, which include enzyme-linked immunosorbent assays and immunochromatographic assays. The diagnosis of rotavirus infection can also be made by genome detection (RT-PCR), which is being increasingly used in diagnostic laboratories in industrialised countries. However, the increased sensitivity of molecular assays means that asymptomatic shedding of rotavirus is detected in addition to symptomatic disease.

TREATMENT

The mainstay of therapy consists of oral rehydration with fluids of specified electrolyte and glucose composition. Intravenous rehydration therapy is reserved for patients with severe dehydration, shock or reduced level of consciousness. Zinc supplementation reduces the duration and severity of diarrhoeal episodes in children in low-income countries. Although specific anti-rotaviral treatment is not indicated routinely, probiotic therapy (e.g., with *Lactobacillus* GG) has been shown in clinical trials to shorten the duration of symptoms of gastroenteritis. In selected clinical situations, antirotaviral immunoglobulin therapy has been used as prophylaxis against and as treatment of rotavirus gastroenteritis.

CONTROL

Attention to hygienic measures such as handwashing, safe disposal of faeces and disinfection of contaminated surfaces is essential in reducing the risk of onward transmission of rotavirus. However, universal vaccination of infants is the most important preventive strategy. The rotavirus vaccines that are licensed for use are live-attenuated, orally administered rotavirus strains. Attenuation of virulence has been achieved either by repeated passage in cell culture or by substitution, through genetic reassortment, of serotype-determining gene segment(s) of a human rotavirus into the backbone of an animal rotavirus (which is both naturally attenuated for humans and attenuated through repeated cell culture passage).

The first licensed rotavirus vaccine, a rhesus monkey rotavirus-based tetravalent human reassortant vaccine (RotaShield), was withdrawn after this live oral vaccine was associated with the development of intestinal intussusception in approximately 1 in 10,000 vaccine recipients in the United States. Two further live-attenuated oral rotavirus vaccines were developed and extensively evaluated and have now entered childhood immunisation programmes following recommendation by the World Health Organisation. These are the monovalent G1P[8] human rotavirus vaccine Rotarix, and the pentavalent human-bovine reassortant rotavirus vaccine RotaTeq, which includes the most common human serotypes G1, G2, G3, G4 and P[8] on a bovine rotavirus background. Both vaccines have demonstrated efficacy against severe rotavirus disease caused by globally common rotavirus strains. A naturally occurring monovalent human-bovine G9P[11] rotavirus vaccine, 116E, has shown efficacy in a clinical trial in India. The number of hospitalisations due to rotavirus infection has dramatically fallen in the United States and in those European countries that have introduced rotavirus vaccine into their national schedules. The greatest potential for impact on child morbidity and mortality lies in the developing countries in Africa and Asia where, although vaccine efficacy was lower than that observed in industrialised settings, universal rotavirus vaccination would result in a large decrease in the number of severe rotavirus episodes because of the high incidence of disease. Rollout of rotavirus vaccine across Africa has been rapid, with early evidence of substantial vaccine impact on rotavirus hospitalisations. While reduction of diarrhoea deaths in Latin America has been attributed to rotavirus vaccination, the full impact of vaccination in reducing infant mortality due to diarrhoea in Africa and Asia is awaited.

RECOMMENDED READING

Staat, M. A., McNeal, M. M., & Bernstein, D. (2014). Rotavirus. In J. D. Cherry, G. J. Harrison, S. L. Kaplan, W. J. Steinbach, & P. J. Hotez (Eds.), *Feigin and Cherry's Textbook of Pediatric Infectious Diseases* (7th ed., pp. 2176–2195). Philadelphia: Elsevier.

Estes, M. K., & Greenberg, H. B. (2013). Rotaviruses. In D. M. Knipe & P. M. Howley (Eds.), *Field's Virology* (6th ed., pp. 1347–1401). Philadelphia: Wolters Kluwer Health/Lippincott Williams & Wilkins.

52 Retroviruses

Acquired immune deficiency syndrome; HTLV-1

YUSRI TAHA

KEY POINTS

- Some retroviruses, including HTLV-I, cause tumours in animal hosts.
- HIV-1 is the cause of the acquired immune deficiency syndrome (AIDS), a persistent infection leading to loss of CD4+ T cells, immunodeficiency and many opportunistic infections and cancers.
- HIV has a global distribution; it is spread by sexual intercourse, mother-to-child transmission and via blood and blood products.
- Disease status can be monitored by sequential changes in CD4+ count and plasma HIV RNA copy number (viral load).
- HIV replication can be inhibited by drugs that block coreceptor binding, membrane fusion, reverse transcription, integration and protein cleavage during maturation.
- Combination antiretroviral therapy (ART) is recommended for all people living with HIV, regardless of their clinical or immunological status.
- ART, combined with control of opportunistic infections, substantially improves survival. It also reduces the risk of transmitting the virus to others.

The family Retroviridae contains many viruses from widely different host species including birds, mice, cattle, pigs and several primates. They have been studied for many years, initially because a wide variety of tumours including leukaemias and lymphomas, sarcomas and breast and brain tumours are caused by oncogenic members of this family. Other retroviruses are associated with a plethora of neurological, autoimmune and blood disorders. The first human retrovirus was isolated from T cells of patients with T-cell leukaemia (human T-cell lymphotropic virus type I or HTLV-I) in 1980. The acquired immunodeficiency syndrome (AIDS) is caused by a different retrovirus, also with a predilection for T cells that is referred to as human immunodeficiency virus type 1 or HIV-1. Infection with

this virus has become pandemic and remains a major cause of morbidity and mortality, particularly among young adults. HIV-2 infection is restricted largely to West Africa and is less pathogenic.

DESCRIPTION

All retroviruses have an outer envelope of lipid and viral proteins; the envelope encloses the core, consisting of other viral proteins, within which lie two molecules of viral RNA (positive single stranded) and the enzymes reverse transcriptase, integrase and protease. The virions have a diameter of about 100 nm (Fig. 52.1) and, in thin sections, characteristic differences can be seen in the appearance and position of the core (e.g., C-type and D-type particles), a feature that was previously used to classify retroviruses. The typical genome size is approximately 10 kb.

CLASSIFICATION

Nucleotide sequencing of a large number of human and animal retroviruses has revealed that viruses cluster in two subfamilies, the Spumavirinae and Orthoretrovirinae, with the latter comprising six distinct genera, the *Alpha-*, *Beta-*, *Delta-*, *Epsilon-* and *Gammaretrovirus* and the *Lentivirus* genus (Fig. 52.2).

The spumaviruses have been detected in various species, including cats, cattle and primates but are not associated with disease. The name is derived from the foamy (vacuolated) appearance of infected cells in culture. There is no evidence for pathogenic human infection with spumaviruses.

The human retroviruses HTLV-I and HTLV-II belong to the genus *Deltaretrovirus* (formerly termed *Oncovirus*). They are related to the simian viruses STLV-I and -II, which are widely distributed in Old World and New World monkeys. STLV-I shows approximately 90% similarity to HTLV-I at the sequence level. The recent identification

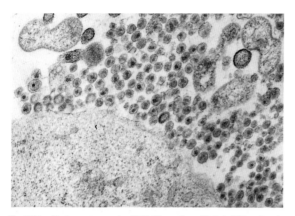

Fig. 52.1 Electron micrograph of HIV. Thin section of infected T lymphocyte. There are numerous virions lying outside the cell membrane.

of two new HTLV types (HTLV-III and HTLV-IV) in a few bush meat hunters in central Africa is believed to represent isolated incidents of primate-to-human virus transmission rather than an established human infection.

The other two human retroviruses HIV-1 and HIV-2 are lentiviruses, closely related to lentiviruses that infect Old World primates. HIV-2 is almost identical to simian immunodeficiency virus (SIV$_{sm}$) found in sooty mangabeys. It is believed that human infection originated through cross-species transmission. Similarly, HIV-1 corresponds closely to SIV$_{cpz}$ variants that infect chimpanzees in Central Africa, the probable source of the human virus. The Visna-Maedi virus of sheep was the first lentivirus to be recognised. Lentiviruses are distinguished from deltaretroviruses by their molecular structure and lack of oncogenic

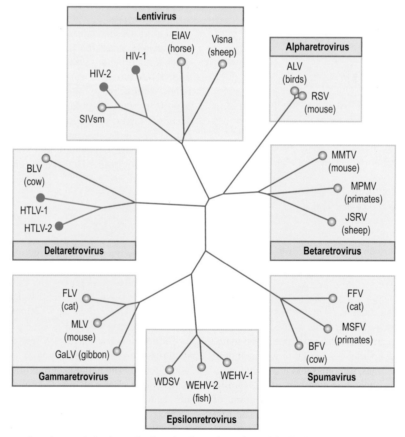

Fig. 52.2 Tree of sequences from the retroviral *pol* gene showing relatedness of retroviruses infecting humans and a range of animal species. Sequences form seven main genera, in which human retroviruses (HTLV and HIV; shown in *blue*) are found in two. For animal retroviruses *(red)*, the host species and names of familiar viruses are indicated. (*ALV*, avian leukosis virus; *BFV*, Bovine foamy virus; *BLV*, bovine leukaemia virus; *EIAV*, equine infectious anaemia virus; *FFV*, feline foamy virus; *FLV*, feline leukaemia virus; *GaLV*, Gibbon ape leukaemia virus; *JSRV*, Jaagsiekte sheep retrovirus; *MLV*, murine leukaemia virus; *MMTV*, mouse mammary tumour virus; *MPMV*, Mason-Pfizer monkey virus; *MSFV*, macaque simian foamy virus; *RSV*, Rous sarcoma virus; *SIV*, simian immunodeficiency virus; *WDSV*, walleye dermal sarcoma virus; *WEHV*, walleye epidermal hyperplasia virus)

capability; however, both genera are capable of establishing prolonged asymptomatic infection.

Both HIV-1 and HIV-2 show considerable sequence variability, allowing their classification into a number of subtypes with marked differences in geographical distribution and association with risk groups. HIV-1 variants are classified into three genotypes or groups: major (M), outlier (O) and non-M, non-O (N). Group M viruses, which dominate the pandemic, are further classified into subtypes A, B, C, D, F, G, H, J and K and several circulating recombinant forms (CRF) that comprise more than one subtype. Former subtypes E and I are now reclassified as CRF01-AE and CRF04-cpx, respectively. Subtype B is most frequently found in Western countries, whereas other subtypes such as C (Africa, parts of Asia), CRF01-AE (Thailand) and F (South America) are the main subtypes responsible for the recent epidemic spread. HIV-1 diversity is greatest in Sub-Saharan African countries such as the Congo, where there is wide cocirculation of most of the current subtypes.

Human endogenous retroviruses, often replication defective, are present in the human germ line and have not been shown to cause disease.

Genome and gene coding assignment

The genome organisation is similar for all retroviruses as their genomes contain in the same order the genes *gag*, *pol* and *env* coding for three groups of structural and enzymatic proteins (Fig. 52.3A). The long terminal repeat (LTR) sequences at both ends of the genome contain promoter and enhancer sequences. However, there are important differences between the viruses in the accessory genes involved in the regulation of replication, which are found only in complex retroviruses (Δ-, ε-, lenti- and spumaviruses). Simple retroviruses (α-, β- and γ-retroviruses) encode only for *gag*, *pol* and *env* genes products. Studies of HTLV genes and gene products provided the basis for understanding of the functional homologues subsequently found in HIV. The HIV transactivating gene, *tat*, which stimulates the synthesis of all viral proteins and *rev*, the gene that mediates the transport of unspliced viral mRNA from the nucleus to the cytoplasm are homologues of the HTLV genes *tax* and *rex*, respectively. HIV-1 has an additional four regulatory genes: *Vif*, *Nef*, *Vpr* and *Vpu*.

The p55 precursor protein coded for by the *gag* gene of HIV is cleaved by viral protease into at least five proteins; including p7, p17 and p24, all of which are found in the virion (see Fig. 52.3B). The *pol* gene products are the protease, reverse transcriptase and integrase enzymes; all required during replication. The *env* gene codes for a large protein that is glycosylated and cleaved by a host protease to gp41, the transmembrane protein, and gp120, present on the envelope as a trimer with many glycosylation sites.

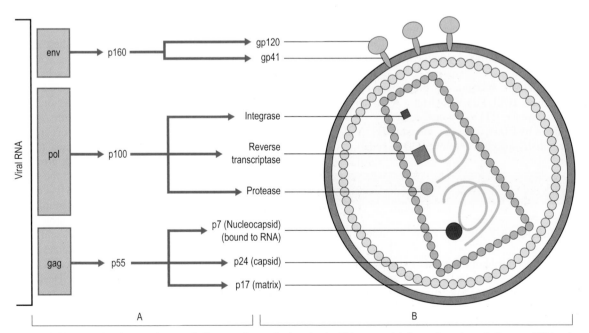

Fig. 52.3 HIV structural and enzymatic genes. A, The genomic organisation of major HIV genes and their protein products. B, Diagram of HIV to show location of structural proteins.

REPLICATION

Retroviruses replicate and produce viral RNA from a DNA copy of the virion RNA (hence their name).

Initial binding of HIV to target cells is by the interaction of the external envelope glycoprotein gp120 with part of the CD4 molecule of T lymphocytes and other cells; the HIV envelope then interacts with a second (co-) receptor. These include the chemokine receptors, CCR5 and CXCR4, expressed on a wide range of lymphoid and nonlymphoid cells. Viruses that use the coreceptor CCR5 are called R5 HIV, those using CXCR4 are called X4 HIV and viruses that can use both chemokine receptors are termed R5X4 HIV (dual tropic). With rare exceptions, only R5 and R5X4 viruses are transmitted between individuals. After this second binding step, entry of the virus occurs by fusion of the viral envelope with the cellular membrane, which requires exposure of a hydrophobic domain in gp41. Once the RNA is released into the cytoplasm, the reverse transcriptase acts to form the double-stranded DNA copy, which is transported to the nucleus and is spliced into the host cell DNA (in which state it is referred to as the integrated provirus). Once inserted into the host DNA, infection with HIV is permanent. The virus may stay latent or enter a productive cycle. Transcription of mRNA from the provirus is by the host RNA polymerase II to produce viral mRNA and genomic RNA. Proteins are synthesised and processed to form the virion components (Fig. 52.3B). Virions are assembled at the cell membrane where envelope and core proteins have located. The internal structure of the virion matures as it buds from the cell; the entire replicative cycle is completed in approximately 24 hours. In the productive growth cycle the host cell is frequently destroyed.

The HTLV-1 receptor is the ubiquitous glucose transporter-1 (GLUT-1), found on a wide range of cell types. However, HTLV-1 propagation in vivo is mainly supported by CD4+ cells, in contrast to HTLV-II, which preferentially infects CD8+ over CD4+ cells.

HIV INFECTION

EPIDEMIOLOGY OF HIV

The extent of spread of infection can be measured by the numbers of cases identified clinically and by serological testing. Much more evidence can be obtained from seroprevalence surveys, for example, of patients attending hospitals, antenatal clinics, sexually transmitted disease clinics and blood donors. Specific groups such as people who inject drugs (PWID) can be targeted; noninvasive

sampling (e.g., collecting saliva or dried blood spots) may make these studies more feasible. Repeat testing over time will give an indication of the trend of infection in that population. Similarly, recent infection testing algorithm (RITA) tests are used in public health surveillance to identify the incidence of recently acquired HIV infection. This can then be used to direct public health interventions and evaluate their effects.

AIDS was first recognised in 1981, with the causative agent, HIV, isolated in 1983; however, the first identified case dates back to 1959. During the 1970s the virus began to spread widely in some populations and groups by the routes described below.

The scale of the HIV-1 epidemic is monitored by coordinated surveillance by the Joint United Nations Programme on HIV/AIDS (UNAIDS). For 2015 estimates, there were 36.7 million individuals living with HIV worldwide, 2.1 million newly infected individuals and 1.1 million AIDS-associated deaths, of whom 110,000 were children under 15 years of age. Although the global number of annual new infections has declined by 19% in comparison to 2000, the total number of individuals living with HIV has actually increased by 27% since 2000. This is contributed to by the significant reductions in annual AIDS-associated deaths brought about by the increased availability of antiretroviral drugs and care afforded to infected patients in developing countries. Ominously, over 5700 new HIV infections occur every day, over a third of whom are young people between 15 and 24 years old. The social and economic consequences of this epidemic have been devastating, with the loss of parents and wage earners.

Frequencies of HIV infection remain highest in Sub-Saharan Africa where 70% of people living with HIV (PLWH) reside and most AIDS-related deaths occur. Exceptional effort is clearly required, at all levels, to curtail the ruinous effects of the epidemic in this region.

In Western and Central Europe and North America, approximately 50% of new HIV infections occur in gay men and other men who have sex with men (MSM). Parenteral drug users are another major risk group particularly in Eastern Europe/Central Asia and the Middle East, where they contributed 28% and 51% of new infections in 2015, respectively. The numbers of infections in risk groups can change as health education programmes are introduced; however, their success varies and advice may be ignored if the perception of risk changes.

Despite the unprecedented expansion of access to ART that has occurred since the United Nations' Declaration of Commitment on HIV/AIDS in 2001, up to two-thirds of PLWH still have no access to the drugs. The UN General Assembly issued a second declaration on HIV/AIDS in 2011, reaffirming the 2001 commitment. More recently, a new ambitious strategy (the UNAIDS 2016–2021) was adopted with an aim to end the AIDS epidemic as a public health threat by 2030.

TRANSMISSION

Virus is present in the blood, semen and cervical and vaginal secretions, and these sources are important in transmission. Virus may also be present in cerebrospinal fluid, saliva, tears and urine but at lower titres than in blood, and there is no epidemiological evidence that these are significant sources for transmission. Free virus is present at high titre during the early stage of infection and increases in titre in the blood in the later stages of the disease; there is evidence of a greater risk of transmission from such patients. With low virus titres, attained naturally or through the use of antiretroviral drugs, the risk is significantly reduced.

To transmit, virus has to reach susceptible cells at the point of entry (e.g., Langerhans cells in mucous membranes) or after entering the circulation.

The three important routes of transmission of HIV are:

1. by unprotected, penetrative sexual intercourse
2. from mother to child
3. by blood and blood products

Sexual intercourse

Heterosexual transfer of virus is the route by which the great majority of infections are spread, accounting for 90% of the global total, mostly in the developing world. Overall, the estimated risk of transmission from one unprotected exposure is 0.1%–0.2% for vaginal intercourse. The probability of transfer is increased if either partner has ulcerative genital or other sexually transmitted disease. Any trauma during intercourse will also facilitate transfer, by allowing direct access of the virus to susceptible cells and the circulation. Transmission may be more likely from male to female.

AIDS was first recognised in men who have sex with men in the United States. Most early studies established that unprotected anal intercourse was a particular risk, especially to the passive, receptive partner. The estimated risk from a single exposure is 0.1%–0.3%.

Male circumcision has been shown to confer a protective effect against HIV in men, possibly through reduction in surface area of disrupted foreskin epithelium teeming with cells permissive for HIV infection, including CD4+ T lymphocytes.

Transmission during oral sexual contact has been documented but is not a major route.

Previously, it has been shown that sharing HLA Class B alleles is independently associated with accelerated intercouple transmissibility of HIV.

Mother to child

Most transmission occurs late in pregnancy or during birth (perinatal). The most likely source is cells and virus in the cervix and vagina, as the baby passes through the birth canal. Maternal plasma viral load is the strongest predictor of the risk of virus transmission from mother to infant; the transmission rate is estimated to be 2% or less in mothers with a viral load of <1000 copies/mL. Clinical factors known to influence the risk of transmission include coinfection with other sexually transmitted diseases and prolonged and difficult labour. Breast milk is another source that is responsible for as many as 40% of new HIV infections in infants occurring in the postnatal period.

Blood and blood products

All blood for transfusion and the preparation of products such as factor VIII for haemophiliacs is screened for HIV by sensitive assays. This eliminates almost all the risk, but it is important to ask donors about possible exposure to risk. Preparation of blood products from large pools of donations was a major factor in contaminating the product as just one infected donation could introduce virus to all the material. Transplanted organs have been implicated in transmission in a few cases.

Intravenous drug use is a major risk factor for acquisition of HIV infection. The risk rises with the volume of blood injected and the frequency of sharing contaminated equipment. The withdrawal of blood before injection increases contamination. By sharing syringes, the virus can spread very rapidly so that most PWID in an area become infected in a few months. Those infected in this way can spread the virus to their sexual partners or children. Drug and sexual routes merge when PWID support their habit by prostitution.

Occupational exposure of health-care workers to infected patients has resulted in transmission in a small number of cases. The route is via accidental penetrating injuries with needles and sharps contaminated with blood. The risk from a needlestick is 1 in 200–300; contamination of eyes and mucous membranes has a lower risk of transmission. Transmission from health-care workers to patients has been suspected in only a few cases.

HIV-2 is transmitted by the same routes as HIV-1. There is no evidence that HIV can spread by casual contact or inhalation.

CLINICAL FEATURES

The different stages of HIV infection are generally reflected in CDC classification (Table 52.1) and WHO clinical staging systems that utilise immunological and/or clinical evidence to classify established HIV infections. Patients are assigned a stage according to the lowest CD4+ T-cell count or worst clinical stage they have ever reached.

Symptomatic primary HIV infection (PHI), often referred to as acute seroconversion illness or acute HIV infection, occurs within 10–30 days of initial exposure to the virus and resolves in the majority of infected individuals within a month. Features described include fever, pharyngitis, headache, malaise, generalised lymphadenopathy and nonpruritic maculopapular rash.

Following resolution of primary infection symptoms, a prolonged, largely asymptomatic phase ensues (Fig. 52.4).

Table 52.1 Staging of laboratory-confirmed human immunodeficiency virus infection (Centers for Disease Control, CDC)

CD4+ cell count categories	Clinical categories		
	(A) Asymptomatic, acute HIV, or PGL*	(B) Symptomatic conditions, not A or C	(C) AIDS-defining conditions
(1) ≥500 cells/μL	A1	B1	C1
(2) 200–499 cells/μL	A2	B2	C2
(3) <200 cell/μL	A3	B3	C3

*PGL, Persistent generalised lymphadenopathy.

This may last as long as 10 years, during which the virus continues to replicate resulting ultimately in significant damage to the immune system in untreated individuals. Persistent generalised lymphadenopathy (PGL) is present in 30%–70% of patients who are otherwise asymptomatic. The rate of progression of patients to AIDS is no greater in these patients than in those without adenopathy.

The inexorable decline in immune function eventually predisposes the patient to the development of the acquired immunodeficiency syndrome (AIDS). This may present in many ways, all due to loss of the ability to respond appropriately to infectious agents and to control tumours. There are over 20 AIDS-defining conditions reflecting the specific agents involved; a diagnosis of AIDS is made if one (or more) of the conditions listed in Box 52.1 is present.

The occurrence of an AIDS-defining illness may be preceded by nonspecific features such as fever, adenopathy and weight loss, and minor opportunistic infections such as reactivation of latent herpes viruses (e.g., herpes zoster), oral candidiasis and oral hairy leucoplakia (secondary to Epstein-Barr virus infection). The latter condition in which the margins of the tongue show white ridges of fronds on the epithelium appears to be unique to HIV-infected patients. Without treatment, such patients progress rapidly to AIDS.

Pneumocystis jirovecii pneumonia was the presenting illness in many of the first AIDS patients. Salient features include fever, unproductive cough and progressive

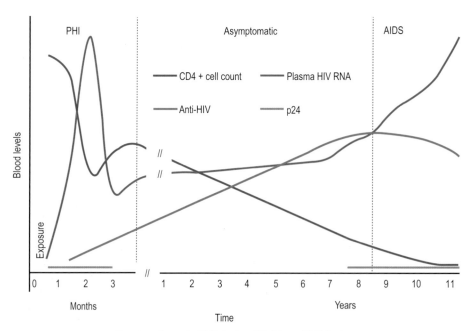

Fig. 52.4 Events in HIV infection. *PHI,* Primary HIV infection.

Box 52.1 AIDS-defining clinical conditions

- Bacterial infections, multiple or recurrent in child aged <13 years
- Candidiasis of oesophagus, bronchi or lungs
- Cervical cancer
- Coccidiomycosis, disseminated
- Cryptococcosis, extrapulmonary
- Cytomegalovirus retinitis
- Encephalopathy, HIV related
- Herpes simples virus for >1 month; or HSV of bronchi, lung or oesophagus
- Histoplasmosis, extrapulmonary or disseminated
- Isosporiasis, chronic
- Kaposi's sarcoma
- Lymphoma, non-Hodgkin's or primary of CNS
- Lymphoid interstitial pneumonia/pulmonary lymphoid hyperplasia in child <13 years
- *Mycobacterium tuberculosis*, any site
- *Mycobacterium* (other species), extrapulmonary or disseminated
- *Pneumocystis jirovecii* pneumonia
- Progressive multifocal leukoencephalopathy
- Salmonella septicaemia, recurrent
- Toxoplasmosis of the brain
- Wasting syndrome

Mycobacterium tuberculosis infections are an enormous problem in many regions, with the development of strains of the organism resistant to many antibiotics. Many patients show profound weight loss, perhaps accompanied by chronic diarrhoea; the term 'slim disease' has been given to this presentation.

Paediatric patients with AIDS suffer from many of the same problems as adults. However, children infected early in life or at birth are at risk of recurring bacterial infections as they have not acquired immunity to microorganisms. Lymphoid interstitial pneumonia and pulmonary lymphoid hyperplasia are presentations seen only in young children.

HIV-associated clinical manifestations, regardless of whether they are AIDS-defining or not, are diverse and affect all body organ systems. The advent of antiretroviral therapy has dramatically decreased the overall incidence of opportunistic infections (OI) owing to the improvement attained in immune function. However, immune recovery may paradoxically worsen underlying OI. This phenomenon, referred to as immune reconstitution inflammatory syndrome (IRIS), is not fully understood. IRIS clinical features vary with the pathogen and the organ system involved (e.g., *Cryptococcus neoformans* in the brain).

PATHOGENESIS OF HIV INFECTION AND AIDS

The major virological and immunological features of the acute and persistent stages of HIV infection are shown in Fig. 52.4. The incubation period in the acute stage is 1–2 months. This is preceded by a period of intense, unrestrained viral replication, reflected in the presence of high numbers of viral RNA genomes and p24 antigen in the circulation. After entering the body, virus is taken up by cells such as dendritic cells that express viral receptors. Within 24–48 hours, infected cells are present in the regional lymph nodes; virus can be detected in the blood and circulating lymphocytes by 5 days; the number of circulating CD4+ T lymphocytes is decreased. As the immune system responds, both p24 antigen and RNA copy number (usually referred to as viral load) decrease, so that by 6–12 months, p24 antigen is usually undetectable and the RNA load has stabilised at a lower level (referred to as the set-point); in some it may be undetectable. The HIV viral load set-point, an indirect reflection of the rate of CD4+ cell death, is a strong predictor of the rapidity of progression to AIDS. Temporary increases in viral load can be seen during intercurrent infections, immunisations and pregnancy. CD4+ cell counts recover, albeit partially, and remain more or less within the normal ranges until progression to AIDS occurs, the count then being <200/µL.

In peripheral blood, lymphoid tissue and other tissues such as brain where HIV replication occurs, HIV targets

shortness of breath. Radiological examination classically shows bilateral lung infiltrates radiating out of the perihilar region on plain chest film and/or ground-glass lung opacities on high-resolution CT scan. Diagnosis is confirmed by detection of fungal cysts in deep respiratory specimens and, increasingly, by fungal DNA detection by PCR (see Ch. 58).

Toxoplasma gondii remains the most common cause of AIDS complications affecting the brain. Toxoplasma encephalitis (TE), which is almost always caused by a reactivation of latent toxoplasma cysts, classically presents with headache, confusion and fever, developing subacutely over a few days to a month. Seizure and focal neurological signs such as hemiparesis are often present, and head MRI (or CT) scans show multiple, ring-enhancing brain lesions in most cases. The imaging findings are characteristic but not diagnostic of TE.

Kaposi's sarcoma was one of the earliest diseases used to define AIDS. This previously rare tumour had been known for many years; it usually occurred at a single site and was not aggressive. In patients with AIDS the tumour arises in many sites, including the skin, mouth, gut and eye. The tumours arise from endothelial cells of blood vessels, causing bluish-purple, raised, irregular lesions. The aetiological agent is human herpesvirus 8 (see Ch. 38). The tumours were mainly seen in homosexual men, presumably reflecting sexual transmission of the causative agent. In developing countries, whilst many of the same infections are seen, there is also an emphasis on local problems.

CD4+ T cells and cells of the monocyte–macrophage lineage; the latter may act as a reservoir of virus. Macrophages are also important in carrying the virus into the central nervous system across the blood–brain barrier.

Destruction of CD4+ T cells is caused by:

- viral replication
- syncytium formation via membrane gp120 binding to cell CD4 antigen
- cytotoxic T cell lysis of infected cells
- cytotoxic T cell lysis of CD4+ cells carrying gp120 released from infected cells
- increased susceptibility of CD4+ cells (infected and uninfected) to apoptosis

Analysis of viral genomes from an individual patient shows that there are several different viral sequences (known as a quasispecies) present at any time and that these change with time. Virus isolated in culture may be different from the predominant variants in the blood. Viruses isolated in the later stages of infection have been shown to grow more rapidly, to higher titres and to form syncytia (giant cells) more readily than virus isolated in the early stages. The switch to syncytium-inducing variants is accompanied by a virus change from R5 to X4. Regions of the envelope glycoproteins show most variation, and this could affect the ability of antibody to react with the viruses. Although this could be relevant to the progression of the infection, it also has important implications for the development of vaccines.

Disease progression

There are host genetic differences influencing the risk of disease progression; for example, human leucocyte antigen (HLA) alleles A24 and A1B8DR3 have been linked to rapid development and severe disease. There is also an age effect, with evidence of fast progression in some infants and in the elderly. Conversely, other host genetic factors, such as HLA B*5701 and heterozygosity for a 32-bp deletion in the chemokine receptor CCR5 *(CCR5-Δ32)* and immune response factors, such as effective CTL responses, are strongly linked to long-term non-progression. Infection with attenuated strains has similarly been implicated as a possible mechanism for long-term non-progression in HIV. Box 52.2 lists a number of laboratory markers that are associated with progression. The most useful marker in assessing the state of a patient's immune system is the absolute CD4+ cell count. When the count reaches 200/μL the patient is severely compromised, and the diagnosis of AIDS is made even in the absence of an AIDS-defining illness. The median time from infection onset to AIDS is approximately 10 years, although the use of ART has fundamentally changed the outlook for people living with HIV.

Box 52.2 Laboratory markers associated with progression of HIV infection

1. Decreasing number of CD4+ T lymphocytes
2. Increasing proportion of infected CD4+ cells
3. High level of set-point HIV RNA in plasma (viral load)
4. Increasing levels of HIV RNA in plasma (viral load)
5. Detectable p24 antigen in plasma
6. Isolation of virus in culture – rapid growth, syncytium formation

Paediatric infection

In most paediatric cases, infection arises from mother-to-child transmission in the perinatal period when the child's immune system is immature. This results in a major difference from the picture seen in older children and adults as the initial replicative phase is not limited by the immune response and thus high levels of viral RNA persist. HIV-infected infants are usually asymptomatic during the first 2 months of life. About 85% of the infants show a slow clinical progression thereafter; however, by age 9–16 years a third of this group are asymptomatic. The other 15% of infants have high levels of viral RNA and develop early-onset disease, with death by 4 years of age without treatment. These babies may have been infected before birth by a mother with advanced disease. This group can be identified by detection within peripheral blood of proviral DNA and viral RNA within 48 hours of birth. Analysis of the child's RNA may show that it differs from that of the mother, suggesting that replication has occurred by the time of sample collection or that a minor maternal variant has been transmitted to the baby.

LABORATORY INVESTIGATION

HIV infection can be diagnosed through detection of antibodies to the virus (anti-HIV), or of the virus itself (e.g., HIV p24 antigen, RNA or proviral DNA) in a peripheral blood sample.

Tests for anti-HIV

The main approach to the diagnosis of infection in patients and for screening populations (e.g., blood donors) has been by testing for anti-HIV. Many different testing formats are available, most using enzyme-linked immunosorbent assay (ELISA). All current tests use HIV antigens derived from cloned recombinant HIV *gag, pol* and *env* genes expressed in *Escherichia coli*, or synthetic peptides. Western or immunoblotting has been used extensively as a confirmatory assay. Most current assays can detect antibody to both HIV-1 and HIV-2 antigens. A first positive result must be confirmed by another assay, ideally two, with different viral antigens, and a second serum sample checked to confirm that the original sample was identified correctly. The confirmatory assay(s) should distinguish between antibodies to HIV-1 and to HIV-2. Most patients will seroconvert within 1–2 months. Thus there is a window before antibody tests can detect infection. Rapid tests are now available to detect antibody in blood and saliva; this format is very useful for point-of-care testing.

Combination assays

Reliable and highly sensitive methods to detect anti-HIV and p24 antigen in a single EIA are now available (so-called fourth-generation assays); these allow improved diagnostic sensitivity of primary HIV infection (PHI) diagnosis by approximately 1 week. Although less sensitive than RT-PCR for HIV RNA, the combination test is now the standard test for diagnosis and for large-scale screening (e.g., blood donors).

PCR

Direct detection methods are required when serological tests are inappropriate, such as during the early acute stage and in infants who still carry maternal anti-HIV, and for monitoring progression.

Both HIV RNA and DNA sequences can be detected in blood. RNA sequences are found in extracellular virus particles in plasma, and the RNA can be accurately quantified as the number of RNA copies to indicate the extent of virus replication in the patient. Measurement of plasma virus load is essential for monitoring disease progression and the response to antiretroviral therapy. A number of commercial assays have been developed to provide accurate and standardised viral load measurements in clinical laboratories.

HIV proviral DNA is present in infected cells and can be detected in peripheral blood mononuclear cells. This method is used principally to diagnose infection in infants born to HIV-infected mothers. The standard procedure involves analysis of serial blood samples collected at birth, 6 weeks and 3 months. The absence of proviral DNA at 3 months of age (or any time later) excludes HIV infection in babies who are not being breast-fed.

TREATMENT

Currently used multiple drug regimens (previously referred to as *h*ighly *a*ctive *a*nti*r*etroviral *t*herapy, or HAART; now known simply as *a*nti*r*etroviral *t*herapy, or ART) have

---

> **Box 52.3** Timing of ART initiation (BHIVA Guidelines, 2015)
>
> 1. Chronic HIV infection:
>   - All recommended to start ART
> 2. Individuals presenting with AIDS or a major infection:
>   - ART recommended within 2 weeks of initiation of specific antimicrobial therapy
> 3. Primary HIV infection (PHI) suspected or diagnosed:
>   - ART offered immediately
>   - Expedited ART initiation recommended in:
>   i. Neurological involvement
>   ii. Any AIDS-defining illness
>   iii. CD4+ cell count <350 cells/µL
>   iv. PHI diagnosed within 12 weeks of a previous negative test
> 4. Treatment to prevent onward transmission:
>   - ART to be offered to all PLWH

---

achieved remarkable success in halting the progression to AIDS and have helped to transform HIV from a deadly infection to a treatable chronic condition in countries with access to therapy.

The aim of antiretroviral therapy is to arrest and reverse the damage to the immune system. This will in turn avert the risks of HIV-related clinical problems, reduce infectivity and prolong survival. The decision on the timing to commence ART was traditionally based on specific clinical and immunological factors; however, it is now universally recommended that all individuals living with HIV should be started on ART, regardless of their CD4+ cell count or clinical disease stage (Box 52.3).

Antiretroviral drugs exert their effects by inhibiting specific steps in the virus replicative cycle that range from virus entry and reverse transcription to integration and protein processing in budding virus (see Ch. 5). To maximise effect and delay or prevent the emergence of viral resistance, three drugs, from at least two different classes, are prescribed together.

The objective of therapy is to achieve continuous suppression of plasma viral RNA to a level below the limits of detection afforded by modern molecular assays, usually around 40 copies/mL. In a patient who has not been treated before, a combination of two nucleoside/nucleotide reverse transcriptase inhibitors (NRTI, e.g., tenofovir/emtricitabine, abacavir/lamivudine) plus one of the following: ritonavir-boosted protease inhibitor (PI/r, e.g., darunavir/ritonavir, atazanavir/ritonavir), nonnucleoside reverse transcriptase inhibitor (NNRTI, e.g., rilpivirine, efavirenz) or integrase inhibitor (INI, e.g., dolutegravir, raltegravir, cobicistat-boosted elvitegravir) is currently recommended. The two NRTI agents, often referred to as the backbone, are preferably given as a coformulated preparation. Testing for HLA B*5701 and viral coreceptor tropism should be performed before initiation of abacavir and CCR5 antagonists, respectively.

The management of HIV infection can be difficult and is ideally delivered by a specialist team with access to a clinical laboratory. Specific clinical guidelines are available from many national and international bodies, including the British HIV Association (BHIVA).

A patient on combination therapy will have to adhere to a strict regimen. This may be a problem in very young and adolescent patients. The drugs chosen may have side effects in a particular patient or interactions with therapy for other conditions such as tuberculosis, toxoplasmosis and *P. jirovecii*. Therapy to prevent or treat these infections, if indicated, must be maintained.

Knowledge of previous antiretroviral therapy is also essential as drug resistance may have arisen. It is now standard practice to test the patient's virus population for drug resistance using genotyping methods, before initiation of ART and in situations of virological failure.

Monitoring progress

The CD4 count and the plasma viral load should be assayed when therapy is started and at 1-month and 3- to 6-month intervals thereafter. If there is a response, the RNA load will decrease within a few days, will drop by 1 $\log_{10}$ at 2–8 weeks and be <40 copies/mL by 4–6 months. If these objectives are not achieved, or the viral load increases after a time on therapy, or the clinical state deteriorates, a new combination regimen should be started (assuming patient compliance with the prescribed regimen). The resistance pattern of the patient's virus should be tested before selecting new drugs. Genotypic resistance testing is accomplished by sequencing of viral target genes and comparing the sequences against an extensive repository of possible resistance mutations such as the Stanford Database (http://hivdb.stanford.edu). The locus and nature of any identified mutations will allow determination of which drug(s) within the combination regimen are failing and therefore rational drug switches/substitution(s) by the attending physician.

It is important to note that drug-related toxicity, a largely unpredictable phenomenon, and potential drug-drug interactions remain significant problems despite the progress made in improving drug efficacy and tolerability.

PREVENTION AND CONTROL

Until a vaccine is available, the emphasis in controlling the spread of infection must be on risk reduction. Antiretroviral therapy to all PLWH is expected to play an important part in the efforts to contain the spread of HIV-1. The 90-90-90 targets, comprising getting 90% of PLWH to know their HIV status, 90% of the people diagnosed to receive sustainable ART and 90% of all people receiving ART to achieve viral suppression, by 2020, represent the first of 10 commitments in the current global strategy to end AIDS by 2030. Furthermore, oral pre-exposure antiretroviral therapy (PrEP), containing at least tenofovir, taken daily, is also recommended as an effective additional prevention choice for HIV-negative people at substantial risk of HIV.

Sexual transmission

The emphasis is on risk reduction by avoiding unprotected penetrative intercourse with partners of unknown status. Despite knowledge of the major routes of infection, there has been only limited success in reducing sexual transmission. Globally the problem is enormous, and efforts are hampered by the poverty and lack of resources of the worst affected countries. The use of condoms could have an impact, but they need to be available and acceptable to the local population.

In the areas of the world with low levels of infection, early efforts to encourage safe practices had an effect on the spread of the virus among MSM in the Americas, Europe and Australia, but this was not always maintained.

HIV transmission rates among circumcised males are lower than for uncircumcised males. Modeling indicated that the population-level impact will be greater than the individual-level gain if a large proportion of men get circumcised. Therefore, a plan for voluntary medical circumcision of 27 million additional men in high-prevalence settings, where heterosexual transmission is the dominant route, is now included as part of the global strategy to end AIDS.

Mother to child transmission

In the absence of any intervention, around 15%–45% of HIV-infected pregnant women transmit the virus to their infants. Rational strategies, based on improved understanding of disease pathogenesis and availability of better antiretroviral drugs and reliable laboratory monitoring methods, have almost eliminated the risk of mother-to-child transmission (MTCT) in high-income nations. The main components of current recommendations are universal antenatal HIV testing to identify infected mothers, use of ART to suppress plasma viral load, planning caesarian delivery when indicated, use of antiretroviral prophylaxis in the newborn and avoidance of breast-feeding.

Traditionally, the timing and components of antiretroviral therapies offered to HIV-infected pregnant and breast-feeding women were determined according to the stage of their disease. However, in 2013 a substantial shift in guidelines, based on clinical and operational research evidence, was issued by WHO recommending that all pregnant and breast-feeding women be initiated on ART regardless of clinical or immunological eligibility. This approach is believed to serve three synergistic functions: improving health outcome of women living with HIV, preventing MTCT and preventing horizontal transmission to any uninfected partner.

Exclusive bottle-feeding may reduce risk of virus transmission; however, that may occur at the expense of increased infant mortality from diarrheal and respiratory infection in developing countries. For HIV-infected women who have chosen to breast-feed their babies, the WHO recommends exclusive breast-feeding for 6 months, in combination with maternal ART and a period of infant prophylaxis, to minimise the risk of HIV transmission while optimising the health benefits of breast-feeding for the infant.

Exposure to blood

Drug injectors can avoid risk by not injecting or can reduce risk by using only clean equipment, e.g., through needle and syringe programmes (NSPs) that ensure the provision of sterile injecting equipment and its safe disposal. Screening of all blood donors should eliminate almost all possibility of transmission through receipt of blood transfusion. Factor VIII and other blood products are heat treated, if possible, to inactivate HIV. All organ donors must be screened.

Occupational risk in the health-care setting can be controlled by the implementation of safe working practices to prevent accidental injury and contamination with blood and body fluids. The use of gloves, masks and eye protection is important in situations such as surgical procedures where bleeding and spattering are possible. The risk must be assessed in other situations. Safe disposal of used needles, scalpel blades and other sharps is an essential requirement. The sensitivity of HIV to heat and various disinfectants is described below.

HIV is inactivated by:

- heat, in an autoclave or hot-air oven
- glutaraldehyde (2%)
- hypochlorite (10,000 ppm); 1 in 10 dilution of domestic bleach
- other disinfectants, including alcohol

The chemicals will inactivate at least 10^5 units of virus within a few minutes, but disinfectants are inactivated in the presence of organic material.

HIV can survive for up to 15 days at room temperature and for 10–15 days at 37°C. At temperatures >60°C, virus is inactivated 100-fold each hour.

If an accidental exposure occurs, any wound should be washed with soap and water, or mucous membranes flushed with water. The accident must be reported so that, if necessary, post-exposure prophylaxis (PEP) can be started as soon as possible. The risk must be assessed through knowledge of the circumstances:

- The HIV status/risk of the source patient; if unknown, can the source be tested?
- The nature of the exposure (e.g., penetrating injury or contamination of skin or mucous membranes)

The risk of infection from splashing onto mucous membranes or skin is hard to quantify but is certainly less than with penetrating injuries. An intact skin is an effective barrier, but abrasions and diseases such as eczema may impair this protection.

If a sharp injury is reported the nature of the injury has to be assessed.

- Needlestick or cut with sharp instrument
- Depth of penetration
- Volume of blood involved
- Whether the needle had entered a blood vessel

If there is an indication of risk, PEP must be started within 1–2 hours, and not later than 48–72 hours. If no professional advice is available, for instance, at night, prophylaxis should be started and advice obtained subsequently. A decision should be made about continuing with the drugs preferably within 12–24 hours. The victim should be involved in the decision, with discussion of the risks and the possible side effects of the drugs.

It is recommended that a triple-agent combination, including tenofovir-emtricitabine with an integrase inhibitor or a ritonavir-boosted protease inhibitor be used for PEP. Alternative combinations can be offered or specifically selected with knowledge of any drug resistance in the source. Therapy should be continued for 4 weeks and the victim followed with testing for virus for the next 6 months.

Vaccines

Much effort has been devoted to the development of a vaccine to provide protection against infection after exposure (prophylactic vaccine) or to boost the immune system of those infected (therapeutic vaccine). Major problems arise because of the antigenic variability of HIV and the difficulty of developing immunogens that elicit protective responses to all variants. In addition, HIV may be transferred by blood-borne or mucosal routes, through transfer of free virus or infected cells. To protect, therefore, it is likely that both cell-mediated and humoral responses need to be stimulated. Whether an HIV vaccine could ever induce fully protective immunity is subject to some doubt because the immune response, although highly active during acute infection, is never capable of fully clearing infection, and lifelong persistence is the norm.

Most efforts have been directed to the development of vaccines containing the viral *env* proteins gp160, gp120 or gp41 prepared by recombinant DNA cloning and expression, or synthetic peptides known to be important epitopes for induction of neutralising antibodies. To date, human trials have shown no conclusive evidence of protection from infection by sexual transmission and injecting-drug use.

HTLV-I AND –II INFECTION

EPIDEMIOLOGY AND TRANSMISSION

There are three lineages of HTLV-I strains, which are linked to Melanesia, Central Africa and various countries (the Cosmopolitan group). The latter includes viruses from Japan, North and West Africa and the Caribbean, which can be distinguished. HTLV-I and the simian virus, STLV-I, are closely related, and it is proposed that human infection occurred many thousands of years ago in Africa and that the presence of the virus in many different parts of the world is related to the migration of ancient peoples. The slave trade may account for foci found in the West Indies and the southern United States.

The virus is endemic in certain communities. In parts of Japan, the prevalence of antibody can be as high as 27%, with a rising trend from 7% to 8% in the 20- to 39-year age group to 52% in females and 32% in males by 80 years. In the Caribbean, the rates are in the range of 5%–10%, with clusters in communities and families. In other regions, infection has been found in parenteral-drug users and sex workers.

The virus is cell associated in the host, so transmission will occur when infected cells are transferred. This can occur during sexual intercourse, blood transfusion and through sharing contaminated injecting equipment. In contrast to HIV, breast-feeding appears to be the dominant route of mother-to-child transmission; maternal retroviral load is the major predictor of transmission. HTLV-II is transmitted by the same routes. The strains found in PWID in different countries are related.

PATHOGENESIS

During the latent period viral proteins are expressed, as there are steady high antibody titres to various proteins, particularly the *gag* proteins. The virus is genetically stable and little cell-free virus is produced. However, during the latent period, virus is present as integrated provirus and is replicated with the cellular DNA as the cell divides. The tumour cells contain monoclonally integrated HTLV-I provirus at random sites. There are no transforming genes. The T-cell proliferation is the result of the action of the viral *tax* gene, which can activate transcription of cellular genes including those for interleukin-2 and its receptor (IL-2R), and cause cell proliferation. The malignant cells are mature CD4+/CD8− with increased IL2-Rα chain (CD25/TAC antigen) expression. It is not known what triggers this effect after the long latency in the 1%–4% of those infected who develop disease. Antibody to the *tax* protein can block the stimulation of cell division; loss or decay of immune control may be important. Interactions with tumour-suppressor genes such as p53 and promotion of S-phase in the cell cycle are other probable mechanisms of oncogenesis.

CLINICAL FEATURES

Primary HTLV-I infection is not associated with a recognisable clinical syndrome or seroconversion illness. Like HIV, up to 8 weeks may elapse following initial exposure for antibody to become detectable. Seroconversion is followed by an asymptomatic period that can last from years to decades. Clinical disease may eventually develop as a direct result of cell transformation by the virus, in 1%–4% of cases (adult T-cell leukaemia/lymphoma, ATL), or as a manifestation of immunological responses to it, in 1%–2% (human T-cell lymphotropic virus-associated myelopathy, HAM, or tropical spastic paraparesis, TSP).

ATL was first recognised in Japan. It is an aggressive T-cell proliferative malignancy; the features are leukaemia, generalised lymphadenopathy and hepatosplenomegaly, skin lesions and metabolic disorders, especially hypercalcaemia (acute ATL). A distinct, aggressive T cell-lymphoma clinical type has also been identified (lymphoma/leukaemia ATL). The two forms have poor prognosis, with median survival time of 6.2 and 10 months, respectively. Other less dramatic forms exist, including a variant that runs a slow course, associated with adenopathy and splenomegaly (chronic ATL) and an indolent form with skin lesions but no visceral involvement (smouldering ATL). Males are at greater risk than females of developing ATL. The T cells involved carry the CD4 antigen.

HTLV-I is also the cause of HAM/TSP, a slowly progressive myelopathy with spastic or ataxic features. Pathologically, areas of demyelination with lymphocytic inflammation and perivascular cuffing are seen.

There are several other recognised virus-associated diseases, notably a form of uveitis in otherwise asymptomatic carriers, and infective dermatitis in children born to HTLV-I–positive mothers.

HTLV-II has not conclusively been shown to cause a particular disease; however, evidence showing a link to HAM/TSP and possibly other neurological manifestations is accumulating.

LABORATORY INVESTIGATION

Current serological assays, incorporating recombinant or synthetic viral peptides, for the detection of antibody to HTLV-I and HTLV-II are highly sensitive and specific. As with HIV, confirmation is achieved by other assays or immunoblotting (e.g., Western blot), although interpretation can be difficult. Confirmatory tests are able to distinguish between antibodies to HTLV-I and HTLV-II. Detection of HTLV proviral sequences by PCR can also be used as a confirmatory test, and to distinguish between types.

TREATMENT

There is no indication for treatment of asymptomatic HTLV carriers. ATL patients are treated with conventional anticancer chemotherapy or, when appropriate, haematopoietic stem cell transplantation. Interferon and inhibitors of reverse transcriptase (e.g., zidovudine and lamivudine) may have a complementary role in treatment of HTLV-related diseases but further evaluation is needed.

CONTROL

Standard preventative measures include screening of blood donations, avoidance of breast-feeding by known infected mothers and using condoms. These measures address the major routes of transmission; however, these are hardly cost effective in developed countries, other than Japan where infection is endemic, or feasible in developing countries. Although effective HTLV-I vaccines have been studied in primates, there are no current plans to develop or market a human vaccine.

RECOMMENDED READING

Knipe, D. M., & Howley, P. M. (Eds.). (2013). Chs. 47–52. *Fields virology* (6th ed., pp. 1424–1632). Philadelphia: Wolters Kluwer/Lippincott Williams & Wilkins.

UK Health Departments. (1998). Guidance for Clinical Health Care Workers; Protection against Infection with Blood-Borne Viruses. Recommendations of the Expert Advisory Group. London: HMSO.

Volberding, P. A., & Deeks, S. G. (2010). Antiretroviral therapy and management of HIV infection. *The Lancet, 376*(9734), 49–62. doi:10.1016/S0140-6736(10)60676-9.

Centers for Disease Control and Prevention, Atlanta, USA. HIV/AIDS. Guidelines and recommendations. Retrieved from http://www.cdc.gov/hiv/guidelines/. (Accessed Nov 2017).

Joint United Nations Programme on HIV/AIDS (UNAIDS). UNAIDS Strategy. (Accessed Nov 2017).

UNAIDS Strategy 2016–2021. Retrieved from http://www.unaids.org/en/goals/unaidsstrategy. (Accessed Nov 2017).

Websites

British HIV Association (BHIVA). Current guidelines. Retrieved from http://www.bhiva.org/Guidelines.aspx. (Accessed Nov 2017).

53 Caliciviruses and astroviruses

DAVID J. ALLEN AND MIREN ITURRIZA-GÓMARA

KEY POINTS

- Norovirus is the most common cause of sporadic cases and outbreaks of diarrhoeal disease globally and is ranked as the principal cause of foodborne disease. Sapoviruses and astroviruses are also commonly associated with sporadic cases and outbreaks of diarrhoea, but they are less prevalent.
- Caliciviruses and astroviruses are transmitted via the faecal-oral route.
- Disease is usually self-limiting, characterised by a brief incubation time (12–72 hours) and short duration of symptoms (24–72 hours).
- Immunity to noroviruses is not fully cross-protective and wanes over time; therefore reinfections and repeated norovirus disease are common.
- Chronic infection can lead to severe and life-threatening disease in immunodeficient or severely immunocompromised patients.
- Astroviruses can be associated with neurological disease.
- The gold standard for detection of caliciviruses and astroviruses is reverse transcription-polymerase chain reaction (RT-PCR), but the extreme sensitivity of this assay can result in the detection of asymptomatic shedding of these viruses.

DESCRIPTION

Acute gastrointestinal disease in all age groups is frequently associated with a viral aetiology. Viruses belonging to the *Norovirus* and *Sapovirus* genera of the Caliciviridae family, and those belonging to the *Mamastrovirus* genus of the Astroviridae family are discussed in this chapter.

MORPHOLOGY AND CLASSIFICATION

Caliciviridae

The Caliciviridae family received its named from the cup-shaped cavities (from the Latin *calyx*) on the virus surface as seen by electron microscopy (EM). They are small nonenveloped viruses, and based on phylogenetic differences, the family is currently divided into five genera: *Lagovirus, Nebovirus, Norovirus, Sapovirus* and *Vesivirus*. These genera include viruses that infect a variety of animals in addition to humans and other mammalian species, birds and reptiles. Two of the five genera, *Norovirus* and *Sapovirus*, are important pathogens of humans and are associated with gastroenteritis in children and adults.

Norovirus

The mature norovirus virion is approximately 27–32 nm in diameter, with 32 cup-shaped cavities across the virus surface. The appearance of norovirus virions as viewed by EM can be more amorphous than that of the sapovirus virion due to differences in the three-dimensional structure of the norovirus capsomere that obscures the cavity of the cup-like structure.

The classification of the *Norovirus* genus is based on sequence diversity in the major capsid protein (VP1). There are currently seven recognised genogroups (GI–GVII) that are further subdivided into genotypes, of which more than 40 have been described across the entire *Norovirus* genus. Amino acid sequence diversity in the VP1 protein between genogroups can be >40%, up to 20% between genotypes, and 3%–5% between strains of the same genotype. Human infection and disease has been associated with three of these genogroups: GI, GII and GIV. The majority of human norovirus diarrhoeal cases are associated with GII, particularly with genotype 4 (GII-4) viruses, which are responsible for 70%–80% of global outbreaks, and >50% of

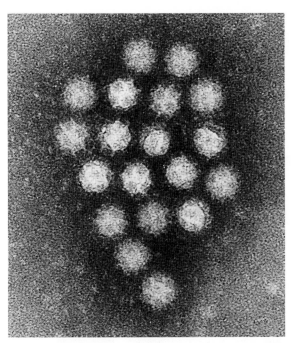

Table 53.1 Amino acid similarity in the capsid protein within astrovirus genotypes associated with infection in humans

	MAstV1	MAstV6	MAstV8	MAstV9
% amino acid similarity within genotype	63–84	74–90	78–79	75–77

Fig. 53.1 Sapovirus, displaying characteristic cupped surface morphology. Original magnification ×300,000. (From Cubitt, W. D., Blacklow, N. R., Herrmann, J. E., Nowak, N. A., Nakata, S., & Chiba, S. (1987). Antigenic relationships between human caliciviruses and Norwalk virus. *Journal of Infectious Diseases*, 156(5), 806-814.)

sporadic cases in all ages. The GII-4 viruses cause periodic epidemics through a mechanism known as epochal evolution; GII-4 variants emerge from time to time, displacing previously circulating virus strains to become dominant globally due to a lack of herd protection in the population, similar to the phenomenon described for influenza viruses.

Sapovirus

Sapovirus virions are 30–38 nm in diameter, with the distinctive typical calicivirus morphology of 32 cup-shaped cavities across the virus surface when visualised by EM along the two-, three-, or fivefold axes of symmetry (Fig. 53.1).

There are currently four formal genogroups within the *Sapovirus* genus (GI–GIV) based on sequence diversity of the sapovirus major capsid protein (VP1). In addition, a fifth genogroup (GV) has been recognised and a further nine (GVI–GXIV) have been proposed.

Astroviridae

The Astroviridae are a family of nonenveloped viruses. Astrovirus particles viewed by EM appear with a smooth margin and a distinct five- or six-pointed star, and are 28–30 nm in diameter. Viruses observed from clinical specimens are reported to be smaller in size than those produced in cell culture, which have an external diameter of approximately 40 nm and distinct surface spikes, but lack the star-shaped appearance.

The Astroviridae are divided into two genera: *Mamastrovirus* (MAstV, comprising viruses of mammals) and *Avastrovirus* (AAstV, comprising viruses of birds). There are 19 species of MAstVs (MAstV1–19): MAstV1, MAstV6, MAstV8 and MAstV9 (see Table 53.1) have been identified in humans, and among MAstV1 astroviruses, also known as classic human astroviruses (HAstV), eight genotypes have been described to date (HAstV1–HAstV8). Genome sequence and phylogenetic analysis correlate tightly with serotypes determined through serological assays. HAstV1 is associated with the majority of cases of astrovirus diarrhoea in children (30%–84% of all HAstV reported globally). Within each HAstV genotype, lineages or subtypes are defined based on nucleotide sequence divergence >7%; so far HAstV1 has been divided into six lineages, and HAstV2, HAstV3 and HAstV4 have been divided into four, two and three lineages, respectively.

MAJOR FEATURES

Norovirus genome organisation

The norovirus genome is a single strand of positive-sense RNA (+ssRNA, Baltimore Class IV) and is approximately 7500 nt in length. The RNA is covalently linked to a virus-encoded protein (VPg) at the 5′ end and is polyadenylated at the 3′ end. The genome is organised into three open reading frames (ORFs) (Fig. 53.2A). The 5′-proximal ORF1 encodes a large polyprotein, which is posttranslationally processed by the virus protease into six nonstructural proteins required for virus replication. These proteins include the VPg, protease, and RNA-dependent RNA polymerase. The remaining ORFs, ORF2 and ORF3, encode the major (VP1) and minor (VP2) capsid proteins, respectively.

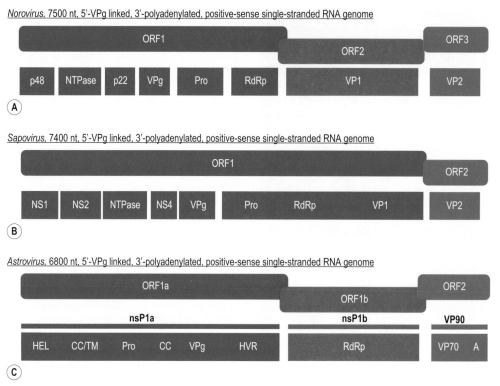

Norovirus, 7500 nt, 5'-VPg linked, 3'-polyadenylated, positive-sense single-stranded RNA genome

Fig. 53.2 Genome organisation of (A) *Norovirus*, (B) *Sapovirus*, and (C) *Astrovirus*. All three genomes are positive-sense, single-stranded RNA, of length 6800–7600 nt. All three genomes have a viral protein linked to the 5'- end of the genome (VPg) and are polyadenylated at the 3' end. (A). The norovirus genome is organised into three open reading frames (ORFs) encoding eight proteins. ORF1 encodes a large polyprotein, which is posttranslationally processed into the nonstructural proteins including the 5'-genome protein (VPg), protease (Pro) and RNA-dependent RNA polymerase (RdRp). ORF2 encodes the major capsid protein (VP1). ORF3 encodes a small basic protein (VP2) of unknown function. (B). The sapovirus genome is organised as two ORFs; ORF1 encodes a large polyprotein, which is posttranslationally processed into the nonstructural and structural proteins, including the 5'-genome protein (VPg), protease (Pro) and RNA-dependent RNA polymerase (RdRp) and the major capsid protein (VP1). ORF2 encodes the small structural protein VP2. (C). The astrovirus genome is organised into three ORFs: ORF1a encodes nonstructural protein nsP1a, which has putative helicase (HEL) domain, coiled-coil (CC), transmembrane (TM) and hypervariable (HVR) domains, a protease domain (Pro) and a VPg-coding sequence. ORF1b encodes nonstructural protein nsP1b, which contains an RdRp motif. ORF2 encodes the virus capsid protein VP90, which is posttranslationally processed into an acidic domain (A) and capsid precursor (VP70), which itself is further processed into structural proteins VP34, VP27/29 and VP25/26.

Sapovirus genome organisation

The sapovirus genome is +ssRNA, approximately 7400 nt in length, and is organised into two ORFs (Fig. 53.2B). ORF1 encodes a large polyprotein, which is posttranslationally processed into the virus nonstructural proteins and the major capsid protein (VP1). Studies in vitro suggest that the virus protease (NS6) and RNA-dependent RNA polymerase (NS7) may remain fused in the infected cell, although both perform their respective functions when expressed individually.

Astrovirus genome organisation

The astrovirus genome is +ssRNA, approximately 6800 nt in length, and is organised into three ORFs (Fig. 53.2C). ORF1a and ORF1b encode the nonstructural virus proteins,

which are involved in replication and provide protease and RNA-dependent RNA polymerase functions, putative helicase function and have a number of coiled-coil, transmembrane domains, and both a death domain and nuclear localisation signal adjacent to the VPg-coding region. The 3'-proximal ORF3 encodes the virus capsid protein VP90, which is posttranslationally processed into the capsid precursor protein VP70, which is further proteolytically processed into the structural proteins VP34, VP27/29 and VP25/26.

Norovirus structure

The norovirus capsid is comprised of 180 copies (as 90 homodimers) of the major capsid protein VP1, which forms an icosahedral particle (T=3 symmetry). The VP1 protein itself is highly organised, with distinct functional domains:

an N-terminal (N) domain, shell (S) domain and a protruding (P) domain. The S domain forms the concentric shell of the virus and encloses the +ssRNA genome. The P domain can be further subdivided into the P1 (P1.1 and P.2) domains and the hypervariable P2 domain. The P domain forms spikelike protrusions extending from the virus surface, and the P2 domain forms the most surface-exposed portion of these protrusions. Receptor-binding and immunoreactivity functions have been associated with the P2 domain.

Sapovirus structure

The complete sapovirus virion is formed of 180 copies of the 60-kDa VP1 protein, produced either by cleavage from the ORF1 polyprotein, or translated from a subgenomic RNA. The capsid is icosahedral and has the same structural arrangement as observed for *Norovirus*. The sapovirus VP1 protein can also be described as a multi-domain protein, with the following domains identified: N-terminal variable region (NVR), N-terminal region (N), central variable region (CVR) and C-terminal region (C). It is likely that the sapovirus CVR corresponds to the norovirus P2 domain in structure and function.

Astrovirus structure

The mature astrovirus virion is icosahedral, assembled from the VP90 precursor following its cleavage by cellular proteases to remove an acidic domain and release the VP70 precursor. The resulting particles formed from the VP70 protein are immature and require further cleavage by trypsin in the extracellular environment that leads to formation of the mature infectious particle comprised of VP70 cleavage products VP34, VP27/29 and VP25/26. The VP34 protein is derived from the N-terminal portion of the VP70 protein and forms the virion shell. The dimeric spikes around the virus surface are comprised of the VP27/29 and VP25/26 proteins, themselves derived by cleavage from the C-terminal portion of the VP70 protein. These proteins are more variable than the VP34 protein (see Table 53.2).

EPIDEMIOLOGY

Caliciviruses and astroviruses are transmitted via the faecal-oral route. Person to person is the main mode of transmission, but environmental, food and water contamination also contribute significantly to the burden of infection.

The reservoir of both human calicivirus and human astrovirus strains is the human population. Animal norovirus, sapovirus and astrovirus strains exist and are associated with disease in their host species, and therefore potential for zoonotic transmission exists. Animals, and in particular pigs, can be infected with human noroviruses, and exposure to human noroviruses has been detected through serology or the detection of RNA in animal stools (pig and dog). It has also been shown that humans can

Table 53.2 Summary of properties of human caliciviruses and human astroviruses

	Norovirus	*Sapovirus*	*Astrovirus*
Family	Caliciviridae	Caliciviridae	Astroviridae
Genus	*Norovirus*	*Sapovirus*	*Mamastrovirus*
Genogroups (species)	7	5	19
Major human genogroups	2 (I & II)	4 (I, II, IV & V)	1 (MAstV1, 6, 8 & 9)
Major human genotypes	GII-4	GIV-1 (since 2007)	HAst 1–4
Nucleic acid	+ssRNA	+ssRNA	+ssRNA
Structural proteins	VP1 (major)	VP1 (major)	VP34, VP27/29, VP25/26
	VP2 (minor)	VP2 (minor)	
Particle size (diameter)	27–32 nm	30–38 nm	28–30 nm
Replication	Cytoplasmic	Cytoplasmic	Cytoplasmic & nuclear
Incubation period	1–2 days	1–3 days	1–5 days
Symptomatic period	1–4 days	1–4 days	1–4 days
Symptoms	Diarrhoea, projectile vomiting	Diarrhoea	Diarrhoea
Asymptomatic shedding	Yes, frequent	Yes, frequent	Yes, frequency unknown
Transmission routes reported			
Person to person	Yes, most frequent	Yes, most frequent	Yes, most frequent
Fomites	Yes	Yes	Yes
Food/water	Yes	Yes	Yes
Epidemiology	Sporadic/endemic in children Outbreaks in all ages	Sporadic/endemic in children Outbreaks all ages, predominantly health and social care associated	Sporadic/endemic in children Outbreaks predominantly in children

mount immune responses to bovine and canine noroviruses, but no animal noroviruses have to date been detected in human stools. Similarly, no direct evidence of zoonotic transmission of animal astroviruses to humans has been documented so far despite growing evidence that animal astroviruses can cross species barriers. However, the detection of antibodies against turkey astroviruses type 2 in a significant proportion of abattoir workers reported in a recent study warrants further investigations in order to determine if exposure to avian astroviruses results in replication and/or disease in humans.

Human noroviruses are the leading cause of gastroenteritis and are associated with 18% of diarrhoeal disease globally, with similar proportions of disease in high-, middle- and low-income countries.

Noroviruses infect people of all ages, but children experience the highest incidence. Severe disease leading to hospitalisation and death is more frequent in children and the elderly. In countries in which rotavirus vaccines have been introduced, *Norovirus* has become the most common cause of medically attended paediatric gastroenteritis. Exposure to norovirus infection occurs early in life, and multiple reinfections are common; it is estimated that on average a person will experience an average of three to eight norovirus disease episodes in their lifetime. Recent estimates ranked *Norovirus* as the number one cause of foodborne illness, fourth most frequent cause of foodborne-associated deaths, and fifth cause of foodborne disability-adjusted life years (DALYs).

In addition, noroviruses are a leading cause of outbreaks of gastroenteritis, and, in high-income countries, health and social care–associated outbreaks are common in the winter months, adding significant pressure to the care systems and the economy.

Several studies have demonstrated that susceptibility to norovirus infection is determined genetically via the expression of histo-blood group antigens (HBGAs). HBGAs have a critical function in norovirus attachment to host cells, and these viruses display a strain-dependent variation in the patterns of HBGA molecular recognition, which may also contribute to host restriction. Furthermore, the presence of antibodies that specifically block norovirus binding to HBGA has been correlated with protection from norovirus disease. More recently, HBGA-driven susceptibility to rotavirus infections in a strain-specific manner has also been identified, but no such genetic determinant of susceptibility to infection has so far been identified for sapoviruses or astroviruses.

Sapovirus- and astrovirus-associated diarrhoea is less prevalent, although both can be detected in sporadic cases and are implicated in causing outbreaks. Sapovirus-associated sporadic diarrhoea can be detected in all ages, and outbreaks are more common among children or associated with elderly care facilities. Astroviruses are

detected in sporadic cases and outbreaks predominantly affecting children.

Asymptomatic shedding either due to prolonged shedding following an acute infection or due to asymptomatic infection has been described for caliciviruses and astroviruses. The contribution of shedding, which in the case of *Norovirus* has been identified in up to 16% of the healthy population, to the burden of transmission is currently not fully understood. However, transmission studies in outbreak situations indicate that most transmission events occur in the early infection phase, during which acute symptoms are apparent (within 12–72 hours postinfection), although shedding may last for several weeks (see Fig. 53.3).

REPLICATION

The cellular processes involved in human calicivirus replication are not well understood, primarily because of the lack of a tractable laboratory culture system in which to study the replication of these viruses until very recently. For astroviruses, the availability of in vitro culture methods means that the basic life cycle and pathogenesis of these viruses is somewhat better understood, although significant gaps remain.

Calicivirus and astrovirus replication is thought to occur predominantly in the small intestine. To date, no viremia or any other evidence of extraintestinal replication sites has been confirmed in human calicivirus infection, although extraintestinal tropism of astroviruses is increasingly being recognised.

CLINICAL FEATURES

Clinical features of symptomatic infection with *Calicivirus* and *Astrovirus* are similar and characterised by watery diarrhoea with or without vomiting. Projectile vomiting is frequently reported in norovirus infections. Other symptoms include low-grade fever, abdominal pain, myalgia and muscular pains.

The incubation period for caliciviruses ranges from 12 to 72 hours, and slightly longer, 24 hours to 5 days, for astroviruses. Generally, symptoms last for 1–4 days, and the illness is self-limiting; however, virus shedding can occur for several days following resolution of symptoms. Norovirus diarrhoea also contributes to mortality in the elderly population, particularly among those in long-term care, and norovirus infections have also been associated with postinfectious irritable bowel syndrome (PI-IBS).

Chronic infection with *Norovirus* can occur in immunodeficient or severely immunosuppressed individuals, and this can be severe and life threatening. Astroviruses

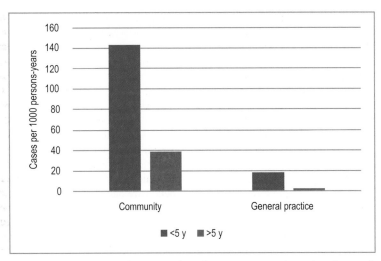

Fig. 53.3 Incidence of norovirus disease in the community or general practice among cases under or above 5 years of age. (Data from the Second Study of Infectious Intestinal Disease Study (IID2), United Kingdom.)

have more recently been detected as the causative agents of encephalitis in immunodeficient patients.

DIAGNOSIS

Clinical

Diagnosis of individual cases of viral gastroenteritis requires laboratory testing; however, clinical diagnosis of outbreaks of *Norovirus* has historically relied on the Kaplan criteria. These state that an outbreak is likely to be caused by *Norovirus* if: (1) no bacterial/parasitic pathogen can be found; (2) >50% of the cases present with vomiting; (3) illness lasts 12–60 hours, and (4) the incubation period is between 24 and 48 hours. Whilst useful in a clinical setting, these criteria can be insensitive to discriminating between outbreaks of norovirus gastroenteritis and outbreaks caused by other (viral) agents.

Cultivation

Caliciviruses are difficult to propagate using in vitro systems and for a long time were regarded as noncultivable. Recently, two systems have been described for the propagation of *Norovirus* in the laboratory, one using peripheral blood B lymphocytes in the presence of microbial or human-derived HBGA molecules, and a second using stem cell–derived human intestinal enteroids. Additionally, two systems have been reported for the propagation of sapoviruses, using either green monkey kidney cells or human embryo kidney cells in the presence of trypsin and actinomycin D. At present, these methods are subject to

reproducibility studies and it remains to be determined whether these are stable and robust systems for the in vitro propagation of caliciviruses.

Astroviruses can be propagated in vitro using human intestinal cell lines Caco-2 and HT-29, requiring trypsin to be incorporated into the growth medium.

Antigen detection assays

Enzyme-linked immunosorbent assays (ELISAs) can be used to detect antigen in patients' stool in cases of calicivirus and astrovirus infection.

Immunological assays have been shown to be useful in investigation of norovirus outbreaks. Sensitivity of ELISAs for norovirus detection is 30%–40% when two specimens from an outbreak are tested; however, this increases to 80% when seven or more samples are tested from an outbreak.

For *Norovirus, Sapovirus* and *Astrovirus*, the usefulness of immunological assays is constantly hindered by the difficulty in detecting the broad antigenic diversity within these virus groups, the emergence of antigenically novel viruses, and the low sensitivity compared to molecular methods. Furthermore, although a number of commercial enzyme-linked immuno assay (EIA) and immunochromatographic tests are available for *Norovirus*, there has been much less effort to make tests for *Sapovirus* and *Astrovirus* commercially available.

Genome detection assays

Polymerase chain reaction (PCR) assays are widely used for the detection of *Calicivirus* and *Astrovirus*, and increasingly, these are based on realtime PCR technology. These methods are fast and relatively inexpensive (following investment in the technology) and produce results with speed and high sensitivity and specificity.

Most PCR assays for these viruses target the conserved regions of the genome within the ORF encoding the major capsid protein (VP1). The sequence diversity here is usually sufficiently low to permit design of primers that are broadly reactive or that may be genogroup (or species) specific.

The high sensitivity of PCR assays raises questions around when detection of the virus genome by PCR is clinically relevant. Population studies have shown that *Norovirus* and *Sapovirus* (and likely, but less well studied, *Astrovirus*) can be asymptomatically carried, and a PCR-positive result cannot always be associated with illness, given that multiple infections with several pathogens are relatively common, particularly in young children. In population case-control studies, attributable fractions have been estimated using odds ratio calculations or quantitative PCR results, under the assumption that symptoms are associated with higher viral loads. Currently these methods are not applicable to routine diagnosis of individual clinical cases, and a syndromic approach by which samples are screened against a battery of likely enteric pathogens simultaneously in order detect other potential co-pathogens is increasingly being employed, particularly in large laboratories in which molecular diagnostic automation is available.

TREATMENT

There is no specific treatment for infections with caliciviruses or astroviruses, and much of the focus is on patient management, providing fluid replacement to mitigate dehydration and instigating good infection control. There have been a small number of studies in which patients with immunological deficiencies and chronic norovirus infection have been treated with ribavirin or nitazoxanide; however, the success of these interventions has been variable, and further work is needed to understand the usefulness of antiviral drugs in treating these infections.

CONTROL

Control of caliciviruses and astroviruses relies on good hygiene measures to prevent spread of the infection. There are various national and regional-level guidelines for the prevention and control of norovirus infections in health- and social-care settings and the catering and holiday/cruise ship industries.

All guidelines are based around common principles designed to identify and isolate cases by applying appropriate diagnostic tools, cohorting patients and/or closing wards in health-care settings, delaying the return to work until 48 hours after the resolution of symptoms, maintaining high levels of personal and environmental hygiene by promoting hand hygiene with soap and water (the use of alcohol-based hand sanitisers alone is not recommended as these are not effective against nonenveloped viruses) and decontaminating surfaces with a bleach solution.

Norovirus vaccines are currently under development, and a nonreplicating vaccine consisting of virus-like particles (VLPs) is currently in early clinical studies (phase II-B). Early results suggest that this prototype vaccine is highly immunogenic and can confer protection from disease in healthy adult volunteers in challenge studies. Further research is still necessary in order to understand the duration of protection, whether the protection is sufficiently broad and prevents disease against a variety of genotypes and the periodically emerging variant strains, and whether the current vaccine design, which is administered intramuscularly, will elicit protection in the two main target groups for vaccination. It remains to be seen whether this vaccine can protect infants without a history of preexposure to *Norovirus* or whether immunosenescence may challenge its effectiveness in the elderly.

RECOMMENDED READING

Bosch, A., Pintó, R. M., & Guix, S. (2014). Human astroviruses. *Clinical Microbiology Reviews, 27*(4), 1048–1074. doi:10.1128/CMR.00013-14.

de Graaf, M., van Beek, J., & Koopmans, M. P. (2016). Human norovirus transmission and evolution in a changing world. *Nature Reviews Microbiology, 14*(7), 421–433. doi:10.1038/nrmicro2016.48.

Ettayebi, K., Crawford, S. E., Murakami, K., Broughman, J. R., Karandikar, U., Tenge, V. R., ... Estes, M. K. (2016). Replication of human noroviruses in stem cell-derived human enteroids. *Science, 353*(6306), 1387–1393.

Kambhampati, A., Payne, D. C., Costantini, V., & Lopman, B. A. (2016). Host genetic susceptibility to enteric viruses: a systematic review and metaanalysis. *Clinical Infectious Diseases, 62*(1), 11–18. doi:10.1093/cid/civ873.

Oka, T., Wang, Q., Katayama, K., & Saif, L. J. (2015). Comprehensive review of human sapoviruses. *Clinical Microbiology Reviews, 28*(1), 32–53. doi:10.1128/CMR.00011-14.

Prasad, B. V., Shanker, S., Muhaxhiri, Z., Deng, L., Choi, J. M., Estes, M. K., ... Atmar, R. L. (2016). Antiviral targets of human noroviruses. *Current Opinion in Virology, 18*, 117–125. doi:10.1016/j.coviro.2016.06.002.

Riddle, M. S., & Walker, R. I. (2016). Status of vaccine research and development for norovirus. *Vaccine, 34*(26), 2895–2899. doi:10.1016/j.vaccine.2016.03.077.

Tam, C. C., Rodrigues, L. C., Viviani, L., Dodds, J. P., Evans, M. R., Hunter, P. R., ... IID2 Study Executive Committee. (2012). Longitudinal study of infectious intestinal disease in the UK (IID2 study): incidence in the community and presenting to general practice. *Gut, 61*(1), 69–77. doi:10.1136/gut.2011.238386.

Websites

Advisory Committee on the Microbiological Safety of Food. An update on viruses in the food chain. Retrieved from https://www.food.gov.uk/sites/default/files/multimedia/pdfs/consultation/viruses-foodchain-acmsf.pdf. (Accessed Nov 2017).

Centers for Disease Control and Prevention. Guideline for the prevention and control of norovirus gastroenteritis outbreaks in healthcare settings. Retrieved from http://www.cdc.gov/hicpac/pdf/norovirus/Norovirus-Guideline-2011.pdf. (Accessed Nov 2017).

Centers for Disease Control and Prevention. Global burden of norovirus and prospects for vaccine development. Retrieved from http://www.cdc.gov/norovirus/downloads/global-burden-report.pdf. (Accessed Nov 2017).

European Centre for Disease Prevention and Control. Prevention of norovirus infection in schools and childcare facilities. Retrieved from http://ecdc.europa.eu/en/publications/Publications/norovirus-prevention-infection-schools-childcare-facilities.pdf. (Accessed Nov 2017).

UK Government. Guidelines for the management of norovirus outbreaks in acute and community health and social care settings. Retrieved from https://www.gov.uk/government/uploads/system/uploads/attachment_data/file/322943/Guidance_for_managing_norovirus_outbreaks_in_healthcare_settings.pdf. (Accessed Nov 2017).

UK Government. Guidance for the management of norovirus infection in cruise ships. Retrieved from https://www.gov.uk/government/uploads/system/uploads/attachment_data/file/362998/2007_guideline_norovirus_cruiseships.pdf. (Accessed Nov 2017).

54 Coronaviruses

J. S. MALIK PEIRIS

KEY POINTS

- Coronaviruses (CoVs) are widespread among mammals and birds, affecting many organ systems and causing a range of diseases.
- Human coronaviruses (HCoV) 229E and OC43 are major causes of the common cold. These, as well as the newly discovered HCoV NL63 and HKU1, cause both upper respiratory tract infection and, sometimes, lower respiratory tract infections in all age groups.
- Severe acute respiratory syndrome (SARS) CoV emerged from bats, adapted in other small wild mammals (e.g., civet cats) and acquired efficient human transmission leading to a global outbreak of a novel disease in 2003. It is no longer circulating in humans.
- Middle East respiratory syndrome (MERS) CoV is endemic in dromedary camels and continues to cause outbreaks of zoonotic origin in the Arabian Peninsula.
- No vaccines or antivirals are in routine clinical use for any HCoV.

Coronaviruses were discovered in the early 1930s when an acute respiratory infection of domesticated chickens was shown to be caused by a virus now known as avian infectious bronchitis virus (IBV). The first human coronaviruses (HCoVs) were discovered in the 1960s. Research with human volunteers at the Common Cold Unit near Salisbury, United Kingdom, showed that colds could be induced by nasal washings that did not contain rhinoviruses, a virus then known to be a cause of the common cold. Subsequent experiments where nasal swabs from these volunteers were inoculated onto organ cultures of the respiratory tract revealed the presence of enveloped viruses with the characteristic morphology of coronaviruses as previously described for IBV. The term *coronavirus* (Latin: *corona*, crown) was adopted for these agents, reflecting their characteristic fringed 'crown-like' appearance in the electron microscope after negative staining. Coronaviruses are now recognised in a range of animal species, causing respiratory, gastrointestinal, neurological and systemic diseases (Box 54.1).

Until the emergence of severe acute respiratory syndrome (SARS) in 2003, only two, HCoV 229E and OC43, were recognised as human pathogens. Both were causes of the common cold, considered a mild and insignificant illness and thus not a high priority for intensive research. Following the recognition that SARS was caused by a novel coronavirus, two other new HCoVs, NL63 and HKU1, were found in association with human respiratory disease. The renewed interest in this group of viruses has led to the discovery of a plethora of other animal coronaviruses in diverse species and stimulated research on their capacity to cross species barriers to infect new animal species. Initially discovered in 2012, Middle East respiratory syndrome (MERS) CoV is enzootic in dromedary camels and causes zoonotic respiratory disease in humans sometimes leading to outbreaks of human respiratory disease, especially within health-care facilities.

TAXONOMY

Coronaviruses and toroviruses are two virus genera within the virus family Coronaviridae, order Nidovirales. Coronaviruses are well-established pathogens of humans and animals, while toroviruses are recognised causes of animal diarrhoea. Toroviruses have also been found in human faeces, but their aetiological role remains unclear.

Coronaviruses are classified into four groups, initially based on antigenic relationships of the spike (S), membrane (M) and nucleocapsid (N) proteins and now reenforced by viral genetic phylogeny (Box 54.1). The HCoVs 229E and NL63 are classified as alphacoronaviruses, while OC43, HKU1, SARS and MERS coronaviruses are betacoronaviruses. Gammacoronaviruses are found in avian species, and the newly defined deltacoronaviruses include viruses found in passerine birds and swine. Genetic recombination readily occurs between members of the same and of

---

Box 54.1 Classification of coronaviruses

Alphacoronaviruses (previously group 1)
- Human coronavirus (HCoV) 229E
- Human coronavirus NL63
- Porcine transmissible gastroenteritis virus (TGEV)
- Canine coronavirus (CCoV)
- Feline infectious peritonitis virus (FIPV)
- Porcine epidemic diarrhoea virus (PEDV)
- Bat coronaviruses (e.g., 1A, HKU2)

Betacoronaviruses (previously group 2)
- Human coronavirus (HCoV) OC43
- Human coronavirus HKU1
- SARS coronavirus
- Rat coronavirus (RCoV)
- Rat sialodacryoadenitis virus (SDAV)
- Porcine haemagglutinating encephalomyelitis virus (HEV)
- Bovine coronavirus (BCoV)
- Mouse hepatitis virus (MHV)
- MERS coronavirus
- Bat coronaviruses (e.g., SARS-like coronavirus Rp3, HKU4, 229E-like bat coronavirus)

Gammacoronaviruses (previously group 3)
- Avian infectious bronchitis virus (IBV)
- Turkey coronavirus (TcoV)

Deltacoronaviruses
- Porcine coronavirus HKU15
- Thrush coronavirus HKU12

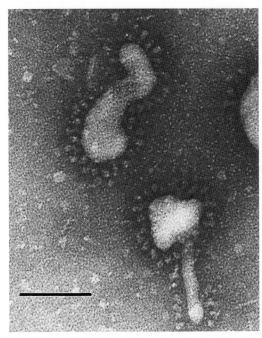

Fig. 54.1 Particles of HCoV 229E grown in human fibroblast cells and stained with 1.5% phosphotungstic acid. Bar = 100 nm.

PROPERTIES

MORPHOLOGY AND STRUCTURE

different coronavirus groups providing the opportunity for increased genetic diversity. Unlike other RNA viruses where an error prone RNA polymerase leads to a high mutation rate, coronaviruses have a proofreading mechanism that reduces mutation.

Efforts to identify the animal reservoir of SARS coronavirus led to the discovery of diverse bat coronaviruses in both alpha- and betacoronaviruses that are closely related phylogenetically to different mammalian coronaviruses. It has been proposed that bat and rodent coronaviruses may indeed have been the ancestors of most mammalian coronaviruses. Recent studies on the comparative evolution of animal and human coronaviruses have led to the conclusion that HCoV 229E and OC43, the causes of the common cold that are now globally endemic in humans, crossed species from their animal reservoirs (bats via dromedary camels in the case of 229E; cattle with OC43) to humans, probably within the past 1000 years or so, illustrating the fact that coronaviruses continue to cross species barriers to give rise to novel human diseases. SARS CoV and MERS CoV are recent examples of human pathogens to arise from the animal reservoir, but neither of them has become an endemic infection of humans so far.

Coronaviruses are pleomorphic and enveloped, varying between 60 and 220 nm in diameter in negatively stained virus particles. Club-shaped surface projections or peplomers (composed of trimers of spike [S] protein) of approximately 20 nm in length are seen in all species, giving the particles their characteristic fringed appearance (Fig. 54.1). Some betacoronaviruses (OC43, bovine coronavirus) have an additional shorter haemagglutinin-esterase protein on the virus surface that forms a distinct inner fringe of short peplomers.

Coronaviruses have a nonsegmented single-stranded positive-sense RNA genome of approximately 30 kb, making these the largest known RNA virus genomes. In the virion, viral RNA is complexed with nucleoprotein (N) in an extended helical nucleocapsid 9–11 nm in diameter. This is enclosed within a lipid-bilayer membrane envelope in association with a transmembrane protein (M), which is the most abundant virus structural protein. The spike (S) glycoprotein, smaller amounts of a nonglycosylated envelope (E) protein and, in some betacoronaviruses, also the haemagglutinin-esterase (HE) protein are also found on the virus envelope.

The S protein is the major inducer of neutralising antibody, although when it is present, the haemagglutinin-esterase protein is also a target for neutralising antibody. Monoclonal antibodies raised against M protein can neutralise infectivity in the presence of complement. Antigenic variation is a feature of the S protein, whereas the N protein is relatively conserved.

REPLICATION

Coronaviruses attach to their glycoprotein receptors on host cells via their S (and when present, HE) proteins. The tissue tropism of coronaviruses is mainly determined by the S1 part of the S protein and by the type and distribution of respective receptors on the cell surface. An illustrative example comes from veterinary virology. Transmissible gastroenteritis virus (TGEV) and porcine respiratory coronavirus (PRCV) are common causes of disease in pigs, the former causing gastrointestinal disease and the latter being a cause of respiratory disease. It has been found that PRCV arose from TGEV through a deletion in part of the S protein that dramatically altered the tropism of the virus from the gastrointestinal to the respiratory tract.

Alphacoronaviruses 229E and NL63 bind to the metalloproteases, human aminopeptidase N and angiotensin converting enzyme 2 (ACE-2), respectively. Some betacoronaviruses bind to 9-O-acetylated neuraminic acid molecules on the cell surface. However, SARS and MERS coronaviruses use ACE-2 and dipeptidyl peptidase (DPP4) (CD26), respectively, as receptors for virus binding and entry. Viral entry is mediated by fusion of the viral envelope with the host cell membrane or by receptor-mediated endocytosis. The fusion of the viral and cell membranes (either at the cell surface or within the endocytic vesicle) is mediated by the S2 portion of the virus spike protein that functions as a class 1 fusion protein.

Once the viral RNA is released into the cytoplasm, an RNA-dependent RNA polymerase translated from the plus-stranded viral genomic RNA makes a negative strand template from which it then synthesises a series of 3′ co-terminal nested genomic mRNAs. The viruses replicate in the cytoplasm with a growth cycle of 10–12 hours. Newly forming virions bud into the rough endoplasmic reticulum (where the M protein localises) and accumulate into intracytoplasmic vesicles (Fig. 54.2). These newly formed virions are transported via the Golgi apparatus to the plasma membrane where they are released by exocytosis. Viral infection may result in cell lysis, or fusion of adjacent cells may lead to the formation of syncytia.

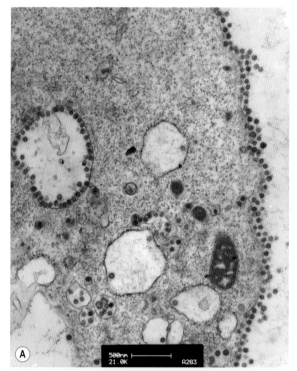

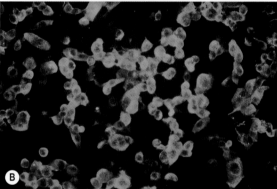

Fig. 54.2 (A) Thin section transmission electron microscopy of cells infected with SARS CoV showing virus particles in intracellular vesicles and on cell surface. Bar = 500 nm. (Courtesy Dr J. M. Nicholls.) (B) Immunofluorescence reaction of a serum from a patient with SARS on SARS CoV-infected cells. (Courtesy Dr K. H. Chan.)

PATHOGENESIS

Infection with the common cold coronaviruses leads to loss of ciliary action (ciliostasis) and degenerative changes affecting the cilia of epithelial cells of the respiratory tract. Direct cell cytolysis is not prominent, although this may also contribute to pathogenesis. The mechanisms of pathogenesis of HKU1 and NL63 are not yet well studied. SARS CoV and MERS CoV target type 1 and type 2 alveolar epithelial cells of the lung and also differentiated bronchial epithelial cells. The desquamation of alveolar epithelial cells leads to hyaline membrane formation within the alveoli and diffuse alveolar damage, the histological hallmark of acute respiratory distress syndrome (ARDS). Innate immune dysregulation contributes to the pathology of SARS and MERS. The severity of SARS and MERS infection increases with age and underlying co-morbidities. Interestingly, severity of SARS CoV in experimentally infected mice and primates also increases with age. The SARS CoV also infects the intestinal epithelium and the virus is shed in the faeces. The diarrhoea associated with SARS infection may be related, in part, to direct infection of the intestinal tract.

A possible link between multiple sclerosis and coronaviruses has been investigated for some time. The genomes of *Coronavirus* 229E and OC43 have been detected in the brain tissue of patients with multiple sclerosis. However, these virus genomes are also detected in persons dying of nonneurological causes, and thus the aetiological link between coronaviruses and neurological disease in humans seems unclear. Some animal coronaviruses, such as variants of mouse hepatitis virus, can cause demyelinating CNS disease following experimental infection in the mouse.

TRANSMISSION

The primary route of transmission of human coronaviruses is via infected respiratory droplets. Experimental transmission of disease was demonstrated by the intranasal inoculation of adult human volunteers with 229E and OC43. These viruses have also caused outbreaks of nosocomial disease. Implementing contact and droplet precautions reduced its transmission in health-care settings suggesting that respiratory droplets and direct or indirect contact was the major route of transmission. There is evidence of small-particle aerosol (long-range) airborne transmission associated with aerosol generating procedures (e.g., use of nebulisers, intubation, high-flow oxygen therapy). SARS coronavirus is also excreted in faeces. Aerosolised faecal material from a faulty sewage system has been proposed as the mechanism of spread in one high-rise housing estate in Hong Kong where one index case led to many hundreds of secondary cases. SARS CoV and MERS CoV retain infectivity on smooth surfaces for longer than some other human respiratory coronaviruses or other respiratory viruses suggesting the potential importance of fomites and indirect contact as additional modes of transmission.

EPIDEMIOLOGY

Studies using virus detection or serology have shown that HCoV 229E, OC43 and NL63 occur worldwide.

Although data on HKU1 are more limited, it too has a global distribution and has been found wherever it has been diligently sought. Initial infections occur early in life, but reinfection continues to occur at all ages. There is no cross-protection between different types of coronavirus and immunity to the same virus type is short lived, with reinfection being documented within a few months. They have a winter-spring seasonality in temperate and subtropical climates. In contrast to viruses such as influenza or RSV, which cause predictable annual outbreaks, the contribution of each HCoV may vary widely from year to year, for example, 229E contributing as little as 1% to acute respiratory infections in the community in 1 year and up to 35% in the next. Furthermore, activity may be heterogeneous in different geographical regions of the same country.

SARS AND MERS CORONAVIRUS

The epidemiology of SARS CoV and MERS CoV deserves special mention because it highlights the emergence and control of novel human infectious diseases arising from zoonotic reservoirs. SARS CoV emerged from a precursor virus, which is endemic in insectivorous bats. The close proximity of different animal species (including bats) within large live game-animal markets that service the restaurant trade for exotic food in southern China allowed the bat SARS CoV-like precursor virus to adapt to other mammalian species (civet cats, raccoon dogs) and, subsequently, to humans. Initial clusters of transmission in late 2002 were not sustained, but the virus finally adapted to efficient human transmission leading to large outbreaks of disease in Guangdong Province, China, in February 2003. One infected patient from Guangdong travelled to Hong Kong and stayed 1 day at a hotel there leading to the infection of 15 other guests who travelled onwards to Toronto, Singapore, Hanoi and elsewhere, seeding chains of secondary transmission in different parts of the world. Within months, the outbreak had spread to 29 countries and regions causing over 8000 human cases and almost 800 deaths. By July 2003, determined and coordinated global public health measures of case identification and isolation had interrupted transmission in humans.

MERS CoV was first recognised in a patient with fatal viral pneumonia in Saudi Arabia in 2012. The virus is enzootic in dromedary camels, and zoonotic transmission continues to be reported in the Arabian Peninsula. Sometimes, transmission between humans can lead to outbreaks, especially within health-care facilities, sometimes involving hundreds of patients. Patients acquiring infection in the Arabian Peninsula have caused disease outbreaks elsewhere; for example, in 2015, a returning traveller who acquired infection in the Middle East gave rise to an outbreak involving 186 patients in the Republic of Korea, with a case fatality ratio of >19%.

CLINICAL FEATURES

Around 25% of common colds are associated with 229E and OC43 and are second only to rhinoviruses as the cause of this syndrome. Human volunteer studies have established that the incubation period is around 2 days, with peak symptoms occurring at 3–4 days postinfection. Subclinical or mild infections are common. The symptoms of nasal discharge, mild sore throat, sneezing, sometimes together with headache and general malaise last for 6–7 days. Fever and cough are found in a minority of cases. Around 10% of children with otitis media have evidence of coronavirus infection. Coronaviruses have also been found in some patients with lower respiratory tract infections but as they may also be found in a proportion of asymptomatic controls, their aetiological role is difficult to establish. HCoV 229E, OC43, NL63 and HKU1 have all been identified in bronchoalveolar lavages in immunocompromised patients with lower respiratory tract disease suggesting that they contribute to severe respiratory illness in these patients. Serological studies have shown an association between coronavirus infections and exacerbations of respiratory symptoms in adults with underlying respiratory diseases or asthma. HCoV infections in the elderly with underlying respiratory disease may lead to lower respiratory tract disease although rarely severe enough to warrant hospitalisation.

NL63 and HKU1 have been associated with a range of symptoms including fever, cough, rhinorrhoea, pharyngitis, bronchiolitis, pneumonia and febrile seizures. NL63 has also been strongly implicated as a cause of croup. Between 50% and 80% of patients with HKU1 infections have other underlying diseases.

SARS AND MERS CORONAVIRUSES

The incubation period of SARS and MERS is estimated to be 2–14 days. The disease presents as fever, myalgia, chills and a cough of acute onset leading to a rapidly progressing viral pneumonia. Upper respiratory symptoms of rhinorrhoea and sore throat are less common. Some patients have watery diarrhoea. Evidence of unilateral or bilateral consolidation of the lungs is seen on radiographic examination. Some patients progress to increasing tachypnoea, oxygen desaturation and respiratory distress syndrome. Moderate liver dysfunction and marked lymphopenia can be seen. The overall case fatality rate of SARS was 9.6%, the severity of disease increasing with age and with the presence of underlying comorbidities. The case fatality

ratio of currently reported MERS patients is around 40% overall, but this is likely skewed by recognition of more severely ill patients who are older and with comorbidities. Infection in young healthy adults can be asymptomatic or mild.

GASTROINTESTINAL DISEASE CAUSED BY CORONAVIRUSES AND TOROVIRUSES

Coronavirus-like particles have been detected by electron microscopy in stool from diarrhoeal as well as healthy subjects and their role in diarrhoeal disease has remained controversial. A few human enteric coronaviruses (HECoVs) have been successfully cultured in human embryonic intestinal organ culture. They appear to be endemic throughout the world, with a higher prevalence in developing countries. In Western countries the prevalence is high in travellers from developing countries and in low socioeconomic groups, and is markedly higher in men who have sex with men (MSM) than in the general population. There is strong circumstantial evidence that HECoVs are spread by the enteric or faecal–oral route. The observed high prevalence among Western MSM may be explained by oral–anal–genital contact.

More recently, HKU1 has been detected in stool as well as the respiratory tract of patients with diarrhoeal syndromes by molecular methods, and it is possible that this virus disseminates beyond the respiratory tract.

Toroviruses (a distinct genus within the family Coronaviridae; see section on TAXONOMY) have also been found in association with gastroenteritis in humans. Clinically, these cases were less likely to manifest with vomiting and more likely to have a bloody diarrhoea and were more common in the immunocompromised.

LABORATORY INVESTIGATION

Respiratory specimens are the specimens of choice. While upper respiratory specimens are optimal in patients with upper respiratory tract infection, lower respiratory specimens (sputum, tracheal aspirates, bronchoalveolar lavage) may be required in patients with severe lower respiratory tract diseases, for example, MERS. Some coronaviruses (HKU1, SARS CoV, enteric coronaviruses) can also be detected in stool specimens. Prior to the emergence of SARS and MERS, coronaviruses were regarded as insignificant pathogens and routine laboratory diagnosis was not regarded as important. Furthermore, isolation of coronaviruses from clinical specimens is technically challenging, some of them requiring inoculation onto organ cultures of human embryonic trachea (e.g., OC43-like viruses) or special cell lines (e.g., human embryonic lung fibroblasts, HUH7, LLC-MK2, Vero E6) together with multiple subpassages for their detection, procedures not readily amenable to routine diagnostic practice. The human hepatoma cell line HUH7 has been recently used for primary isolation of OC43, 229E and HKU1 viruses from clinical specimens, and NL63 has been isolated in LLC-MK2 and Vero B4 cells. SARS and MERS CoVs are best isolated in Vero E6 cells. Some avian and mammalian (not human) coronaviruses can be cultivated readily in embryonated eggs. Some coronaviruses have the ability to haemagglutinate red blood cells, a property that has been used to detect their growth in cell cultures. Direct antigen detection of virus-infected cells in clinical specimens is feasible, but validated reagents are not commercially available and the method is not frequently used.

Detection of CoV viral RNA by RT-PCR is now the most widely used method for diagnosis. Specific primers for detecting 229E, OC43, NL63, HKU, SARS and MERS CoV have been reported. There are also consensus coronavirus-specific primers that are broadly reactive with many human and animal coronavirus types and these have been used to detect novel coronaviruses (for example, HKU1 was initially detected this way), but they are typically less sensitive than good type-specific primers.

Electron microscopy of negatively stained stool specimens is useful for the detection of enteric coronaviruses and toroviruses. The two types of viruses are similar in size and may be difficult to distinguish by electron microscopic morphology, but toroviruses typically exhibit a doughnut-like or rodlike appearance unlike typical coronaviruses.

Complement fixation, ELISA assays, immunofluorescence or virus neutralisation tests have been used for serological diagnosis and for seroepidemiology of coronavirus infections.

CASE STUDY OF THE DISCOVERY OF A NEW HUMAN PATHOGEN, SARS CORONAVIRUS

Although SARS is no longer circulating in the human population, its emergence and control are summarised because this is illustrative of the challenges posed by novel emerging infections. In 2003, a novel severe progressive 'viral-like pneumonia' emerged in Guangdong Province, southern China. There were no pathognomonic features except a propensity to lead to clusters of disease in close contacts including health-care workers. Initial investigations of suspected cases did not find conclusive evidence of known respiratory pathogens. Clusters of cases were also reported in Hong Kong, Hanoi, Singapore and Toronto, leading World Health Organization (WHO) to issue a global alert. The disease was named severe acute respiratory syndrome (SARS), and a case definition was established. WHO set up a worldwide network of virological laboratories investigating SARS cases that discussed their results in daily teleconferences. Approaches taken to identify a novel pathogen included virus isolation (including cell lines not typically used to grow respiratory pathogens) and electron microscopy (EM) on respiratory specimens including lung tissue obtained at open-lung biopsy or autopsy. Immunological methods for virus detection require specific antibodies reactive with the virus and PCR or RT-PCR methods predicate knowledge of the viral genetic sequence upon which PCR primers are based, information and reagents not available in the context of the emergence of a novel pathogen. However, "consensus primers" targeting regions of the viral genome conserved across viral genera or families, low stringency PCR and PCR using random primers are feasible approaches to detect novel pathogens and were deployed in the hunt for the aetiological agent of SARS. Technologies such as NexGen 'deep' sequencing that can now be deployed to detect novel viral genetic sequences in clinical specimens were not available in 2003. The initial findings independently came from three laboratories within the WHO network isolating a cytopathic effect–causing agent in fetal rhesus kidney cell lines or Vero E6 cells. Thin section EM revealed that these cells were indeed infected with a virus (Fig. 54.2A), and immunofluorescence tests showed that this agent was not reactive with antibodies to previously known respiratory pathogens. EM of negatively stained preparations of ultracentrifuged deposits of infected cells showed particles that were compatible in size and morphology to coronaviruses. EM of lung-biopsy tissue also revealed virus-like particles of comparable size. PCR amplicons generated by random primer-based RT-PCR assays on infected and noninfected cells were compared, and those unique to virus-infected cells were genetically sequenced. Some sequences were found to have homology to those of the family Coronaviridae. In immunofluorescent tests using virus-infected cells, sera collected early in the course of illness from these patients (acute sera) failed to react, whereas convalescent sera from patients with suspected SARS gave a strong reaction (Fig. 54.2B), suggesting seroconversion to the novel virus in patients with this novel disease. Control sera from an uninfected population had no antibody to this newly isolated virus. Taken together, these provided strong circumstantial evidence of an association between the coronavirus isolated in cell culture and SARS. The partial virus genetic sequence was then used to design specific RT-PCR assays, and the virus-infected cells were used as substrates for serological diagnosis in immunofluorescence tests and enzyme-linked immunosorbent assays (ELISAs). Koch's postulates were fulfilled by infecting macaques with the isolated virus and reproducing a disease similar to SARS. A short while later, the full genome of the novel pathogen was elucidated, confirming thereby that the aetiological agent of SARS was indeed a novel pathogen within betacoronaviruses.

CONTROL

Given the sheer number of common cold episodes, their inconvenience and economic impact, prophylactic strategies that target coronaviruses and rhinoviruses (the two common aetiological agents of this syndrome) would be attractive. The recognition that coronaviruses, especially SARS and MERS coronavirus, can cause severe lower respiratory illnesses re-enforces this need. However, there are no validated antiviral drugs or vaccines to treat or prevent coronavirus infections so far.

TREATMENT

During the outbreak of SARS, given its severity and high mortality rates, a number of therapeutic options including ribavirin, interferon alpha, lopinavir/ritonavir, and nucleoside analogue protease inhibitor combination therapy were all tried. While there is evidence of activity in vitro, these drugs were not evaluated in controlled clinical trials and their therapeutic benefit remains uncertain. Some of these therapeutic modalities have also been tried with MERS, but, again, controlled clinical trial data of efficacy are not available. Passive immunotherapy using convalescent human plasma was evaluated in SARS and, more recently, with MERS. Monoclonal or polyclonal antibodies that neutralise MERS CoV are also being developed and evaluated in experimental animal models.

PREVENTION

Attempts to control transmissible gastroenteritis virus of pigs and feline coronavirus of cats through the use of vaccines have not been successful. Vaccines for the avian disease infectious bronchitis virus are available but have modest benefit. The fact that natural infections with 229E or OC43 do not provide long-lasting immunity is instructive in this regard. Thus, so far, there is no vaccine for a HCoV that is in clinical use. The severity of SARS led to a concerted effort to develop vaccines for SARS CoV, and a range of vaccine strategies including inactivated whole-virus vaccines, spike-subunit vaccines, DNA vaccines and vaccinia or parainfluenza virus type 3 vectored vaccines have all been tried in experimental animal models, with some providing evidence of efficacy. It has been established that antibody to the spike protein is the key correlate of protection in animal models. However, as there is perceived to be no imminent public health threat from SARS, few of these vaccines have been taken to human clinical trials.

A number of vaccine strategies for MERS are currently being evaluated in experimental animal models and in phase 1 clinical trials. Since dromedary camels are the source of zoonotic human infection, experimental vaccines for use in dromedaries are also in development. While such vaccines have been effective in reducing virus shedding in experimental studies in camels, it remains to be seen if they will prevent MERS CoV reinfection in field settings.

RECOMMENDED READING

Bradburne, A. F., Bynoe, M. L., & Tyrrell, D. A. (1967). Effects of a 'new' human respiratory virus in volunteers. *British Medical Journal*, *3*(5568), 767–769.

Coleman, C. M., & Frieman, M. B. (2014). Coronaviruses: important emerging human pathogens. *Journal of Virology*, *88*(10), 5209–5212. doi:10.1128/JVI.03488-13.

Falsey, A. R., Walsh, E. E., & Hayden, F. G. (2002). Rhinoviruses and coronavirus infection-associated hospitalization among older adults. *The Journal of Infectious Diseases*, *185*(9), 1338–1341.

Peiris, J. S. M. (2017). Coronaviruses. Ch. 52. In D. D. Richman, R. J. Whitley, & F. G. Hayden (Eds.), *Clinical virology* (4th ed.). Washington DC: ASM Press.

Perlman, S., & Netland, J. (2009). Coronaviruses post-SARS: update on replication and pathogenesis. *Nature Reviews. Microbiology*, *7*(6), 439–450. doi:10.1038/nrmicro2147.

van der Hoek, L. (2007). Human coronaviruses: What do they cause? *Antiviral Therapy*, *12*(4 Pt. B), 651–658.

55 Rhabdoviruses

GUANGHUI WU, ASHLEY C. BANYARD AND ANTHONY R. FOOKS

KEY POINTS

- Rabies should be made notifiable in endemic regions with notifiability driving the development of diagnostic capability.
- Rabies has the highest case-fatality rate (100%) of any infectious disease once clinical signs are observed. There are at least 60,000 cases annually worldwide.
- Over 99% of human rabies infections are due to bites from a rabid dog. Most of these occur in developing countries, and almost 50% occur in children.
- Vaccination of people in high-risk groups (laboratory workers, animal handlers and those travelling to rabies-endemic areas) is recommended.
- Pre- and post-exposure vaccination (PEP) is available and both are extremely effective; however, PEP is expensive, and scarce in areas where it is needed most.
- Reducing the risk of rabies virus transmission to humans means implementation of vaccination schemes for both domestic animals and wildlife.
- In high-risk areas, rabies control efforts must focus on the elimination of rabies in domestic dog populations.

The rhabdoviruses belong to the order Mononegavirales, family Rhabdoviridae, and as such they contain a single stranded negative-sense RNA as their genome. The Rhabdoviridae comprise 13 genera including: *Ephemerovirus, Lyssavirus, Tibrovirus* and *Vesiculovirus* that infect mammals, *Cytorhabdovirus, Dichorhavirus, Nucleorhabdovirus* and *Varicosavirus* that infect plants, *Novirhabdovirus, Perhabdovirus* and *Sprivivirus* that infect fish, *Tupavirus* that infects birds and *Sigmavirus* that infects insects. There are also four species not yet assigned to a genus. All have nonsegmented genomes, with the exception of viruses in the genera *Dichorhavirus* and *Varicosavirus*, which have bipartite genomes. Only viruses within the

Lyssavirus and *Vesiculovirus* genera are known to infect both animals and humans and cause clinical disease. The lyssaviruses include one of the most notable viruses known to humans, rabies virus (RABV). Because of the importance of rabies virus in shaping modern virology from ancient beginnings, this virus will be the main focus of the remainder of this chapter. First described in Mesopotamia in 2300 BC, rabies has been recognised for many centuries as an almost invariably fatal disease once clinical signs have developed. Disease presents with an acute encephalomyelitis, often preceded by periods of excitement or agitation, and is quickly followed by coma and death. Hypersalivation, hydrophobia and aerophobia are also prominent features.

VIRUS STRUCTURE AND LIFE CYCLE

Virion morphology

The *Lyssavirus* genus includes rabies virus and 13 other recognised species, differentiated according to their genomic sequence. Two further isolates Gannoruwa bat lyssavirus (GBLV) and Lleida virus (LLEIV) are awaiting official classification (Table 55.1). First established by Pierre Galtier as a transmissible agent in 1879, the rabies virion is bullet shaped in appearance, with an average diameter of approximately 75 nm (60–110 nm), an average length of 180 nm (130–200 nm) and a helical symmetry (Fig. 55.1).

Virus genome structure

The *Lyssavirus* genome is composed of approximately 12,000 nucleotides of RNA (Fig. 55.2). This contains all the information necessary to produce five viral proteins: nucleoprotein (N), phosphoprotein (P), matrix protein (M), glycoprotein (G), and large polymerase protein (L). The viral ribonucleoprotein core (RNP) consists of the viral RNA encapsulated by the N protein and associated with the P and L proteins. This RNP is the minimal replicative

Table 55.1 Lyssaviruses

Virus	Phylogroup (Location)	Species from which isolated
Aravan Virus (ARAV)	I (Eurasia)	Insectivorous bats
Australian Bat Lyssavirus (ABLV)	I (Australia)	Frugivorous and insectivorous bats, horses and humans
Bokeloh Bat Lyssavirus (BBLV)	I (Europe)	Insectivorous bats
Duvenhage Virus (DUVV)	I (Africa)	Insectivorous bats and humans
European Bat Lyssavirus Type-1 (EBLV-1)	I (Europe)	Insectivorous bats, sheep, a stone marten and humans
European Bat Lyssavirus Type-2 (EBLV-2)	I (Europe)	Insectivorous bats and humans
Gannoruwa Bat Lyssavirus (GBLV)[a]	I (Asia)	Frugivorous bats
Ikoma Lyssavirus (IKOV)	III (Africa)	African civet
Irkut Virus (IRKV)	I (Eurasia)	Insectivorous bats
Khujand Virus (KHUV)	I (Eurasia)	Insectivorous bats
Lagos Bat Virus (LBV)	II (Africa)	Frugivorous bats, dogs and cats
Lleida Bat Lyssavirus (LLEIV)[a]	III (Europe)	Insectivorous bat
Mokola Virus (MOKV)	II (Africa)	Shrews, cats, dogs, rodents and humans
Rabies Virus (RABV)	I (Global)	Wide range of mammals
Shimoni Bat Virus (SHIBV)	II (Africa)	Insectivorous bats
West Caucasian Bat Virus (WCBV)	III (Europe)	Insectivorous bats

[a]Not yet formally recognised as species.

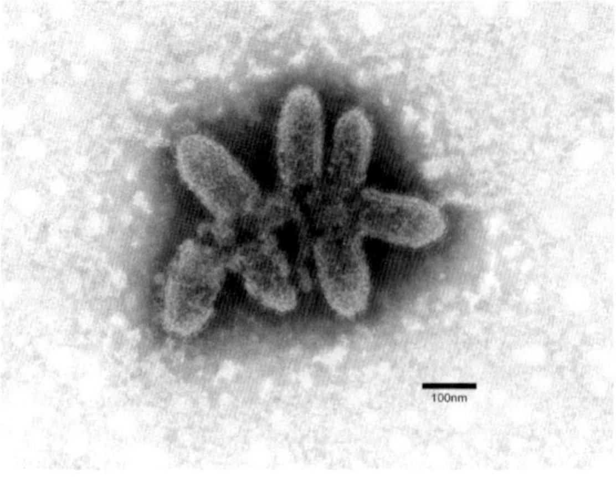

Fig. 55.1 Electron micrograph of RABV virions.

unit for these viruses. The other viral proteins, M and G, are involved in maintaining virion structure and attachment to cellular receptors, respectively.

Viral life cycle

Infection is initiated when the virus envelope glycoprotein (G) attaches to a cell receptor on the host cell. This process, known as adsorption, involves the interaction of the glycoprotein spikes, the major determinants for virus neuropathogenicity, with cell surface receptors. The virus may then enter the cell through a number of mechanisms. Experimental studies show that RABV may or may not replicate at the inoculation site before it invades the central nervous system (CNS). When a rabies virus enters a neuronal cell, the G protein, in combination with undefined host cell and viral proteins, mediates the retrograde transportation of virus along the axon to the cell body where uncoating is triggered by a change in local pH. Transcription and replication occurs in the cell body.

The RNP complex contains all of the components to activate viral transcription. The virion RNA polymerase (L) can both transcribe and replicate the viral RNA while it is in the RNP form. The five viral proteins are encoded on individual monocistronic messenger RNAs (mRNA). These mRNAs are transcribed, capped, methylated and polyadenylated by enzymes packaged within the virion. Transcription proceeds following attachment of the polymerase complex to the genome promoter at the terminal 3' end of the genome. The transcriptase complex produces transcripts of each gene with a transcriptional gradient arising from polymerase dissociation with viral template at specific gene boundaries. This results in a much greater expression of 3' proximal genes. Following transcription, the mRNAs are processed using the host cell translational machinery. Dense areas of the cell, referred to as 'Negri bodies', represent inclusion bodies where viral transcription and replication take place.

Following the accumulation of viral proteins, the composition of the viral polymerase complex alters, resulting in a switch from transcription to replication. Once the polymerase is in a replicative mode, the complex initially drives the production of full-length antigenome (positive) sense strands of RNA, ignoring the transcriptional signals present at each of the gene boundaries. The positive-sense antigenome strand serves as a template for the formation of nascent genome (negative) sense RNA. Because of the relative strength of genome and antigenome promoter regions at genome termini, the ratio of negative-stranded RNA and positive-stranded RNA is approximately 50:1.

The negative-sense genomic RNA encapsulated by the N protein forms the RNP core. Interactions between M

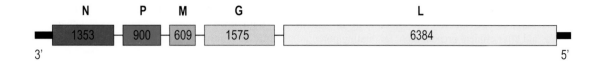

		3' UTR*	N protein	N–P	P protein	P–M	M protein	M–G	G protein	G–L	L protein	5' UTR	Genome
Phylogroup I	RABV	70	1353	90-1	894	87-89	609	211-5	1575	516-522	6384	130-133	11,923-8
	ABLV	70	1353	94	894	89	609	207-209	1578-81	508-509	6384	131	11,918
	GBLV	70	1353	92	894	88	609	212	1581	505	6384	131	11,919
	EBLV-1	70	1356	90	897	83	609	211	1575	560	6384	131	11,966
	EBLV-2	70	1356	101	894	88	609	210 (205)	1575	512	6384	131	11,930
	BBLV	70	1356	93	894	86	609	210	1575	496	6384	129	11,902
	DUVV	70	1356	90	897	83	609	191	1602	562-563	6384	130-131	11,975-6
	ARAV	70	1356	85	894	85	609	210	1581	514	6384	130	11,918
	KHUV	70	1356	95	894	72	609	208	1581	504	6384	130	11,903
	IRKV	70	1356	92	897	83	609	214	1575	569	6384	131	11,980
Phylogroup II	SHIBV	70	1353	98	918	76	609	205	1569	613	6384	150	12,045
	LBV	70	1353	101-103	918	73-76	609	204	1569	574-588	6384	143-146	12,003-16
	MOKV	70	1353	100-102	912	80-81	609	203-204	1569	546-563	6384	112-114	11,940-57
Phylogroup III	WCBV	70	1353	64	894	133	609	206	1578	862	6384	125	12,278
	IKOV	70	1353	66	870	74	609	209	1575	569	6381	126	11,902
	LLEBV	70	1353	68	870	74	609	198	1578	608	6381	122	11,931

Fig. 55.2 Schematic representation of rabies virus genome, with approximate genome sizes (in nucleotides) for representatives of all proposed lyssavirus species. *UTR, untranslated region.

and the RNP are thought to enable relocation of nascent RNPs to areas of the plasma membrane in which the glycoprotein is embedded. Once associated with the glycoprotein, the condensed M-RNP forms a complete virion that buds from the plasma membrane and is released from the cell.

VIRUS TRANSMISSION, PATHOGENESIS AND TREATMENT

The inability of RABV to penetrate the dermal barrier means that it has to gain entry through broken skin (often as a result of a bite) or through mucous membranes (eyes, nose and mouth). In many developing countries, where canine immunisation programs are minimal or nonexistent, dogs are the predominant source of human infection, and dog-derived rabies accounts for 99% of human rabies cases worldwide. In regions where canine rabies has been controlled by vaccination, wild animal bites represent the main source of human infection. Bat bites are also a source of concern throughout the world, as these are often small and may go unnoticed.

There have also been reports of rabies infection due to aerosolised virus, either following exposure in caves containing large numbers of potentially infected bats or

following accidental laboratory exposure. Experimental aerosol transmission has been reported using a murine model, although such transmission is most likely through infection of external mucosae. Transfer of infection via infected corneal transplants and other organs has also been reported. In 2004 in the United States, transplantation of kidneys, liver and an arterial segment from a donor who died from unexplained encephalitis resulted in the deaths of the transplant recipients from RABV. A history of bat bite was subsequently identified in the donor. Another death from rabies happened in 2013 after an organ transplantation in 2011. Both donor and recipient had the same raccoon strain of rabies virus. A similar situation occurred in Germany in 2005. In 2015, two rabies deaths in China were probably the result of receiving kidneys from the same donor who was diagnosed with possible viral encephalitis. Even though virus has been shown to be excreted in both saliva and conjunctival exudates, direct transmission of virus following person-to-person spread is extremely rare, although vertical transmission from mother to child has been reported.

After entering the body, lyssaviruses spread through the chain of neuronal connections via synaptic junctions within the CNS. Once the brain is infected, high levels of virus replication occur, and typically the virus spreads centrifugally to the peripheral and autonomic nervous system reaching all innervated organs including the salivary glands. Virus can be detected intermittently in saliva both before and after clinical presentation, facilitating potential transmission to another host.

The precise cause of death following lyssavirus infection is often not fully established. Overwhelming virus replication in the nervous system leads to many systemic complications, including multiorgan failure. Heart failure is often cited as the cause of death. No effective treatment is available once virus has reached the brain.

Antibodies induced by preimmunisation alone can mediate viral clearance from the CNS, although in cases of late-stage disease, the detection of neutralising antibodies in cerebrospinal fluid is not enough to prevent death. Other immune effector mechanisms, such as innate immune responses, also play a role in virus clearance, although such responses are largely undefined. An immune response is not usually detected until the virus has entered the CNS. It is not clear how the virus avoids immune surveillance in the periphery, but this might be due to low-level replication early in infection as well as virus-mediated immune suppression. The P protein is known to play a role in evading the immune system by acting as an interferon (IFN) antagonist

Despite having a case fatality rate nearing 100%, there are only a few reported cases of recovery from rabies once clinical signs have developed. Of these, four were treated with the Milwaukee protocol or variations thereof. This procedure includes the induction of a therapeutic coma and administration of a cocktail of drugs including ketamine, midazolam, ribavirin and amantadine to reduce both viral replication and host responses that might be detrimental to recovery. However, in the majority of cases, the application of the Milwaukee protocol has been unsuccessful. Most documented survivors had received one or more doses of rabies vaccine prior to the onset of the disease and this most likely contributed to survival. Currently, several new treatments are being developed and evaluated, including antiviral molecules (e.g., favipiravir, RNA interference, and molecules that target viral components and their activities), immunotherapy, neuroprotective therapy, substances for opening up the blood–brain and blood–spinal cord barriers, and the application of therapeutic hypothermia.

CLINICAL FEATURES

The incubation period following infection can vary considerably. For dogs and cats it is generally between 2 and 12 weeks, although longer incubation periods have been reported. In humans, it is typically 2–8 weeks, but may vary from weeks to, on rare occasions, several years. The first neurological symptoms in humans include pain, paraesthesia, or pruritus at the site of infection due to

viral replication in local dorsal root ganglia and associated ganglionitis. As the disease progresses, either the encephalitic or paralytic forms of the disease may be observed. Clinical forms of the disease often present with agitation and hypersalivation. In animals, clinical signs vary considerably, though two forms typically present. The aggressive form may include sudden behavioural changes, aggression, lack of inhibition and excessive salivation. Alternatively, a docile, paralytic or flaccid form of disease may present, where the principal symptoms include depression, unusual docile behaviour, facial paralysis extending to the throat and neck, causing abnormal facial expressions, drooling and an inability to swallow. Regardless, all established infections lead to a progressive paralysis of the entire body and ultimately death.

EPIDEMIOLOGY

Rabies is present on all continents, with the exception of Antarctica. Extensive control measures including vaccination campaigns in both dog and terrestrial wildlife populations have reduced the incidence of rabies across the globe and eliminated rabies in domestic carnivores in North America and Western Europe. However, the virus remains endemic across much of the developing world, where the majority (99%) of human deaths due to rabies occur, mainly in Africa and Asia where the WHO estimates an annual death toll of 59,000. Importantly, a high proportion of infections occur in children under the age of 16, often in poor rural areas where vaccine and postexposure prophylaxis are not readily available.

The epidemiological knowledge regarding rabies infection in endemic areas is sparse, and data are usually based on clinical reports and test results from material submitted to public health or veterinary diagnostic laboratories. A general lack of diagnostic capability in endemic regions means that the actual number of rabies infections is likely to be a gross underestimate. Figures for the infection of both domestic and wildlife species are not available.

In endemic areas across Africa and Asia, unowned, unlicensed free-roaming dogs are the main reservoir for rabies, causing fatalities in both humans and animals. Sylvatic rabies, which refers to the spread of disease amongst wildlife, generally poses less of a threat to the human population in endemic areas where dog-derived rabies predominates. Although rabies can infect all mammals, sylvatic spread is usually confined to particular species depending on the region. For example, rabies is reported in red foxes *(Vulpes vulpes)* in continental Europe, Canada and southern states of the United States, in arctic foxes *(Vulpes lagopus)* in Arctic areas, in the yellow mongoose *(Cynictis penicillata)* populations of the West

Indies and Africa, in raccoon dogs *(Nyctereutes procyonoides)* and ferret badgers *(Melogale moschata)* in China, and in African wild dogs *(Lycaon pictus)* and Ethiopian wolves *(Canis simensis)* in Africa.

In areas free of terrestrial rabies, reintroduction of the disease from endemic areas can occur. Recent examples of incursions of disease into the European Union include the illegal importation of a rabid Algerian dog into France in 2015, and a rabid dog attacking several people in Spain in 2013 after being smuggled in from Morocco. From a UK perspective, 26 human cases of rabies were reported between 1946 and 2016. The majority of these cases were acquired abroad. However, the death in 2002 of a bat conservationist in Scotland due to infection with an indigenous bat lyssavirus, European bat lyssavirus type-2 (EBLV-2), was a notable exception.

Terrestrial rabies has been eliminated from most regions of Western Europe. During the last 10 years approximately 80,000 cases of rabies were reported across Europe, the majority being reported in Eastern European countries including the Russian Federation (34.3%), Ukraine (24.5%), Belarus (10.3%), Croatia (6.0%), Romania (5.8%), Lithuania (5.6%) and Turkey (5.0%). Of these, 45% of cases were detected in domesticated animals, 55% in wildlife species, with a comparatively low number of human and bat cases. There has been a substantial decrease in reported rabies cases in these countries in recent years, apart from the Russian Federation and Turkey.

Having eliminated terrestrial rabies in domesticated animals, more than 90% of all animal cases reported in the United States occur in wildlife species. In 2014, 6033 rabies cases were reported to the Centers for Disease Control and Prevention (CDC). The sylvatic rabies included cases in racoons (30.2%) along the US eastern seaboard, bats (29.1%), skunks (26.3%) in the Midwestern states and foxes (4.1%) in southern states. As there is limited contact between these wild species and humans, spread is mostly to susceptible wildlife. US cases in domestic animals accounted for 7.37% (n = 445) of the total, including 59 from dogs, 272 from cats, 78 from cattle and 25 from horses and mules during 2014. On average, two or three cases of human rabies are reported in the United States each year.

In contrast to RABV, other lyssaviruses have been detected on fewer occasions, with only a handful of genetically confirmed detections. All lyssaviruses, with the exception of Mokola Virus (MOKV) and Ikoma Lyssavirus (IKOV), have been isolated from bat species (Table 55.1). An unexplained epidemiological conundrum is that RABV is present in both terrestrial carnivores and bat species across the Americas, whilst no other lyssaviruses have been detected there. In contrast, RABV is present in terrestrial carnivores across the Old World, but has never been detected in bats, whilst the other 13 lyssavirus species have been detected exclusively in the Old World, predominantly in bat species. Importantly, across the European Union the threat to the human population from these viruses is considered to be low. However, because of the inability to prevent infection in bat populations, and the protected nature of European bat species, the threat of spillover events into humans or terrestrial carnivores remains ever present.

In Central and Western Europe, although fox rabies has been eliminated through oral vaccination, four lyssaviruses have been detected within bat populations. European bat lyssavirus type-1 (EBLV- 1) is present in Europe as two distinct genetic lineages, EBLV-1a and EBLV-1b. Most of the EBLV-1 cases in European bats have been identified in one bat species, *Eptesicus serotinus,* which habituates both the United Kingdom and mainland Europe and is generally regarded as the host species for EBLV-1. European bat lyssavirus type-2 (EBLV-2) was first isolated in 1985 from a Swiss bat biologist who had been working with bats in Finland, Switzerland and Malaysia. A year later this virus was isolated from bats in Denmark *(Myotis daubentonii* and *M. dasycneme)* and from *M. daubentonii* in Germany, the only known natural wild host for this virus (apart from a single case in *N. noctula).* Both EBLV-1 and EBLV-2 cause disease in mammals, including companion animals, wildlife and domestic livestock. EBLV-1 has been shown to cause disease in sheep, foxes, a stone marten, ferrets, cats and dogs. In contrast, EBLV-2 has not been detected naturally in mammals other than bats and humans. Two novel lyssaviruses have also been included within the genus—Bokeloh bat virus (BBLV) was isolated from Natterer's bats *(Myotis nattereri)* in Germany in 2010, and an unclassified virus, Lleida bat lyssavirus (LLEBV), was discovered in a common bent-wing bat *(Miniopterus schreibersii)* in Spain in 2012. The relevance of these discoveries for lyssavirus infection in the European Union is high as the ability of rabies vaccines to afford protection has been questioned where more divergent lyssaviruses are involved.

Australia was thought to be completely free of lyssaviruses until Australian bat lyssavirus (ABLV) was isolated from fruit bats in 1996. Since then, ABLV has been discovered in both frugivorous and insectivorous bats in Australia and has been associated with three human fatalities. Antibodies against this, or an antigenically related virus, have been detected in 9.5% of bat serum samples collected from the Philippines; therefore, it is likely that this, or a related virus, has a wider geographical distribution.

LABORATORY INVESTIGATION

Diagnosis of rabies infection may be difficult, especially if there is no recorded history of animal bite or travel to a rabies-endemic area. A number of diagnostic techniques can be used to test for the presence of virus antigen, virus genome or live virus. Tests on CSF for specific antibodies and on skin biopsies from the nape of the neck (nuchal skin biopsy) are the only reliable assays that can be used antemortem. Postmortem diagnosis of rabies infection in brain samples is reliable and is used as a confirmatory test following death.

Diagnostic methods

Historically, rabies was diagnosed through the detection of Negri bodies in the cytoplasm of infected nerve cells, most notably where infection of Ammon's horn within the hippocampus was present. Because of its low sensitivity, especially in the case of autolysed specimens, this test is no longer recommended by the Office International des Epizooties (OIE) for primary diagnosis.

Rabies virus antigen detection techniques

The gold standard OIE and World Health Organization (WHO)-approved diagnostic test is the fluorescent antibody test (FAT), which detects virus antigen in brain samples (hippocampus, brainstem or cerebellum) using fluorescently labelled antirabies antibodies. This test can provide results within 2 hours. Sensitivity, however, is dependent on the quality of the sample received. The general expense of the FAT, mainly through the requirement of fluorescein isothiocyanate (FITC)-conjugated polyclonal antibody preparations and the need for a fluorescent microscope, has driven the development of cheaper alternative tests to detect virus antigen in brain samples.

As an alternative to FAT, immunoperoxidase methods using low-cost light microscopy have been developed, such as the direct rapid immunohistochemistry test (dRIT). This method can detect RABV antigen in fresh brain impressions within 1 hour. An enzyme-linked immunosorbent assay (ELISA) has also been developed and is both simple and cost effective. However, it cannot be used with specimens that have been fixed with formalin and is generally considered to be less sensitive than FAT.

Rabies virus isolation

The mouse inoculation test (MIT), involving intracranial inoculation of homogenised sample and observation of the animal for 28 days or until clinical signs develop, is an OIE-recommended assay for rabies virus isolation. This has now been superseded and replaced by tissue culture methods where available as an ethically more acceptable assay. However, the lack of sterile tissue culture facilities in many rabies-endemic countries means that the MIT is still regularly performed as a confirmatory test for the FAT.

The rabies tissue culture isolation test (RTCIT) is used to isolate lyssaviruses in a range of clinical specimens from a number of host species, including dogs, cats, bats, wild carnivores and humans. Samples are inoculated onto a murine neuroblastoma monolayer. Following a 4-day incubation period, the plates are fixed and stained using fluorescein-labelled monoclonal antibodies (mAbs) and the presence or absence of viral antigen is determined.

Histopathological examination

Histopathological analysis of tissue samples is often used postmortem as a confirmatory test. The sample is fixed, blocked and stained with eosin and haematoxylin before the application of a rabies-specific antibody, which detects the presence of rabies virus nucleoprotein.

Serological assays

Rabies virus neutralising antibodies can be detected using the fluorescent antibody virus neutralisation assay (FAVN), a rapid fluorescent focus inhibition test (RFFIT) or an ELISA-based detection system. The FAVN is one method for assessing both human and animal antibody titres following preexposure vaccination. The basic premise for both the RFFIT and FAVN is that a known quantity of virus is mixed with different dilutions of test serum and the neutralising limit dilution is determined. The non-neutralised virus is then detected using a fluorescence-conjugated virus-specific antibody. The results are then calibrated from standard reference sera and expressed as international units (IU). Because of the use of live virus in these assays, the test must be undertaken in high-containment facilities.

Molecular methods for the detection of rabies viral RNA

The use of molecular-based assays to detect the presence of virus nucleic acid is becoming more commonplace. These techniques are not currently accepted as diagnostic techniques by the OIE or WHO, but are useful as screening tools and are also used for the generation of sequence data for the phylogenetic analysis of samples. Molecular methods have the highest sensitivity, and they can detect positive samples that may be negative by FAT, an important use when assessing samples that are partially decomposed. Furthermore, they can be used antemortem (e.g., skin biopsies, saliva, cerebrospinal fluid, tears and urine) where the current OIE approved methods are inappropriate. There are further complications as the virus can be shed intermittently in these samples and nucleic acids may be degraded in samples. For antemortem diagnostic assessments, a combination of tests should be considered before drawing conclusions from results yielded.

The heminested reverse transcriptase–polymerase chain reaction (RT-PCR) and various other similar techniques are being utilised routinely in laboratories worldwide for rabies virus detection. Other assays include the Taqman PCR, a realtime assay that can distinguish between some lyssavirus species, and also a PCR ELISA. The SYBR Green PCR that detects amplified double-stranded DNA is more sensitive than the Taqman PCR, but the specificity of the amplification needs to be determined by melting curve analysis or gel electrophoresis.

The detection of rabies virus antemortem is more difficult, as the virus is only excreted intermittently in saliva samples and antibodies are not always detectable in CSF. The use of nucleic acid sequence-based amplification (NASBA) is more sensitive than RT-PCR when assessing antemortem samples. This technique amplifies viral RNA directly in an isothermal reaction and therefore does not require expensive thermocycling equipment.

Next-generation sequencing (NGS) of suspect samples is expected to play an increasingly important role in viral diagnostics. Currently it is mainly used to analyse positive samples and generate full genome nucleotide sequence data as well as assess viral heterogeneity. However, in the future it may prove a useful tool in the diagnosis of viral diseases of the CNS, for which rabies virus detection will form part of the differential diagnosis.

PREVENTION

Vaccination

It was the French chemist Louis Pasteur, working with Laurent Roux and following the distinguished work of Pierre Galtier, who first introduced vaccination following rabies virus exposure. In 1885 the original vaccine was a crude extract of infected rabbit spinal cord, which had been desiccated and passaged several times to produce a fixed strain of the virus. The successful treatment of a young boy who experienced multiple bites from a rabid animal subsequently established this approach. The Semple vaccine, a modification of Pasteur's original vaccine, was a suspension of infected goat or sheep brain inactivated with phenol or beta-propiolactone. This was used in the United Kingdom between 1919 and 1966, but because of the high rate of allergic encephalitis following its administration, it was replaced by a duck-embryo–derived vaccine in 1966. This type of vaccine has since been replaced by cell-culture–derived vaccines, several types of which are currently available, including human diploid cell vaccine (HDCV), purified chick embryo cell vaccine (PCEV), purified duck embryo vaccine (PDEV), Vero cell vaccine

and primary hamster kidney cell vaccine (PHKCV). While each of these current vaccines has proven to be both safe and immunogenic, they are not necessarily available in developing countries.

Preexposure prophylaxis

In the United Kingdom, the HDCV and PCEV vaccines are licensed and available. These are normally administered to those who require preexposure vaccination, for example laboratory staff working directly with the virus, and bat handlers. For those people travelling to rabies-endemic countries, preexposure vaccination may be recommended depending on the local incidence of rabies in the country to be visited, the availability of appropriate antirabies biologicals, and the intended activity and duration of stay of the traveller. The protocol requires administration of three intramuscular doses of vaccine at days 0, 7 and day 21 or 28, following which the levels of neutralising antibody are assessed using a certified test. Response to these vaccines can persist for at least 2 years postvaccination. These vaccines are safe and well tolerated, with adverse reactions being extremely rare.

There are a number of different animal vaccines available, mostly live-attenuated preparations that are not currently acceptable for human use due to fears of reversion to virulence. Animals are generally inoculated intramuscularly, with boosters being required every 1–3 years depending on the vaccine type.

Postexposure prophylaxis (PEP)

Wound cleansing and immunisations, undertaken as soon as possible after suspected contact with an animal and following WHO recommendations, can prevent the onset of rabies in virtually 100% of exposures, although some exceptions to this have been recorded. The wound should be washed immediately with copious amounts of water and preferably cleansed with soap. Alcohol, quaternary ammonium compounds, iodine or povidone should be used, if available. The level of treatment or care required depends on the category of the contact as outlined by the WHO (category 1, 2 or 3; see Table 55.2). Postexposure antirabies vaccination should always include administration of both passive antibody (human or equine rabies immunoglobulin, RIG) and vaccine in patients without any history of rabies prevaccination, for both bite and nonbite exposures, regardless of the interval between exposure and initiation of treatment. HRIG provides immediate availability of neutralising antibodies at the site of exposure before the patient elicits an endogenous antibody response following vaccination.

Depending on vaccine type, the postexposure schedule requires four to five intramuscular doses over 4 weeks.

Table 55.2 WHO categories of rabies exposure

Category	Exposure	Treatment
1	Touching, feeding of animals or licks on unbroken skin	No treatment if history is reliable
2	Minor scratches or abrasions without bleeding, or licks on broken skin and nibbling of uncovered skin	Treat with vaccine
3	Single or multiple transdermal bites, scratches or contamination of mucous membrane with saliva (i.e., licks); exposure to bat bites or scratches	Treat with immunoglobulin and vaccine

Data from World Health Organization, Guide for postexposure prophylaxis http://www.who.int/rabies/human/postexp/en/. Accessed Mar 2017.

According to the WHO, two intramuscular doses of a cell-derived vaccine separated by 3 days are sufficient for patients who have previously undergone complete pre-vaccination. Rabies immune globulin treatment is not necessary in such cases.

CONTROL

Control of the spread of rabies would require elimination of infection from all reservoir species throughout the world, which is unlikely because of its broad host range, and its urban and sylvatic circulation. Methods involving termination of reservoir host species, such as shooting or gassing animals, only have short-term effects on the circulation of the virus. Therefore the principal aim of current strategies is to eliminate rabies in domestic dogs worldwide, thus breaking the transmission cycle and reducing the risk of human infection acquired from dogs.

A number of countries are considered to be free of terrestrial rabies, including much of Western and Central Europe. This has been achieved by a combination of strict quarantine laws and vaccination programmes. Although achieving a rabies-free status is more difficult in countries that share borders with rabies-endemic regions, the control of sylvatic rabies throughout Eastern Europe and North America is underway. This has largely been possible through the vaccination of domestic animals as well as oral bait vaccination schemes for wild animals. As most cases of rabies in humans are due to contact with a rabid dog or cat, these vaccination programmes, together with PEP for those individuals exposed in specific incidents to suspected rabid animals, have notably reduced the number of human fatalities due to rabies virus infection in the developed world. This approach, together with vaccination of specific individuals who may come into contact with rabies virus or rabid animals during the course of their work (e.g., laboratory workers, those individuals handling animals at quarantine centres, veterinarians, animal health inspectors, bat handlers and travellers to areas where rabies is still endemic), has reduced the number of incidents in developed countries that have adopted this scheme.

The OIE has targeted the global elimination of dog-mediated rabies by 2030 with the concomitant reduction in human rabies cases; however, the presence of lyssaviruses in bats means that rabies is unlikely to ever be eradicated globally.

RECOMMENDED READING

Websites

Global alliance for rabies control (GARC). Retrieved from https://rabiesalliance.org. (Accessed Aug 2016).
UK Government. Rabies: risk assessment, post-exposure treatment, management. Retrieved from https://www.gov.uk/government/collections/rabies-risk-assessment-post-exposure-treatment-management. (Accessed Aug 2016).
World Health Organization. Rabies. Retrieved from http://www.who.int/rabies/en. (Accessed Aug 2016).
World Organisation for Animal Health (OIE). Retrieved from http://www.oie.int. (Accessed Aug 2016).

56 Togaviruses

Rubella

LUDMILA PERELYGINA AND JOSEPH P. ICENOGLE

KEY POINTS

- Rubella (German measles) is caused by infection with a single-stranded, enveloped RNA virus of a single serotype. It is characterised by a widespread maculopapular rash.
- In the first 3 months of pregnancy, rubella virus can infect the foetus, causing congenital rubella syndrome (CRS) in 70% or more of maternal infections. Clinical signs of CRS include multiple abnormalities of the eye, ear and heart as well as a range of other problems such as mental handicap and purpura.
- Clinical diagnosis is unreliable. Serological detection of specific immunoglobulin M (IgM) and molecular detection of viral genomes are the laboratory confirmation methods of choice.
- Rubella is now eliminated in the Americas and uncommon in most developed countries in the world owing to widespread immunisation with a live-attenuated vaccine.

DESCRIPTION

The Togaviridae family is comprised of two genera, the *Alphavirus* genus, which contains arthropod-borne viruses (see Ch. 47), and the *Rubivirus* genus, which contains rubella virus as its sole member. Rubella was first recognised as a disease in the mid-18th century by two German physicians who described it as a modified form of measles (German measles, later named rubella). Little attention was paid to rubella until 1941 when an Australian ophthalmologist, Sir Norman Gregg, described the association between maternal rubella in pregnancy and congenital cataract and heart defects in infants. The isolation of rubella virus in 1962 led to the development of several live-attenuated vaccines.

EPIDEMIOLOGY

Rubella has a worldwide distribution, and transmission is endemic in countries that have not had a successful immunisation policy. Infection spreads via droplet transmission or direct contact with infected individuals and is common in childhood. Outbreaks can occur in all seasons, with major epidemics occurring every 5–9 years. Attack rates in susceptible individuals are between 50% and 90%. In countries without vaccination programs, 5%–20% of women of childbearing age remain susceptible to rubella.

Rubella is an important cause of preventable congenital defects and neonatal death. The infant mortality rate can be as high as 33%, and disability-adjusted life years (DALYs) lost per CRS case was estimated to be between 19 and 38. The global burden of CRS is around 110,000 cases annually.

REPLICATION (VIROLOGY)

Rubella virus has a genomic organisation similar to alphaviruses, but little sequence homology. It has a single-stranded positive-sense RNA genome, and replication occurs in the cytoplasm of infected cells. There are three virion polypeptides: capsid protein, and the envelope glycoproteins E1 and E2. Rubella particles assemble in an association with the Golgi complex. The mature infectious virions are released from infected cells via the secretory pathway of the trans-Golgi network without cell destruction. Haemagglutination inhibition and neutralising epitopes are localised predominantly on the E1 protein.

The virus is stable at 4°C for over 7 days, but can be heat-inactivated at 56°C for 20 minutes. Because it is an enveloped virus, ionic and nonionic detergents and lipid solvents effectively inactivate infectious particles. UV irradiation is another means for inactivation as it induces damage to viral RNA.

The virus can be isolated in a variety of primary and continuous cell lines (e.g., Vero). Many cell cultures support persistent rubella infection, which could not be eliminated by treatment with rubella-specific antibody. The World Health Organization (WHO) has subdivided rubella viruses into two clades currently comprised of 13 genotypes. There is no evidence that immunity to the vaccine virus (genotype 1a) does not cross-protect for the other 12 genotypes. Only genotypes 1E, 1G, 1J and 2B are currently observed worldwide. Rubella virus can be experimentally transmitted to laboratory animals, but humans are the only naturally infected species.

CLINICAL FEATURES

Postnatal primary rubella

The incubation period for postnatal primary rubella is 12–21 days. Virus may be excreted in the throat for up to a week before and after the rash, and this covers the period of infectivity. Close contact is needed for onwards transmission. Infection has several characteristic clinical features.

- A maculopapular rash (Fig. 56.1) with low fever, which usually lasts 3 days and appears first on the face and then spreads to the trunk and limbs. In childhood the rash may be fleeting, and perhaps 50% of infections in children are asymptomatic. In adults, asymptomatic rubella is less common.
- Minor pyrexia, malaise, mild conjunctivitis and lymphadenopathy also occur, with the suboccipital nodes sometimes being enlarged and tender.
- Arthralgia is uncommon in children but may occur in up to 60% of women. The joints commonly involved are the fingers, wrists, ankles and knees. Arthralgia usually lasts for a few days, but may occasionally persist for months.

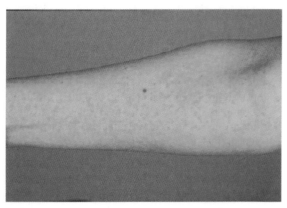

Fig. 56.1 Rubella rash.

- Encephalitis (1 in 6000 cases) and thrombocytopenia (1 in 3000 cases) are rare complications of rubella. Recovery is usually complete.

Rubella is difficult to diagnose clinically as other mild virus infections can present with identical clinical features. Hence laboratory confirmation is essential. In many countries, rubella is a legally notifiable infection.

Rubella reinfection

Clinically apparent reinfection, although extremely rare, can result in viremia and may be a concern in pregnant women. Although difficult to evaluate, the risk of asymptomatic reinfection in pregnancy appears to be negligible. Only a few cases have been described in the literature, most of them lack compelling evidence of maternal immunity prior to pregnancy.

Congenital rubella

If the foetus is infected following a primary maternal infection during the first trimester of pregnancy, miscarriage, stillbirth or CRS can occur. CRS includes the following spectrum of abnormalities in a newborn:

- Bilateral or unilateral sensorineural deafness is the most common defect; it may increase in severity as the child gets older.
- Bilateral or unilateral abnormalities of the eyes include cataracts, microphthalmia, glaucoma and pigmentary retinopathy, which may result in blindness.
- There are many possible heart defects, with patent ductus arteriosus, pulmonary artery and valvular stenosis and ventricular septal defect being the most common.
- The baby often has a low birth weight. A purpuric rash sometimes develops due to thrombocytopenia, but this usually resolves as does hepatosplenomegaly.
- Microcephaly, psychomotor retardation, behavioural disorders and developmental delay occur. Rarely, there may be a persistent infection of the central nervous system (progressive rubella subacute panencephalitis) similar clinically to subacute sclerosing panencephalitis due to measles virus infection.
- Other problems that may present later in life include pneumonitis, diabetes mellitus, growth hormone deficiency, and thyroid function abnormalities.

Single birth defects can be caused by genetic disorders, environmental factors, or various congenital infections. However, combinations of defects in CRS are very specific.

The classical CRS triad consists of abnormalities of the eyes, ears and heart.

If maternal infection occurs in the first trimester, babies have one or more developmental defects and the risk of CRS is 70% or more. The risk of congenital defects drops to about 20% or less between 12 and 16 weeks of pregnancy and the only abnormality likely to be seen is sensorineural deafness. After 16 weeks, although foetal infection still occurs, congenital abnormalities are rarely observed. Such cases would be classified as congenital rubella infection (CRI).

PATHOGENESIS

Postnatal rubella

The virus first replicates in the epithelium of the buccal mucosa and the lymphoid tissue of the nasopharynx and upper respiratory tract. Towards the end of the incubation period a viremia occurs and seeds target organs such as skin, joints and placenta. Most of the clinical features are probably due to the host's immune response; for example, virus can be demonstrated in both unaffected skin and the macules of the rash, suggesting that the presence of virus per se is not sufficient to cause the rash.

Congenital rubella

During viremia the virus establishes persistent infection in the placenta and then crosses the placenta (in early gestation this is an ineffective barrier to infection) to infect the differentiating cells of the foetus. Since the foetus is incapable of mounting an immune response and transplacental transfer of maternal IgG is blocked during the first trimester, foetal infection often results in viral persistence in multiple organs in the foetus until term and then in infants. Different, multiple cell types can be affected including endothelial cells, neurons, cardiac and interstitial fibroblast and epithelial cells of lung, kidney and ciliary body of the eye. Rubella infection of each cell type is consistent with abnormalities that have been identified in patients with CRS. The congenital abnormalities arise from the direct effects of rubella virus on infected cells as well as due to the placental damage and vascular insufficiency (general growth retardation and neurodegenerative damage). Persistent infection may result in the clinical problems presenting later in life, possibly caused by direct damage, such as in late onset deafness or because of immunopathological mechanisms such as in pneumonitis.

DIAGNOSIS

Postnatal rubella

Given the unreliability of clinical diagnosis, laboratory investigation is required to diagnose rubella and this is of paramount importance for the pregnant patient. As subclinical rubella may occur, pregnant women should also be investigated for prior evidence of immunity, if they have had a contact with someone who has rubella. In the near and postelimination era, it is desirable to collect both serum and virological specimens for all suspected rubella cases.

The relationship among the timing of clinical signs, virus isolation and serological markers is shown in Fig. 56.2. For primary rubella infection, detection of rubella IgM antibody is the most commonly used diagnostic method. Several commercial assays are available, with capture ELISA typically having lower background. Most sera collected between 5 and 40 days of rash onset are positive for rubella IgM, whereas only about 50% of the sera collected on the day of rash onset contain detectable levels of rubella IgM. If specimens collected too soon after rash onset were negative for IgM, a convalescent sample should be obtained 2–3 weeks later and tested in parallel with the acute sera. Rubella IgG antibody appears about a week after rash onset and persists for life. IgG seroconversion or at least a four-fold rise in IgG antibody titre in convalescent sera (taken at 2–3 weeks after rash onset) relative to acute sera is another method for diagnosis of recent rubella infection. Rubella IgG avidity (the strength of the bond between antibody and antigen) can also be used to differentiate between recent (low avidity) and remote (high avidity) infection.

The diagnosis of recent rubella can also be made by detection of the infectious virus or viral genomes in clinical specimens. Throat washings and oral fluids are excellent specimens for this type of diagnosis, although urine and serum can be used as well. For successful rubella virus detection, the specimens should be collected within 3–4 days after rash onset. Detection of rubella RNA directly from clinical specimens can be achieved by reverse transcription–polymerase chain reaction (RT-PCR). A 739-nucleotide sequence of the *E1* gene is used for virus genotyping, which can also help to determine the epidemiological source of the virus. Virus titre in clinical samples is typically low and virus amplification in a cell culture is often required to obtain sufficient RNA amounts for genotyping. Cell culture is more time consuming than RT-PCR for virus detection. Moreover, clinical strains often do not produce a cytopathic effect in Vero cells, and thus the presence of virus in such cultures is demonstrated by detection of viral genomes

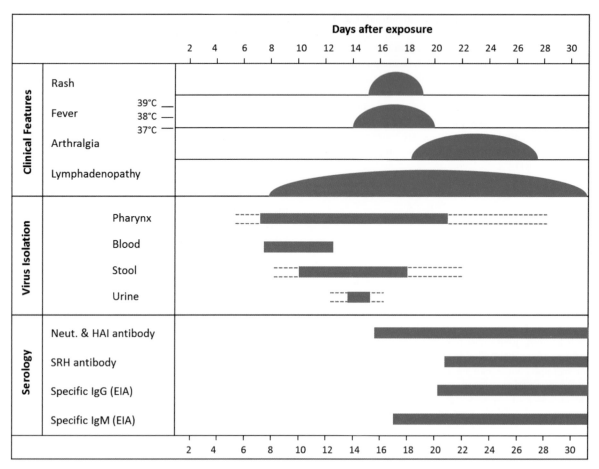

Fig. 56.2 The relationship among clinical signs, virus isolation and serological markers of postnatal rubella infection. *EIA*, enzyme immunoassay; *HAI*, haemagglutination inhibition; *Neut.*, neutralising; *SRH*, single radial haemolysis.

using RT-PCR or viral proteins using immunological methods.

Congenital rubella

Laboratory testing methodology for CRS-suspected cases is the same as for postnatal rubella cases, although timing of CRS biological markers is different. IgM ELISA is the most common method for confirmation of CRS cases in the newborns. Maternal IgM does not cross the placenta, so the detection of rubella-specific IgM in a newborn baby is diagnostic of intrauterine infection. IgG crosses the placenta so its detection in the first few months of life is of no help. Maternal IgG has a half-life in the infant of 3–4 weeks, and so, in the absence of rubella or vaccination against rubella, IgG at age of 9–12 months is diagnostic of CRS. The reliable diagnosis of congenital infection in older children is currently impossible as any rubella-specific IgM generated by

congenital infection will have disappeared and virus shedding stopped, while rubella-specific IgG in the patient's serum may have arisen from postnatal infection or immunisation.

RT-PCR is another reliable and sensitive method for CRS case confirmation. CRS infants excrete virus at birth and some continue to excrete virus for months after birth. After 4 months the proportion of CRS infants shedding virus decreases to 50%–60%. Virus persists for different times in different body sites—up to 6 months in urine and blood, up to 18 months in nasopharyngeal secretions and cerebrospinal fluid and sometimes for decades in lenses. At birth, virus titres in CRS babies can be 100–1000 times higher than in postnatal rubella cases and subsequently decline. However, virus titres have been reported to sharply increase with waning of maternal antibody. CRS infants are highly contagious and have caused several outbreaks among health-care workers; thus, virus shedding should be monitored closely. To prevent outbreaks, persons in contact with CRS infants should be immune to rubella; those that are not immune should be vaccinated or avoid contact. Two negative cultures (or RT-PCR) of samples collected 1 month apart are required to document termination of rubella virus shedding in CRS patients.

Screening for rubella antibody

The 10 IU/mL IgG antibody level was defined in many countries as sufficient to provide adequate protection from rubella. Screening for rubella IgG in pregnant women identifies individuals who are susceptible and who should be offered vaccine postpartum. Sometimes preconceptual screening is performed, especially in those undergoing in vitro fertilisation. Rubella antibody screening is usually performed by IgG ELISA or latex agglutination tests, which are sensitive and easily automated. IgM ELISA should not be used for screening for rubella immunity. Some individuals do not produce the accepted protective levels of antibody, even after several vaccinations, and they should be considered immune if they have had two documented doses of vaccine.

TREATMENT

No scientifically proven cure exists for rubella. There is little evidence that administering normal human immunoglobulin or interferon after contact reduces the risk of maternal rubella and foetal infection, although it may attenuate the illness.

CONTROL

Attenuated, live rubella vaccines are commonly used in combinations with measles (MR), measles and mumps (MMR), or measles, mumps and varicella (MMRV) vaccines. The most widely used rubella vaccine, RA27/3, is safe, effective and only has minimal side effects such as a transient rash, low grade fever and arthralgia. Vaccine virus can be isolated from the throat of vaccinees, but there is no evidence of onwards transmission to susceptible contacts. The vaccine is contraindicated in pregnancy, which should be avoided in the month after vaccination. Although vaccine virus has been shown to infect the foetus, there is no evidence of teratogenicity. Thus, if a susceptible woman is immunised inadvertently whilst pregnant, she can be reassured that any risk to the baby is remote. Live rubella vaccine is also not recommended for children with certain types of primary immune deficiencies, for example, severe antibody deficiency, T-lymphocyte deficiencies or innate immune defects. Immunisation of these children may result in persistence of vaccine virus in patient's tissues possibly causing pathologies. For example, an association between RA27/3 vaccine persistence in skin and formation of cutaneous granulomas in children with primary immune deficiencies has been recently reported.

The 2020 WHO Global Vaccine Action Plan established the measles and rubella/CRS elimination goal in at least five out of six WHO regions. The action plan provides strategies and guiding principles with the following key elements:

- childhood immunisation with two doses of vaccine supplemented by immunisation campaigns to close immunization gaps
- achievement and maintenance of >95% vaccination coverage
- establishment of an effective surveillance programme
- development of an outbreak response programme
- building public confidence in immunisation
- research and development of improved vaccination and diagnostic methodologies

Rubella and CRS were officially declared eliminated in the Region of Americas in 2015 following implementation of these vaccination strategies. This achievement shows that with political commitment and sufficient financial support this vaccine-preventable disease could be eliminated worldwide.

RECOMMENDED READING

Banatvala, J. E., & Peckham, C. A. (2007). *Rubella viruses. Perspectives in medical virology* (Vol. 15). Amsterdam, Netherlands: Elsevier.

Bellini, W. J., & Icenogle, J. P. (2015). Measles and rubella viruses. *Manual of clinical microbiology* (11th ed.). American Society of Microbiology.

McLean, H. Q., Fiebelkorn, A. P., Temte, J. L., Wallace, G. S., & Centers for Disease Control and Prevention. (2013). Prevention of measles, rubella, congenital rubella syndrome, and mumps, 2013: summary recommendations of the Advisory Committee on Immunization Practices (ACIP). *Morbidity and Mortality Weekly Report, Recommendations and Reports, 62*(RR04), 1–34.

Plotkin, S., Reef, S., Cooper, L., & Alford, C. A. (2011). Rubella. In J. Remington, J. Klein, C. Wilson, V. Nizet,& Y. Maldonato (Eds.), *Infectious diseases of the fetus and newborn infant* (pp. 861–898). Philadelphia, PA: Elsveier.

Websites

Centers for Disease Control and Prevention. Ch. 14: Rubella. Retrieved from http://www.cdc.gov/vaccines/pubs/surv-manual/chpt14-rubella.html. (Accessed Aug 2017).

Centers for Disease Control and Prevention. Ch. 15: Congenital Rubella Syndrome. Retrieved from http://www.cdc.gov/vaccines/pubs/surv-manual/chpt15-crs.html. (Accessed Aug 2017).

Red Book Online. Rubella. Retrieved from http://redbook.solutions.aap.org/chapter.aspx?sectionid=88187232&bookid=1484.

World Health Organization. Rubella. Retrieved from http://www.who.int/topics/rubella/en/. (Accessed Aug 2017).

57 Prion diseases (transmissible spongiform encephalopathies)

Creutzfeldt–Jakob disease; Gerstmann–Sträussler–Scheinker syndrome; fatal familial insomnia; iatrogenic Creutzfeldt–Jakob disease; kuru; variant Creutzfeldt–Jakob disease; bovine spongiform encephalopathy; scrapie and chronic wasting disease

JAMES W. IRONSIDE AND MARK W. HEAD

KEY POINTS

- Prion diseases are fatal neurodegenerative disorders with very lengthy incubation periods caused by unconventional agents. They are transmitted by inoculation or ingestion; the intracerebral route of transmission results in the shortest incubation period.
- Prion diseases occur in mammals, including scrapie in sheep, bovine spongiform encephalopathy (BSE) in cattle, chronic wasting disease in deer and Creutzfeldt–Jakob disease (CJD) in humans.
- The infectious agents are known as prions, which lack a nucleic acid genome and appear to consist entirely of a disease-associated protein (PrP^{Sc}), which is derived from misfolding of the normal cellular form of the prion protein (PrP^{C}).
- Prion diseases do not elicit conventionally detectable immune responses. Asymptomatic or subclinical infections are very difficult to detect.
- Human prion diseases occur in sporadic, genetic and acquired forms, all of which are rare diseases. In 1996 a new form of human prion disease known as variant CJD was identified, which results from infection with the BSE agent, probably via the oral route.

Prion diseases (also known as transmissible spongiform encephalopathies) are a unique group of fatal neurodegenerative disorders occurring in human beings and animals and possess two major characteristics:

1. All are transmissible to a variety of mammals, either experimentally or by natural exposure. The precise nature of the transmissible agents involved is unknown (see later in the chapter), but they possess physical and chemical properties that are quite distinct from those of conventional viruses and bacteria. The prion hypothesis states that the infectious agent is composed entirely of protein, without any nucleic acid, for which the term *prion* (*pr*oteinaceous *in*fectious particle) is used. No evidence of a conventional host immune reaction has been found in prion diseases.

2. The diseases caused by these agents are characterised in all species by neurodegeneration in the central nervous system (CNS), usually with spongiform change. This consists of numerous small vacuoles (10–200 μm) that are formed within neuronal cell bodies and their processes (Fig. 57.1A), probably through dilatation of neuronal lysosomal, Golgi and endoplasmic reticulum structures. Ultimately, neuronal death occurs accompanied by reactive proliferation of astrocytes and microglia. The normal cellular form of the prion protein (PrP^{C}) is converted by misfolding into an abnormal disease-associated form (PrP^{Sc}) and accumulates within the CNS, occasionally in the form of amyloid plaques.

THE TRANSMISSIBLE AGENT: A PRION

Although the precise composition and structure of prions are uncertain, they are subviral in size and notoriously resistant to inactivation by many physical and chemical agents, including:

- heat
- exposure to ionizing or ultraviolet radiation
- deoxyribonuclease (DNase) and ribonuclease (RNase)
- formaldehyde and glutaraldehyde.

Prions have been studied by experimental transmission to mice and hamsters; this has identified around 20 strains of scrapie, a naturally occurring prion disease in sheep. Strains are defined by their biological properties—the disease incubation period and the nature and distribution

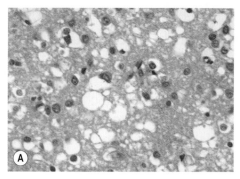
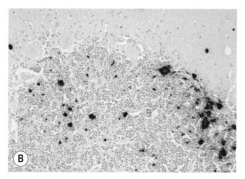

Fig. 57.1 (A) Spongiform change in the cerebral cortex in a case of sporadic CJD consists of numerous small cystlike spaces that tend to coalesce in the neuropil and around neurones (centre). Haematoxylin and eosin stain, original magnification ×400. (B) In this case of sporadic CJD, prion protein (PrP) accumulation in the cerebellum has occurred in the form of numerous amyloid plaques that stain intensely on immunohistochemistry for PrP. Original magnification ×200.

of the pathology in the CNS. Incubation periods range from 60 days to >2 years, which is close to the natural lifespan of mice and hamsters, and cases of asymptomatic infection have been recorded. The incubation period is influenced by:

- the route of inoculation—intracerebral inoculation is the most efficient mode of infection; oral or parenteral routes are often less efficient
- the dose of the injected inoculum and its infective titre
- host genetic factors, particularly polymorphisms in the prion protein gene.

PrP^C is expressed in a variety of cells, including neurones in the CNS, where it is thought to be involved in differentiation and neuronal maintenance. This protein has a mass weight of 33–35 kDa and is highly conserved through a wide range of species, but its amino acid sequence varies from one species to another. This variation is thought to influence the species barrier, a factor that regulates the success of disease transmission from one species to another under experimental and natural conditions.

During prion infection, PrP^C undergoes a conformational change to convert to PrP^{Sc}. This abnormal isoform has increased β-sheet content, which renders it partially resistant to digestion with proteinases and confers a propensity to aggregate as amyloid fibrils. In the prion hypothesis, conversion of the PrP^C to PrP^{Sc} occurs by a direct interaction, which initiates autocatalytic conversion. This has been replicated experimentally using purified prion protein that has been misfolded in a cell-free system to produce infectious PrP^{Sc}. These findings support the prion hypothesis; however, it is not known whether this biochemical change alone accounts for all the biological properties of prions. Deposition of other proteins in misfolded forms or as amyloid is a characteristic of a number of common noninfectious neurodegenerative diseases, such as Aβ and tau proteins in Alzheimer's disease and α-synuclein in Parkinson's disease. A major strand in current research in this area is to try to understand whether the conversion mechanisms and spread of neuropathology in these diseases is by a prion-like mechanism.

PATHOGENESIS

Experimental transmission of prions to hamsters and mice can be achieved by inoculation of infected brain tissue into a number of sites. After oral inoculation, prions cross the gut wall to replicate in the gut-associated lymphoid tissue (Peyer's patches). Spread of infection may then occur either along the vagus nerve to the brainstem, or by blood spread to the other lymphoid tissues in the body. In the spleen, prions can spread via the splanchnic plexus to the CNS.

HUMAN PRION DISEASES

The most common form of human prion disease was first described in the 1920s and is known as Creutzfeldt–Jakob disease (CJD) after the authors of these reports. Since then, a widening spectrum of human prion diseases has been identified (Table 57.1), with three main subgroups comprising:

- idiopathic disorders, where the cause is unknown
- genetic disorders, occurring as autosomal dominant diseases
- acquired disorders, following accidental infection by inoculation or ingestion.

The identification of the prion protein and sequencing of the human prion protein gene on chromosome 20 have

Table 57.1 Human spongiform encephalopathies classified by aetiology

Aetiology	Encephalopathy
Idiopathic disorders	Sporadic CJD (around 90% of all cases)
Genetic disorders	Familial CJD (around 10% of all cases) Gerstmann–Sträussler–Scheinker syndrome Fatal familial insomnia
Transmitted from person to person	Kuru Iatrogenic CJD (<1% of all cases)
Transmitted from bovines to humans	Variant CJD

CJD, Creutzfeldt–Jakob disease.

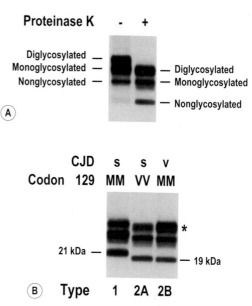

Fig. 57.2 Western blot analysis of prion protein (PrP) in postmortem CJD brain. PrP from CJD brain occurs in three glycoforms resulting in diglycosylated, monoglycosylated or nonglycosylated PrP, which can be separated by Western blotting into distinct bands. Proteinase K treatment (+) destroys the normal form of the prion protein, but in CJD it only partly denatures the disease-associated protein, which has an increased mobility (shown in A). Two main subtypes of the abnormal protein can be identified: (B) types 1 and 2 are found in sporadic CJD (s) irrespective of the genotype at codon 129. Examples of two types (MM1 and VV2) are shown here. Almost all cases of variant CJD (v) thus far tested are methionine homozygotes (MM) and have had a type 2 PrP characterised by the predominance of the diglycosylated glycoform (*), termed type 2B. The type 2 cases found in sporadic CJD, in which the monoglycosylated glycoform predominates, are termed type 2A.

greatly increased our understanding of human transmissible spongiform encephalopathies.

DIAGNOSIS

The diagnosis of human prion diseases requires a range of clinical, biochemical, genetic and pathological studies. Careful assessment of the clinical features (see later in the chapter) by an experienced neurologist allows a presumptive diagnosis of CJD to be made with a high level of accuracy (at least 70%). Analysis of the prion protein gene is essential to identify pathogenic mutations in cases of familial CJD. Genetic studies have also demonstrated a naturally occurring polymorphism at codon 129 in the prion protein gene, which is important in determining disease susceptibility (see later in the chapter). At present, there is no screening test for human prion diseases, although the detection of prion protein seeding activity in the cerebrospinal fluid appears promising as a clinical diagnostic test for sporadic CJD. There is no specific treatment currently available. A definitive diagnosis depends on examination of the brain at autopsy. Brain biopsy is not a routine investigation, as the procedure can compromise an already ill patient and if the diagnosis is confirmed the neurosurgical instruments used have to be destroyed to prevent accidental iatrogenic infection via subsequent neurosurgical procedures.

NEUROPATHOLOGY

It is recommended that all suspected CJD cases should be investigated by autopsy, with appropriate permission for retention and examination of the brain to allow

confirmation of the clinical diagnosis and accurate subclassification of the case. The principal neuropathological features of human prion diseases are:

- spongiform change (Fig. 57.1A)
- neuronal loss
- astrocytosis
- accumulation of PrP^{Sc}
- amyloid plaque formation (Fig. 57.1B).

PrP^{Sc} can be detected by immunocytochemistry in the CNS in a variety of patterns, including amyloid plaques (see Fig. 57.1B) and perivacuolar, perineuronal and axonal deposition. PrP^{Sc} can also be detected by Western blot techniques, which allow further study of the PrP^{Sc} isotype in terms of its glycosylation and molecular weight following digestion with proteinase K (Fig. 57.2). Detecting PrP^{Sc} in patient body fluids, such as blood, urine and cerebrospinal fluid, is more challenging, but progress is being made with the aid of in vitro protein misfolding assays.

SPORADIC CJD

CJD occurs most commonly as a sporadic disorder, affecting around one person per million population per year worldwide. Sporadic CJD usually presents as a rapidly progressive dementia, often accompanied by other neurological abnormalities, including cerebellar dysfunction, pyramidal and extrapyramidal signs, cortical blindness and akinetic mutism. The peak incidence is in the seventh decade of life, but the disease has been described in teenagers, and even in the ninth decade. The disease is untreatable and invariably fatal; most patients survive for only 4 months after the onset of major symptoms.

The naturally occurring methionine/valine polymorphism at codon 129 in the prion protein gene is of major influence in determining susceptibility to sporadic CJD (Table 57.2). The mechanism for this influence is unclear. The precipitating event leading to development of sporadic CJD remains unknown; it might possibly reflect stochastic changes in prion protein conformation, a somatic mutation involving the prion protein in the CNS or other unknown genetic susceptibility factors (Fig. 57.3). No occupational or dietary risk factors exist for sporadic CJD.

GENETIC PRION DISEASES

Around 10% of cases of CJD occur as autosomal dominant inherited disorders; these are associated with mutations or insertions in the open reading frame of the human prion protein gene on chromosome 20 (see Fig. 57.3). Gerstmann–Sträussler–Scheinker syndrome (GSS) is the best known example of an inherited human prion disease. This very rare disorder affects middle-aged adults, causing cerebellar ataxia, nystagmus and gait abnormalities with dementia occurring only towards the end of the illness. Numerous multicentric PrP amyloid plaques are present throughout the CNS. GSS was the first human disease linked to a mutation in the *PrP* gene; a codon 102 proline-to-leucine mutation was identified in 1989. Fatal familial insomnia is an extremely rare

inherited disorder, characterised clinically by disturbances of sleep and autonomic function with relative intellectual preservation. This disorder is associated with a unique PrP genotype (codon 178 asparagine, 129 methionine/ methionine) and neuropathological changes mainly in the thalamus.

ACQUIRED PRION DISEASES

IATROGENIC CJD

CJD can occur by accidental transmission from one person to another (see Fig. 57.3). Iatrogenic CJD was first described in 1974 in a corneal graft recipient. Other examples of iatrogenic CJD have involved accidental inoculation of contaminated CNS tissue from a CJD patient to another patient, for example, following the implantation of inadequately decontaminated intracerebral electrodes, or via human dura mater grafts. In the United Kingdom the most common form of iatrogenic CJD occurs in recipients of human growth hormone derived from cadaveric pituitary glands, at an approximate incidence of 1 in 10,000 at-risk individuals. Although the use of cadaveric pituitary human growth hormone was abandoned in the United Kingdom in 1985, rare cases of associated iatrogenic CJD still occur, evidence of the prolonged incubation periods possible in prion diseases.

KURU

Kuru was a disease occurring in the Fore tribe of Papua New Guinea, apparently in association with practices related to ritualistic cannibalism. In the local dialect the name kuru means shivering or trembling, and reflects the predominant clinical manifestations of a progressive cerebellar syndrome with dementia. The incubation period was variable, ranging from around 5 to over 40 years. Its increasing prevalence made it a common cause of death within the tribe in the 1960s. The disease is now extinct since cannibalistic practices were abandoned.

VARIANT CJD

The emergence of bovine spongiform encephalopathy (BSE) as a new epidemic in British cattle raised the possibility that this disorder might be transmitted to humans through the food chain. A National CJD Surveillance Unit was established for the United Kingdom in May 1990, based in Edinburgh. In 1996 the unit identified a new

Table 57.2 Prion protein gene codon 129 polymorphism in CJD			
Codon 129 genotype	Methionine/ methionine	Methionine/ valine	Valine/ valine
Normal population	44%	45%	11%
Sporadic CJD	60%	20%	20%
Variant CJD	99%	1%	0%
CJD, Creutzfeldt–Jakob disease.			

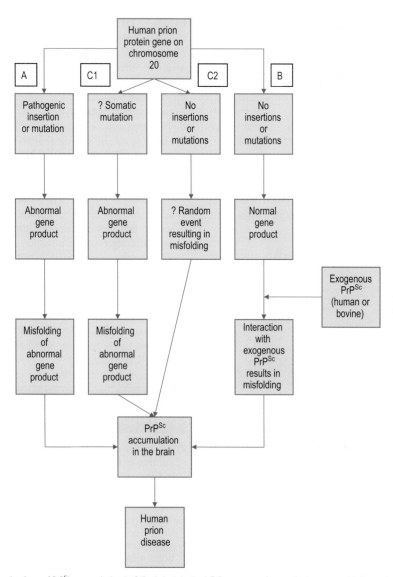

Fig. 57.3 Postulated mechanisms of PrP^{Sc} accumulation in CJD. *A,* An inherited *PrP* gene mutation results in an unstable form of prion protein that misfolds to cause familial CJD. *B,* Exogenous PrP^{Sc} interacts with the normal host prion protein, resulting in PrP^{Sc} accumulation. This mechanism is thought to operate in iatrogenic CJD (exposure to human PrP^{Sc}) and variant CJD (exposure to bovine PrP^{Sc}). The cause of sporadic CJD is unknown, but proponents of the prion hypothesis have suggested that a somatic mutation in a neurone *C1,* might initiate the process of PrP^{Sc} accumulation in the brain, or alternatively a rare random event results in spontaneous misfolding of the normal prion protein *C2.* These rare events might also explain the low incidence of sporadic CJD.

form of human prion disease, now known as variant *CJD,* which by 2016 had affected 178 people in the United Kingdom, and 53 in other countries including France, Ireland, the Netherlands, Spain, Portugal, the United States, Canada, Japan and Saudi Arabia.

- The age of onset is unusually young (mean age 28 years), with a range from 12 to 74 years.
- The clinical illness is prolonged, with an average duration of 14 months (range 6–39 months).

- The clinical features are also unusual, with psychiatric and sensory symptoms at onset, followed by ataxia and myoclonus, with dementia only in the final stages of the illness.
- Until recently, all patients with definite variant CJD have been found to be methionine homozygotes at codon 129 in the prion protein gene (see Table 57.2).

The neuropathological features are relatively uniform, with massive accumulations of PrP^{Sc} in the CNS and the formation of multiple amyloid plaques surrounded by spongiform change (Fig. 57.4). Variant CJD differs from other forms of human prion disease in that PrP^{Sc} can be detected in lymphoid tissues (in follicular dendritic cells) both during the clinical illness (Fig. 57.5) and in the late preclinical illness. This is consistent with variant CJD being acquired by the oral route (see later in the chapter) and has implications for the possible transmission of the variant CJD agent by surgical instruments used on lymphoid tissues (e.g., in tonsillectomies).

The variant CJD prion is also present in the blood of individuals in the preclinical incubation phase of the illness. Four cases of variant CJD transmission by blood transfusion have been reported in the United Kingdom. Many steps have been taken in the United Kingdom to prevent further transmission by this route, including filtration of whole blood to remove white cells (which may carry the highest levels of infectivity), sourcing of plasma products from overseas and banning recipients of blood transfusions from themselves becoming blood donors.

Experimental strain-typing studies in mice have shown that the transmissible agent in variant CJD is identical to the BSE agent. Biochemical analysis of PrP^{Sc} from cases of variant CJD shows a similar banding pattern in Western blot preparations to PrP^{Sc} from BSE in cattle, but is distinct from sporadic CJD (see Fig. 57.2). These findings provide strong support for the hypothesis that variant CJD is causally linked to BSE, and there is epidemiological evidence that dietary exposure through beef products is the most likely route of infection.

The incidence and death rate for variant CJD in the United Kingdom peaked in the year 2000 and has continued to fall since. However, continuing surveillance is required because the incubation period for variant CJD is unknown, and the appearance of a definite case of variant CJD in a *PRNP* codon 129 heterozygous individual in 2016 suggests that future cases may emerge in other genetic subgroups in the UK population.

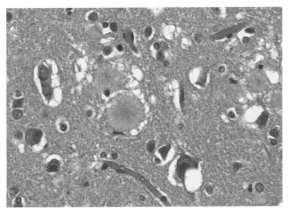

Fig. 57.4 The cerebral cortex in variant CJD contains numerous aggregates of PrP^{Sc} in the form of fibrillary amyloid plaques (centre), surrounded by spongiform change. Haematoxylin and eosin stain, original magnification ×200.

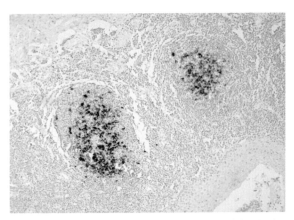

Fig. 57.5 Section of a tonsil from a patient with variant CJD stained to show the prion protein by immunohistochemistry. The dark stain demonstrates accumulation of the prion protein in the follicular dendritic cells within germinal centres of the tonsil. Accumulation of prion protein in lymphoid tissues does not occur in sporadic CJD. Original magnification ×100.

BOVINE SPONGIFORM ENCEPHALOPATHY AND OTHER ANIMAL PRION DISEASES

Prion diseases have been recorded in an increasing number of captive or domesticated animals (Table 57.3), the most significant of which is BSE. This was identified in 1985 in the United Kingdom and spread rapidly throughout the cattle population to affect around 1% of all adult cattle by 1992. It appears that this epidemic resulted from:

- oral ingestion of a prion via contaminated meat and bone meal in cattle feed
- recycling of contaminated cattle carcasses in the meat and bone meal fed to cattle.

The incidence of BSE has declined markedly as a result of a ban on the use of bovine organs as foodstuffs for other animals. Experimental studies on BSE indicate that it represents a single prion strain spread to humans, giving rise to variant CJD (see earlier in the chapter). Other, possibly sporadic, bovine prion diseases unrelated to BSE do occur worldwide, but whether these pose a risk to human health is not known.

SCRAPIE

Scrapie is an endemic disorder of sheep and goats that has been present in Europe for at least 2 centuries.

Table 57.3 Animal diseases caused by scrapie and related agents

Disease	Occurrence	Hosts
Scrapie	Common in many countries worldwide	Sheep and goats
Transmissible mink encephalopathy	Very rare, mostly in farms in the United States	Mink
Chronic wasting disease	Spreading widely across North America; now also found in Korea and Norway	Deer and elk
Bovine spongiform encephalopathy	Widespread epidemic in dairy cattle in the United Kingdom; smaller outbreaks in other countries	Domestic cattle
Exotic ungulate spongiform encephalopathy	Small number of exotic ungulates in zoos fed with BSE-contaminated animal feed	Nyala, gemsbok, greater kudu, Arabian oryx, eland
Feline spongiform encephalopathy	Small numbers of domestic cats in the United Kingdom fed with BSE-contaminated animal feed and a few large cats in UK zoos fed with BSE-contaminated animal carcasses	Domestic cats, cheetah, lion, puma, ocelot, tiger

BSE, Bovine spongiform encephalopathy.

Affected animals become ataxic and wasted and often rub or scrape the fleece off the sides of their bodies, hence the name. The first experimental transmission of scrapie was reported in 1936. Natural transmission is thought to occur at parturition or via the oral route. The placenta from an infected ewe is one known source of infection that can contaminate the farm environment. There is no epidemiological evidence that scrapie is pathogenic to humans.

CHRONIC WASTING DISEASE

Chronic wasting disease (CWD) is a contagious prion disease of cervids, endemic in large parts of North America and recently reported in Northern Europe. Whilst there is no direct evidence of CWD transmission to humans, its status, whether zoonotic (like BSE) or nonzoonotic (like scrapie), is a matter of current public health concern.

RECOMMENDED READING

Bruce, M. E., Will, R. G., Ironside, J. W., McConnell, I., Drummond, D., Suttie, A., ... Bostock, C. J. (1997). Transmissions to mice indicate the 'new variant' CJD is caused by the BSE agent. *Nature, 389*(6650), 498–501.

Collinge, J., & Clarke, A. (2007). A general model of prion strains and their pathogenicity. *Science, 318*(5852), 930–936.

Goedert, M. (2015). Neurodegeneration. Alzheimer's and Parkinson's disease: the prion concept in relation to assembled Aβ, tau and α-synuclein. *Science, 349*(6248), 1255555. doi:10.1126/science.1255555.

Head, M. W., Ironside, J. W., Ghetti, B., Jeffrey, M., Piccardo, P., & Wil, R. G. (2015). Prion diseases. In S. Love, H. Budka, J. W. Ironside, & A. Perry (Eds.), *Greenfield's Neuropathology* (9th ed., Vol. 2, pp. 1016–1086). London: CRC Press.

Peden, A. H., Head, M. W., Ritchie, D. L., Bell, J. E., & Ironside, J. W. (2004). Preclinical vCJD after blood transfusion in a *PRNP* codon 129 heterozygous patient. *Lancet, 364*(9433), 527–529.

Prusiner, S. B. (1998). Prions. *Proceedings of the National Academy of Sciences of the USA, 95*(23), 13363–13383. doi:10.1073/pnas.95.23.13363.

Will, R. G., Ironside, J. W., Zeidler, M., Estibeiro, K., Cousens, S. N., Smith, P. G., ... Hofman, A. (1996). A new variant of Creutzfeldt–Jakob disease in the UK. *Lancet, 347*(9006), 921–925.

Websites

BSE: How to spot and report the disease. Retrieved from https://www.gov.uk/guidance/bse. (Accessed Jul 2017).

Creutzfeldt-Jakob disease surveillance (CJD): biannual updates. Retrieved from https://www.gov.uk/government/publications/creutzfeldt-jakob-disease-cjd-surveillance-biannual-updates. (Accessed Jul 2017).

Medical Research Council Prion Unit. Retrieved from http://www.prion.ucl.ac.uk/. (Accessed Jul 2017).

Minimizing transmission risk of CJD and vCJD in healthcare settings. Retrieved from https://www.gov.uk/government/publications/guidance-from-the-acdp-tse-risk-management-subgroup-formerly-tse-working-group. (Accessed Jul 2017).

The transfusion medicine epidemiological review (TMER). Retrieved from http://www.cjd.ed.ac.uk/all-projects/transfusion-medicine-epidemiology-review-tmer. (Accessed Jul 2017).

UK CJD Research & Surveillance Unit. Retrieved from http://www.cjd.ed.ac.uk/. (Accessed Jul 2017).

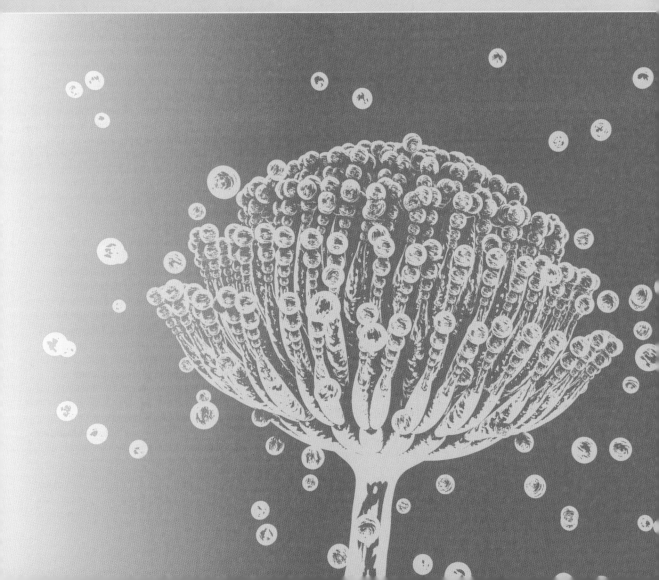

PART 5

FUNGAL PATHOGENS, PARASITIC INFECTIONS AND MEDICAL ENTOMOLOGY

58 Fungi

Superficial; subcutaneous and systemic mycoses

DAVID W. WARNOCK

KEY POINTS

- Most infections are caused by fungi that grow as saprophytes in the environment. Superficial, subcutaneous and systemic patterns of infection are recognised.
- Fungi take the form of yeasts, which grow by budding; moulds, which grow as filamentous extensions called hyphae, forming a mycelium; or dimorphic fungi, which can grow as yeast or mould forms.
- Pathogenic fungi can establish an infection in all exposed individuals; others are opportunist pathogens that cause disease only in a compromised host.
- Many fungal diseases have a global distribution, but some are endemic to specific geographical regions.
- Subcutaneous fungal infections are acquired by traumatic implantation; systemic infections are usually acquired by inhalation.
- Only dermatophytosis, a common superficial infection of the skin, nails and scalp hair, is truly contagious.
- Some yeasts are human commensals and cause endogenous infection when there is some imbalance in the host.
- The most frequently encountered fungal agents in the United Kingdom are *Candida* spp., dermatophytes, *Aspergillus* spp., *Cryptococcus* spp. and *Pneumocystis jirovecii*.
- Diagnosis of fungal infections is based on a combination of clinical observation and laboratory investigation, which may include direct microscopy, histology, culture, PCR and serology. Early recognition of systemic infections in immunocompromised persons is a major challenge.

Fungi constitute a large, diverse group of heterotrophic organisms, most of which are found as saprophytes in the soil and on decomposing organic matter. They are eukaryotic, with a range of internal membrane systems, membrane-bound organelles, and a well-defined cell wall composed largely of polysaccharides (glucan, mannan) and chitin. They show considerable variation in size and form, but can be divided into three main groups:

1. Moulds (multicellular filamentous fungi), which are composed of branching filaments, termed hyphae, grow by apical extension to form an intertwined mass termed a mycelium. In most fungi the hyphae have regular cross-walls (septa) but in lower fungi these are usually absent. Moulds reproduce by means of spores produced, often in large numbers, by an asexual process (involving mitosis only) or as a result of sexual reproduction (involving meiosis, preceded by fusion of the nuclei of two haploid cells). Many fungi can produce more than one type of spore, depending on the growth conditions. The precise method of spore production and the type(s) of spore produced are unique to each individual fungal species. In some higher fungi the sexual spores are produced in macroscopic structures such as mushrooms and toadstools. In laboratory cultures, moulds produce mainly asexual spores.
2. Yeasts are predominantly unicellular and oval or round in shape. Most propagate by an asexual process called budding in which the cell develops a protuberance, which enlarges and eventually separates from the parent cell. Some yeasts produce chains of elongated cells (pseudohyphae) that resemble the hyphae of moulds; some species also produce true hyphae. A small number of yeasts reproduce by fission. Yeasts are neither a natural nor a formal taxonomic group, but are a growth form shown by a wide range of unrelated fungi.
3. Dimorphic fungi are capable of changing their growth to either a mycelial or yeast phase, depending on the growth conditions.

Historically, fungal classification has largely been based on their morphological characteristics, although physiological and biochemical tests have been important in yeast identification. Molecular sequence analysis has demonstrated that many of the phenotypic characteristics used to classify fungi do not predict phylogenetic relatedness, and its use has led to major changes in fungal classification and nomenclature. Many laboratories today employ DNA sequencing as part of their routine protocol for fungal identification.

FUNGAL DISEASES OF HUMANS

FUNGAL PATHOGENS

There are at least 100,000 named species of fungi. However, <1000 have been recognised to cause disease (mycosis) in humans or animals. Most are moulds, but there are a number of pathogenic yeasts, and some are dimorphic. Dimorphic fungi usually change from a multicellular mould form in the natural environment to a budding single-celled yeast form when causing infection. In the laboratory the tissue form can be induced by culture at 37°C on rich media such as blood agar, whereas the mould form develops when incubated at a lower temperature (25–30°C) on a less rich medium such as Sabouraud dextrose agar.

Some fungi, such as the systemic pathogens *Histoplasma capsulatum* and *Blastomyces dermatitidis*, can establish an infection in all exposed individuals. Others, such as *Candida* and *Aspergillus* species, are opportunist pathogens that ordinarily cause disease only in a compromised host. In some mycoses the form and severity of the infection depend on the degree of exposure to the fungus, the site and method of entry into the body and the level of immunocompetence of the host.

Some fungi may cause serious, occasionally fatal, toxic effects in humans, following either ingestion of poisonous toadstools or consumption of mouldy food that contains toxic secondary metabolites (mycotoxins). Allergic disease of the airways may result from inhalation of fungal spores.

EPIDEMIOLOGY

Most human fungal infections are caused by fungi that grow as saprophytes in the environment. Infection is acquired by inhalation, ingestion or traumatic implantation. Some yeasts are human commensals and cause endogenous infections when there is some imbalance in the host. Only dermatophyte infections are truly contagious.

Many fungal diseases have a worldwide distribution, but some are endemic to specific geographical regions, usually because the causal agents are saprophytes restricted in their distribution by soil and climatic conditions.

TYPES OF INFECTION

Superficial mycoses

Diseases of the skin, hair, nail and mucous membranes are the most common of all fungal infections and have a worldwide distribution.

- Dermatophytosis (ringworm) is a complex of diseases affecting the outermost keratinized tissues of hair, nail and the stratum corneum of the skin. it is caused by a group of closely related mould fungi called dermatophytes, which can digest keratin. Dermatophyte infections occur in both humans and animals.
- Yeast infections affect the skin, nail and mucous membranes of the mouth and vagina, and are usually caused by commensal *Candida* species, notably *C. albicans*. Infection is generally endogenous in origin, but genital infection can be transmitted sexually. The yeast *Malassezia furfur*, a skin commensal, can cause an infection of the skin called pityriasis versicolor.

Subcutaneous mycoses

Mycoses of the dermis, subcutaneous tissues and adjacent bones that show slow localised spread occur mainly in the tropics and subtropics, and they usually result from the traumatic inoculation of saprophytic fungi from soil or vegetation into the subcutaneous tissue. The principal subcutaneous mycoses are mycetoma, chromoblastomycosis and sporotrichosis.

Systemic mycoses

Deep-seated fungal infections generally result from the inhalation of airborne spores produced by the causal moulds, present as saprophytes in the environment. Initially there is a pulmonary infection, but the organism may become disseminated to other organs. The organisms that cause systemic mycoses can be divided into two distinct groups: the true pathogens and the opportunistic pathogens. The first of these groups is comprised mostly of dimorphic fungi, and infections occur mainly in the Americas. The principal diseases are:

- blastomycosis (caused by *Blastomyces dermatitidis*)
- coccidioidomycosis (*Coccidioides immitis* and *C. posadasii*)
- histoplasmosis *(H. capsulatum)*
- paracoccidioidomycosis *(Paracoccidioides brasiliensis).*

Systemic mycoses caused by opportunistic pathogens such as *Aspergillus, Candida* and *Cryptococcus* species have a more widespread distribution. These infections are being seen with increasing frequency in patients compromised by disease or drug treatment. In transplant patients, for example, these fungi are among the most frequent causes of death due to infection.

INCIDENCE

The incidence of all the mycoses is related directly to factors that affect the degree of exposure to the causal fungi, such as living conditions, occupation and leisure activities.

- Dermatophytosis of the foot (athlete's foot), with associated infections of nails and groin, occurs most commonly in swimmers, sportspersons and industrial workers who use communal bathing facilities.
- Animal dermatophytosis is an occupational hazard for farmers, veterinarians and others closely associated with animals.
- Agricultural workers in warm climates who wear little protective clothing frequently contract subcutaneous infections following minor injuries from vegetation.
- In developed countries the incidence of infections due to opportunistic fungal pathogens has increased following major advances in health care that have led to increases in the size of the population at risk.
- In many developing countries the acquired immune deficiency syndrome (AIDS) pandemic has been associated with a marked increase in the rate of opportunistic fungal infections. High mortality rates have been reported from countries where adequate treatment is often unavailable.
- The incidence of several of the systemic mycoses that are endemic in the Americas has increased as a result of urban development and changing land use in the endemic areas. Increased international travel and tourism has also led to a rise in the number of cases of disease among individuals who normally reside in countries far from the endemic areas.

DIAGNOSIS

Diagnosis of fungal infections is based on a combination of clinical features and laboratory investigations.

Clinical features

Superficial and subcutaneous mycoses often produce characteristic lesions, but they may also closely resemble and be confused with other diseases. In addition, the appearance of lesions may be modified beyond recognition by previous therapy, for example, with topical steroids.

The first indication that a patient may have a systemic mycosis is often their failure to respond to antibacterial antibiotics. As early diagnosis considerably increases the chances of successful treatment, it is important that the possibility of fungal infection be considered from the outset, particularly in those known to be at risk of developing a fungal infection. Computed tomography is widely used to help diagnose *Aspergillus* and other invasive mycoses.

Laboratory investigation

Laboratory diagnosis depends on:

- recognition of the pathogen in tissue by microscopy
- isolation of the causal fungus in culture
- detection of fungal antigens
- detection of fungal DNA by the polymerase chain reaction (PCR)
- detection of fungal antibodies.

It is important that the correct type of specimen, together with adequate clinical data, is sent to the laboratory so that the appropriate investigations can be carried out. Information on factors such as travel or residence abroad, animal contacts and the occupation of the patient enables the laboratory staff to direct their investigations towards a particular fungus or group of fungi when appropriate.

Types of specimen

Skin scales, nail clippings and scrapings of the scalp that include hair stubs and skin scales are the most suitable specimens for the diagnosis of ringworm; these are collected into folded paper squares for transport to the laboratory. Swabs should be taken from suspected *Candida* infections from the mucous membranes and preferably sent to the laboratory in clear transport medium. For subcutaneous infections the most suitable specimens are scrapings and crusts, aspirated pus and biopsies. In suspected systemic infection, specimens should be taken from appropriate sites.

Direct microscopy

Most specimens can be examined satisfactorily in wet mounts after partial digestion of the tissue with 10%–20% potassium hydroxide. Addition of Calcofluor white and subsequent examination by fluorescence microscopy enhances the detection of most fungi as the fluorescent hydroxide–Calcofluor binds to the fungal cell walls. Gram films may also be used for the diagnosis of yeast infections of mucous membranes. Giemsa staining of smears is advised for detection of the yeast cells of *H. capsulatum* because of their small size.

Histology

Invasive procedures are required to obtain specimens for histological examination. Although sometimes necessary to provide firm evidence of invasive disease, such procedures are often impracticable on patients who are already seriously ill. Haematoxylin and eosin staining is seldom of value for demonstrating fungi in tissue, and specific fungal stains such as periodic acid–Schiff and Grocott–Gomori methenamine–silver are widely used.

Culture

Most pathogenic fungi are easy to grow in culture. Sabouraud dextrose agar and 4% malt extract agar are most commonly used. These may be supplemented with chloramphenicol (50 mg/L) to minimise bacterial contamination and cycloheximide (500 mg/L) to reduce contamination with saprophytic fungi. Many fungal pathogens have an optimum growth temperature below 37°C. Consequently, cultures are incubated at 25–30°C and at 37°C. With some dimorphic pathogens, enriched media such as brain–heart infusion or blood agar are used to promote growth of the yeast phase.

Many fungi grow relatively slowly, and cultures should be retained for at least 2–3 weeks (in some cases up to 6 weeks) before being discarded; yeasts usually grow within 1–5 days. Moulds are traditionally identified by their macroscopic and microscopic morphology. Yeasts are identified by sugar fermentation and their ability to assimilate carbon and nitrogen sources. Commercial kits are available for the identification of medically important yeasts. When traditional phenotypic tests are unhelpful (e.g., when a mould fails to sporulate in culture), DNA sequencing may be required.

Culture may provide unequivocal evidence of fungal infection when established pathogens are isolated or when fungi are recovered from normally sterile sites. However, when commensals such as *Candida* species are isolated from nonsterile sites (e.g., sputum samples), results must be correlated with clinical evidence and other investigations (e.g., imaging) and interpreted accordingly.

Serology

Detection of fungal antigens and antibody are increasingly used in diagnosis because of ease of detection compared to finding the organism directly in clinical specimens. They can be found in large amounts in body fluids (blood, cerebrospinal fluid, urine and bronchoalveolar lavage).

The most common tests for fungal antibodies are:

- immunodiffusion
- countercurrent immunoelectrophoresis (CIE)
- whole cell agglutination
- complement fixation
- enzyme-linked immunosorbent assay (ELISA).

For antigen detection the following are used:

- latex particle agglutination
- ELISA
- lateral flow assay

Polymerase chain reaction

Detection of fungal DNA in clinical material, principally blood, serum, bronchoalveolar lavage fluid and sputum, is increasingly used for diagnosis. Comparison of results is limited because of lack of standardisation of tests.

TREATMENT

There are relatively few therapeutically useful antifungal agents compared with the large number of antibacterial agents that are available (see Ch. 5). As fungi and human beings are both eukaryotes, most substances that kill or inhibit fungal pathogens are also toxic to the host. Antifungal agents vary considerably in their spectrum of activity (see Ch. 5). Most exploit differences in the sterol composition of the fungal and mammalian cell membranes, although the echinocandins (anidulafungin, caspofungin and micafungin) interfere with β-glucan synthesis in the fungal cell wall.

Most antifungal agents are available only for topical use. Relatively few can be administered systemically.

- Amphotericin B and the echinocandins (anidulafungin, caspofungin, micafungin) are given parenterally because of poor absorption from the gastrointestinal tract.
- The azoles (fluconazole, itraconazole, posaconazole, voriconazole, isavuconazole) and flucytosine are available for oral and/or parenteral administration.
- Terbinafine and griseofulvin are usually administered orally.
- Amphotericin B is the historical treatment of choice in life-threatening disease, despite its toxicity; liposomal and lipid complex formulations are less toxic but much more expensive.
- A combination of amphotericin B and flucytosine reduces the likelihood of the emergence of resistance to flucytosine. Combinations of azole drugs and amphotericin B are seldom used therapeutically.

- New antifungals are being evaluated for use in systemic mycoses. Posaconazole or isavuconazole is used as step-down therapy in invasive aspergillosis and mucormycosis for patients who have responded to amphotericin B or as salvage therapy for patients who do not respond or cannot tolerate amphotericin B.
- Antifungal prophylaxis is often used to help prevent opportunistic infections in patients undergoing solid organ or stem cell transplants and in those with haematological malignancies. Oral or topical antifungals are also used to prevent recurrent vaginal candidosis.

Acquired resistance to antifungal drugs has not been a major problem. It is sometimes encountered, especially after prolonged azole or echinocandin therapy of invasive candidosis. Azole-resistant *Aspergillus fumigatus* infection, acquired from the environment as an unintended consequence of agricultural fungicide use, has recently been identified in many countries worldwide. Consequently, susceptibility testing is often carried out for any drug that fails to produce the expected therapeutic response.

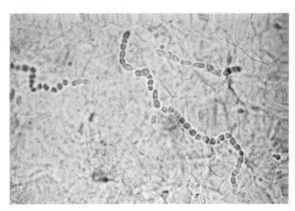

Fig. 58.1 Microscopical appearance of infected skin scrapings showing the development of arthroconidia. (Reproduced with permission from Richardson, M. D., Warnock, D. W., & Campbell, C. K. (1995). *Slide Atlas of Fungal Infection: Superficial Fungal Infections.* Oxford: Blackwell Science. ISBN 0-86542-930-8. Figure 16.)

SUPERFICIAL INFECTIONS

DERMATOPHYTOSIS

Dermatophyte infections are common diseases of the stratum corneum of the skin, hair and nail. They are also referred to as ringworm or as tinea, a name that is qualified by the site affected, for example tinea pedis or tinea capitis for infections of the feet or scalp, respectively. These infections are caused by about 20 species of fungi that are grouped into three genera: *Trichophyton, Microsporum* and *Epidermophyton*. Some species are worldwide in distribution, whereas others are restricted to, or are more common in, particular parts of the world.

Many dermatophyte species produce two types of asexual spore—multicelled macroconidia and single-celled microconidia. Classification into the three genera *Trichophyton, Microsporum* and *Epidermophyton* is based on the morphology of the macroconidia, although the identification of species is also based on the shape and disposition of the microconidia and the macroscopic appearance of the colonies. Molecular sequence analysis supports the ongoing classification of the dermatophytes into the three traditional genera.

The clinical appearances of dermatophyte infections are the result of a combination of direct tissue damage caused by the fungus and of the immune response of the host. The damage to tissue is due to a combination of mechanical pressure and enzymatic activities. In tissue the dermatophytes take the form of branching hyphae, which may eventually break up into arthroconidia, particularly in infected hair (Fig. 58.1).

Epidemiology

The dermatophytes can be divided into three groups depending on whether their normal habitat is the soil (geophilic species), animals (zoophilic species) or humans (anthropophilic species). Members of all three groups can cause human infection, but their different natural reservoirs have important epidemiological implications in relation to the acquisition, site and spread of human disease.

Although geophilic dermatophytes occasionally cause infection in both animals and man, their normal habitat is the soil. Members of the anthropophilic and zoophilic groups are thought to have evolved from these and other keratinophilic soil-inhabiting fungi, different species having adapted to different natural hosts. Individual members of the zoophilic group are often associated with a particular animal host, for instance *M. canis* with cats and dogs and *T. verrucosum* with cattle. However, these organisms can also spread to humans. The anthropophilic species are the most highly specialised group of dermatophytes. They rarely infect other animals and often show a strong preference for a particular body site, only occasionally being found in other regions. For instance, *M. audouinii* commonly infects scalp hair, whereas *E. floccosum* is usually found on the skin.

Infections are spread by direct or indirect contact with an infected individual or animal. The infective particle is usually a fragment of keratin containing viable fungus. Indirect transfer may occur via the floors of swimming pools and showers, or on brushes, towels and animal grooming implements. Dermatophytes can remain viable for long periods of time, and the interval between deposition and transfer may be considerable. In addition to exposure to the fungus, some abnormality of the epidermis, such as slight peeling or minor trauma, is probably necessary for the establishment of infection.

In industrialised countries, tinea capitis is relatively uncommon and is caused by dermatophytes of both human and animal origin, although infections with the anthropophilic species *T. tonsurans* are on the increase among urban populations in Europe and the Americas. However, the use of communal bathing facilities has resulted in a considerable increase in the incidence of tinea pedis and associated nail and groin infections. These now constitute about 75% of all dermatophyte infections diagnosed in temperate zones.

In developing countries, particularly in warm climates, scalp, body and groin infections predominate, with *T. rubrum* and *T. violaceum* among the most common causes.

Clinical features

Lesions vary considerably according to the site of the infection and the species of fungus involved. Sometimes there is only dry scaling or hyperkeratosis, but more commonly there is irritation, erythema, oedema and some vesiculation. More inflammatory lesions with weeping vesicles, pustules and ulceration are usually caused by zoophilic species.

In skin infections of the body, face and scalp, spreading annular lesions with a raised, inflammatory border are usually produced (Fig. 58.2). Lesions in body folds, such as the groin, tend to spread outwards from the flexures. In tinea pedis, infection is often confined to the toe clefts, but it can spread to the sole, and sometimes painful secondary bacterial infection occurs in the toe clefts.

In nail infection, the nail becomes discoloured, thickened, raised and friable. Most nail infections are due to *T. rubrum* and involve the toenails (Fig. 58.3).

In scalp infections there is scaling and hair loss, the extent of which depends on the causal fungus. Some zoophilic species give rise to a highly inflammatory, raised, suppurating lesion called a kerion; kerions may also occur in the beard area of adults. It is important that tinea capitis is recognised and treated promptly because it can lead to scarring and permanent hair loss.

In scalp infection the fungus invades the hair shaft and the hyphae then break up into chains of arthroconidia. In some species (e.g., *T. tonsurans, T. violaceum*) the arthroconidia are retained within the hair shaft (endothrix invasion), whereas in others (e.g., *Microsporum* species, *T. verrucosum*) they are produced in a sheath

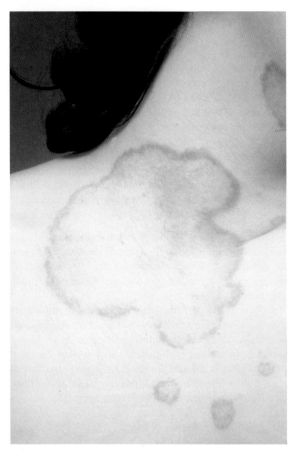

Fig. 58.2 Tinea corporis due to *Microsporum canis*.

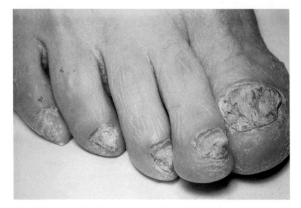

Fig. 58.3 Toenail infection due to *Trichophyton rubrum*. (Reproduced with permission from Richardson, M. D., Warnock, D. W., & Campbell, C. K. (1995). *Slide Atlas of Fungal Infection: Superficial Fungal Infections*. Oxford: Blackwell Science. ISBN 0-86542-930-8. Figure 3.)

surrounding the hair shaft (ectothrix invasion). The pattern of hair invasion affects the clinical appearance of the lesion.

- In endothrix infection the hair breaks off at, or just below, the mouth of the follicle to give what is described as a black dot appearance.
- In ectothrix infection the hair usually breaks off 2–3 mm above the mouth of the follicle, leaving short stumps of hair.
- In favus, caused by *T. schoenleinii*, fungal growth within the hair is minimal. The hair remains intact, but intense fungal growth within and around the hair follicle produces a waxy, honeycomb-like crust on the scalp (Fig. 58.4).

Infections of the groin, hands and nails are nearly always secondary to infection of the feet and are usually (except in developing countries) caused by *T. rubrum, T. mentagrophytes* or *E. floccosum*. Mixed infections also occur.

Occasionally, patients with inflammatory infections develop a secondary rash known as an id reaction, which is thought to be an immunological reaction to fungal antigens. In patients with tinea pedis this takes the form of a vesicular eczema of the hands, whereas patients with tinea capitis (especially kerion) develop a follicular rash, usually on the trunk or limbs. These secondary lesions do not contain viable fungus and they disappear spontaneously when the infection subsides.

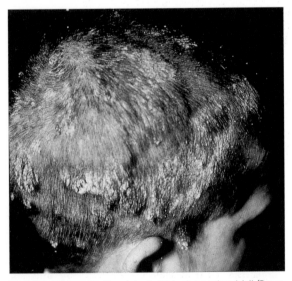

Fig. 58.4 Tinea capitis (favus) due to *Trichophyton schoenleinii*. (Reproduced with permission from Richardson, M. D., Warnock, D. W., & Campbell, C. K. (1995). *Slide Atlas of Fungal Infection: Superficial Fungal Infections*. Oxford: Blackwell Science. ISBN 0-86542-930-8. Figure 16.)

Laboratory investigation

Dermatophyte infections may be reliably diagnosed in the laboratory by direct microscopical examination and culture of skin, crusts, hair and nail.

Collection of samples

Skin, hair and nail samples are best collected into folded squares of black paper or card, which can be fastened with a paper clip. The use of paper allows the specimen to dry out, which helps reduce bacterial contamination and provides conditions under which specimens can be stored for 12 months or more without appreciable loss in viability of the fungus.

Nail samples should be collected by taking clippings from any discoloured, dystrophic or brittle parts of the nail and, importantly, by scraping material from underneath the nail. The sample should be taken from as far back as possible from the free edge of the nail.

Scales from skin lesions should be collected by scraping outwards with a blunt scalpel from the edges of the lesions, where most viable fungus is likely to be. Specimens from the scalp should include hair stubs, the contents of plugged follicles and skin scales. Infected hairs are usually easy to pluck from the scalp with forceps. Cut hairs are unsatisfactory because the focus of infection is usually below or near the surface of the scalp.

Wood's lamp

This is a source of long-wave ultraviolet light that can be used to detect fluorescence in infected hair. It is especially useful for the detection of inconspicuous scalp lesions and to select infected hairs for laboratory investigation.

Hairbrush sampling

Adequate material from minimal lesions may be obtained by brushing the scalp with a sterilised plastic hairbrush or scalp massage pad; this is then used to inoculate an appropriate culture medium by pressing the brush or pad spines into the agar.

Processing of specimens

If there is insufficient material for both microscopy and culture, the sample should be used for culture, since this is generally the more sensitive procedure (except for nails).

The specimen should first be examined macroscopically; hair samples are examined under a Wood's lamp. Material from representative parts, and any fluorescent hairs, are divided up into 1–2-mm fragments with a sterile scalpel blade before microscopical examination and culture.

Direct microscopy

Microscopy of wet mounts of keratinous material in potassium hydroxide is simple and reliable. The preparation is allowed to stand for 15–20 minutes to digest and clear the keratin. Dermatophytes are seen in skin and nail as branching hyphae, which often appear slightly greenish in colour and run across the outlines of the colourless host cells (Fig. 58.1). With Calcofluor (see earlier in the chapter) the cell outlines fluoresce white.

Culture

Small fragments of keratinous material are planted or scattered on Sabouraud dextrose or 4% malt extract agar and incubated at 28–30°C for up to 2 weeks; room temperature is adequate but the dermatophytes grow more slowly. Only *T. verrucosum* grows well at 37°C.

Identification is based on colonial appearance and colour, pigment production, and the micromorphology of any spores produced. Special tests exist for differentiating certain morphologically similar species. Thus, the ability of *T. mentagrophytes* to produce urease within 2–4 days distinguishes it from *T. rubrum*, and the ability to grow on rice grains distinguishes *M. canis* from *M. audouinii*.

Treatment and prevention

Topical therapy is satisfactory for most skin infections, although oral antifungals are required to treat infections of the nail and scalp and severe or extensive skin infections.

Topical agents include azole compounds, terbinafine, amorolfine and ciclopirox olamine. Oral griseofulvin is useful for scalp, skin and fingernail infections, but gives poor results in toenail infections, even after 18 months' therapy. Terbinafine and itraconazole have largely replaced griseofulvin for the treatment of nail infections because of their much better cure rates and shorter periods of treatment (around 85% cure for toenails after 3 months' therapy).

Relatively little has been done to control the spread of dermatophyte infections. Use of antifungal foot powder after bathing as prophylaxis has helped reduce the spread of infection among swimmers. Foot baths containing antiseptic solutions, which are commonplace in swimming pools, are of no value.

SUPERFICIAL CANDIDOSIS

Superficial *Candida* infections involving the skin, nails and mucous membranes of the mouth and vagina are very common throughout the world. *Candida albicans* accounts for 80%–90% of cases, but other species, notably *C. glabrata, C. parapsilosis, C. tropicalis, C. krusei* and *C. guilliermondii*, may occur.

On Sabouraud dextrose agar *Candida* species grow predominantly in the yeast phase as round or oval cells 3–8 mm in diameter. A mixture of yeast cells, pseudohyphae and true hyphae is found in vivo and under microaerophilic growth conditions on nutritionally poor media. *C. glabrata* does not form either hyphae or pseudohyphae.

Epidemiology

Candida species, usually *C. albicans*, are found in small numbers in the commensal flora (mouth, gastrointestinal tract, vagina, skin) of about 20% of the normal population. The carriage rate tends to increase with age and is higher in the vagina during pregnancy. Commensal yeasts are more prevalent among patients in hospital. Yeast overgrowth and infection occur when the normal microbial flora of the body is altered or when host resistance to infection is lowered by disease.

In most cases, infection is derived from an individual's own endogenous reservoir. In some instances, however, transmission from person to person can occur; for example, neonatal oral candidosis is more common in infants born of mothers with vaginal candidosis. The hands of healthcare workers are another potential source of neonatal infection.

Individuals colonised with *Candida* species possess numerous nonspecific and immunological defences to prevent infection. In superficial candidosis the nonspecific inhibitory factors include inhibitors in serum, such as unsaturated transferrin, and epithelial proliferation. Specific defence largely depends on the development of active T cell–mediated immunity.

Both general and local predisposing factors are important in the development of oropharyngeal candidosis. Debilitated and immunosuppressed individuals, such as persons with diabetes mellitus, stem cell transplant recipients and those with human immunodeficiency virus (HIV) infection, are more susceptible to infection. Local factors, such as xerostomia and trauma from unhygienic or ill-fitting dentures, are also important. Local tissue damage is also a critical factor in the development of cutaneous forms of candidosis. Most infections occur in moist, occluded sites and follow maceration of tissue.

Vaginal candidosis is more common during pregnancy. The lower prevalence of this infection after menopause emphasises the hormonal dependence of the infection. Most cases of vaginal candidosis in older women are associated with uncontrolled diabetes mellitus or the use of exogenous oestrogen replacement treatment.

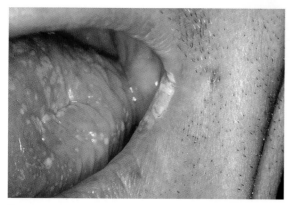

Fig. 58.5 Pseudomembranous oral candidosis with associated angular cheilitis.

Clinical features

Mucosal infection

This is the most common form of superficial candidosis. Discrete white patches develop on the mucosal surface, and may eventually become confluent and form a curdlike pseudomembrane (Fig. 58.5).

In oropharyngeal candidosis, white flecks appear on the buccal mucosa, tongue and the hard and soft palate; although these are adherent, they can be removed. The surrounding mucosa is red and sore. This form of oropharyngeal candidosis occurs most frequently in infancy and old age, or in severely immunocompromised patients, including those with AIDS. Other forms of oral candidosis occur:

- lesions in the occluded area under the denture in those who wear dentures
- painful infection of the tongue in some individuals receiving antibiotic therapy
- chronic infection with extensive leucoplakia and infection of the angles of the mouth (angular cheilitis)

In vaginal candidosis, itching, soreness and a nonhomogeneous white discharge accompany typical white lesions on the epithelial surfaces of the vulva, vagina and cervix. Sometimes the mucosa simply appears inflamed and friable. The perivulval skin may become sore, and small satellite pustules may appear around the perineum and natal cleft. Some women suffer recurrent episodes.

Chronic, intractable oropharyngeal candidosis, which may extend to give oesophageal infection, is common in persons with HIV infection, although the use of combinations of antiretroviral drugs has reduced its incidence. The appearance of this infection can be the indicator of the transition from HIV-positive status to AIDS.

Skin and nail infection

Cutaneous candidosis is less common than dermatophytosis. The lesions usually develop in warm, moist sites such as the axillae, groin and submammary folds. In infants, *Candida* species are often secondary invaders in napkin dermatitis. Infection of the finger webs, nail folds and nails is associated with frequent immersion of the hands in water.

Chronic mucocutaneous candidosis

This is a rare form of candidosis that usually becomes apparent in childhood and takes the form of a persistent, sometimes granulomatous, infection of the mouth, scalp, hands, feet and nails. In some cases, disfiguring hyperkeratotic lesions develop on the scalp and face. Some of those who develop this condition have subtle defects in lymphocyte function.

Laboratory investigation

Specimens of skin and nail are collected in the same way as for suspected dermatophytosis. For infections of the mouth or vagina, scrapings taken with a blunt scalpel or a spatula from areas with white plaques or erythema are better than swabs if the material is to be processed immediately. However, swabs are more convenient for transport to the laboratory, and they are better for collecting vaginal discharge. Swabs should first be moistened with sterile water or saline before taking the sample and should be sent to the laboratory in clear transport medium.

In Gram-stained smears of mucous membrane samples the fungus is seen as budding Gram-positive yeast cells; pseudohyphae are usually present except in the case of *C. glabrata* (Fig. 58.6). Contrary to popular belief, the presence of *Candida* pseudohyphae in clinical material does not confirm infection with the organism, particularly as it may have developed in the period between collection and processing of the sample.

Candida species grow well on Sabouraud medium or on blood agar at 25–37°C; typical yeast colonies appear within 1–2 days. *C. albicans* isolates can be identified by the germ tube test: after incubation in serum at 37°C for 1.5–2 hours, *C. albicans* produces short hyphae known as germ tubes. Other yeasts may be identified with one of the commercial kits, or by fermentation and assimilation tests. Many laboratories today employ MALDI-TOF mass spectrometry and DNA sequencing as part of their routine protocol for yeast identification.

Quantification of growth, especially in the case of vulvovaginal samples, may help the clinician to distinguish between commensal carriage and infection.

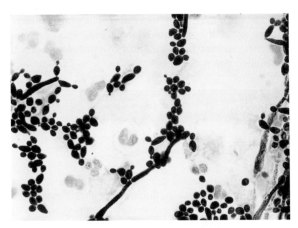

Fig. 58.6 Microscopical appearance of *Candida albicans* yeast cells and pseudohyphae in a Gram-stained vaginal smear.

Detection of *Candida* mannan, a cell wall polysaccharide and 1, 3 β-D-glucan by EIA offers alternative methods of diagnosis. Commercial tests detecting anti-*Candida* antibody by EIA is also available. These tests are associated with false-positive results, particularly with colonisation, and false-negative results in immunocompromised individuals.

Treatment and prevention

Most superficial infections respond well to topical therapy with an imidazole. In oral candidosis, nystatin, amphotericin B or miconazole may be effective in lozenge or gel form. Most patients with vaginal candidosis can be treated successfully with a single application of a topical imidazole, or with oral fluconazole or itraconazole. Intermittent prophylaxis with an oral azole or vaginal pessaries is of benefit in controlling recurrent vaginal candidosis.

Treatment of chronic paronychia involves a combination of antifungal therapy, nail care and avoidance of prolonged exposure to water by use of protective gloves; patients should dry their hands carefully after washing. Regular application of an azole lotion or an azole given orally, sometimes in conjunction with a topical steroid and an antibacterial agent, is the most appropriate therapy, but it may take several months to cure the condition; antifungal creams or ointments are less effective.

Oral therapy is essential for the treatment of intractable chronic *Candida* infections; treatment is given until remission is achieved but in some patients, for instance those with AIDS, relapse is common, and intermittent or prolonged therapy may be required. This may, however, lead to the development of resistance, as occasionally happens with fluconazole.

PITYRIASIS VERSICOLOR

This is a common, mild and often recurrent infection of the stratum corneum that produces a patchy discoloration of the skin caused by lipophilic yeasts of the genus *Malassezia*. These organisms require lipids for growth, and special media containing Tween and lipid supplements have been developed.

On normal skin and in conditions such as dandruff and seborrhoeic dermatitis (in which its precise role is uncertain), *Malassezia* occurs as oval or bottle-shaped yeast, which characteristically produces buds on a broad base. In pityriasis versicolor the organism produces predominantly round yeast cells and short hyphae.

Epidemiology

Malassezia species are common members of the normal skin flora, and most infections are thought to be endogenous. The incidence of skin colonisation rises from around 25% in children to almost 100% in adolescents and adults. Disease is probably related to host and environmental factors. It is very common in hot, humid tropical climates, where 30%–40% of adults may be affected.

Clinical features

Small patches of well demarcated, noninflammatory scaling are usually present on the upper trunk or neck; these may appear hypopigmented or hyperpigmented, depending on the degree of pigmentation of the surrounding skin. The lesions tend to spread and coalesce, and occasionally they spread to other sites.

Laboratory investigation

The diagnosis can be confirmed reliably by direct microscopy of skin scales; culture is unnecessary. Demonstration of clusters of the characteristic round yeast cells (5–8 μm in diameter) with short, stout hyphae, which may be curved and occasionally branched, is diagnostic.

Treatment

Pityriasis versicolor responds well to topical therapy with 2% selenium sulphide or azoles such as ketoconazole in cream, lotion or a shampoo. Oral azole therapy is sometimes used for recalcitrant or widespread infections. Relapse is common, particularly in hot climates.

OTHER SUPERFICIAL INFECTIONS

Skin and nail

Certain nondermatophyte moulds may cause infection of skin and nail. It is important that these are recognised because they are often resistant to the agents used to treat dermatophytosis and superficial candidosis.

In the United Kingdom, about 5% of fungal nail infections are caused by nondermatophyte moulds. *Scopulariopsis brevicaulis*, a ubiquitous saprophyte of soil, is the most common, although other saprophytic moulds such as *Fusarium, Aspergillus* and *Acremonium* species are also occasionally implicated. There is some debate as to whether these moulds are primary pathogens of nails—infection usually follows trauma, and in many cases they are found in nails along with a dermatophyte.

Nondermatophyte mould infections do not respond to existing antifungal agents. Attempts may be made to remove the nail with topical 40% urea paste.

Otomycosis

About 10%–20% of chronic ear infections are due to fungi. The disease has a worldwide distribution, but is more common in warm climates. Topical antibiotics and steroids are predisposing factors. The most common causes are species of *Aspergillus*, in particular *A. niger*. The fungi are easy to see in material from swabs or scrapings and grow readily in culture.

Treatment with topical antifungals is usually successful, although relapse is common. Any concurrent bacterial infection or other underlying abnormality should also be treated.

Mycotic keratitis

Fungal infections of the cornea usually follow traumatic implantation of spores. Topical antibiotics and steroids are important predisposing factors. These infections occur most often in hot climates and are caused by common saprophytic moulds, in particular *Aspergillus* and *Fusarium* species. Culture results should be interpreted with care as these opportunist pathogens are also encountered as contaminants. Superficial swabs are of no value for laboratory investigation, and scrapings should be taken from the base or edge of the ulcer. The branched, septate hyphae may be rather sparse in potassium hydroxide mounts, and some of the material should also be stained with periodic acid–Schiff or Grocott–Gomori methenamine–silver.

Management entails surgical debridement of infected tissue, discontinuation of topical corticosteroids, and topical or oral treatment with an antifungal drug. Topical treatment with natamycin is often successful, but oral treatment with an azole drug is required in patients with severe or worsening lesions. Even with intensive treatment, corneal perforation can occur.

SUBCUTANEOUS INFECTIONS

MYCETOMA

Mycetoma is a chronic granulomatous infection of the skin, subcutaneous tissues, fascia and bone that most often affects the foot or the hand. It may be caused by one of a number of different actinomycetes (actinomycetoma) (see Ch. 28) or moulds (eumycetoma). The disease is most prevalent in tropical and subtropical regions of Africa, Asia, and Central and South America. In 2016, it was added to the World Health Organization's official list of neglected tropical diseases.

A large number of organisms have been implicated in this disease, including species of *Madurella, Trematosphaeria, Falciformispora (Leptosphaeria), Fusarium, Scedosporium, Actinomadura, Nocardia* and *Streptomyces*. Within host tissues the organisms develop to form compacted colonies (grains) 0.5–2 mm in diameter, the colour of which depends on the organism responsible; for example, in unstained preparations, *Trematosphaeria grisea* grains are black and *Actinomadura pelletieri* grains are red (Fig. 58.7).

Epidemiology

Infection follows traumatic inoculation of the organism into the subcutaneous tissue from soil or vegetation, usually

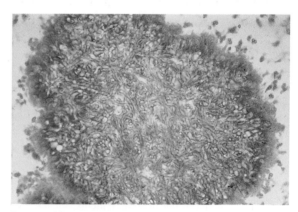

Fig. 58.7 Microscopical appearance of *Trematosphaeria (Madurella) grisea* in a stained mycetoma grain. (Reproduced with permission from Richardson, M. D., Warnock, D. W., & Campbell, C. K. (1995). *Slide Atlas of Fungal Infection: Subcutaneous and Unusual Fungal Infections.* Oxford: Blackwell Science. ISBN 0-86542-932-4. Figure 24.)

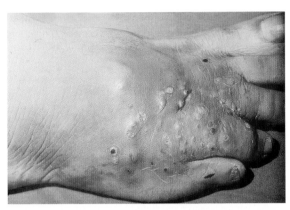

Fig. 58.8 Mycetoma of the foot.

on thorns or wood splinters. Consequently, the disease occurs most frequently in agricultural workers in whom minor penetrating skin injuries are common.

Clinical features

Localised swollen lesions that develop multiple draining sinuses are usually found on the limbs, although infections occur on other parts of the body (Fig. 58.8). There is often a long period between the initial infection and formation of the characteristic lesions; spread from the site of origin is unusual but may occur, particularly from the foot up the long bones of the leg.

Laboratory investigation

The presence of grains in pus collected from draining sinuses or in biopsy material is diagnostic. The grains are visible to the naked eye, and their colour may help to identify the causal agent. Grains should be crushed in potassium hydroxide and examined microscopically to differentiate between actinomycetoma and eumycetoma; material from actinomycetoma grains may be Gram stained to demonstrate the Gram-positive filaments. Samples should also be cultured, at both 25–30°C and 37°C, on brain–heart infusion agar or blood agar for actinomycetes and on Sabouraud agar (without cycloheximide) for fungi. The fungi that cause eumycetoma are all septate moulds that appear in culture within 1–4 weeks, but their identification requires expert knowledge.

Treatment

The prognosis varies according to the causal agent, so it is important that the identity is established. Actinomycetoma responds well to medical treatment; combinations of streptomycin with co-trimoxazole or dapsone are often effective, but an average of 9 months' therapy is required. Posaconazole has been licensed for salvage treatment of eumycetoma, but the cost is prohibitive in most endemic regions. Other drugs are ineffective, and radical surgery is usually necessary.

CHROMOBLASTOMYCOSIS

This disease, also known as chromomycosis, is a chronic, localised infection of the skin and subcutaneous tissues, characterised by slow-growing verrucous lesions usually involving the limbs. The disease is encountered mainly in the tropics, in Central and South America, and Madagascar. The principal causes are *Fonsecaea pedrosoi*, *Phialophora verrucosa* and *Cladophialophora carrionii*. Like mycetoma, infection follows traumatic inoculation of the organism into the skin or subcutaneous tissue and is seen most often among those with outdoor occupations.

Laboratory investigation

The characteristic clusters of brown-pigmented, thick-walled fungal cells are relatively easy to see on microscopical examination of skin scrapings, crusts and pus. Culture on Sabouraud agar at 25–30°C yields slow-growing, greenish grey to black, compact, folded colonies. Cultures should be incubated for 4–6 weeks. Specific identification of these closely related fungi is usually left to a reference laboratory.

Treatment

There is no ideal treatment for this disease, but promising results have been obtained with terbinafine and itraconazole, both of which can be combined with flucytosine in difficult cases. Early, solitary lesions may be excised.

SPOROTRICHOSIS

Sporotrichosis is a chronic, pyogenic, granulomatous infection of the skin and subcutaneous tissues that may remain localised or show lymphatic spread. It is caused by *Sporothrix schenckii*, which is found in the soil and on plant materials, such as wood and sphagnum moss. The disease is worldwide in distribution, but occurs mainly in Central and South America, parts of the United States and Africa, and Australia; it is rare in Europe.

S. schenckii is a dimorphic fungus. In nature and in culture at 25–30°C, it develops as a mould with septate hyphae. The yeast phase is formed in tissue and in culture at 37°C and is composed of spherical or cigar-shaped cells (1–3 × 3–10 μm).

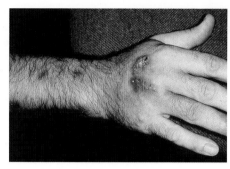

Fig. 58.9 Sporotrichosis of the hand showing local lymphatic spread.

Epidemiology

Minor trauma, such as abrasions or wounds due to wood splinters, is often sufficient to introduce the organism. Infection occurs mainly in adults and is more common among individuals whose work or recreational activities bring them into contact with soil or plant materials, such as gardeners and florists. Zoonotic sporotrichosis occurs with exposure to infected animals, most commonly cats.

Clinical features

Sporotrichosis presents most frequently as a nodular, ulcerating disease of the skin and subcutaneous tissues, with spread along local lymphatic channels (Fig. 58.9). Typically, the primary lesion is on the hand with secondary lesions extending up the arm. The primary lesion may remain localised or disseminate to involve the bones, joints, lungs and, in rare cases, the central nervous system. Disseminated disease usually occurs in debilitated or immunosuppressed individuals.

Laboratory investigation

Diagnosis is confirmed by isolation of the causative organism by culture of swabs from moist, ulcerated lesions or pus aspirated from subcutaneous nodules; biopsy specimens may be necessary in some cases. Direct microscopy is of little value as so few of the small *S. schenckii* yeast cells are present in diseased tissue. The mycelial phase develops within 7–10 days on Sabouraud agar or blood agar at 25–30°C; the yeast phase develops in 2 days at 37°C. Identification depends on the micro-morphology of the mould phase and its conversion to the yeast phase at 37°C.

Treatment

Prolonged therapy is usually required. For the lymphocutaneous form, treatment with itraconazole is recommended; potassium iodide is an alternative in resource-limited settings. In disseminated disease, intravenous amphotericin B is required.

OTHER SUBCUTANEOUS MYCOSES

Phaeohyphomycosis is a general term used to describe solitary subcutaneous lesions caused by any brown-pigmented mould. If left untreated, these lesions slowly increase in size to form a painless abscess. Diagnosis is often made at surgery, and treatment is by excision.

Several other fungi, including *Lacazia loboi*, *Basidiobolus ranarum* and *Conidiobolus coronatus*, occasionally cause subcutaneous infections, usually in the tropics. Surgical excision is often curative in *L. loboi* infections; antifungal therapy may be of use for the other infections, but the newer drugs have not been properly evaluated.

SYSTEMIC MYCOSES

COCCIDIOIDOMYCOSIS

This is primarily an infection of the lungs caused by *Coccidioides immitis* and *C. posadasii*, two closely related dimorphic fungi found in the soil of semiarid regions of the western hemisphere. In the United States, the endemic region includes parts of California, Arizona, Nevada, New Mexico, Utah and Texas. The endemic region extends southwards into the desert regions of northern Mexico, and parts of Central and South America.

In culture and in soil *Coccidioides* grows as a mould, producing large numbers of barrel-shaped arthroconidia (4 × 6 μm diameter), which are easily dispersed in wind currents (Fig. 58.10). In the lungs the arthroconidia form spherules (up to 120 μm in diameter) that contain numerous endospores (2–4 μm in diameter) (Fig. 58.11). Endospores are released by rupture of the spherule wall and develop to form new spherules in adjacent tissue or elsewhere in the body. In culture, the mould colonies are initially moist and white but change within 5–12 days to become floccose and pale grey or brown.

Epidemiology

Infection is acquired by inhalation; the incubation period is 1–3 weeks. The major risk factor for infection is environmental exposure. Outbreaks have been associated with ground-disturbing activities, such as building construction and archaeological excavation, as well as with natural events that result in the generation of dust clouds, such as earthquakes and dust storms. The most serious

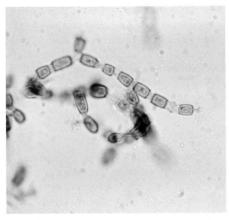

Fig. 58.10 Microscopical appearance of *Coccidioides* arthroconidia.

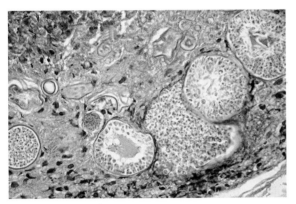

Fig. 58.11 Microscopical appearance of *Coccidioides* spherules in tissue.

disseminated forms of the disease are more common among those of black, Asian or Filipino ethnicity, and among pregnant women in the third trimester.

Clinical features

Coccidioides causes a wide spectrum of disease, ranging from a transient pulmonary infection that resolves without treatment, to chronic pulmonary infection, or to more widespread disseminated disease. About 40% of newly infected persons develop an acute symptomatic and often severe influenza-like illness. However, most otherwise healthy persons recover without treatment, their symptoms disappearing in a few weeks. In some cases, primary infection may result in chronic, cavitating, pulmonary disease.

Fewer than 1% of infected individuals develop disseminated coccidioidomycosis. This is a progressive disease that usually develops within 3–12 months of the initial infection, although it can occur much later following reactivation of a quiescent infection in an immunosuppressed individual. The clinical manifestations range from a fulminant illness that is fatal within a few weeks if left untreated, to an indolent chronic disease that persists for months or years. One or more sites may be involved, but the skin, soft tissue, bones, joints and central nervous system are most commonly affected. Meningitis is the most serious complication of coccidioidomycosis, occurring in 30%–50% of patients with disseminated disease. Without therapy, it is almost always fatal.

Laboratory investigation

Microscopical examination of sputum, pus and biopsy material is helpful as the relatively large size and numbers of mature spherules present makes their detection and identification comparatively straightforward. Material for culture should be inoculated onto screw-capped slopes of Sabouraud agar and incubated at 25–30°C for 1–2 weeks. The fungus can be identified by its colonial morphology and the presence of numerous thick-walled arthroconidia formed in chains from alternate cells of the septate hyphae.

The arthroconidia are highly infectious and are a serious danger to laboratory staff. Consequently, Petri dishes should never be used for isolation of the organism, and all procedures should be carried out in a biological safety cabinet under Category 3 containment. Preparations for microscopy should be made only after wetting the colony to reduce spore dispersal.

Serological tests play an important part in diagnosis. The immunodiffusion test is most useful for detection of early primary infection or exacerbation of existing disease; antibodies appear 1–3 weeks after infection but are seldom detectable after 2–6 months, or in patients with disseminated coccidioidomycosis. The latex agglutination test gives similar results to the immunodiffusion test, but is less specific. Complement-fixing antibodies appear 1–3 months after infection and persist for long periods in individuals with chronic or disseminated disease. In most cases the titre is proportional to the extent of infection; failure of the titre to fall during treatment of disseminated coccidioidomycosis is an ominous sign.

Treatment

The historical standard of treatment is intravenous amphotericin B, but oral fluconazole is now used to treat many patients with skin, soft tissue, bone or joint infections. Itraconazole is also effective, but less well tolerated. Because oral fluconazole is so much more benign than intrathecal amphotericin B, it is now the drug of choice for coccidioidal meningitis.

HISTOPLASMOSIS

This disease is caused by *H. capsulatum*, a dimorphic fungus found in soil enriched with the droppings of birds and bats. Histoplasmosis is the most common endemic mycosis in North America, but also occurs throughout Central and South America. In the United States, the disease is most prevalent in states surrounding the Mississippi and Ohio Rivers. Other endemic regions include parts of Africa, Australia, India and Malaysia. *H. capsulatum* var. *duboisii* is restricted to the continent of Africa.

H. capsulatum var. *capsulatum* grows in soil and in culture at 25–30°C as a mould and as an intracellular yeast in animal tissues. The small oval yeast phase cells (2–4 μm diameter) can also be produced in vitro by culture at 37°C on blood agar or other enriched media containing cysteine. In culture the mould colonies are fluffy, white or buff-brown; the mycelium is septate and two types of unicellular asexual spores are usually produced—large round, tuberculate macroconidia (8–15 μm in diameter) are most prominent and are diagnostic, but smaller, broadly elliptical, smooth-walled microconidia (2–4 μm in diameter) are also present in primary isolates (Fig. 58.12). *H. capsulatum* var. *duboisii* is morphologically identical to *H. capsulatum* var. *capsulatum* in its mycelial phase, but in the yeast phase has larger cells (10–15 μm in diameter).

Epidemiology

Infection results from the inhalation of spores; the incubation period is 1–3 weeks. The major risk factor is environmental exposure; longer and more intense exposures usually result in more severe pulmonary disease. Most reported outbreaks have been associated with exposures to sites contaminated with *H. capsulatum* or have followed activities that disturbed accumulations of bird or bat guano, such as building demolition, soil excavation and caving.

The most serious disseminated forms of the disease are more common among individuals with underlying cell-mediated immunological deficiencies, such as persons with HIV infection, transplant recipients, and those receiving immunosuppressive treatments.

Clinical features

There is a wide spectrum of disease, ranging from a transient pulmonary infection that subsides without treatment, to chronic pulmonary infection, or to more widespread disseminated disease. Many healthy individuals develop no symptoms when exposed to *H. capsulatum* in an endemic setting. Higher levels of exposure result in an acute symptomatic and often severe flulike illness, with fever, chills, nonproductive cough and fatigue. The symptoms usually disappear within a few weeks, but patients are frequently left with discrete, calcified lesions in the lung.

Disseminated histoplasmosis may range from an acute illness that is fatal within a few weeks if left untreated (often seen in infants, persons with AIDS and solid organ transplant recipients) to an indolent, chronic illness that can affect a wide range of sites. Hepatic infection is common in nonimmunosuppressed individuals, and adrenal gland destruction is a frequent problem. Mucosal ulcers are found in >60% of these patients; central nervous system disease occurs in 5%–20% of patients.

The clinical features of *H. capsulatum* var. *duboisii* infection differ from those of var. *capsulatum* infection. The illness is indolent in onset, and the predominant sites affected are the skin and bones. Those with more widespread infection involving the liver, spleen and other organs have a febrile wasting illness that is fatal within weeks or months if left untreated.

Laboratory investigation

Microscopy of smears of sputum or pus should be stained by the Wright or Giemsa procedure. Blood smears may be positive for *H. capsulatum*, especially in persons with AIDS. Liver or lung biopsies stained with periodic acid–Schiff or Grocott–Gomori methenamine–silver may provide a rapid diagnosis of disseminated histoplasmosis in some patients. *H. capsulatum* is seen as small, oval yeast cells, often within macrophages or monocytes (Fig. 58.13).

Specimens should be cultured on Sabouraud agar at 25–30°C to obtain the mycelial phase. Mycelial colonies develop within 1–2 weeks, but cultures should be retained for 4 weeks before discarding. The fungus is identified by its colonial morphology and the presence of the

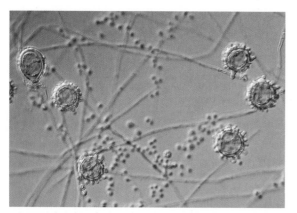

Fig. 58.12 Microscopical appearance of *Histoplasma capsulatum* microconidia and macroconidia.

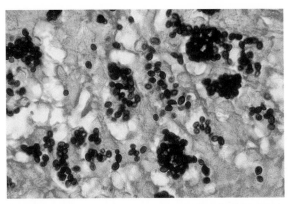

Fig. 58.13 Microscopical appearance of *Histoplasma capsulatum* yeast cells in tissue.

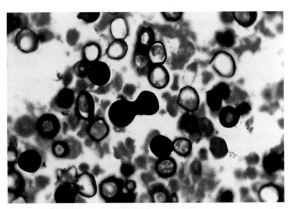

Fig. 58.14 Microscopical appearance of *Blastomyces dermatitidis* yeast cells in tissue, showing broad-based budding.

characteristic macroconidia and microconidia. Culture at 37°C for the yeast phase is not used for primary isolation, although conversion from the mould to yeast phase is useful to confirm the identity of isolates. Mould cultures of *H. capsulatum* are a hazard to laboratory staff, and consequently screw-capped slopes rather than Petri dishes should be used for isolation.

Serological tests are useful, but cross-reactions can occur, mainly with *Coccidioides*. Antibody tests fail to detect antibodies in up to 50% of immunosuppressed individuals. Tests for antigen detection in the urine by ELISA are useful in disseminated histoplasmosis but are not widely available outside the United States.

Treatment

Intravenous amphotericin B is recommended for treatment of the most severe forms of disseminated histoplasmosis. Itraconazole is widely used in nonimmunocompromised patients with milder forms of disseminated disease and for the continuation of treatment in those who have responded to amphotericin B.

BLASTOMYCOSIS

This disease is caused by *B. dermatitidis*, a dimorphic soil-inhabiting fungus. The largest number of cases of blastomycosis has been reported from North America, but the disease is also endemic in Africa and parts of Central and South America. In the United States the organism is most commonly found in states surrounding the Mississippi and Ohio Rivers; in Canada the disease occurs in the provinces that border the Great Lakes.

In culture at 25–30°C, *B. dermatitidis* grows as a mould with a septate mycelium. The colony varies in texture from floccose to smooth and from white to brown in colour. Asexual conidia are produced on lateral hyphal branches of variable length; the oval or pear-shaped conidia are 2–10 μm in diameter. In tissue and in culture at 37°C the fungus grows as a large round yeast (5–15 μm in diameter) that characteristically produces broad-based buds from a single pole on the mother cell (Fig. 58.14).

Epidemiology

Infection results from inhalation of spores; the incubation period is 4–6 weeks. The disease is more commonly seen in adults than in children, and often occurs in individuals with an outdoor occupation or recreational interest.

Clinical features

Acute pulmonary blastomycosis usually presents as a nonspecific influenza-like illness, similar to that seen with histoplasmosis or coccidioidomycosis. Most otherwise healthy persons recover after 2–12 weeks of symptoms, but some return months later with infection of other sites. Other patients with acute blastomycosis fail to recover and develop chronic pulmonary disease or disseminated infection.

The skin and bones are the most common sites of disseminated disease. The skin is involved in >70% of cases; the characteristic lesions are typically raised, with a well-demarcated edge. It is from these skin lesions that the diagnosis is most often made. Osteomyelitis occurs in about 30% of patients, with the spine, ribs and long bones being the most common sites of infection. Arthritis occurs in about 10% of patients. Meningitis is rare, except in immunocompromised individuals.

Laboratory investigation

Direct microscopy of pus, scrapings from skin lesions, or sputum usually shows thick-walled yeast cells 5–15 μm in diameter that characteristically produce buds on a broad base; the buds remain attached until they are almost the size of the parent cell, often forming chains of three or four cells. In biopsy material the yeasts are best seen in stained sections.

B. dermatitidis will grow in culture on Sabouraud agar (or blood agar) without cycloheximide, to which the fungus is sensitive. The mycelial phase develops slowly at 25–30°C, and cultures must be retained for 6 weeks before discarding. Test-tube slopes rather than Petri dishes are used for culture. Identification is usually confirmed by subculture at 37°C to convert it to the yeast phase.

The most useful serological test is the immunodiffusion test using the A antigen of *B. dermatitidis*. However, a negative result does not rule out the diagnosis because the sensitivity ranges from 30% for localised infections to 90% for cases of disseminated blastomycosis.

Treatment

Intravenous amphotericin B is used to treat all forms of blastomycosis and is the drug of choice in serious life-threatening infection. Itraconazole follow-on therapy is given once the patient improves. Itraconazole is also the drug of choice in less serious infection that does not involve the central nervous system.

PARACOCCIDIOIDOMYCOSIS

This is a chronic granulomatous infection caused by the dimorphic fungus *P. brasiliensis* that may involve the lungs, mucosa, skin and lymphatic system. The disease may be fatal if untreated. Although *P. brasiliensis* has been isolated from soil, understanding of its precise environmental reservoir remains limited. The endemic region extends from Mexico to Argentina, but the disease is seen most frequently in Brazil, Colombia and Venezuela.

P. brasiliensis grows in the mycelial phase in culture at 25–30°C and in the yeast phase in tissue or at 37°C on brain–heart infusion or blood agar. The mould colonies are slow growing with a variable colonial morphology, although most are white and velvety to floccose in texture with a pale brown reverse. Spore production is usually sparse and best seen in 4–6-week-old cultures. Asexual conidia may be produced but are not characteristic, and identification depends on conversion from the mycelial to the yeast phase. The yeast phase consists of oval or globose cells 2–30 μm in diameter, with small buds attached by a narrow neck encircling the parent cell (Fig. 58.15).

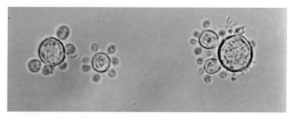

Fig. 58.15 Microscopical appearance of *Paracoccidioides brasiliensis* yeast cells in sputum, showing multipolar budding.

Epidemiology

Infection is usually acquired by inhalation; the incubation period is unknown. More than 90% of cases of symptomatic disease occur in men, most of whom have agricultural occupations; oestrogen-mediated inhibition of the mould to yeast transformation could help to account for this.

Clinical features

The lungs are the usual initial site of *P. brasiliensis* infection, but the organism then spreads through the lymphatics to the regional lymph nodes. In most cases the primary infection is asymptomatic. There is evidence of prolonged latent infection before overt disease develops, and a mild, self-limiting pulmonary form of paracoccidioidomycosis probably exists. Children and adolescents sometimes present with an acute disseminated form of infection in which superficial and/or visceral lymph node enlargement is the major manifestation. This presentation is also seen in immunocompromised patients. It has a poor prognosis.

In adults, paracoccidioidomycosis usually presents as an ulcerative granulomatous infection of the oral and nasal mucosa and adjacent skin. In 80% of cases the disease involves the lungs. In some, the liver and spleen, intestines, adrenals, bones and joints, and central nervous system are also involved. The disease is slowly progressive and may take months or even years to become established.

Laboratory investigation

Microscopy of sputum or pus, crusts and biopsies from granulomatous lesions usually reveals numerous yeast cells showing the characteristic multipolar budding, which is diagnostic. In culture the mycelial and yeast phases both develop slowly, and cultures must be retained for 6 weeks before discarding. The mould phase can be isolated on Sabouraud agar supplemented with yeast extract at 25–30°C, but colonies may take 2–4 weeks to appear. Serological tests are useful for diagnosis and for monitoring the response to therapy.

Treatment

The choice of therapy depends on the site of infection and its severity. Oral itraconazole is the drug of choice, although amphotericin B remains useful for severe or refractory infections. Oral ketoconazole is almost as effective, but less well tolerated than itraconazole.

ASPERGILLOSIS

There are >200 species of *Aspergillus,* but <20 have been implicated in human disease; the most important are *A. fumigatus, A. flavus, A. terreus, A. niger* and *A. nidulans.* In immunocompromised individuals, inhalation of spores can give rise to life-threatening invasive infection of the lungs or sinuses and dissemination to other organs often follows (invasive aspergillosis). In nonimmunocompromised persons, these moulds can cause localised infection of the lungs, sinuses and other sites. Human disease can also result from noninfectious mechanisms—inhalation of spores can cause allergic symptoms in both atopic and nonatopic individuals.

Aspergillus species are ubiquitous in the environment, growing in the soil, on plants, and on decomposing organic matter. These moulds are often found in the outdoor and indoor air, in water, on food items, and in dust. All grow in nature and in culture as moulds with septate hyphae and distinctive asexual sporing structures, termed conidiophores, that bear long chains of conidia (Fig. 58.16).

Epidemiology

Inhalation of *Aspergillus* conidia is the usual mode of infection; less frequently, infection follows the traumatic implantation of spores as in corneal infection (see Ch. 62), or inadvertent inoculation as in endocarditis.

Invasive aspergillosis has emerged as a major problem in several groups of immunocompromised patients, including those with acute leukaemia, stem cell and solid organ transplant recipients, and children with chronic granulomatous disease. The likelihood of aspergillosis developing in these individuals depends on a number of host factors, the most important of which is the level of immunosuppression. The mortality rate is high, ranging from 50% to 100% in almost all groups of immunocompromised patients.

Clinical features

Invasive aspergillosis

This form occurs in severely immunocompromised individuals who have a serious underlying illness. *A. fumigatus* is the species most frequently involved. The

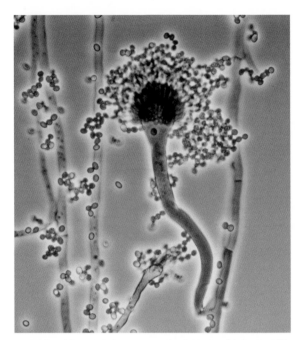

Fig. 58.16 Microscopical appearance of an *Aspergillus fumigatus* conidiophore. (Reproduced with permission from Richardson, M. D., Warnock, D. W., & Campbell, C. K. (1995). *Slide Atlas of Fungal Infection: Systemic Fungal Infections.* Oxford: Blackwell Science. ISBN 0-86542-931-6. Figure 2.)

most common initial presentation in the neutropenic patient is an unremitting fever (>38°C), without any respiratory tract symptoms, that fails to respond to broad-spectrum antibiotics.

The lung is the sole site of infection in 70% of patients, but dissemination of infection to other organs often occurs; the central nervous system is involved in 10%–20% of cases. There is widespread destructive growth of *Aspergillus* species in lung tissue, and the fungus invades blood vessels, causing thrombosis and infarction; septic emboli may spread the infection to other organs. Invasive aspergillosis has a poor prognosis; early diagnosis is essential for successful management.

Aspergilloma

In this form of aspergillosis, also referred to as fungus ball, the fungus colonises preexisting (often tuberculous) cavities in the lung and forms a compact ball of mycelium, eventually surrounded by a dense fibrous wall (Fig. 58.17).

Aspergillomas are usually solitary. Patients are either asymptomatic or have only a moderate cough and sputum production. Occasional haemoptysis may occur, especially when the fungus is actively growing, and haemorrhage following invasion of a blood vessel is one of the fatal

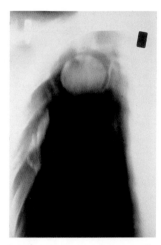

Fig. 58.17 Radiological appearance of an aspergilloma. (Reproduced with permission from Richardson, M. D., Warnock, D. W., & Campbell, C. K. (1995). *Slide Atlas of Fungal Infection: Systemic Fungal Infections.* Oxford: Blackwell Science. ISBN 0-86542-931-6. Figure 4.)

complications. Surgical resection is most often used to treat this condition.

Chronic pulmonary aspergillosis

This is a slowly progressive condition that usually occurs in immunocompetent individuals with underlying lung disease, such as bronchiectasis or sarcoidosis. There are several clinical forms.

Sinusitis

Aspergillus species, particularly *A. flavus* and *A. fumigatus*, may colonise and invade the paranasal sinuses; the infection may spread through the bone to the orbit of the eye and brain. Acute invasive sinusitis is a rapidly progressive disease, most commonly seen in immunocompromised persons. There are also several forms of slowly progressive chronic *Aspergillus* sinusitis that occur in immunocompetent individuals.

Allergic bronchopulmonary aspergillosis

Allergy to *Aspergillus* species is usually seen in atopic individuals with raised immunoglobulin (Ig) E levels; about 10%–20% of asthmatics react to *A. fumigatus*. The condition is a form of asthma with pulmonary eosinophilia that manifests as episodes of bronchial obstruction and lung consolidation; the fungus grows in the airways to produce mucous plugs of fungal mycelium that may block off segments of lung tissue and that, when coughed up, are a diagnostic feature.

Laboratory investigation

The value of the laboratory in diagnosis varies according to the clinical form of aspergillosis; the diagnosis of invasive disease is particularly difficult.

Direct microscopy

In potassium hydroxide preparations (preferably with Calcofluor to enhance detection) of sputum the fungus appears as nonpigmented septate hyphae, 3–5 μm in diameter, with characteristic dichotomous branching and an irregular outline; rarely the characteristic sporing heads of *Aspergillus* species are present.

- In allergic aspergillosis there is usually abundant fungus in the sputum, and mycelial plugs may also be present.
- In aspergilloma, fungus may be difficult to find on microscopy.
- In invasive aspergillosis, microscopy is often negative.

Biopsy may provide a definitive diagnosis, although many clinicians are reluctant to undertake this procedure because of the associated risk in immunosuppressed patients. In tissue sections, *Aspergillus* species are best seen after staining with periodic acid–Schiff or methenamine–silver.

Culture

Aspergillus species grow readily at 25–37°C on Sabouraud agar without cycloheximide; colonies appear after 1–2 days. Isolates can be identified by their colonial appearance and micromorphology. The ability of *A. fumigatus* to grow well at 45°C can be used to help identify this species or to isolate it selectively.

As aspergilli are among the most common laboratory contaminants, quantification of the amount of fungus in sputum helps to confirm the relevance of a positive culture. However, all isolates from immunocompromised patients must be taken seriously and acted on.

Large quantities of fungus are usually recovered from the sputum of patients with allergic aspergillosis, but cultures from those with aspergilloma or invasive disease are commonly negative or yield only a few colonies. Blood cultures are negative in invasive disease.

Skin tests

Skin tests with *A. fumigatus* antigen are useful for the diagnosis of allergic aspergillosis. All patients give an immediate type I reaction, and 70% of those with pulmonary eosinophilia also give a delayed type III Arthus reaction.

Serological tests

Immunodiffusion, CIE and ELISA are widely used for the detection of antibodies in the diagnosis of all forms of aspergillosis, particularly aspergilloma and allergic bronchopulmonary aspergillosis. Tests for *Aspergillus* antibodies are seldom helpful in the diagnosis of invasive infection in immunocompromised patients.

Galactomannan antigen detection in serum and bronchoalveolar lavage fluid by ELISA is used successfully for diagnosis of invasive aspergillosis. Nucleic acid amplification methods are also available for diagnosis of invasive aspergillosis.

Treatment

In invasive aspergillosis, the historical standard of treatment is intravenous amphotericin B (conventional or liposomal). Voriconazole is now the preferred agent for this disease.

Aspergilloma is treated by surgical excision because antifungal therapy is of little value, but because of the significant morbidity and mortality with this procedure it is reserved for patients with episodes of life-threatening haemoptysis. Long-term treatment with voriconazole is recommended for chronic pulmonary aspergillosis, but relapse is common when therapy is stopped. Allergic forms of aspergillosis are treated with corticosteroids.

INVASIVE CANDIDOSIS

In addition to causing mucosal and cutaneous infections, *Candida* species can cause acute or chronic invasive infections in immunocompromised or debilitated individuals. This may be confined to one organ or become widespread (disseminated candidosis).

Epidemiology

In most cases, invasive candidosis is endogenous in origin, but transmission of organisms from person to person can also occur. Hospital outbreaks of infection have sometimes been linked to contaminated medical devices, such as vascular catheters, and/or parenteral nutrition. There are also reports of cross-infection due to hand carriage by health-care workers.

Invasive candidosis is a significant problem in several distinct groups of hospitalised patients:

- neutropenic cancer patients
- stem cell and liver transplant recipients
- patients receiving intensive care

Invasive candidosis is now more common in patients in intensive care than among neutropenic individuals. The reduced incidence of the disease among the latter group has been attributed to the widespread use of fluconazole prophylaxis. More than 90% of cases are caused by five species: *C. albicans*, *C. glabrata*, *C. tropicalis*, *C. parapsilosis* and *C. krusei*.

Many risk factors for invasive candidosis have been identified. These can be divided into host-related and health care–related factors:

- underlying immunosuppression
- low birth weight
- intravascular catheterisation
- broad-spectrum antibiotic use
- total parenteral nutrition
- haemodialysis

Among adult patients cared for in surgical intensive care units, *Candida* bloodstream infection has a case fatality rate of about 40%.

Clinical features

Infection may be localised, for instance in the urinary tract, liver, heart or meninges, or may be widely disseminated and associated with a septicaemia (candidaemia). Invasive candidosis is difficult to diagnose and treat, and for some forms the prognosis is poor.

Disseminated infection is most commonly seen in seriously ill individuals who usually have one or more indwelling vascular catheters, although these are not necessarily the source of the infection. Many cases are thought to arise from translocation of organisms across the wall of the intestinal tract.

Adults with candidaemia usually present with a persistent fever that fails to respond to broad-spectrum antibiotics, but with few other symptoms or clinical signs. One sign of invasive candidosis is the presence of white lesions within the eye (*Candida* endophthalmitis) (Fig. 58.18). These are found in up to 45% of patients in the intensive care unit, but are seldom seen in neutropenic individuals. Other useful signs are the nodular cutaneous lesions that occur in about 10% of neutropenic individuals with disseminated *Candida* infection. Other manifestations include:

- meningitis
- renal abscess
- myocarditis
- osteomyelitis
- arthritis.

Invasive candidosis is a common complication in infants of low birth weight (<1000 g) requiring prolonged neonatal intensive care. Meningitis occurs more frequently than in older patients and is sometimes associated with arthritis and osteomyelitis.

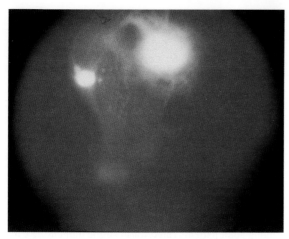

Fig. 58.18 Fundoscopic appearance of *Candida* endophthalmitis. (Reproduced with permission from Richardson, M. D., Warnock, D. W., & Campbell, C. K. (1995). *Slide Atlas of Fungal Infection: Systemic Fungal Infections.* Oxford: Blackwell Science. ISBN 0-86542-931-6. Figure 22.)

Laboratory investigation

Candida species may be present as commensals in the absence of infection, so that isolation from clinical material, except from sites that are normally sterile, is of little significance. Similarly, antibodies to *Candida* species can be detected in uninfected individuals because of their exposure to commensal yeasts, although a rise in antibody titre or high titres may be of diagnostic significance. In suspected invasive candidosis, samples from as many sources as possible should be examined by direct microscopy and culture. Results should always be interpreted in the light of clinical findings.

Direct microscopy

Appropriate samples are examined microscopically in potassium hydroxide or after Gram staining. In tissue sections, the fungus is seen best in stained preparations. Hyphae are often abundant, but their presence in sputum or urine does not confirm that the yeast is present as a pathogen.

Culture

Candida species grow readily in culture at 37°C on common isolation media, such as Sabouraud dextrose agar. Blood cultures provide the most reliable evidence of invasive infection, although repeated attempts to isolate the organism may be required.

Isolation of the yeast from otherwise sterile sites provides reliable evidence for the diagnosis, but cultures obtained from urine, faeces and sputum are of less value unless done quantitatively over a period of time. Cell counts of the yeast in urine in excess of 10^4 per mL are usually taken to indicate urinary tract infection, except in those with an indwelling urinary catheter. As *Candida* species multiply rapidly in clinical material it is important that specimens are processed as soon as possible after collection.

Serological tests

Currently available tests lack specificity and sensitivity, and the results must be interpreted with care. A positive test does not necessarily indicate infection because the antigens used do not differentiate between antibodies formed during mucosal colonisation and those produced during deep infection. Similarly, a negative antibody test does not necessarily rule out the possibility of invasive candidosis in immunocompromised patients who are incapable of mounting an adequate antibody response.

Antigen tests, based mainly on ELISA or latex agglutination, that detect cell wall mannan or cytoplasmic components have been developed and are used for diagnosis. Nucleic acid detection methods are increasingly being used to diagnose invasive candidosis, although their place in diagnosis is still being evaluated.

Treatment

The treatments of choice for most forms of invasive candidosis are:

- intravenous echinocandin (anidulafungin, caspofungin or micafungin)
- intravenous amphotericin B (conventional or liposomal)
- intravenous or oral fluconazole.

Amphotericin B can be used in combination with flucytosine, but flucytosine is not used alone as resistance may develop during treatment.

Removal of existing intravenous catheters is desirable if feasible, especially in nonneutropenic patients.

The choice of antifungal treatment depends on both the clinical status of the patient and the species of infecting organism.

- Almost all *Candida* species are susceptible to echinocandins.
- *C. albicans*, *C. parapsilosis* and *C. tropicalis* are susceptible to amphotericin B and fluconazole.
- *C. glabrata* often becomes resistant to fluconazole during therapy. *C. krusei* is intrinsically resistant to fluconazole.

CRYPTOCOCCOSIS

Cryptococcosis, caused by the encapsulated yeasts *Cryptococcus neoformans* and *C. gattii*, is most frequently recognised as a disease of the central nervous system, although the primary site of infection is the lungs. The disease occurs sporadically throughout the world, but it is currently seen most often in persons with AIDS.

There are four serotypes of *Cryptococcus* (A–D) that represent two distinct species of the organism, namely, *C. neoformans* (A & D) and *C. gattii* (B & C). Most infections are caused by *C. neoformans*, which is commonly found in the droppings of wild and domesticated birds throughout the world. Pigeons carry *C. neoformans* in their crops, but do not appear to become infected, probably because of their high body temperature. *C. gattii* has been isolated from decaying wood in various species of trees including Eucalyptus. These trees are indigenous to Australia, but have been planted in numerous other countries. *C. gattii* infection has been reported from subtropical regions and from temperate parts of the world, including western Canada and the Pacific North West Region of the United States.

Epidemiology

Infection is acquired by inhalation; the incubation period is unknown. The likelihood that an infection with *C. neoformans* will develop after inhalation depends largely on host factors. Even before the advent of AIDS, infections with *C. neoformans* tended to occur in individuals with abnormalities of T lymphocyte function, such as are found in persons with lymphoma, and those receiving corticosteroid therapy. The major risk factor for development of infection with *C. gattii* appears to be environmental exposure, although there is indirect evidence that unidentified host factors contribute to the higher incidence of disease in Australian Aboriginals.

With the advent of the AIDS epidemic, cryptococcosis became the most common cause of meningitis in hospitals in which persons with HIV infection are treated. Although the incidence of the disease has declined in developed countries where combination antiretroviral treatment is available, the incidence is rising in many developing countries afflicted with large epidemics of HIV infection.

Clinical features

A mild self-limiting pulmonary infection is believed to be the most common form of cryptococcosis. In symptomatic pulmonary infection there are no clear diagnostic features. Lesions may take the form of small discrete nodules, which may heal with a residual scar or may become enlarged, encapsulated and chronic (cryptococcoma form). An acute pneumonic type of disease has also been described.

The meningeal form of cryptococcosis can occur in apparently healthy individuals, but occurs most frequently in immunocompromised persons. Chronic meningitis or meningoencephalitis develops insidiously with headaches and low-grade fever, followed by changes in mental state, visual disturbances and eventually coma. The disease may last from a few months to several years, but the outcome is always fatal unless it is treated. Patients with AIDS and cryptococcosis generally develop a chronic meningeal form with milder symptoms.

Although predominantly a disease of the central nervous system, lesions of the skin, bones and other deep sites may also occur; in its disseminated form, the disease may resemble tuberculosis. Rarely, lesions of skin and bones may occur without any evidence of infection elsewhere.

Laboratory investigation

Cryptococcus is readily demonstrated in cerebrospinal fluid (CSF) or other material by direct microscopy, culture or serological tests for capsular antigen. The yeast load is generally higher in patients with AIDS. The cellular reaction and chemical changes in CSF usually resemble those seen in tuberculous meningitis. The yeast cells of *Cryptococcus* are round, 4–10 μm in diameter and surrounded by a mucopolysaccharide capsule. The width of the capsule varies and is greatest in vivo and on rich media in vitro.

In unstained wet preparations of CSF mixed with a drop of India ink or nigrosine, the capsule can be seen as a clear halo around the yeast cells (Fig. 58.19). Capsulate yeasts are seen in the CSF of about 60% of patients with cryptococcosis (higher in AIDS), but the capsule may be difficult to visualise in some cases. Sputum, pus or brain tissue should be examined after digestion in potassium hydroxide, and here the capsulate yeasts are often delineated by the cellular debris. For examination of tissue sections it is best to use a specific fungal stain such as periodic acid–Schiff; alcian blue and mucicarmine stain the capsular material, enabling the organisms to be differentiated from *H. capsulatum* and *B. dermatitidis*.

The yeast is easily cultured from CSF, although large volumes or multiple samples may be required in some cases; in patients with AIDS it is also useful to culture blood. On Sabouraud agar (without cycloheximide) cultured at 25–30°C and 37°C, colonies normally appear within 2–3 days, but cultures should not be discarded for 3 weeks. In culture, *Cryptococcus* appears as creamy white to yellow-brown colonies, which are mucoid in strains with well-developed capsules and dry in strains that lack prominent capsules. Buds appear at any point on the cell surface, but hyphae or pseudohyphae are not normally produced. Preliminary identification depends

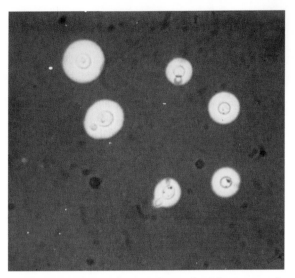

Fig. 58.19 Microscopic appearance of encapsulated *Cryptococcus* cells in an India ink preparation of CSF. (Reproduced with permission from Richardson, M. D., Warnock, D. W., & Campbell, C. K. (1995). *Slide Atlas of Fungal Infection: Systemic Fungal Infections.* Oxford: Blackwell Science. ISBN 0-86542-931-6. Figure 25.)

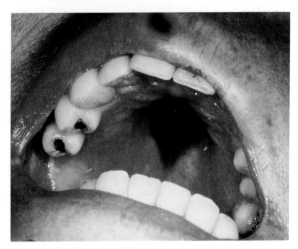

Fig. 58.20 Necrotic palatal lesion in a case of rhinocerebral mucormycosis. (Reproduced with permission from Richardson, M. D., Warnock, D. W., & Campbell, C. K. (1995). *Slide Atlas of Fungal Infection: Systemic Fungal Infections.* Oxford: Blackwell Science. ISBN 0-86542-931-6. Figure 32.)

on demonstration of the capsule, but this may be absent or difficult to see. *Cryptococcus* can be identified with commercial kits or distinguished from other yeasts by its lack of fermentative ability, its ability to produce urease, to grow at 37°C and to assimilate inositol.

The latex agglutination test for the detection of cryptococcal polysaccharide antigen in CSF or blood is highly sensitive and specific for the diagnosis of cryptococcal meningitis and disseminated forms of the disease and gives better results than microscopy and culture. In AIDS, the test is positive in well over 90% of infected patients; titres of over 10^6 may be detected.

Treatment

Intravenous amphotericin B in combination with flucytosine is usually the treatment of choice for individuals with meningeal or disseminated cryptococcosis. Oral fluconazole is widely used for the continuation of treatment in those who have responded to amphotericin B. Patients with AIDS commonly relapse after the initial course of therapy, and many require lifelong maintenance treatment with fluconazole.

MUCORMYCOSIS

Mucormycosis, formerly known as zygomycosis, is a relatively rare, opportunistic infection caused by saprophytic mould fungi, notably species of *Rhizopus* and

Lichtheimia (Absidia). These moulds are ubiquitous in the soil and on decomposing organic matter. They are characterised by having broad, aseptate hyphae, with large numbers of asexual spores inside a sporangium that develops at the end of an aerial hypha.

Epidemiology

Most infections follow inhalation of spores; less frequently, infection follows traumatic inoculation into the skin and soft tissue. Major risk factors include:

- prolonged or profound neutropenia
- uncontrolled diabetes mellitus
- other forms of metabolic acidosis
- burns.

Certain predisposing conditions seem to be more commonly associated with particular clinical forms of disease; for example, persons with diabetic ketoacidosis often develop rhinocerebral mucormycosis, whereas neutropenic individuals often develop pulmonary or disseminated disease.

Clinical features

The best known form of the disease is rhinocerebral mucormycosis. There is rapid and extensive tissue destruction, most commonly spreading from the nasal mucosa to the turbinate bone, paranasal sinuses, orbit and brain (Fig. 58.20). The condition is fatal if untreated, and, although the prognosis has improved over recent years, many diagnoses are still made at necropsy.

Pulmonary and disseminated infections can occur in severely immunocompromised individuals. Primary

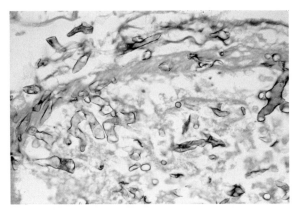

Fig. 58.21 Microscopic appearance of mucormycosis. (Reproduced with permission from Richardson, M. D., Warnock, D. W., & Campbell, C. K. (1995). *Slide Atlas of Fungal Infection: Systemic Fungal Infections.* Oxford: Blackwell Science. ISBN 0-86542-931-6. Figure 35.)

cutaneous infections have also been reported; these are uncommon, but often result in extensive necrotising fasciitis or disseminated disease. They usually occur in patients with burns or other forms of local trauma.

Laboratory investigation

Recognition of the fungus in tissue by microscopy is considerably more reliable than culture, but material such as nasal discharge or sputum seldom contains much fungal material and examination of a biopsy is usually necessary for a firm diagnosis. Direct examination of curetted or biopsy material in potassium hydroxide may reveal the characteristic broad, aseptate, branched and sometimes distorted hyphae. However, they are seen much more clearly when stained with methenamine–silver; the hyphae of these fungi do not stain with periodic acid–Schiff (Fig. 58.21).

The fungi are readily isolated on Sabouraud dextrose agar at 37°C, but isolation is of little diagnostic significance in the absence of strong supporting clinical evidence of infection. There are no established serological tests.

Treatment

Successful treatment depends on early diagnosis of the infection to allow prompt therapy with high doses of intravenous amphotericin B (conventional or liposomal), control of any underlying disorder, such as diabetes, and aggressive surgical intervention.

PNEUMOCYSTOSIS

Pneumocystis is an opportunistic pathogen with some of the features of protozoa, but comparative DNA sequence analysis showed it to be more closely related to the fungi. The organism was originally described as a cause of atypical pneumonia in malnourished infants, but came to prominence in the 1980s as a common cause of pneumonia, which was commonly fatal, in patients with AIDS. With the advent of reliable antiretroviral therapy, the incidence of the disease in HIV-positive individuals has declined.

Based on its morphology, which is similar to that of protozoa, the life cycle of *Pneumocystis* is divided into three stages:

1. the cyst, a spherical or crescent-shaped form (5–7 μm in diameter)
2. the sporozoite, up to eight of which develop within each cyst
3. the trophozoite, found outside the cyst.

When openings appear in the cyst wall, the excysted sporozoites become trophozoites. All of these forms reside within the alveoli of the lungs. As the organism is not cultivatable in vitro, its life cycle has not been fully elucidated.

The finding that *Pneumocystis* organisms from different mammalian hosts are genetically quite dissimilar has led to a name change from *P. carinii* (which infects rats) to *P. jirovecii* for the organisms that infect humans.

Epidemiology

Infection is probably acquired by inhalation. Serological and PCR studies indicate that most human beings become subclinically infected with *Pneumocystis* during childhood and that this infection is usually well contained by an intact immune system. The occurrence of clinical disease is related to the extent of immunosuppression, especially impairment of cell-mediated immunity. It may be due to primary infection, reinfection or reactivation. Pneumocystosis has a global distribution.

Clinical features

The clinical presentation of *Pneumocystis* pneumonia is nonspecific. Symptoms include:

- fever
- nonproductive cough
- shortness of breath.

Patients with AIDS have a more indolent course with longer duration of symptoms than do patients receiving immunosuppressive drugs. Without treatment the course is progressive and usually ends in death.

In addition to pneumonia, *Pneumocystis* infection may disseminate to the lymph nodes, liver, spleen, bone marrow, adrenal gland, intestines and meninges. Extrapulmonary disease occurs predominantly in patients with advanced

HIV infection and in those not taking co-trimoxazole prophylaxis or receiving aerosolised pentamidine.

Laboratory investigation

Diagnosis usually depends on the identification of typical octonucleate cysts or trophozoites in tissues or body fluids. Organisms are detected by immunofluorescent staining of bronchoalveolar lavage fluid or induced sputum smears. Molecular diagnosis by PCR is also available. 1, 3, β-D-glucan a cell wall polysaccharide found in fungal cell wall is also found in large quantities in the cell wall of *Pneumocystis*.

Treatment

Co-trimoxazole and intravenous pentamidine are the most effective therapies. The former is as potent as the latter, but less toxic. Other regimens include atovaquone, trimetrexate, the combination of trimethoprim and dapsone and the combination of clindamycin and primaquine.

Co-trimoxazole is the preferred prophylactic agent, but patients with AIDS or those undergoing solid organ or bone marrow transplantation may suffer unacceptable side effects to the high doses used. Aerosolised pentamidine is also used for prophylaxis.

OTHER OPPORTUNIST FUNGI

Talaromyces (Penicillium) marneffei causes serious disseminated disease with characteristic papular skin lesions in patients with AIDS in Southeast Asia. The fungus is dimorphic, forming yeastlike cells that are often intracellular, resembling histoplasmosis, in infected tissues. Treatment is with amphotericin B, followed by itraconazole to prevent relapse.

Almost any fungus may invade a severely immunocompromised host, and infections with many common fungi, including *Fusarium* species, *Scedosporium* species and *Trichosporon asahii*, have been reported. Diagnosis is made by culture of the causative organism from clinical specimens, and serological tests play little part. Tissue sections are often not very helpful, either because the causal fungi have no special features to enable identification or because they resemble other fungal pathogens.

Infections are usually treated speculatively, and sometimes successfully, with amphotericin B.

RECOMMENDED READING

Anaissie, E. J., McGinnis, M. R., & Pfaller, M. A. (Eds.). (2009). *Clinical Mycology* (2nd ed.). New York: Elsevier.

Campbell, C. K., Johnson, E. M., & Warnock, D. W. (2013). *Identification of Pathogenic Fungi* (2nd ed.). Oxford: Wiley Blackwell.

Dismukes, W. E., Kauffman, C., Pappas, P. G., & Sobel, J. D. (Eds.). (2010). *Clinical Mycology* (2nd ed.). New York: Springer.

Hospenthal, D. R., & Rinaldi, M. G. (Eds.). (2008). *Diagnosis and Treatment of Human Mycoses*. Totowa, New Jersey: Humana Press.

Richardson, M. D., & Johnson, E. M. (2006). *Pocket Guide to Fungal Infection* (2nd ed.). Oxford: Wiley Blackwell.

Richardson, M. D., & Warnock, D. W. (2012). *Fungal Infection: Diagnosis and Management* (4th ed.). Oxford: Wiley Blackwell.

Websites

Centers for Disease Control and Prevention. Fungal Diseases: Resources and Educational Materials for Health Professionals. Available at http://www.cdc.gov/fungal/resources.html. (Accessed Aug 2017).

Mycetoma Research Center. Available at http://www.mycetoma.edu.sd.

The Aspergillus Website. Available at http://www.aspergillus.org.uk/. (Accessed Aug 2017).

University of Adelaide Mycology Online. Available at http://www.mycology.adelaide.edu.au/. (Accessed Aug 2017).

Valley Fever Center for Excellence. http://www.vfce.arizona.edu/about. (Accessed Aug 2017).

59 Protozoa

Malaria; toxoplasmosis; cryptosporidiosis; amoebiasis; trypanosomiasis; leishmaniasis; giardiasis; trichomoniasis

NADIRA D. KARUNAWEERA

KEY POINTS

- Protozoa are unicellular eukaryotic organisms.
- Most protozoal infections require laboratory confirmation for diagnosis; toxoplasmosis is diagnosed serologically.
- Malaria kills over 400,000 people each year—the vast majority are children.
- Acute malaria is a medical emergency demanding immediate diagnosis and treatment; quinine or artemisinin derivatives, usually in combination with other antimalarial drugs, are effective.
- African trypanosomiasis (sleeping sickness) is treated with toxic arsenical drugs; the West African form responds to eflornithine.
- South American trypanosomiasis (Chagas' disease) is a chronic condition that is difficult to treat.
- Leishmaniases are considered as a group of diseases; the most dangerous is visceral leishmaniasis (kala azar). Atypical presentations of leishmaniasis, resistance to regular therapy and presence of reservoir hosts pose challenges to its containment. Antimonial compounds, antifungal drugs or miltefosine is used for treatment.
- Amoebiasis, giardiasis and trichomoniasis occur worldwide; they usually respond to 5-nitroimidazole drugs such as metronidazole.

Infection with pathogenic protozoa exacts an enormous toll of human suffering, notably, but not exclusively, in the tropics. Numerically the most important of the life-threatening protozoan diseases is malaria, which is responsible for over 400,000 deaths a year, mostly in young children in Africa.

Pathogenic protozoan parasites are conveniently dealt with by placing them in four groups: sporozoa, amoebae, flagellates and a miscellaneous group of other protozoa that may cause human disease (Table 59.1).

SPOROZOA

This group includes the malaria parasites and related coccidia, which exhibit a complex life cycle involving alternating cycles of asexual division (schizogony) and sexual development (sporogony). In malaria parasites, the sexual cycle takes place in the female anopheline mosquito (Fig. 59.1).

MALARIA PARASITES

Description

Four species are commonly encountered in human disease: *Plasmodium falciparum*, which is responsible for most fatalities; *P. vivax* and *P. ovale*, both of which cause benign tertian malaria (febrile episodes typically occurring at 48-hour intervals); and *P. malariae*, which causes quartan malaria (febrile episodes typically occurring at 72-hour intervals). The appearances of trophozoites of the four species as seen in Romanowsky-stained films of peripheral blood are illustrated in Figs 59.2–59.7 (Fig. 59.2 is available online). *P. knowlesi*, a natural parasite of long-tailed macaque, monkeys is now recognised as the fifth *Plasmodium* species that causes human malaria. Malaria due to *P. knowlesi* has been reported from countries in the Southeast Asian region, where the parasite is found, and may be present elsewhere though unreported, particularly since the blood forms (Fig. 59.8) can be easily confused with *P. falciparum* or *P. malariae*.

Life cycle

When an infected mosquito bites, sporozoites present in the salivary glands, enter the bloodstream and are carried to the liver, where they invade liver parenchyma cells. They undergo a process of multiple nuclear divisions, followed by cytoplasmic division (schizogony); when this is complete, the liver cell ruptures, releasing several thousand

Table 59.1 Principal protozoan pathogens of humans

Group	Species	Disease
Sporozoa	Plasmodium falciparum	Malignant tertian malaria
	P. vivax	Benign tertian malaria
	P. ovale	Benign tertian malaria
	P. malariae	Quartan malaria
	P. knowlesi	Zoonotic malaria
	Toxoplasma gondii	Toxoplasmosis
	Isospora belli	Diarrhoea
	Cryptosporidium parvum	Diarrhoea
	Cyclospora cayetanensis	Diarrhoea
Amoebae	Entamoeba histolytica	Amoebic dysentery; liver abscess
	Naegleria fowleri[a]	Meningoencephalitis
	Acanthamoeba spp.[a]	Keratitis
	Balamuthia mandrillaris[a]	Encephalitis
	Blastocystis hominis[b]	Pathogenicity doubtful
Flagellates	Giardia lamblia	Diarrhoea, malabsorption
	Trichomonas vaginalis	Vaginitis, urethritis
	Trypanosoma brucei gambiense	Sleeping sickness
	Trypanosoma brucei rhodesiense	Sleeping sickness
	Trypanosoma cruzi	Chagas' disease
	Leishmania spp.	See Table 59.4
Others	Babesia microti[a]	Babesiosis
	Babesia divergens[a]	Babesiosis
	Balantidium coli[a]	Balantidial dysentery
	Encephalitozoon cuniculi[a]	Microsporidiosis
	Enterocytozoon bieneusi[a]	Microsporidiosis
	Nosema connori[a]	Microsporidiosis

[a]Organisms rarely encountered in human disease.
[b]Taxonomic status uncertain.

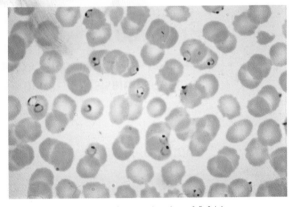

Fig. 59.3 Ring form trophozoites of *P. falciparum*.

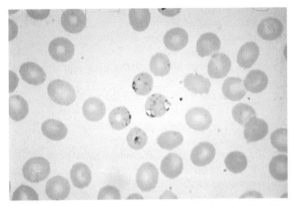

Fig. 59.4 Trophozoites of *P. falciparum*. Note peripheral location of the parasites (*appliqué* or *accolé* forms) and light stippling of the red cells (Maurer's spots).

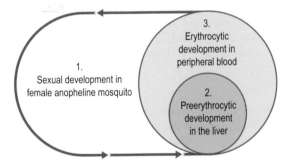

Fig. 59.1 Schematic representation of the life cycle of malaria parasites.

1. Sexual development in female anopheline mosquito
2. Preerythrocytic development in the liver
3. Erythrocytic development in peripheral blood

individual parasites (merozoites) into the bloodstream. The merozoites penetrate red blood cells and adopt a typical signet-ring morphology (see Fig. 59.3).

In the case of *P. vivax and P. ovale*, some parasites in the liver remain dormant (hypnozoites) and the cycle of preerythrocytic schizogony is completed only after a long delay. Such parasites are responsible for the relapses of tertian malaria that may occur, usually within 2 years of the initial infection.

In the bloodstream the young ring forms (trophozoites) develop and start to undergo nuclear division (erythrocytic schizogony). Depending on the species, about 8–24 nuclei are produced before cytoplasmic division occurs, and the red cell ruptures to release the individual merozoites, which then infect fresh red blood cells (see Fig. 59.2).

Instead of entering the cycle of erythrocytic schizogony, some merozoites develop within red cells into male or female gametocytes. These do not develop further in the human host, but when the insect vector ingests the blood, the nuclear material and cytoplasm of the male gametocytes

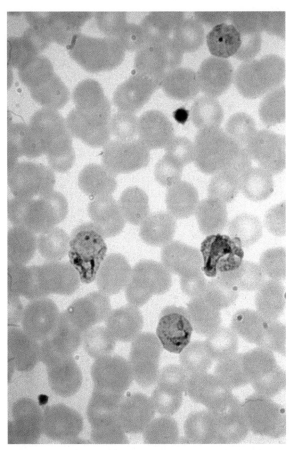

Fig. 59.5 Amoeboid trophozoites of *P. vivax*. Note the marked enlargement of the parasitized red cells and the intense stippling (Schüffner's dots).

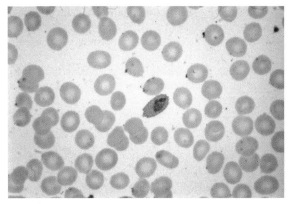

Fig. 59.6 Trophozoite of *P. ovale*. Note the fimbriate, oval-shaped red cell and marked stippling (James' stippling).

P. knowlesi

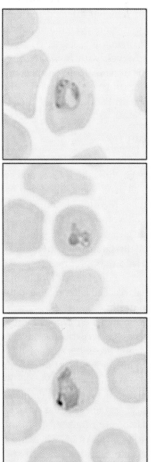

Fig. 59.8 Thin smears of a *P. knowlesi* stained with Giemsa in ×1000 original magnification.

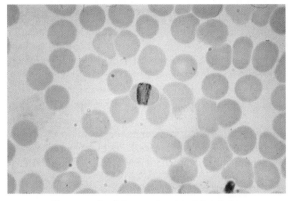

Fig. 59.7 Band-form trophozoite of *P. malariae*.

differentiate to produce several individual gametes, which give it the appearance of a flagellate body (exflagellating male gametocyte). The gametes become detached and penetrate the female gametocyte, which elongates into a zygotic form, the ookinete. This penetrates the midgut wall of the mosquito and settles on the body cavity side as an oocyst, within which numerous sporozoites are formed. When mature, the oocyst ruptures, releasing the sporozoites into the body cavity, from where some find their way to the salivary glands.

P. falciparum differs from the other forms of malaria parasite in that developing erythrocytic schizonts form aggregates and adhere to the endothelium of the capillaries of the brain and other internal organs (phenomenon known as sequestration), so that normally only relatively young ring forms or gametocytes (which are typically crescent shaped) are found in peripheral blood.

The cycle of erythrocytic schizogony takes 48 hours, except in *P. malariae*, where the cycle is 72 hours, and in *P. knowlesi* is 24 hours. Febrile episodes occur shortly after rupture of schizont-infected red cells and the rise and fall of the pyrogenic cytokine tumour necrosis factor-alpha, which explains the characteristic periodic fevers (Fig. 59.9). However, with *P. falciparum*, the cycles of different broods of parasite do not become synchronised as they do in other forms of malaria; therefore typical tertian fever pattern is not usual in falciparum malaria.

Clinical features

Malaria in its typical form is characterised by periodic episodes of severe chills, high fever and sweating, which are referred to as paroxysms, the duration of which may vary. Paroxysms are often accompanied by headache, muscle pain and vomiting. Paroxysms are particularly prominent in *P. vivax* infections, while they may not be well delineated in falciparum infections. Furthermore, falciparum malaria may progress (especially in primary infections) to severe disease with multiorgan dysfunction and cerebral malaria. The latter may lead to coma, convulsions and even death.

Individuals who are heterozygous for the sickle cell and thalassaemia genes have a particular advantage over others in malaria endemic areas because of the much-reduced susceptibility to infection with *P. falciparum*, and this has provided a selective advantage for the maintenance of these blood cell disorders in holoendemic areas. Similarly, individuals whose red cells lack the surface antigen known as the Duffy factor are protected from infection with *P. vivax*. In parts of tropical Africa, where most of the population are Duffy factor negative, *P. vivax* is rare, although the related *P. ovale* is found, especially in West Africa. Malaria due to *P. knowlesi*, a form of zoonotic infection in humans, has been reported in considerable numbers,

particularly from Malaysia. Though young parasitic stages of *P. knowlesi* appear very similar to those of *P. malariae*, the latter multiplies every 3 days (quartan) and generally achieves only low parasitaemias. In contrast, *P. knowlesi* has a daily cycle (quotidian) and if left untreated parasitaemias can rise to dangerously high levels.

Laboratory investigation

Immediate laboratory confirmation of malaria is important because early treatment of malaria can save lives, particularly in the case of acute falciparum malaria. None of the symptoms or signs of malaria are specific, which makes clinical diagnosis unreliable. Therefore, laboratory confirmation of malaria through demonstration of parasites, its antigens or products in a patient's blood plays an important role in patient management. Microscopic examination of stained thick and thin blood smears is the gold standard in malaria diagnosis. A blood sample obtained through a finger prick is sufficient to make the smears on a glass slide. While two or three blood spots are required to make the thick smear, a single drop is used to make the thin smear. The smears are allowed to dry thoroughly, and only the thin smear is fixed in absolute methanol. Both smears are then stained using Giemsa (or Leishman's or any other appropriate stain), which stains the cells and the parasites in the thin smear and also haemolyses the red cells in the thick smear, so that the parasites are easy to detect despite the thickness of the film.

With experience, the species of malaria can usually be determined from a thick blood film, but some of the characteristic features used to establish the identity of the parasites (Table 59.2), such as the typical stippling and the enlargement of the red cell that accompany infection with *P. vivax* or *P. ovale*, are better observed in a conventional thin blood film. Examination of the thin film also enables quantification of parasites in the blood (parasitaemia), an index that assists clinicians in patient management. The water used to dilute the stain should be at pH 7.2 (not 6.8 as used for haematological purposes).

Various other diagnostic tests have been devised for the rapid diagnosis of malaria including simple dipstick tests (RDTs), which are sufficiently reliable to be used by inexperienced staff or under field conditions where microscopy is not available. RDTs have become more and more popular, particularly in low malaria transmission settings because of the relative ease in performance and interpretation. Some RDTs detect a single species (either *P. falciparum* or *P. vivax*), some detect multiple species (*P. falciparum*, *P. vivax*, *P. malariae* and *P. ovale*) and some further distinguish between *P. falciparum* and non–*P. falciparum* infection or between specific species. Blood for the test is commonly obtained from a finger prick, and results are available within 15–30 minutes. They are

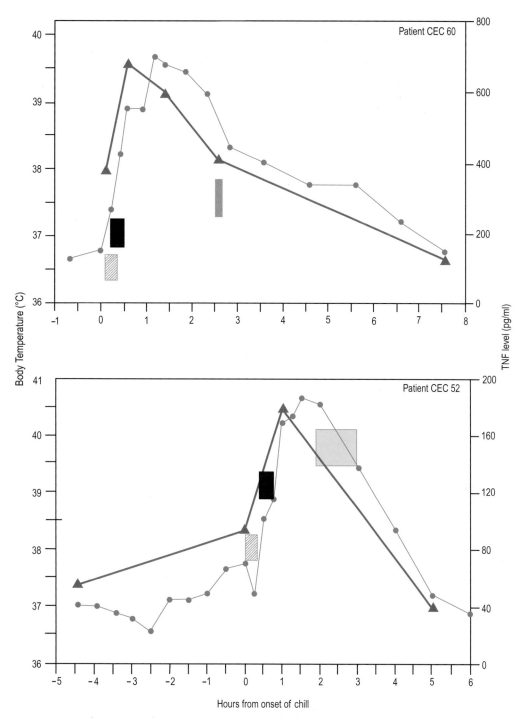

Fig. 59.9 Body temperature (measured orally), plasma tumour necrosis factor (TNF) level, and the period and duration of the chill (hatched box), rigor (black box), and sweating (grey box) during the course of a single paroxysm in two *P. vivax* patients. (Figure modified and reproduced with permission from the Proceedings of the National Academy of Sciences, USA.)

Table 59.2 Differential characteristics of human malaria parasites as seen in Romanowsky-stained thin films of peripheral blood (see also Figs 59.2–59.7)

Species	Morphology of trophozoite	Morphology of red cell	Stippling of red cell	Morphology of gametocyte	No. of merozoites in mature schizont
P. falciparum	Ring forms only	Normal	Maurer's spots[a]	Crescentic	(16–24)[b]
P. vivax	Rings, becoming amoeboid during development	Enlarged	Schüffner's dots	Large, round	16–24
P. ovale	Rings, becoming compact during development	Slightly enlarged; sometimes oval with fimbriate edge	James' stippling[c]	Round	8–12
P. malariae	Rings, becoming compact, stretched across red cell	Normal or slightly shrunken	(Ziemann's dots)[d]	Small, round	8–12
P. knowlesi	Rings, becoming compact, occasional band forms	Normal or slightly shrunken	Sinton and Mulligan's stippling[e]	Normal or small, round to oval	Up to 16

[a]Maurer's spots (or clefts) are relatively scanty and accompany more mature ring forms.
[b]Mature schizonts of P. falciparum are rarely seen in peripheral blood.
[c]James' stippling is similar to the intense stippling of Schüffner's dots.
[d]Ziemann's dots are rarely seen, except in intensely stained preparations.
[e]Sinton and Mulligan's stippling are rarely seen under certain staining conditions.

not fool proof, and may remain positive for some time after successful treatment.

Molecular diagnosis that has superior levels of sensitivity also plays a role in malaria diagnosis in selected settings. However, such ultrasensitive methods are generally not used in routine diagnosis of malaria in endemic areas because of the high cost and the need for established laboratories. Therefore, its usefulness as a diagnostic tool is largely limited to settings with no malaria transmission, cases with mixed infections and for detection of submicroscopic levels of parasitaemias.

Treatment

For many years the standard treatment for acute malaria was chloroquine. However, resistance to that drug in *P. falciparum* (and, less commonly, in *P. vivax*) is now widespread and other agents have to be used. Derivatives of artemisinin (a natural product from the plant *Artemisia annua*), including artemether and sodium artesunate, are quick acting and effective. They have become the drugs of choice for treatment of uncomplicated falciparum malaria in endemic areas; combination therapy with other antimalarial agents that target different functions in the parasite and have different half-lives in blood are recommended.

Alternatively, quinine (or quinidine), which has been available for centuries derived from cinchona bark, remains effective. Some antibiotics, including tetracyclines and clindamycin, exhibit antimalarial activity and are used as an adjunct to quinine therapy. Mefloquine and halofantrine are active against chloroquine-resistant strains, but resistance is

increasing. The combination of atovaquone and proguanil offers a safer alternative.

Treatment of acute malaria with chloroquine, quinine or other antimalarials will not eliminate parasites in the liver. Similarly, gametocytes or sexual stages of parasites of *P. falciparum* are resistant to the regular antimalarials. Therefore, in order to achieve radical cure in both *P. vivax* (where parasites can remain dormant in the liver as hypnozoites) and *P. falciparum* the 8-aminoquinoline drug primaquine is used. This agent carries the risk of precipitating haemolysis in individuals who are deficient in the enzyme glucose-6-phosphate dehydrogenase.

Prophylaxis

Antimalarial prophylaxis is essential for nonimmune travellers to malarious areas. Chloroquine and the antifolate drugs pyrimethamine (often combined with sulfadoxine or dapsone) and proguanil were formerly used widely, but the widespread occurrence of resistance to these agents has made it difficult to offer definitive advice to travellers, particularly those going to regions in which *P. falciparum* is prevalent. Common recommendations include:

- the combination of atovaquone and proguanil daily
- the combination of daily proguanil and weekly chloroquine
- mefloquine, once a week.

Others recommend daily doxycycline or even primaquine. Whatever prophylactic guidance is given, it should be combined with advice to bring any fever to medical attention; to avoid exposure to mosquito bites by wearing long clothing in the evening when the insects are most active; to use insect repellents; and to sleep under mosquito netting impregnated with insecticide.

Because parasites in the preerythrocytic stage of development escape the action of most prophylactic drugs, prophylaxis should continue for at least 4 weeks after leaving a malarious area. This will effectively prevent the development of malaria, although relapses of malaria may occur (commonly in the case of *P. vivax*) up to several years after exposure.

An effective vaccine has long been sought, but is still awaited.

COCCIDIA

The coccidia are related to malaria parasites and share alternating sexual and asexual phases of development. They are not, however, transmitted by insects, and infection is usually acquired by ingesting mature oocysts.

Toxoplasma gondii

This is a coccidian parasite of the intestinal tract of the cat that is transmissible to many other mammals. It occurs worldwide. Serological evidence suggests that human infection is common, presumably as a transient febrile illness or a subclinical attack in most cases. Occasionally, more severe infection can result, such as:

- intrauterine toxoplasmosis; an important cause of stillbirth and congenital abnormality
- cerebral toxoplasmosis; in immunocompromised patients, due to reactivation of latent infection.

Mature oocysts excreted by infected cats contain two sporocysts, within which tachyzoites develop. On ingestion of oocysts, the tachyzoites are released and enter the bloodstream and lymphatics to invade macrophages, in which they multiply (Fig. 59.10). As the immune response develops, other cells are infected and tissue cysts containing slowly metabolizing bradyzoites are formed. Infection is acquired by ingestion of oocysts through contaminated food or tissue cysts in undercooked meat or via inhalation. Intrauterine infection is acquired transplacentally following a primary infection in the mother. A particularly vulnerable period is the first trimester during which organogenesis of the foetus occurs.

It is difficult to find *Toxoplasma* organisms in clinical material. Diagnosis of acute infection is made often by demonstration of a rising titre of serum antibodies to *T. gondii*. The Sabin–Feldman dye exclusion test recognises the ability of serum antibody to kill viable toxoplasmas. Other serological tests, including an enzyme-linked

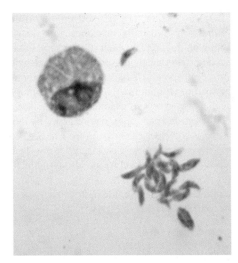

Fig. 59.10 Tachyzoites of *Toxoplasma gondii* in a macrophage *(top left)* and lying free *(bottom right)*.

immunosorbent assay (ELISA), are available and have the advantage that they avoid the use of live parasites. The polymerase chain reaction (PCR) is useful in the diagnosis of intrauterine and cerebral infections.

Treatment is indicated in symptomatic patients with evidence of active infection. The combination of pyrimethamine and a sulphonamide is effective against active tachyzoites. Spiramycin is also effective and may be preferred during pregnancy. Clindamycin, azithromycin and atovaquone, usually in combination with pyrimethamine, offer alternatives in patients with cerebral toxoplasmosis.

Isospora belli

This coccidian parasite usually causes mild self-limiting diarrhoea, but is occasionally associated with more severe infection, particularly in patients with acquired immune deficiency syndrome (AIDS). It is more common in areas of poor sanitation. The characteristic oocysts can be seen in faecal wet mounts, but are poorly refractile and easily missed. Co-trimoxazole is usually effective if antimicrobial treatment is necessary.

Cryptosporidium parvum

Cryptosporidium is a common animal parasite associated with gastrointestinal disease in all classes of vertebrates. There are about 20 species that have been characterised by molecular methods. *C. parvum* is the main species responsible for clinical disease in humans, especially in infants and children.

Infection is usually waterborne, and outbreaks related to contaminated water sources are common.

The majority of infection is a self-limiting mild diarrhoeal illness and usually responds to symptomatic treatment, with fluid replacement if necessary. In severely immunocompromised patients, particularly those with HIV infection, cryptosporidia may cause severe life-threatening diarrhea with or without involvement of the biliary tract.

Large numbers of oocysts are often present in faeces; they are partially acid-fast and can be demonstrated by modifications of the Ziehl–Neelsen method (see Ch. 63). Enzyme immunoassays and polymerase chain reaction tests that detect *Cryptosporidia* in faecal samples are also available.

In severe disease, it is reasonable to consider antimicrobial therapy. Nitazoxanide has been shown to offer some benefit.

Cyclospora cayetanensis

Unlike *Cryptosporidia*, *Cyclospora* develops intracellularly in the gut mucosa. The immature oocysts are excreted in the faeces as round bodies about 10 μm in diameter, with a characteristic mulberry appearance. They are more variably acid-fast than are *Cryptosporidia*.

Cyclospora cayetanensis causes diarrhoea and is associated with poor sanitation. As with other coccidian parasites, infection is more severe in the immunocompromised. Mild infection is treated symptomatically, with rehydration if necessary. Co-trimoxazole appears to be effective in serious infection.

Sarcocystis species

The animal parasites *Sarcocystis bovihominis* and *S. suihominis* occasionally invade the human intestinal tract or muscle. Infection is usually subclinical and discovered accidentally.

AMOEBAE

ENTAMOEBA HISTOLYTICA

This is the most important amoebic parasite of humans. The amoebae invade the colonic mucosa, producing characteristic ulcerative lesions and a profuse bloody diarrhoea (amoebic dysentery). Systemic infection may arise, leading to abscess formation in internal organs, notably the liver. Such disease may arise in the absence of a past history of frank dysentery.

Laboratory investigation

In acute amoebiasis, blood-stained mucus or colonic scrapings from ulcerated areas are examined by direct microscopy. The material should be examined within 2 hours of collection. *Entamoeba histolytica* may be recognised by its active movement, pushing out finger-like pseudopodia and, sometimes, progressing across the microscope field. If mucosal invasion has occurred, the amoebae usually contain ingested red blood cells, but these may be absent if infection is confined to the gut lumen. The nucleus is not usually visible in unstained wet preparations, but in fixed smears stained with haematoxylin it is seen as a delicate ring of chromatin with a central karyosome (Fig. 59.11A).

Typical amoebic trophozoites may also be seen in aspirates of a liver abscess. The pus often has a distinctive red-brown anchovy sauce appearance. As the amoebae actively multiply in the walls of the abscess, they are most likely to be found in the last few drops of pus drained from the lesion.

In the intestinal carrier state, active amoebae are usually absent, but the encysted form, by which infection is spread, may be found. They are spherical, about 10–15 μm in diameter, and contain one to four of the nuclei typical of *Entamoeba* species—a circular ring with a central dot. Young uninucleate cysts may also contain a large glycogen vacuole, and, in fresh specimens, cysts of all stages of development may exhibit one or more thick, blunt-ended chromatoidal bars (Fig. 59.11B).

Although demonstration of active amoebae or cysts is the best way to make a definitive diagnosis, serology is also sometimes helpful, particularly in systemic disease. Various immunodiagnostic tests have been described, but they are usually performed only in reference centres. Culture of *E. histolytica* is unhelpful as a diagnostic procedure in most cases.

Treatment

Metronidazole and tinidazole have superseded older drugs such as emetine and dehydroemetine for the treatment of amoebic dysentery and amoebic liver abscess.

Not all strains of *E. histolytica* are invasive, and some (now classified as *E. dispar*) never cause disease. However, since cysts of pathogenic and nonpathogenic strains are indistinguishable, it is prudent to treat all asymptomatic cyst excreters, particularly if they are food handlers, at least in areas of the world in which amoebiasis is uncommon. For this purpose, diloxanide furoate is often used.

NONPATHOGENIC INTESTINAL AMOEBAE

Although there are occasional reports of diarrhoea associated with other intestinal amoebae, notably *Dientamoeba fragilis* (an amoeba flagellate), most are commensals and are important only because of potential confusion with

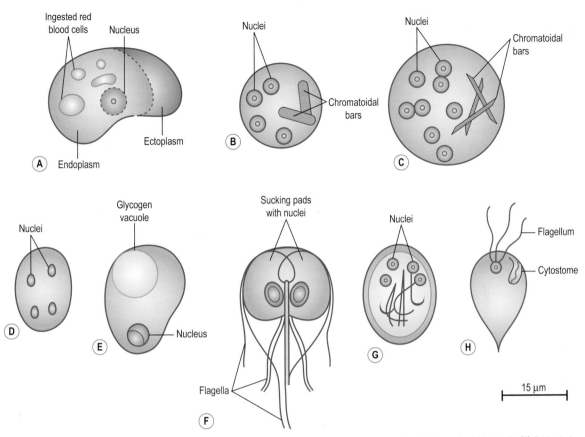

Fig. 59.11 Diagrammatic representation of some intestinal parasites: (A) *Entamoeba histolytica*, trophozoite with ingested red blood cells; (B) *E. histolytica*, mature cyst; (C) *E. coli*, mature cyst; (D) *Endolimax nana*, mature cyst; (E) *Iodamoeba bütschlii*, mature cyst; (F) *Giardia lamblia*, trophozoite; (G) *G. lamblia*, mature cyst; (H) *Chilomastix mesnili*, trophozoite.

E. histolytica. The differential characteristics of non-pathogenic intestinal amoebae are compared with those of *E. histolytica* in Table 59.3. The greatest risk of confusion arises with the other intestinal *Entamoeba* species, *E. hartmanni* and *E. coli*. *E. hartmanni* is morphologically identical to *E. histolytica*, but is smaller and the trophozoite never contains ingested red blood cells. *E. coli* is somewhat larger than *E. histolytica*, particularly in the cyst form. The trophozoites are more sluggish than those of *E. histolytica*, and mature cysts contain up to eight nuclei; chromatoidal bars, if present, are fine and pointed, rather like slivers of broken glass (Fig. 59.11C). Cysts of related intestinal amoebae *Endolimax nana* (Fig. 59.11D) and *Iodamoeba bütschlii* (Fig. 59.11E) are smaller and lack chromatoidal bars; they can create confusions in laboratory diagnosis of *E.histolytica* infections.

Blastocystis hominis, an organism commonly found in faeces and formerly thought to be a yeast, is probably an amoeba. Any pathogenic role is the subject of dispute, but it has been associated with diarrhoea in the absence of other known pathogens. Metronidazole is believed to be useful if true infection is suspected.

FREE-LIVING AMOEBAE

Environmental amoebae belonging to the genus *Naegleria* (usually *N. fowleri*) are occasionally implicated in meningoencephalitis. Rare cases of granulomatous encephalitis caused by *Balamuthia mandrillaris* and *Acanthamoeba* species have also been described, often, but not exclusively, in immunocompromised patients. The outcome in all kinds of amoebic encephalitis is generally fatal, although amphotericin B has been successfully used in infections with *N. fowleri*.

Acanthamoeba spp. more commonly cause keratitis, sometimes following use of contaminated cleaning fluids for soft contact lenses. Optimal antimicrobial chemotherapy remains to be defined, but topical treatment with propamidine, biguanides or voriconazole has been used.

Table 59.3 Differential characteristics of intestinal amoebae

Species	Trophozoites		Cysts			
	Size (μm)	Ingested red blood cells	Size (μm)	No. of nuclei[a]	Chromatoidal bars	Nuclear morphology
Entamoeba histolytica[b]	10–40	+	10–15	4	Solid, blunt ended	Fine ring of chromatin with central karyosome
E. hartmanni	4–10	–	6–10	4	As above	As above
E. coli	10–40	–	15–25	8	Slender, pointed	As above, but karyosome may be eccentric
E. gingivalis[c]	10–25	–	No cyst stage			
Iodamoeba bütschlii	10–20	–	10–15	1	None	Chromatin massed at one end of ring
Endolimax nana	5–12	–	5–8	4	None	Small shadowy masses of chromatin
Dientamoeba fragilis	5–10	–	No cyst stage			Ring containing several chromatin granules

[a]Refers to mature cyst.
[b]Including *E. dispar*.
[c]*E. gingivalis* is a commensal of the mouth.

FLAGELLATES

GIARDIA LAMBLIA (SYN. *G. INTESTINALIS*, *G. DUODENALIS*)

This intestinal parasite lives attached to the mucosal surface of the upper small intestine. Vast numbers may be present, and their presence may lead to malabsorption of fat and chronic diarrhoea. Young infants may be particularly severely affected. Infection is usually waterborne.

The trophozoite is kite shaped, with two nucleated sucking pads and four pairs of flagella (Fig. 59.11F). Trophozoites may be found in duodenal aspirate, but examination of faeces usually reveals the cyst form by which the disease is transmitted. This is oval, about 10×8 μm, and contains up to four nuclei as well as the remains of the skeletal structure of the trophozoite (Fig. 59.11G).

Cysts of other, nonpathogenic, intestinal protozoa, including *Chilomastix mesnili*, *Enteromonas hominis* and *Retortamonas intestinalis*, may be mistaken for *G. lamblia*, but they are usually smaller and lack the regular oval shape and characteristic internal morphology. These nonpathogenic protozoa may also be found as trophozoites during microscopy of diarrhoeic faeces, but the most common intestinal flagellate is *Trichomonas hominis*, which is recognisable by its undulating membrane. There is no cyst form.

Giardiasis can be treated with 5-nitroimidazoles such as metronidazole or, on the rare occasions when this fails (and reinfection is excluded), with albendazole or mepacrine (quinacrine).

TRICHOMONAS VAGINALIS

T. vaginalis is a flagellate protozoan with four anterior flagella and one lateral flagellum that is attached to the surface of the parasite to form an undulating membrane. There is no cyst form; the parasite is transmitted by sexual intercourse.

As the name suggests, *T. vaginalis* is predominantly a vaginal parasite, although urethritis may occur in the male consorts of infected women. The organism causes vaginitis, with discharge, which ordinarily responds to treatment with metronidazole or tinidazole.

T. vaginalis is readily identified by its characteristic motility in untreated wet films of vaginal discharge and can be cultivated in appropriate culture media.

TRYPANOSOMES

In contrast to the flagellates already described, trypanosomes have a complex life cycle involving an insect vector. The diseases that are caused in humans, African trypanosomiasis (sleeping sickness) and South American trypanosomiasis (Chagas' disease), are restricted in distribution according to the habitat of the insect host.

African trypanosomiasis

African sleeping sickness is caused by trypanosomes that are subspecies of *Trypanosoma brucei*, an important aetiological agent of the fatal disease nagana in cattle in tropical Africa. Tsetse flies (see Ch. 61) act as the insect vector. The human parasites are *T. brucei gambiense*, which occurs in riverine areas of West and Central Africa, and *T. brucei rhodesiense*, a parasite of the savannah plains of East Africa, where cattle and wild antelope act as reservoirs of infection.

Pathogenesis

Following the bite of an infected tsetse fly, a localized trypanosomal chancre may appear transiently, but invasion of the bloodstream rapidly occurs. The parasites multiply in blood, and at this stage there may be nonspecific symptoms with occasional febrile episodes and some lymphadenitis. Swollen lymph glands in the posterior triangle of the neck (Winterbottom's sign) are often present in *T. brucei gambiense* infection. If untreated, the disease progresses inexorably to involve the central nervous system with the classical signs of sleeping sickness and, ultimately, death.

Infection with *T. brucei rhodesiense* tends to follow a more acute, fulminating course over a period of a few months, whereas *T. brucei gambiense* infection usually progresses slowly, sometimes over several years.

Laboratory investigation

During the parasitaemic stage, sparse trypanosomes may be found in peripheral blood in unstained wet mounts or in smears stained by the Giemsa or Leishman methods. Examination of lymph node exudate may be helpful. Once the disease has progressed to involve the central nervous system, examination of cerebrospinal fluid reveals a lymphocytic exudate, often with morula cells (plasma cells) and sparse motile trypanosomes.

The parasites have a characteristic morphology—they are elongated, about 20–30 μm in length, with a single anterior flagellum arising via an undulating membrane from a basal body situated near a posteriorly placed kinetoplast (Figs 59.12 & 59.13).

In vitro cultivation is unreliable, but animal inoculation is sometimes useful, particularly with *T. brucei rhodesiense*, which infects laboratory mice more readily than *T. brucei gambiense*. Various immunodiagnostic tests have been described, but they are not as reliable as direct microscopy in establishing a definitive diagnosis.

Treatment

In the early parasitaemic stage, the infection is amenable to treatment with suramin or pentamidine, but once the disease has progressed to sleeping sickness the trivalent arsenicals, melarsoprol or tryparsamide, are used. Less toxic alternatives are clearly required; eflornithine is effective in *T. brucei gambiense* infections, but not in disease caused by *T. brucei rhodesiense*.

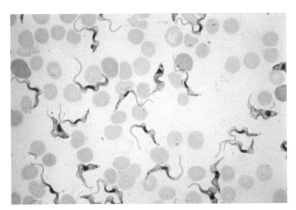

Fig. 59.12 Trypomastigotes of *Trypanosoma brucei rhodesiense* in mouse blood.

South american trypanosomiasis

Chagas' disease, caused by *T. cruzi*, is quite different from African trypanosomiasis. The insect vectors are various species of reduviid bugs (see Ch. 61). The trypanosomes are present in the bug's faeces, which the unwitting sleeper rubs into the bite wound. They do not multiply in the bloodstream, but invade cells of the reticuloendothelial system and muscle, where they lose their flagellum and associated undulating membrane and adopt a more rounded shape (Fig. 59.13). This morphological form is called an amastigote and suggests a phylogenetic relationship with *Leishmania* species (see later in the chapter). The amastigotes multiply in muscle and are liberated from ruptured cells as trypanosomal forms (trypomastigotes), which disseminate the infection and provide the parasitaemia needed to infect fresh reduviid bugs when they next feed.

Trypomastigotes are shorter than those of the *T. brucei* group and have a characteristically large kinetoplast (Fig. 59.14). The appearance of amastigotes in heart muscle is shown in Fig. 59.15.

Pathogenesis

Chagas' disease is a chronic condition characterised by extensive cardiomyopathy, sometimes with gross distension of other organs (e.g., megaoesophagus and megacolon). Death is usually from heart failure.

Laboratory investigation

PCR methods and various immunoassays have been described for serological diagnosis and are now preferred to older tests. These include direct microscopy of peripheral blood, in which small numbers of trypomastigotes may be found; culture in the rich blood agar medium also used

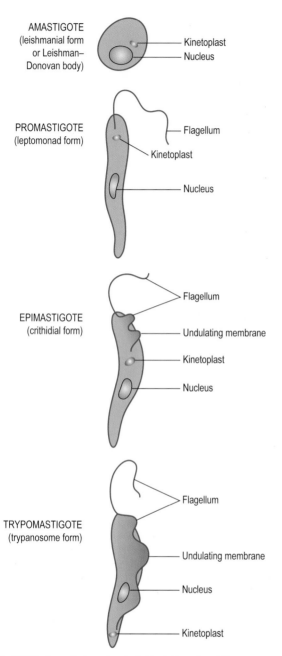

AMASTIGOTE
(leishmanial form
or Leishman–
Donovan body)
— Kinetoplast
— Nucleus

PROMASTIGOTE
(leptomonad form)
— Flagellum
— Kinetoplast
— Nucleus

EPIMASTIGOTE
(crithidial form)
— Flagellum
— Undulating membrane
— Kinetoplast
— Nucleus

TRYPOMASTIGOTE
(trypanosome form)
— Flagellum
— Undulating membrane
— Nucleus
— Kinetoplast

Fig. 59.13 Forms that may be adopted by *Leishmania* and *Trypanosoma* spp. In parentheses are given the terms for the forms under the old nomenclature now superseded.

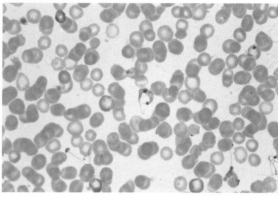

Fig. 59.14 Trypomastigote of *T. cruzi* in blood. Note the prominent kinetoplast and the 'C' shape adopted by the parasite.

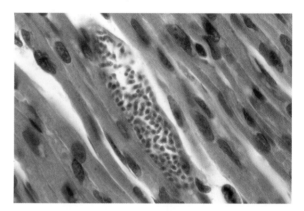

Fig. 59.15 Amastigotes of *T. cruzi* in heart muscle.

Treatment

There is no reliable chemotherapy for Chagas' disease. The nitrofuran derivative nifurtimox and the imidazole compound benznidazole have been used with modest success.

Leishmania species

Leishmania species are intracellular parasites of the reticuloendothelial system. They are related to trypanosomes, but exist in only two morphological forms: amastigotes (nonflagellate forms), which occur in the infected lesion, and promastigotes (flagellate forms that lack an undulating membrane), which occur in the insect vector or in laboratory culture (Figs 59.13, 59.16 & 59.17).

The parasites are transmitted by sandflies (see Ch. 61) in various parts of the world, including the Middle East,

to isolate *Leishmania* (see later in the chapter); mouse inoculation; and xenodiagnosis, in which uninfected reduviid bugs are allowed to feed on the patient and after about 3–4 weeks the gut contents of the bug are examined for trypanosomes.

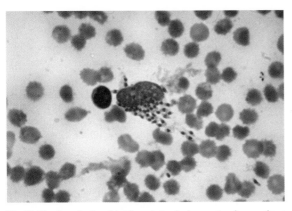

Fig. 59.16 Amastigotes of *Leishmania tropica* in a ruptured macrophage from a cutaneous lesion (oriental sore).

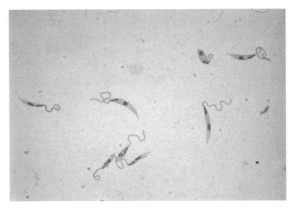

Fig. 59.17 Promastigotes of *L. tropica* from laboratory culture in Novy, MacNeal and Nicolle's (NNN) medium.

Table 59.4 *Leishmania* species involved in human disease

Species	Form of disease		Common names	Main geographical distribution
Leishmania tropica	Cutaneous	⎱	Oriental sore, Baghdad	Middle East, central Asia
L. major	Cutaneous	⎰	boil, Delhi boil, etc.	Africa, Indian subcontinent, central Asia, Ethiopia, Kenya
L. aethiopica	Cutaneous, DCL			
L. donovani	Visceral	⎫		Middle East, Africa, Indian subcontinent
	Occasionally cutaneous	⎬	Kala azar, Dum-dum	
L. infantum[a]	Visceral		fever	Mediterranean coast, Middle East, China
L. chagasi	Visceral	⎭		Tropical South America
L. mexicana complex	Cutaneous, DCL		Chiclero's ulcer	Central America, Amazon basin
L. braziliensis complex	Mucocutaneous		Espundia	Tropical South America
L. peruviana	Cutaneous		Uta	Western Peru

DCL, Disseminated cutaneous leishmaniasis.
[a]*L. infantum* may be a subspecies of *L. donovani*.

India, South America, the Mediterranean Littoral and parts of Africa.

Pathogenesis

Several distinct types of disease are recognised that range from asymptomatic infections or uncomplicated skin lesions to potentially fatal visceral disease. Therefore it is not considered as a single disease entity but as a spectrum of diseases referred to as leishmaniases. Varying disease forms in leishmaniases are distributed in defined geographical areas and caused by specific *Leishmania* species (Table 59.4), which are morphologically identical. However, the more recent identification of *L. donovani* (a usually visceralising parasite) as the causative agent of the cutaneous form of disease in a south Asian country, Sri Lanka, has blurred the picture of the traditionally accepted phenotypic characteristics of this causative agent. Cutaneous leishmaniasis (oriental sore) is the least troublesome, causing a boil-like swelling on the face or other exposed part of the body (Fig. 59.18). The central part of the lesion may become secondarily infected with bacteria, but the *Leishmania* organisms reside in the raised, indurated edge of the lesion. The sore usually heals spontaneously, leaving a scar, but with some species a more severe disseminated cutaneous leishmaniasis may occur. Parasites of the *Leishmania mexicana* complex may cause a destructive lesion of the outer ear (Chiclero's ulcer).

In mucocutaneous leishmaniasis (espundia), which is associated with the *L. braziliensis* complex, disfiguring lesions of the mouth and nose may be caused. However, the most serious form of leishmaniasis is visceral leishmaniasis (kala azar), which is a life-threatening disease involving the entire reticuloendothelial system. There are estimated to be around 500,000 new cases a year in the world, with the greatest burden in northeast India and Bangladesh. A late complication of kala azar, post–*kala*

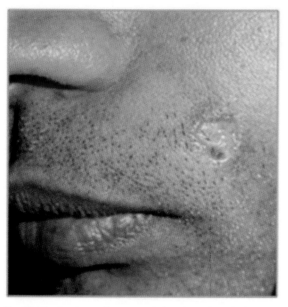

Fig. 59.18 An ulcerated cutaneous lesion observed on the face of a cutaneous leishmaniasis patient.

azar dermal leishmaniasis, may be confused with leprosy or other skin conditions.

Laboratory investigation

In the cutaneous or mucocutaneous form of the disease, typical intracellular amastigotes may be recognised in Giemsa-stained smears of material obtained from tissues at the margin of the lesion (Fig. 59.16). Free amastigotes are commonly seen because of rupture of the macrophage host cell. Material should also be cultured in Novy, MacNeal and Nicolle's (NNN) medium or a modification thereof. This is a rabbit blood agar containing antibiotic to prevent bacterial contamination and a buffered salt overlay solution in which the parasites grow as promastigotes (Fig. 59.17). Incubation is maintained approximately at 25°C for up to 3 weeks.

In kala azar, spleen puncture is the most reliable method to obtain tissue material for parasite isolation and confirmation of diagnosis. This could be performed with minimal risks using ultrasound scan guidance by a trained clinician. Alternatively, sternal marrow aspirate or lymph node biopsies also could be used for confirmation of diagnosis, though chances of isolating parasites are not so high. Smears and cultures are made and examined as for cutaneous leishmaniasis. Various serological tests have been designed with the rapid diagnostic test based on rK39 *L. donovani* amastigotes antigen probably being the most widely used. However, demonstration of the parasite by microscopy or culture is preferable whenever possible.

Treatment

The pentavalent antimony compounds, sodium stibogluconate and meglumine antimoniate, have been used traditionally in all forms of leishmaniasis, but they are toxic and therapy often fails. In cutaneous leishmaniasis, antimony compounds could be administered intralesionally with less chance of toxicity. Amphotericin B is effective, but poorly tolerated, and the less toxic lipid-based formulations are preferred. Antifungal azoles and paromomycin (aminosidine) have been used with some success in cutaneous forms of disease. Thermotherapy is yet another alternative in the management of cutaneous leishmaniasis that has been tried with success in some settings. A phosphocholine derivative, miltefosine, introduced more recently, offered considerable promise in kala azar because of its availability as an oral drug. However, the appearance of drug resistance has hindered its use in some endemic areas.

OTHER PATHOGENIC PROTOZOA

BABESIA SPECIES

Babesiae are predominantly animal parasites related to the piroplasmas that cause theileriasis in wild and domestic animals in many parts of the world. They are intracellular parasites living within red blood cells and are transmitted by ixodid ticks (see Ch. 61). In stained-blood films they superficially resemble young ring forms of plasmodia.

Human infection is uncommon. European cases have mostly been in patients whose resistance was impaired by lack of a functioning spleen; the causative parasite was usually *Babesia divergens*. In contrast, babesiosis caused by *B. microti* has been reported in otherwise healthy persons in parts of the United States.

In immunocompetent individuals the disease is usually self-limiting, so specific treatment is not required. Optimal treatment for more serious cases has not been properly defined, but the combination of quinine with clindamycin has been used successfully.

BALANTIDIUM COLI

The ciliate protozoan *Balantidium coli* is a common parasite of the pig, and human infections have usually been traced to contact with these animals. The infective form is a large (about 50 μm in diameter) thick-walled cyst. The trophozoite inhabits the lumen of the gut and may attack the colonic mucosa in much the same way as *E. histolytica*, to cause balantidial dysentery. Many highly motile ciliate trophozoites are readily seen in untreated wet films of diarrhoeic faeces. Tetracyclines and metronidazole are said to offer effective treatment.

MICROSPORIDIA

These animal and insect parasites are now thought to be fungi and are represented by several genera, including *Encephalitozoon*, *Enterocytozoon* and *Nosema*. They are, on rare occasions, implicated in opportunistic infections of immunocompromised patients, especially those with AIDS. Infections of the eye, meninges and other organs have been reported. Albendazole may be useful in treatment, but is not always curative.

RECOMMENDED READING

Cook, G. C., & Zumla, A. (Eds.), (2008). *Manson's tropical diseases* (22nd ed.). London: Elsevier, Saunders.

Croft, S. L. (2008). Kinetoplastida: New therapeutic strategies. *Parasite (Paris, France)*, *15*(3), 522–527.

Farthing, M. J. (2006). Treatment options for the eradication of intestinal protozoa. *Nature Clinical Practice. Gastroenterology and Hepatology*, *3*(8), 436–445.

Greenwood, B. M., Bojang, K., Whitty, C. J. M., & Targett, G. A. T. (2005). Malaria. *The Lancet*, *365*(9469), 1487–1498.

Guerrant, R. L., Walker, D. H., & Weller, P. F. (2011). *Tropical infectious diseases* (3rd ed.). Philadelphia: Elsevier, Saunders.

Jacquerioz, F. A., & Croft, A. M. (2009). Drugs for preventing malaria in travellers. *Cochrane Database Systematic Review*, (4), CD006491. doi:10.1002/14651858.CD006491.

Kantele, A., & Jokiranta, T. S. (2011). Review of cases with the emerging fifth human malaria parasite, *Plasmodium knowlesi*. *Clinical Infectious Disease*, *52*(11), 1356–1362. doi:10.1093/cid/cir180.

Karunaweera, N. D. (2009). *Leishmania donovani* causing cutaneous leishmaniasis in Sri Lanka: A wolf in sheep's clothing? *Trends in Parasitology*, *25*(10), 458–463.

Karunaweera, N. D., Grau, G. E., Gamage, P., Carter, R., & Mendis, K. N. (1992). Dynamics of fever and serum levels of tumor necrosis factor are closely associated during clinical paroxysms in *Plasmodium vivax* malaria. *Proceedings of the National Academy of Sciences USA*, *89*(8), 3200–3203.

Nosten, F., & White, N. J. (2007). Artemisinin-based combination treatment of falciparum malaria. *American Journal of Tropical Medicine and Hygiene*, *77*(6 Suppl.), 181–192.

Peters, W., & Pasvol, G. (2006). *Atlas of tropical medicine and parasitology* (6th ed.). London: Elsevier, Mosby.

Rosenblatt, J. E. (2009). Laboratory diagnosis of infections due to blood and tissue parasites. *Clinical Infectious Diseases*, *49*(7), 1103–1108.

Stanley, S. L., Jr. (2003). Amoebiasis. *The Lancet*, *361*(9362), 1025–1034.

White, N. J. (2008). *Plasmodium knowlesi*: The fifth human malaria parasite. *Clinical Infectious Diseases*, *46*(2), 172–173. doi:10.1086/524889.

World Health Organization. (1991). *Basic Laboratory Methods in Medical Parasitology*. Geneva: WHO.

CD-ROMs

The CD-ROMs produced by the Wellcome Trust, London are available from the Wellcome Trust (http://www.wellcome.ac.uk) and (for developing countries) from TALC (Teaching-aids at Low Cost; http://www.talcuk.org/).

Wellcome Trust. (2000). Leishmaniasis (Topics in International Health series).

Wellcome Trust. (2007). Human African Trypanosomiasis (Topics in International Health series).

Wellcome Trust. (2007). Malaria (3th ed.). (Topics in International Health series).

World Health Organization and Centers for Disease Control, USA. (2009). The microscopic diagnosis of malaria. Available at http://www.who.int/malaria/areas/diagnosis/microscopy_cd_rom/en/.

Websites

Centers for Disease Control and Prevention. Division of Parasitic Diseases, Professional Information. Parasites. Retrieved from http://www.cdc.gov/parasites. (Accessed Aug 2017).

Centers for Disease Control and Prevention. Malaria. Retrieved from https://www.cdc.gov/dpdx/malaria/dx.html. (Accessed Aug 2017).

Malaria Centre, London School of Hygiene and Tropical Medicine. Retrieved from http://malaria.lshtm.ac.uk/. (Accessed Aug 2017).

National Travel Health Network and Centre. Retrieved from http://nathnac.net/. (Accessed Aug 2017).

World Health Organization. Basic Laboratory Methods in Medical Parasitology. Retrieved from http://whqlibdoc.who.int/publications/9241544104_%28part1%29.pdf. (Accessed Aug 2017).

World Health Organization. Malaria Rapid Diagnostic Tests. Retrieved from http://www.who.int/malaria/areas/diagnosis/rapid-diagnostic-tests/en/. (Accessed Aug 2017).

World Health Organization. World Malaria Report 2015. Retrieved from www.who.int/malaria/publications/world-malaria-report-2015/report/en/. (Accessed Aug 2017).

60 Helminths

Intestinal worm infections; filariasis; schistosomiasis; hydatid disease

NILANTHI R. DE SILVA AND NELUN PERERA

KEY POINTS

- Helminths are multicellular parasitic worms that often have complex life cycles.
- Intestinal nematodes (roundworms) are extremely common, especially in conditions of poor sanitation.
- Heavy infections with hookworm cause severe anaemia; benzimidazoles offer effective therapy.
- Serious infections caused by tissue nematodes include bancroftian filariasis (elephantiasis) and onchocerciasis (river blindness); they are treated with ivermectin or diethylcarbamazine.
- Trematodes (flukes) cause schistosomiasis (bilharzia) and other diseases such as Chinese liver fluke infection.
- Adult cestodes (tapeworms) usually cause little pathology, but larval infections cause more serious disease.
- Most trematode and cestode infections respond to praziquantel.
- Hydatid disease is caused by a dog tapeworm. Mainstay of treatment is surgery.

Medical helminthology is concerned with the study of worms that parasitise humans. These creatures are responsible for an enormous burden of infection throughout the world and, although few helminthic infections are life threatening, their impact on human health is incalculable. Most medically important helminths have no independent existence outside the host and are therefore truly parasitic. As they rely on the host for sustenance, it is not in their interest to cause the host harm; consequently, they do not usually exhibit great virulence and are characterised more by the strategies that they have evolved to prevent rejection by the host defences. The pathogenic manifestations of helminthic disease, which can nonetheless be considerable, are ordinarily due to physical factors related to the location of the worms, their lifestyle or their size and only occasionally due to the host's immune response to the worms (see Ch. 11).

There are two major groups of medically important helminths: nematodes, or roundworms, and platyhelminths, or flatworms. Flatworms are, in their turn, represented by two classes: trematodes (flukes) and cestodes (tapeworms).

NEMATODES

The principal nematode parasites of humans are conveniently considered under two headings: intestinal nematodes and tissue nematodes.

INTESTINAL NEMATODES

Infection with intestinal roundworms (Table 60.1) is generally associated with conditions of poor sanitation and hygiene. Such infections are extremely common, particularly throughout the tropics and subtropics, although several are also found in temperate regions. Low worm burdens are generally asymptomatic, but heavy infections may cause problems, especially in young children in whom they have been associated with impaired development.

Ascaris lumbricoides

This is the common roundworm, which infects about 800 million people in the world. The adults are large and fleshy and, as with many nematodes (other than the hookworm group), the smaller male can be recognised by his characteristically curled tail. The eggs (ova) are produced in huge numbers; they are thick walled, bile stained and typically exhibit a corrugated albuminous coat (Fig. 60.1A). In the absence of a male worm, the female produces infertile eggs, which are more elongated and irregular than the fertile variety (Fig. 60.1B).

In warm, moist conditions, infective larvae develop within fertile eggs but do not hatch. Under favourable conditions, such eggs can survive for several years in soil. If ingested, the infective eggs hatch in the duodenum and the larvae penetrate the gut mucosa to reach the bloodstream.

They are carried to the pulmonary circulation, where they gain access to the lung and undergo two moults before migrating via the trachea to the intestinal tract. Having completed their round trip, they mature in the gut lumen and live for about a year.

Ascaris lumbricoides is a well-adapted parasite that is usually not pathogenic in the ordinary sense. However, pneumonic symptoms may accompany the migratory phase, and infection with these large worms may result in stunting of growth in young children. The adult worms may invade the biliary and pancreatic ducts, while heavy infections (with 50 or more worms) can cause intestinal obstruction. Allergy is also sometimes a problem.

The dog ascarid, *Toxocara canis*, may accidentally infect humans. Larvae hatch in the small intestine and penetrate the gut wall, but they are unable to complete their migratory phase. Instead, they find their way to visceral organs such as the liver and lungs, a condition known as visceral larva migrans. Occasionally the larvae reach the eye and cause serious retinal lesions. Larvae of several other roundworms, including *Angiostrongylus*, *Gnathostoma* and *Anisakis* species, are occasionally implicated in visceral larva migrans in some parts of the world.

Trichuris trichiura

This is the common whipworm, often found together with *Ascaris*. The adults live with the head (the whip end of the worm) embedded in the colonic mucosa. Each female lays thousands of characteristic tea-tray eggs (Fig. 60.1C) every day. Like those of *Ascaris*, they develop infective larvae in warm, moist conditions, but the ova do not hatch outside the body. However, after ingestion and hatching, there is no migratory phase and adult worms develop directly in the large intestine.

Infection is usually trivial, although massive infections can cause rectal prolapse in young children, and a form

Table 60.1 Principal intestinal nematodes of humans

Species	Common name	Relevant examination
Ancylostoma duodenale	Hookworm	Faecal concentration (ova)
Ascaris lumbricoides	Common roundworm	Faecal concentration (ova)
Enterobius vermicularis	Threadworm	Perianal swab (ova), adult worms on stool
Necator americanus	Hookworm	Faecal concentration (ova)
Strongyloides stercoralis	–	Faecal culture (larvae)
Toxocara canis[a]	Dog roundworm	Serology
Trichostrongylus spp.	Hookworm	Faecal concentration (ova)
Trichuris trichiura	Whipworm	Faecal concentration (ova)

[a]Not an intestinal parasite of humans; causes visceral larva migrans (see text).

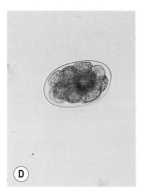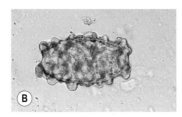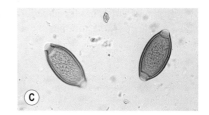

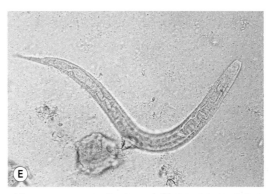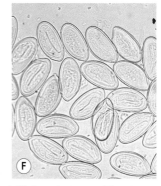

Fig. 60.1 Eggs of intestinal helminths: (A) *Ascaris lumbricoides* (fertile eggs); (B) *A. lumbricoides* (infertile egg); (C) *Trichuris trichiura*; (D) Hookworm; (E) *Strongyloides stercoralis* (larva); (F) *Enterobius vermicularis*.

of dysentery combined with severe growth retardation is described.

Hookworm

The two human hookworms, *Ancylostoma duodenale* and *Necator americanus*, are widely distributed throughout the tropics and subtropics. The two species produce indistinguishable thin-walled eggs (Fig. 60.1D) that hatch in soil. Infection is usually acquired by walking barefoot in soil contaminated with human faeces. The larvae undergo two moults before infective larvae are produced. These are capable of penetrating unbroken skin, and in this way they gain access to the bloodstream to begin a migratory phase similar to that of *A. lumbricoides*. When they reach the gut they attach by their mouthparts to the mucosa of the small intestine. The adult worms, which are about 1 cm long, are similar, but the buccal capsule of *A. duodenale* bears two pairs of teeth, whereas *N. americanus* has two so-called cutting plates. Unlike most nematodes, the tail of male hookworms has a membranous bursa used for attachment to the female during copulation.

Hookworms ingest blood and move from site to site in the gut mucosa, leaving behind small bleeding lesions. These two facts are responsible for the chief pathological manifestation of heavy infection with hookworms—iron deficiency anaemia.

Larvae of animal hookworms, notably the dog hookworm, *A. caninum*, may penetrate human skin, but do not migrate further. They do, however, cause local irritation by wandering through subcutaneous tissue, a condition called cutaneous larva migrans.

Trichostrongylus species

Various species of *Trichostrongylus* have been associated with human disease, particularly in the Middle East. Like the hookworms, they are bursate nematodes with similar but more elongated, eggs.

Strongyloides stercoralis

This parasite is also related to the hookworms but differs in several important respects. There is a distinct free-living phase in the life cycle, during which males and females reproduce. Human infections arise after penetration of infective larvae through skin and there is a migratory phase involving the lungs. However, human infection appears to be restricted to female worms, which embed themselves in the gut mucosa and produce eggs that contain fully developed larvae; these hatch within the intestinal lumen so that larvae, not eggs, are found in faecal samples (Fig. 60.1E). Infection can persist for many years because some larvae can develop sufficiently within the body to initiate a fresh cycle of development and cause autoinfection.

Symptoms are usually benign, but in debilitated individuals, larvae may be activated to penetrate the gut wall and invade other organs, a serious condition known as hyperinfection.

Enterobius vermicularis

This is the common threadworm, which infects children throughout the world. It has the simplest life cycle of all intestinal worms. Adults live in the large intestine and are occasionally found in the appendix. Mature, gravid females crawl through the anus at night and lay their eggs in the perianal area. The eggs are characteristically flattened on one side (Fig. 60.1F) and usually contain fully developed larvae. Ingestion of these eggs initiates a fresh infection. Symptoms are restricted to itching (pruritus ani) associated with the deposition of eggs.

As eggs are not discharged by the worm into faeces, faecal examination is not appropriate in the laboratory diagnosis of threadworm infection. The diagnosis is established by finding the characteristic threads on the surface of formed stools, or by examination of swabs (or cellophane strip impressions) of unwashed perianal skin for the characteristic ova.

Treatment of intestinal nematode infections

The range of options is listed in Table 60.2. Most effective are the benzimidazole derivatives, especially albendazole and mebendazole. In endemic areas, where 20% or more children are likely to be infected with roundworm, whipworm or hookworm, mass deworming programmes, where all children are treated annually or biannually with a single dose of albendazole or mebendazole, are recommended by WHO because these anthelmintics are safe, effective and cost little. In all other situations, anthelmintic treatment should follow confirmation of infection by laboratory diagnosis.

TISSUE NEMATODES

This group includes the filarial worms, the Guineaworm *(Dracunculus medinensis)* and *Trichinella spiralis* (Table 60.3).

Filarial worms

Filarial worms have a complex life cycle involving developmental stages in an insect vector. They vary considerably in their pathogenic effects, but some are

Table 60.2 Spectrum of activity of drugs used in the treatment of intestinal nematode infections

Drug	Ancylostoma duodenale	Necator americanus	Ascaris lumbricoides	Strongyloides stercoralis	Trichuris trichiura	Enterobius vermicularis
Levamisole	++	++	+++	−	−	−
Pyrantel pamoate	++	++	+++	+	++	+++
Thiabendazole	++	++	++	++	−	++
Mebendazole	++	++	+++	+	++	+++
Albendazole	+++	++	+++	++	++	+++
Ivermectin	−	−	+	++	+	+

+++, highly effective; +, poorly effective; −, no useful activity.
Adapted from Greenwood, D., Finch, R. G., Davey, P. G., & Wilcox, M. H. (2007) *Antimicrobial Chemotherapy* (5th ed.). Oxford: Oxford University Press.

Table 60.3 Principal tissue nematodes of humans

Parasite species	Vector	Geographical distribution	Relevant examination
Wuchereria bancrofti	Mosquitoes	Tropical belt	Night blood
Brugia malayi	Mosquitoes	Southeast Asia	Night blood
Loa loa	Chrysops spp.	West and Central Africa	Day blood
Mansonella perstans	Culicoides spp.	Tropical Africa, South America	Blood
M. ozzardi	Culicoides spp.	West Indies, South America	Blood
Onchocerca volvulus	Simulium spp.	Tropical Africa, Central America	Skin snips
M. streptocerca	Culicoides spp.	West and Central Africa	Skin snips
Dracunculus medinensis	Water fleas	Africa	Adult worm when mature
Trichinella spiralis	None[a]	Worldwide	Muscle biopsy, serology

[a]Pork forms the chief reservoir.

responsible for disabling diseases that have a major impact on communities living in endemic areas.

Wuchereria bancrofti

This worm is transmitted through the bite of various species of mosquito (mostly *Culex* or *Anopheles* spp.) throughout the tropical belt of the world. Over 100 million people are thought to be infected. The larvae invade the lymphatics, usually of the lower limbs, where they develop into adult worms. The presence of adult worms, the immune response to their presence and recurrent bacterial infections of the skin results in lymphatic blockage and gross lymphoedema, which sometimes leads to the bizarre deformities associated with bancroftian filariasis, elephantiasis.

Embryonic forms (microfilariae) are liberated into the bloodstream. They retain the elastic egg membrane as a sheath, which covers the whole larva (Fig. 60.2A). Microfilariae remain in the pulmonary circulation during the day, emerging into the peripheral circulation only at night, to coincide with the biting habits of the insect vector. The physiological basis of this nocturnal periodicity is not understood, but it is also known that strains of *W. bancrofti* encountered in some Pacific islands, where the parasite is transmitted by day-biting mosquitoes of *Aedes* spp., do not exhibit a nocturnal periodicity. Aside from these exceptions, blood for examination for *W. bancrofti* must be taken during the night, optimally between midnight and 2 a.m. Commercially available rapid diagnostic test strips, which detect circulating parasite antigen, are useful because they do not require night blood.

Brugia malayi

This parasite is transmitted by mosquitoes in parts of India, the Far East and Southeast Asia. Adult worms inhabit the lymphatics and, like *W. bancrofti*, can cause elephantiasis. Microfilaraemia usually shows a nocturnal periodicity.

Loa loa

This worm is restricted in distribution to central and western parts of tropical Africa, where it is transmitted

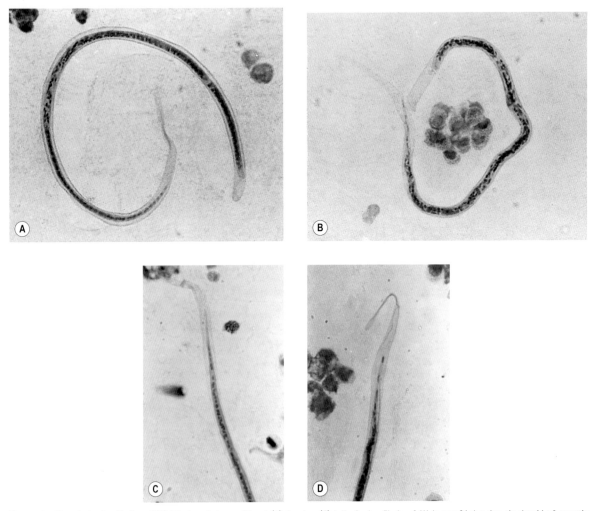

Fig. 60.2 Sheathed microfilariae of (A) *Wuchereria bancrofti* and (B) *Loa loa*; (C) tail of microfilaria of *W. bancrofti* showing tip devoid of somatic nuclei; (D) tail of microfilaria of *L. loa* showing nuclei extending to tip of tail.

by biting flies (*Chrysops* spp., see Ch. 61). The adult worms live in subcutaneous tissue and wander round the body, provoking localised reactions known as Calabar swellings and sometimes migrating across the front of the eye.

The sheathed microfilariae of *Loa loa* (Fig. 60.2B) exhibit diurnal periodicity, so that, unlike those of *W. bancrofti*, they appear in peripheral blood only during the day.

Onchocerca volvulus

This filarial worm is common in parts of tropical Africa and Central America. It is transmitted by blackflies of the *Simulium* spp. (see Ch. 61). Adult worms develop in subcutaneous and connective tissue, and often become encapsulated in nodules, which form on bony parts of the body such as the hip, elbow and (particularly in Central America) the head. The microfilariae are not found in blood, but live in the superficial layers of the skin and provoke an intense inflammatory reaction, especially on dying, which results in itching and, in heavy chronic infections, gross thickening of the skin. The eye is commonly invaded by microfilariae, which may cause corneal and retinal lesions that lead to blindness. Because the vector breeds by rivers, the condition is known as river blindness.

If nodules are present, diagnosis can be made by finding macroscopic worms within an excised nodule. Otherwise, skin snips taken from calves, buttocks and shoulders are suspended in a drop of saline and examined microscopically for motile microfilariae.

Mansonella species

Mansonella perstans is widespread throughout tropical Africa and parts of South America; the related *M. ozzardi* is restricted to parts of the West Indies and South America. They are transmitted by biting midges (*Culicoides* species; see Ch. 61). The unsheathed microfilariae appear in the bloodstream and exhibit no periodicity. They are generally regarded as non-pathogenic.

M. streptocerca causes skin infections similar to those of *Onchocerca volvulus*, although the symptoms are usually milder. It is restricted to parts of Western and Central Africa.

Differential characteristics of microfilariae

The microfilariae of filarial worms can be differentiated in stained preparations of clinical material by various criteria, the most useful of which are the presence or absence of a sheath and the disposition of the somatic nuclei in the tip of the tail (Table 60.4 and Fig. 60.2). Giemsa stain is suitable for the demonstration of somatic nuclei, but hot (60°C) haematoxylin is necessary to stain the sheath.

Treatment of filarial infections

Diethylcarbamazine (DEC) has been used for many years for the treatment of all forms of lymphatic filariasis. It effectively kills microfilariae but is not reliably lethal to adult worms. It is relatively nontoxic, but death of the microfilariae may be accompanied by a severe allergic reaction (Mazzotti reaction), especially in onchocerciasis.

The treatment of onchocerciasis has been revolutionised by use of the veterinary anthelminthic ivermectin. This drug is effective in a single oral dose and is less likely than DEC to elicit a severe reaction. Periodic administration of ivermectin, together with vector control measures, has had an important impact on controlling onchocerciasis transmission in endemic areas.

Ivermectin and albendazole are effective in other forms of filariasis, although neither drug kills adult worms. As they exhibit activity against intestinal nematodes, including *A. lumbricoides*, these may be incidentally expelled during treatment. Albendazole is used in combination with ivermectin or DEC, in campaigns aimed at eradicating lymphatic filariasis.

Surprisingly, tetracyclines also have an effect in filariasis, apparently by inhibiting endosymbiotic bacteria (*Wolbachia* species) that are essential for the fertility of the worms.

Dracunculus medinensis

This parasite, also known as Guinea worm, is now near eradication and is found only in a few Sub-Saharan countries. Human infection is normally acquired through drinking water containing infected water fleas of the *Cyclops* spp. The larvae penetrate the gut mucosa and grow to maturity in connective tissue, usually of the lower limbs. The female worm incubates larvae to maturity and, when ready to give birth, emerges to the skin surface to provoke an intensely irritating blister. When the sufferer immerses the blister in water, the uterus of the female worm bursts, liberating up to 1 million larvae, which are ingested by water fleas, to continue the cycle.

Attempts can be made to wind out the dead worm over several days, but breakage of the worm often occurs, and pyogenic cocci may be carried into the tissues to cause a cellulitis. Chemotherapy is not usually helpful, other than to treat secondary bacterial infection. Prevention is the best approach; health education campaigns and the provision of safe water have greatly reduced the prevalence of this disease.

Trichinella spiralis

Unlike most parasitic worms, *Trichinella* spp. (of which *T. spiralis* is the most common) has an extremely wide host range. Human infections are usually acquired by

Table 60.4 Differential features of human microfilariae

Species	Site in human host	Periodicity	Sheath	Nuclei in tip of tail	Length (µm)
Wuchereria bancrofti	Blood	Nocturnal[a]	Present	Absent	250–300
Brugia malayi	Blood	(Nocturnal)[b]	Present	Present[c]	200–250
Loa loa	Blood	Diurnal	Present	Present	250–300
Mansonella perstans	Blood	Nonperiodic	Absent	Present	150–200
M. ozzardi	Blood	Nonperiodic	Absent	Absent	180–220
Onchocerca volvulus	Skin	Nonperiodic	Absent	Absent	250–300
M. streptocerca	Skin	Nonperiodic	Absent	Present	180–240

[a]Subperiodic forms occur in the Pacific Islands.
[b]Partial nocturnal periodicity.
[c]Two small, well-separated nuclei in the tip of the tail.

eating undercooked pork products. The infected larvae lie dormant in skeletal muscle (Fig. 60.3) and are released when the meat is digested. Male and female worms develop to maturity attached to the mucosa of the small intestine. The female is viviparous, producing numerous larvae during a life span of only a few weeks. The larvae penetrate the gut wall and migrate to skeletal muscle, where they enter the quiescent phase. Most of the symptoms of trichinosis, which can be severe, even life threatening, are associated with the migration of larvae.

Treatment with large doses of albendazole or mebendazole early in the infection can kill the adult worms and prevent further release of larvae and progression to the invasive stage.

TREMATODES

The flukes (Table 60.5) are a diverse group of worms that share a similar life cycle involving a snail host and, often, a second intermediate host that provides the vehicle for the transmission of infection. Most flukes have a restricted geographical distribution that reflects the habitat of the appropriate type of snail.

Most trematodes are hermaphroditic, but the most important human flukes, the schistosomes, are differentiated into separate sexes.

Life cycle

When excreted, trematode eggs often contain a fully developed ciliated stage called a miracidium, although in some species immature eggs are produced that require a period of development before the miracidium is formed. In water, the miracidium escapes, either through a lidlike operculum in the egg shell or (in the case of the schistosomes) by osmotic rupture of the egg. The miracidium penetrates the appropriate species of snail and undergoes several stages of asexual reproduction before emerging as a free-swimming body called a cercaria. The cercariae encyst in the muscle of fish *(Clonorchis sinensis)*, crabs and crayfish *(Paragonimus westermani)*, water chestnuts *(Fasciolopsis buski)* or vegetation *(Fasciola hepatica)*, and humans become infected by ingesting the encysted metacercariae. In the case of *Schistosoma* species, the cercariae remain in water and penetrate unbroken skin to gain access to the body.

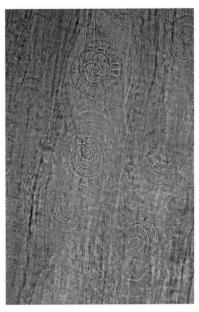

Fig. 60.3   Larvae of *Trichinella spiralis* in muscle.

Table 60.5   Principal trematode parasites of humans

Species	Common name	Intermediate host First[a]	Second	Geographical distribution	Relevant examination
Clonorchis sinensis	Chinese liver fluke	Bithynia sp.	Freshwater fish	Far East	Stool concentration
Fasciola hepatica	Sheep liver fluke	Lymnaea sp.	Vegetation	Worldwide	Stool concentration, serology
Fasciolopsis buski	Giant intestinal fluke	Segmentina sp. etc.	Water chestnut	Far East	Stool concentration
Paragonimus westermani	Lung fluke	Semisulcospira sp.	Crabs and crayfish	Chiefly Far East	Sputum
Schistosoma mansoni	Bilharzia	Biomphalaria sp.	None (water)	Africa, West Indies, South America	Stool concentration, rectal biopsy
S. haematobium	Bilharzia	Bulinus sp.	None (water)	Africa	Terminal urine (midday)
S. japonicum	Bilharzia	Oncomelania sp.	None (water)	Far East	Stool concentration, rectal biopsy

[a]The first intermediate host is a snail in each case.

Clonorchis sinensis (syn. Opisthorchis sinensis)

This is the Chinese liver fluke. Infection is acquired from uncooked freshwater fish, notably carp. The metacercariae excyst in the small intestine and pass into the bile ducts, where they mature. Typical small, flask-shaped eggs with a prominent operculum (Fig. 60.4A) are excreted in large numbers into the faeces.

Infection is commonly asymptomatic, but fibrosis of the bile ducts with impairment of liver function may occur in heavy, chronic infections. Long-standing untreated infections are known to increase the risk of cholangiocarcinoma. As with most fluke infections, praziquantel is the drug of choice for treatment.

A closely related fluke, *Opisthorchis felineus*, which is a parasite of the cat, has been associated with human disease in parts of Eastern Europe.

Fasciola hepatica

This is the cosmopolitan liver fluke of sheep. Human infections have usually been associated with eating wild watercress from infected sheep pastures. The adult worm is larger than *C. sinensis*, and lighter infections can cause biliary fibrosis and obstructive jaundice. The large, immature eggs with an indistinct operculum (Fig. 60.4B) may be found in faeces but are usually sparse.

Unlike other trematode infections, fascioliasis does not reliably respond to praziquantel, and the veterinary anthelminthic triclabendazole is the drug of choice for treatment of this infection.

Paragonimus westermani

This is the lung fluke, which is found in parts of the Far East. Closely related species have occasionally been implicated in human disease in parts of Africa and South America. Human infection follows ingestion of raw, infected muscle of freshwater crabs and crayfish. The metacercariae penetrate through the gut wall and diaphragm to reach the lung, where they develop to maturity. Occasionally the larvae find their way to the brain. Pulmonary infection usually provokes the production of sputum, in which the characteristic large eggs (Fig. 60.4C) can be found, often associated with flecks of altered blood. Praziquantel is used for treatment.

Intestinal flukes

Several genera of intestinal flukes cause human infection, particularly in the Far East. *Fasciolopsis buski* is found in restricted foci in China and Southeast Asia. Infection is often acquired by the habit of opening water chestnuts with the teeth. The adult flukes live attached to the wall

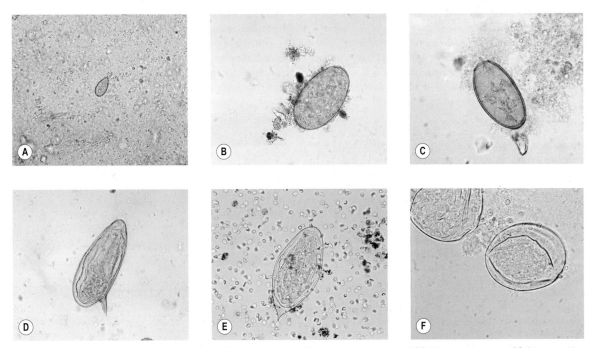

Fig. 60.4 Eggs of trematodes: (A) *Clonorchis sinensis*; (B) *Fasciola hepatica*; (C) *Paragonimus westermani*; (D) *Schistosoma mansoni*; (E) *S. haematobium*; (F) *S. japonicum*.

of the small intestine and produce a large number of eggs that resemble those of *F. hepatica*.

Schistosoma species

The schistosomes, or blood flukes, also known as bilharzia, after the discoverer Theodor Bilharz, are the most important of the pathogenic trematodes. At least 200 million people are infected, principally in Africa, where *S. mansoni* and *S. haematobium* are widespread, and *S. intercalatum* is encountered in some areas. *S. mansoni* is also found in parts of the West Indies and South America; *S. japonicum* and the related *S. mekongi* are restricted to the Far East.

Human infection follows exposure to cercariae in water harbouring infected snails. The cercariae penetrate the skin, often causing a transient dermatitis called swimmer's itch. Once in the bloodstream, the schistosomula migrate to the liver, where they develop into adult worms. The integument of the mature male worm is adapted in the form of two long flaps, the gynaecophoral canal, in which the female is held. The mature worms migrate to the small veins of the rectum *(S. mansoni, S. intercalatum, S. japonicum* and *S. mekongi)* or the bladder *(S. haematobium)*. Eggs, which contain a fully developed miracidium, are passed through the rectal mucosa onto the surface of colonic faeces or through the bladder wall into the urine.

The ova of *S. mansoni* (Fig. 60.4D) are large (about 140 μm long) and possess a characteristic lateral spine, whereas those of *S. haematobium* (Fig. 60.4E) and *S. intercalatum* have a terminal spine. The smaller, more rounded, eggs of *S. japonicum* and *S. mekongi* do not have a prominent spine, but may exhibit a rudimentary nipple-like appendage (Fig. 60.4F).

Pathogenesis

The adult worms adopt the subterfuge of coating themselves with host antigens to evade attack by host defences; in themselves, the adults are innocuous. Most of the serious manifestations of schistosomiasis arise from the deposition of eggs, with resultant formation of granulomata and fibrotic lesions of the liver, bladder or other organs. Such effects may herald malignant changes. Heavy infection with *S. mansoni* may give rise to schistosomal dysentery, whereas *S. haematobium* infections are commonly accompanied by a marked haematuria (visible in Fig. 60.4E).

Laboratory investigation

Ova of rectal schistosomes can be sought on the surface of formed faeces. Blood-stained mucus should be examined, if present. Alternatively, microscopic examination of snips of rectal mucosa teased out in a drop of saline on a microscope slide may reveal viable or calcified eggs.

For the diagnosis of infection with *S. haematobium*, the last few drops of urine at the end of micturition (terminal urine) are most likely to be rich in ova. Excretion is said to be maximal around midday.

Various serodiagnostic tests, including enzyme-linked immunosorbent assay (ELISA), are available but are no substitute for demonstration of the ova.

Treatment

Praziquantel is effective against all the human schistosomes and is the drug of choice. Because of its lack of toxicity and simplicity in administration, praziquantel has been used together with molluscicides and water purification in control programmes.

Other compounds are more selective in their action: metrifonate (an organophosphate compound) is active against *S. haematobium*; oxamniquine is effective in *S. mansoni* infection.

CESTODES

The species of tapeworm most commonly involved in human infection are listed in Table 60.6.

Table 60.6 Principal cestode parasites of humans

Species	Common name	Intermediate host	Relevant examination
Taenia saginata	Beef tapeworm	Cattle	Mature segments on
T. solium	Pork tapeworm	Pig	stool
Diphyllobothrium latum	Fish tapeworm	*Cyclops* spp./fish	Ova in stool
Hymenolepis nana	Dwarf tapeworm	None	Ova in stool
Echinococcus granulosus[a]	Hydatid worm	Sheep, humans	Radiology, serology

[a]Dog tapeworm; human is one of the intermediate hosts.

TAENIA SPECIES

Taenia saginata, the beef tapeworm, is much more prevalent than the related *T. solium*, the pork tapeworm. Both have a relatively simple life cycle, alternating between humans and the intermediate host. Human infection is acquired by eating raw or undercooked beef or pork containing the encysted larval stage, the cysticercus. The larvae hatch in the small intestine and attach to the mucosal surface by four suckers on the head (scolex) of the worm. The scolex of *T. solium* additionally carries a crown of hooklets. The worm grows backwards from the head, first producing immature segments (proglottids), which continue to develop as they become more distant from the head. When sexually mature, the proglottids, which exhibit both male and female characteristics (hermaphroditic), cross-fertilise one another, and eggs start to be produced in the uterine canal. This becomes grossly distended as more eggs are produced, so that the fully gravid segments at the end of the worm become nothing more than bags full of eggs. The complete chain of segments is known as a strobila and may measure 10 m or more.

Eggs are not laid. They are retained within the proglottids, which become detached from the end of the worm and are passed with the faeces. Animals become infected by ingesting the eggs from pastures contaminated with inadequately treated sewage or by the droppings of birds that scavenge in untreated sewage.

Considering the size of the worm, infection is usually remarkably asymptomatic. However, in the case of *T. solium*, eggs may hatch in the human host and develop into cysticerci. When these form in the brain, they may cause neurocysticercosis, a common cause of epilepsy in endemic countries.

Laboratory investigation

Taenia infection is usually diagnosed by finding the typical segments in faeces. Since eggs are not laid, faecal examination for ova is inappropriate. *T. saginata* can usually be differentiated from *T. solium* if the segment is pressed between two microscope slides and examined macroscopically. In the case of *T. saginata*, numerous branchings of the central uterine canal are evident, whereas there are usually far fewer branchings with *T. solium* (Fig. 60.5). The eggs (Fig. 60.6A) are thick walled and contain an oncosphere with six hooklets. The eggs of *T. saginata* and *T. solium* are indistinguishable.

Treatment

A single dose of praziquantel is usually successful. Niclosamide is also used, but this drug causes the worm to disintegrate, with the consequent theoretical (but unproven) risk of autoinfection in the case of *T. solium* through the intraluminal release of eggs. Treatment of cerebral cysticercosis is problematical, but albendazole and praziquantel have been used successfully.

DIPHYLLOBOTHRIUM LATUM

This is the fish tapeworm, which is prevalent in lakeland areas where freshwater fish is eaten raw. The life cycle resembles that of the trematodes. The mature adult worm, which may attain a length of 10 m, lays numerous operculate eggs within which a ciliated body called a coracidium develops. This hatches in water and is ingested by the water flea (*Cyclops* species). After a period of development, the larva awaits ingestion by a freshwater fish in which it invades the muscle as an infective plerocercoid larva or sparganum.

Human infection is usually asymptomatic, although a form of pernicious anaemia caused by competition for dietary vitamin B_{12} has been described.

The characteristic immature eggs have an indistinct operculum (Fig. 60.6B) and are usually present in large numbers in faeces. Occasionally a length of the worm may break off and be passed in the stool.

Niclosamide or praziquantel is used for treatment.

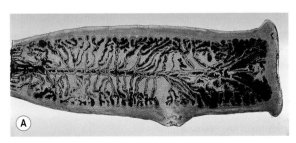
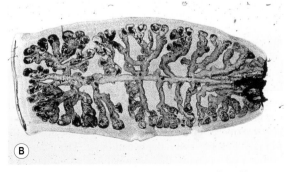

Fig. 60.5 Segments of (A) *Taenia saginata* and (B) *T. solium*. The uterine canal has been injected with Indian ink to show the branchings.

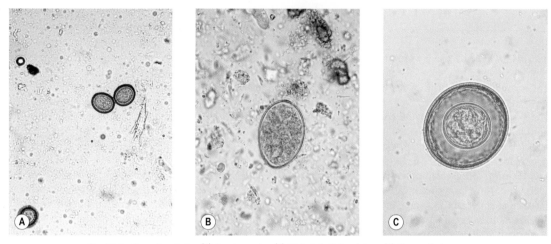

Fig. 60.6 Eggs of cestodes: (A) *Taenia* species; (B) *Diphyllobothrium latum*; (C) *Hymenolepis nana*.

HYMENOLEPIS NANA

In contrast to the enormous length of *Taenia* species and *D. latum, Hymenolepis nana* is only 2–4 cm long and is consequently known as the dwarf tapeworm. It has a very simple life cycle with no known intermediate host. The characteristic poached egg ova (Fig. 60.6C) are directly infective, and it is surprising that infection is not more common.

Infection is usually asymptomatic; heavy infections can be treated with praziquantel or niclosamide.

A slightly larger species, *H. diminuta*, is occasionally found in humans. This is a parasite of small rodents and is transmitted by their fleas.

ECHINOCOCCUS GRANULOSUS

This is the tapeworm of the dog and other canine species, and, unusually, humans are an intermediate host. It is a small worm, consisting usually of just four segments and measuring less than a centimetre. Sheep are the usual intermediate hosts. Other animals, including humans, may become infected, especially in sheep-farming areas, where the cycle of transmission is maintained between sheep and dogs.

After ingestion of the eggs, which resemble those of *Taenia* species, larvae hatch in the small intestine, penetrate the gut mucosa and are carried by the bloodstream to various organs (commonly the liver), where they are filtered out. The larva starts to grow, eventually forming a cystic cavity, the hydatid cyst. The inner wall of the cyst contains the germinal layer, from which develop brood capsules that bud off and fall into the cyst cavity. Within these brood capsules new scolices develop, and some of these may initiate the formation of daughter cysts within the main cavity. The young cyst may die and calcify, but it often continues to grow inexorably, eventually seriously compromising the function of the organ in which it is situated. The cysts can also infiltrate the surrounding tissue and metastasizes to other sites (i.e., lungs), making it difficult to remove surgically.

In certain parts of the world, notably the arctic regions of North America, Mongolia and Siberia, infection with a related canine tapeworm, *E. multilocularis*, is encountered. Many infections are acquired in childhood but do not cause clinical manifestations until adulthood. Symptoms depend on the site and size of the cysts. Symptoms are due to mass effect on organs, obstruction to blood and lymphatic flow, rupture of cysts and secondary bacterial infection.

Laboratory investigation

Imaging techniques supported by serological tests offer the best means of diagnosis. Examination of the cyst fluid (hydatid sand) reveals the typical invaginated scolices (Fig. 60.7), but diagnostic puncture of cysts is not recommended because of the risk of spillage (see later in the chapter).

Serological tests have varying sensitivity and specificity. Enzyme-linked immunosorbent assay (ELISA) is the most widely used method for the detection of anti-Echinococcus antibodies (immunoglobulin G). Detection of cestode specific antibodies available in specialised laboratories is useful to exclude cross reactions caused by non-cestode parasites. The ELISA test is also useful in follow-up to detect recurrence.

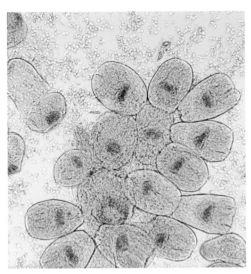

Fig. 60.7 Scolices of *Echinococcus granulosus* from hydatid cyst.

A skin test with antigen derived from hydatid fluid (Casoni test) is now largely abandoned because of low sensitivity and potential for severe local allergic reactions.

Treatment

Cysts of *E. granulosus* can often be removed surgically, but accidental spillage of viable scolices into body cavities may cause an anaphylactic reaction and, moreover, is likely to lead to the development of fresh cysts. For this reason the hydatid cyst is first injected with a scolicidal agent, such as hypertonic saline or ethanol.

The relative impermeability of the cyst militates against successful chemotherapy, but some success has been obtained with benzimidazole derivatives, notably albendazole with praziquantel.

RECOMMENDED READING

Colley, D. G., Bustinduy, A. L., Secor, W. E., & King, C. H. (2014). Human schistosomiasis. *The Lancet, 383*(9936), 2253–2264. doi:10.1016/S0140-6736(13)61949-2.

Farrar, J., Hotez, P., Junghanss, T., Kang, G., Lalloo, D., & White, N. J. (Eds.). (2014). *Manson's tropical diseases* (23rd ed.). London: Elsevier, Saunders.

Fürst, T., Sayasone, S., Odermatt, P., Keiser, J., & Utzinger, J. (2012). Manifestation, diagnosis and management of foodborne trematodiasis. *BMJ: British Medical Journal, 344*, e4093. doi:10.1136/bmj.e4093.

Guerrant, R. L., Walker, D. H., & Weller, P. F. (2011). *Tropical infectious diseases* (3rd ed.). Philadelphia: Elsevier, Saunders.

Knopp, S., Steinmann, P., Keiser, J., & Utzinger, J. (2012). Nematode infections: soil-transmitted helminths and trichinella. *Infectious Disease Clinics of North America, 26*(2), 341–358. doi:10.1016/j.idc.2012.02.006.

Knopp, S., Steinmann, P., Hatz, C., Keiser, J., & Utzinger, J. (2012). Nematode infections: filariases. *Infectious Disease Clinics of North America, 26*(2), 359–381. doi:10.1016/j.idc.2012.02.005.

Peters, W., & Pasvol, G. (2006). *Atlas of tropical medicine and parasitology* (6th ed.). London: Elsevier, Mosby.

Websites

Centers for Disease Control and Prevention. DPDx – Laboratory Identification of Parasitic Diseases of Public Health Concern. Retrieved from http://www.cdc.gov/dpdx/. (Accessed Aug 2017).

UpToDate. An evidence-based clinical decision support resource. Available at http://www.uptodate.com. (Accessed Aug 2017).

World Health Organization. Neglected Tropical Diseases. Retrieved from http://www.who.int/neglected_diseases/en/. (Accessed Aug 2017).

61 Arthropods

Arthropod-borne diseases; ectoparasitic infections; allergy

RICHARD C. RUSSELL

KEY POINTS

- Medically important arthropods include insects (e.g., bugs, flies, gnats, lice and fleas) and arachnids (e.g., spiders, ticks and mites).
- Many arthropods act as accidental or obligatory vectors of bacteria, viruses, protozoa or helminths.
- Certain fleas, lice and mites are human ectoparasites.
- Some arthropods cause allergies (e.g., house dust mites); others may cause painful bites or stings.
- Myiasis is a condition caused by invasion of the body by insect larvae.

Arthropods are invertebrate animals with jointed legs, segmented bodies and chitinous exoskeletons. They are hugely diverse and incredibly numerous, with more than a million described species (perhaps only one-tenth of the true number) and represent approximately three-quarters of all described animal species. Strictly speaking, the term arthropod includes the crustaceans (e.g., lobsters and crabs), the myriapods (e.g., millipedes and centipedes) and some minor groups, but these seldom cause much serious mischief, and most medical interest centres on the insects (e.g., mosquitoes, fleas and lice) and the arachnids (e.g., mites, ticks and spiders). A simplified classification and relevance scheme is shown in Table 61.1.

MEDICAL IMPORTANCE OF ARTHROPODS

Insects and other arthropods are mainly of importance in human disease in three ways:

1. as vectors of the agents of bacterial, viral or parasitic infection
2. as parasites in their own right, spending part or all of their life span on humans
3. as instigators of allergic responses that vary in severity

In addition, many arthropods have a considerable nuisance effect because of their biting or stinging habits, and these occasionally give rise to serious, even life-threatening, reactions.

The larvae (maggots) of some common flies that feed on decomposing matter have been used for centuries to treat infected lesions. There is renewed interest in this phenomenon as wound therapy, as the maggots not only scavenge dead tissue but also appear to secrete factors conducive to wound healing.

Abnormal fear of insects or other arthropods (e.g., arachnophobia, excessive fear of spiders) is well recognised, as are delusions of infestation with these creatures. The mere mention of head lice can make people scratch their scalps. Distinguishing between the real and the imaginary can test the diagnostic acumen of the attending physician. Persistent cases may need psychiatric referral.

ARTHROPODS AS DISEASE VECTORS

Mechanical transmission

Insects such as flies, ants and cockroaches that are attracted by food can transmit pathogenic microorganisms passively. The common house fly, *Musca domestica*, is a particular nuisance because of its predilection for decaying matter, its mobility and its habit (shared by a number of other flies) of regurgitating gut contents and defecating on food. While such flies can undoubtedly play a role in the transmission of enteric diseases, and also trachoma, along with cockroaches they are of lesser importance in modern urban settings than in poorer communities where lower standards of sanitation and hygiene prevail.

Intermediate hosts

A wide variety of arthropods act as obligatory hosts in the transmission of viral, bacterial, protozoal and helminthic agents of human disease. Their association with particular vectors is mentioned below and their role in individual

Table 61.1 Simplified classification of arthropods of medical importance

Class	Members of class	Medical importance
Insects	Ants, bees, wasps (Hymenoptera)	Venomous bites and stings
	Beetles (Coleoptera)	Some secrete fluids causing blisters
	Bugs (Hemiptera)	Bites; vectors of Chagas' disease
	Butterflies and moths (Lepidoptera)	Urticaria (caterpillars)
	Cockroaches (Dictyoptera)	Mechanical vectors of disease
	Fleas (Siphonaptera)	Ectoparasites; vectors of plague and endemic typhus
	Flies and gnats (Diptera)	Bites; vectors of many viral and parasitic diseases; myiasis
	Lice (Phthiraptera)	Ectoparasites; vectors of epidemic typhus, trench fever, relapsing fever
Arachnids	Spiders and scorpions	Venomous bites and stings
	Ticks	Ectoparasites; vectors of rickettsiae, borreliae, viruses
	Mites	Ectoparasites; scabies; respiratory and dermatological allergies; vectors of scrub typhus and rickettsial pox
Pentastomes	Tongue worms	Animal parasites; human infestations rare
Myriapods	Centipedes and millipedes	Some cause painful bites or secrete fluids causing blisters
Crustacea	Crabs, crayfish	Intermediate host of lung fluke
	Copepods	Intermediate host of fish tapeworm and Guinea worm

diseases is dealt with in appropriate chapters elsewhere in the book.

ARTHROPODS AS ECTOPARASITES

Many insects, ticks and mites pester humans to obtain a blood meal or spend part or all of their life in association with human beings. Several fleas, lice and mites are among those that are adapted in various ways for life on humans. Occasionally, humans act as the host of the larval stages of certain insects, and this invasive condition is known as myiasis.

ARTHROPODS AS ALLERGENS

Stinging insects and other venomous arthropods can give rise to severe reactions in hypersensitive individuals, and anaphylactic reactions need immediate treatment with adrenaline (epinephrine). The hairs of several caterpillar species found in various parts of the world are irritating and may give rise to urticaria if brushed against. The irritating reactions to the bites of mosquitoes, midges, fleas and some other insects are immunological reactions to the salivary secretions that are injected at the bite site. However, the degree of reaction can vary remarkably between individuals, from little or no reaction to quite severe dermal and systemic affects and may need medical attention in the latter cases.

Various domestic arthropods, such as dust mites and cockroaches have been incriminated as a cause of asthma in atopic subjects; their allergens can be present in dead bodies as well as in the live individuals and also secreted in the faeces.

INSECTS

Insects are the most numerous and familiar form of arthropod life. They are characterised by having six legs and segmented bodies. The legs (and wings, if present) are carried on the thoracic segments between the head, which bears sucking or biting mouthparts, and the abdomen. Most insects of medical importance, apart from lice and bugs, undergo complete metamorphosis, developing from eggs to adults through morphologically distinct active larval but often inactive pupal stages inside which the adult is developing.

ANTS, BEES AND WASPS (HYMENOPTERA)

These insects have little medical relevance apart from their propensity to retaliate to disturbance with defensive bites or stings. These can be serious if the subject is hypersensitive but are usually trivial. Particularly notorious are the African honey bees *(Apis mellifera scutellata)*, the European wasp *(Vespula germanica)* and the South American fire ants *(Solenopsis* spp.), all of which have been introduced into various countries, and also the bull ants *(Myrmecia* spp.) of Australia. Other ants also forage in urban areas wherever food is to be found and frequently infest kitchens and food stores; they have some potential to mechanically transfer pathogenic organisms (particularly in hospitals).

BEETLES (COLEOPTERA)

Some beetles act as intermediate host of the dwarf tapeworm *Hymenolepis diminuta*, an uncommon human parasite of minor importance (see Ch. 60). Otherwise, their only real medical significance lies in the fact that the body fluids of certain beetles (e.g., *Meloid* and *Staphylinid* species) can cause blistering of the skin. One such blister beetle, *Lytta vesicatoria*, known as Spanish fly, is the source of cantharidin, a vesiculating agent.

BUGS (HEMIPTERA)

The true bugs of importance in human medicine are blood-sucking species. Most familiar throughout the world is the common bed bug, *Cimex lectularius*, which in recent years has been undergoing a widespread international resurgence in distribution and abundance. There is also a tropical species, *C. hemipterus*, which is confined to warmer climes. They have a body that is flattened dorsoventrally and from a distance they resemble brown lentils. Bed bugs live in cracks and crevices of walls, floorboards and furniture, from where they emerge to take a blood meal whenever it is on offer. The adults are long-lived and can survive up to a year without a blood meal. They are usually spread between premises in infested furniture or personal baggage. There is no evidence that they transmit disease.

Reduviid bugs (colloquially known as kissing bugs or assassin bugs) transmit the protozoan *Trypansoma cruzi* that causes Chagas' disease in Central and South America (see Ch. 59). Various species of *Triatoma*, *Rhodnius* and *Panstrongylus* are implicated. They are about 2.5 cm in length, much larger than bed bugs and, unlike them, they have wings (Fig. 61.1). They are usually active at night, settling on the face of an unsuspecting sleeper to take a blood meal and to defecate on site. The infective trypanosomes are in the hindgut

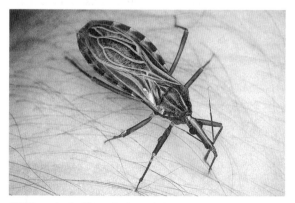

Fig. 61.1 A reduviid bug feeding on human skin. These insects transmit Chagas' disease in South America. (Photograph courtesy H-J Grundmann.)

and the bitten person becomes infected by rubbing the bug's faeces into the irritating bite wound or mucous membranes.

BUTTERFLIES AND MOTHS (LEPIDOPTERA)

Adult butterflies and moths are of no great medical significance (although there is one species that feeds on the blood of large mammals in Southeast Asia, and some that feed on the discharge from the eyes of mammals, including humans), but certain caterpillars can cause skin rashes through contact with either fine urticarial body hairs or stronger barbed hairs and spines that have associated venom glands.

COCKROACHES (DICTYOPTERA, BLATTARIA)

Cockroaches are of little medical significance. They can harbour various pathogens (viruses, bacteria and protozoans), but, as with house flies, they are of lesser significance in modern urban settings than in developing regions with less sanitary conditions. In modern cities, however, they are also known to be responsible for allergy-related conditions including asthma.

FLEAS (SIPHONAPTERA)

Fleas are small blood-sucking parasites. Their laterally flattened bodies and lack of wings enable them to negotiate the hairs and feathers of their animal hosts. Well-developed hind legs enable them to jump from host to host (Fig. 61.2). Many fleas will feed on humans if given the opportunity as those who have been attacked by the common cat flea *Ctenocephalides felis* can bear witness. However, the species that is adapted for life on humans is the human flea, *Pulex irritans*, which is still common throughout the world. Female fleas of another species, *Tunga penetrans*, known as chigoes or jiggers, attack humans by burrowing into the underside skin of the foot, or under the toenails, and the abdomen of the gravid female becomes grossly distended with eggs, causing pain, irritation and, sometimes, secondary infection. These fleas are common in dry, sandy soil, mainly in Africa and parts of Central and South America.

Human or cat fleas are seldom implicated in the transmission of disease, but some other species are important disease vectors. Most notorious is the rat flea, *Xenopsylla cheopis*, which is the most important, but not the sole, vector of the bacterium *Yersinia pestis* that is responsible for plague (see Ch. 19, and Fig. 61.2). Some forms of rickettsial typhus (*Rickettsia typhi*–murine or

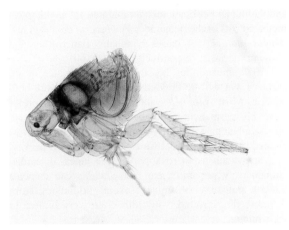

Fig. 61.2 The rat flea *Xenopsylla cheopis*, vector of plague.

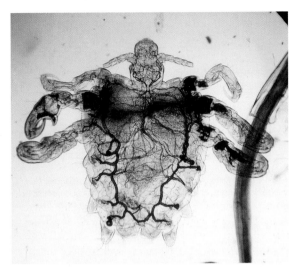

Fig. 61.3 *Pthirus pubis*, the human crab louse.

endemic typhus) are also transmitted by rodent fleas (see Ch. 36).

LICE (PHTHIRAPTERA, ANOPLURA)

Lice are wingless insects that undergo incomplete metamorphosis during their development. The ones that parasitise humans are blood-sucking species with flattened bodies and short legs that are adapted to cling to hairs or clothing. Body lice and head lice are variants of the same species, *Pediculus humanus*. Although the body louse, *P. humanus corporis*, is somewhat larger than the head louse, *P. humanus capitis*, and there are other minor differences, they are not readily distinguishable. A third species, *Pthirus pubis*, is quite distinct morphologically, living up to its common description as the crab louse (Fig. 61.3). Head lice are usually confined to the hairs of the scalp, but body lice live in clothing covering the body, rather than on the skin itself. *P. pubis*, as the name suggests, is usually found on pubic hairs, but may also infest other hairy parts, including body and axillary hair in adults and eyelashes in children. All types attach their characteristic eggs (often called nits) to body hairs (head and crab louse) or clothing fibres (body louse), and effective treatment involves removal of the eggs as well as dealing with the adults.

Body lice are the classic vectors of the rickettsia *Rickettsia prowazekii* that causes epidemic typhus (see Ch. 36) and the spirochaete *Borrelia recurrentis* that causes relapsing fever (see Ch. 32), but head and pubic lice are generally not involved as vectors of pathogens. Lice also cause irritation, and continuous scratching may lead to various forms of infective dermatitis.

Lice are very common throughout the world and head lice, in particular, often spread quickly between school children, even in affluent areas. Treatment with insecticides such as permethrin, malathion and carbaryl may be effective, but chemical resistance is widespread, and because of concern for toxic side effects of the insecticides, unnecessary repeat treatments should be avoided. Repeated wet-combing with a fine-tooth comb after shampooing the hair and applying conditioner can succeed in eliminating an infestation, although reinfection from untreated family members or school contacts is common. The same insecticidal treatments can be effective against pubic lice but all body hair should be treated and, as the infestation is transmitted by intimate contact, sexual partners should also be treated.

FLIES (DIPTERA)

Dipterous insects are usually active flyers as adults, with a pair of wings used for flying and an additional vestigial pair, known as halteres, which are used as organs of balance. The developmental cycle from egg to adult fly involves complete metamorphosis. As well as being among the most annoying of insect pests, many biting flies have an obligate role in the transmission of a wide variety of important infections (Table 61.2). The larvae of certain flies may also infest wounds or body orifices, and others are able to penetrate intact skin, causing myiasis (see later in the chapter).

Mosquitoes

Mosquitoes are readily recognised by a long needle-like proboscis (Fig. 61.4). Adult males and females both feed

Table 61.2 Principal infections associated with biting flies, mosquitoes and midges

Type of insect	Diseases transmitted
Biting midges (*Culicoides* spp.)	Filariasis (*Mansonella* spp.)
Black flies (*Simulium* spp.)	Onchocerciasis
Deer flies (*Chrysops* spp.)	Loiasis
Mosquitoes	
Anopheline (*Anopheles* spp.)	Malaria; bancroftian filariasis
Culicine (*Culex, Aedes, Mansonia* spp., et al.)	Bancroftian and Brugian filariasis; chikungunya, dengue, Japanese encephalitis, yellow fever, Zika, and other arbovirus infections
Sandflies (*Phlebotomus, Lutzomyia* spp.)	Leishmaniasis; Oroya fever; sandfly fever
Tsetse flies (*Glossina* spp.)	African trypanosomiasis

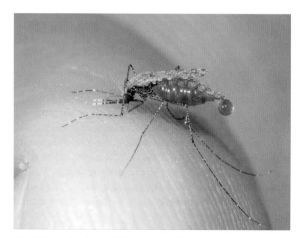

Fig. 61.4 A female anopheline mosquito, the vector of human malaria. (Photograph courtesy S Doggett.)

on plant juices, but the female needs blood for the development of her eggs and is a voracious predator on a wide variety of vertebrate animals throughout the world. Mosquitoes of importance in human medicine are divided into two broad types: anopheline mosquitoes, numerous *Anopheles* species of which transmit the *Plasmodium* protozoans that cause malaria in humans and result in great mortality in tropical countries (see Ch. 59), and culicine mosquitoes (e.g., *Culex* and *Aedes* spp.), which are the vectors of many so-called arboviruses (arthropod-borne viruses), such as yellow fever, dengue, Zika, West Nile, Japanese encephalitis, chikungunya, Ockelbo and Ross River viruses, that can cause various encephalitis, haemorrhagic and polyarthritic symptoms in both tropical and temperate regions (see Ch. 47). Some species of both

anopheline and culicine mosquitoes also act as the intermediate hosts of the nematodes *Wuchereria bancrofti* and *Brugia malayi* that cause lymphatic Bancroftian and Brugian filariasis, respectively. (see Ch. 60).

Female mosquitoes lay their eggs on water or on surfaces that will be flooded; larvae and pupae are both aquatic. Most *Anopheles* and *Culex* mosquitoes prefer relatively permanent water bodies that do not dry up, but *Aedes* spp. will utilise temporary habitats, such as created by flood and tidal waters, and also small pockets of water, such as in rock pools, tree holes, discarded containers, water butts, etc. Some adults can disperse widely and may be found several kilometres from their breeding ground, while others are very limited in their range.

Biting midges

Biting midges are tiny flies that are able to cause a nuisance out of all proportion to their size. They arise from mostly aquatic or semiaquatic habitats and the females attack in swarms, usually in the evening, and may give rise to painful and intensely itchy reactions. These midges are more important in veterinary than human medicine as vectors of arboviruses, although some *Culicoides* spp. transmit filarial nematodes of *Mansonella* spp. to humans in parts of Africa and Central/South America (see Ch. 60).

Sandflies

Sandflies are small enough to penetrate most mosquito netting. They have terrestrial (not aquatic) habitats and utilise dark, humid natural hollow areas, such as rodent burrows or termite mounds, but are often also found in or around human earthen dwellings and associated animal shelters. Female flies suck blood, usually at night, but have limited flight range, so that the diseases they transmit—the protozoal *Leishmania* visceral (kala azar) and cutaneous (e.g., oriental sore) infections (see Ch. 59), the bacterial *Bartonella* infections (see Ch. 31) and the viral sandfly fevers (see Ch. 47)—tend to be localised in distribution. Species associated with disease transmission in Africa, the Middle East, Asia and the Mediterranean belong to the genus *Phlebotomus*, while in Central and South America the vectors of the various pathogens are species of *Lutzomyia*.

Other biting flies

Although flies that are capable of inflicting a painful bite, such as the stable fly *Stomoxys calcitrans*, various black flies and tabanids are found throughout the world and can be serious nuisance pests in temperate regions, species that are important vectors of human disease are restricted in distribution to areas of the tropics.

Black flies (*Simulium* species) are the vectors of *Onchocerca volvulus* the filaria that causes onchocerciasis (river blindness; see Ch. 60) in parts of tropical Africa, and also Central and South America, and are associated with flowing rivers where the immature stages are attached to vegetation or rock substrates. The adults are small hump-backed flies that often attack in swarms, but only the females feed on blood. Species in the *Simulium damnosum* complex and the *S. neavei* group are important vectors in western and eastern regions of Africa, respectively, while other species such as *S. ochraceum* and *S. metallicum* transmit the infection in the Americas.

Tsetse flies, *Glossina* spp., are large flies found only in Africa, where they transmit *Trypanosoma brucei gambiense* and *Trypanosoma brucei rhodesiense*, the protozoans responsible for African trypanosomiasis (known as sleeping sickness) in humans, as well as carrying other trypanosome species that infect cattle and other animals (see Ch. 59). The immature stages are associated with dry terrestrial habitats where mature larvae are deposited on friable soil that they penetrate for pupal development. Both male and female adults feed on blood, and the vectors of human trypanosomiasis in areas of West Africa are riverine species belonging to the *Glossina palpalis* group, whereas the principal vectors in the eastern part of the continent are species in the *G. morsitans* group that prefer savannah plains and woodlands.

Tabanids (sometimes known as deer flies) are large flies that can act as vectors of the filarial worm *Loa loa* (see Ch. 60) in tropical West and Central Africa, where *Chrysops dimidiatus* and *C. silaceus* breed in aquatic or semiaquatic muddy or marshy areas of the rainforests. Other tabanid species, known throughout the world by various common names such as horse flies, clegs and March flies, have very painful bites but generally are not involved in disease transmission (although some have been associated with tularaemia and anthrax).

Myiasis

Given the chance, many common flies that usually lay their eggs or larvae on carrion, will deposit eggs or first-stage larvae on exposed human tissues of ulcers and sores, which consequently become infested with the maggots. The condition is known as semispecific or facultative myiasis to distinguish it from specific or obligatory myiasis, in which humans and other animals act as obligate hosts for the larval stage of development of certain species. Accidental myiasis is said to occur when larvae are ingested with food, or incidentally invade orifices such as the urogenital tract.

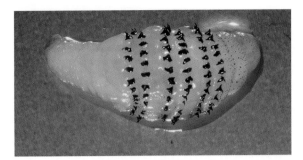

Fig. 61.5 Larva of *Dermatobia hominis*, from a case of human myiasis.

Myiasis is of great economic importance in animal husbandry throughout the world, but human infestation is largely a problem of the tropics. Obligatory myiasis in Africa is most commonly caused by *Cordylobia anthropophaga* (the tumbu fly) or *C. rodhaini* (Lund's fly). In Central and South America *Dermatobia hominis* (the human bot fly) is the usual culprit. *Cordylobia* lays its eggs in soil or dust contaminated with urine or faeces and humans are infested when contacting that substrate, but *Dermatobia* attaches its eggs to other insects (including mosquitoes) that are attracted to humans. When the carrier insect visits a human the larvae hatch and burrow into the skin of the individual with whom they are in contact and remain there, breathing through spiracles at the posterior end until they are ready to pupate and emerge. This is also termed cutaneous myiasis and is a transient condition resulting in boil-like lesions in the skin. The body of the larva is furnished with spines (Fig. 61.5), which make it difficult to remove, but covering the lesion (and thus the posterior spiracles) with an occlusive substance (such as petroleum jelly, Vaseline) prevents the larva from breathing and encourages it to emerge with the help of digital pressure. There should be no subsequent problem with the lesion, providing care is taken not to allow it to become secondarily infected.

Larvae of another African fly, *Auchmeromyia luteola* (the Congo floor maggot), also parasitise humans, but they do not penetrate the skin, preferring instead to suck the blood of unsuspecting sleepers.

ARACHNIDS

Of most importance in this group are spiders, scorpions, ticks and mites. Unlike insects, the adult forms have eight legs and are invariably wingless. They have two main body regions—cephalothorax and abdomen—which in mites and ticks are fused to give the appearance of a single segment. They develop by incomplete metamorphosis, from egg to larva to nymph to adult, and immature forms resemble small versions of adults. However, the larval stages of ticks and mites have only three pairs of legs and acquire the full complement of eight legs only when they become nymphs during their progression to adulthood.

MITES

Despite their name, mites are variable in size, although many, including those commonly implicated in human disease, are so small as to be almost invisible to the naked eye. The only strictly human parasites are *Sarcoptes scabiei* (the itch mite), and *Demodex folliculorum* and *Demodex brevis* (the follicle mites).

The human itch mite, *Sarcoptes scabiei*, is related to mites causing mange in various animals (Fig. 61.6). It is the cause of scabies, an infestation of the skin that is still very prevalent in many countries. After fertilisation on the surface of the skin, the gravid female mite burrows into the epidermis, eventually leaving behind a trail of about 40 eggs. The larvae usually hatch in 3–4 days, leave the burrow and pass through nymphal stages to reach adulthood in hair follicles. Burrowing females cause intense itching. There may be a rash on the trunk but this is unrelated to the distribution of the mites, which are most often found in folds of thin skin, especially between the fingers, often on the wrists and elbows, the axillae, and penis in men and breasts in women. There may be secondary bacterial infection that complicates diagnosis and treatment, and elderly and immunocompromised patients may develop a severe keratotic crusting infestation known as crusted scabies (previously Norwegian scabies), which can cause outbreaks in institutions and may be misdiagnosed as psoriasis. Application of an aqueous solution of malathion or permethrin is often successful therapy, but household contacts should also be treated. Crusted scabies can be treated systemically with the anthelminthic agent ivermectin, which is widely used in animal husbandry for the control of ectoparasites.

Demodex spp., the follicle mites, have an elongated body adapted for life in hair follicles and sebaceous glands on the face, commonly around the nose, on the cheeks or eyelashes. They seldom cause much pathology (although they have been associated with acne and other skin conditions) but can be treated with permethrin application or sulphur preparations.

Other species that impact on human health occupy a wide variety of habitats that humans enter or create, and human contact with certain species may lead to an intense pruritus or dermatitis. Mites associated with commensal birds and rodents (*Ornithonyssus* spp.), and stored grains or dry foodstuffs (e.g., *Tyrophagus putrescentiae* and related spp.), can cause serious dermatological irritation.

Dust mites (*Dermatophagoides* spp. and *Euroglyphus* spp.) have attracted considerable attention as a precipitating cause of atopic disease, including asthma and eczema. The *Dermatophagoides* species (usually *D. pteronyssinus* in Europe and more commonly *D. farinae* in North America) flourish in centrally heated homes with wall-to-wall carpeting and feed on flakes of skin and other organic matter. They have been incriminated as a cause of asthma in atopic subjects, and the allergens are also present in the dead bodies and secreted in the mites' faeces.

The most important mite-borne pathogenic disease is the rickettsial (*Orientia tsutsugamushi*) scrub typhus (see Ch. 36), a potentially fatal infection with a localised but widespread distribution in eastern and south-eastern Asia to northern Australia; the mites responsible for scrub typhus in Asia (e.g., *Leptotrombidium deliense*), have relatives in Europe and North America known as harvest mites (e.g., *Neotrombicula autumnalis*) and chiggers (e.g., *Eutrombicula alfredduggesi*), respectively, that cause a pruritic dermatitis.

TICKS

Ticks are essentially large mites, but they are much more important as vectors of human disease. They are conveniently classified into two main families: hard (ixodid) ticks, which have a chitinous shield (scutum) on the back (Fig. 61.7), and soft (argasid) ticks, which lack this feature. In addition, the head parts of soft ticks are hidden on the ventral surface and are not visible from above. Ticks are obligate blood feeders. They parasitise a very wide variety of animals in nature and many species will attack humans, given the opportunity. The initial bite is usually painless, but it can give rise to a serious reaction and, in some countries (notably Canada, the United States and Australia), ixodid ticks are responsible for tick paralysis, a potentially

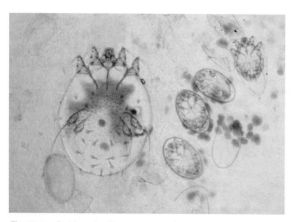

Fig. 61.6 Scabies mite *(Sarcoptes scabiei)*, female with eggs/embryos.

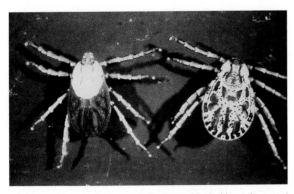

Fig. 61.7 *Dermacentor andersoni*, the vector of Rocky Mountain spotted fever and a cause of tick paralysis. These are known as hard ticks because of the presence of the dorsal scutum, prominent in the male *(right)*, but much reduced in the female *(left)*.

fatal condition caused by a neurotoxin injected while the tick feeds.

Ixodid ticks also transmit many rickettsiae of the spotted fever group (e.g., *Rickettsia conorii* and *R. rickettsii*; see Ch. 36), as well as the agents of Q fever *(Coxiella burnetti)*, spirochaetal Lyme disease (e.g., *Borrelia burgdorferi*; see Ch. 32), bacterial tularaemia (*Francisella tularensis*; see Ch. 19), protozoan babesiosis (*Babesia microti*; see Ch. 59) and various arboviruses (e.g., tick-borne encephalitis virus, Crimean–Congo haemorrhagic fever virus; see Ch. 47) that can cause encephalitis. Adults, especially the females, gorge on blood for long periods, and efforts to remove them manually often leave the head embedded in the skin. However, the developmental stages (larvae, nymphs and adults) are not necessarily on the same host and some of the most important species involved in disease transmission, such as *Dermacentor andersoni* and *Ixodes ricinus*, are known as three-host ticks. Larvae that acquire microorganisms remain infected through the nymphal and adult stages (transstadial transmission); the adult can, in turn, pass on infection to the next generation through the eggs (transovarial transmission). Thus, spread of infection to new hosts may be very efficient.

Argasid ticks tend to be nest ticks, preferring to attack a resting or sleeping host at night, and do not remain attached to the host after feeding. They are relatively long-lived and inhabit dry, dusty environments, mainly in hot countries. The most important species from a medical point of view is *Ornithodoros moubata*, the main vector of tick-borne borreliosis (*Borrelia duttoni* or relapsing fever) in tropical Africa (see Ch. 32). Other species of *Ornithodoros* transmit American forms of relapsing fever, and some are notorious for their voracious feeding habits and extremely painful bites.

SPIDERS AND SCORPIONS

Although all spiders kill their prey by injecting venom, the toxin is usually innocuous to humans, and the mouthparts (chelicerae) are seldom robust enough to allow penetration of human skin. The sting of scorpions, which is carried at the end of an elongated extension of the abdomen, can penetrate human skin, but the venom is usually of low potency (although it can be sufficient to make children ill).

However, some spiders and scorpions have painful bites or stings, and a few can cause serious, occasionally fatal, illness by virtue of powerful neurotoxins. The most dangerous spider is the Australian funnel web spider, *Atrax robustus*, but species of *Latrodectus* (including types of black widow spider, found in many areas of the world, and the Australian redback spider) can also inflict a serious bite. The venom of some *Loxosceles* spiders encountered in the United States and South America may cause tissue necrosis.

The most dangerous scorpions belong to the large Buthidae family. Buthid scorpions with dangerous stings are most commonly found in parts of Africa, the Middle East, the southern states of the United States and Central America. They are nocturnal creatures and sting as a defensive reaction. Most human cases of scorpion sting occur when the arthropod seeks shelter in shoes or other clothing.

Spider and scorpion wounds seldom need more than supportive treatment. Antivenoms are sometimes available in areas where the more dangerous species are prevalent.

OTHER ARTHROPODS

Some centipedes can inflict a painful bite and some millipedes can secrete a fluid capable of raising blisters. Crustaceans (crabs and crayfish) are of interest in human medicine mainly as intermediate hosts of *Paragonimus westermani*, the lung fluke (see Ch. 60). Copepods (water fleas) are similarly important only as hosts of the Guinea worm, *Dracunculus medinensis* (see Ch. 60) and the fish tapeworm, *Diphyllobothrium latum* (see Ch. 60).

RECOMMENDED READING

Goddard, J. (2007). *Physician's guide to arthropods of medical importance* (5th ed.). Boca Raton: CRC Press.

Kettle, D. S. (1995). *Medical and veterinary entomology* (2nd ed.). Wallingford: CABI Publications.

Mullen, G., & Durden, L. (2009). *Medical and veterinary entomology* (2nd ed.). Burlington: Academic Press.

Russell, R. C., Otranto, D., & Wall, R. L. (2013). *The encyclopedia of medical and veterinary entomology*. Wallingford: CABI Publications.

Service, M. W. (2008). *Medical entomology for students* (4th ed.). Cambridge: Cambridge University Press.

Website

Iowa State University Entomology Index of Internet Resources. Available at http://www.ent.iastate.edu/list/directory/114/vid/5. (Accessed Aug 2017).

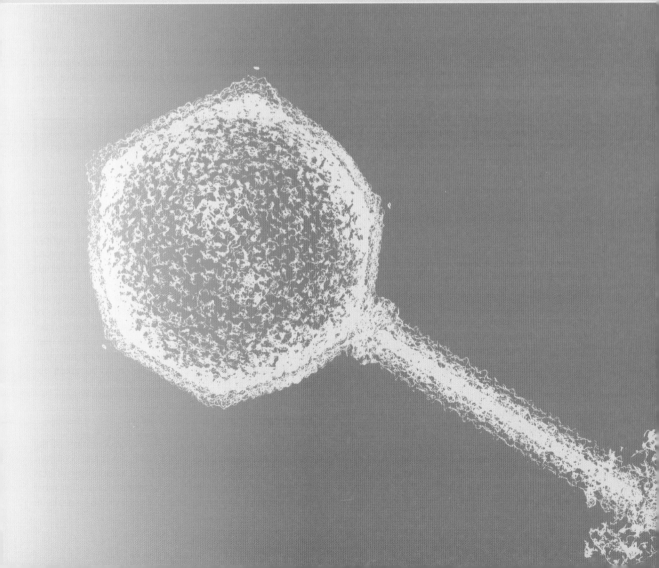

PART 6

DIAGNOSIS, TREATMENT AND CONTROL OF INFECTION

NELUN PERERA

KEY POINTS

- Clinically distinct infective syndromes can generally be caused by several different organisms. Sometimes the specific microbial aetiology may be apparent on clinical grounds alone (e.g., several viral exanthems). More usually a systematic and hierarchical approach is necessary.

- Whether a local or generalised (systemic) process is involved, the medical history, clinical signs (especially temperature) and nonmicrobiological investigations (e.g., white cell count, inflammatory markers and radiological findings) are often used to determine whether infection should be considered in the differential diagnosis.

- In further establishing the differential diagnosis, the time course of symptoms (acute, subacute, chronic) and potential exposure of the patient to endogenous (e.g., surgery) or exogenous (e.g., travel) sources of infection are critical factors.

- Key localised infective syndromes in which a microbiological aetiology is commonly attempted include: pharyngitis; lower respiratory tract infections; gastrointestinal infections; urinary and genital tract infections; meningitis and other central nervous system infections; cardiovascular infections; eye, skin, soft tissue, bone and joint infections.

- Important systemic and general syndromes that may demand extensive microbiological investigation include fever of unknown origin and sepsis.

Throughout this book, infections have been dealt with as appropriate according to the microorganisms involved. In this chapter, infection is considered by syndromes associated with the major organs, to emphasise the variety of microbes that infect different body systems. This will be presented in broad outline, and the reader should refer back to earlier chapters for a more detailed account of specific infections.

In infectious diseases, as in other branches of clinical medicine, a diagnosis may be obvious and require little investigation, for example, a case of chickenpox, or may be established only after laboratory and radiological examination as with a patient with fever of unknown origin (FUO). Fig. 62.1 shows a flow diagram of a rational approach to investigation and management of a patient with infection. In practice, treatment is often started based on the best guess of most likely organism, before isolating and identifying the pathogen. The availability of rapid laboratory methods and new chemotherapeutic agents has made the accurate diagnosis of infectious disease even more important.

SPECIFIC SYNDROMES

UPPER RESPIRATORY TRACT

The upper respiratory tract is frequently the site of general and localised infections. It is one of the most common infections presenting to domiciliary practice. The majority of infections are caused by viruses, which are spread by sneezing, coughing or direct contact with materials contaminated by respiratory secretions. Secondary bacterial infection may follow, particularly in the very young and elderly and are commonly caused by the microbiota of the upper respiratory tract such as *Haemophilus influenzae, Moraxella catarrhalis* and *Streptococcus pneumoniae.* Fig. 62.2 shows the anatomical sites of respiratory infection and the appropriate specimens that may be taken for microbiological investigations.

Pharyngitis

Pharyngitis is a common inflammatory condition of the pharynx that manifests as a sore throat, fever and occasionally with cervical lymphadenitis. It commonly affects children and young adults. In temperate countries most cases occur in winter months and correspond to peaks in

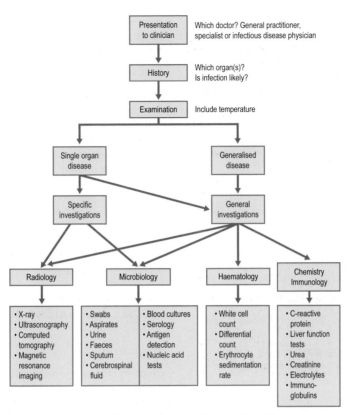

Fig. 62.1 Flow diagram for the diagnosis of infection.

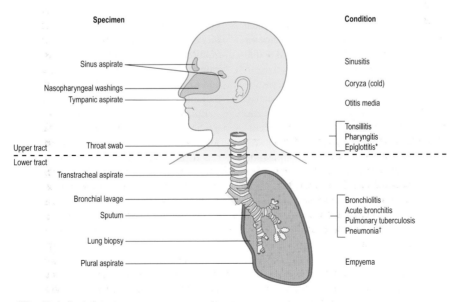

*Take a blood culture to diagnose
†Blood culture and serology may be useful

Fig. 62.2 Microbial infections of the respiratory tract and the appropriate specimens for laboratory investigation.

respiratory viral infections. The common cause of pharyngitis is viruses, with adenovirus being commonly identified. *Strep. pyogenes* is a bacterial cause that is commonly offered antibiotic treatment to prevent complications such as peritonsillar abscess and postinfectious immunological complications such as rheumatic fever and acute glomerulonephritis. Group C and G streptococci commonly found as microbiota of the human pharynx are also increasingly recognised as causes of pharyngitis. However, they have not been associated with rheumatic fever and acute glomerulonephritis.

Pharyngitis due to viruses is commonly self-limiting. Recognising patients with *Strep. pyogenes* pharyngitis who require laboratory investigations and treatment is challenging.

This has led to three approaches:

1. Treat all children with a penicillin, or erythromycin if allergic. Adults are treated if the throat looks very inflamed or if there is pus on the tonsils.
2. Swabs are taken for culture of streptococci, and antibiotics are started as above but stopped if *Strep. pyogenes* is not found.
3. Swabs are taken for rapid diagnosis (by antigen detection), and penicillin commenced only if the throat swab is positive.

There are pros and cons to each method. One drawback to the early use of antibiotics is that the patient may react to the drug. If ampicillin is used, there is a strong chance of a skin reaction if the sore throat is the harbinger of glandular fever. In defence of the antibiotic lobby, there is no doubt that complications of streptococcal disease are seen far less commonly where there is access to medical service and pharmacies. However, these improvements have occurred in concert with better housing and social conditions.

Fusobacterium nechrophorum is a cause of pharyngitis that commonly affects young adults that can be associated with severe complications (i.e., peritonsillar abscess and Lemierre syndrome). It has also been implicated in recurrent or chronic sore throat syndrome.

In an unvaccinated severely ill child with toxaemia and a membrane in the throat, diphtheria must be considered and treatment should be commenced while awaiting laboratory investigations. Moreover, the laboratory needs to do special tests to isolate and identify *Corynebacterium diphtheriae*, and communication (by telephone, if possible) between the clinician and laboratory is essential. Other corynebacteria such as *Corynebacterium ulcerans* and *Arcanobacterium haemolyticum* (formerly *Corynebacterium haemolyticum*) may rarely cause ulcerated sore throats. Pharyngitis caused by gonorrhoea should be considered in sexually active adolescents and young adults. *Mycoplasma pneumoniae* and *Chlamydia*

pneumoniae should also be considered as a less common cause of pharyngitis.

Sinusitis and otitis media

Direct extension of a viral or bacterial infection from the nasopharynx into frontal and maxillary sinuses in adults and into the middle ear in children is not uncommon. Obtaining adequate material for microbiology is difficult and requires the expertise of ear, nose and throat specialists. In most cases of acute sinusitis or otitis media the microbial cause is not found. It is assumed that severe pain and discharge of pus from the nose or ear is suggestive of bacterial infection and antibiotics are usually given to cover streptococci (mainly *Strep. pneumoniae*) and *H. influenzae*. In adults with recurrent or chronic sinusitis, anaerobes *(Peptostreptococcus* or *Bacteroides)* are often found in sinus washings.

LOWER RESPIRATORY TRACT

Epiglottitis

Epiglottitis is an invasive cellulitis of the epiglottis and its adjacent supraglottic (supraglottitis) structures. In its severe form it can cause abrupt, complete airways obstruction. Before routine infant immunisation with *H. influenzae* type B conjugate vaccine, epiglottitis occurred in children 1–4 years of age and was almost always a bacteraemic invasive disease. The cases of epiglottitis, nowadays, are predominantly in older children and adults. In these patients, *Strep. pneumoniae, Strep. pyogenes* and *Staphylococcus aureus* are occasionally isolated from surface cultures of the epiglottitis and, rarely, from blood. Unusual causes of epiglottitis include *Pseudomonas aeruginosa* and *Candida albicans*, especially in immunocompromised patients.

Epiglottitis in children presents with acute onset fever, irritability and rapidly progressive respiratory distress. These children frequently appear toxic, with drooling oral secretions and a hoarse voice. In contrast, epiglottitis in older children and adults is a less severe illness (subacute) and predominantly presents as a sore throat and pain on swallowing.

The diagnosis of epiglottitis is established by visualisation of an oedematous cherry-red epiglottis by direct or indirect laryngoscopy. Because of the risk of sudden airways obstruction, this procedure is not recommended outside an intensive care setting. Blood cultures were useful in children, which invariably grew *H. influenzae* type B. Lateral radiographs of the neck are useful in older children and adults with subacute epiglottitis, and will show an enlarged and swollen epiglottis (thumb sign).

Maintenance of an adequate airway should be the primary concern when a diagnosis of epiglottitis is suspected. In most cases, antibiotic therapy with a third-generation cephalosporin such as ceftriaxone or cefotaxime directed at the most likely organisms is recommended.

Acute bronchitis is a clinical syndrome characterised by a self-limiting inflammatory process of the large and medium-sized bronchi, without involvement of the lung parenchyma. It is characterised by a dry or productive cough of <3 weeks duration, is most common in winter, and is predominantly caused by viruses. Secondary bacterial infection may follow in susceptible individuals. It should be distinguished from acute bronchiolitis—a clinical syndrome involving small airways, associated with respiratory syncytial virus and human metapneumovirus infection in infants.

Acute exacerbation of chronic obstructive pulmonary disease (COPD) characterised by increased sputum purulence, volume and dyspnea are commonly associated with higher bacterial loads of *Strep. pneumoniae, H. influenzae* and *Moraxella catarrhalis*. In individuals with greater functional impairment, recent antibiotic use and systemic corticosteroid therapy, Gram-negative bacteria such as *Ps. aeruginosa* and Enterobacteriaceae have also been isolated. Amongst the viruses, rhinovirus is the most frequently isolated. Coinfection with bacteria and viruses is associated with severe presentations and poor outcome. Because of stable colonisation of the airways with bacteria, routine examination of sputum in the laboratory is not recommended. Antibiotic treatment has shown to improve quality of life in hospitalised patients.

Cystic fibrosis patients have frequent exacerbations and, in those situations, sputum examination is valuable because the causative bacteria *(Staph. aureus, H. influenzae, Ps. aeruginosa* or *Burkholderia cepacia)* may show variable antimicrobial resistance, and appropriate therapy is essential.

Pneumonia

Pneumonia is a respiratory infection characterised by inflammation of the alveoli, which can be a mild outpatient infection to a severe illness requiring hospitalisation and intensive care. It is arbitrarily divided into community-acquired pneumonia (CAP) when the infection occurs in patients living in the community, and hospital-acquired pneumonia (HAP) when infection is acquired in a health-care institution. Ventilator-associated pneumonia (VAP) is a particular subgroup of HAP. If the alveolar infection involves an entire anatomical lobe of the lung, it is termed lobar pneumonia. If the inflammatory process is patchy and adjacent to bronchi it is termed a bronchopneumonia. This division has some correlation to aetiology and in guiding treatment, although not all cases always follow the textbook.

The most common pathogen for CAP in all patient populations is *Strep. pneumoniae*. Other organisms include, *H. influenzae, Moraxella catarrhalis*, atypical pathogens like *Mycoplasma pneumoniae, Chlamydophila pneumoniae, Legionella pneumophila* and viruses such as influenza, parainfluenza, adenovirus and respiratory syncytial virus. Enteric Gram-negative organisms are less common in CAP. There are also clinical associations with specific pathogens (Table. 62.1).

HAP follows aspiration into the lungs of bacteria that colonise the upper respiratory tract. Enteric Gram-negative bacteria are therefore the most common organisms causing HAP.

Chest radiography is the standard investigation for pneumonia.

Blood cultures and examination of good-quality expectorated sputum by microscopy and culture are laboratory investigations that should be performed to aid diagnosis. Also available are urine antigen detection tests for *Strep. pneumoniae* and *Legionella pneumophila* and respiratory nucleic acid amplification tests for atypical pathogens and viruses.

Empiric treatment should be focused on the pathogens most likely to be present for a given type of patient. Readers are encouraged to refer to guidelines of professional societies for more details.

Table 62.1 Clinical associations with specific pathogens (see individual chapters for details)

Condition	Commonly encountered pathogens
Alcoholism	*Streptococcus pneumoniae,* anaerobes, *Klebsiella pneumoniae*
COPD/smoker	*Streptococcus pneumoniae, Haemophilus influenzae, Moraxella catarrhalis, Legionella* spp., enteric Gram-negative bacteria
Bat exposure	*Histoplasma capsulatum*
Bird exposure	*Chlamydia psittaci, Cryptococcus neoformans, Histoplasma capsulatum*
Rabbit exposure	*Francisella tularensis*
Travel (i.e., southwest United States)	Coccidioidomycosis, hantavirus in selected areas
Exposure to farm animals	*Coxiella burnetii* (Q fever)
Travel to Southeast Asia	*Mycobacterium tuberculosis, Burkholderia pseudomallei,* SARS virus
Suspected bioterrorism	Anthrax, smallpox, pneumonic plague
Postinfluenza pneumonia	*Streptococcus pneumoniae, Staphylococcus aureus*
Structural disease of the lung (bronchiectasis, cystic fibrosis, etc.)	*Pseudomonas aeruginosa, Burkholderia cepacia* or *Staphylococcus aureus*

GASTROINTESTINAL INFECTION

Acute diarrhoea

Acute diarrhoea is a syndrome difficult to differentiate clinically by aetiological agent. An array of bacterial, viral and parasitic organisms is implicated (Table 62.2). The diarrhea is a result of damage to the intestinal epithelium either directly by multiplying organisms or due to toxins. The clinical manifestations vary from self-limited disease to death. Death is primarily due to dehydration, which is common in children in developing countries. Most cases are foodborne. Water-borne illness due to contaminated treated water (*Cryptosporidium*), fresh water (toxigenic *Escherichia coli* and norovirus) and aquarium water (*Aeromonas* spp.) has been reported. Acute diarrhoea due to travel (toxigenic *E. coli*) and cruising (norovirus) are also increasingly reported.

The source of acute diarrhoea in hospitals is commonly an infectious patient or staff member. On occasion it has also followed contaminated food (*Salmonella* spp.) and inanimate hospital environment (*Clostridium difficile* and norovirus).

A search for all causes involves extensive and expensive laboratory effort, and this is often considered unnecessary for a condition that is usually self-limiting and relatively harmless.

Toxin-mediated disease of microbial origin ranges in severity from relatively trivial episodes of food poisoning caused by:

- enterotoxin-producing strains of *Staph. aureus*
- *Clostridium perfringens*
- *Bacillus cereus*

to the life-threatening systemic diseases:

- botulism caused by *Cl. botulinum*
- severe pseudomembranous colitis caused by *Cl. difficile* (often antibiotic-associated)

Table 62.2 Common microbial causes of infectious intestinal disease (see individual chapters for details)

Viruses	Bacteria	Protozoa
Norovirus (SRSV)	*Salmonella enterica* serotypes	*Cryptosporidium parvum*
Rotavirus	*Campylobacter* spp.	
Astrovirus	*Clostridium difficile*	*Entamoeba histolytica*
Calicivirus (SRSV)	*Shigella* spp.	*Giardia lamblia*
	E. coli (ETEC, VTEC)	
	Vibrio cholerae	
	Vibrio parahaemolyticus	
	Yersinia enterocolitica	

ETEC, Enterotoxigenic *E. coli*; *SRSV*, small round structured viruses; *VTEC*, verotoxigenic *E. coli*.

There are, in addition, many nonmicrobial causes of food poisoning, such as that caused by the ingestion of certain toadstools, undercooked red kidney beans or various types of fish (ciguatera toxin, scombrotoxin); most notorious is the puffer fish, which, during part of its reproductive cycle, produces a neurotoxin that is responsible for >100 deaths a year in Japan, where the delicacy *fugu* is enjoyed.

Intraabdominal sepsis, peritonitis, biliary sepsis and pancreatitis

The peritoneum is the largest cavity within the body. Peritonitis follows contamination of the peritoneal cavity with the microbiota of the stomach and intestine. Anaerobic bacteria (*Bacteroides* spp.) and aerobic Gram-negative bacilli of the Enterobacteriaceae family (*E. coli* and others) are predominant causes of community-acquired peritonitis (appendicitis, diverticular disease) and spontaneous bacterial peritonitis.

Postoperative peritonitis follows abdominal surgery and is due to a leak from a suture line. In these patients, in addition to the above organisms, *Ps. aeruginosa,* Enterococci and *Candida* spp. may be implicated.

Surgical drainage (washout) is the mainstay of management. Antimicrobial therapy and resuscitation complement the surgical management.

Peritonitis caused by chronic ambulatory peritoneal dialysis (CAPD) is most commonly due to coagulase-negative staphylococci, *Staph. aureus*, Gram-negative bacilli and fungi. The most common route of infection is colonisation of the peritoneal dialysis catheter and infection of the exit site. Initial empiric treatment should cover Gram-positive and Gram-negative organisms. Intraperitoneal (IP) administration is superior to the parenteral route. A combination of IP vancomycin and gentamicin is commonly used. Early removal of the peritoneal dialysis catheter should occur with infection due to *Ps. aeruginosa*, fungi, mycobacteria and recurrent peritonitis with the same organism.

Biliary sepsis is usually cause by bile duct obstruction associated with gallstones, pancreatic and bile duct malignancy and previous bile duct surgery. Organisms involved are usually Enterobacteriaceae.

Although acute pancreatitis is a chemical inflammation of the pancreas, progression to severe necrotising pancreatitis is commonly associated with secondary bacterial infection, which is almost always polymicrobial.

URINARY TRACT INFECTIONS

Urinary tract infections (UTIs) are a common infectious cause of presenting to general practice. Most infections are limited to the lower urinary tract but may be complicated by pyelonephritis and bacteraemia. Other than in the first 3 months, where UTIs are common in males,

Table 62.3 Common causes of urinary tract infection (approximate %)

Organism	Domiciliary (%)	Hospital (%)
E. coli	70–80	50
Proteus mirabilis	10	1–5
Klebsiella spp.	1–5	5–10
Staph. saprophyticus	10–15	0
Staph. epidermidis	1–5	10–20
Enterococci	1–5	10–20
Other coliforms	<1	5–10
Pseudomonas aeruginosa	1–2	5–10

in all other age groups, females are more commonly affected. Uncomplicated cystitis is common in healthy nonpregnant females and responds well to antimicrobial treatment.

Anatomical and functional abnormalities of the urinary tract are associated with complicated infections. Asymptomatic bacteriuria in pregnancy is associated with increased risk of acute pyelonephritis, preeclampsia, low foetal birth weight, prematurity and perinatal mortality. Many elderly patients have asymptomatic bacteriuria. Uncomplicated UTIs are commonly monomicrobial and are most commonly caused by E. coli (Table 62.3). Urease-producing organisms (Proteus, Providencia and Morganella spp.) are associated with stones in the urinary tract.

The diagnosis of UTIs can only be proven by culture of an adequately collected urine sample. This is essential in all suspected UTIs in males, infants, children and complicated UTIs in women.

The cornerstone of management is effective antimicrobial therapy. There is no convincing evidence that treatment of asymptomatic bacteriuria in the elderly benefits the patients. Chemoprophylaxis should be considered in complicated UTIs with recurrent episodes.

Readers are encouraged to refer to local guidelines for detailed treatment.

INFECTIONS OF THE CENTRAL NERVOUS SYSTEM

Meningitis

Throughout the world the epidemiology of community-acquired bacterial meningitis has changed significantly in the past 2 decades because of changes made to childhood vaccination programmes. The routine vaccination of children against H. influenzae type B has virtually eradicated H. influenzae meningitis in the developed world. The introduction of the conjugate vaccine against 13 serotypes of Strep. pneumoniae has reduced the incidence

of invasive pneumococcal disease in young children and older people. The integration of the meningococcal protein-polysaccharide conjugate vaccine into vaccination programmes in several countries has further reduced the disease burden of bacterial meningitis.

Worldwide Strep. pneumoniae affects all ages and causes the most severe disease in the very young and the very old. There is increasing resistance to penicillin in certain parts of the world, with important consequences for treatment.

Neisseria meningitidis is mainly responsible for bacterial meningitis in young adults. Small outbreaks due to spread among close contacts is common among school contacts, etc. Group B streptococcus and E. coli are pathogens of neonates and often cause devastating sepsis and meningitis. They colonise the maternal birth canal and are transmitted to the newborn.

Listeria monocytogenes causes meningitis primarily in neonates, in adults with alcoholism, immunosuppression and iron overload and in pregnant women. Usually there is an encephalitic component to the presentation. Bacterial meningitis can follow neurosurgical procedures and focal infections of the head. The common organisms implicated are Staph. aureus, coagulase-negative staphylococcus, streptococci and Gram-negative bacilli (E. coli, Klebsiella spp., Pseudomonas spp. and others).

Because of the high mortality of acute bacterial meningitis, starting antimicrobial therapy and the diagnostic process should be initiated simultaneously. Blood cultures and cerebrospinal fluid (CSF) should be collected in all patients with suspected meningitis. In some patients, lumbar puncture has to be delayed because of severe sepsis with accompanying disseminated intravascular coagulopathy or requiring prior cranial imaging.

CSF analysis for cells, protein and glucose provide valuable information to guide treatment. Gram stain and culture can identify the organism in most untreated patients. Antigen and DNA detection tests are increasingly used to detect small numbers of viable and nonviable organisms.

Empirical antibiotic treatment is directed at the most likely bacterial pathogens according to the age of patient. A third-generation cephalosporin (cefotaxime or ceftriaxone) plus penicillin (or ampicillin) to treat L. monocytogenes is commonly recommended. Close contacts of N. meningitidis and H. influenzae meningitis should be offered antibiotic prophylaxis. Table 62.4 shows some of the other causes of meningitis.

Enteroviruses are the common cause of acute viral meningitis. CSF analysis of patients with viral meningitis typically shows raised leukocytes (10–500) and slightly raised proteins. Availability of molecular techniques has provided rapid and reliable tests to identify most viruses.

Table 62.4 Other causes of meningitis

Viruses	Enteroviruses (echoviruses, polioviruses, coxsackieviruses)
	Mumps (including postimmunisation)
	Herpes (herpes simplex and varicella-zoster)
	Arboviruses
Spiral bacteria	Syphilis *(Treponema pallidum)*
	Leptospira *(Leptospira canicola)*
Other bacteria	Partially treated with antibiotics
	Tuberculous *(Mycobacterium tuberculosis)*
	Brain abscess
Fungi	*Cryptococcus neoformans*
Protozoa	*Acanthamoeba, Naegleria, Toxoplasma gondii*
Noninfective	Lymphomas, leukaemias
	Metastatic and primary neoplasms
	Collagen-vascular diseases

Table 62.5 Causes of neurological damage in HIV-infected patients

Direct HIV infection	Subacute encephalomyelitis (AIDS-dementia complex)
Opportunist infections	
Viruses	Cytomegalovirus
	Herpes simplex
	Varicella-zoster
	Papovavirus
Bacteria	*Treponema pallidum* (syphilis)
Fungi	*Cryptococcus neoformans*
Protozoa	*Toxoplasma gondii*
Malignancy	
Primary	Brain lymphoma
Secondary	Kaposi's sarcoma
	Systemic lymphoma

In the immunocompromised, listeria meningitis may be seen in the adult and *Cryptococcus neoformans* in all age groups, but particularly those with human immunodeficiency virus (HIV) infection. Central nervous system disease in patients with acquired immune deficiency syndrome (AIDS) is complex and has a range of differential diagnoses (Table 62.5).

Cerebral infections

Encephalitis is inflammation of the brain parenchyma. Often it is associated with meningeal inflammation referred to as meningoencephalitis.

In addition to fever and headache, there is often altered level of consciousness and varying neurological manifestations. Viruses are the common cause. There are also noninfectious conditions that mimic encephalitis.

In Western Europe, herpes simplex or varicella-zoster viruses are the most common causes of encephalitis, but in many parts of the world, arboviruses, such as Japanese B encephalitis virus, are important (see Ch. 51).

Abscesses in the brain or subdural space may arise from haematogenous spread during bacteraemia or by direct extension, either through the cribriform plate from the nasopharynx or from sinuses or the middle ear. They may be clinically silent or present as a space-occupying lesion accompanied by fever and systemic upset. Scanning by computed axial tomography (CAT) or magnetic resonance imaging (MRI) and early neurosurgical intervention will reduce complications and with appropriate systemic antibiotics given for a prolonged period, the success rate is good.

CARDIOVASCULAR INFECTIONS

Infective endocarditis

In spite of global improvements in health-care, the incidence of infective endocarditis (IE) has not decreased. Whilst rheumatic heart disease remains an important risk factor in developing countries, there is an expansion of at-risk groups such as people who inject drugs (PWID), elderly people with degenerative valve lesions and patients with intravascular devices. More patients are also diagnosed because of advances in diagnostic criteria, including echocardiography and molecular biology.

Infecting microorganisms are also evolving. The most prevalent organisms are listed in Table 62.6. Oral streptococci are still the predominant organisms causing native valve IE. *Staph. aureus* and coagulase-negative staphylococci have become predominant in PWID, in prosthetic valve IE and in patients with device-related IE. *Strep. gallolyticus* is common in the elderly and is often associated with colonic tumours.

Acute IE can be devastating. It is often caused by *Staph. aureus, Staph. lugdunensis* and certain streptococci (*Strep. pyogenes, Strep. pneumoniae* and the streptococci milleri group). Patients are acutely ill with high fever, hypotension and shock. Oral streptococci, enterococci and coagulase-negative staphylococci usually cause subacute IE. The clinical manifestations are commonly nonspecific and can mimic a chronic wasting disease.

Blood cultures and echocardiography are the two most important investigations performed to confirm a diagnosis and guide therapy. Blood cultures are not always positive in IE. Bacteria of the HACEK group (Table 62.6) usually grow after prolonged incubation of the blood cultures. A very common cause of blood culture negative IE is prior antimicrobial therapy. IE associated with *Brucella* spp., *Coxiella burnetii, Bartonella* spp., *Chlamydia* spp., *Mycoplasma* spp., *Legionella* spp. and *Topheryma whipplei* is invariably blood culture negative.

Table 62.6 Microbiological causes of infective endocarditis (approximate %)

Organisms	(%)
Streptococci	45.2
Viridans streptococci	22.9
Streptococcus pneumoniae	3.6
Streptococcus bovis	3
Other streptococci	6.3
Enterococci	9.5
Staphylococci	34.5
Methicillin-sensitive staphylococci	18.5
Methicillin-resistant staphylococci	0.6
Coagulase-negative staphylococci	15.5
Enterobacteriaceae	0.9
HACEK*	3
Coxiella burnetii	0.3
Other bacteria	9.5
Fungi	1.8
Polymicrobial	11.3
No organism identified	14.6

*HACEK, Haemophilus, Actinobacillus, Cardiobacterium, Eikenella, Kingella.
D.J.B Marks et al. *International Journal of Medicine*, 2015, Vol. 108(3), pp. 219-229 [Peer Reviewed Journal].

Table 62.7 Likely aetiology of skin and soft tissue infections associated with specific risk factors

Risk factor or setting	Likely organisms
Cat bite	*Pasteurella multocida*
Dog bite	*Pasteurella multocida* and *Capnocytophaga canimorsus*, *Staphylococcus intermedius*
Tick bite	*Borrelia burgdoferi*
Hot tub exposure	*Pseudomonas aeruginosa*
Diabetes mellitus and peripheral vascular disease	Group B streptococci
Periorbital cellulitis	*Haemophilus influenzae*
Saphenous vein donor site cellulitis	Group C and G streptococci
Freshwater lacerations	*Aeromonas hydrophila*
Sea-water exposure, cirrhosis, raw oysters	*Vibrio vulnificus*
Cellulitis associated with stasis and dermatitis	Groups A, C and G streptococci
Lymphoedema	Groups A, C and G streptococci
Cat scratch	*Bartonella henselae*
HIV-positive patient with bacillary angiomatosis	*Bartonella henselae* and *Bartonella quintana*
Fishmongering	*Erysipelothrix rhusiopathiae*
Fish tank exposure	*Mycobacterium marinum*
Compromised host with ecthyma gangrenosum	*Pseudomonas aeruginosa*
Human bite	*Eikenella corrodens*, *Fusobacterium* spp.

If the patient undergoes valve surgery the valve should be sent to the laboratory for culture and other microbiological tests. Polymerase chain reaction amplification of 16S ribosomal RNA genes has become a valuable method for bacterial identification in tissue samples.

Readers are encouraged to refer to published guidelines for more detail on antibiotic treatment.

INFECTIONS ASSOCIATED WITH INTRAVASCULAR LINES

Bacteraemia associated with intravascular lines is becoming increasingly common because of their widespread use for administration of fluids, medication, blood products, nutrition, haemodynamic monitoring and haemodialysis.

The most common organisms implicated are skin microbiota such as staphylococci (coagulase-negative staphylococci and *Staph. aureus*), yeasts and Gram-negative bacilli. Formation of a biofilm on the surface of the catheter promotes persistence of the infection.

Differential time to positivity of paired blood cultures is a technique that measures the differences in blood culture load between a blood culture taken from a line and peripherally. The time to positivity is available in laboratories that use automated blood culture machines. When a blood culture taken from a line becomes positive at least 2 hours earlier than that taken peripherally it is highly likely infection is associated with the line. Removing

the line is considered the best approach to manage the infection.

SKIN AND SOFT TISSUE INFECTIONS

Skin is a common site of infection for a large number of bacteria (including rickettsiae), viruses, fungi, parasites and spirochaetes. They may occur as a single or recurrent episode. Many are mild infections, but some may progress to severe infection, loss of limbs or digits or even death.

Impetigo, cellulitis and abscesses are common bacterial skin and soft tissue infections. *Staph. aureus* and *Strep. pyogenes* are the two most common organisms causing these infections. Some skin infections are associated with specific risk factors or settings (Table 62.7).

Necrotising fasciitis is a life-threatening form of soft tissue infection. It can occur in association with gas gangrene as part of a generalised tissue necrosis caused by *Clostridium* spp. or as a separate entity. Two types are recognised. Type I occurs in patients who have diabetes mellitus or severe peripheral vascular disease, or both, and is usually caused by mixed aerobic and anaerobic bacteria. Type II is caused by *Strep. pyogenes*. Despite antibiotics, appropriate surgical debridement and intensive supportive care mortality of Type II necrotising fasciitis remains high. This is thought to be due to highly virulent strains of the organisms. Penicillin plus clindamycin should be administered for suspected cases. Administration of intravenous immunoglobulin to neutralise circulating streptococcal toxins has shown to affect mortality and morbidity in fulminant infections.

Fournier's gangrene is a form of Type 1 necrotising fasciitis involving the anterior abdominal wall, gluteal muscles and in male the scrotum and the penis, caused by aerobic Gram-negative bacteria, enterococci and anaerobic bacteria such as *Bacteroides* spp. and *Peptostreptococcus*. Surgical debridement is always necessary for diagnosis and treatment. An appropriate empiric antibiotic regiment would be piperacillin and tazobactam combination plus clindamycin.

Skin lesions are a feature of some virus infections, such as warts, herpes simplex and molluscum contagiosum. In other virus diseases, including rubella and measles, chickenpox (and, before its eradication, smallpox), a characteristic rash follows the viraemic phase of the illness.

Cutaneous ulcers follow direct destruction of dermal cells by bacterial enzymes and toxins, or secondary to an intense inflammatory reaction.

Cutaneous anthrax follows direct inoculation of *Bacillus anthracis* spores into the skin of animal handlers or as a result of deliberate bioterrorism. Cutaneous diphtheria presents as a chronic nonhealing ulcer with an overlying grey membrane. Cutaneous tularemia follows a tick bite or handling infected rodents or rabbits and commonly presents as a suppurating ulcer with an eschar and enlarged draining lymph nodes. Buruli ulcer caused by *Mycobacterium ulcerans,* common in tropical climates, presents as a slowly progressive shallow ulcer of the limbs.

Cutaneous leishmaniasis caused by *Leishmaniasis tropica* presents as a shallow ulcer with an expanding margin and should be suspected in patients residing in or returning from central or South America.

Cutaneous ulcers in the genital area should include syphilis, lymphogranuloma venereum, chancroid and herpes simplex virus infection.

GENITAL TRACT INFECTIONS

In the male, acute urethritis is a common condition, usually caused by a sexually transmitted microbe such as *N. gonorrhoeae, Ch. trachomatis* or *Ureaplasma urealyticum*. If untreated, these organisms can cause prostatitis or epididymitis, and gonorrhoea may produce unpleasant consequences such as urethral stricture or sterility. Genital ulcers in both sexes may be due to herpes simplex virus, syphilis or chancroid *(H. ducreyi)*.

The more complicated female reproductive organs are subjected to many more infections with a greater scope for sequelae. Vaginitis may present as vaginal discharge or irritation, and often these symptoms are due to infections that are not always exogenously acquired. *Trichomonas vaginalis* is the most common sexually acquired microbe, although both *N. gonorrhoeae* and *Ch. trachomatis* may also present as discharge. Thrush caused by *Candida* species is especially common in pregnancy and in diabetics. It is usually an endogenous condition due to disturbances in the normal microbiota. Another cause of vaginal discharge, but usually without inflammatory cells and irritation, is associated with an alteration of local pH with proliferation of *Gardnerella vaginalis* and anaerobic spiral bacteria, now termed *Mobiluncus* species. The alkaline conditions and characteristic amines found in bacterial vaginosis allow a diagnosis to be easily made on examination of the patient. This condition, which used to be called nonspecific vaginitis, is a common condition in sexually active women, although probably not a venereal disease in the usual sense.

The endocervical canal is the site of infection with *N. gonorrhoeae* and *Ch. trachomatis* in the sexually mature woman. During parturition, both organisms may be passed to the baby's eyes to give rise to ophthalmia neonatorum. The cervix may also be infected with human papillomavirus (HPV), the cause of genital warts. Some types are associated with a high risk of cervical cancer (see Ch. 45).

Ascending genital infection may present as acute salpingitis with fever and pelvic pain. On vaginal examination, there is referred lower abdominal pain on moving the cervix (cervical excitation) and tenderness in the iliac fossa on abdominal palpation. Signs and symptoms in cases due to *Ch. trachomatis* are much less pronounced than those due to *N. gonorrhoeae*. Some women may develop chronic pelvic inflammatory disease (PID) without having suffered a recognisable acute episode. PID, although most often initiated by these two common sexually transmitted pathogens, is usually a polymicrobial infection, in which endogenous commensals, particularly anaerobes, play an important role.

EYE INFECTIONS

Various microbes may cause acute conjunctivitis. During birth, *N. gonorrhoeae* and *Ch. trachomatis* may be passed to the baby's eyes from the maternal genital tract to give rise to ophthalmia neonatorum. In the newborn, *Staph. aureus* is commonly found in sticky eyes, either as a primary cause of conjunctivitis or after infection with another pathogen. In older infants and children, *H. influenzae* and *Strep. pneumoniae* are common. Chlamydiae give rise to trachoma, the most common cause of blindness

Table 62.8 Causes of choroidoretinitis

Viruses	Cytomegalovirus, rubella
Bacteria	*Treponema pallidum*
Protozoa	*Toxoplasma gondii*
Helminths	*Toxocara canis, Onchocerca volvulus*

in the world, and to a milder form of inclusion blennorrhoea in sexually active individuals.

Primary viral conjunctivitis often occurs in epidemics when certain types of adenovirus are implicated. This is usually a mild condition with few sequelae compared with the keratitis caused by herpes simplex virus or in shingles when the ophthalmic division of the trigeminal nerve is infected with varicella-zoster virus.

Corneal damage due to fungi as well as herpesviruses is seen in immunosuppressed patients, and keratitis caused by free-living amoebae (*Acanthamoeba* species), though rare, is becoming more common, particularly in wearers of contact lenses.

Penetrating injuries of the eye and ophthalmic surgery may introduce a wide range of bacteria and fungi into the chambers of the eye, which may give rise to hypopyon (pus in the eye). This condition requires prompt surgical drainage and instillation of appropriate antibiotics such as gentamicin. *Ps. aeruginosa* and *Proteus* species are among the more common organisms isolated.

Infections of the back of the eye (choroidoretinitis) are seen in many diverse infectious diseases (Table 62.8).

INFECTION OF BONE AND JOINTS

Infective arthritis

Infective arthritis is inflammation of the joint space by invasion of the joint space by organisms. Arthritis in children is often due to contiguous spread from osteomyelitis. Bacteraemia secondary to an infection elsewhere in the body (pneumonia, cellulitis), injection drug use and direct inoculation of organisms into the joint space due to trauma and arthroscopy, etc. are common routes of infection in adults.

The common causes of infective arthritis are *Staph. aureus*, *Strep. pyogenes*, other β haemolytic streptococci and *Strep. pneumoniae*. Patients with disseminated gonococcal infection are at risk of gonococcal arthritis. Coagulase-negative staphylococci, aerobic Gram-negative bacilli and enterococci are recognised causes of prosthetic joint infections.

Culture of synovial fluid for organisms is the definitive method for diagnosing bacterial arthritis.

Prompt drainage of the joint and prolonged antimicrobial therapy is required for satisfactory resolution of infection.

Acute osteomyelitis

Acute haematogenous osteomyelitis is a disease of children. Chronic osteomyelitis is more frequently associated with trauma and instrumentation than haematogenous infection.

With the elimination of *H. influenzae,* osteomyelitis through immunisation, *Staph. aureus* is the most common causative organism. Infection due to mixed organisms is common in diabetic foot osteomyelitis. *Mycobacterium tuberculosis* and *Brucella* spp. are causes of spondylodiscitis, while *Salmonella typhi* and nontyphoidal *Salmonella* have been implicated with sickle cell disease and HIV infection.

GENERAL SYNDROMES

Fever of unknown origin

Failure to establish a cause for a persistent fever despite a standard diagnostic workup is commonly referred as a fever of unknown origin (FUO). The principal disease categories of FUO are undiagnosed infection, malignancy and collagen diseases.

Infections that commonly present as FUO are tuberculosis, endocarditis, intraabdominal, retroperitoneal and pelvic abscesses, occult osteomyelitis and mycotic aneurysms, brucellosis, Epstein–Barr virus, cytomegalovirus and parvovirus infection (Table 62.9).

Drug fever can occur with any medication. Despite common belief, eosinophilia and rash are not always present. Correction of fever upon discontinuation of the drug confirms the diagnosis.

A thorough and repeated history and physical examination for potential diagnostic clues with a baseline set of laboratory tests and imaging is essential. Particular attention should be paid to:

1. travel (recent and remote)
2. exposure to animals and pets
3. occupation
4. sick contacts
5. family history of significant illness (tuberculosis)
6. immunisation (BCG)
7. drug list

Patients should be admitted to hospital for verification of temperature. A factitious fever should not be overlooked. Therapeutic interventions are discouraged in stable patients.

Table 62.9 Some common sites of infection in pyrexia of unknown origin

Abdomen	Subphrenic abscess
	Appendiceal abscess
	Ileal tuberculosis
	Pelvic abscess
Liver and	Intrahepatic abscess
biliary tract	Empyema of gallbladder
	Ascending cholangitis
	Cholecystitis
	Viral hepatitis
Kidney and	Perinephric abscess
urinary tract	Renal tuberculosis
	Pyelonephritis (especially children)
Bones	Vertebral osteomyelitis
	Tuberculosis
	Prosthetic infections
Cardiovascular	Endocarditis
	Graft infections
Respiratory	Tuberculosis
	Empyema and lung abscess
Nervous system	Cryptococcal or tuberculous meningitis
	Brain or spinal abscess

Sepsis

Sepsis is a heterogeneous condition resulting from the interaction of host, pathogen and environmental factors. Sepsis-induced organ dysfunction or tissue hypoperfusion is referred to as severe sepsis. Sepsis-induced hypotension not responding to fluid resuscitation is called septic shock.

Mortality from sepsis is high. Factors determining mortality are the number of organ systems involved, acidosis, shock, medical comorbidities, underlying illness and sources of infection. *Ps. aeruginosa, Candida* spp. and mixed infections have been associated with higher attributable mortality.

Bacteria are the most common pathogens causing sepsis. Fungi, rickettsiae, protozoa and some viruses have been rarely implicated. A proportion of patients with sepsis will be bacteraemic, with pulmonary, abdominal, skin and urinary tract as the most common sites of infection.

A variety of exotoxins and endogenous cell wall products released by bacteria producing local or distant proinflammatory effects and immune activation are central to the pathogenesis of sepsis (see Ch. 13). Widespread activation of coagulation pathways is common and leads to disseminated intravascular coagulation.

Sepsis has a dynamic and evolving clinical picture, and frequent evaluation of the patient is essential to identify progression to severe sepsis and septic shock. Occasionally, physical signs are helpful as in the purpuric rash or peripheral gangrene in meningococcaemia, peripheral emboli in endocarditis, the erythematous rash or desquamation in staphylococcal or streptococcal toxic shock syndrome or ecthyma gangrenosum in patients who have neutropenia and *Ps. aeruginosa* bacteraemia.

Microbiological investigations are needed to identify the causative organism and to direct antimicrobial therapy, particularly with reports of increased antimicrobial resistance in patients with severe sepsis. Blood cultures are the most important, and two or three blood culture sets should be collected before initiating antimicrobial treatment.

Prompt and effective antimicrobial therapy and, where indicated, source control are essential. Delay in administering antibiotics has shown to worsen survival. Readers are encouraged to refer to the Surviving Sepsis Campaign Guidelines for understanding the approach to management.

Travel-associated infections

Travellers may be exposed to infection either during the journey or at the destination, they may also be exposed to gastrointestinal and respiratory infections during travel.

Gastrointestinal infections caused by contaminated food and water have been reported in aeroplanes and ships. Common organisms are viruses (astrovirus, norovirus and rotavirus) and nontyphoidal *Salmonella*. Respiratory viruses (influenza virus, SARS virus and corona virus) and *My. tuberculosis* have been transmitted in aeroplanes.

Whilst at the destination, travellers are commonly exposed to respiratory and gastrointestinal infections. The destination and the type of activities undertaken determine other infections.

Depending on the duration of travel, infections may manifest in the country of travel or after returning to the home country.

Knowledge of medical geography is useful, but conditions vary greatly within one country and with time. Up-to-date information is held, often on computer, by communicable disease centres and tropical disease hospitals and schools. The World Health Organization and the Centers for Disease Control and Prevention (CDC) publish international notification data and maps. Undoubtedly the most important condition to diagnose is malaria due to *Plasmodium falciparum*, which may be rapidly fatal without appropriate treatment in the nonimmune subject. The wide distribution of drug resistance in *P. falciparum* has led to difficulties in giving adequate prophylaxis and in treating an acute attack. Other common febrile illnesses acquired in developing countries are typhoid and paratyphoid. These do not usually present with diarrhoea, so the possibility of an enteric fever may not be considered. It is also obvious, but sometimes overlooked, that the fever may not be related to the travel history and that the cause is a microbe that could have been caught at home.

Table 62.10 Some important infective conditions imported to temperate regions from the tropics

Causative organism	Tourists[a]	Expatriates[a]	Immigrants[a]
Viruses	Hepatitis A	HIV	Hepatitis B
	Influenza	Yellow fever (other arboviruses)	Haemorrhagic fever
Rickettsiae and chlamydiae	Tick typhus	Q fever	Trachoma
Bacteria	Legionnaires' disease	Brucellosis	Tuberculosis, enteric fever
	Toxigenic *E. coli*	Shigellosis	Cholera
Protozoa	Cryptosporidiosis	Giardiasis	Amoebiasis
	Falciparum malaria	Malaria (all)	Vivax malaria
	Cutaneous leishmaniasis	Schistosomiasis	Kala azar (visceral leishmaniasis)
Helminths	–	Tapeworm	Roundworm
		Filariasis	Hookworm
		Stronglyloidiasis	
Ectoparasites (ticks, mites and insects)	Ticks	Myiasis jigger flea	Scabies
Fungi	–	Dermatophytosis Histoplasmosis	Mycetoma

[a]These categories are not mutually exclusive.

Table 62.10 lists some of the common infections imported from developing countries to developed countries.

There are three groups of patients that are considered separately, but the separation of diseases and microbes is not exclusive:

1. Short-term travellers or tourists who usually visit major cities or special holiday areas, stay in good accommodation and have minimal contact with the indigenous population.
2. Long-term visitors who may be engaged in lengthy overland trips or be working abroad as expatriates.
3. Immigrants who were brought up abroad and visit or have residence in the host country; also settled immigrants who pay short-term visits to their country of origin.

Generally, advice given by travel operators, tourist offices, embassies and medical sources has greatly improved in the past few years. Companies sending out expatriate workers tend to look after their staff well. Nevertheless, many tourists (up to 50% in some studies) have episodes of travellers' diarrhoea, which in some cases results in admission to hospital. The major groups who are missed in preventative programmes are overland travellers and immigrants returning to their homeland, often with young families who have never been exposed to the infectious risks of their parents' home. Immigrants returning for visits to malarious areas seldom take prophylactic advice, believing themselves to be immune, but protective immunity wanes with prolonged absence.

RECOMMENDED READING

Armstrong, D., & Cohen, J. (Eds.). (2011). *Infectious Diseases*. St. Louis: Mosby, Elsevier.

Conlon, C., & Snydman, D. (2000). *Color Atlas and Text of Infectious Diseases*. St. Louis: Mosby, Elsevier.

Long, S. S., Pickering, L. K., & Prober, C. G. (Eds.). (2009). *Principles and Practice of Paediatric Infectious Diseases*. Philadelphia: Saunders, Elsevier.

Mandell, G. L., Bennett, J. E., & Dolin, R. (2009). *Principles and Practice of Infectious Diseases* (6th ed.). Philadelphia: Churchill Livingstone, Elsevier.

Rhodes, A., Evans, L., Alhazzani, W., Levy, M., Antonelli, M., Ferre, R., ... Dellinger, R. P. (2017). Surviving sepsis campaign: international guidelines for management of sepsis and septic shock: 2016. *Critical Care Medicine, 45*(3), 486–552. doi:10.1097/CCM.0000000000002255.

Warrell, D. A., Cox, T. M., & Firth, J. D. (2010). *Oxford Textbook of Medicine* (5th ed.). Oxford: Oxford University Press.

63 Laboratory investigations

NELUN PERERA

KEY POINTS

- The microbiology laboratory plays a pivotal role in the management of patients with infections.
- The primary function is to process clinical specimens appropriately, and interpret and communicate results to positively influence antimicrobial treatment.
- Even with the best available methods, the laboratory can only detect organisms that are in specimens at the time they are received in the laboratory; hence, it is imperative that the clinical specimens are of high quality, transported rapidly and accompanied by the necessary information.
- In the United Kingdom, laboratories follow standard operating procedures (SOPs) for all clinical specimens. The SOPs are fully validated, and there are quality control measures for quality assurance of results.
- Laboratory methods detect microorganisms or their products or evidence of a patient's immune response to the organism. Although new methods such as polymerase chain reaction (PCR) are increasingly used to detect organisms rapidly, antimicrobial susceptibility can only be reliably determined and appropriate treatment information provided by isolating the organism in culture.
- The application of molecular techniques has the potential of increasing the sensitivity, specificity and speed of laboratory results. With the unprecedented advances in technology, it is likely that there will be techniques sufficiently versatile to allow a hunt for all 'unknown' organisms in patients' specimens in the not so distant future.
- In spite of advances in laboratory investigations that could inform the clinician of the infective process, clinicians and microbiologists must show mutual respect and cooperation, and communicate with each other, in the best interest of the patients.

The microbiology laboratory in a hospital plays a central role in the management of patients with infections. It assists clinicians to collect the most appropriate clinical specimens from patients, selects the relevant investigations for the specimens received in the laboratory and communicates results of investigations to the clinician to make a judicious decision on antimicrobial treatment. In addition, it also plays an important role in antimicrobial stewardship, in infection prevention and control and in epidemiological surveillance of infection and antimicrobial resistance.

The role of the laboratory is to:

- provide accurate information on the presence or absence of microorganisms in specimens sent to the laboratory
- provide information on in vitro antimicrobial susceptibility of microorganisms isolated
- engage clinicians in the discussions on the relevance of demonstrating microorganisms in clinical specimens to the patient's disease process
- guide clinicians on selecting the most appropriate antimicrobial agent to treat the patient's infection.

Detecting microorganisms in clinical specimens is achieved in the laboratory by one of several methods:

- direct demonstration of microorganisms by microscopy
- isolation of microorganisms by culture
- demonstration of microbial products such as structural components (e.g., cell wall antigens), extracellular products (e.g., toxins) and nuclear material (DNA or RNA)
- demonstration of specific antibodies or sensitised T lymphocytes to microorganisms (e.g., patient's immune response to infection).

This chapter focuses on the fundamentals of preanalytical, analytical and postanalytical steps in laboratory investigations (Fig. 63.1). For more detailed information on laboratory methods, including specimen containers and culture media, the readers are encouraged to refer to the recommended reading section at the end of the chapter.

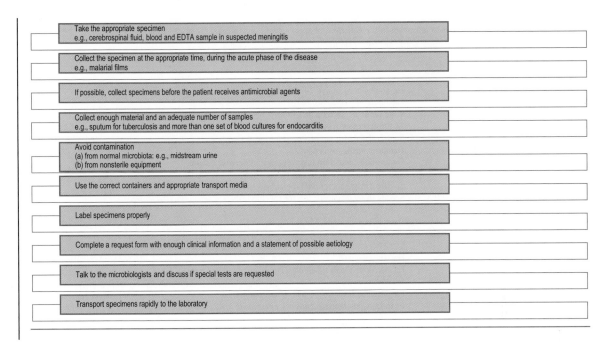

Fig. 63.1 Preanalytical steps in laboratory investigation.

COLLECTION OF SPECIMENS

A fundamental step in all laboratory investigations is the correct choice of an appropriate specimen. This requires a good understanding of the pathogenesis of infective syndromes (Ch. 62).

Collecting specimens is the clinician's responsibility, but the laboratory should provide the correct instructions and sterile containers. If a patient is asked to collect a specimen (e.g., urine or sputum), similarly, the patient should be given clear instructions. In all instances, specimens should be of appropriate volume, good quality and represent the infective process.

Selection of the appropriate specimens depends on diagnostic tests performed on the specimen. Some points to remember with individual specimens are shown in Table 63.1.

If the test is culture of the organism then the specimen must contain viable organisms. Care must be taken to avoid contamination of specimens from the patient's microbiota or from the environment. Wherever possible, specimens should be collected before commencing antimicrobial therapy. An adequate volume of specimen should be collected to increase the chances of growing the organism in culture, and adequate number of specimens should be collected if the organisms are transiently present (e.g., more than one blood culture set for endocarditis).

Collecting a large enough volume of the sample increases the chances of isolation of organisms and helps maintain the viability of organisms during transport. Whenever possible, actual fluid (e.g., wound exudate or pus) should be collected into sterile containers instead of collecting as swabs. Tissue samples should be collected into sterile containers devoid of histological preservatives (e.g., formalin). If the diagnostic test is antigen detection or nucleic acid detection the appropriate specimen is determined by the suspected pathogens (e.g., cerebrospinal fluid for cryptococcal meningitis, urine for *Legionella pneumophila*, and throat swab for influenza virus).

'Paired serum' samples from acute and convalescent phases of the disease (14 days apart) should be collected to detect host antibody responses to diseases. To avoid errors in specimen identification, all specimens must be properly labeled and accompanied by a request form providing the necessary information about the patient, the clinical diagnosis and current antimicrobial therapy. In addition, to avoid laboratory transmission of hazardous organisms (e.g., *Mycobacterium tuberculosis*, *Salmonella typhi*) the laboratory should be appropriately notified by labeling the specimens and the request form 'high risk'.

All clinical specimens from patients with blood-borne virus infections (hepatitis B, C and HIV) should also be clearly labeled as 'high risk' both on the specimen and request form.

Table 63.1 Some important points to remember in the collection of specimens for microbiological examination

Type of specimen	Comments
Respiratory secretions	
Nasal swab (anterior)	For staphylococcal and streptococcal carriage
Nasopharyngeal swab	For *Bordetella pertussis*, *Neisseria meningitidis* and viruses
External ear swab	Wide range of bacteria and fungi
Myringotomy and sinus samples	As for abscesses – including anaerobes
Throat (pharyngeal) swab	Specify if only for streptococci; inform if *Corynebacterium diphtheriae* is suspected; use virus transport media for viruses
Saliva	For antibody detection (e.g., measles); otherwise discard
Laryngeal swab	Specify if for *Mycobacterium tuberculosis*
Expectorated sputum	Specify if *Mycobacterium tuberculosis* is suspected
Transtracheal aspirate, bronchoscopy specimens, lung biopsy	Specify likely diagnosis; ask for specific tests (e.g., *Pneumocystis jeroveci*)
Pleural fluid	Treat as pus
Gastrointestinal specimens	
Vomitus	For viruses only
Gastric washings	For *Mycobacterium tuberculosis* (particularly in children)
Gastric biopsy	For *Helicobacter pylori*
Duodenal/jejunal aspirates	For protozoa (*Giardia lamblia*, Microsporidia, etc.)
Liver aspirates	As for pus (anaerobes); consider *Entamoeba histolytica*
Spleen puncture	For *Leishmania* spp.
Rectal biopsy	For *Schistosoma* spp.
Rectal swab	For *Neisseria gonorrhoea* and *Chlamydia trachomatis*
Colonic biopsy	Histopathological diagnosis of amoebiasis *(Entamoeba histolytica)*, pseudomembranous colitis *(Clostridium difficile)*
Colonic scrapings	For protozoa; *Entamoeba histolytica* trophozoites (deliver to laboratory immediately)
Faeces	Specify possible diagnosis; specify *Clostridium difficile* toxins, parasite examination
Perianal swab	For eggs of threadworm
Urine	
Midstream (MSU)	Suitable for most patients
Clean catch	Infants and elderly – increased contamination
Suprapubic aspirate	Infants and neonates
Ureteric/bladder washout	To localise infection
Prostatic massage	Collect samples before, during and at end of micturition
Terminal urine	For *Schistosoma* spp. ova, *Chlamydia trachomatis* DNA amplification
Complete early morning or 24-h urine	For *Mycobacterium tuberculosis*
Central nervous system	
Cerebrospinal fluid by spinal tap	For meningitis, collect sample for protein and glucose – test blood sugar simultaneously, specify virology, fungi or syphilis serology
Ventricular tap	Specify if through an indwelling shunt or catheter
Brain abscess	As for pus – including anaerobes
Skin and soft tissue	
Skin scraping/nail clipping	For dermatophyte fungi
Skin swab	Rarely valuable without pus
Skin snips	Onchocerciasis – seek advice
Vesicle fluid	Suitable for electron microscopy for viruses, HSV and VZV PCR
Wound swab	Obtain pus if possible; record site
Pus, tissues, aspirates	Describe site and any relevant operative details
Genital	
Urethral swab	For *Neisseria gonorrhoea* and *Chlamydia trachomatis*
Vaginal swab (adult)	For *Candida* spp., *Trichomonas vaginalis*, bacterial vaginosis
Vaginal swab (prepubertal)	State age; caution required if abuse possible
Cervical swab	For *Neisseria gonorrhoea* and *Chlamydia trachomatis* DNA
Ulcer scrape	Immediate dark-ground microscopy; in viral transport medium for viruses or *Haemophilus ducreyi* (chancroid)
Uterine secretions	Specify puerperium or postabortion
Pelvic aspirates	As for pus – include anaerobes
Laparoscopy specimens	Include *Chlamydia trachomatis* specimen

Table 63.1 Some important points to remember in the collection of specimens for microbiological examination—cont'd

Type of specimen	Comments
Eye	
Conjunctival swab	Separate virology; scrape for chlamydia
Aspirates	As for pus – include anaerobes
Blood	
Culture	Strict aseptic technique; take large sample in special media before antibiotics
Bone marrow	For *Leishmania* spp., *Mycobacterium tuberculosis*, nontuberculous mycobacteria and *Brucella* spp.
Film	For malaria (thick and thin), filaria, borrelia, trypanosomes
Whole blood	For filaria (day or night samples as appropriate)
Serum antigen	Rapid diagnosis of many microbial diseases (e.g., hepatitis B)
Serum antibody	Retrospective diagnosis of common viral diseases, syphilis and other selected infections; need rising titer or specific IgM
Blood	Interferon gamma assays for *Mycobacterium tuberculosis*

HSV, herpes simplex virus; *VZV*, varicella zoster virus.

TRANSPORT

When collecting specimens for laboratory investigations, the ideal situation is to bring the patient to the laboratory or take the laboratory to where the patient is. Both approaches are used in special situations but are obviously inconvenient for many patients and inappropriate and costly for complicated techniques that need specialised (and safe) facilities.

Many microbes may perish on transit from the host's body to a laboratory incubator. Some contaminants, especially coliforms, may overgrow the pathogen and so mask its presence. To overcome these constraints, specimens should be transported to the laboratory as quickly as possible to protect the viability of any pathogen.

To overcome any drawbacks due to delay in reaching the microbiology laboratory, the following methods may be used:

1. *Transport media.* See Table 63.2.
2. *Boric acid.* The addition of boric acid to urine at a concentration of 1.8% (v/w) will stop bacterial multiplication, but lower concentrations are ineffective and higher ones may kill the pathogen.
3. *Refrigeration.* Storage at 4°C before processing will prevent multiplication of most bacteria. However, delicate microbes such as *Neisseria meningitides* may not survive, whereas certain organisms, notably *Listeria* sp., flourish at low temperatures.
4. *Freezing.* Temperatures of −70°C or below, which can be achieved in liquid nitrogen or special deep freezes, will preserve many microbes, provided they

Table 63.2 Types of transport medium

Type of organism	Medium	Comments
Bacteria	Stuart's semisolid agar	Contains charcoal to inactivate toxic material
Anaerobic bacteria	Various systems, including gassed-out tubes and anaerobic bags	Not widely used, but essential for some strict anaerobes
Viruses	Buffered salts solution containing serum	Contains antibiotics to control bacteria and fungi
Chlamydiae	Similar to viral transport medium, but without agents that inhibit chlamydiae	Chlamydial antigen media contain detergent to lyse infected cells
Protozoa, helminths	Merthiolate–iodine–formalin	Kills active protozoa, but preserves cysts and ova in a form suitable for concentration and microscopy

are protected by a stabilising fluid such as serum or glycerol.

RECEPTION

The importance of good documentation cannot be overstressed. No matter how well the specimen was taken, transported and processed in the laboratory, the end result depends on communication between people. The clinician making the request must give complete details on the request card and specimen to reduce errors. Staff receiving specimens in the laboratory must match them with the cards and record them into a book or computer. This is usually done by assigning a unique number to each specimen and labelling both the specimen and the request. When parts of the specimen are separated from the original bottle (e.g., after centrifugation of serum), the laboratory number becomes the only recognisable identification. Transcription errors are far more common than is supposed and are especially important for requests for blood-borne virus investigations, which may have disastrous consequences and medicolegal implications if reported incorrectly.

SPECIMEN PROCESSING IN THE LABORATORY

Looking at clinical material with the naked eye or hand-lens should be part of the examination of a patient at the bedside. Many unnecessary laboratory tests could be avoided if unsuitable specimens were rejected on the ward or in the general practitioner's surgery. These would include crystal-clear urine from patients with 'cystitis'; well-formed stools from patients with 'diarrhoea'; and mouth washings or saliva from patients with respiratory symptoms.

The standard approach in most laboratories is to process specimens by specimen type (e.g., urine, wound swab). The aim is to examine specimens for frequently encountered pathogens in each specimen type. If the laboratory is provided with additional clinical information, steps are taken to look for fastidious or unusual organisms (e.g., prolong incubation of blood culture bottles for *Brucella* spp.).

Specimen processing methods can be divided into culture and nonculture methods. In addition, there are methods to detect antibody response to organisms and sensitised T lymphocytes in the patient's blood.

MICROSCOPY

Microscopy is an important part of the examination of many specimens. For bacteriology, wet material (e.g., cerebrospinal fluid [CSF]) and dried, stained smears are examined under the bright-field light microscope. The differential Gram stains and acid-fast (Ziehl–Neelsen) stains that exploit the differences in structure of the bacterial cell wall are used for demonstrating bacteria and mycobacteria. The demonstration of fungi or parasites requires special stains or concentration techniques. 'Wet' mounts (i.e., unstained preparations of fluid material) are widely used in examining cells in urine, CSF, faeces and vaginal secretions. None of these procedures takes >5 or 10 minutes, and they are inexpensive in reagent costs and capital equipment. They are therefore useful

rapid methods, and new diagnostic techniques have to be judged against microscopy. An initial report, such as 'Gram-negative diplococci and pus cells seen' in a purulent CSF, can be issued within a few minutes of receiving the specimen in the laboratory and will aid the clinician in supporting the clinical diagnosis and starting appropriate antibiotics.

Similarly, examination of stained blood films for malaria parasites (e.g., *Plasmodium falciparum*) can be lifesaving. Indeed, suspected bacterial meningitis and falciparum malaria are among the few conditions for which it is clearly justifiable to call upon emergency laboratory services outside normal working hours.

Electron microscopy (EM) is used to detect virus particles in specimens (e.g., diarrhoeal stool for rotavirus or vesicle fluid for varicella zoster virus). EM has been largely replaced by nucleic acid detection methods in routine laboratories. However, unlike culture or antigen/nucleic acid methods, EM is an entirely nonselective method of detecting any virus that can lead to the detection of novel viruses (e.g., discovery of SARS virus). Fluorescent microscopy detects organisms that have been stained with fluorescent dyes (e.g., auramine stained mycobacteria or calcofluor stained fungal filaments). It is also used in detecting microbial antigens and antibody using specific antibodies tagged with fluorescent dyes (immunofluorescence).

NONCULTURE METHODS

There are many situations where isolation of microbes in vitro or in tissue culture is difficult or is insufficiently sensitive. The isolation of many viruses requires laborious tissue culture methods that are too slow to influence patient management. Microscopy is usually of low sensitivity; for example, the threshold of detection of acid-fast bacilli in sputum is about 10^5 microbes per millilitre. Microscopy also has low specificity; for example, Gram staining of faeces would yield millions of Gram-negative rods, but it is not possible to recognise those that are pathogenic by this means.

Nonculture-based methods detect microbial products and do not rely on viable organisms in the specimen. Methods detecting microbial antigens, toxins and nucleic acids are available.

Antigen detection

Detection of microbial antigens offers a rapid method of detecting microorganisms in specimens. A number of commercial antigen tests for detection of bacteria, fungi, viruses, parasites or their toxins in clinical specimens are available (e.g., pneumococcal antigen in blood and CSF,

Legionella antigen in urine, Rotavirus in faeces, and *Clostridium difficile* toxin in faeces). The tests have variable sensitivity and specificity and are not available for detecting all microorganisms. Different detection methods are employed, for example enzyme-immunoassays (EIA), immunofluorescence, latex particle agglutination etc.

Nucleic acid–based tests

In the last few years there has been a significant increase in commercial nucleic acid–based tests for detection of microorganisms in clinical specimens. Particularly noteworthy are the multiplex tests developed for detection of common pathogens in CSF, respiratory gastrointestinal and genitourinary specimens. A number of different testing platforms that are automated, sensitive and specific and allow testing single samples or multiple samples for high throughput testing with minimal trained technologist are available. With further refinement of the technology, it is likely that there will be more tests menus that are less expensive and easy to perform and that can be incorporated into most clinical laboratories in the future.

DETECTION OF HOST IMMUNOLOGICAL RESPONSE TO MICROORGANISMS

Microorganisms contain a wide array of molecules capable of eliciting an immune response in the host. The polyclonal activation of lymphocytes can be demonstrated in vivo (e.g., tuberculin skin test) or in vitro (detection of antibodies and sensitised T cells). Detecting IgM and IgG antibodies in serum or plasma (serology) using specific antigens has the advantage of demonstrating indirect evidence to infection, particularly where the microorganisms are either difficult to culture or impossible to culture (e.g., EIA for hepatitis C virus, *Treponema pallidum*). Methods detecting antibodies in other body fluids are also available (e.g., saliva, CSF and urine). The interferon gamma releasing assays detect sensitised T lymphocytes to microorganisms (e.g., *Mycobacterium tuberculosis*).

The major drawback of serology is it takes 10–14 days for antibodies to appear after an infection. In some infections (e.g., HIV, hepatitis B virus and hepatitis C virus), it can take weeks to months to demonstrate detectable antibodies. Immunocompromised patients may not always mount an immune response. False-positive tests are observed due to cross-reactive antibodies.

Other than tests designed to measure IgM-specific antibody in a single sample, it is generally necessary to demonstrate a four-fold increase in antibody titer between an acute and a convalescent serum sample to support a recent infection.

LABORATORY CULTURE OF MICROORGANISMS

The basis of the study of medical microbiology was laid over a century ago by culture of microbes in pure culture in the laboratory. The methods used by the fathers of bacteriology have been adapted, simplified and, in some cases, automated for the modern diagnostic laboratory. The principles remain the same: use sterile equipment and media (with cell lines if necessary) and add clinical material. After incubation at 37°C, for a variable time, from a few hours for enterobacteria to weeks for mycobacteria and some viruses and fungi, a visible effect will be produced. This might be colonies growing on agar or a cytopathic effect (CPE) in tissue culture. The skill of microbiology is in identifying the microbes responsible for the effect.

Solid and liquid nutrient media are available to grow bacteria and fungi in the laboratory. On solid media, bacteria and fungi produce colonies composed of thousands of cells derived from a single cell. It takes up to 12–48 hours for bacteria and yeast to produce macroscopically visible colonies, but some organisms that divide slowly can take several weeks (e.g., *Mycobacterium tuberculosis*, dermatophytes). Selective media incorporating substances such as antibiotics are available for specimens collected from body sites with microbiota.

The majority of bacteria and fungi of medical importance can be grown on laboratory culture media, but there is no one culture medium that will support the growth of all organisms.

There are limits to the methods that can be used in a routine hospital laboratory to culture microorganisms. The choice of media used is dictated by the specimen and by the clinical condition of the patient. For example, in some areas of the world there is little value in looking for *Corynebacterium diphtheriae* in every throat swab, so the specific media needed are not routinely used. It is therefore incumbent on the attending clinician to make sure that the laboratory is alerted to look for diphtheria bacilli in any suspicious case. Similarly, clinicians need to know which microbes are routinely sought from particular specimens so that they can make a special request if they suspect the unusual.

Parasites such as *Trichomonas*, *Leishmania* and *Trypanosoma* are grown in liquid media to allow the parasites to multiply and thus make it easier to detect by microscopy. Some microorganisms (e.g., *Mycobacterium leprae* and *Treponema pallidum*) have only been grown in experimental animals. Viruses, *Chlamydia* and *Rickettsia* can only be grown in cell or tissue culture because these organisms are incapable of a free-living existence.

'New' causes of illness are often found, and new methods of investigating old diseases regularly appear on the market. It is a difficult decision for the laboratory manager to assess at what point a 'new' pathogen becomes sufficiently important to be routinely sought, or to balance the advantages of new (and expensive) technology against cheap and well-tried techniques, especially in resource-poor countries.

IDENTIFICATION

The full identification of each microbe isolated in a clinical laboratory is both uneconomic and unnecessary. A presumptive identification of common bacteria is usually possible based on microscopic morphology and characteristics of the colonies on culture media. In most laboratory settings, the experienced microbiologists will offer a reliable identification based on these characteristics and certain preliminary tests (e.g., catalase, coagulase, oxidase, motility tests). This offers timely laboratory information to influence clinical decision making.

Most UK laboratories will attempt a definitive identification of bacteria and fungi isolated in blood and other fluids (e.g., CSF) using additional laboratory methods. These include:

- biochemical methods (metabolic profile)
- serological methods (i.e., using antiserum)
- genomic techniques
- proteomic methods.

Identifying bacteria based on biochemical reactions has been in use for a long time. A number of commercial manual multitest identification systems (e.g., analytical profile index [API]; bioMerieux systems) and automated identification systems (e.g., Vitek AutoMicrobic System) for bacteria and fungi are available. The 'metabolic profile' generated is compared against an established database for the most likely organism identification.

Certain microorganisms isolated in culture can be identified employing specific commercially prepared antisera (Table 63.3).

Genomic techniques have become the method of choice for rapid and accurate identification of a variety of bacteria and fungi grown in culture. Probe-based and DNA–sequence-based methods are available. Commercial and in-house sequence-based assays that detect ribosomal ribonucleic acid genes (e.g., 16S and 18S rRNA) and other housekeeping genes are used widely in resource-rich countries. In addition, genomic techniques offer genotyping organisms in investigation of outbreaks. It is now possible to identify organisms with whole genome sequencing (e.g., *Mycobacterium tuberculosis*). The precise genomic identification allows discriminating strains to single-base differences (Ch. 64).

Table 63.3 Identification of common bacteria using antisera

Bacteria	Antisera identification
β haemolytic *Streptococcus*	Lancefield grouping based on cell wall carbohydrates; A, B, C, D, F and G most common
Streptococcus pneumoniae	>90 capsular polysaccharides; polyvalent antisera used to identify *S. pneumoniae* in blood and CSF cultures
Neisseria meningitidis	Thirteen capsular polysaccharides; A, B, C, Y and W135 most common
Haemophilus influenzae	Capsular polysaccharides classify into six subtypes; subtype B most invasive
Salmonella enterica	Subtyped using cell wall (O) polysaccharides; >2500 subtypes
Shigella spp.	Cell wall (O) polysaccharides divide into 45 subtypes
Escherichia coli	Cell wall (O) 157 polysaccharide associated with haemorrhagic colitis
Legionella pneumophila	Polyvalent antisera subdivide into 16 serogroups; serogroup 1 most important

Table 63.4 Examples of bacterial identification in medical laboratories

Reason for request	Extent of identification	
	Example 1	Example 2
Test of sterility	Bacteria present	
Initial blood culture report	Gram-negative rod	Gram-positive cocci
Urine examination	'Coliforms'	Staphylococci
Wound swab	*Escherichia coli*	*Staphylococcus aureus*
Outbreak epidemiology	*E. coli* O157	*Staph. aureus* phage type 80/81
Pathogenicity tests	*E. coli* O157 vero toxin–producing	*Staph. aureus* enterotoxin A-positive

Proteomics, the study of protein expression at the cellular level, is another laboratory identification method. The method employs mass spectrometry. There are two commercial identification methods widely used in resource-rich countries. They are MALDI-TOF and VITEK MS. Both systems have very large databases that can offer the identification of a large number of organisms. They are fully automated systems and can significantly improve workflow in the laboratory.

Typing of isolates is performed for epidemiological or other special reasons, and this is usually done in national reference centres using standardised methods.

Examples of the extent of identification are shown in Table 63.4. This shows that the same organism may not be identified even to the genus level, or it may have extensive genetic investigation depending on the reason for the request. In a cost-conscious climate you get what you pay for and what the service thinks you need!

Point-of-care testing

Accurate and rapid detection of microorganisms in the clinical environment (i.e., point-of-care testing [POCT]) has the potential to influence clinical decisions in real time. It has the potential to improve patient care pathways by reducing turnaround times, reducing utilisation of resources (e.g., antimicrobial consumption) and bringing in cost benefits. Methods employing antigen detection (e.g., *Streptococcus pyogenes,* respiratory syncytial virus and influenza virus in throat swabs, *Streptococcus pneumoniae* in urine), nucleic acid detection (e.g., influenza virus in throat swabs), antibody detection (HIV in blood) and enzyme detection (*Helicobacter pylori* in gastric biopsies) are available. Introduction of POCT requires careful consideration of test validation, quality assurance, training of staff, safety measures and cost.

ANTIMICROBIAL SUSCEPTIBILITY TESTING

Antimicrobial susceptibility testing should be performed on a bacterial or fungal isolate from a clinical specimen, if the isolate is thought to be a probable cause of the patient's infection. One advantage of good identification of microorganisms is that it can help choose the most appropriate antimicrobial agent, and in some situations, in vitro tests of susceptibility may be unnecessary. However, the widespread occurrence of bacterial resistance, even in genera such as *Neisseria* and *Haemophilus* in which sensitivity to β-lactam antibiotics was previously assumed, has meant that tests are usually performed on all significant clinical isolates of bacteria and fungi. The relevance of information generated from susceptibility testing in the extremely artificial conditions of the laboratory is discussed in Ch. 64.

As there are technical problems in carrying out susceptibility tests at the same time as the primary culture, the report will be delayed for at least 24 hours after isolation of the pathogen. Tests of slow-growing bacteria such as mycobacteria take much longer, and tests involving viruses and protozoa are not ordinarily available. In general, all patients with acute symptoms will receive treatment before the report returns to the doctor, so the result will merely confirm that correct treatment had been chosen. Sometimes, the laboratory report will allow empirical antimicrobial therapy to be modified, for example, by allowing one or more drugs in a combination to be discontinued.

A frequent difficulty facing microbiologists is which, out of a rapidly increasing number of agents, should be tested and, of those tested, which should be reported. Most laboratories test a few representative compounds from among the many penicillins, cephalosporins, aminoglycosides, tetracyclines, quinolones, etc., and restrict those reported to the clinician to two or three agents selected for their appropriateness in the particular infection. In this way, institutional antibiotic policies are reinforced and the impact of the promotional activities of pharmaceutical companies is lessened.

COMMUNICATION OF RESULTS OF LABORATORY INVESTIGATIONS

The postanalytical phase of the laboratory investigation consists of communication of results to the clinician treating the patient. The fundamental premise is to ensure accurate and timely information. The reports should be clear and free of microbiology jargon and abbreviations. The clinician may be unfamiliar with the laboratory procedures or the taxonomic status of the organism involved. Where appropriate, it may be necessary to include interpretative statements.

In these days of computers and emails, it is attractive to use these latest technologies to transfer results. The telephone is a satisfactory substitute in many cases and is far preferable to a report form printed by a computer and arriving after the crisis is over. It behoves us all to communicate better and faster.

Certain microbiology results are considered 'urgent' and must be reported to the clinician immediately. These are results that indicate situations that need a prompt clinical response (Box 63.1).

As in so many spheres of health care, a spirit of mutual respect and cooperation is in the best interests of the patients, and this is most likely to happen if microbiologists regularly visit the wards and if clinicians are encouraged to discuss problems with laboratory staff.

Box 63.1 'Urgent' results in microbiology

- Positive blood culture
- Positive cerebrospinal fluid Gram-stain and culture
- Positive cryptococcal antigen test or culture
- Positive blood smear for malaria
- *Streptococcus pyogenes* from a sterile site
- Positive acid-fast smears or positive *Mycobacterium* culture
- *Streptococcus agalactiae* or herpes simplex virus from genital tract of a pregnant woman at term
- Other significant pathogens (i.e., *Legionella* sp., *Bordetella pertussis*)

Box 63.2 List of notifiable diseases in England and Wales

- Acute encephalitis/meningitis
- Acute infectious hepatitis
- Acute poliomyelitis
- Anthrax
- Botulism
- Brucellosis
- Cholera
- Diphtheria
- Dysentery (amoebic or bacillary)
- Enteric fever (paratyphoid/typhoid)
- Food poisoning
- Haemolytic uraemic syndrome
- Infectious bloody diarrhoea
- Invasive group A streptococcal disease and scarlet fever
- Legionnaires' disease
- Leprosy
- Malaria
- Measles
- Meningococcal septicaemia
- Mumps
- Plague
- Rabies
- Rubella
- SARS
- Smallpox
- Scarlet fever
- Tetanus
- Tuberculosis
- Typhus
- Viral haemorrhagic fever
- Whooping cough
- Yellow fever

Health Protection Regulations 2010.

NOTIFICATION OF INFECTIOUS DISEASES

In addition to making a clinical diagnosis and treating the individual, there is a need with some infectious diseases to determine the source and prevent further spread. In some countries there are public health laws specifying the method of reporting these. The list of notifiable diseases in England and Wales is shown in Box 63.2. This reporting system requires a clinical diagnosis, with or without laboratory confirmation, which is notified separately. In England and Wales, each health district has a consultant responsible for communicable disease control who is usually the 'proper officer' for the local government authority. Notifications are sent to Public Health England (PHE).

There is also an obligation, which in some circumstances may be statutory, for laboratories to report isolates of certain pathogens to central authorities for surveillance purposes. For HIV/AIDS infection, the system is voluntary and confidential, yet over 90% of cases are reported in the United Kingdom. In an outbreak, or where the pathogen is highly infectious, it is essential to inform both the clinician looking after the patient and local Public Health England staff. In this way, a coordinated approach can be made to prevent further spread of infection. In particular, if there is any indication that staff working in the laboratory have been exposed to hazard group 3 and above organisms this must be reported to the relevant authority; in the United Kingdom that is the Health and Safety Executive.

RECOMMENDED READING

Forbes, B. A., Sahm, D. F., & Weissfeld, A. S. (2002). *Bailey and Scott's diagnostic microbiology* (10th ed.). St. Louis: Mosby.

Johnson, F. B. (1990). Transport of viral specimens. *Clinical Microbiology Reviews*, *3*(2), 120–131.

Mahon, C. R., Lehman, D. C., & Manuselis, G. (2015). *Textbook of diagnostic microbiology* (5th ed.). Missouri: Elsevier.

Mandell, G. L., Bennett, J. E., & Dolin, R. (2009). *Principles and practice of infectious diseases* (6th ed.). Philadelphia: Churchill Livingstone, Elsevier.

Versalovic, J., Carrol, K. C., Funke, G., et al: American Society for Microbiology. (2011). *Manual of clinical microbiology* (10th ed.). Washington, DC: American Society for Microbiology.

64 Molecular methods in diagnostic microbiology

MATHEW A. DIGGLE

KEY POINTS

- With a history only starting in the early 1980s, molecular techniques are fast developing to become an integral part of the diagnostic pathway.
- Molecular techniques can be divided into two main groups, either gel based or sequence based, and are used to identify a wide range of bacteria, viruses, parasites and fungi.
- Polymerase chain reaction (PCR) has provided an invaluable technique and is considered one of the most important tools in the advance of molecular technology.
- Sequence-based tools are now used as highly sensitive and specific detection tools and as specialised characterisation tools.
- Quality, not quantity, should be the mainstay of any molecular advances.

INTRODUCTION

When a patient is suspected of having a life-threatening infectious disease it is important to obtain as much microbiological information as possible. The pace with which developments have occurred in molecular techniques and characterisation tools makes it seem increasingly likely that molecular techniques will play some role with virtually all disease investigations in the future. It is important to utilise molecular techniques and realise their tremendous value not only in the investigation of basic scientific questions but also by their application to a wide variety of problems and limitations affecting all agents that can affect the human condition.

Such stimuli have helped this area progress and develop so that investigators can adequately address the genetic basis of biological function. This had slowly emerged over the latter half of the 20th century and has continually gathered pace over the last decade. The development of genetics, specifically molecular genetics, has incorporated newly evolving techniques and resulted in the start of the genetic revolution, which has led to a greater understanding of basic mechanisms of disease-causing pathogens. The primary motivation behind this unprecedented growth of molecular genetics was initially to benefit the understanding of human genetics. This has ultimately benefited other areas of molecular science including microbial genetics. Virtually all major scientific disciplines will find molecular techniques increasingly necessary in areas such as research, laboratory investigation, prognosis and clinical management. This chapter will provide an insight into the origins of and an up-to-date introduction into the molecular techniques used for the laboratory investigation of infection. It attempts to highlight the constant evolution and continual need for diagnostic procedures and molecular characterisation. The techniques required for the laboratory investigation and characterisation of infection and the future prospects for the role of new technologies in such environments are described.

MOLECULAR DIAGNOSTICS—THE HISTORICAL PERSPECTIVE

The field of molecular biology grew in the late 20th century, as did its clinical application. In the early 1980s, genetic testing did not rely upon genotypic DNA sequencing, but rather on gel-based techniques that relied upon fragmenting DNA using specalised enzymes producing different lengths that could be profiled. As a consequence, during the 1990s, the identification of newly discovered genes and new techniques for DNA sequencing led to the appearance of a distinct field of molecular and genomic laboratory medicine.

Moreover, as a commercial application, molecular techniques have become increasingly important and so has the debate about selected targets, performance specificity, sensitivity and interpretation of increasingly complex amounts of data. This has led to the recent developments in semiautomated and fully automated molecular platforms, which include sample processing, extrations, amplification and basic analysis.

MOLECULAR TECHNIQUES—THE GOLD STANDARDS

Molecular techniques are used to identify a wide range of bacteria, viruses, parasites, and fungi such as *Chlamydia*, influenza virus, *Mycobacterium tuberculosis* and *Pneumocystis jiroveci*. Genetic identification can now be swift; for example, a loop-mediated isothermal amplification test detects the malaria parasite and is reliable enough for low-income countries. But despite these advances in genome analysis, in 2013 infectious organisms were still more often identified by other means such as culture, their proteome, bacteriophage, or biochemical profile. Molecular techniques are also used to characterise specific strains of a pathogen, for example, its antimicrobial resistance capabilities by detecting which drug resistance genes it possesses and therefore optimising therapy.

GLOBAL TRENDS IN MOLECULAR TECHNIQUES

The continuing commercial development of molecular techniques and platforms has made it practical to use them in various settings, such as in centralised high throughput laboratory testing or smaller near-patient testing. Platform developments, automation and miniaturisation have brought medical diagnostics into a wide range of primary and secondary care settings. In addiation, clinical laboratory testing requires high standards of reliability; molecular techniques may require accreditation or fall under medical device regulations. Nevertheless, while there is still demand for bespoke molecular techniques, clinical laboratories will continue to use assays labeled as "research use only" in combination with those that are fully accredited.

In modern molecular testing, laboratory processes need to adhere to a wide range of regulations and standards—for example, Good Laboratory Practice, UK Accreditation Service (UKAS), Clinical Laboratory Improvement Amendments, Health Insurance Portability and Accountability Act, and Food and Drug Administration specifications. Supporting these standards involves a wide range of tools, including a laboratory information management system (LIMS), which as an informatics and more recently a bioinformatics tool helps the tracking and processing of samples. In addition, regulation applies to both staff and supplies. For a number of years, many countries have required health care scientists and laboratory technicians from a specific seniority to be licensed by their national professional bodies and organisations; the Health Care Professions Council (HCPC), the American Board of Medical Genetics, The Royal College of Pathologists, and the American Board of Pathology certify technologists, supervisors and laboratory directors.

MOLECULAR TECHNIQUES: POLYMERASE CHAIN REACTION (PCR)

The PCR method has been available for over a decade and has been applied in many different ways for the detection of a wide range of infectious organisms. During the past decade, the PCR has provided an invaluable tool and is considered a key advance in molecular technology. There are a number of different methods available for the detection or amplification of specific DNA sequences. The fundamental PCR method has found a home in many areas that utilise molecular techniques in research and nonresearch environments including microbiology, animal and human genetics and clinical diagnostics. Traditionally PCR products are amplified in a commercial thermocycler followed by visualisation of PCR products either on a gel-based system or via fluorescence of probes associated with amplified products (Fig. 64.1).

Because of the nature of PCR detection within clinical samples, inhibitors can sometimes be present such as immunoglobulin G in human plasma, hemoglobin and lactoferrin in erythrocytes and leukocytes, respectively. They have been identified as major inhibitors of diagnostic PCRs, which can decrease their efficacy. PCR-based detection and characterisation is especially useful when treatment has been given and a culture has proven negative. The success of positive nonculture detection and characterisation can be as little as 31% of suspected cases of infection.

The clinical value of PCR-based detection methods is sometimes limited due to low sensitivity, lack of specificity, high cost or their laborious methodology. However, various technologies are now available to exploit the PCR method beyond its basic concept and are now an invaluable tool in investigating infections.

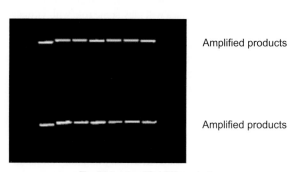

Amplified products

Amplified products

Fig. 64.1 Amplified PCR products.

Within routine microbiology laboratories it is still common to use a combination of both gel-based and probe-based PCR detection systems. Although similar genes are routinely used for the detection and characterisation of common infections (e.g., *Staphlococcus aureus, Clostridium difficile*), the specific gene sequence targets can vary in different laboratories but the principle remains the same.

In principle there are three main areas where PCR is used: disease investigation, determination of bacterial load, and amplification of genetic material for sequencing. PCR allows the in vitro amplification of specific target DNA sequences by a factor of 10^6 and is thus an extremely sensitive technique. It is based on an enzymatic reaction involving the use of synthetic oligonucleotides flanking the target nucleic acid sequence of interest. These oligonucleotides act as primers for the thermostable Taq polymerase. Repeated cycles (usually 25 to 40) of denaturation of the template DNA (at 94°C), annealing of primers to their complementary sequences (50°C), and primer extension (72°C) result in the exponential production of the specific target fragment (Fig. 64.2). Further sensitivity and specificity may be obtained by nested PCR, which

in essessce is the PCR process repeated twice, whereby the first stage amplifies a DNA fragment large enough to allow the second PCR process to amplify a smaller fragment from the existing fragment (e.g., nested). Detection of the PCR product is usually carried out by one of two methods: either agarose gel electrophoresis or fluorescent probe techniques such as real-time PCR. Real-time PCR is a tool now widely used in clinical diagnostics. This is when there are two initial compounds attached to the probe, one the fluorophore and the other the quencher. When free in the reaction, the two components are sufficiently close to each other and fluorescence is quenched. When in a reaction where a target sequence is identified, the probe hybridises to its complementary sequence, during extension, Taq polymerase exerts its exonuclease activity, cleaving the fluorophore from the probe and allowing it to fluoresce. The hybridised primer continues with its extension of the selected target. Further analysis of the PCR product can be performed by hybridisation with a specific oligonucleotide probe, restriction enzyme analysis or DNA sequencing. There are numerous advantages but also disadvantages to PCR. Advantages include extremely high sensitivity, the ability to detect down to one bacterial

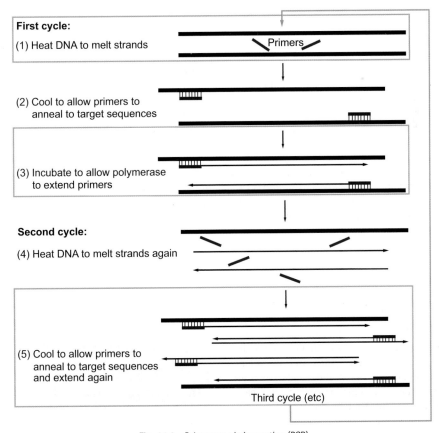

Fig. 64.2 Polymerase chain reaction (PCR).

genome per sample volume, its easy setup, and fast turnaround time compared to other investigation methods. Disadvanges include that it can be easily liable to contamination, for manual support it requires a high degree of operator skill, and it is not easy to set up fully quantitative assays.

Molecular characterisation

There are many ways with which molecular techniques are used in the laboratory investigation of infection. Detection of infectious organisms is the primary function of any clinical microbiology service; however, further characterisation is also valuable when we look at details of the infecting organism or how we ascertain its presence and spread within a closed setting or wider population.

Selective fragment amplification typing methods

In recent years, a range of PCR-based approaches have been developed and used with varying degrees of success for characterising infection. These molecular methods tend to be relatively quick and can be sensitive and specific. A typical test can take only a few hours before a definitive result is known.

An increasing number of methods for nonculture diagnosis that detect and type infection are available. These are based on the amplification of genes specific to a certain organism or species such as 16S rRNA genes. The vast majority of reported methods only identify the presence of organisms without detailed characterisation.

There are initial trends towards the development of comprehensive diagnostic nonculture characterisation methods based on PCR, which can identify group, type and subtype, and in some cases further analysis of the appropriate genes (e.g., shotgun sequencing). However, a good example of the limited techniques available is the lack of a test to detect the expression of antimicrobial resistance, rather than simply presence and absence of genes responsible for resistance.

Developments in selective fragment amplification typing methods

The initial growth in molecular techniques started with the first licensed kit using nucleic-acid–based technology (Roche Diagnostics, Indianapolis) and has continued with yet another important growth in molecular typing techniques including real-time detection of PCR products and the move toward automation. New chemicals, such as TaqMan® and molecular beacons, have been developed commercially to provide real-time PCR that is also more sensitive than the equivalent gel-based system because it is fluorescence based. These chemistries have also allowed the further expansion of the applications of PCR into areas such as single nucleotide polymorphism (SNP) analysis whilst standard PCR has been developed into providing amplicons for microarray analysis. Automation has also recently become more affordable and therefore more accessible to standard laboratories. It is now used heavily in the pharmaceutical industry and more recently in academic research and clinical diagnostics.

The three probe chemistries currently used for real-time detection of PCR products are as follows:

- Hybridisation probes, a process of hybridisation of small oligonucleotide probes to specific target DNA
- Hydrolysis probes, which rely on the 5′-3′ exonuclease activity of Taq polymerase, which degrades a hybridised nonextendible DNA probe during the extension step of the PCR
- Hairpin probes, which contain a duplex region adjacent to a single-stranded target capture region

The basis of these three chemistries allows the elimination of post-PCR processing while allowing real-time anaylsis of PCR products produced during amplification. Hairpin probe chemistry includes molecular beacons, which are oligonucleotide probes that can report the presence of specific nucleic acid sequences. Molecular beacons are molecules with an internally quenched fluorophore whose fluorescence is restored when they bind to a target DNA sequence. They are designed in a way that allows the loop portion of the molecule to be the probe sequence for the target DNA.

The loop is attached to a stem formed by the annealing of complementary sequences of the probe sequence. On one arm of this stem is a fluorescent moiety, and a quenching moiety is attached to the end of the other arm. The function of the stem is to maintain the close proximity of both the fluorescent and quencher moieties. The quencher prevents fluorescence by converting the absorbing fluorescent energy into heat. Only when the target probe encounters a complementary target molecule will it form a hybrid that is long and stable enough to maintain a conformational reorganisation that forces the stem apart. This causes the two moieties to separate, leading to the reestablishment of fluorescence, which can be detected. This technology is continuing to develop and expand in the diagnostic field, and given the value of this technology combined with the potential value of automation it will continue to expand.

Gel-based characterisation methods

Systems that utilise various types of gels are commonly used for characterisation and population genetics; consequently isolates from infections can be characterised into limited numbers of genetically related types or clones each thought to contain strains with a common ancestry. A number of alternative techniques for the determination of the clonal types present in bacterial populations have been investigated, and these include but are not limited to pulse-field gel electrophoresis (PFGE), restriction fragment length polymorphism (RFLP), multiple-locus enzyme electrophoresis (MLEE), amplified fragment length polymorphism (AFLP) and fluorescent amplified fragment length polymorphism (FAFLP).

Pulsed-field gel electrophoresis

PFGE uses chromosomal DNA isolated from strains of target organisms and digested with restriction endonucleases that cut the chromosome into 10 to 40 fragments that are resolved into fingerprint patterns by the process of PFGE.

PFGE involves embedding your organism in agarose, lysing it, and digesting the DNA with restriction endonucleases that cleave occasionally. The resulting DNA fragments are reloaded into agarose wells, and the various fragments are resolved into a specific pattern within the gel by an apparatus that switches the direction of the current in a predetermined pattern. Consequently, it can be difficult when comparing similar strains from different laboratories. Although patterns produced are interpreted rather simply and quickly, they are stable for at least eight passages of the strain in vitro. PFGE is used for comparison of these fingerprints enabling distinction and identification of clonal subgroups of isolates and allows evaluation of genetic relationships between strains belonging to the same clonal subgroup.

Restriction fragment length polymorphism

RFLP is a technique in which organisms may be differentiated by analysis of patterns derived from cleavage of their DNA. If two organisms differ in the distance between sites of cleavage of a particular restriction endonuclease, the length of the fragments produced will differ when the DNA is digested with a restriction enzyme. The similarity of the patterns generated can be used to possibly differentiate strains from one another.

An example of an RFLP typing method was developed for *Neisseria meningitidis* in which a cloned *Eco*RI fragment from a serogroup B strain was used to probe Southern blots of total chromosomal DNA restriction fragments (enzyme *Ava*I). A group of 75 apparently unrelated organisms gave rise to 26 different RFLPs and two different groups of epidemiologically related strains had RFLP patterns that were distinct for each group. The technique was highly reproducible and discriminatory. The RFLP data were compared with the results of serotyping and subtyping and isoenzyme electrophoretic typing. These data were consistent with those from alternative typing methods. The use of RFLP typing technology has proven to be of considerable epidemiological value.

Multiple-locus enzyme electrophoresis

MLEE was long considered the gold standard for the molecular characterisation of disease-causing organisms. MLEE has been used for the genotyping of organisms of interest, to identify specific clones and to study the genetic diversity of selected species. Although the correlation between the electrophoretic migration of individual enzymes and the genotype may be disrupted by horizontal gene transfer, the use of multiple enzymes makes MLEE a moderately robust typing method.

MLEE was first described in 1966 as a molecular approach to the study of genetic variation in eukaryotic systems, and microbiologists have as described been able to incorporate MLEE as a highly useful molecular typing tool. MLEE is fundamentally based around the different electrophoretic mobilities of constitutive enzymes from different amino acid changes. These enzymes were chosen on the basis of their powers to discriminate and type all strains and therefore allow enhanced population and evolutionary studies. Although only a small number of variants are detected at each locus, analysing 20 or more loci can obtain a high level of resolution. MLEE does have many attractive features for global epidemiology and epidemic-associated strain characterisation. Nowadays this procedure is considered labour intensive, and it can be subjective, relying on uncharacterised genomic differences between isolates while producing results that are difficult to compare between different laboratories. Given the emphasis on global epidemiology, due to the ability of infections to spread over whole countries and continents, tools are now being developed that not only maintain the same level of discrimination but also are easy to compare between far-reaching laboratories.

Amplified fragment length polymorphism

AFLP is based on the selective PCR amplification of restriction fragments from a total digest of genomic DNA. Fingerprints are produced without prior sequence knowledge using a limited set of generic primers. This technique can be considered as a combination of the robustness and reliability of RFLP and the relative power of the PCR technique. The genomic fingerprinting process can be separated into three appropriate steps: (1) the restriction of the DNA and ligation of oligonucleotide adapters, (2) selective amplification of sets of restriction fragments, and (3) gel analysis of the amplified fragments using semiautomated scoring software of AFLP images. Additionally the PCR primers can be labeled fluorescently, and the dye-labeled fragments can be separated by capillary electorphoresis, which is still considered a suitable method of fragment analysis. Using a capillary electrophoresis system with appropriate size standards enables FAFLP with a usual fragment accuracy of +/− 1 bp. FAFLP can be used as a genotyping tool with a high resolution and accurate size determination.

Single-stranded conformational polymorphism analysis

Single-stranded conformational polymorphism (SSCP) was developed to obtain the subspecific typing information on organisms present in clinical samples such as blood and CSF. SSCP analysis of post-PCR products allows detection of single nucleotide point mutations within target DNA. This has been used to demonstrate the identities and nonidentities of infections between clinical specimens. The principle of this method is similar to the different SNP methods. SNPs can be considered highly abundant within bacterial genomes and, along with the tools available to determine the exact variant present in a DNA target sequence, are useful molecular investigation and typing tools.

Sequence-based detection and typing methods

Given the disadvantages of relying on uncharacterised genomic differences between isolates, sequence-based approaches have become the alternative to overcome this. DNA sequencing has many advantages over other methods that are used for local diagnostics and national and global epidemiology as well as to distinguish apparently identical strains identified by other methods. In recent years nucleotide sequencing has been applied to a wide range of diagnostic tools, genotyping and whole genomic sequencing and is now considered a gold standard in its own right. As with any high-profile application, nucleotide sequencing has received both praise and criticism, and certain nucleotide sequencing methods are still considered prohibitively expensive for routine diagnostic testing. This could be considered a misconception, as cost may have been justified over a decade ago when the development of molecular technology and recombinant DNA technology promised breakthroughs of an unprecedented level. Since these initial developments, the attitude of scientific thought has encouraged nucleotide sequencing to develop in many different areas. Unfortunately, certain perceptions have not evolved with the same vigor and accomplishment. Nucleotide sequencing systems now have many attractive features, such as high throughput, relative low consumable costs and not only good intralaboratory reproducibility but also interlaboratory reproducibility. After initial capital startup costs of £50,000 to £150,000, depending on

throughput requirements, the nucleotide sequencing costs are low. Examples include multilocus sequence typing (MLST), a method which has gained much credibility for bacterial population biology analysis since it was first described in 1998. Novel techniques often require high levels of specialisation and complexity and when compared to older and more familiar techniques may fuel skepticism; therefore, initial concerns are justified. Not surprisingly, as nucleotide sequencing has become widely used and the chemistry cheaper, the actual costs involved have been reduced dramatically. Some costs have been reduced by over 60%; for example, the average cost for sequencing 600 nucleotides on both strands is as low as £2. This includes all processes involved in sample preparation, sequence setup, and data handling. In conclusion, nucleotide sequencing should now be accepted as a cost-effective method for molecular investigations and bacterial typing that is readily available, affordable and as easily utilized as any technique presently available.

Multilocus sequence typing

MLST was developed as a method for the differentiation of strains that appear identical by standard phenotypic typing methods. The method can be used during outbreaks of infection, and at a time when sequencing has become a valuable tool, a number of laboratories already have started using molecular techniques as a way of detection and detailed characterisation. MLST produces nucleotide sequence data of approximately 500 base-pair segments from seven housekeeping genes providing results that are digital and therefore highly portable between laboratories.

MLST was first validated on *N. meningitidis* by Maiden and colleagues. This method was originally evaluated on *N. meningitidis* because it provides a good example in which genetic recombination events are considered common. Originally MLST for *N. meningitidis* centered on 10 loci from isolates that had been previously characterised. The *N. meningitidis* MLST housekeeping genes were subsequently reduced to use 7 loci on the basis of its discriminatory power. This unique method was applied to a collection of 107 *N. meningitidis* isolates from invasive disease and healthy carriers that had been previously characterised by MLEE. MLST has now been validated for a wide range of important bacteria and fungi including *Bordetella pertussis*, *Campylobacter jejuni*, *Candida albicans*, *Enterococcus faecalis*, *Enterococcus faecium*, *Escherichia coli*, *Haemophilus influenzae*, *Listeria monocytogenes*, salmonella, *Staphylococcus aureus*, *Streptococcus pneumoniae*, *Streptococcus pyogenes* and *Streptococcus suis*. The method is based on the well-tested principle of MLEE that, as mentioned, assigns a gel-based profile indirectly from the electrophoretic mobilities of gene products.

This can be incorporated with similar enhanced systems in most laboratories as a routine method and consequently can provide data that are useful for the public health management of clusters or outbreaks in institutions such as schools, and also for general disease surveillance on a regional and national basis.

Molecular techniques, sequencing, and interpretation of sequence data can be considered holistically as multilocus sequence analysis (MLSA). MLSA can be a useful diagnostic and epidemiological tool and provide greater knowledge to the genetic variation that can occur with a species population. The sequence data obtained from such systems as MLST and subsequent analysis can determine population structures by analysing the extent of linkage disequilibrium between alleles and observing the recombination by the noncongruence of gene trees and by the presence of significant mosaic structures. For highly clonal species, the phylogenetic relationship between isolates can be inferred from the dendrogram derived from the pairwise differences between sequence types (STs) and independently from a consensus tree constructed from the gene sequence. MLSA (Fig. 64.3) is valuable for the identification of currently circulating hypervirulent lineages as these are recognised as clusters of isolates with identical or very similar sequence types. Although nucleotide differences between alleles can go unscrutinised with just a simple allocation of an allele number and an ST, these nucleotide differences can determine the evolution of given alleles using nucleotide sequence analysis programs.

ST	Frequency	Single locus variants	Double locus variants	Satellites
352	1	1	2	0
275*	4	2	0	1
269	8	0	1	2
1273	1	1	1	1

Summary view:

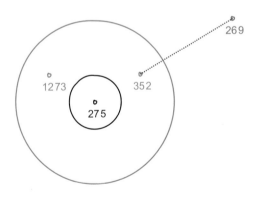

SLV ST
DLV ST
SAT ST
.... SLV Link
.... DLV Link

SLV – Single locus variant
DLV – Double locus variant
SAT – satellite isolate

Fig. 64.3 Comparison of 14 meningococcal isolates with a range of sequence types.

Matrix-assisted laser desorption/ionisation time-of-flight (MALDI-TOF) analysis

MALDI-TOF mass spectrometry has become, in recent years, a tool of choice for large-molecule analysis. Essentially MALDI-TOF is a technique for measuring large molecular masses precisely and is accurate enough to detect the differences between single nucleotides. The principle of using bacterially identified reference strains as a marker could be used to detect differences in specific DNA sequences and is a technique now widely used in many diagnostic microbiology services.

Pyrosequencing

Fundamentally, pyrosequencing involves the synthesis of a number of different chemicals, which enables a fast and accurate analysis of DNA sequences. After DNA amplification and subsequent single-stranded DNA formation, a sequencing primer is hybridised to its complement sequence on the template prior to the sequence of interest. Incubated enzymes are added with substrates to catalyse the incorporation of deoxynucleotide triphosphates (dNTP) into the DNA strand if it is complementary. Each incorporation event is accompanied by release of pyrophosphate (PPi) in a quantity equimolar to the amount of incorporated nucleotide. A complex cascade reaction follows that results in the generation of visible light in amounts proportional to the amount of dNTP originally incorporated. This is detected by a charged coupled device (CCD) camera and finally represented as a peak in a pyrogram displayed on a computer screen (Fig. 64.4). As the process continues, the complementary DNA strand is built up and the nucleotide sequence is determined from the collection of signal peaks in the pyrogram. The reaction is simple and robust and the technology can be adapted to create dedicated tools for specific applications (Fig. 64.4).

There are a few limitations in the function of pyrosequencing for sequence typing. The initial concerns are the limitation in read length. Most typing systems use nucleotide sequences, which are longer than those currently achieved with pyrosequencing (range of 50–200 bp). However, with the development of improved enzymes and substrates, this limiting factor could be overcome and the possibility of using this system to produce hundreds of base-pairs of high-quality sequence would bring this technology closer towards other well-established sequence systems. The development of different instrument versions has increased the current capacity, with the utilisation of both 96-well and 384-well formats.

Currently, pyrosequencing is used in a wide range of applications investigating polymorphisms, point mutations, identification, and characterisation studies. These use either single nucleotide polymorphisms or short nucleotide sequence to identify and differentiate. The main areas that have utilised pyrosequencng are pharmacogenomics and microbial typing. Common themes arising from these areas include the analysis of genes, proteins and single nucleotide polymorphisms. This can include genotyping and characterising microorganisms and their drug-resistant profiles, detailed analysis of genes responsible for housekeeping functions such as transport and drug metabolism, and the

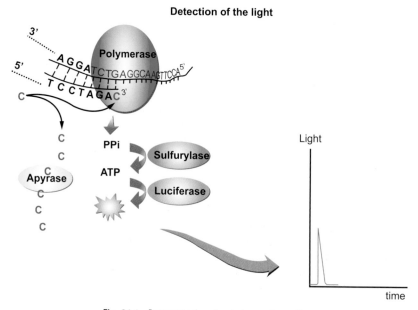

Fig. 64.4 Pyrosequencing chemical cascade reaction.

assessment of patient susceptibility. These applications can provide a greater insight into the identification, characterisation and treatment of both causative organisms and the corresponding susceptible host. The anticipated benefits of using sequencing technology within pharmacogenomics could include more powerful medicines based on the proteins, enzymes, DNA and RNA molecules associated with genes of disease; better, safer drugs the first time, instead of the standard trial-and-error method of matching patients with the right drugs; more accurate methods of determining appropriate drug dosages based on an individual person's genetics rather than dosages based on weight and size; advanced screening of disease through DNA or RNA vaccines that would be tailormade for a population; and a decrease in the overall cost of health care if the number of adverse drug reactions were decreased and effective treatment was increased.

Microarrays

Microarray expression analysis has become one of the most widely functional genomics tools. Microarrays are DNA segments representing a collection of genes or the various combinations of a single gene to be assayed. These are amplified by PCR and mechanically spotted at high density on glass microscope slides using simple x-y-z stage robotic systems. This results in a microarray containing thousands of elements. These microarrays can easily be constructed within a relatively short period of time. Using fluorescent-based technology, hybridisation of complement DNA segments upon the microarray with target DNA can be detected and immediately identified. This has already been reported for the discrimination of six gene sequences, which are representatives of different bacterial identification assays for *Escherichia coli gyrA, Salmonella gyrA, Campylobacter gyrA, E. coli parC, Staphlococcus mecA* and *Chlamydia* cryptic plasmid. It was also reported to have the ability of discriminating strains carrying antibiotic resistance single-nucleotide polymorphism mutations. Microarrays are simple characterisation processes, allowing minimal processing of samples and required practical experience after system setup. The limitations with such a new technology include cost and the practicality within laboratories with limited resources and technical support. The challenge with such a technology is to find ways in which it can be used to study different aspects of the bacterial population—for example, the comparison of selected genes expressed by a pathogenic strain compared with that expressed by a nonpathogenic strain by hybridisation to an array made from the genome of the pathogenic strain. In this way, this method could be used to develop DNA arrays that are suitable for both diagnosis and typing of bacterial species commonly associated with infection.

Whole genome sequencing

In recent years, there has been an increase in the use of next generation sequencing (NGS), which for some epidemiological situations could be considered the gold standard in its own right. As with any high-profile application, NGS has received both praise and criticism, with common themes mainly around cost of testing and complexity in interpretation. Currently within the diagnostic laboratory setting this may well be justified; however, breakthroughs of an unprecedented scale have encouraged both academic and industrial research to develop different areas in an attempt to mitigate these common challenges. Unfortunately, clinical institutions have not evolved with the same vigour or accomplishment and it's reasonable to summarise, more clinical facilities do not have these techniques within their services than those that do. However, this does not mean little exposure to such technology, as there is increasing evidence clinical services are collaborating with academic and industrial partners in utilising such technology with increasing regularity.

Novel techniques often require high levels of specialisation and complexity and when compared to older and more familiar techniques may fuel scepticism; therefore, initial concerns are justified. Not surprisingly, as NGS becomes more widely used, the chemistry cheaper, and interpretation quicker the actual costs in time and money will reduce further. Thus NGS like many other novel molecular techniques in the past will eventually become a cost-effective method for the profiling of sample types and characterisation of isolates, as well as readily available, affordable and as easily utilised as any technique presently available.

KEY CHALLENGES FOR THE FUTURE

We've seen huge developments in molecular diagnostics in the past decade. Many technologies that were originally exclusively used within research have now become more refined and user friendly. At the same time, there has been a marked decrease in the cost of those technologies, a combination that has made them more applicable to the needs of a routine clinical laboratory. When these changes were new, clinical virology laboratories were natural early adopters because the advantages (in terms of time, cost and labor savings) offered by molecular techniques were so overwhelming when compared to traditional techniques such as cell culture. But since then, the other areas of clinical microbiology have also begun using genetic and molecular testing to inform their conclusions. The technology is useful: it shows increased sensitivity and specificity over traditional phenotypic diagnostic methods and often yields better reproducibility. In fact, "black box" technologies that automate laboratory tasks have shown advantages in reduced hands-on time, quick turnaround time to result and reliability. These advantages have real benefits for patient care and the quality of the support we can provide. The data also help us to better understand infection and prevention in hospital and community settings, as well as provide the tools to continually improve and challenge ourselves. However, if we opt to employ new technologies, especially ones that automate laboratory tasks that were previously our responsibility, we need to ensure that we aren't sacrificing a complete and detailed understanding of the diagnostic process.

More information, even with regard to identifying and characterising disease, doesn't always mean a better outcome for us or the patient. It forces us to ask ourselves, "What does this information mean?" And sometimes, having so much data to interpret can even be a disadvantage. Where we might previously have obtained a negative test result, we might now get a positive one; where we might previously have had a single positive result, we now have multiple results to interpret and weigh against one another. In adopting new technologies, we risk reducing our understanding of the reasons we conduct a given test. The initial stages of clinical diagnosis, especially the selection of appropriate tests, have been an important part of the diagnostic role. But if people don't fully understand how and why certain testing is done, it becomes much harder to identify what's truly needed, and we run the risk of "screen" testing, which if inappropriate can be as dangerous as not testing at all. Risks like these might make laboratory professionals want to return to older methods where results were more familiar and interpretation simpler.

Rather than sacrifice the technological gains we've made since molecular diagnostics came to the fore, it's important to work out a balance and there's no one right way of doing this.

It's true that the costs of molecular diagnostics are dropping rapidly. For some time, they followed a Moore-law-esque trend of steady decrease; however, after next-generation sequencing eclipsed Sanger-based methods in 2008, the drop was precipitous. However, our priorities shouldn't be focused on getting as much data as possible because with that as our goal, we may end up getting so much information that we can't translate it all into clinical services. It's important to ask ourselves what clinical value any given piece of information might have—and then to make the case for acquiring that information to the people responsible for funding its acquisition. This is especially true when these costs go beyond a single test (for instance, buying a new piece of equipment or hiring a new staff member with specialised skills).

Moreover, these challenges are not unique to any one lab. It's difficult to establish strategies for advancement when there's no good one-size-fits-all solution to present, but there's a lot to be gained by communicating with other pathologists and learning what they're doing. For labs that are trying to increase or improve their use of molecular diagnostics, one should stop the "silo mentality" we tend to prefer and instead develop strong networks. Share best practices, collaborate with other pathology centers and break down the divisions between clinical and academic environments. The same applies to liaisons between health care, academia and industry, three sectors that have historically treated one another with some trepidation. There's a lot we can learn from one another, and a lot of opportunities to be gained from making connections between different professional groups.

The rise of molecular diagnostics, and our need to manage and streamline large amounts of information, has presented us with unique challenges we're still learning to address. But this isn't the first time pathology has tackled such a radical change. In the beginnings of the profession, even identifying the organism associated with a clinical presentation was difficult and confusing, but we didn't step back; we carried on, trying to understand. We can see the same process happening today. As long as we remember that more doesn't always mean better, and focus on using collaboration and prioritisation to make things better for our patients, then molecular diagnostics will prove to be not only an impressive but also a useful tool.

RECOMMENDED READING

Dolinger, D. L., & Whalen, A. M. (2016). Molecular diagnostics and the changing face of point-of-care. *Molecular Microbiology* (ASM) Jan 1, 545–555.

Ledeboer, N. (2016). Automation advances microbiology to operational excellence. *MLO Med Lab Obs*, 2016 May;48(5):8–11.

Peruski, L. F., Jr., & Peruski, A. H. (2016). Molecular diagnostic approaches in infectious disease. *Nucleic Acid Testing for Human Disease*, Ch13, 331.

Spitzer, E. D. (December 2012). Molecular microbiology: Diagnostic principles and practice. In D. H. Persing, F. C. Tenover, Y.-W. Tang, F. S. Nolte, R. T. Hayden, & A. van Belkum (Eds.), *The quarterly review of biology* (Vol. 87, no. 4, pp. 393).

Russell, M., & Dixon, C. (2016). Using case studies as a tool to teach laboratory techniques and principles in a clinical molecular diagnostics laboratory. *Clinical Laboratory Science: Journal of the American Society for Medical Technology*, 29(2).

Yusuf, E., & Goossens, H. (2017). Capturing rapidly evolving molecular medical microbiology. *Lancet*, 17(4), 379.

65 Management of antimicrobial chemotherapy

DAVID R. JENKINS

KEY POINTS

- Antimicrobials exploit differences in microbial and host structures and produce toxicity to the microbes, which is referred to as 'selective toxicity'.
- There are four broad classes of antimicrobials: antibacterial, antiviral, antifungal and antiparasitic, and it is generally the case that agents active against one class of microbe are inactive against other classes.
- Given the distinct differences between prokaryotes and eukaryotes, the antibacterial class of antimicrobials contains the widest range of drugs.
- A major function of clinical microbiology laboratories is to perform antibacterial susceptibility testing on the causative organisms of infection.
- Antibacterial susceptibility testing combines antibacterial pharmacokinetics (the entry, distribution and elimination of drugs in the patient's body) and pharmacodynamics (the effect of the drug on the microorganism) and provides a result that indicates the likelihood that an infection at a specific site with a given bacterium treated with a stated drug will result in cure of the infection.
- The aim of antimicrobial therapy is to cure the patient. The causative organism, patient factors (i.e., age, renal and hepatic function etc.) and the processes (i.e., local and national antimicrobial guidelines) determine choice of antimicrobial agent.
- The ability of some bacteria to collect resistance genes on transferable DNA has led to clinically important bacteria becoming multidrug-resistant (MDR). Concurrent with the rise in MDR bacteria, there has been a virtual halt in the development and introduction into clinical practice of new antibacterial classes.
- Antimicrobial stewardship through the development and implementation of a coherent set of actions aims to extend the effectiveness of antibiotics for as long as possible.

PRINCIPLES OF ANTIMICROBIAL THERAPY

The discovery and clinical exploitation of antimicrobials is based on the selective toxicity of antimicrobials for target microbes. That is, antimicrobials have a lethal action on clinically important viruses, bacteria, fungi or parasites, while having no or little harmful effect on human cellular metabolism or physiology (or animal cells in the case of veterinary medicine). The basis for selective toxicity is the difference between the molecular structures and biochemical pathways of microbes and host cells.

Antimicrobials primarily work by binding to microbe macromolecules, either reversibly or irreversibly, thereby interfering with microbial physiology by distorting microbial molecular structures. This can either result in an impaired cellular structure, for example, in the case of a protein essential for cell wall synthesis and integrity, or impaired cellular function, if the antimicrobial distorts the active site of an enzyme, for example.

The challenge posed to antimicrobial development by selective toxicity is to exploit differences between microbial and host structures in a way that produces worthwhile toxicity in microbes while leaving the host sufficiently unharmed as to make the antimicrobial clinically acceptable. To illustrate how hard this challenge is, consider that, at the time of writing in 2017, no novel antibacterial has been developed since 1987 that has progressed to established clinical use. Then consider that antibacterial development should be the easiest class of antimicrobials to develop, given the major differences between the prokaryotic cells of bacteria and the eukaryotic cells of hosts.

Antivirals have relatively few opportunities to target, given the stripped-down nature of viral metabolism and the major reliance of viral replication pathways on host biochemistry. The development of antifungal and antiparasitic agents is also problematic because microbes have eukaryotic cell structures and are consequently identical in many ways to the host. The fact that effective and safe antimicrobials exist for an extensive range of microbes is an impressive achievement.

Not all antimicrobials are the same. Reference has already been made to the classification of antimicrobials into the broad division of antivirals, antibacterials, antifungals and antiparasitic agents, and it is generally the case that agents active against one class of microbe are inactive against other classes. Within these classes, there are further subdivisions; antivirals are only effective against certain groups of viruses, and there are similar subdivisions for antibacterials, antifungals and antiparasitic agents, so the clinical use of antimicrobials requires a knowledge of both the identity of the infecting organism and its susceptibility to different classes of antimicrobials. The basis of this selectivity is again structural—antimicrobials can be categorised into chemically related structural families, and it is broadly true that chemically related antimicrobials have a similar antimicrobial action. However, although molecular studies have provided many insights into the actions of antimicrobials, it is still the case that designer drugs, synthesised from first principles to have specific actions, are a distant aspiration.

Given the distinct differences between prokaryotes and eukaryotes, it is perhaps not surprising that the antibacterial class of antimicrobials contains the widest range of drugs so that all the major classes of clinically important bacteria are covered. To a large extent, the range of activity of antibacterials is coterminous with the most frequently used ways of classifying bacteria. Thus, antibacterials can be grouped according to their actions against Gram-positive or Gram-negative bacteria, against Enterobacteriaceae or Pseudomonads and against aerobes or anaerobes. This convenient finding is not entirely serendipitous; categorisation of bacteria in the 19th and 20th century was predominantly on the basis of structure (Gram stain) or metabolic activity (lactose fermentation, aerobic/anaerobic activity), and these properties are exactly those that underlie the basis of antibacterial action. The clinical importance of different bacteria has also driven antibacterial development; major Gram-positive pathogens such as *Staphylococcus aureus* and beta-haemolytic streptococci were early targets of antibacterial development, mostly using naturally occurring antibacterials—antibiotics—as a starting point. A major function of clinical microbiology laboratories is to perform antibacterial susceptibility testing on the causative organisms of infection. A major function of clinical microbiologists is to provide advice to clinicians on the best antibacterial to use to treat or prevent significant bacterial infections, based on susceptibility testing of isolated pathogens or inferred susceptibility based on knowledge of the common causative organisms of infectious conditions.

PRINCIPLES OF IN VITRO SUSCEPTIBILITY TESTING AND THE DIFFERENT METHODS

As implied earlier in the chapter, antibacterials have selective activity against different bacterial species. Bacteria susceptible to one class of antibacterial may be resistant to another. Resistance can be innate, expressed as a wild-type phenotype (for example, all enterococci are resistant to all cephalosporins), or can develop through either spontaneous mutation of bacterial chromosomal DNA or by the acquisition of preexisting resistance genes on transferable DNA, notably plasmids. Mechanisms of acquired resistance include changes in the molecular structure of antibacterial targets; overproduction of the target molecule; reduced uptake of the antibacterial into the bacterial cell; increased elimination of the antibacterial from the bacterial cell; increased breakdown of the antibiotic by bacterial enzymes; and by-passing of antibacterial-inhibited metabolism through new pathways.

Consequently, while general statements can be made regarding the usual susceptibility of a specific wild-type bacterial species to a chosen antibacterial, the possibility of acquired resistance can never be discounted. While acquired resistance may be a rare event for some bacterial species, *Neisseria meningitidis*, for example, acquired resistance to a wide range of antibiotics is a frequent and serious problem in other species, *Neisseria gonorrhoeae* being a clinically important instance of this. A consequence of the possibility of unpredictable resistance is the need to test empirically the susceptibility of bacteria cultured from clinical specimens if antibacterial treatment of an infection is required.

The primary aim of antibacterial susceptibility testing (AST) is to provide a guide to the appropriate clinical use of antibacterials in the treatment of infections. AST combines antibacterial pharmacokinetics (the entry, distribution and elimination of drugs in the patient's body) and pharmacodynamics (the effect of the drug on the microorganism) and provides a result that indicates the likelihood that an infection at a specific site with a given bacterium treated with a stated drug will result in cure of the infection.

A key parameter that is foundational to AST is the minimal inhibitory concentration (MIC) of a bacterium–drug pairing. The MIC is the minimal concentration of the antibacterial required to inhibit (note: not kill) the growth of the microorganism in a defined in vitro setting. For example, the MIC of vancomycin and an isolate of *Staph. aureus* may be 0.5 mg/L, indicating that a concentration of vancomycin of 0.5 mg/L inhibits the growth of this particular isolate of *Staph. aureus* in these test conditions. The MIC is not a fixed value for a given species-antibacterial pair because it may vary between different isolates of the same species of bacteria. It is typically the case that a population of independent isolates of the same species tested against the same antibacterial will have slightly different MICs so that an MIC frequency plot will have the appearance of a normal curve. Consequently, MICs can be described for populations of a bacterial species by adding a subscript such as 50 or 99 (MIC_{50}, MIC_{99}) to indicate the MIC for 50% or 99% of the population. MICs can also vary in value for the same isolate–antibiotic pairing due to differences in measurement methodology, culture media and measurement error, and this variation should be taken into account when using the result for clinical purposes.

The standard approach to MIC measurement is based on growing the test isolate in a series of doubling dilutions of the antibiotic, as exemplified by the microbroth dilution method. As a consequence, MIC measurements are commonly distributed along a doubling or halving scale with the origin at 1 mg/L. Microbroth dilution is not a convenient method for MIC measurement in routine clinical laboratories, so alternative, simpler methods have been developed. These include placing a commercially prepared strip containing a gradient of antibiotic along its length onto an agar plate seeded with a suspension of the test isolate and incubating the plate for an appropriate duration, usually overnight (Fig. 65.1A). Antibiotic diffuses from the strip in such a way as to create a concentration gradient in the agar alongside the strip. At antibiotic concentrations greater than the MIC, bacterial growth abutting the strip will be inhibited and there will be a zone of no growth. At antibiotic concentrations less than the MIC, bacterial growth will occur up to the strip. The concentration at which this occurs, and which is taken as the MIC, can be read off a scale printed on the strip (Fig. 65.1B).

Automated, machine-based methods for providing MIC methods are also available. These methods, which usually provide an identification of the isolate too, are often aimed at providing MIC measurements for large numbers of isolates with minimal user involvement. They offer a reproducible, standardised and often faster approach to MIC measurement compared with manual methods, but depend on expensive machinery that must be either bought or hired.

It should be emphasised that MIC measurements carried out by different methodologies can provide results that vary considerably, and the differences can be clinically significant. For example, MIC measurements for *Staph. aureus*–vancomycin can vary between microbroth and gradient strip methods to an extent that the gradient strip method would indicate a successful outcome to treatment, while the microbroth method would indicate likely failure. These concerns also affect automated methods of

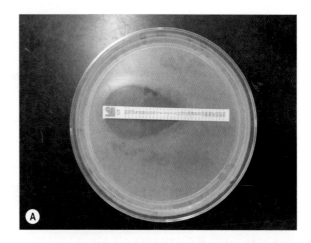

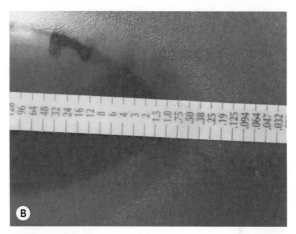

Fig. 65.1 A, E-test determination of ceftolozane-tazobactam/*Pseudomonas aeruginosa* MIC. B, Close-up.

susceptibility testing. Generally, the microbroth method is taken as the gold-standard approach and is recommended if knowing an accurate MIC is critical, even if this means referring the isolate to a specialist laboratory for testing.

1. While MICs underlie susceptibility testing, in practice, the large majority of antibiotic sensitivity testing carried out in clinical laboratories aims to categorise an isolate as either sensitive, intermediate or resistant to an antibiotic, without providing a numerical value, through the use of commercially prepared paper discs accurately loaded with the test antibiotic. These discs are placed on an agar plate freshly seeded with a suspension of bacteria and incubated overnight (Figs. 65.2 and 65.3).

   After incubation, there should be confluent bacterial growth over the entire surface of the

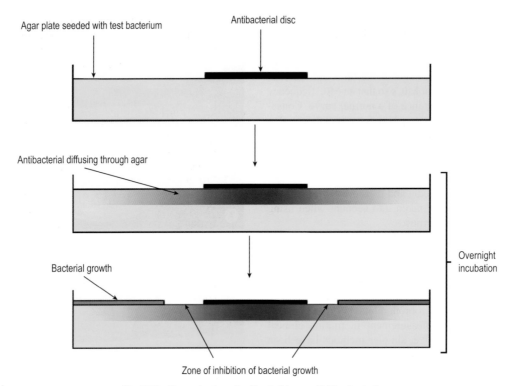

Agar plate seeded with test bacterium

Antibacterial disc

Antibacterial diffusing through agar

Overnight incubation

Bacterial growth

Zone of inhibition of bacterial growth

Fig. 65.2 The mechanism of antibacterial susceptibility disc testing.

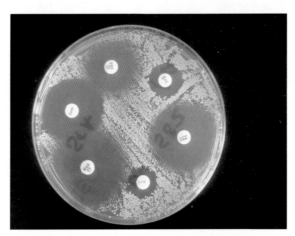

Fig. 65.3 Antibacterial susceptibility disc testing of *Staph. aureus*.

plate except in areas where the antibiotic concentration in the agar is such that it prevents growth. This is typified by clear circular zones of no growth around the antibiotic discs. The diameters of the no-growth zones are determined by the susceptibility of the bacterial isolate to the antibiotic. Bacteria with greater susceptibility to a particular antibiotic have a larger zone of no growth compared to more resistant bacteria. Bacteria can be categorised as sensitive, intermediate or resistant by measurement of the zone size and comparison of this measurement to diameters known as breakpoints.

Breakpoints are parameters that are derived from MICs and so depend on bacterial species–antibiotic pairings. They also take into account pharmacokinetic and pharmacodynamic considerations that are designed to ensure that, when an isolate is described as sensitive, licensed doses of antibiotics are likely to produce clinically effective tissue concentrations in the large majority of infected patients despite variation in body mass, hepatic metabolism and renal excretory function. Conversely, a zone size that is less than the breakpoint indicates that the isolate is resistant to the test antibiotic, meaning that licensed antibiotic doses are unlikely to provide effective therapy of infections caused by this isolate.

2. Zone sizes are not comparable between different bacteria–antibiotic combinations. Some bacteria–antibiotic combinations have small diameter breakpoints, while others are far larger. A small zone size does not necessarily mean resistance, and, conversely, a large zone size does not

automatically infer sensitivity. In each case, the zone size must be compared with the stated breakpoint for the specific bacterial species–antibiotic combination.

3. Breakpoints are set to avoid splitting wild-type MIC distributions into resistant and sensitive groups. Accordingly, breakpoints are not the same as the highest MIC of organisms lacking phenotypically expressed resistance, a value known as the epidemiological cut-off value (ECOFF). In routine clinical laboratory work, the breakpoint is the workhorse of the susceptibility-testing bench. However, not all bacterial species–antibiotic combinations have a defined breakpoint. This may be due to insufficient isolates of a particular species to allow a breakpoint designation, a new antibiotic only recently becoming available or changes in the formulation or dose presentation of an antibiotic or inherent phenotypic resistance to an antibiotic class. Consequently, occasions arise when it may be wished to use an unorthodox antibiotic because of patient factors (allergy to other more usual choices, problems with access for administration or metabolism/elimination) or bacterial features (resistance to alternatives) but where no breakpoint exists to support alternative antibiotic choices. In such circumstances, MIC measurement, and possibly comparison to the ECOFF, may provide guidance as to the suitability of an antibiotic.

4. Various schemes have been developed over the years that provide laboratories with catalogues of zone sizes for different bacteria–antibiotic combinations that allow this categorisation. The two preeminent schemes currently are the Clinical and Laboratory Standards Institute (CLSI) and European Committee on Antimicrobial Susceptibility Testing (EUCAST) schemes. Though similar in principle, they are not identical, differing in structure of their governing bodies, access (the EUCAST methodology is open access, but access to CLSI requires a subscription) and their interpretation of zone sizes. As a consequence, some bacteria–antibiotic combinations with identical zone sizes are categorised differently between the two schemes, although there are ongoing discussions aimed at eliminating these disparities.

Empiric and directed therapy

1. Susceptibility testing provides guidance for the treatment of the individual patient from whom the bacterial isolate was collected. Typically, up to six antibiotic-containing discs are placed on an agar plate freshly seeded with a suspension of the bacterial isolate and the resultant zones of no growth are interpreted through comparison with breakpoints to indicate whether the organism is sensitive or resistant to the antibiotic. For some bacterial species–antibiotic pairings, there is a third alternative—intermediate—that can be interpreted as indicating likely susceptibility to increased doses of the antibiotic.

2. The choice of antibiotic discs to use in susceptibility testing is primarily driven by the treatment protocols for specific infectious conditions that are, in turn, based on the usual susceptibility patterns of the most likely pathogens to cause these infections. Thus, the selection of antibiotic discs is an iterative process that relies on the outcome of previous susceptibility testing and clinical response to local treatment protocols. The local availability of antibiotics for treatment will also play an important part in the selection of antibiotic discs. Another factor in the choice of discs is the requirement to detect changes in patterns of resistance. Expert rules have been developed that set out patterns of expected intrinsic resistance and provide alerts for the flagging of new, exceptional resistance instances. Mechanisms of resistance can also be inferred from the results of disc testing. This highlights a role for antibiotic susceptibility testing in infection control and public health—alerting a hospital's infection control service to the presence of new resistance patterns can prevent spread of resistant bacteria, and contributing to regional and national surveillance systems can help identify wider spread, emerging problems in resistance.

3. The process of antibiotic susceptibility testing is completed by the provision of a report to the requesting clinician. Typically, this identifies the pathogen and its susceptibility to a number of antibiotics. Not all the antibiotics tested need necessarily be reported. As highlighted earlier in the chapter, some susceptibility testing might be carried out in order to detect resistance mechanisms, and the antibiotics used for this purpose may not be clinically available or relevant. In addition, there is increasingly a desire to use the susceptibility testing report to drive clinical use of antibiotics in a particular direction, as part of an antibiotic stewardship process. Accordingly, many laboratories routinely suppress some of the antibiotic results, releasing

the results of only a few of the antibiotic tests carried out.

4. Using the antibacterial susceptibility results of a bacterial isolate to determine treatment choice for the patient from whom the isolate was cultured is termed *directed therapy* and increases the probability of a successful outcome. However, most antibiotic treatment in both primary and secondary care is empirical, in that treatment is commenced before the susceptibility of the causative pathogen is established or, frequently, even before its identity is known. Empirical treatment is therefore less assured of success, but in practice most empirical antibiotic choices lead to cure. This does not devalue antibiotic susceptibility testing since empirical prescribing is based on the accumulated results of microbiological examination of specimens from previous patients with similar clinical presentations. Thus, antibiotic susceptibility testing supports the development of local empirical prescribing guidelines, providing clinicians faced with a specific clinical picture with informed conjecture of the probable identity and susceptibility of bacterial pathogens. The development of local empirical prescribing guidelines based on up-to-date results of susceptibility tests is a vital part of a modern clinical microbiology laboratory's duties.

Selecting the right agent

1. Whether antibiotic treatment is guided by susceptibility testing or empirically chosen, usually there is more than one antibiotic that can be reasonably selected as a suitable choice. Proof of this can be had by comparing antibiotic guidelines from different but similar health-care organisations, something that is facilitated by the ready availability of guidelines on websites and smartphone apps; virtually no two organisations' guidelines are identical. Given that the identity of pathogens causing identical clinical conditions does not vary significantly around the world, the reasons for variation in recommended antibiotic choices fall into the following categories: pathogen (variation in susceptibility profiles, e.g., locally high prevalence of meticillin-resistant *Staph. aureus* [MRSA] as a cause of skin and soft tissue infection); patient (case mix variation, e.g., high proportion of patients with renal or liver failure); and process (e.g., variation in availability of antibiotics due to cost, licensing or manufacturer supply restrictions, and ability to

carry out therapeutic drug monitoring). Restrictions may fall into more than one category, for example, local (process) restrictions on cephalosporin availability in order to reduce *Clostridium difficile* infections (pathogen). Finally, variation may also be accounted for by the personal, not always rational, views and experience of individuals or committees who compile antibiotic guidelines.

2. Given the potential for choice, prescribers and those clinicians in charge of constructing guidelines should ideally work advised by a number of principles when selecting antibiotic therapy. First and foremost, the antibiotic should be reliably active against the likely pathogens causing a specific infection, which means that, in addition to in vitro activity of the antibiotic against the target organisms, the pharmacokinetics of the antibacterial consistently predict effective concentrations at the site of infection. This can be a particular challenge for some infection types where barriers to diffusion of the antibacterial from the bloodstream to the infected tissue prevent attainment of effective concentrations. Examples of such infections include meningitis, endophthalmitis and bone infections, all of which occur behind hard-to-penetrate anatomical-physiological barriers.

3. Routes of administration are an important consideration. Although there is a growing enthusiasm for providing intravenous antibiotics in an outpatient setting, or even in the patient's own home, through the establishment of outpatient parenteral antibiotic therapy (OPAT) services, most outpatient or community antibiotic prescribing is practically limited to orally administered antibiotics. This restriction means that some entire antibiotic families, including aminoglycosides, glycopeptides and carbapenems, are completely removed from consideration for inclusion in primary care or outpatient prescribing guidelines because they require intravenous administration.

4. Another important consideration is the propensity of antibiotics to cause adverse effects. These can be predictable, dose-related toxicities, including nephrotoxicity associated with aminoglycosides; idiosyncratic adverse effects, notably allergic reactions; drug–drug interactions, particularly affecting drugs that compete with antibiotics for metabolic pathways such as the cytochrome P450 enzyme system; and ecological effects, especially those affecting the large bowel microbiota where a significant risk is the selection of *Clostridium*

difficile by antibiotics, or antibiotic metabolites with residual antibacterial activity, entering the gut lumen as a consequence of hepatic metabolism and biliary excretion.

5. Some adverse effects are only relevant to certain age groups or physiological states (e.g., bone and dental discolouration by tetracyclines in foetuses and children). Other adverse effects are more likely in patients with abnormal liver or renal function when impaired organ function can lead to accumulation of antibiotics to toxic levels.

6. Some antibiotics have a narrow therapeutic index, meaning that there is a narrow range of drug concentrations where therapeutic efficacy can be expected without unacceptable risks of toxicity. Prime examples of such antibiotics include the aminoglycosides and vancomycin. When such drugs are prescribed, it is standard and necessary practice to monitor blood drug levels to ensure the patient is receiving a sufficient amount, but not too much, of the medication. An example of such therapeutic drug monitoring (TDM) is pre-dose (trough) assay of vancomycin.

   Standard approaches to gentamicin TDM include the use of a nomogram that relates the serum concentration of gentamicin to the frequency of subsequent doses, although the reliability of nomograms has been questioned. Advances in population pharmacokinetics have led to sophisticated software packages that, given serum assay results and renal function parameters, can accurately predict drug clearance and so calculate optimum doses for maximum efficacy and minimal toxicity. Such approaches are increasingly being introduced into the care of critically ill patients, where such optimisation may make a difference between survival and death.

7. Other factors to consider include patient acceptability of an antibiotic. For example, flucloxacillin syrup and other drugs with unpleasant tastes are unlikely to be accepted by infants. Multiple daily doses and long courses of antibiotics are less likely to be taken as prescribed than single daily doses or short courses of treatment.

8. An important consideration is the price of the antibiotic. Many older antibiotics are remarkably cheap given their life-saving properties. However, newer antibacterials can be extremely expensive. Health-care payers are frequently reluctant to fund placement of these drugs onto local antibiotic guidelines unless these medicines offer substantial benefits over existing treatments.

Pharmacodynamics

1. In addition to the choice of antibiotic, guidelines should also advise on dose and frequency of administration. These parameters are determined by pharmacodynamic considerations, that is, the time-dependent effects of antibiotics on the infecting pathogen. Antibiotic pharmacodynamics can be broadly grouped into either time-dependent or concentration-dependent killing effects, although evidence is emerging of an intermediate group, with features of the two other categories.

2. Time-dependent antibacterials have microbicidal effects that depend on the presence of antibiotic above a threshold concentration at the site of infection for a minimum percentage of the interval between doses. The threshold concentration equates to the MIC, and the minimum between-dose interval is around 50%. Notably, concentrations greater than the MIC do not contribute to markedly greater killing effect. Beta-lactam antibiotics and glycopeptides possess time-dependent pharmacodynamics. Given these properties, the optimal way to administer time-dependent antibacterials would appear to be through continuous infusion titrated to achieve concentrations above the MIC, and no more, at the site of infection, thereby maximising the microbicidal effect while minimising concentration dependent toxicity. In practice, continuous intravenous infusions are often inconvenient because they require the use of continuous infusion pumps and dedicated access to an intravascular cannula, and so intermittent dosing remains the standard approach to administration of time-dependent antibacterials.

Concentration-dependent antibacterials have a killing effect that is related to the ratio of the maximum antibiotic concentration (C_{max}) to the MIC. The greater the ratio the greater the killing effect. A bolus injection of an intravenous antibiotic will rapidly attain a C_{max}, followed by a gradual reduction in concentration. Depending on clearance and the timing of the next dose, drug levels may fall below the MIC and even become undetectable before subsequent doses. However, concentration-dependent antibacterials characteristically demonstrate a postantibiotic effect (PAE), where inhibition of bacterial growth persists despite the absence of antibiotic. This phenomenon is exploited by the once-daily administration regimens of aminoglycosides, where the large single daily intravenous dose produces a C_{max} that is many multiples of the MIC, followed by several hours of low or undetectable amounts of aminoglycoside. Other concentration-dependent killing antimicrobials include fluoroquinolones, daptomycin and metronidazole.

The intermediate antibacterial pharmacodynamics group has time-dependent features combined with a PAE, where the best predictor of microbicidal success is the ratio of the area under the concentration-time curve over a 24-hour dosing interval divided by the MIC (AUC_{24}/MIC). The efficacy of macrolides, tetracyclines and linezolid seems best described by this parameter.

PRINCIPLES OF USING ANTIMICROBIALS AGENTS IN PROPHYLAXIS

Surgical site infections were such a frequent complication of surgery in the preantibiotic era that, in 1921, Lord Moynihan, the then-president of the Royal College of Surgeons, remarked that, "Every operation in surgery is an experiment in bacteriology." The discovery that antibacterials given at the time of surgery could dramatically reduce infection rates was a major breakthrough in surgical practice and has allowed many important advances, including prosthetic joint and transplant surgery.

The important principles guiding the use of antibacterials in surgical practice include choosing antibacterial agents that are likely to cover the bacterial pathogens found at the surgical site; administering prophylaxis to ensure that antibacterial activity is present at the surgical site from the moment of incision to the closure of the wound; with few exceptions (prolonged surgery, major blood loss, specific procedures, e.g., cardiac surgery), prophylaxis consisting of a single dose of antibiotic; and establishing prophylaxis guidelines and monitor compliance. Antibiotic prophylaxis of surgical site infections is an adjunct to good surgical technique and other surgical infection prevention practices and not a substitute for these.

ANTIMICROBIAL STEWARDSHIP

A unique feature of antimicrobials is that their efficacy is jeopardised by the risk of development of transferable resistance. While other, nonantimicrobial, drug classes may lose their activity in individual patients, through receptor up or downregulation, for example, this loss of action does not affect the prospect of successful treatment in other patients. However, bacteria can exchange resistance genes, even across species boundaries, and human hosts can exchange resistant bacteria, even across national boundaries. Resistance is an ancient phenomenon, probably contemporaneous with the evolution of the capacity of certain bacteria and moulds, millions of years ago, to produce antibiotic substances. However, the clinical (and veterinary and agricultural) use of antibacterials has been overwhelmingly important in selecting for and promoting the emergence of resistant bacteria. The ability of some bacteria to collect resistance genes on transferable DNA has led to clinically important bacteria becoming multidrug-resistant (MDR—resistant to antibiotics from at least three different antibiotic classes), extensively drug resistant (XDR—sensitive to antibiotics from, at most, two antibiotic classes) or pan-drug resistant (PDR—resistant to all known antibacterials). While some resistance mechanisms carry a fitness cost to the host bacterium, this is not universally true, and so it cannot be assumed that an absence of antibiotics in the bacterial environment will necessarily lead to resistant bacteria being "cured" of their resistance or being supplanted by sensitive bacteria. For practical purposes, resistance should be considered a permanent, irreversible event. Concurrent with the rise in MDR bacteria, there has been a virtual halt in the development and introduction into clinical practice of new antibacterial classes, so that relying on new antibiotics is not a prudent strategic response to the challenge of resistance.

Consequently, clinicians are facing the unavoidable certainty that their use of antibacterials to treat current patients undermines their ability to treat future patients. Antibacterial efficacy should be considered as a limited resource that, at best, is only partially renewable. This realisation has prompted the development of the concept of antimicrobial stewardship, an idea that aims to extend the effectiveness of antibiotics for as long as possible through the development and implementation of a coherent set of actions designed to use antimicrobials responsibly.

In the sense that good stewardship requires every dose of antimicrobial to be justified, at the level of the individual patient, stewardship can be summed up in the phrase, *the right antibacterial at the right dose by the right route for the right duration.* Right antibacterial implies that treatment is indicated. In practice, this means that the patient has either a confirmed bacterial infection or that there are reasonable grounds to suspect a bacterial infection and that the future health of the patient would be improved by treatment. This rules out the use of antibacterials to treat nonbacterial infections and also highlights that not all bacterial infections warrant antibiotic treatment. Infections such as otitis media in children, *Streptococcus pyogenes* pharyngitis and bacterial gastroenteritis normally resolve spontaneously in a time course that is not made significantly shorter by antibiotics. Assuming antibacterial treatment is indicated, antibiotic choice, dose and frequency should be based on local empirical treatment guidelines, as discussed earlier in the chapter, or determined by culture and susceptibility results.

The route of administration is often dictated by the antibiotic choice because many drugs are only available by one route of delivery. However, when a choice of oral or intravenous administration is available, deciding which route to use will be driven by the patient's ability to take drugs by mouth; the reliability of absorption from the gut, which may be compromised by vomiting or diarrhoea; and the bioavailability of the drug, set against the availability of intravascular access, the differential costs of the different drug presentations and patient preference.

The next question to address is the duration of treatment. This is possibly the least studied aspect of antibacterial therapy. Clinical trials tend to compare the clinical efficacy of different drugs, not the impact of different durations of treatment of the same drug. However, treatment duration is of increasing interest because of the realisation that courses of treatment beyond that necessary to successfully treat an infection confer no additional therapeutic benefit but continue to expose host microbiota to resistance-selecting pressure. On the other hand, too short a duration of treatment increases the likelihood of treatment failure, albeit with the original sensitive bacteria, prompting a further course of antibiotics with the accompanying impact on resistance selection.

One approach that is best suited to the management of inpatients is to not set a specific treatment length, but instead implement a process of regular review of the patient, asking every day the question, should the patient stop antibiotics, continue current treatment or change to another antibacterial? The approach to answering this question is based on the standard clinical method of history taking, patient physical examination and the result of investigations. For some infection types, published or local guidelines may be available, including online resources, which can be used to support decision making. The route of administration can also be reviewed during treatment in line with the patient's clinical response, switching from intravenous to oral administration of antibiotics if this is appropriate.

In primary care, the option for regular review tends not to be practicable, and so usual practice is to follow prescribing guidelines, which should cover the large majority of infections seen.

Patients with severe, acute infections that threaten to be rapidly fatal pose a special stewardship problem. Patient survival often depends on immediate effective antibiotic treatment, but the identity of the infecting organism and its antibacterial susceptibility are rarely known at the time treatment must be commenced. The stewardship issue is that the broad-spectrum treatment that offers the best guarantee of successful therapy is liable to cause disruption of the patient's microbiota, especially in the large bowel, and promote the emergence of resistance, when a narrow-spectrum agent could be just as clinically effective without the ecological disruption, if only it was known which narrow-spectrum agent should be given. A compromise between effective treatment and minimising microbiota disruption is to start with a broad-spectrum antibiotic and

focus on the pathogen, once identified, by de-escalating to narrow-spectrum treatment.

In addition to the review of the response of individual patients to treatment, most interpretations of antimicrobial stewardship require regular review of antibiotic prescriptions and resistance at an organisational or population level, including audit of the indications for antibiotic prescriptions; the appropriateness of prescriptions; and evidence that clinical progress is monitored and used to guide decisions on continuing, changing or terminating treatment.

Overall antibiotic consumption, broken down by class, should be measured and monitored to pick up trends in prescribing. A useful index of consumption is the defined daily dose (DDD), a measure of the standard total daily adult dose of a drug. The total weight of antibacterial prescribed or administered in a clinical setting, such as a ward or clinical service, over a time period, such as a month or year, divided by the DDD, will give the number of daily doses of the drug in the time period. Dividing this figure by a measure of clinical activity, such as admissions or patient bed-days, will give a rate of antibiotic use that can be compared with previous rates within the clinical unit or with other similar clinical units or benchmark figures. High rates of antibiotic consumption should be a prompt to look for reasons for the high use, which may include important differences in case mix including changes in infection rates or case ascertainment, or might be due to changes in prescribing practice, which may need to be challenged.

The analysis and reporting of bacterial antibiotic susceptibility data is a valuable complement to antibiotic consumption surveillance. This should be reported syndromically, so that prescribers are given an insight into which antibacterials are the most effective treatments of clinical presentations such as wound, urinary or respiratory tract infections.

While prescribers retain the responsibility to review antibiotic prescribing at the patient level, it is increasingly common for hospitals to have antimicrobial stewardship teams who have the remit to gather the organisational-level data and provide expert analysis and interpretation of it. Stewardship teams typically include infection specialists such as medical microbiologists and infectious disease physicians, antimicrobial pharmacists, data analysts and IT specialists. Stewardship teams work closely with infection prevention and control teams, developing joint action plans aimed at the prevention, detection and removal of resistant bacteria.

Stewardship strategies have been classed into three major categories—persuasive, restrictive and structural. Persuasive approaches include providing prescribers with guidelines, audit and feedback, leaving reminder notes on prescription charts, promotion of best practice by key opinion leaders and prescribing champions. Restrictive approaches include restricting the reporting of antibiotic results on microbiology reports, limiting the availability of antibiotics on the local formulary, or requiring permission before certain antibiotics can be prescribed or before courses can be extended beyond a specified duration. Structural approaches are aimed at supporting best practice prescribing, for example, through computer-supported diagnosis and treatment advice, and algorithm-supported dose adjustment aimed at optimising antibiotic concentrations.

There is good evidence that antibiotic stewardship achieves the aim of reducing duration of antibiotic treatment. Stewardship also improves the rate of appropriate treatment and likely delivers other patient benefits, such as reduced hospital stay. However, unintended consequences of stewardship, such as delays in treatment and negative effects on professional culture through breakdown in trust and communication, have been reported. Antimicrobial stewardship is a complex matter and requires substantial further research.

RECOMMENDED READING

Abdul-aziz, M. H., Lipman, J., Mouton, J. W., Hope, W. W., & Roberts, J. A. (2015). Applying pharmacokinetic/pharmacodynamic principles in critically ill patients: optimizing efficacy and reducing resistance development. *Seminars in Respiratory and Critical Care Medicine, 36*(1), 136–153. doi:10.1055/s-0034-1398490.

Craig, W. A. (1998). Pharmacokinetic/pharmacodynamic parameters: rationale for antibacterial dosing of mice and men. *Clinical Infectious Diseases, 26*(1), 1–10.

Davey, P., Brown, E., Charani, E., Fenelon, L., Gould, I. M., Holmes, A., ... Wilcox, M. (2013). Interventions to improve antibiotic prescribing practices for hospital inpatients. *Cochrane Database of Systematic Reviews*, (4), CD003543. doi:10.1002/14651858.

Davey, P., Marwick, C. A., Scott, C. L., Charani, E., McNeil, K., Brown, E., ... Michie, S. (2017). Interventions to improve antibiotic prescribing practices for hospital inpatients. *Cochrane Database of Systematic Reviews*, (2), CD003543. doi:10.1002/14651858.

Dyar, O. J., Huttner, B., Schouten, J., *et al.* (2017). What is antimicrobial stewardship? *Clinical Microbiology and Infection.*

Nielsen, E. I., & Friberg, L. E. (2013). Pharmacokinetic-pharmacodynamic modelling of antibacterial drugs. *Pharmacological Reviews, 65*(3), 1053–1090. doi: 10.1124/pr.111.005769.

Scottish Intercollegiate Guidelines Network. Healthcare Improvement Scotland. SIGN 104 Antibiotic prophylaxis in surgery. Updated 2014. Available at: http://www.sign.ac.uk/assets/sign104.pdf. (Accessed Sep 2017).

Wallace, A. W., Jones, M., & Bertino, J. S., Jr. (2002). Evaluation of four once-daily aminoglycoside dosing nomograms. *Pharmacotherapy, 22*(9), 1077–1083.

Websites

Clinical and Laboratory Standards Institute. Standards. Microbiology. Available at: https://clsi.org/standards/products/microbiology/. (Accessed Sep 2017).

The European Committee on Antimicrobial Susceptibility Testing. Available at: http://www.eucast.org/. (Accessed Sep 2017).

The European Committee on Antimicrobial Susceptibility Testing. Expert rules and intrinsic resistance. Available at: http://www.eucast.org/expert_rules_and_intrinsic_resistance/. (Accessed Sep 2017).

The European Committee on Antimicrobial Susceptibility Testing. Instruction videos from EUCAST. How to perform antimicrobial susceptibility testing. Available at: http://www.eucast.org/videos_from_eucast/#c19324. (Accessed Sep 2017).

WHO Collaborating Centre for Drug Statistics Methodology. Definition and general considerations. Available at: https://www.whocc.no/ddd/definition_and_general_considera/. (Accessed Sep 2017).

66 Epidemiology and control of community infections

MANISH PAREEK AND ANDREW ROSSER

KEY POINTS

- The surveillance of infection provides the basis for appropriate investigation and preventive action.
- The infectious process involves three main factors: the microorganism, the host and the environment.
- Infection is spread in five ways: from person to person, from healthy carriers, from animal sources, from environmental sources and as a result of an organism situated in an area of the body where it is harmless gaining access to a more dangerous site.
- Infection may manifest itself as a sporadic case, an outbreak, an epidemic or a pandemic.
- The epidemiological investigation of an outbreak involves an analysis concerning the persons involved, the place it occurred and the time those infected became ill.
- Vigilance and high-quality surveillance are necessary in order to have an early warning of emerging infections.

INTRODUCTION

Attempts to observe and record diseases to understand their causation and to devise control strategies have a long history. Hippocrates (460–361 BC), the father of medical science, and Herodotus (484–425 BC), the father of history, both related environmental factors to health. Hippocrates, when writing of the occurrence of diseases, distinguished between the 'steady state', the 'endemic state' and the abrupt change in incidence, the 'epidemic'.

Probably the first public health measures based on case reports of infectious diseases were instituted in 1348, when the Republic of Venice excluded ships carrying persons with a plague-like illness on board in order to control outbreaks of pneumonic plague (the black death). Fifty years later, again in Venice, the concept of quarantine was introduced when ships from plague-stricken areas had to stay outside the harbours for 40 days *(quaranta giorni)*.

Later, in 1592, the fear of a plague epidemic spurred the publishing of the *Bills of Mortality* in London, within which the causes of death were recorded. In 1662, John Graunt (1620–1674), in his book *Natural and Political Observations Made Upon the Bills of Mortality*, was the first to count the number of persons dying in London from specific illnesses such as consumption (pulmonary tuberculosis) and to advocate the collation of numerical data on a population to study the causes of disease (Table 66.1). Following this, in 1837, the office of the Registrar General was established to develop the work started by John Graunt; the English physician William Farr (1807–1883) added reports to those of the Registrar General that dealt with infectious diseases, occupational diseases, accidents or hazardous work conditions.

The importance of the careful observation of disease to determine the likely cause has been shown on many occasions. In 1849, 34 years before the identification of *Vibrio cholerae* by Robert Koch (1843–1910), John Snow (1813–1858), a London physician, proved by epidemiological observation that cholera was mainly spread by drinking infected water and not through the air in the form of miasmas (noxious air emanating from rotting organic material) as was thought at the time. More recently, William Pickles (1885–1969), a general practitioner in Wensleydale, Yorkshire, elucidated many of the epidemiological characteristics of hepatitis and other infections well before microbiological advances confirmed his observations.

From these beginnings, the surveillance of infection has assumed national and international proportions. National surveillance is carried out in most countries, for example at the Centers for Disease Control and Prevention (CDC) in Atlanta, Georgia, USA. In the United Kingdom, information on infectious diseases and environmental hazards is collated for each devolved administration by different public health agencies. At a Pan-European level, the European Centre for Disease Prevention and Control in Stockholm collects such data for each European country and, on a worldwide basis, the World Health Organization maintains surveillance

Table 66.1 Selection of causes of death in London taken from the Bills of Mortality, 1632

Causes of death	No. of deaths
Chrisomes[a] and infancy	2268
Consumption[b]	1797
Fever	1108
Aged	628
Smallpox	531
Teeth	470
Abortive and stillborn	445
Bloody flux[c], scouring[d] and flux	348
Dropsy[e] and swelling	267
Convulsions	241
Childbed	171
Measles	80
Ague[f]	43
King's evil[g]	38

[a]A child who died during the first month of life or a child who died unbaptised.
[b]Usually pulmonary tuberculosis
[c]Dysentery
[d]Diarrhoea
[e]Oedema
[f]Malaria
[g]Tuberculosis of the skin

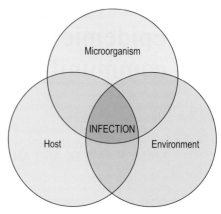

Fig. 66.1 The three main factors involved in the infectious process.

on specific infectious diseases such as tuberculosis (TB) as well as responding to emerging infections such as the Zika virus. This international cooperation is vital because germs do not recognise boundaries.

EPIDEMIOLOGICAL PRINCIPLES

DEFINITIONS

Epidemiology is defined as 'the study of the occurrence and distribution of health-related events, states, and processes in specified populations, including the study of the determinants influencing such processes, and the application of this knowledge to control relevant health problems.' (Porter M, 2014). Although particularly appropriate to the study of infectious diseases, epidemiological principles are also used to elucidate the causes of noncommunicable diseases.

Closely linked with the study of epidemiology is the concept of surveillance, which is probably the most effective infection control technique available. Surveillance is defined as: 'the epidemiological study of a disease as a dynamic process involving the ecology of the infectious agent, the host, the reservoirs, the vectors as well as the complex mechanisms concerned in the spread of infection and the extent to which this spread will occur' (Greenwood, 18th ed.).

For the surveillance of infectious diseases to be effective, three main elements must occur: (1) the systematic collection of pertinent data; (2) the orderly consolidation and evaluation of data and (3) the prompt dissemination of findings, particularly to those who can take appropriate action.

Surveillance provides for the recognition of acute problems requiring immediate local, national or international action and for further assessment by revealing trends or facilitating forecasts. It also provides a rational basis for planning and implementing efficient control measures and for their evaluation and continuing assessment.

The infectious process is a dynamic state involving three interconnected main factors: the microorganism, the host and the environment (Fig. 66.1).

THE MICROORGANISM

Relatively few microorganisms cause disease in humans. This propensity is described by two terms, *pathogenicity* and *virulence,* which are often used interchangeably. Pathogenicity is a qualitative description of the ability of a pathogen to cause disease in a particular host, whereas virulence is a quantitative term, which describes the amount of damage caused to the host. Virulence should not just be thought of as an inherent microbial property, it actually represents an interaction between the organism and host. Organisms considered virulent are avirulent in hosts with specific immunity, and those considered avirulent may cause disease in hosts who are immunodeficient. Specific bacterial factors also contribute to the level of virulence displayed. Whilst there are many, several are consistently noted, including:

• Invasiveness: the capacity of an organisms to spread widely throughout the body.

- Toxigenicity: the toxin-producing property of the organism.
- Adherence: the ability to attach to host tissues.
- Antigenic variation: alteration of organism proteins to evade host defences.

THE HOST

The reaction of the host to a microorganism will depend on its ability to resist infection. A pathogen may overcome a host's innate immunity leading to the contraction of infection. Alternatively, the individual may possess specific protective antibodies or cellular immunity from a previous infection or immunisation. However, immunity is relative and may be overwhelmed by an excessive dose of the pathogen or if the person is infected via an unusual portal of entry; it may also be impaired by immunosuppressive drug therapy, concurrent disease such as cancer or the ageing process.

Herd immunity

Individuals who lack specific immunity to a pathogen may nonetheless be protected against infection when a significant proportion of the population possesses active immunity, either from immunisation or previous infection. The lack of susceptible hosts hinders spread through the community. This form of collective immunity is known as herd immunity.

Herd immunity can be measured:

- Indirectly from the age distribution and incidence pattern of the disease if it is clinically distinct and reasonably common. This is an insensitive technique and inadequate method for infections that manifest subclinically.
- Directly from assessments of immunity in defined population groups by antibody surveys (seroepidemiology) or skin tests; these may show immunity gaps and provide an early warning of susceptibility in the population.

The decision of whether to introduce herd immunity artificially by immunisation against a particular disease will depend on several epidemiological principles.

- The disease must carry a substantial risk.
- The risk of contracting the disease must be considerable.
- The vaccine must be effective at reducing disease incidence in the target population.
- The vaccine must be safe.

The effectiveness and safety of immunisation programmes are monitored by observing the expected and actual effects of such programmes on disease transmission patterns in the community by appropriate epidemiological techniques.

THE ENVIRONMENT

Socioeconomic development and infection

The environment plays a major role in the causation, spread and control of infection. In the United Kingdom, the disappearance of plague and cholera, the rarity of indigenous typhoid fever and the relative infrequency of bacillary dysentery all indicate environmental conditions have improved.

In particular, the decrease in overcrowding and infestation, together with the demand for cleaner water supplies and better sanitation, has been instrumental in producing these dramatic advances. This is highlighted by the case of TB, which was declining before the availability of antituberculous drugs and mass bacille Calmette–Guérin (BCG) vaccination in countries where socioeconomic conditions were improving (Fig. 66.2).

It is noteworthy that despite the socioeconomic improvements that have been made, in many developed countries, urban deprivation is intransigent. Communities are at increased risk of infectious diseases including human immunodeficiency virus, TB and hepatitis C. It is clear that tackling the social determinants of disease is integral to successful disease control.

Climate change

Changes in climatic conditions can significantly affect pathogens, hosts, vectors and their living environments, changing the incidence and geographical spread of infectious diseases. Alterations in conditions can be both advantageous and deleterious to pathogens and vectors. For example, higher ambient temperatures hinder the development of the malaria parasite, whereas rising temperatures may expand the *Aedes* mosquito vector geographical range, contributing to spread of the Zika virus. Climate change is expected to modify the epidemiology of infectious diseases requiring new policies to prevent, prepare for and to respond to outbreaks.

THE SPREAD OF INFECTION

EFFICACY OF TRANSMISSION

The transmissibility of a pathogen can be measured by its basic reproductive number R_0, defined as 'the mean

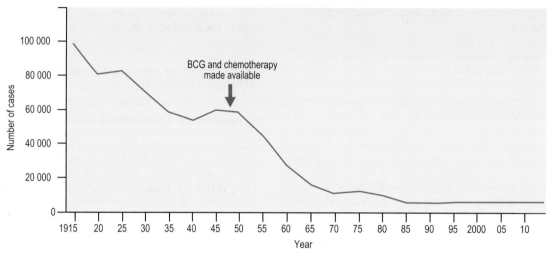

Fig. 66.2 Notifications of tuberculosis in United Kingdom, 1915–2014.

number of secondary infections seeded by a typical infective into a completely susceptible (naïve) host population' (Cintrón-Arias A et al., 2009). If the R_0 is >1, the organism will spread in the population, and if R_0 is <1, the disease will eventually die out. Frequently a population is non-naïve, such as in the case of influenza, where previous infections confer a degree of immunity to subsequent strains. Thus transmissibility is better characterised by the effective reproductive R_n, which accounts for this reduced susceptibility. Ultimately, exhaustion of the susceptible host population leads to the infection dying out.

SPREAD OF INFECTIONS

When an infection is transmitted in a population, spread occurs in a well-defined epidemiological pattern. By understanding these patterns, the extent can be predicted, and measures to control, or in some cases to eradicate, disease can be implemented.

Infection spread directly from one person to another

Infections in this category include highly contagious diseases such as measles. The pathogen is passed directly from a person with the disease to a susceptible contact. Diseases in this category are usually clinically apparent, and healthy carriers are not commonly a feature.

Infection in which healthy carriers are involved

Individuals may carry the bacilli responsible for diseases such as typhoid and diphtheria for long periods of time after they were infected and yet remain free from symptoms. These carriers may transmit infections to others but the source remains undetected. For blood-borne viral infections such as human immunodeficiency virus and hepatitis B and C, the healthy carrier state may last for many years before complications ensue. In malaria endemic areas, high rates of asymptomatic carriage occur. These cases represent a reservoir of infection transmissible to susceptible hosts via the female *Anopheles* mosquito vector.

Infection in which persons harbour the organism before the onset of clinical illness

Organisms such as *Streptococcus pneumoniae*, which normally colonises the nasopharynx, may not be harmful until an event such as a skull fracture allows for the transfer of the bacterium from the nasopharynx to the cerebrospinal space where it can cause potentially fatal meningitis.

Infection derived from animal sources

Diseases derived from animals, such as Lyme disease, leptospirosis, anthrax, rabies and brucellosis, are known as zoonoses. These diseases are spread by direct contact with the animal concerned, indirectly by such means as the ingestion of infected milk or by a vector such as a tick.

Infections derived from environmental sources

The spread of *Legionella* bacteria from cooling towers and air conditioning units to cause Legionnaires' disease is an example of illness derived from an infected environment.

OUTBREAKS OF INFECTION

The crowding together of human beings provides the necessary conditions to allow microorganisms to multiply and spread. When human beings led nomadic lives there were fewer opportunities for outbreaks to occur; the main opportunities came when large numbers gathered, for example for a pilgrimage. These clusterings facilitated the spread of infection, resulting in outbreaks; the subsequent dispersal of the group carried the causative organism elsewhere.

The impact of close living conditions on the transmission of infections is well illustrated by the military. Even outside times of war, compared to their civilian counterparts, military personnel remain at greater risk of infection. Outbreaks of respiratory infections caused by adenovirus, influenza A, *Streptococcus pneumoniae*, *Streptococcus pyogenes* and *Bordetella pertussis* are especially problematic. Fortunately, strategies to control outbreaks by vaccination, targeted antibiotic prophylaxis and surveillance have greatly enhanced disease control.

NOMENCLATURE OF OUTBREAKS

The term *outbreak* is often confused with other epidemiological terms used to enumerate infection which include:

- Sporadic case: A person whose illness is not apparently connected with similar illnesses in another person.
- Outbreak: The occurrence of cases of a disease associated in time or location among a group of persons. A household outbreak involves two or more persons resident in the same private household and not apparently connected with any other case or outbreak. A general outbreak involves two or more persons who are not confined to one private household. A single case of an infectious disease either long absent from a community, not previously recognised in that community or of an unknown aetiology may also constitute an outbreak.
- Epidemic: The large-scale temporary increase in the occurrence of a disease in a community or region that is clearly in excess of normal expectancy.
- Pandemic: An epidemic occurring worldwide, or over a very wide area, crossing international boundaries and usually affecting a large number of people.

TYPES OF OUTBREAKS

By constructing an epidemic curve consisting of the number of cases against time, several patterns of outbreak may be revealed that can indicate the likely mode of spread.

Point source outbreak

This form of common-source outbreak occurs when a group of susceptible hosts are briefly exposed to a single pathogen source such as undercooked chicken at a buffet. Within a short period of time there is a sharp rise followed by a more gradual fall in the number of infected persons (Fig. 66.3).

Continuous common-source outbreak

Exposure to a single pathogen source occurs over an extended time period, for example when a contaminated water source is not tackled. There is a quick rise in the

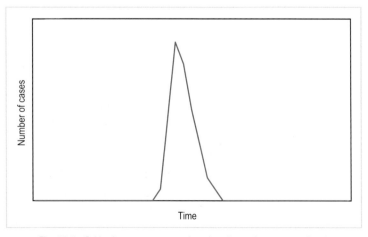

Fig. 66.3 Epidemic curve apparent when there is a point source outbreak.

number of cases and new cases keep occurring as demonstrated by the plateau shape of the curve (Fig. 66.4).

Intermittent common-source outbreak

These occur when a common source is not fully controlled so that repeated outbreaks occur. A staff member colonised with methicillin-resistant *Staphylococcus aureus* (MRSA) on a neonatal intensive care unit could cause this pattern (Fig. 66.5).

Propagated outbreak

There is person-to-person spread of an infectious agent such as the measles virus. The epidemic curve is characterised by increasingly larger peaks (Fig. 66.6) until such time as the pool of susceptible individuals in the population is depleted and/or control measures are implemented and the epidemic abates. Such outbreaks are protracted, taking longer than common-source outbreaks to build up and to subside.

Mixed outbreak

There is a common-source outbreak with subsequent propagation to subjects not exposed to the original source. This is typical of many foodborne pathogens such as norovirus and *Shigella*.

ANALYSIS OF OUTBREAKS

The investigation of an outbreak should be approached in a logical and methodical way. The cause may be elucidated by determining details of the persons involved, the place where they had been and the time when they became ill.

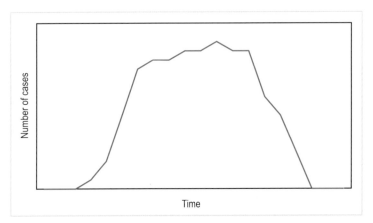

Fig. 66.4   Epidemic curve apparent when there is a continuous common-source outbreak.

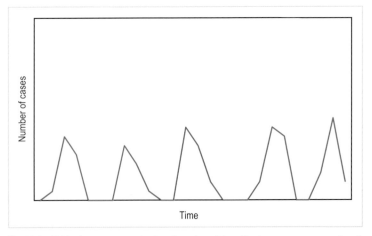

Fig. 66.5   Epidemic curve apparent when there is an intermittent common-source outbreak.

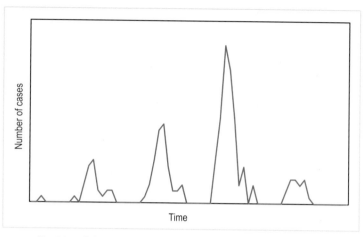

Fig. 66.6 Epidemic curve apparent when there is a propagated outbreak.

The fundamental pieces of information that should be sought whenever an outbreak occurs are as follows:

- **WHO** gets infected? What is their age? For example, if a possible foodborne outbreak affects mainly children, could the source be milk or ice cream?
- **WHERE** were those who became infected? Where have they recently been? For example, in a hospital outbreak, were they all in the same surgical ward? Could a member of the operating staff be a carrier of a pathogen? In a community outbreak of Legionnaires' disease, were those affected living downwind from a source of infection (Fig. 66.7)?
- **WHEN** did the infection occur? By knowing the incubation period of the infection and the date of onset of symptoms, it may be possible to trace back to an event that was attended by all those affected.
- **WHAT** was the common factor? For example, in a food poisoning episode, the ingestion of an article of food by most of those affected but not by those unaffected may be a vital piece of evidence.
- **HOW** did those involved become infected? For example, abscess formation among recently immunised persons might be due to contaminated vaccine.
- **WHY** did the infection occur? For example, the reheating of meat may be the cause of a *Clostridium perfringens* food-poisoning outbreak.

INVESTIGATION OF OUTBREAKS

In the investigation of outbreaks, it is important to have a standardised approach to the various steps

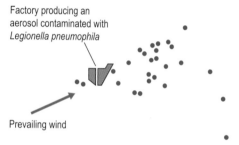

Fig. 66.7 Occurrence of Legionnaires' disease in persons living downwind from a factory with an evaporative condenser contaminated with *Legionella pneumophila*.

involved. Such an approach might have the following as a basis:

1. Preparation. At the beginning of an outbreak investigation, the members of the outbreak team and the resources required should be identified.
2. Establish the presence of an outbreak. The baseline rates of disease can be determined from surveillance data. An increase in the frequency of disease above that expected may indicate an outbreak. However, an apparent outbreak can actually be due to a change in case definition, improvements in diagnostic testing or a change in the mechanism of reporting, which may increase the number of reports of illness.
3. Verify the diagnosis. It is always prudent to confirm that the clinical history is compatible with the diagnosis. Laboratory testing can be useful; for example, hepatitis A serology can distinguish recent from past infection.

4. Establish a case definition. Patients are designated as cases using criteria laid out in the case definition. These include clinical information, the personal characteristics of the cases, the location of the suspected exposure and the specified time period for the outbreak.

5. Case finding. Often the number of cases notified is only a proportion of the total number of those affected. It is necessary to seek out the additional cases, or vital information may be lost.

6. Perform descriptive epidemiology. It is useful to characterise the outbreak by time, person and place. The time course of an epidemic can be represented using an epidemic curve. It can suggest the pattern of disease transmission and the stage the outbreak has reached, for example, if the outbreak is tailing off. Assessment of the outbreak by place indicates the extent of the disease and can identify clusters or patterns of disease, such as those grouped around a restaurant. Describing the outbreak by person indicates who the cases are and who the at-risk population is. This information is used to generate hypotheses about the source of infection, the mode of transmission and the exposures causing disease.

7. Evaluation of hypotheses. Epidemiological studies can be used to test hypotheses. Cohort studies compare the incidence of disease amongst those who were and were not exposed to various factors such as certain foods. Case-control studies compare prior exposures between those with and without the disease.

8. Refine hypotheses and perform additional studies as required. Sometimes analytical studies are unrevealing. If this is the case, hypotheses should be reexamined and further studies of cases to identify common links undertaken. Laboratory testing can support hypotheses such as matching *Salmonella* from confirmed cases with suspected food items by typing methods such as whole genome sequencing.

9. Implementation of control measures. As soon as the source is identified, preventative measures can be instituted expeditiously.

The application of new technologies to outbreak investigations

The development of new diagnostic technologies and analytical approaches promises to transform the detection and investigation of outbreaks, no more so than for tuberculosis. At present, mycobacterial genotyping is used to identify cases in the chain of transmission, to detect additional cases linked to the outbreak and to determine the completeness of contact investigations. Currently the genotyping methods in common use lack sufficient discriminatory power, which is particularly problematic where highly conserved genotypes are prevalent. Whole genome sequencing is a much more discriminatory technique with the power to resolve single nucleotide differences between isolates. This means false clustering of isolates with identical profiles from other genotyping methods can be resolved and transmission events ruled out. Additionally, transmission events missed by conventional methods can be detected and linked to an outbreak, better profiling the outbreak. However, this is a rapidly evolving field and the optimal use of this technology remains to be determined.

Once contacts in a TB outbreak are identified, they are evaluated for latent TB infection (LTBI) and those found to be infected are treated to prevent progression to active disease. Interferon gamma assays are a relatively new diagnostic test for LTBI, which measure the cell-mediated immune response to TB antigens. Unlike the tuberculin skin test, they are unaffected by BCG vaccination status and are highly specific, so treatment can be better targeted.

Further refinement of these technologies promises to further improve disease control and ultimately may help eliminate TB.

CONTROL OF OUTBREAKS

The investigation of an outbreak should be carried out as swiftly as possible so that adequate control measures can be started without delay to prevent spread amongst the at-risk population. Knowledge of the source of infection, the route of transmission and the persons at risk should allow appropriate action to be taken.

Sources of infection

Infection may be acquired endogenously from one's own flora or exogenously from sources including other humans, animals or from the environment.

When humans represent the source of infection, if the initial cases have readily identifiable clinical features (e.g., chickenpox) then control is often easier as it is much more likely that the index case will be located. Prompt diagnosis and effective patient management reduce patient sequelae and prevent onward transmission.

On the other hand, it is more difficult to control diseases in which apparently healthy carriers are responsible as it is necessary to search for an infected person who may be asymptomatic.

It may be important to isolate the case or carrier, and possibly to institute appropriate treatment, until the patient

Table 66.2 Isolation procedures for cases during outbreaks

Infection control precautions	Mode of transmission	Ease of spread	Protective actions	Aetiology
Strict isolation	Airborne or direct contact with infected fluids or tissue	Extremely infectious	Single room, dedicated medical equipment	Viral haemorrhagic fever
Enteric precautions	Direct or indirect contact with infected faeces or fomites	Highly infectious	Contact precautions and disposal of excreta	Hepatitis E, cholera, rotavirus
Respiratory isolation	Direct contact with patients, their secretions or airborne droplets	Highly infectious	Single room, masks/respirator, contact precautions	Measles, tuberculosis, diphtheria
Standard contact precautions	Direct or indirect contact with all bodily fluids, blood, excretions and secretions	Moderately infectious	Gloves, gowns, handwashing, disposal of contaminated objects	Most infectious diseases

is no longer infectious. The degree of isolation will depend on the type of disease as not all infections require strict isolation. For example, a patient with a highly infectious disease such as a viral haemorrhagic fever requires very strict isolation and safe disposal of biohazardous material, whereas a salmonella excreter will usually need only to cease food-handling activities and observe a high standard of personal hygiene until free from infection (see Table 66.2). In contrast to isolation, the term *quarantine* applies to restrictions on the healthy contacts of an infectious disease.

If an animal reservoir is responsible, action has to be directed at ensuring that the source of infection is eradicated, withdrawn from consumption or rendered harmless, for example, by the pasteurisation of milk or the adequate cooking of meat.

When the environment is the source of an outbreak the control measures required will depend on the nature of infection and the mode of spread. Legionnaires' disease is contracted when patients inhale mist or vapour containing the bacilli. This can come from environmental sources including shower heads, air-conditioning systems or from cooling towers (Fig. 66.8). Environmental measures, such as the use of biocides, can destroy the causative legionellae at the source and so prevent further cases.

The hospital setting is particularly dangerous as the presence of compromised patients can result in serious consequences, such as in a haematology/oncology setting. Moreover, the increasing use of invasive techniques and the appearance of antibiotic-resistant strains of microorganisms further compound the problem. The early detection of infection by effective surveillance, the emphasis on the cleanest possible environment and awareness among the staff of potential problems are among the measures that need to be stressed to control infection among hospital patients (see Ch. 67).

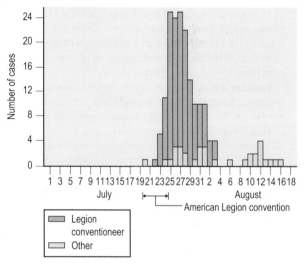

Fig. 66.8 Legionnaires' disease among those associated with a convention in a hotel in Philadelphia (July–August 1976); an example of an explosive outbreak.

Route of transmission

Infection may be spread by various routes including:

- direct or indirect contact
- airborne transmission
- food- and water-borne transmission
- insect-borne (vector) transmission
- percutaneous transmission
- sexual transmission
- transplacental (vertical) transmission

During an outbreak, measures to interrupt the spread of a pathogen are most effective when targeted to the route(s) of transmission involved. General measures may include effective hand-washing and disinfection or disposal, if necessary, of the patient's belongings. Strict adherence to high standards of personal hygiene by the contacts of a case is also an important measure.

When the disease is airborne, overcrowding should be avoided and beds well spaced. If suspected cases are admitted to hospital, the failure to implement sufficient infection control measures such as strict quarantine and adequate personal protective equipment use can lead to serious nosocomial outbreaks as illustrated by the South Korean outbreak of the Middle Eastern respiratory syndrome (MERS) coronavirus in 2015, which affected 186 persons, resulting in 38 deaths. In certain instances, major isolation measures, such as those adopted to control the outbreak of severe acute respiratory syndrome (SARS) coronavirus in 2003, need to be implemented. Indeed, the spread of the coronavirus, the airborne infection responsible for SARS, throughout regions of the Far East (China, Vietnam and Singapore) and North America (Toronto), before it was brought under control, demonstrates how effectively international travel and overcrowding in major cities can facilitate the transmission of serious airborne infections.

Food and water should be as free as possible from infection; otherwise their consumption can cause major outbreaks. To prevent insect-borne transmission, insect eradication policies and repellents should be considered. HIV is an infection that, commonly, is transmitted through the percutaneous, sexual and transplacental routes; the elimination of infected blood donations by blood donor testing, the provision of sterile needles and syringes for infected drug users, the use of condoms, the treatment of HIV-infected pregnant women with antiretroviral therapy and pre-emptive administration of antiretrovirals to those considered at high-risk of infection are measures that prevent the spread of this infection through these routes.

Persons at risk

Where indicated and feasible, susceptible persons at risk should be protected as soon as possible. Among the measures available, the following may need to be considered:

- immunisation
- chemoprophylaxis for close contacts

Immunity against several infectious diseases can be obtained by either active or passive immunisation (see Ch. 68). An example of rapid effective protection of communities by active immunisation is the ring vaccination policy used to protect close contacts of poliomyelitis to stop more widespread dissemination of poliovirus. Passive immunisation, usually by means of human specific immunoglobulin, gives rapid protection to contacts of certain infections, such as hepatitis B, although protection is short lived. Chemoprophylaxis is effective in the protection of close contacts of meningococcal infections and diphtheria.

MATHEMATICAL MODELS

Mathematical modelling techniques attempt to define, by use of relatively simple estimates and assumptions, the dynamic conditions governing transmission of communicable agents.

Details of the multiplication and growth rates of microorganisms and the spread of infection under natural or experimental conditions need to be known to simulate spread in defined communities.

Measurable factors include:

- the number of infective persons or sources of introduction of infection
- the proportion of susceptible persons in a community at risk
- the duration of immunity
- the introduction of new susceptibles
- the removal rate of infective persons (by isolation, immunity or death)
- the response to vaccines and chemotherapeutic agents

Mathematical models can be used to predict the outcome of epidemics and to determine optimal control strategies.

ASSOCIATION AND CAUSATION OF INFECTION

A problem commonly encountered by microbiologists and epidemiologists is the attribution of an infectious disease to a particular microorganism. How do we determine whether the relationship is one of causation or merely a chance association?

Koch addressed this when he formulated his postulates in 1891. These state that:

1. The organism must always be found in the given disease.
2. The organism must be isolated in pure culture.
3. The organism must reproduce the given disease after inoculation of a pure culture into a susceptible animal.
4. The organism must be recoverable from the animal so inoculated.

The postulates are commonly not applicable to organisms that cannot be grown in culture or to viral and parasitic diseases. They are not applicable to the study of the transmission of infection within a population. For this purpose, it is more appropriate to consider the following factors, suggested by the medical statistician Austin Bradford Hill, to establish whether a disease is caused by a particular infectious agent:

1. **Strength.** What is the strength of the association? During the cholera epidemic in London in 1854, John Snow compared the death rates among persons drinking the sewage-polluted drinking water of the Southwark and Vauxhall Company with those receiving the purer water of the Lambeth Company; he discovered that the rate in the former was 14 times greater. This strength of association allowed Snow to consider that polluted water was a cause of cholera, although at that time the causative organism itself had not been identified.
2. **Consistency.** Similar observations, made by different people at different times in different places, add confidence to a conclusion that causation is likely.
3. **Specificity.** If the association is limited to a specific group of persons, with a specific type of illness, who have all been subjected to the same specific infection, then a cause-and-effect relationship can be more strongly suspected.
4. **Temporality.** This can be of especial importance when persons in particular occupations become infected (e.g., leptospirosis in sewer workers). The history of working in a particular environment before infection rather than vice versa is particularly relevant.
5. **Biological gradient.** If a dose–response curve is apparent, then the evidence for causation is much stronger.
6. **Plausibility.** Is the possibility biologically plausible? The likelihood of veterinary surgeons becoming ill with a zoonotic infection from affected cattle that they have recently been treating seems biologically plausible.
7. **Coherence.** If all the evidence is coherent (e.g., if the same microorganism is isolated from the index case, the vehicle of transmission and from the victims), this is strong support for causation.
8. **Experiment.** Is the frequency of infection reduced if certain preventive measures are taken? The benefit of milk pasteurisation to reduce milk-borne salmonellosis is presumptive evidence of a zoonotic relationship.
9. **Analogy.** Has there been similar evidence in the past? The known capacity of the rubella virus to cause congenital abnormalities in the infants of infected mothers makes it easier to accept other viruses such as the Zika virus causing similar problems, if maternal infection occurs.

CONCLUSION

Because of the multifactorial causation of infection, it is usually necessary to study the epidemiology of infection in a multidisciplinary manner. The microbiologist, the clinician, the epidemiologist, the infection control nurse, the veterinarian, the environmental health officer and other appropriate personnel must all be involved; the extent of the involvement will depend on the nature of the infection. Success will depend on the expertise and cooperation of these members of the team.

ACKNOWLEDGMENTS

Funding statement: This report is supported by the National Institute for Health Research (NIHR Post-Doctoral Fellowship, Dr Manish Pareek, PDF-2015-08-102). The views expressed in this publication are those of the author(s) and not necessarily those of the NHS, the National Institute for Health Research or the Department of Health.

RECOMMENDED READING

Cintrón-Arias, A., Castillo-Chávez, C., Bettencourt, L. M., Lloyd, A. L., & Banks, H. T. (2009). The estimation of the effective reproductive number from disease outbreak data. *Math Biosci Eng, 6*(2), 261–282.

Detels, R., Beaglehole, R., Lansang, M. A., & Gulliford, M. (2009). *Oxford textbook of public health.* Oxford: Oxford University Press.

Donaldson, L. J., & Scally, G. (2009). *Essential public health* (3rd ed.). Oxford: Radcliffe.

Ekdahl, K. (2012). *Communicable disease control and health protection handbook.* Chichester: Wiley Blackwell.

Heymann, D. L. (2014). *Control of communicable diseases manual* (20th ed.). Washington, DC: American Public Health Association.

Mandell, G., Douglas, R. G., & Bennet, J. (2014). *Principles and practice of infectious diseases* (8th ed.). Philadelphia: Elsevier, Churchill Livingstone.

Nelson, K. E., & Williams, C. (2013). *Infectious disease epidemiology: theory and practice* (3rd ed.). Jones and Bartlett Learning.

Porter, M. (2014). *A dictionary of epidemiology* (6th ed.). Oxford: Oxford University Press.

Websites

Centers for Disease Control and Prevention. Available at http://www.cdc.gov/. (Accessed Nov 2017).

European Centre for Disease Prevention and Control. Available at http://www.ecdc.europa.eu/. (Accessed Nov 2017).

Health Protection Scotland. Available at http://www.hps.scot.nhs.uk/. (Accessed Nov 2017).

Iechyd Cyhoeddus Cymru / Public Health Wales. Available at http://www.publichealthwales.wales.nhs.uk. (Accessed Nov 2017).

Public Health Agency Northern Ireland. Available at http://www.publichealth.hscni.net. (Accessed Nov 2017).

Public Health England. Available at http://www.gov.uk/government/organisations/public-health-england. (Accessed Nov 2017).

World Health Organization. Available at http://www.who.int/en/. (Accessed Nov 2017).

67 Healthcare–associated infections

NELUN PERERA

KEY POINTS

- Health-care institutions constitute a special environment where the epidemiology of infection is distinct. The chief contributing factors are the accumulation of patients with particular features, the special activities undertaken in the health-care setting and the special environment created by the patients and the activities.
- Healthcare-associated infections are infections acquired while in health-care institutions.
- Urinary tract infections are the most common healthcare-associated infection in most health-care settings, and *Escherichia coli* and *Staphylococcus aureus* are the most common organisms causing these infections.
- Sources of health-care infections are people and contaminated objects, and the most common routes of spread are airborne and contact spread.
- Patients may constitute a special hazard because they are infectious, or they may be unusually susceptible to infection because they have particular conditions or are receiving immunosuppressive treatments.
- Many healthcare-associated infections are preventable.
- Careful and detailed attention must be paid to controlling the routes of transmission of infection, through the establishment and maintenance of an *infection control policy*.

The battle between humans and the microbe is at its most obvious in institutions where vulnerable people are crowded together. Amassing sick people under one roof has many advantages; however, it has some disadvantages, notably the ease of transmission of infection from one person to another. Historically, hospitals have a notorious reputation for infection. The hazards of puerperal sepsis and the horrors of septic infection in the pre-Listerian era have been well documented; admission to hospital in the mid-19th century was associated with the fear of gangrene and death.

Since then, surgical and medical techniques have developed dramatically, basic standards of building and hygiene have greatly improved, and the identification and treatment of most infecting microorganisms have become possible. Despite such changes, infection acquired in health-care institutions remains a major cause of morbidity and mortality, leading directly or indirectly to an enormous increase in the cost of hospital care and to the emergence of new health hazards for the community. In the past two decades enormous advances in biomedical technology and therapeutics have produced greater numbers of highly susceptible patients requiring treatment in hospitals, and this is aggravated by the occurrence of transferable resistance to antibiotics in pathogenic bacteria and the emergence of new pathogens transmitted by a variety of routes. In spite of these advances in medical care, in many countries pressures on health-care facilities and shortages of trained staff make it difficult to practice adequate infection prevention and control. There has also been a mistaken view among many health professionals that the advent of the antibiotic era made such precautions unnecessary, and many studies have shown poor compliance with simple hygiene.

DEFINITION AND CLASSIFICATION

Healthcare-associated infection is defined as any infection acquired in a health-care setting. The majority of infections usually become apparent in the health-care settings, but some (e.g., postoperative wound infections) may manifest in the community. With early discharges to reduce institutional costs, the number of these infections is likely to increase, although in principle there are less chances of exposure to infection.

To measure the extent of infections and conduct surveillance the following definitions should be considered:

Community-acquired infections: Infections acquired and developing outside institutions requiring admission to a health-care institution (e.g., pneumococcal pneumonia) or infections acquired outside institutions that become clinically apparent within 48 hours of admission or when a patient has been admitted to hospital for other reasons (e.g., chickenpox or zoster).

Healthcare-associated infections (HAIs):

1. Infections acquired and developing within a health-care setting as a direct result of treatment or contact with the health-care setting (e.g., device-associated bacteraemia).
2. Infections acquired in a health-care setting and becoming clinically apparent after discharge from the institution (e.g., postoperative wound infections).
3. Infections acquired outside a health-care setting (e.g., in the community) and brought into a health-care setting by patients, staff or visitors and transmitted to others within that setting (e.g., norovirus).
4. Infections acquired by health-care staff as a consequence of their work, whether or not this involves direct contact with patients (e.g., hepatitis B).

EPIDEMIOLOGY

HAIs pose a serious risk to patients, staff and visitors in health-care settings and can result in significant harm to those infected. Over 4 million people in Europe get a HAI every year, and around 37,000 die as a direct result of the infection. In England it is estimated that 300,000 patients a year acquire a HAI as a result of care within the National Health Service (NHS). Each one of these infections means additional use of NHS resources, greater patient discomfort and a decrease in patient safety.

HAI can occur in people of all ages. The very young and the elderly suffer a greater risk of infection due to the immaturity of the immune system in the former and underlying disease and treatments in the latter (Table 67.1). HAI can occur in otherwise healthy people, especially if invasive procedures or devices are used. Health-care workers, family members, and caregivers are also at risk of acquiring infections when caring for patients.

HAI can result in the following:

- Serious illness or death
- Exacerbation of existing or underlying conditions, delay in recovery and prolonged hospital stay, which in turn affect adversely the quality of life and economic consequences to patients and their family
- A need for additional antimicrobial therapy (as well as its additional cost), which exposes patients to additional risks of toxicity and increases selective pressure for resistance to emerge among hospital pathogens
- The infected patient becoming a source of infection for other patients in the hospital and community

Various risk factors, alone or in combination, influence the frequency and nature of HAIs. When comparing rates of HAI it is important to be aware of the frequencies of risk factors such as age, drug treatment or preexisting diseases in the population surveyed as well as the medical or surgical procedures used.

SOURCES

HAI may be exogenous or endogenous in origin. The exogenous source may be another person in the hospital (*cross-infection*) or a contaminated item of equipment or building service (*environmental infection*). A high

Table 67.1 Factors that predispose patients to healthcare-associated infection

Age	Extremes of age are more susceptible
Specific immunity	Lack of protective antibodies to specific infections (e.g., measles, chickenpox, whooping cough)
Underlying disease	Chronic diseases that lead to increased susceptibility (e.g., diabetes, cancer, hepatic and renal diseases, neutropenia)
Other infections	HIV and other immunosuppressive conditions, primary viral infections leading to secondary bacterial infections (e.g., influenza and herpes infections leading to *Staphylococcus aureus* pneumonia)
Specific medications	Cytotoxic drugs and steroids that reduce immunity to infection and broad-spectrum antibiotics that alter gut microbiota predisposing to *Clostridium difficile* diarrhoea
Trauma	
Accidental	Burn, stabbing, and gunshot wounds / Road traffic accidents ⎤
Intentional	Surgery, intravenous and urinary catheters, peritoneal dialysis catheters ⎦ Alters natural host defenses

proportion of clinically apparent HAI are endogenous *(self-infection)*, the infecting organism being derived from the patient's own skin, gastrointestinal microbiota or upper respiratory microbiota.

Patients and staff as a source of infection

In common with any large institution or workplace, the patients and staff of health-care settings share many facilities in close or crowded conditions. Outbreaks of diarrhoea and foodborne disease may be traced to a common source via the water or food supplies. Patients with comparable vulnerability to infection tend to be concentrated in the same area (e.g., in neonatal units, burns units or urological wards), where infected and noninfected patients may be cared for by the same staff, thus creating numerous opportunities for the spread of microorganisms by direct contact. The more susceptible patients usually require the most intensive care with far more daily contacts with staff who act as a vehicle in the transmission of microbes like insects spreading parasites.

The infectious period of a human source varies with the disease. Carriers of transmissible strains (e.g., *Staphylococcus aureus* or *Streptococcus pyogenes*) may act as a source of infection, although they themselves do not develop disease. Carrier states may persist for long periods and go unnoticed unless there is an outbreak of infection that is traced to the carrier.

Inanimate reservoirs of infection

Equipment and materials in use in health-care settings often become contaminated with microorganisms that may subsequently be transferred to susceptible body sites on patients. Gram-positive cocci, derived from skin scales, are found in the air, in dust and on surfaces where they may survive along with fungal and bacterial spores of environmental origin. Gram-negative aerobic bacilli are common in moist situations and in fluids, where they often survive for long periods, and may even multiply in the presence of minimal nutrients. An important example of this is legionellae in domestic water supplies of health-care settings. Awareness of the common reservoirs of environmental and contaminating microorganisms provides the basis for maintaining standards of hygiene (cleaning, disinfection, sterilisation) throughout the health care settings as well as good engineering and buildings.

Role of antibiotic treatment

At least 30% of patients receive antibiotics during their stay in hospital, and this exerts strong selective pressures on the microbiota, especially of the gastrointestinal tract, leading to the development of antibiotic-associated diarrhoea

due to *Clostridium difficile* (see Ch. 29), one of the most causes of outbreaks of HAI. Sensitive species or strains of microorganisms that normally maintain a protective function on the skin and other mucosal surfaces tend to be eliminated, whereas those that are more resistant survive and become endemic in health-care settings. This may restrict the range of agents available for treatment and may lead to the transmission of antibiotic resistance genes into strains that show increased virulence, survival and spread within the hospital.

COMMON INFECTIONS

Infections most commonly acquired in health-care settings are:

* Surgical site infections
* Respiratory tract infections (e.g., ventilator-associated infection)
* Urinary tract infections
* Bloodstream infections
* Gastroenteritis

The relative frequency of different HAIs varies in different patient populations, but, overall, urinary tract infections are the most common. Bloodstream infections may be primary (e.g., contaminated device or intravenous fluid) or secondary to a focus of infection already present (e.g., urinary tract infection or pneumonia).

COMMON ORGANISMS

Almost any organism can cause HAI. Over the years the microorganisms causing HAI have shown significant changes. In the preantibiotic era the most common organisms were *Streptococcus pyogenes* and *Staphylococcus aureus*. Before the advent of penicillinase-stable penicillins such as methicillin in the early 1960s, outbreaks of *S. aureus* infection had been reported in surgical wards and maternity units. With the advent of penicillins active against staphylococci and streptococci, Gram-negative organisms such as *Escherichia coli* and *Pseudomonas aeruginosa* emerged as important organisms causing HAI. Subsequently, epidemic or pandemic strains characterised by resistance to methicillin [methicillin-resistant *Staphylococcus aureus* (MRSA)] were found in many health-care settings worldwide, presenting a daunting challenge. More recently, the development of broad-spectrum antibiotics such as second- and third-generation cephalosporins has led to an increase in incidence of multiresistant Gram-negative organisms, such as extended spectrum β-lactamse–producing organisms and carbapenemase-producing organisms (e.g., *E. coli*, *Klebsiella pneumonia*,

P. aeruginosa and *Acinetobacter baumanii*), and Gram-positive organisms (e.g., vancomycin-resistant enterococci). Similarly, the development of invasive medical techniques has been accompanied by an increase in incidence of Gram-positive organisms and fungi. The common organisms associated with medical devices (e.g., intravenous catheters, prosthetic heart valves and pacemakers, hip and knee joints) are coagulase-negative staphylococci, *S. aureus*, *P. aeruginosa* and *Candida* spp.

The most common viruses associated with HAIs are influenza virus, respiratory syncytial virus, varicella zoster virus and norovirus.

ROUTES OF TRANSMISSION

The common routes of spread of microorganisms in healthcare settings are airborne, contact and common vehicle. Understanding the sources and spread of infection enables planning effective preventive measures.

Common routes of transmission for different microorganisms are shown in Table 67.2.

Airborne transmission

Microorganisms may spread:

- By airborne transmission from the respiratory tract (talking, coughing, sneezing)
- From the skin by natural shedding of skin scales during wound dressing or bedmaking
- By aerosols from equipment such as respiratory apparatus and air-conditioning plants

Infectious agents may be dispersed as small particles or droplets over long distances (Fig. 67.1). Staphylococci survive well on mucosal secretions, skin scales and dried pus and may be redistributed in the air after initial

settlement during periods of increased activity (Fig. 67.2). Gram-negative bacilli do not generally survive desiccation in air, and this route of transmission is therefore limited to conditions of high humidity such as ventilatory equipment, showers or other fine water aerosols.

Contact spread

The most common routes of transmission of microorganisms causing HAI are:

- By *direct* contact spread from person to person
- By *indirect* contact spread via contaminated hands or equipment

Human secretions as well as contaminated dust particles or fluids may be carried on thermometers, bedpans, bed linens, cutlery or other shared items. Hands and, to a lesser extent, clothing of hospital staff serve as vectors of

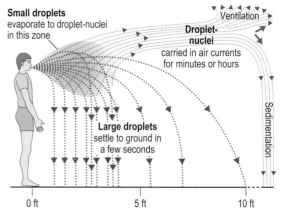

Fig. 67.1 Spread of respiratory infections by droplets and droplet nuclei.

Table 67.2 Healthcare-associated infection: sources and spread

Route	Source	Examples of disease
1. Aerial (from persons)	Mouth	Measles, tuberculosis, whooping cough
Droplets	Nose	Staphylococcal sepsis
Skin scales	Skin exudate, infected lesion	Staphylococcal and streptococcal sepsis
2. Aerial (from inanimate sources)	Respiratory equipment	Gram-negative respiratory infection
Particles	Air-conditioning plant	Legionnaire disease
3. Contact (from persons)		
Direct spread	Respiratory secretions	Staphylococcal and streptococcal sepsis
Indirect via equipment	Faeces, urine, skin and wound exudate	Enterobacterial and viral diarrhoea, *Pseudomonas aeruginosa* sepsis
4. Contact (environmental source)	Equipment, food, medicaments, fluids	Enterobacterial sepsis (*Klebsiella*/*Serratia*/*Enterobacter* spp.) *P. aeruginosa* and other pseudomonads
5. Inoculation	Sharps injury, blood products	Hepatitis B, HIV, malaria

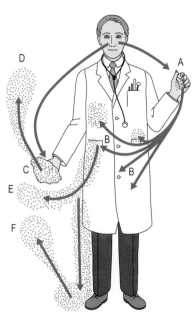

Fig. 67.2 Infection of the air with dust particles derived from nasal and oral secretions contaminating hands, handkerchief, clothing and surrounding surfaces. (A) Hand soiled with secretions from lips or nose-picking. (B) Clothing contaminated by hand. (C) Soiled handkerchief. (D) Infected dust from handkerchief. (E) Dust from clothing (e.g., from near handkerchief pocket). (F) Infected dust raised after settling on floor.

Gram-negative and Gram-positive infection. Procedures involving contact with mucosal surfaces (e.g., insertion of a urinary catheter) may introduce microorganisms from the contaminated hands of the operator or from the patient's own urethral microbiota into the normally sterile bladder.

Foodborne spread

Infection may originate in the hospital kitchen, or in special diets, infant feeds and kitchen or commercial supplies. Deteriorating hygiene standards may support the proliferation of flies, cockroaches and other insects or rodents that damage stored products and act as carriers of microbes.

Bloodborne spread

The accidental transmission of infections such as human immunodeficiency virus (HIV), hepatitis B or hepatitis C by needlestick or contaminated "sharps" injuries has been well documented. In areas of high prevalence of bloodborne viruses, malaria or syphilis stringent precautions should be taken to minimise transmission between patients and from health-care workers by strict use of single-use items and screening blood products.

PREVENTION AND CONTROL

Prevention of HAI should be a high priority in every health-care institution. There are three main strategies:

1. Exclusion of sources of microorganisms from health-care settings
2. Interrupting transmission of microorganisms from source to susceptible hosts
3. Enhancing the host's ability to resist infection

The common preventative measures for HAI are shown in Fig. 67.3. For more detailed information on methods of infection prevention and control, readers are encouraged to refer to Ch. 4 and the references at the end of this chapter.

Exclusion of sources of microorganisms from health-care settings

Exclusion of environmental (inanimate) sources of microorganisms such as the provision of sterile instruments and dressings, sterile medication and sterile intravenous fluids and the screening of blood and blood products, organs and tissues for infectious agents to a large extent is achievable and is known to reduce HAI. Sometimes the source may become contaminated from an environmental reservoir of organisms—for example, contaminated antiseptic solution distributed for use into sterile containers. In such situations, exclusion of the source will require elimination of the reservoir.

Elimination of human sources of microorganisms (e.g., patients, staff or rarely visitors) and objects that become contaminated by human sources is not always straightforward and can be challenging.

Human sources of microorganisms may include:

- People who are symptomatic with infection
- People who are incubating an infection
- Healthy carriers

Identifying healthy carriers is challenging. For example, identifying carriers of MRSA is difficult unless bacteriological screening is undertaken. In the United Kingdom, most health-care institutions screen patients admitted to "high risk" areas (e.g., intensive care units, general surgery, orthopaedic and vascular wards) for carriage of MRSA and offer such patients decolonisation medication to eliminate MRSA carriage. Routine screening of staff for carriage of infectious organisms is neither feasible nor cost-effective. In addition, staff is a source of opportunistic organisms such as coagulase-negative staphylococci and enterobacteria, which are part of their normal microbiota. A more pragmatic approach is to offer a preemployment screen for selected infectious diseases and immunisation

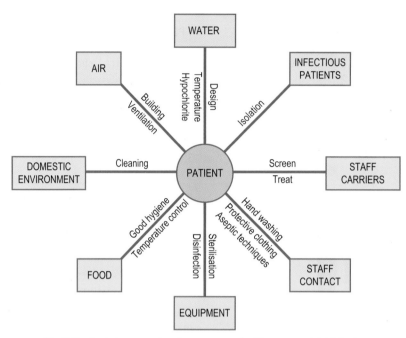

Fig. 67.3 Control measures to reduce exogenous health care–associated infection.

status by occupational health services (e.g., tuberculosis, hepatitis B, etc.). Staff with infections should be encouraged to report to occupational health services and should be relieved from direct contact with patients. Similarly, kitchen staff should be relieved from duty if they are suffering from diarrhoea or hepatitis A, or have infected lesions on their hands. Healthcare institutions with effective immunisation programmes for staff (e.g., peer vaccination programmes for seasonal influenza) have shown significant reduction in HAI.

Interrupting spread of microorganisms from source to susceptible hosts

The two most important routes of transmission of microorganisms in health-care settings are the airborne route and contact spread. Wards comprising separate rooms for patients have been shown to offer some protection against airborne spread. Source isolation of patients and protecting susceptible hosts from exposure to pathogenic microorganisms can significantly reduce airborne spread. Source isolation also helps prevent spread by other routes, by limiting access to the patient and reminding staff of the importance of contact in the spread of microorganisms. Maintaining the air-conditioning systems in hospitals is important to prevent *Legionella* infection there. Similarly, attention to airflow especially when building work is going on in the locality is important to reduce the airborne spread of *Aspergillus* infection in haematology and stem cell

transplant wards. Ventilation systems in operating theatres must be properly installed and maintained to prevent the inflow of contaminated air and to minimise air currents carrying organisms from the staff in the operating theatre to the operation site. "Ultraclean" air delivered through high-efficiency filters to remove bacteria has been shown to reduce postoperative wound infections after prolonged orthopaedic and vascular operations.

The general hospital environment should be kept clean by attention to basic cleaning, waste disposal and laundry. The use of chemical disinfectants for walls, floors and furniture is necessary only in special instances, such as spillages of body fluids from patients with bloodborne virus infections and when there are periods of increased activity of infections leading to outbreaks (e.g., *C. difficile*, norovirus).

The hands of staff can carry microorganisms to patients from other patients, from contaminated equipment and from staff themselves.

Staff should wash their hands:

- Before any procedure for which gloves or forceps are necessary
- After contact with an infected patient or one who is colonised with a multiresistant organism
- After touching infective material

Soap and water are adequate in most instances, with antiseptic liquids reserved when dealing with infected patients. Drying of hands after washing is important. A "surgical scrub" is recommended before commencing surgery. There has been a high degree of sophistication of design of taps, soap dispensers, and other washing facilities; however, human compliance with such facilities has been disappointing. Therefore training and regular reinforcement in appropriate behavior is essential.

Enhancing the host's ability to resist infection

Eliminating sources of miroorganisms and preventing their spread to susceptible hosts is not always failsafe. They, too, may not protect the host from endogenous infection.

A host's ability to resist infection can be enhanced by the following:

- Boosting specific immunity by active or passive immunisation (Ch. 68)
- Using appropriate prophylactic antibiotics (Ch. 65)
- Taking care of invasive devices (e.g., urinary catheters and intravenous lines)
- Reducing risks predisposing to postoperative infections

INFECTION CONTROL POLICY

The establishment of an effective infection control organisation is the responsibility of good management of any health-care institution. There will normally be two parts:

1. An *infection control committee*, meeting regularly to formulate and update policies on matters having implications for infection control, and to manage outbreaks of HAI.
2. An *infection control team* of workers, headed by the *infection control doctor*, to take day-to-day responsibility for this policy.

The functions of this team include surveillance and control of HAI, establishment and monitoring of policies and procedures designed to prevent HAI (e.g., hand hygiene practices, decontamination and disinfection, catheter care and antibiotic prescribing), investigating outbreaks and training and educating all staff in the microbiologically safe performance of procedures (e.g., donning of personal protective equipment when caring for patients with suspected Ebola). The *infection control nurse* is a key member of this team. Close working links between the microbiology laboratory, infection control nurse and the different clinical specialties and support services (including sterile services, laundry, pharmacy and engineering) are important to establish and maintain the infection control policy and to ensure that it is rationally based and that the recommended procedures are practicable. It is important for all members of the committee to ensure that everyone in the organisation makes infection control and hospital hygiene their

responsibility. Some of the control measures with which the infection control team should be involved are shown in Fig. 67.3.

Surveillance and the role of the laboratory

To establish normal trends and to recognise any change in the number or type of infections it is important to maintain accurate records of incidence and prevalence of HAI. In addition, there are also mandatory surveillance schemes for HAIs of national importance (e.g., MRSA and Gram-negative bacteraemia, *C. difficile* disease).

Sources of surveillance data are:

- Microbiology laboratory reports—general surveillance and monitoring "alert" organisms such as MRSA, *C. difficile, Mycobacterium tuberculosis*
- Ward rounds—reviewing patients (e.g., postoperative wound infections)
- Autopsy reports, staff health records

When routine surveillance highlights an increase in incidence of HAI, the infection control committee should initiate an investigation.

It is the role of the microbiology laboratory to show that all patients in the outbreak are infected with an organism that is indistinguishable. This is achieved by epidemiological typing methods. A variety of phenotypic and genotypic characterisation methods are available that offer a "fingerprint" for the organism (Ch. 3).

The identity of the organism provides clues to the possible source; for example, an outbreak of wound infection with MRSA is likely to be associated with contact spread from staff in the theatre or on the ward, whereas an outbreak of *Salmonella* gastroenteritis is more likely to originate in the kitchen.

While the investigation is proceeding, infected patients must be isolated and treated appropriately, and staff who are infected and carriers of infection must be removed from contact with patients. At the end of the investigation the relevant procedures must be reviewed to try and prevent a similar outbreak occurring again.

EFFICACY OF INFECTION CONTROL

The evidence base in the literature for acceptable proof of efficacy for infection control measures is limited. These include sterilisation, hand washing, closed-drainage systems for urinary catheters, intravenous catheter care, perioperative antibiotic prophylaxis for contaminated wounds, and techniques for the care of equipment used in respiratory therapy. Isolation techniques are assumed to be reasonable as suggested by experience or inference. Measures that are now considered to be ineffective include regular chemical disinfection of floors, walls and sinks, and routine environmental monitoring.

Effective surveillance and action by the infection control team have been shown to reduce infection rates. One important role of the team is to monitor compliance with practices known to be effective and to eliminate the many rituals or less effective practices that may even increase the incidence or cost of cross-infection. As further advances occur in medical care and limited health-care resources are spread across hospital and community needs, innovations in infection control will need to be evaluated for efficacy and cost-effectiveness. With this understanding it is possible that hospital infection can be controlled and largely prevented. The dictum of Florence Nightingale, made over a century ago, that "the very first requirement in a hospital is that it should do the sick no harm," remains the goal.

RECOMMENDED READING

Department of Health. (2013). The UK 5 year antimicrobial resistance strategy 2013-2018.

Department of Health. (2015). The Health and Social Care Act 2008: code of practice for health and adult social care on the prevention and control of infections and related guidance. Department of Health, London.

Fraise, A. P., & Bradley, C. (Eds.). (2009). *Ayliffe's control of hospital infection* (5th ed.). London: Hodder Arnold.

Fraise, A. P., Lambert, P., & Maillard, J.-Y. (Eds.). (2004). *Russell, Hugo and Ayliffe's principles and practice of disinfection, preservation and sterilization* (4th ed.). Oxford: Blackwell.

Loveday, H., Wilson, J., Pratt, R., et al. (2014). Epic 3: National evidence-based guidelines for preventing healthcare-associated infections in NHS hospitals in England. *Journal of Hospital Infection*, 86, S1–S70.

NHS England. (2013). Everyone counts: planning for patients 2014/15 to 2018/19.

NHS England. (2013). Commissioning for quality and innovation (CQUIN): 2013/14 guidance.

Wenzel, R. P. (Ed.). (2002). *Prevention and control of nosocomial infection* (4th ed.). Baltimore: Lippincott, Williams and Wilkins.

Websites

Centers for Disease Control. Healthcare-associated Infections (HAIs). http://www.cdc.gov/hai/.

Department of Health (England). Reducing Healthcare Associated Infection. http://hcai.dh.gov.uk/.

Health and Safety Executive. http://www.hse.gov.uk/.

Hospital Infection Society. http://www.his.org.uk/.

Infection Prevention Society (formerly Infection Control Nurses Association). http://www.ips.uk.net/.

Medicines and Healthcare Products Regulatory Agency. http://www.mhra.gov.uk/.

National Resource for Infection Control (NRIC). http://www.nric.org.uk/.

NICE (2012) CG 139 Prevention and Control of Healthcare-Associated Infections in Primary and Community Care. http://www.nice.org.uk/guidance/cg139/chapter/1-guidance.

Thames Valley University Evidence Based Guidelines. http://www.wolfson.tvu.ac.uk/research.

68 Immunisation

IAIN STEPHENSON

KEY POINTS

- Immunisation is a major means by which infections may be controlled and, in some cases, eradicated.
- Passive immunisation involves transfer of antibodies from immune individuals by use of immunoglobulin-containing preparations. Preparations providing protection against tetanus, diphtheria, hepatitis B, hepatitis A, rabies, and varicella-zoster are available.
- Active immunisation induces long-lasting immunity by stimulation of antibody responses in the recipient. Live-attenuated, killed (inactivated), subunit (e.g., toxoid or capsular antigen) and recombinant vaccines are used widely.
- The use of particular vaccines can be contraindicated in certain individuals, such as the use of live vaccines in immunocompromised individuals.
- Where immunisation prevents onward transmission, immunisation programmes can achieve herd or population immunity, reducing transmission within the community.
- The standard immunisation schedule in the United Kingdom provides for active immunisation in childhood against diphtheria, tetanus, pertussis, 13 serotypes of pneumococci, *Haemophilus influenzae* type B (Hib), *Neisseria meningitidis* groups A, B, C, W and Y, polio, influenza, four types of human papillomavirus, rotavirus and measles, mumps and rubella.
- Additional active immunisation may be considered against hepatitis B, varicella (shingles), tuberculosis and influenza for specific groups, and travellers are routinely offered additional vaccines specific to the locations visited.

It is appropriate that the last chapter of this book should be devoted to immunisation. Although only one of the measures deployed to control infectious diseases, immunisation has eliminated smallpox from the world and is well on the way to eradicating poliomyelitis. With advances in understanding of host responses to antigens, more efficient vaccine production and delivery methods, the future is exciting for combating other communicable diseases. The cost-effectiveness of immunisation programmes needs to be evaluated against alternative control methods (Box. 68.1) including environmental sanitation, safe sewage disposal, secure water supply, food hygiene, clean air and adequate ventilation, good animal husbandry with effective quarantine arrangements where necessary, insect vector control and improved nutrition.

Much of the morbidity and mortality caused by infectious diseases remains nonpreventable by immunisation. Many parasitic, diarrhoeal and respiratory infections that pose health burdens among young children in poor and overcrowded communities are not currently vaccine preventable; nor are the common bacterial infections associated with haemolytic streptococci, staphylococci and coliform bacilli.

RATIONALE OF IMMUNISATION

The primary aim of a vaccine is to induce, without harm to the recipient, protective immune responses against an attack of the natural infection. An immunised individual is less likely to be a source of infection, so onward transmission to other susceptible people in the community should be reduced (herd or population immunity).

PASSIVE IMMUNIZATION

Artificial passive immunisation is used to rapidly protect an individual. Antibodies, which may be antitoxin, antibacterial or antiviral, in preparations of human or animal serum can be injected or transfused into a recipient. Human preparations are referred to as homologous and are better tolerated than the injection of animal (heterologous) sera, which are associated with hypersensitivity reactions. The duration of protection from homologous antisera may last 3–6 months, whereas protection afforded by heterologous serum is likely to last for only a few weeks. The use of monoclonal antibodies against specific pathogens, such as respiratory syncytial virus, may increase the role for passive immunisation in future.

Antiserum raised in the horse against diphtheria toxin (equine diphtheria antitoxin) is available for the treatment of diphtheria. A similar heterologous antiserum is available for treatment of suspected botulism and to protect those thought to be at risk.

POOLED IMMUNOGLOBULINS

Protective levels of antibody to a range of diseases prevalent in the general population are present in pooled donor human serum. Human normal immunoglobulin (HNIG) may be used to protect nonimmune individuals after exposure to acute hepatitis A or immunocompromised children exposed to measles.

SPECIFIC IMMUNOGLOBULINS

Preparations of specific immunoglobulins are available for passive immunisation against tetanus, hepatitis B, rabies and varicella-zoster from pooled serum from donors who have been recently immunised, are recovering from recent infection or have high antibody titres to the target organism.

ACTIVE IMMUNISATION

Vaccines confer longer lasting protection by inducing the recipient's own immune system (by a combination of both antibody-mediated and cellular responses) including immunological memory.

TYPES OF VACCINES

Toxoids

Where a single bacterial toxin is responsible for a disease process, a modified or inactivated toxin (toxoid) that preserves its antigenicity, but loses its toxicity, can offer successful active immunisation. This approach has been successful with tetanus and diphtheria toxoid vaccines.

Inactivated killed vaccines

It is possible to induce protective levels of antibody by vaccines developed from chemically disrupted or formaldehyde killed (inactivated) organisms. For example, this is achieved with vaccines against pertussis (whooping cough) and poliovirus (inactivated Salk vaccine).

Attenuated live vaccines

For some organisms, the inactivation process can disrupt the antigenic components required to induce a protective immune response, so the resulting vaccine components lose their immunogenicity. Live vaccines use suspensions of organisms that are reduced or weakened in virulence (attenuated), but retain the ability to replicate in the recipient and therefore stimulate broad immune responses similar to those seen in natural infection. This strategy has produced mumps, measles, rubella (combined), varicella-zoster, polio, influenza, rotavirus and yellow fever vaccines.

Sometimes it is possible to use a related organism with shared antigens as vaccines. The vaccinia virus vaccine was used to eradicate smallpox, and a modified bovine tubercle bacillus (bacille Calmette–Guérin, BCG) is used to protect humans against tuberculosis and leprosy.

Special procedures

Some vaccines, such as those derived from influenza and pertussis are purified by processes to remove unwanted protein and other reactive materials, whilst retaining important antigens. Some purified polysaccharide antigens (meningococcal and pneumococcal organisms) must be conjugated to carrier proteins such as toxoids, or added to immune stimulating chemicals (adjuvants) to enhance immunogenicity. Increasingly, vaccines such as hepatitis B are molecularly engineered or developed from recombinant antigens.

IMMUNE RESPONSE

Specific antibodies directed against some bacterial and viral infections may be present in maternal blood and are passively acquired by the baby. This offers some protection to the infant at a time when its own immune system is underdeveloped but could interfere with the infant's capacity to respond to the stimulus of injected or ingested vaccines in the very early months of life. Although the capacity of an infant to produce specific antibody to injected antigens is poorly developed in the first few months of life, this may be overcome by addition of adjuvants such as aluminium hydroxide and conjugation to toxoids. Combination of toxoids, pertussis antigen and conjugated polysaccharide antigens creates an effective immunising complex (diphtheria, tetanus, pertussis, polio and *Haemophilus influenzae* type b vaccine: DTP/IPV/Hib) given in the United Kingdom at 2, 3 and 4 months of age to cover the period when the lethal potential of these infections is high.

To develop a durable specific antibody response to toxoid or to killed antigen, the usual procedure is administration of multiple vaccine doses at spaced intervals. The response to the first or priming dose is dominated by IgM antibody, but the second dose, typically separated by an interval of a month or two, induces a greater secondary IgG response. A third reinforcing dose is generally recommended at some time thereafter, and further booster doses may be needed to maintain immunity.

Live-attenuated virus vaccines usually promote a broad immune response similar to that seen after natural infection as the vaccine organism replicates at the site of inoculation in the recipient. In addition to serum antibody responses, both cellular and mucosal IgA responses are induced following live-attenuated influenza or rotavirus vaccines that may confer more durable immunity, but these are more difficult to measure by laboratory tests.

DURATION OF IMMUNITY

After effective primary immunisation, protective serum antibody levels may persist for months or years. The duration of the response varies and depends on recipient and vaccine. Conjugated vaccines and live-attenuated vaccines tend to give broader and more durable responses, and even if detectable antibody titres wane, the immune system remains primed and subsequent reinforcing injections will boost immunity. The measurement of antibody levels following immunisation does not necessarily correlate to immune protection as serological antibody assays vary in sensitivity, and furthermore, the functional role of postvaccination antibody is poorly characterised.

AGE OF COMMENCEMENT OF ACTIVE IMMUNISATION

This must consider the immaturity of the antibody-forming system in the early months of life and the likely timing of infectious challenges that a person may encounter in early and later years. Immunisation schedules are adjusted to the known epidemiology of the diseases that are prevalent in the country in which it is be to instituted, but also consider serious infective challenges that may be imported from time to time. Poliomyelitis is a good example of a disease that has been largely eradicated from many communities but can rapidly reemerge if the immunisation shield is lowered.

CONTROLLED STUDIES OF VACCINES

Combined field and laboratory studies aim to provide confidence in the efficacy of vaccines (efficacy: how well the vaccine prevents an attack of actual infection). A field trial only shows whether or not the actual preparation of vaccine used in the trial was successful under the circumstances prevailing at the time. Accordingly, trials require careful design and implementation, and in order to satisfy the requirement for reproducibility, vaccine preparation methods must be meticulously described and controlled. Work is ongoing to better characterise laboratory testing of serum antibody to a particular vaccine, (antigenicity or immunogenicity: how much antibody is produced after vaccine administration) and to determine how this might be correlated with its efficacy. If levels of protective antibody can be established, and serological antibody tests to measure them are reproducible and standardised, these could be adopted to predict if future new vaccines are likely to be efficacious.

Manufacturers of commercial vaccines are required to satisfy certain standards relating to the purity, safety, potency, stability and testing of their products, agreed at national and international level (World Health Organization, WHO). Many countries, including the United Kingdom, have surveillance systems in place for notifying cases of communicable diseases so that estimates of vaccine efficacy can be made but also for suspected vaccine-related adverse reactions.

CONTRAINDICATIONS TO THE USE OF VACCINES

Immunisation schedules need to be widely accepted to be optimally beneficial, but there is a balance between individual rights (often the parent or carer, not the person being immunised) and public health benefits. It is necessary not to take a too legalistic view of theoretical hazards and thus err on the side of opting out. The risk of opting out of immunisation schedules should be appreciated and shown to be greater than the adverse effects. There are useful general principles about contraindications that include: do not give a vaccine to a patient with an acute illness, ensure any postponed immunisation is subsequently given, do not give live vaccines in pregnancy unless there is a clear balance of risk in favour of immunisation, avoid vaccine during the first trimester and do not administer live vaccines to immunosuppressed patients.

HAZARDS OF IMMUNISATION

Possible adverse reactions to immunisation are:

- mild or moderate pain, redness or induration at the site of injection (local reactions)
- fever and malaise for several days (systemic reactions)
- anaphylactic reactions are very rare, but as they may be fatal, vaccine administrators should be aware of the possibility and have access to resuscitation equipment at all immunisation sessions

During the first few years of life when many vaccines are given, children tend to have various health problems including occasional febrile convulsions and, very rarely, unexplained cot death or other tragedy. It is inevitable that some events will coincide with the period shortly after a vaccine was given to a child and the possibility of a causal relationship will be entertained. The probability of such a link must be considered, but it is also important to bear in mind that the issue can become emotive and that ill-informed adverse publicity can do significant harm to an immunisation programme. For example, annual notifications of whooping cough in England and Wales dropped from >120,000 in the early 1950s to some tens of thousands in the late 1950s as immunisation was introduced. By 1972, whooping cough was largely controlled, with about 80% of children immunised. Following adverse publicity regarding safety, vaccine uptake fell to 30%, and this was followed by epidemics of whooping cough in 1978 and 1982, with over 65,000 annual notifications including a number of deaths. As a result of efforts to restore confidence in the vaccine, coverage increased in the 1980s and the disease was brought back under control.

More recently, autism and inflammatory bowel disease were claimed to be associated with MMR vaccine. Although subsequent studies failed to confirm the findings, which were later discredited, heightened

---

Box 68.2   Safety considerations

- Use a separate sterile syringe and needle
- Avoid errors: check the vial personally and sign
- Check cold chain
- Consider the patient's history: note pregnancy and various contraindications
- Keep careful records, including batch number

---

media coverage and anxiety resulted in falling vaccine coverage to the point when measles cases and deaths reemerged. Mathematical models of the dynamics of measles show that if the number of susceptible individuals in a population exceeds 5%, there is a possibility of transmission.

Children who are most vulnerable are often likely to be least protected. Pertussis, polio and measles spread effectively in overcrowded living conditions and almost rely on population density for their spread. Some underprivileged groups in a community are at increased risk when overall population vaccine uptake falls because they often have the lowest vaccine coverage and heightened epidemiological risk.

Because of strong regulation and control of vaccine quality and efficacy, vaccine errors more often lie with the vaccinator than with the producer. Vaccine administrators are obliged to ensure that vaccines are properly stored, reconstituted (if relevant) and correctly administered (Box 68.2). Many preparations lose their potency if frozen and thawed, or exposed to temperature variation. It is essential to maintain the cold chain in which vaccines are held between 2°C–8°C. Appropriate instructions and local protocols should be available and followed in detail. An injectable vaccine must always be given with a separate sterile syringe and needles, and equipment disposed of properly. The dangers of contamination with blood-borne viruses such as HIV and hepatitis B and C in some parts of the world have led to alternative delivery methods by air jets or via mucosal surfaces (nasal or oral).

SITE OF INJECTION

This will vary between vaccines, and specific instructions should be followed. In general, and with the exception of BCG, injectable vaccines are given by intramuscular or deep subcutaneous injection. The anterolateral aspect of the thigh or upper arm is the preferred site for infants. Alternative delivery methods to injections such as oral ingestion, nasal inoculation or air jet delivery are likely to improve the immunisation clinics feared by countless school children.

HERD IMMUNITY

When most people in a community are immune to a particular infection that is transmitted from person to person, the natural spread is effectively limited. Thus, if most children in a residential school have been immunised against measles, the school is unlikely to suffer a measles outbreak, so even the few who have not been immunised will benefit from the general herd immunity and will not be exposed within the school. This will apply as long as the school population is composed largely of immune pupils and a nonimmune pupil does not encounter a measles-infected visitor. However, if there is an influx of susceptible individuals, herd immunity will fall and the general protection will be lost. When the pupils travel to other communities at holiday times, the nonimmune individuals are at risk of measles at their first contact with an infective case.

For herd immunity to be effective in a community or country, vaccine uptake rates must exceed 90%. For highly transmissible infections, such as measles, uptake rates of >95% are targeted. Herd immunity works only for infections transmitted from person to person. As tetanus is acquired by direct inoculation from a contaminated source, a nonimmune individual remains vulnerable even if surrounded by fully immunised colleagues in a closed community (Fig. 68.1).

IMMUNISATION PROGRAMMES

A national immunisation campaign needs to be planned as an ongoing continuous programme to fulfil its aim of disease reduction, unless eradication of the infection is achieved. Thus, in planning immunisation schedules, the general public must be receptive and supportive. Securing and maintaining the trust of parents to bring their children to clinics for a series of inoculations are required, so they must be assured that the benefits are considerable and the risks negligible. Appropriate consent must be obtained for each immunisation.

In the planning and execution of an immunisation programme, immunological points that merit special attention include:

- the use of combined vaccines and simultaneous administration of killed and live vaccines
- the incorporation of adjuvants in killed vaccines and toxoids
- the age of commencement of the schedule
- the number of vaccine doses required and dosing intervals between vaccines

IMMUNISATION SCHEDULES

The provision of active immunisation should be governed by need, vaccine efficacy, vaccine safety and ease of administration. National considerations must also include cost, the availability of manpower to administer vaccine and reliable and robust vaccine supplies. Circumstances and priorities vary widely in different countries. The WHO Global Vaccine Action Plan (GVAP) 2011 has been adopted by most countries as a minimum schedule to protect children in parts of the world where transmission rates are particularly high. Global eradication of poliomyelitis is close, and targets are set for regional elimination of measles, rubella and neonatal tetanus.

In the United Kingdom it is generally agreed that protection of the susceptible population against diphtheria, pertussis, tetanus, polio, *H. influenzae* type b (Hib) (combined as DTaP/IPV/Hib), *Neisseria meningitidis* groups B and C, common serogroups of *Streptococcus pneumoniae*, rotavirus, and mumps, measles and rubella (within a combined live vaccine) merit priority in the first few years. Older children are offered protection from influenza (by intranasal live-attenuated influenza vaccine), four types of human papillomavirus (HPV types 6, 11, 16 and 18) and *N. meningitidis* groups A, C, W and Y. Older adults (>65 or 70 years of age) are offered protection against influenza, several serogroups of *S. pneumoniae* and shingles (zoster) (Table 68.1).

NOTES ON COMMON VACCINES IN USE

ADSORBED TETANUS AND DIPHTHERIA TOXOID

Tetanus and diphtheria vaccine preparations are composed from purified toxins extracted from strains of *Clostridium tetani* and *C. diphtheriae*, respectively, inactivated by formaldehyde to form toxoids and absorbed onto aluminium adjuvant salt to improve immunogenicity. They are only available as a part of combined products with inactivated polio, and often pertussis and *H. influenzae* type B (Hib) vaccine (DTaP/IPV/Hib, DTaP/IPV or Td/IPV). A total of five doses at appropriate intervals, three injections given at 2, 3 and 4 months, with boosters prior to, and on leaving school, should protect for life.

PERTUSSIS VACCINE

Acellular pertussis vaccines have replaced earlier whole-cell vaccines that, whilst strongly immunogenic, were

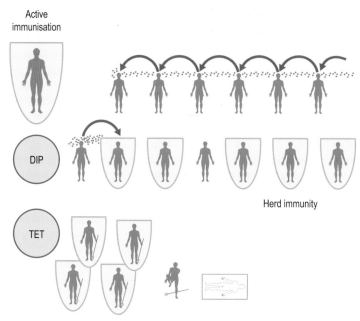

Active immunisation

DIP

TET

Herd immunity

Fig. 68.1 If almost all of the members of a community receive active immunisation against a disease that is normally transmitted from person to person, the resulting herd immunity confers some advantage even upon an occasional nonimmune member because rapid transmission of the disease through the community is prevented. This is true for diphtheria, but not for tetanus, which is not dependent on person-to-person spread.

Table 68.1 Schedule of immunisation for children and adults in the United Kingdom (August 2016)

Age	Vaccine required	Route of administration
2 months	DTaP/IPV/Hib*	Intramuscular injection
	Pneumococcal conjugate vaccine (PCV)	Intramuscular injection
	Meningococcal group B conjugate (MenB)	Intramuscular injection
	Rotavirus (live attenuated)	Oral dose
3 months	DTaP/IPV/Hib*	Intramuscular injection
	Rotavirus (live attenuated)	Oral dose
4 months	DTaP/IPV/Hib*	Intramuscular injection
	Meningococcal group B conjugate (MenB)	Intramuscular injection
	Pneumococcal conjugate vaccine (PCV)	Intramuscular injection
1 year	Hib/MenC conjugate vaccine	Intramuscular injection
	Meningococcal group B conjugate (MenB)	Intramuscular injection
	Pneumococcal conjugate vaccine (PCV)	Intramuscular injection
	Measles, mumps, rubella (MMR)	Intramuscular injection
2–17 years	Annual influenza (live attenuated)	Nasal spray, both nostrils
3 years, 4 months	Diphtheria, tetanus, pertussis, polio (DTaP/IPV)	Intramuscular injection
	Measles, mumps, rubella (MMR)	Intramuscular injection
Girls		
12–14 years	Human papillomavirus types 6, 11, 16 and 18	Intramuscular injection (two doses, 6–24 months apart)
14 years	Diphtheria, tetanus, polio (Td/IPV)	Intramuscular injection
	Meningococcal A, C, W, Y conjugate (MenACWY)	Intramuscular injection
65 years	Pneumococcal polysaccharide vaccine (PPV)	Intramuscular injection
≥65 years	Annual influenza (inactivated)	Intramuscular injection
70 years	Shingles	Intramuscular injection

*Diphtheria, tetanus, pertussis, polio and *Haemophilus influenzae* type B (Hib).

associated with a relatively high incidence of local and systemic reactions. Acellular vaccines are made from purified antigens of formaldehyde killed *Bordetella pertussis* organisms that are adsorbed onto aluminum adjuvant and are only available as part of combination products with at least diphtheria, tetanus, inactivated polio and sometimes Hib.

The combination (tetanus, diphtheria, pertussis) products used for boosting in older individuals contain a lower antigen content for tetanus/diphtheria toxoid and pertussis antigen than in the formulations used for primary boosting (diphtheria content denoted by D or d in the vaccine abbreviation). It is important to ensure the correct product is used as higher doses are required in young children to ensure adequate priming. The lower dose is recommended in those >10 years of age because of adequate immunogenicity and fewer adverse reactions.

POLIOMYELITIS VACCINES

The control of poliomyelitis is one of the great success stories of active immunisation, and the worldwide eradication of poliomyelitis is a WHO goal that has almost been achieved. In the United Kingdom, inactivated polio vaccine (IPV) is only available as a combination product with diphtheria, tetanus, pertussis and Hib and is made from three types of killed polio strains (Salk 1, 2 and 3). An oral live-attenuated polio vaccine (OPV) was initially favoured as promotion of gut mucosal antibody formation offered additional protection against wild virus infection. In addition, faeces contains live vaccine virus for some time after ingestion, so acquisition to nonimmunised contacts of recently immunised children provided community benefit. However, poliomyelitis caused by vaccine virus is a rare but recognised risk of OPV, which is why now, so close to global eradication, IPV is recommended.

HAEMOPHILUS INFLUENZAE TYPE B (HIB) VACCINE

Encapsulated strains of *H. influenzae*, usually serotype b, are associated with invasive infection including meningitis, bacteraemia, epiglottitis and osteomyelitis, particularly among young children, with peak incidence during the first year of life. Early polysaccharide vaccines were poorly immunogenic in the youngest children, but development of conjugate vaccines has overcome this problem. Hib polysaccharide antigen is conjugated to diphtheria or tetanus toxoid and is only available as part of a combined product in the standard childhood primary immunisation schedule or with meningococcal group C antigen.

MENINGOCOCCAL VACCINES (MENC, MEN B, MENACWY)

Meningococci are gram-negative diplococci classified into at least 12 capsular groups based on the types of antigenically distinct polysaccharide capsules. Invasive meningococcal disease occurs in all countries, with group A predominantly in the Sub-Saharan African meningitis belt; group W infections associated with annual Hajj pilgrimages to Saudi Arabia; and groups B, C, W and Y, historically the most prevalent in the United Kingdom. Following the introduction of routine meningococcal C (MenC) vaccines in the United Kingdom, group B and W capsular groups have formed an increasing proportion of infections. Early plain polysaccharide vaccines provided only short-term protection in adults and were poorly immunogenic in children. Conjugate MenC, MenC/Hib and quadrivalent MenACWY vaccines have overcome this issue by linking capsular group polysaccharides with tetanus or diphtheria toxoid inducing high levels of bactericidal antibody.

In 1999 the United Kingdom was the first country to introduce MenC vaccine into routine primary childhood immunisation schedules (with catch-up campaigns for older children, adolescents and young adults), resulting in a significant reduction (>90%) in invasive MenC disease, but also in nasopharyngeal carriage of *N. meningitidis*, leading to herd protection by reducing the potential for further exposure. In order to sustain high antibody levels when meningococcal carriage rates would be expected to increase again in young adults, a MenC booster (within quadrivalent conjugate MenACWY vaccine) in adolescence (around 14 years of age) maintains herd immunity, thus ensuring that the risk of exposure and infection in infants remains low. Consequently, childhood MenC immunisation was phased out in 2016 and was replaced with a recombinant MenB vaccine. A combined MenC/Hib vaccine at 1 year of age will provide protection to toddlers.

PNEUMOCOCCAL VACCINES

Invasive pneumococcal disease is a major cause of morbidity and mortality in the youngest, the elderly and those with immunosuppression. *Streptococcus pneumoniae* is an encapsulated Gram-positive coccus with over 90 antigenically distinct capsular types, although the majority of infections are caused by 8–10 common serotypes.

There are two pneumococcal vaccines. Polysaccharide vaccine (PPV) contains purified polysaccharide antigen from 23 capsular types accounting for >95% pneumococcus isolates in the United Kingdom. The vaccine is immuno-genic in healthy adults, but exhibits poor immunogenicity in children and those with immunosuppression, and is ineffective in preventing noninvasive (nonbacteraemic) pneumococcal disease (e.g., pneumonia, otitis media). Conjugation of the polysaccharide antigen with diphtheria toxoid enhances immunogenicity. Following the introduction in 2006 of the first pneumococcal conjugate vaccine (PCV7) containing capsular antigens from seven serotypes into routine childhood immunisation schedules, there was a significant reduction in invasive and noninvasive disease caused by vaccine serotypes in children and, to a lesser extent, also in the elderly, suggesting some degree of herd immunity. However, there was a corresponding increase in disease caused by nonvaccine serotypes (called serotype replacement), but these replacement infections have been largely covered by the addition of six other capsular types to the conjugate vaccine (PCV13).

MEASLES, MUMPS AND RUBELLA (MMR) VACCINE

MMR vaccines are a mixture of live-attenuated strains of these three viruses in freeze-dried form, so they have to be stored at 2°C–8°C (not frozen), reconstituted and used within 1 hour in accordance to the manufacturer's instructions. The aim of the immunisation programme is to provide two MMR vaccine doses at appropriate intervals. The first dose, given at 12–15 months of age, confers protection in >90% of recipients against measles and rubella, and 65% against mumps. The second dose can be given any time from 3 months after the first but is routinely administered before school entry at 3 years 4 months. It is generally well tolerated, but is associated with mild local and systemic reactions including thrombocytopenia. Single immunisation against each disease component is not recommended as appropriately spaced single vaccine doses would significantly delay onset of protective immunity.

It was hoped that high vaccine coverage with two doses of MMR vaccine in the United Kingdom schedule would eradicate measles, mumps and rubella as it has almost done in North America. Much depends upon public faith in the immunisation programme, which was significantly undermined in the 1990s following media-led speculation over MMR safety and links to autism and inflammatory bowel disease. Prior to adverse publicity in 1996, MMR vaccine uptake among 2 year olds approached 92%, with much reduced cases, but vaccine coverage declined to <80% in 1997. Localised and regional outbreaks of measles and mumps have reemerged, mainly affecting nonimmunised children and teenagers.

Rotavirus

Rotavirus is a highly contagious RNA virus, transmitted mainly by faecal-oral route. Whilst significant morbidity and mortality occurs mainly in resource-poor countries (as a result of severe dehydration), rotavirus gastroenteritis is still a common cause of hospitalisation in children in the United Kingdom. A live-attenuated virus vaccine is derived from an attenuated rotavirus that has undergone multiple passages in cell culture and is administered through an oral applicator. It can cause minor GI symptoms but may be associated with a very small increased risk of intussusception within a week of administration and it is not given to infants below the age of 6 weeks old.

HUMAN PAPILLOMAVIRUS VACCINE TYPES 6, 11, 16 AND 18 (HPV)

There are over 100 types of human papillomavirus (HPV) that infect squamous epithelia including mucosa of the oral and anogenital tracts. Most HPV infections are self-limiting, but types 6 and 11 are responsible for the majority of genital warts, and 85% of invasive cervical cancers are associated with HPV types 16 and 18. HPV subunit vaccines contain virus-like particles (for types 6, 11, 16 and 18) that consist of recombinant HPV viral coat proteins expressed in cell culture. Two doses, separated by 6–24 months intervals, were added to United Kingdom's immunisation schedule in 2014.

HEPATITIS B VACCINE

For the protection of groups of people considered to be at increased risk of acquiring hepatitis B virus, a recombinant vaccine containing hepatitis B surface antigen adsorbed onto aluminium adjuvant is available. A course of three intramuscular injections, at intervals of 1 and 5 months, is needed; thus, it takes 6 months to complete. Following known contact with the virus (including needlestick injury), an accelerated vaccine course can be used, although efficacy is reduced. Protective antibody titres are generally achieved in about 85% of recipients, but there are a number of nonresponders (10%–15% in those over 40 years of age), so antibody responses are routinely checked at least 6 weeks after completion, as a booster dose or a repeat full course may be needed. Vaccine nonresponders are particularly worrying among individuals at continuing risk (health-care staff, those on maintenance haemodialysis, sex workers), and repeat immunisation with higher dose preparations can be tried. For healthy adults, the protection afforded following a vaccine response is considered to last for about 5 years, when a booster dose may be given.

BCG

The attenuated strain of bovine tubercle bacillus known as bacille Calmette–Guérin (BCG) produces cross-immunity to human tuberculosis and has contributed to the control of that disease and to the other important mycobacterial disease, leprosy, in many countries. An intradermal injection of the live-attenuated vaccine is given on the lateral aspect of the arm at the level of the deltoid insertion, but not higher, or on the upper lateral surface of the thigh. Instruction on the reconstitution of the freeze-dried vaccine, the dosage and the detailed technique of giving a truly intradermal injection, should be most carefully observed. With the exception of newborn children, any recipient of BCG vaccination should have been tested for hypersensitivity to tuberculin (Mantoux, Heaf test or IGRA) and found to be negative.

OTHER VACCINES

Various vaccines are available for the protection of special groups of people or for individuals in special circumstances (Box 68.3). The reader is referred to the appropriate chapters for more detailed consideration of such topics as:

- the prevention of tetanus in wounded patients (Ch. 29)
- the indications for pneumococcal vaccine (Ch. 13)
- the management of rabies (Ch. 55)
- the protection of those at special risk from chickenpox or hepatitis B (Chs 49 and 52)
- the protection of the immunocompromised such as HIV/AIDS patients (Ch. 52)

Box 68.3 Vaccines for active immunisation of people at special risk

- Anthrax
- Hepatitis A
- Hepatitis B
- Influenza
- Japanese B encephalitis
- Meningococcal infection
- Plague
- Pneumococcal infection
- Q fever
- Rabies
- Tick-borne encephalitis
- Typhoid
- Typhus
- Varicella-zoster
- Yellow fever

Box 68.4 Properties of an ideal vaccine

- Promotes effective immunity
- Confers lifelong protection
- Safe (no side effects)
- Stable
- Cheap
- Seen to be good and effective by the public

Central Africa or Central America may need protection against yellow fever, or to Mecca for the Hajj pilgrimage to include meningitis and influenza vaccine. Other specific vaccines may be indicated such as those against rabies, hepatitis A, typhoid and encephalitis. Some of the special vaccines listed in Box 68.3 may also merit inclusion, especially if the traveller's activities when abroad are likely to expose him or her to the relevant diseases. Travellers to rural tropical areas must always consider insecticides and antimalarials at the top of their list for health prevention.

PROTECTING THE TRAVELLER

An intending traveller to another country should seek advice in advance about the prevailing diseases and the precautions that should be taken. Advice on immunisation is unlikely to be of benefit if the traveller takes the risk of drinking raw water or eating uncooked salads and vegetables in an area where sanitation is inadequate. In advising travellers, do not forget that diseases uncommon in developed countries may still be common in countries that lack such services. A travelling health-care worker may need to include diphtheria, tuberculosis, hepatitis A and B, measles and poliomyelitis. A traveller going to

UNRESOLVED PROBLEMS

No product is perfect (Box 68.4). Some vaccines are more imperfect than others, and some circumstances pose special problems. Inactivated cholera vaccines have been available, but without any evidence of efficacy for the traveller who is much better protected by a basic knowledge of hygiene. Developments in oral recombinant vaccines appear more promising and may protect against ETEC (enterotoxigenic *E. coli*) as well as cholera.

The influenza virus frequently changes its antigenic pattern (seasonal drift, pandemic shift), so vaccines must be revised and updated to protect against the prevalent circulating strains. Then decisions have to be made on the patients who merit the vaccine. As this includes those people over 65 years of age, and other patients with chronic medical conditions, the logistics of mass immunisation in a short time period are challenging. Most temperate climate countries immunise the elderly and those vulnerable against influenza before winter as this is associated with reductions in mortality and hospital admissions during the influenza season.

Several vaccine candidates have been developed against various herpesviruses, including herpes simplex, varicella-zoster and Epstein–Barr viruses. There have been many difficulties, but live-attenuated varicella vaccine introduced into practice for susceptible staff who work in paediatric or maternity wards has now entered national childhood immunisation programmes in some countries.

Vaccines effective against malaria and HIV infection are being urgently sought. There have been many disappointments as organisms display antigenic variation, possess various techniques to invade cells and promising vaccine candidates have proved to be poorly immunogenic or non-efficacious in field trials. Advances in molecular technology are likely to lead to recombinant protein and DNA vaccines, but standardisation of content, production and assessments of their efficacy are complex. Delivery of vaccine products without using traditional needles and syringes will save infections caused by the reuse of unsterile equipment.

RECOMMENDED READING

Anonymous. Immunological products and vaccines. In *British national formulary*. London (revised at intervals of about 6 months, March 2017, latest): British Medical Association and Royal Pharmaceutical Society of Great Britain.

Centers for Disease Control and Prevention. (2011). G. W. Brunette (Ed.), *CDC Health Information for international travel 2012*. Oxford and New York: Oxford University Press.

Department of Health, Welsh Office, & Scottish Home and Health Department. (2001). *Health information for overseas travel*. London: HMSO.

Department of Health, Welsh Office, Scottish Home and Health Department, & DHSS (Northern Ireland). (2006). *Immunisation against infectious disease*. London: HMSO.

Kassianos, G. C. (2001). *Immunization: childhood and traveller's health* (4th ed.). Oxford: Blackwell.

Mackett, M., & Williamson, J. D. (1995). *Human vaccines and vaccination*. Oxford: Bios Scientific Publications.

Plotkin, S., Orenstein, W., & Offit, P. (Eds.). (2008). *Vaccines* (5th ed.). Philadelphia: WB Saunders.

World Health Organization. (2000). *International travel and health. vaccination requirements and travel advice*. Geneva: WHO.

Websites

British National Formulary. Available at http://www.bnf.org/

Centers for Disease Control and Prevention. Travelers' Health. Retrieved from http://www.cdc.gov/travel/

Centers for Disease Control and Prevention. Vaccines & Immunizations. Retrieved from https://www.cdc.gov/vaccines

Department of Health. The Green Book. Immunisation against infectious disease. Retrieved from https://www.gov.uk/government/collections/immunisation-against-infectious-disease-the-green-book

Health Protection Scotland. Available at http://www.hps.scot.nhs.uk/

National Travel Health Network and Centre. Available at http://www.nathnac.org/

NHS (Scotland). Fit For Travel. Available at http://www.fitfortravel.nhs.uk/

World Health Organization. Immunization, Vaccines and Biologicals. Validating information on vaccine safety. Retrieved from http://www.who.int/immunization/

World Health Organization. International travel and health. Available at http://www.who.int/ith/

Index

Page numbers followed by '*f*' indicate figures, '*t*' indicate tables, '*b*' indicate boxes, and "*e*" indicate online content.